CRITICAL CARE NURSING CERTIFICATION REVIEW

CRITICAL CARE NURSING CERTIFICATION REVIEW

CCRN Prep and Practice Exams

Eighth Edition

Alexander P. Johnson, MSN, RN, ACNP-BC, CCNS, CCRN
Critical Care Clinical Nurse Specialist
Manager of Professional Practice & Development
Northwestern Medicine
Huntley Hospital
Huntley, Illinois

Hillary S. Crumlett, DNP, RN, NEA-BC
Vice President of Operations and Chief Nursing Executive
Northwestern Medicine
Huntley Hospital
Huntley, Illinois

Mc Graw Hill

Critical Care Nursing Certification Review: CCRN Prep and Practice Exams, Eighth Edition

1 2 3 4 5 6 7 8 9 LON 29 28 27 26 25 24

ISBN 978-1-260-47022-2
MHID 1-260-47022-9

This book was set in Minion Pro by KnowledgeWorks Global Ltd.
The editors were Sydney Keen Vitale and Christina M. Thomas.
The production supervisor was Catherine H. Saggese.
Project management was provided by Tasneem Kauser, KnowledgeWorks Global Ltd.

Library of Congress Cataloging-in-Publication Data

Names: Johnson, Alexander P., author. | Crumlett, Hillary S., author.
Title: Critical care nursing certification review : CCRN prep and practice exams / Alexander P. Johnson, Hillary Crumlett.
Other titles: Critical care nursing certification
Description: Eighth edition. | New York : McGraw Hill, [2024] | Preceded by Critical care nursing certification / Alexander P. Johnson, Hillary S. Crumlett. Seventh edition. New York : McGraw-Hill Education, [2018] | Includes bibliographical references and index. | Summary: "In this edition of Critical Care Nursing Certification Review: CCRN Prep and Practice Exams, we have updated the content while honoring the vision and format of previous editions. We hope that you'll find this text serves as a comprehensive critical care reference text using short, easy to read chapters. we have provided some general test-taking strategies at the beginning of each chapter, as well as an estimated amount of questions that you will be likely to see from that chapter on the exam. Another new addition to this edition has been answer rationales for each review question that help provide and reinforce test-taking information, tactics, and techniques that are designed to increase success on future exam questions"—Provided by publisher.
Identifiers: LCCN 2023032285 (print) | LCCN 2023032286 (ebook) | ISBN 9781260470222 (paperback) | ISBN 9781260470239 (ebook)
Subjects: MESH: Critical Care Nursing | Critical Illness—nursing | Test Taking Skills | Examination Questions
Classification: LCC RT120.I5 (print) | LCC RT120.I5 (ebook) | NLM WY 18.2 | DDC 616.02/8076—dc23/eng/20230906
LC record available at https://lccn.loc.gov/2023032285
LC ebook record available at https://lccn.loc.gov/2023032286

McGraw Hill books are available at special quantity discounts to use as premiums and sales promotions, or for use in corporate training programs. To contact a representative please visit the Contact Us pages at www.mhprofessional.com.

To my parents:

Norma ~ for reinforcing to me a love of reading, writing, and a passion for nursing

Philip ~ for encouraging me to further my education, being my bench coach in life, a calming influence, and a voice of reason

Sandra ~ for unconditional love and support, and for always reinforcing God in my life ♦

John ~ for being a steady presence, and modeling the value of persistence, sophistication, style, & insightfulness

Alexander P. Johnson, MSN, RN, ACNP-BC, CCNS, CCRN

To Dr. Jeffrey Huml

Thank you for making the world a better place.

Hillary S. Crumlett, DNP, RN, NEA-BC

Contents

Reviewers

Lori Brien, DNP, ACNP
Assistant Professor
Georgetown University, School of Nursing
Washington, District of Columbia

Patricia Dierks, MS, RN
Clinical Practice Specialist
Northwestern Medicine—Delnor Hospital
Geneva, Illinois

Melissa Golombek, DNP, MS-HCM, RN, NE-BC, CPN
Vice President
TGH Children's Hospital and The Women's Institute
Tampa General Hospital
Tampa, Florida

Natalie Lee, PharmD
Clinical Pharmacist
Department of Pharmacy
Northwestern Medicine—Central DuPage Hospital
Winfield, Illinois

Judy Pasternack, BSN, RN, NPD-BC
Clinical Practice Specialist
Northwestern Medicine—McHenry Hospital
McHenry, Illinois

Kajal Patel, PharmD, BCPS, BCCP
Clinical Specialist—Critical Care
Department of Pharmacy
Northwestern Medicine—Central DuPage Hospital
Winfield, Illinois

Radhika Polisetty, PharmD, FIDSA, BCIDP, AAHIVP
Clinical Specialist, Infectious Diseases
Northwestern Medicine—Central DuPage Hospital
Associate Professor, Department of Pharmacy Practice
Midwestern University College of Pharmacy
Downers Grove, Illinois

Tonya Powell, DNP, ACNP-BC
Adjunct/Clinical Faculty
Adult-Gerontology Acute Care Nurse Practitioner Program
Georgetown University, School of Nursing & Health Studies
Washington, District of Columbia

Heather Roppel, RN, MSN, AGACNP, CCNS, CCRN, CNRN
Critical Care Clinical Nurse Specialist
Northwestern Medicine—Huntley Hospital
Huntley, Illinois

Justin Shiau, PharmD
Clinical Pharmacist
Department of Pharmacy
Northwestern Medicine—Central DuPage Hospital
Winfield, Illinois

Catherine Tierney, DNP, ACNP-BC
Assistant Professor, Clinical Faculty Director
Adult-Gerontology Acute Care Nurse Practitioner Program
Georgetown University School of Nursing
Washington, District of Columbia

Charleen Yeager, MSN, RN, CNL
Staff Nurse
Rush University Medical Center
Chicago, Illinois

Contributors

Bryan Boling, DNP, AGACNP-BC, FCCM
Advanced Practice Provider, Director of Simulation, & POCUS Training
Department of Anesthesiology, Division of Critical Care Medicine
Adjunct Assistant Professor, Adult-Gerontology Acute Care Nurse Practitioner Program
Georgetown University
Washington, District of Columbia
Chapter 42: Anatomy and Physiology of the Renal System
Chapter 43: Renal Regulation of Electrolytes
Chapter 44: Diagnosis and Treatment of Acute Renal Failure
Chapter 45: Renal Trauma

Angela Campbell, MSN, APRN, FNP-BC, PMHNP-BC
Clinical Practice Specialist
Northwestern Medicine—Central DuPage Hospital
Winfield, Illinois
Chapter 50: Behavioral and Psychologic Factors in Critical Care

Angela Craig, MS, APN, CCNS, CCRN-K
Clinical Nurse Specialist for ICU and Sepsis Coordinator
Cookeville Regional Medical Center
Cookeville, Tennessee
Chapter 46: Sepsis and Multiorgan Syndrome
Chapter 47: Toxic Emergencies
Chapter 48: Airway Obstruction

Melissa Golombek, DNP, MS-HCM, RN, NE-BC, CPN
Vice President
TGH Children's Hospital and The Women's Institute
Tampa General Hospital
Tampa, Florida
Chapter 49: Professional Caring and Ethical Practice

Alison M. Keck, MSN, APRN, AGCNS-BC, CCRN-K
Cardiac and Medical–Surgical Clinical Nurse Specialist
Northwestern Medicine—Central DuPage Hospital
Winfield, Illinois
Chapter 1: Cardiovascular Anatomy and Physiology
Chapter 2: Diagnosis and Treatment of Cardiovascular Disorders
Chapter 3: The Normal ECG
Chapter 4: The 12-Lead ECG
Chapter 6: Acute Coronary Syndrome (Angina Pectoris and Myocardial Infarction)
Chapter 7: Conduction Blocks
Chapter 8: Congestive Heart Failure, Pulmonary Edema, and Hypertensive Crisis
Chapter 11: Interpreting Dysrhythmias
Chapter 12: Cardiomyopathies and Pericarditis

Anne C. Lindstrom, DNP, APRN, FNP-BC, NEA-BC, SCRN
Advanced Practice Nurse
Director of Operations
Northwestern Medicine—Marianjoy Rehabilitation Hospital
Wheaton, Illinois
Chapter 29: Anatomy and Physiology of the Nervous System
Chapter 30: Intracranial Pressure
Chapter 31: Acute Head Injuries and Craniotomies
Chapter 32: Stroke
Chapter 33: The Vertebrae and Spinal Cord
Chapter 34: Encephalopathies, Coma, and Brain Herniation
Chapter 35: Meningitis, Guillain–Barré, Muscular Dystrophy, and Myasthenia Gravis
Chapter 36: Seizures and Status Epilepticus

Jennifer MacDermott, MS, RN, NP-C, ACNS-BC, CCRN
Nurse Practitioner
St. Luke's Medical Center
Boise, Idaho
Chapter 20: Introduction to the Endocrine System
Chapter 21: Anatomy, Physiology, and Dysfunction of the Pituitary Gland
Chapter 22: Anatomy, Physiology, and Dysfunction of the Thyroid and Parathyroid Glands
Chapter 23: Anatomy, Physiology, and Dysfunction of the Pancreas
Chapter 24: Anatomy, Physiology, and Dysfunction of the Adrenal Glands

Donna Schweitzer, APRN, CCNS, CCRN
Critical Care Clinical Nurse Specialist
Carle BroMenn Medical Center
Normal, Illinois
Chapter 14: Pulmonary Anatomy and Physiology
Chapter 15: Diagnosis and Treatment of Pulmonary Disorders
Chapter 16: Alternative Methods of Ventilatory Support
Chapter 17: Acute Respiratory Dysfunction
Chapter 18: Acute Pulmonary Embolism and Aspiration
Chapter 19: Thoracic Trauma and Air-Leak Syndromes

Ashley N. Thompson, DNP, AGACNP-BC
Clinical Assistant Professor, Acute Care Track Coordinator
University of Florida College of Nursing
Acute Care Nurse Practitioner
Surgical Critical Care Medicine
University of Florida Health Hospital
Gainesville, Florida
Chapter 25: Physiology of the Immunologic and Hematologic Systems
Chapter 26: Diagnosis and Treatment of Immunologic and Hematologic Problems
Chapter 27: Hematologic and Immunologic Failure and its Effects on Other Organ Systems
Chapter 28: Life-Threatening Coagulopathies

Kelly A. Thompson-Brazill, DNP, ACNP-BC, RN, CCRN-CSC, PCCN, FCCM
Associate Professor; Assistant Dean for APRN Programs
Georgetown University School of Nursing
Washington, District of Columbia
Chapter 5: Hemodynamic Monitoring
Chapter 9: Cardiogenic Shock
Chapter 10: Hemorrhagic (Hypovolemic) Shock
Chapter 13: Treatment of Cardiac, Valvular, and Vascular Insufficiency, and Trauma
Chapter 37: Anatomy and Physiology of the Gastrointestinal System
Chapter 38: Gastrointestinal Hemorrhage and Esophageal Varices
Chapter 39: Acute and Chronic Hepatic Failure, Cirrhosis, Hepatitis, and Acute Pancreatitis
Chapter 40: Intestinal Infarction, Obstruction, Perforation, and Trauma
Chapter 41: Management of the Patient with a Gastrointestinal Disturbance

Preface

In this edition of *Critical Care Nursing Certification Review: CCRN Prep and Practice Exams*, we have updated the content to align with the most recent CCRN exam changes. We hope that this edition may serve as a comprehensive critical care reference text (using short, easy to read chapters), as well as a certification preparation book. In this edition, we have added new features to support learning by providing key highlights, more bolded and italicized content, callout sections, test questions embedded in the text and at the end of each section, provided some general test-taking strategies, and an estimate on the number of questions for each content area on the CCRN exam. Additionally, in this new edition, we have increased the number of test questions and expanded answer rationales to help provide and reinforce test-taking information, tactics, and techniques. We hope these changes increase success on future exam questions.

The CCRN exam generally reflects what you see every day in your practice. A focus is placed on the 80/20 rule, and unusual concepts and conditions are not emphasized on the exam. In other words, "obscure" techniques or procedures, or practices only observed in tertiary medical centers do not appear on the exam. Focus on addressing the root causes in scenario questions, and remember that a strong understanding of the rationale or theory driving a clinical problem on the test will more than outweigh any lack of clinical experience that you may feel. The content of the exam is something that you will generally see in your practice. In fact, one of the best ways to study for the exam is to use this book in your clinical practice.

Passing the exam is a major milestone in your career and helps validate your knowledge, your commitment, and your practice. To paraphrase a famous quote, "We are not telling you it will be easy, but we can tell you it is going to be worth it."

Good luck on your CCRN exam.

Alexander P. Johnson, MSN, RN, ACNP-BC, CCNS, CCRN

Hillary S. Crumlett, DNP, RN, NEA-BC

Acknowledgments

We are indebted to our friends, team members, and leaders at Northwestern Medicine—Central DuPage and Huntley Hospitals. Without their patience, strength, support, and excellent care delivered daily, an endeavor such as this may not have been possible.

Test-Taking Tips

The following are some general test-taking tips. Follow them as you prepare for the examinations in this text and on the CCRN examination. They can make the difference in several points on the examination.

1. **Answer all questions**. Unanswered questions are counted as incorrect. Use your knowledge to rule out incorrect answers whenever in doubt.
2. **Be well-rested before the examination**. Get a good night's sleep before the examination. Do not try to "cram" on the morning of the test: You may confuse yourself if you study right before the test.
3. **Have a good but light breakfast**. The exam is 150 total questions [125 are scored] to be answered within the 3-h timeframe). Eat food that is not all carbohydrates so that you can make it through the examination without becoming hungry or getting a headache.
4. **Do not change answers—<u>unless absolutely sure of your change</u>.** Many first impressions are accurate.
5. **"Flag" questions as you go through the test**. Mark on a piece of scrap paper the questions that are difficult. Then go back and review the difficult questions. Do not be discouraged if there are many hard questions.
6. **Do not expect to answer all questions correctly**. If you do not know the answer to a question, make an educated guess and go on. Do not let it bother you that you missed a few questions. You will not have a good perception of how you did until you get the results. However, bear in mind that in 2022, the first time pass rate of the CCRN was 81.3% which is very strong?
7. **Achieving approximately >70% on practice examinations indicates readiness and adequate preparedness for the examination**. Similarly, a raw score of 88 of 125 (70%) is what is required to pass the examination. So again, do not be too discouraged by questions that may seem challenging.

In addition, general practice trends in critical care nursing are reflected on the exam (such as the overall decreased use of pulmonary artery catheters). However, more focused information reflective of regional or institutional trends are not covered, such as the technical specifications of an esophageal Doppler monitor or stop-cock functionality. Remain mindful of this when considering "obscure" questions to anticipate:

1. Do not let the fact that other people finish early (or that you finish before others) disturb you. People work at different rates without necessarily a difference in results.
2. If you feel thirsty or need to go to the restroom, ask permission from the monitor. Always try to maintain your physiological status at optimal levels. An aspirin (or similar analgesic) may be in order if a headache develops during the test. Consider having ear plugs to reduce ambient noise if you feel this may help you.
3. Do not try to establish patterns in how the items are written (eg, "Two B's have occurred, now some other choice is likely"). The AACN Certification Corporation has excellent test-writing mechanisms. Patterns in test answers, if they occur, are coincidental.

PART I

CARDIOVASCULAR

Alison M. Keck and Kelly A. Thompson-Brazill

1

Cardiovascular Anatomy and Physiology

CHAPTER OVERVIEW AND OBJECTIVES

Although basic anatomy is not commonly addressed in the CCRN exam, an understanding of the principles of anatomy may help your perception of more specific questions regarding cardiovascular concepts. The following chapter is a brief review of key anatomic and physiologic cardiovascular concepts while also addressing background information on cardiovascular concepts. If you do not have a strong background in anatomy and physiology, study this section closely.

The CCRN exam places the most emphasis on the cardiovascular component, with approximately 17% of the test questions in this content area. While many nurses are relatively strong in cardiovascular concepts, do not take this part of the exam lightly. The better you perform in any one area, the greater your chances of overall success on the exam.

After studying this chapter, you should be able to:

- Understand normal anatomy and physiology of the heart and circulatory system.
- Appreciate effects of the cardiac cycle on the mechanics of the heart.
- Appreciate effects of the pressure gradients on the flow of blood within the heart.

1.1 NORMAL LOCATION AND SIZE OF THE HEART

The heart lies in the mediastinum, above the diaphragm, surrounded on both sides by the lungs. If one looks at a frontal (anterior) view, the heart resembles a triangle (**Fig. 1-1**). The base of the heart is parallel to the right edge of the sternum, whereas the lower right point of the triangle represents the apex of the heart. The apex is usually at the left midclavicular line at the fifth intercostal space (ICS). The average adult heart is about 5 in. long and 3½ in. wide, about the size of an average man's clenched fist. The heart weighs about 2 g for each pound of ideal body weight.

1.2 NORMAL ANATOMY OF THE HEART

The heart is supported by a fibrous skeleton (**Fig. 1-2**) composed of dense connective tissue. This skeleton connects the four valve rings (annuli) of the heart: the tricuspid, mitral, pulmonic, and aortic valves. Attached to the superior (top) surface of this skeleton are the right and left atria, the pulmonary artery, and the aorta. Attached to the inferior (lower) surface of the skeleton are the right and left ventricles and the mitral and tricuspid valve cusps.

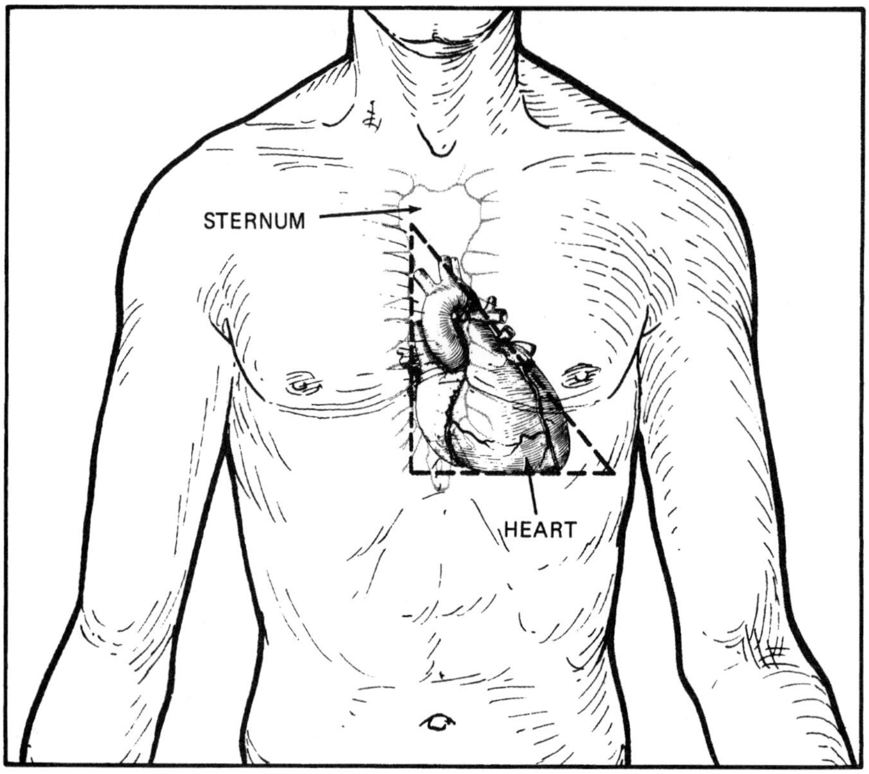

Figure 1-1. Frontal view of the heart.

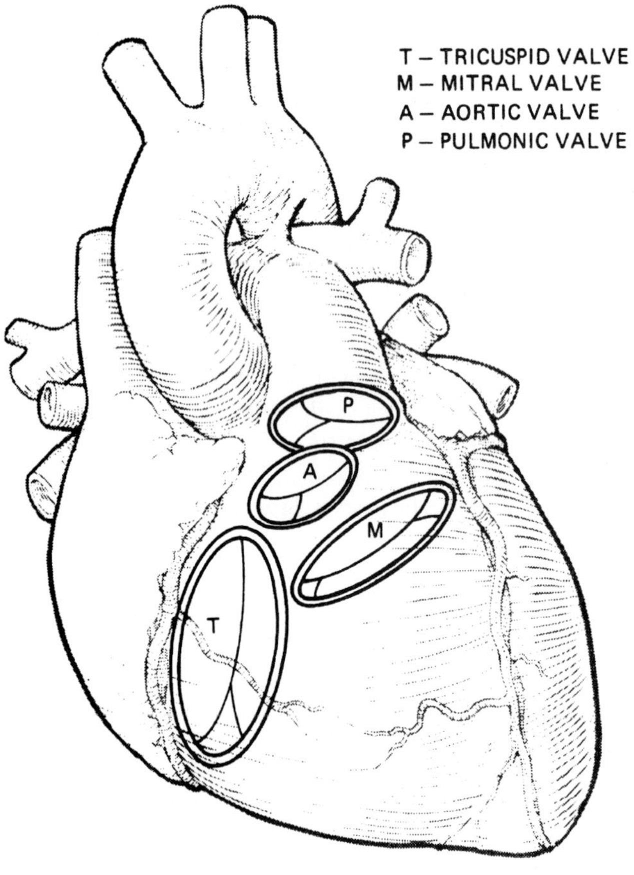

Figure 1-2. Fibrous skeleton of the heart (frontal view).

The heart can be studied as two parallel pumps: the right pump (right atrium and ventricle) and the left pump (left atrium and ventricle). Each pump receives blood into its atrium. The blood flows from atria through a one-way valve into the ventricles. From each ventricle, blood is ejected into a circulatory system. The right ventricle ejects blood into the pulmonary circulation, while the left ventricle ejects blood into the systemic circulation. Although there are differences between the right and left sides of the heart, the gross anatomy of each side is similar. Structural features of each chamber are discussed below.

1.3 STRUCTURE OF THE HEART WALL

The heart is enclosed in a fibrous sac called the pericardium. The pericardium is composed of two layers: the fibrous and parietal pericardia. The fibrous pericardium is the outer layer that helps support the heart. The parietal pericardium, the inside layer, is a smooth fibrous membrane.

Next to the parietal serous layer of the pericardium is a visceral layer, which is actually the outer heart surface. It is most often termed the "epicardium." Between the epicardium and the parietal pericardium is 10 to 20 mL of fluid, which prevents friction during the heart's contraction and relaxation.

The myocardium, or muscle mass of the heart, is composed of cardiac muscle, which has characteristics of both smooth and skeletal muscles. The endocardium is the inner surface of the heart wall. It is a membranous covering that lines all of the heart's chambers and the valves.

Papillary muscles originate in the ventricular endocardium and attach to chordae tendineae (**Fig. 1-3**). The chordae

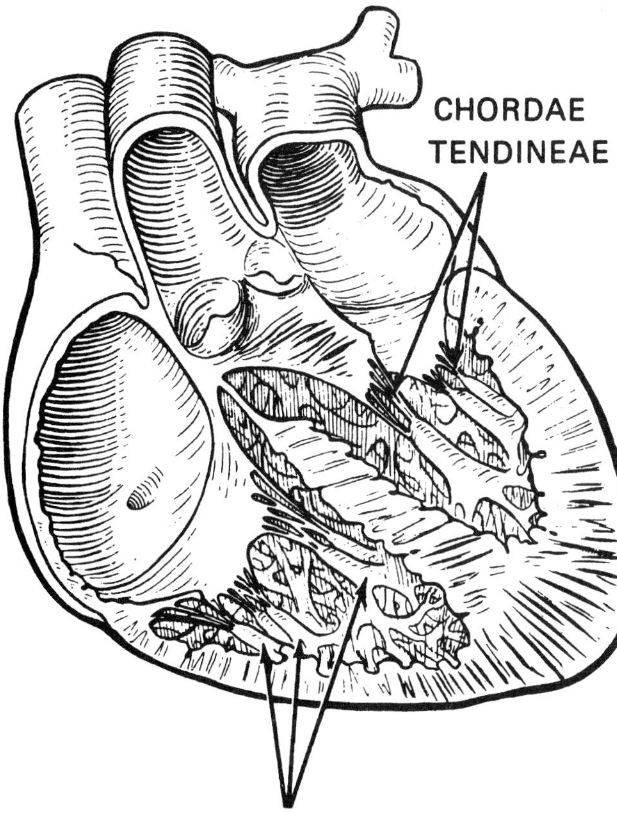

Figure 1-3. Papillary muscles and chordae tendineae.

tendineae attach to the inferior surface of the tricuspid and mitral valve cusps, enabling the valves to open and close. The papillary muscles are in parallel alignment to the ventricular wall.

1.4 CARDIAC MUSCLE CELLS

QUICK TIP! The information in this section regarding cellular aspects of cardiac muscle anatomy and physiology is not likely to be on the CCRN exam. Questions on this area are rare. However, the concepts addressed in this section form the basis for understanding myocardial dysfunction and pharmacological intervention. Read this section to become familiar with the concepts, but not necessarily to memorize specific details.

The sarcomere (**Fig. 1-4**) is the contracting unit of the myocardium. The outer covering of the sarcomere is the sarcolemma, which surrounds the muscle fiber. The sarcolemma covers a muscle fiber that is composed of thick and thin fibers often collectively called myofibrils. Sarcomeres are separated from each other by a thickening of the sarcolemma at the ends of the sarcomere. These thickened ends, called intercalated discs, are actively involved in cardiac contraction. Each sarcomere has a centrally placed nucleus surrounded by sarcoplasma.

Myofibrils are thick and thin parts of the muscle fiber. Thick fibrils are myosin filaments. They have regularly placed projections that form calcium gates to the thick myofibrils. The thin myofibrils are actin. The myosin and actin myofibrils are arranged in specific parallel and hexagonal patterns (**Fig. 1-5**). This arrangement of fibers forms a syncytium that causes all of the fibers to depolarize when even one fiber is depolarized. This is known as the **"all or none" principle**—all fibers depolarize or no fibers depolarize. Troponin and tropomyosin are regulatory proteins attached to or affecting actin. These thick and thin myofibrils slide back and forth over each other, resulting in contraction and relaxation of the sarcomeres and, thus, the heart.

The study of the cardiac cycle's physiology examines the means by which the heart pumps blood and the various mechanisms that control the heart pump. Before looking at the heart as a whole, let us examine the contraction of a single sarcomere.

1.5 CONTRACTION OF THE SARCOMERE

The sarcomeres are much like striated muscles, but they have more mitochondria than do striated or smooth muscles. The mitochondria provide the energy that sarcomeres need to contract. This energy is released by converting adenosine triphosphate (ATP) into adenosine diphosphate (ADP). In addition, the mitochondria are crucial in the storing of energy through the formation of ATP from ADP. The addition of a phosphate molecule to ADP to form ATP is called phosphorylation. This formation of ADP from ATP normally takes place in the presence of oxygen (aerobic metabolism) and is referred to as oxidative phosphorylation. Energy can be produced without oxygen (anaerobic metabolism), but not as efficiently as during aerobic metabolism. Cardiac muscle cells are highly dependent on constant blood flow to maintain adequate supplies of oxygen for the formation of ATP.

In the sarcomere, thick (myosin) and thin (actin) fibrils are arranged side by side in parallel rows. The myosin fibrils have projections that contact actin at specific points. These contact points are referred to as calcium gates (**Fig. 1-6**). During cardiac contraction, myosin and actin slide together and overlap to as great an extent as possible (**Fig. 1-7**). (In the normal resting state, there is some overlapping of the myosin and actin fibrils.) Troponin and tropomyosin are protein rods interwoven around the actin fibril, having a regulatory effect on the actin and its ability to connect with the calcium gates in the presence of calcium ions.

At the start of cellular excitation leading to a contraction, calcium ions (Ca^{2+}) attach to troponin molecules around the actin fibril. This enables the projections (calcium gates) of the myosin fibril to attach to the actin. These projections twist around, causing a sliding of the fibers over each other. The calcium is removed from the calcium gates by calcium pumps located throughout the sarcoplasmic reticulum. As soon as the calcium is removed, the myosin and actin fibers slide back to their original position. This process is repeated, causing the cardiac cell to contract and relax.

KEY CLINICAL CONCEPT

Consider how the physiology described here explains how calcium can augment the cardiac output. For example, this is why calcium chloride IVP augments cardiac output and blood pressure, whereas calcium-channel blockers decrease inotropic effect.

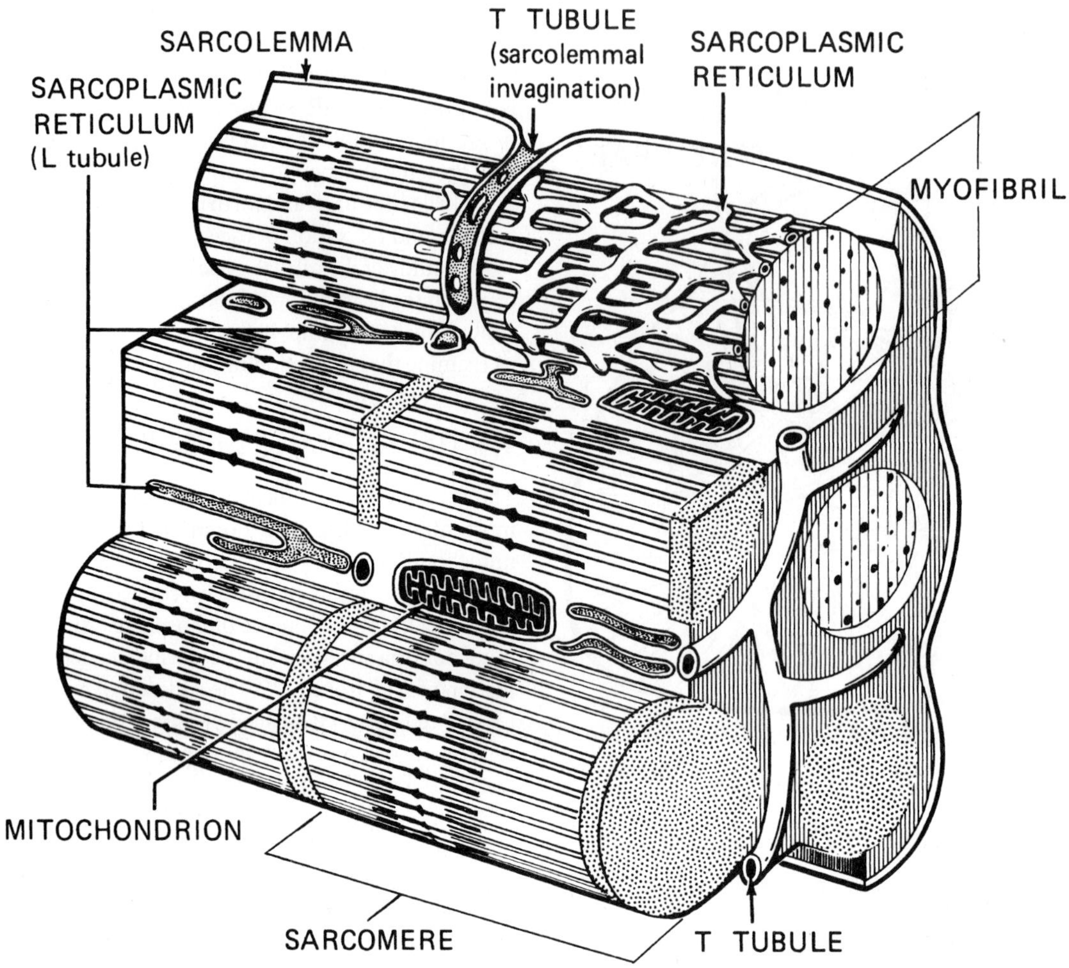

Figure 1-4. The sarcomere.

It is important to remember that calcium initiates and regulates the sarcomere's depolarization and repolarization. The role of calcium in the contraction and relaxation of the cardiac muscle cell serves as the basis for several cardiac therapies, including the use of calcium channel-blocking agents and the potential inotropic (strength) value in administering calcium. Even though calcium ions initiate the sliding movement of the fibrils, calcium alone is not able to cause the contraction. In addition to the presence of calcium, an exchange of ions (creating electrical energy) must occur during phases of depolarization and repolarization. This ionic exchange is mainly between sodium and potassium and creates an ionic action potential. The exchange of chemical elements occurs across the semipermeable cell membrane in three ways: filtration, osmosis, and diffusion (active or passive).

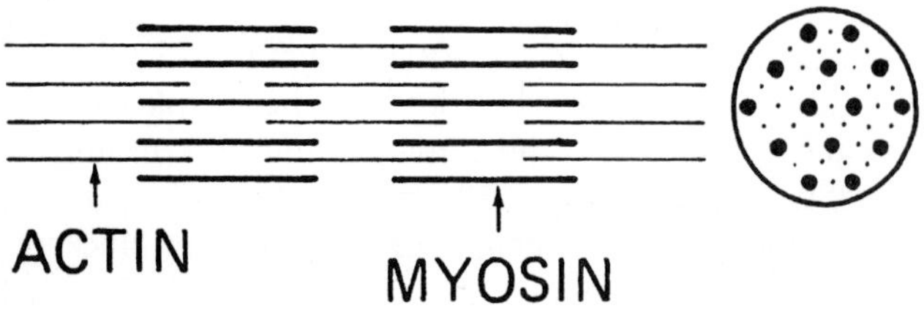

Figure 1-5. Arrangement of myosin and actin myofibrils.

1.6 ACTION POTENTIAL OF THE CARDIAC CELL

There are five phases of activity during the cardiac cell cycle; each phase is described below. The exchange and concentration of ions differ in each phase. Mainly four ions are involved: sodium (Na^+), potassium (K^+), calcium (Ca^{2+}), and chloride (Cl^-). Normally, there is more sodium, calcium, and chloride outside the cell and more potassium inside it. Since all ions have an electrical charge, an electrical gradient is established. When a state of ionic electrical neutrality exists, the cell membrane is relatively impermeable—a period known as the resting potential. The presence of an electrical and chemical (ion) gradient plus membrane selectively establishes an action potential consisting of five phases: 0 through 4.

QUICK TIP! It is not uncommon for one question on the exam to ask what happens in any of the five phases of the action potential of the cardiac cell (in general terms).

Phase 0

As a result of the presence of sodium and potassium outside and inside the cell, respectively, there is an electronegative gradient. A depolarizing stimulus is caused by efflux of potassium from the cell, increasing the cell permeability for sodium. Calcium ions in the T- and L-tubule systems of the sarcomere

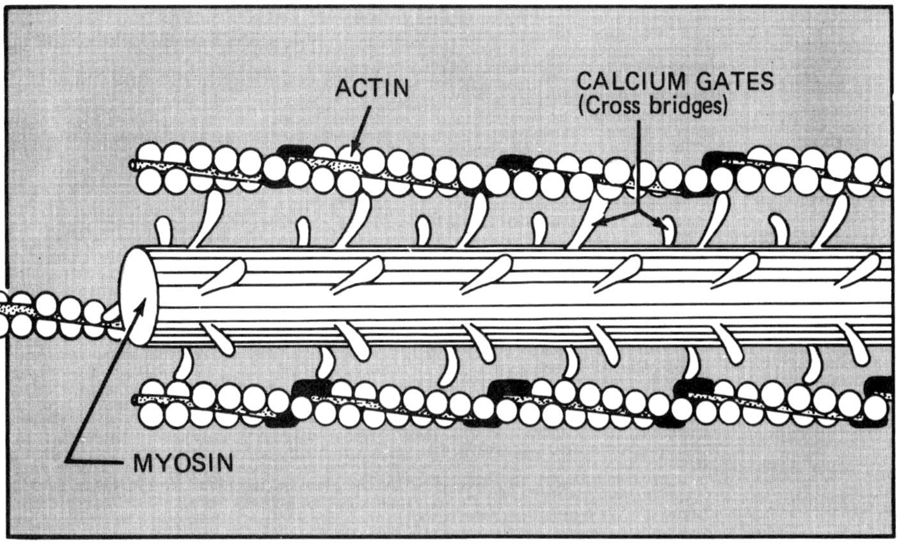

Figure 1-6. Myosin and actin fibrils with calcium gates.

are at Ca^{2+} gates on the cell membrane and "open" the gates for the influx of sodium (see Fig. 1-4). When this gradient reaches about −90 mV inside the cell (resting membrane potential), there is a rapid increase of the action potential (zero in **Fig. 1-8**). The result of the depolarization stimulus is an increase in the cell's permeability to sodium. As the sodium threshold (the point at which sodium moves most freely) is reached (about −55 mV), sodium rushes into the cell and depolarizes it. The cell becomes electropositive at about +20 to +30 mV, causing a spike on the action potential diagram.

Phase 1

This is the spike phase of positive electrical charge. There is a period of initial rapid repolarization (tip of spike to "phase 1" in Fig. 1-8), which is probably due to a flow of chloride ions into the cell.

Phase 2

This is a plateau phase of repolarization. Calcium entering the cell and potassium leaving the cell balance each other, so there is no net electrical change; thus, a flat line (plateau) appears. Sodium entry into the cell is almost completely inactivated. A slow movement of calcium into the cell and potassium out of the cell begins (phase 2 in Fig. 1-8).

Phase 3

This is a rapid decline phase of repolarization (phase 3 in Fig. 1-8). Potassium loss from the cell is greatest in this phase.

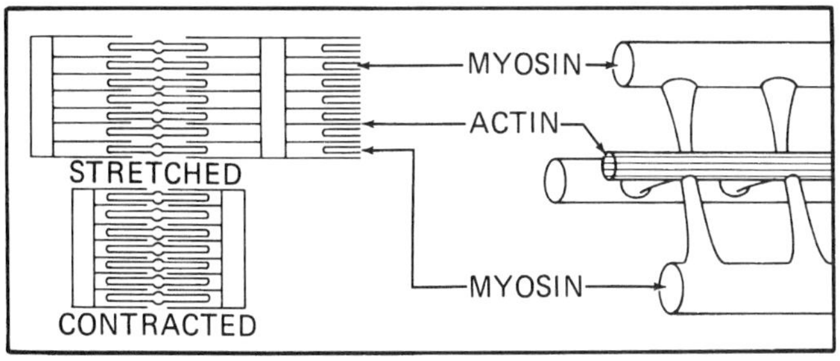

Figure 1-7. Contraction of the myosin and actin fibrils.

This potassium loss returns the cell to electronegativity. Sodium and calcium currents are completely inactivated.

Phase 4

This is the resting interval between action potentials (phase 4 in Fig. 1-8). The sodium/potassium pumps are the most active here in effecting an exchange of potassium for sodium across the cell membrane. Potassium continues to leave the cell, and when electronegativity reaches −90 mV, phase 0 starts again if a stimulus occurs.

1.7 HEART CHAMBERS

There are four chambers in the heart (**Fig. 1-9**). The atria are superior to the ventricles and are separated from the ventricles by valves. The right atrium and ventricle are separated from the left atrium and ventricle by the atrial and ventricular septa.

Right Atrium

The right atrium is a thin-walled chamber exposed to low blood pressures. Systemic venous blood enters the right atrium from the superior and inferior venae cavae. Venous blood from the heart enters the right atrium via the Thebesian veins, which drain into the coronary sinus. The coronary sinus is located on the medial right atrial wall, just about the tricuspid valve.

Right Ventricle

The right ventricle is the pump for the right side of the heart. The right ventricle contracts pumping venous blood into the pulmonary artery and the lungs. The lungs are normally a low-pressure system. The right ventricle is shaped and functions like a bellow to propel blood out during contraction.

Left Atrium

The left atrium, just like the right, is thin walled. Blood flowing passively from the low-lung-pressure area does not stress the walls of the left atrium. The left atrium receives oxygenated blood from the four pulmonary veins.

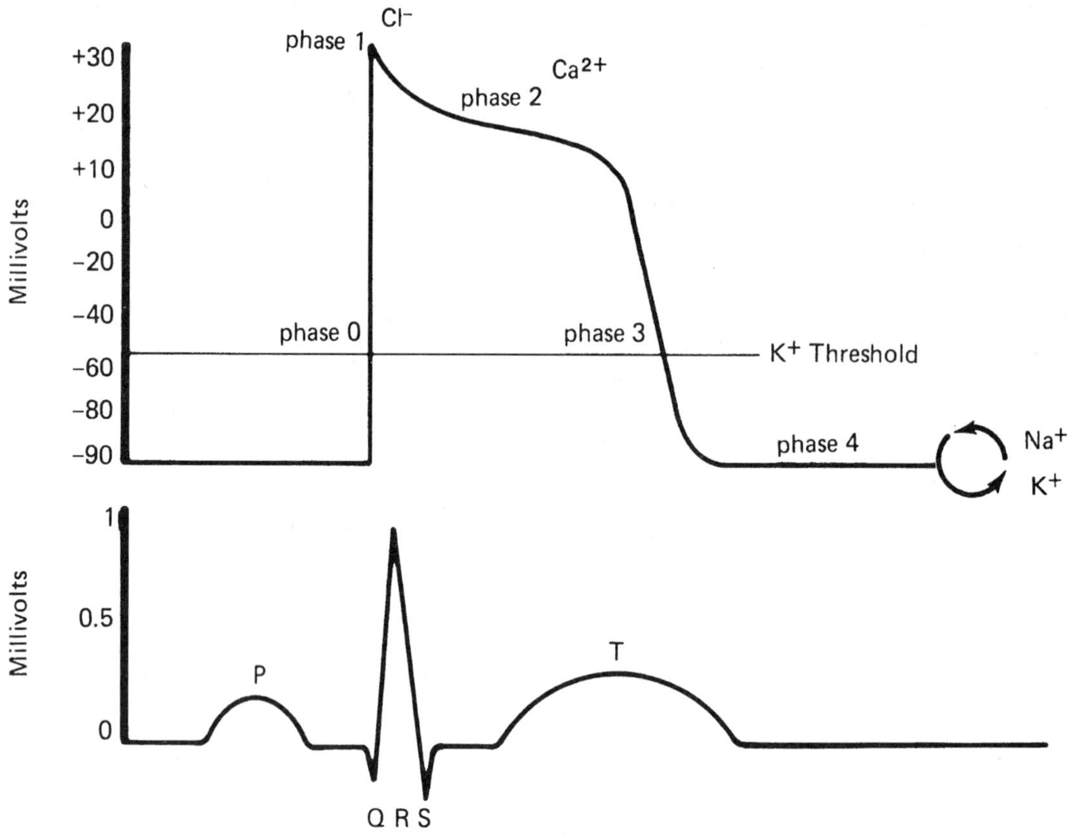

Figure 1-8. Phases of the cardiac potential and ion movement correlated with the ECG tracing.

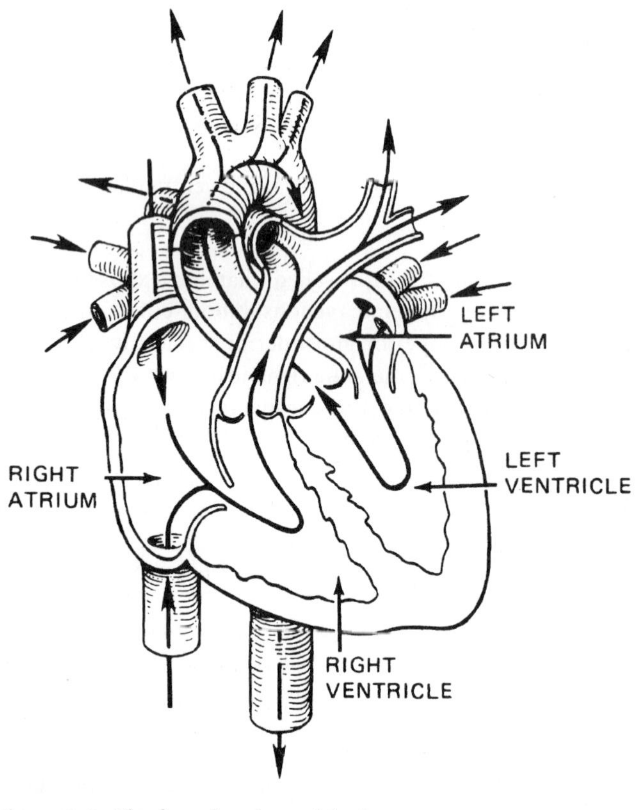

Figure 1-9. The four chambers of the heart.

Left Ventricle

The left ventricle is the major pump for the entire body. As such, it must have thick, strong walls. To overcome the high pressure of the systemic circulation, the left ventricle is shaped like a cylinder. As it contracts (starting from the apex), it also narrows somewhat. This cylindrical shape provides a physical force strong enough to propel blood into the aorta and to overcome the high systemic pressure (resulting from the requirement to pump the blood to distant body areas).

1.8 HEART VALVES

There are two types of valves in the heart: the atrioventricular (AV) and the semilunar valves. All valves in the heart are unidirectional unless they are diseased or dysfunctional. Normally the valves provide very little resistance to cardiac contractions. If the valves become narrow (stenotic) or allow blood to flow past when they should be closed (regurgitation), the work of the heart will substantially increase.

Atrioventricular Valves

The AV valves of the heart are the tricuspid and the mitral valves. These allow blood to flow from the atria into the ventricles during atrial contraction and ventricular diastole. Both the mitral and the tricuspid valves have two large opposing leaflets and small intermediary leaflets at each end.

QUICK TIP! Mnemonics may help you remember which valve is on which side of the heart. Consider the following: "L" and "M" come together in the alphabet and in the heart. The left heart contains the mitral valve. Likewise, "R" and "T" are close in the alphabet. The right heart contains the tricuspid valve.

Mitral Valve. The mitral valve's two large leaflets are not quite equal in size (**Fig. 1-10**). The chordae tendineae from adjacent leaflets are inserted on the same papillary muscles. This physical feature helps to ensure complete closure of the valve. When the mitral valve is open, the valve, chordae tendineae, and papillary muscle look like a funnel. Of all the valves, the mitral is most commonly involved in clinical conditions of valvular dysfunction with mitral regurgitation being one of the most common clinical valvular disturbances. Clinically, mitral regurgitation may be insignificant (subclinical) or represent a life-threatening situation (papillary muscle rupture). The key factor influencing the significance of any valvular disturbance is the effect on stroke volume (SV, amount of blood the heart pumps with each contraction).

Tricuspid Valve. The tricuspid valve differs from the mitral valve in that it has three leaflets and three papillary muscles instead of two. Otherwise, the structures and functions of the two valves are similar. Tricuspid dysfunction is not as much of a clinical problem as is mitral dysfunction.

Semilunar (Pulmonic and Aortic) Valves

The semilunar valves (**Fig. 1-11**) of the heart are the aortic and pulmonary valves. Each has three symmetrical valve cusps to provide for complete opening without stretching the valve. The pulmonary valve is located between the right ventricle and the pulmonary artery. The aortic valve is located between the left ventricle and the aorta.

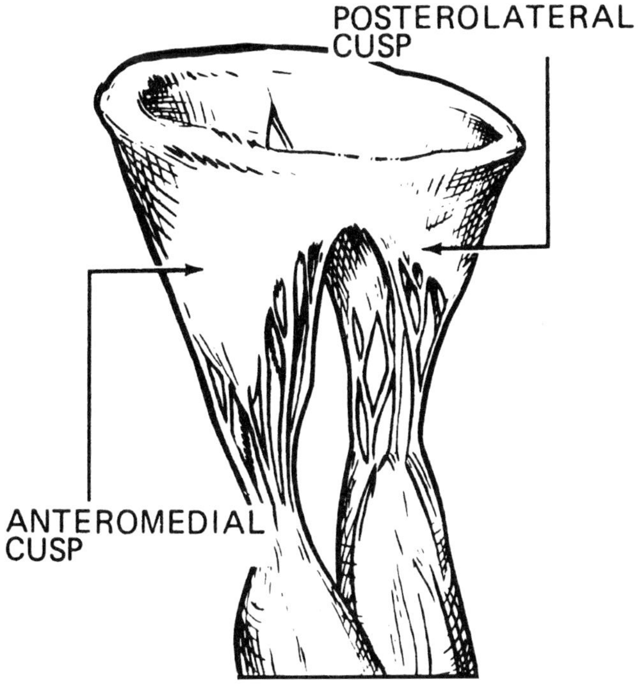

Figure 1-10. Side view of the mitral valve.

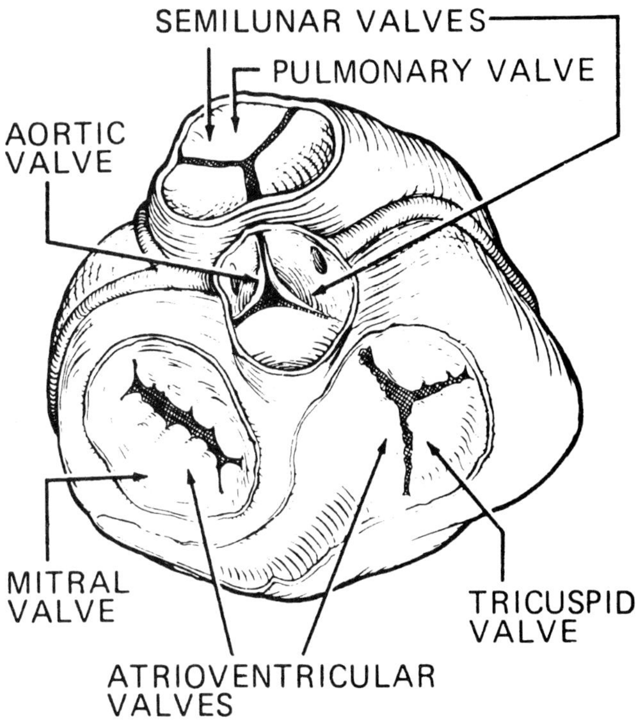

Figure 1-11. The semilunar valves and AV valves (posterior view).

Pulmonary valve dysfunction will potentially affect the performance of the right ventricle. Aortic valve disturbance can affect the performance of the left ventricle.

Physical Assessment of the Cardiac Valves

Cardiac valves can be assessed to some extent through auscultation. Heart sounds can be identified partially based on specific valve functioning. The heart normally generates two sounds, referred to as S_1 and S_2. S_1 is the sound generated through the closure of the mitral (M_1) and tricuspid (T_1) valves. M_1 is best heard at the fifth ICS in the left midclavicular line. T_1 is best heard at the fourth ICS at the left sternal border. S_1 is produced during ventricular contraction. S_1 can be identified by listening (it normally is the louder of the two cardiac sounds at the fourth ICS, left sternal border or the fifth ICS, left midclavicular line) or by comparing the sounds to the electrocardiogram (ECG). The S_1 sound occurs immediately after the QRS complex (which indicates ventricular depolarization and contraction).

S_2 is produced by the closure of the aortic (A_2) and pulmonic (P_2) valves. A_2 is best heard at the second ICS, just to the right of the sternum. The P_2 sound is heard best at the second ICS, just to the left of the sternum. S_2 can also be identified by listening (it is loudest in the locations described above) or by comparing it to the ECG. Normally, the S_2 sound occurs during diastole (when aortic and pulmonary blood pressures are higher than ventricular pressures, forcing the aortic and pulmonary valves to close). The S_2 sound normally appears during the T wave or slightly before the QRS complex.

Abnormal Heart Sounds

Heart valves normally produce sound during closure. There are four situations when other abnormal sounds might develop that are relatively common. These are valve regurgitation, stenosis, ventricular or atrial failure, and disturbances of electrical conduction.

> **QUICK TIP!** Questions regarding normal heart sounds will not likely show up on the exam. However, be ready to recognize S3 (often associated with fluid overload or pulmonary edema) or S4 (suggests a "stiff" ventricle, such as s/p MI).

Valve Regurgitation

When a valve becomes regurgitant (sometimes referred to as insufficient), blood flows past the valve, which is normally closed. This produces a sound usually described as a murmur. Murmurs may be described in several ways, such as blowing and swishing. Murmurs are graded in degree from I to VI. A grade I murmur (written as I/VI) is a very soft sound. A grade VI murmur (written as VI/VI) is so prominent that it can be heard with the stethoscope held about 1 in. from the chest wall. The other grades of murmurs are subjectively described by the clinician as somewhere between I and VI as there is no clear objective criteria for doing this.

Mitral and tricuspid regurgitation will produce a murmur that occurs during systole (normally the mitral and tricuspid valves close during systole). Aortic and pulmonic regurgitation will produce a diastolic murmur.

Valvular Stenosis

A stenosis of a valve produces a murmur that may sound like a regurgitant murmur. However, the reasons for the murmur are different. A mitral or tricuspid stenosis produces a murmur during diastole (normally atrial contraction does not meet resistance to pushing blood past the mitral or tricuspid valve). An aortic or pulmonic stenosis can produce a systolic murmur. Valves can be dysfunctional in isolation (such as a mitral regurgitation) or in multiples. The clinician attempts to identify the cause of the murmur through auscultation and clinical history.

Ventricular and Atrial Failure

During ventricular failure, pressure levels build in the ventricles and atrium. After systole, when blood enters the ventricles from the atrium, the high atrial pressure may force blood into the ventricles with considerable force. This increased, rapid flow of blood into the ventricles may produce a sound, the S_3 sound. The S_3 sound occurs immediately after the S_2 sound. S_3 sounds are not always abnormal but should be considered significant, particularly in the presence of tachycardia. **The combination of a tachycardia and S_3 produces a characteristic "gallop" sound associated with left ventricular (congestive heart) failure. Another sound associated with high pressures is the S_4. It is thought to be an atrial sound, associated with high atrial pressures.**

Electrical Conduction Defects

When there is an electrical conduction defect, such as a bundle branch block, the potential exists for the valves to fail to function in unison. When this happens, a split in the heart sound will occur. For example, a right bundle branch block causes a delay in right ventricular contraction. The result is that the pulmonic valve closes slightly after the aortic valve. The S_2 sound now becomes softer and produces two sounds instead of one. The S_2 can aid in the diagnosis of a right bundle branch block.

> **QUICK TIP!** Clinically speaking, being able to differentiate between right vs. left bundle branch block is important. This level of ECG tracing analysis is usually out of scope for the exam. However, recognizing the ***clinical significance*** is important for the exam.

Pulsus Paradoxus and Change in Heart Sounds

Heart sounds can be ***diminished in intensity*** if air (as in chronic obstructive pulmonary disease) or fluid **(pericardial effusion or tamponade)** is between the heart and the stethoscope. In tamponade, fluid fills the pericardial sac and limits sound transmission. In addition, the increased fluid restricts ventricular expansion and can dangerously drop the cardiac output (CO). If **tamponade** occurs, the inability of the ventricle to distend will produce **diminished heart sounds, equalizing chamber pressures (eg, central venous and pulmonary capillary wedge pressures begin to equalize), venous distention develops, and pulsus paradoxus may occur. Pulsus paradoxus is the decrease of blood pressure during inspiration. A decrease in systolic blood pressure during inspiration of more than 10 mm Hg is characteristic of pulsus paradoxus**. The blood pressure decreases because of the increase in blood entering the atrium during inspiration, further increasing the pericardial pressure. The added pericardial pressure further decreases SV and systolic blood pressure.

Heart sounds can be useful clinical parameters, but the clinician requires frequent practice to become proficient in recognizing them. More accurate tests are replacing the clinical use of heart sounds. If valve dysfunction is thought to exist, echocardiography is the test of choice. If conduction defects exist, electrocardiography is more accurate than echocardiography in detecting abnormalities.

> **QUICK TIP!** For the purpose of the CCRN test, the basic information provided above will help to identify the essential information. Be prepared for questions in which a heart sound is given and you must then identify an associated clinical condition. However, be aware of the more accurate methods for assessing cardiac function, as they may also be addressed on the test.

1.9 THE NORMAL CONDUCTION SYSTEM OF THE HEART

The conduction of an electrical impulse normally follows an orderly, repetitive pattern from the right atrium, through the ventricles, and into the myocardium, where the impulse usually results in ventricular contraction (**Fig. 1-12**).

The sinoatrial (SA) node is at the junction of the superior vena cava and the right atrium. The SA node is a group of specialized heart cells that are self-excitatory. All self-excitatory cells have automaticity; that is, if the cells can excite themselves, they require no stimulus and may excite themselves at will. This is termed inherent automaticity or spontaneous depolarization. The SA node excites itself faster than any other cardiac cells

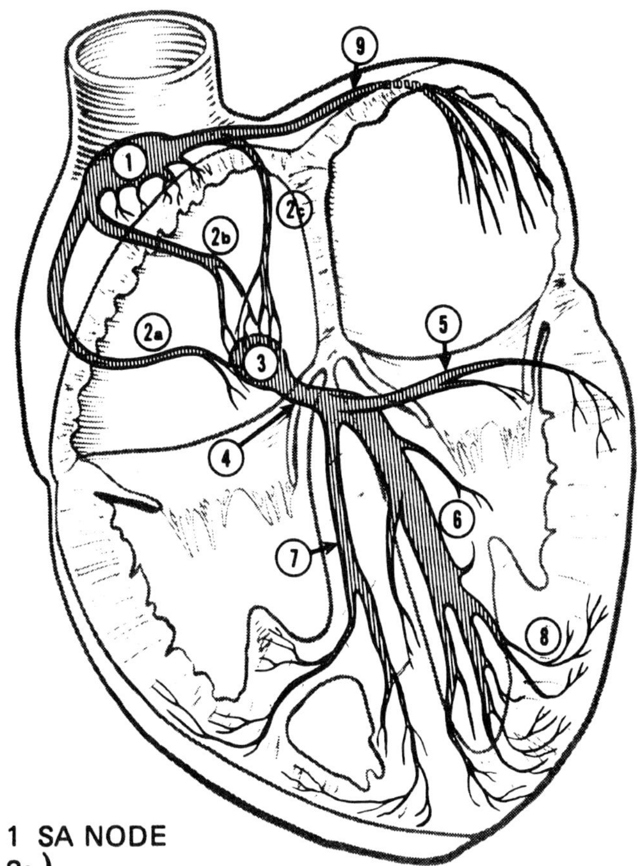

1 SA NODE
2a
2b INTRAATRIAL TRACTS
2c
3 AV NODE
4 BUNDLE OF HIS
5 LEFT BUNDLE BRANCH (anterior fascicle)
6 LEFT BUNDLE BRANCH (posterior fascicle)
7 RIGHT BUNDLE BRANCH
8 PURKINJE FIBERS
9 BACHMANN'S BUNDLE

Figure 1-12. Conduction system of the heart.

under normal conditions. For this reason, the SA node becomes the heart's normal pacemaker. Once the impulse originates in the SA node, it spreads through the atria along three paths, called internodal tracts. The impulse continues from the internodal tracts into the AV junction. The AV node is located at the superior end of the junctional tissue, near the tricuspid valve ring just above the ventricular septum. There is a slight pause in the impulse at the upper portion of the AV node to allow for completion of atrial contraction. The impulse traverses the AV node and the junctional tissue, and then reaches the bundle of His. The bundle of His carries the impulse to the right and left bundle branches.

The left bundle branch continues along the ventricular septum, dividing into two subdivisions called fascicles. The anterior fascicle excites the anterior and superior surfaces of the left ventricle. The posterior fascicle excites the posterior and inferior surfaces of the left ventricle. The right bundle branch continues as a single branch to innervate the right ventricle. Having passed through the bundle of His and the bundle branches, the impulse arrives at the Purkinje fibers, which spread into the ventricular myocardium. The impulse spread is usually followed by ventricular contraction, and thus the cycle is repeated. Disturbances in this conduction system are reviewed as to the specific resulting dysrhythmias.

KEY CLINICAL CONCEPT

The current CCRN format requires a good understanding of the electrical system of the heart and the ability to interpret dysrhythmias and 12-lead ECGs. Whereas specific sections are provided on dysrhythmias and 12-lead analysis, it is important to understand the basic anatomy and physiology of the electrical conduction system. However, actual 12-lead ECG tracings to interpret rarely appear on the CCRN exam. Any questions regarding ECG tracings are more likely to appear within a clinical scenario.

1.10 CIRCULATORY SYSTEMS OF THE BODY

Circulatory paths can be remembered by the mnemonic, "a" for *artery* means "a" for *away*. All arteries carry blood, either oxygenated or deoxygenated (pulmonary), away from the heart. Conversely, all veins carry blood, either oxygenated or deoxygenated, to the heart.

There are two circulatory systems in the body, the pulmonary and the systemic. The heart must pump blood through these two systems in the amount needed by the body to maintain optimal function. In addition, the coronary circulation (a branch of the systemic circulation), the pulmonary circulation, and the systemic circulation have some features that it is helpful to note for the purpose of the CCRN exam.

The Pulmonary Circulation

The pulmonary system is unique in that it is the only system (excluding the fetal) in which the pulmonary artery carries unoxygenated blood away from the heart to the lungs, and the four pulmonary veins carry oxygenated blood from the lungs to the left atrium. The right ventricle sends venous blood into the main pulmonary artery, which divides into the right and left pulmonary arteries. These arteries follow the normal blood vessel path, that is, arteries to arterioles to capillaries (where the blood becomes oxygenated) to venules to veins.

The Systemic Circulation

The aorta is the only artery into which the left ventricle normally ejects blood; it arches over the pulmonary artery and supplies oxygenated blood to the entire body via many branches including the subclavian, carotid, and iliac arteries. In the capillaries, the blood surrenders oxygen and picks up carbon dioxide. The inferior and superior venae cavae are the final veins returning blood to the right atrium.

The Coronary Circulation

The coronary circulatory system begins with the inflow of oxygenated blood into the coronary arteries. The openings of these arteries are called ostia. They are located near the cusps of the aortic valve. These arteries fill during ventricular diastole.

The *right coronary artery* supplies the posterior and inferior myocardium with oxygenated blood. The left coronary artery starts at the valve cusp as the *left main coronary artery* and bifurcates to form the left anterior descending (LAD) and the circumflex arteries. The *LAD artery* supplies the anterior and septal myocardium. The *circumflex artery* supplies the lateral myocardium. These arteries then follow the normal sequence of becoming arterioles, capillaries, venules, and veins as they course through the myocardium. The veins empty into Thebesian veins, which in turn empty into the coronary sinus. Blood from the coronary sinus joins the venous blood in the right atrium.

Autonomic Regulation of Peripheral Vessels

The **sympathetic nervous system** has an *adrenergic effect* on peripheral vessels. The **norepinephrine** released by the sympathetic system causes *vasoconstriction*. This vasoconstriction prevents pooling of blood in the peripheral vessels and augments the return of blood to the heart.

The **parasympathetic nervous system** has a *cholinergic effect* on peripheral vessels. Acetylcholine (ACH) is released by the parasympathetic nervous system. This causes a *vasodilation* of peripheral vessels. With dilation, more blood can remain in the peripheral vessels, and less blood is returned to the heart.

Baroreceptor Control

Baroreceptors are receptors located in the aortic arch, carotid sinus, atria, venae cavae, and pulmonary arteries that are sensitive to the stretching of the arterial and venous vessel walls. This means these specialized cells can be responsive to changes in blood pressure. **These receptor sites are responsive to mean arterial pressure greater than 60 mm Hg.** When stimulated by an elevated pressure, these receptors send signals to the medulla oblongata in the brain. *The medulla then inhibits sympathetic nervous system activity, which allows the vagus nerve of the* ***parasympathetic nervous system*** *to assume control.* This results in vasodilation of peripheral vessels and a *decreased heart rate (HR).* Under normal circumstances, this will allow the blood pressure to return to normal.

Conversely, if pressure is low, vagal tone is decreased, which allows the ***sympathetic nervous system*** *to assume control.* This results in *vasoconstriction* of the peripheral vessels and an increased HR. Under normal circumstances, this will allow the blood pressure to return to normal.

Vasomotor Center of Regulation

There are two areas of vasomotor control in the medulla oblongata: a vasoconstrictor area and a vasodilator area. *The vasomotor center responds to baroreceptors and chemoreceptors in the aortic arch and carotid sinus.*

> **KEY CLINICAL CONCEPT**
>
> The physiology described here explains how when patients are in Trendelenburg position while in shock, the increased flow to the baroreceptors in the carotid and aortic bodies sends a "false message" to the vasomotor center that compensatory vasoconstriction is responding better than it actually is. This is why Trendelenburg in shock resuscitation is no longer considered evidence-based.

If the vasoconstrictor area is stimulated, normally an increased HR, SV, and CO will result because of peripheral vasoconstriction. As the peripheral vessels constrict, more blood is forced from these vessels and returned to the heart. This normally restores arterial blood pressure.

If the vasodilator area is stimulated (by inhibition of the vasoconstrictor area), a decrease in SV and CO will normally occur. The vasodilation allows for more blood to remain in peripheral vessels; therefore, less blood is returned to the heart. The normal end result will be a decrease in blood pressure. This partially explains the bradycardia seen in hypertensive patients.

Chemoreceptors are activated by decreased oxygen pressures, an increased carbon dioxide level, and/or a decreased pH. Once activated, the chemoreceptors stimulate the vasoconstrictor area. The events that normally occur with such stimulation are then set into action.

1.11 HEART RATE

The HR is a valuable diagnostic tool in that it is the first compensatory response to a decrease in SV. A sinus tachycardia is frequently the result of a decrease in SV. The other reason an increase in the HR may occur is an increase in metabolic rate. This requires an increase in CO, which is generally met by increasing both HR and SV. This relationship is often illustrated by the formula:

$$\mathbf{CO = HR \times SV}$$

As one of the regulators of CO, HR, can be used as a guide to therapy and assessment. The HR is regulated by the autonomic nervous system through **sympathetic (adrenergic) and parasympathetic (cholinergic)** mechanisms. *Sympathetic regulation occurs through alpha and beta receptors* located in the cardiovascular system. There are two types of alpha and beta cells: $alpha_1$ and $alpha_2$, and $beta_1$ and $beta_2$. *Parasympathetic effect* is primarily through the *vagus nerve*.

When a bradycardia exists, treatment is based on the factors that control the HR. For example, parasympathetic stimulation has a stronger effect on the heart than does sympathetic stimulation. The stronger parasympathetic effect is the reason **atropine** is the first drug given to treat a bradycardia. **Atropine** is an *anticholinergic* (a.k.a. parasympatholytic) and counteracts the effects of ACH released by the peripheral nervous system (PNS).

HR elevations—for example, sinus tachycardia—by themselves are not generally dangerous. Although the increase in HR will increase myocardial oxygen consumption (MVo_2), the reason for the development of tachycardia is more important. A clinical clue to investigate is the origin of a sinus tachycardia, followed by treating the cause of the tachycardia rather than the tachycardia itself.

1.12 RELATIONSHIP OF BLOOD FLOW AND PRESSURE IN THE CARDIAC CYCLE

The pressure of a fluid in a chamber depends on the size of the chamber, the amount of fluid, the distensibility of the chamber, and whether the chamber is open or closed.

The atria (both right and left) are open chambers. The venae cavae in the right atrium and the pulmonary veins in the left atrium are always open. Thus, pressures in these chambers will

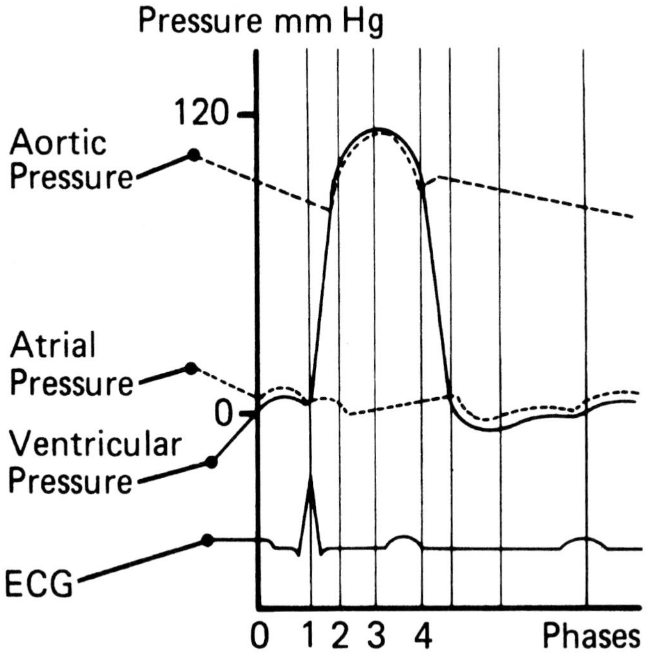

Figure 1-13. Blood flow and pressure during the cardiac cycle.

remain low unless something occludes the openings or prevents them from emptying.

The anatomic structure of the right ventricle contributes to its low pressure. The right ventricle normally empties into a low-pressure system, the lungs.

The left ventricle has a high pressure. Its anatomic structure contributes to the high pressure. It empties into a high-pressure, closed system, the aorta. Trace the flow of blood through the chambers and examine its relationship to the cardiac valves and the chamber pressures. These relationships are shown in **Fig. 1-13**.

Atrial Pressure Curve

Throughout diastole, pressure slowly increases in the atria because of the influx of blood. The volume of blood increases in relation to the chamber size (resulting in a V wave on the atrial waveform). With atrial contraction (first curve on the atrial line in Fig. 1-13), there is a sudden increase in pressure (producing an A wave in the atrial waveform) since the contraction decreases the size of the atrium. During atrial contraction, pressure is greater in the atrium than in the ventricle. This higher pressure causes the AV valves to open. Atrial blood flows through the open AV valves into the ventricles.

> **QUICK TIP!** Interpretation of the atrial pressure curve is important for clinical practice. Be aware of the clinical significance of the atrial pressure, however, actual waveform analysis of the tracing will not be a skill required for the exam.

As the ventricles begin the systolic phase, pressure in the ventricles increases, resulting in closure of the AV valves. The increase in ventricular pressure is so sudden that the AV valves bulge into the atria, increasing the intra-atrial pressure (second curve on atrial pressure wave in Fig. 1-13). Following this second curve, there is a sharp fall in atrial pressure. Gradually, the atrial pressure rises again during the next period of diastole, and the cycle is repeated.

The normal atrial pressures generate three waves: A, C, and V (**Fig. 1-14**). The A wave is the result of atrial contraction and can be found in the PR interval. One exception to the location of the A wave is in regard to the pulmonary capillary wedge pressure, or pulmonary artery occlusive pressure (PAOP). The PAOP is found slightly later, in the QRS, because of the time it takes the wave to travel from the left atrium to the pulmonary catheter. The importance of the A wave is that the mean of the A wave is the parameter used to estimate the central venous pressure (CVP) and PAOP values.

The C wave is due to closure of the tricuspid and mitral valves. The V wave is due to atrial filling and the bulging of the tricuspid and mitral valves into the atrium. Large V waves can develop with noncompliant atria and mitral or tricuspid regurgitation (**Fig. 1-15**).

Ventricular Pressure Curve

During diastole, the ventricular pressure is less than the atrial pressure. Just before atrial systole occurs, the AV valves open and blood flows into the ventricles. As soon as the ventricles fill, the blood flow reverses and closes the AV valves. At this point, the ventricles become closed chambers. The ventricle walls contract against the volume of blood in the ventricle. Since the ventricle is a closed chamber, pressure rises rapidly. Aortic pressure during diastole has fallen to about 80 mm Hg. The period during which ventricular pressure builds from near

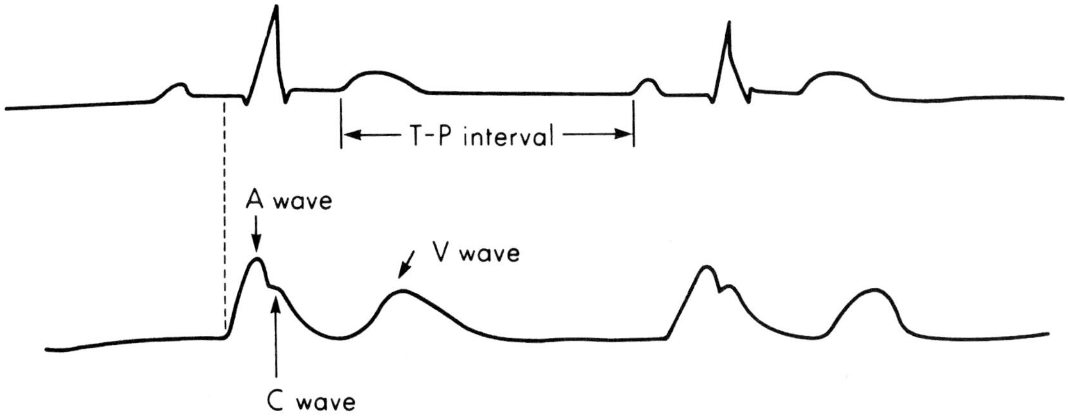

Figure 1-14. Normal atrial waveforms.

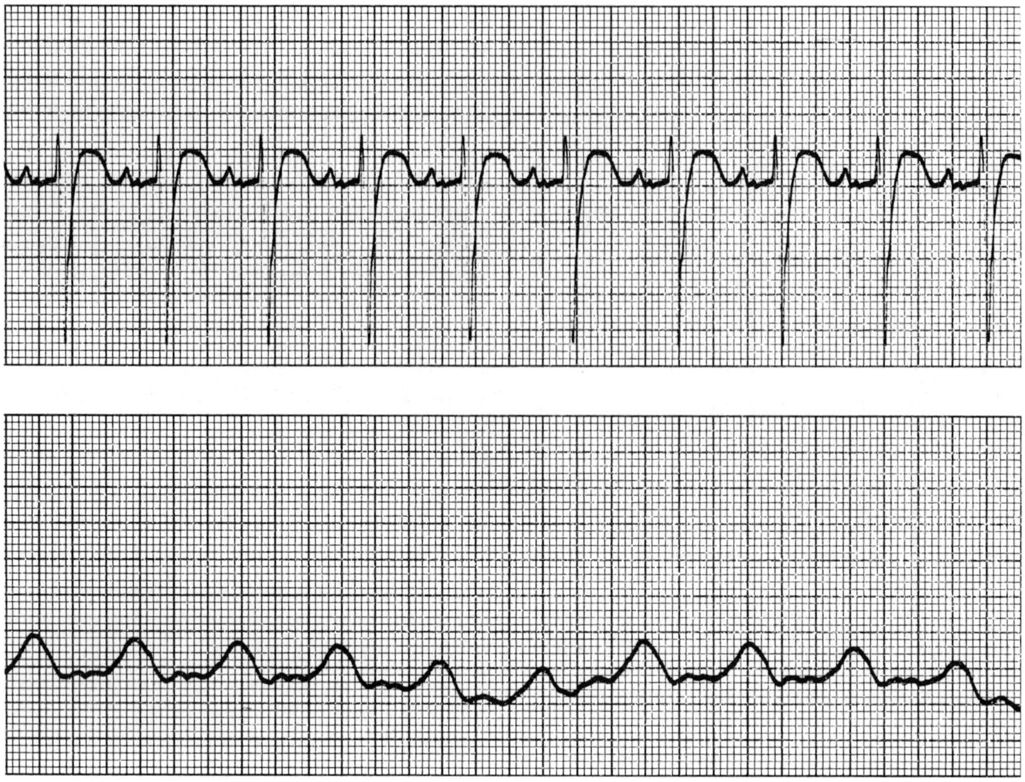

Figure 1-15. Giant V waves in a PAOP tracing.

zero to 80 mm Hg is termed the isometric contraction phase (ventricle curve between lines 1 and 2 in Fig. 1-13). The left ventricle continues to contract strongly, and the pressure rises to about 110 mm Hg. Since left ventricular pressure exceeds the aortic pressure of 80 mm Hg, the aortic valve is forced open, and blood is ejected into the aorta. These same mechanisms are occurring concurrently in the right ventricle, only under much lower pressures. This is called the rapid ejection phase (ventricle curve between lines 2 and 3 in Fig. 1-13). Pressure begins to drop in the ventricle because blood is being ejected faster than the ventricle is contracting. This is called the reduced ejection phase (ventricular curve between lines 3 and 4 in Fig. 1-13). Ventricular contraction ceases, and the ventricle relaxes. Since the ventricular pressure has dropped rapidly, the blood flow starts to reverse at about 80 mm Hg in the aorta. This backward flow closes the aortic valve. The ventricle again becomes a closed chamber, but since no blood is entering, the pressure does not rise. The pressure in the ventricle continues to fall until it is less than the atrial pressure. Then the cycle begins again.

KEY CLINICAL CONTENT CHECKLIST

- ❒ Know basic anatomy and physiology of the heart and electrical conduction system.
- ❒ Know the five phases of the action potential of the cardiac cell.
- ❒ Heart sounds may help you identify a clinical condition. Know what sounds are associated with various clinical conditions, such as S_3 and S_4.
- ❒ The cellular aspects of cardiac muscle A and P are not likely to be on the CCRN exam; however, the concepts can help give you foundational knowledge for understanding myocardial dysfunction and pharmacologic intervention.
- ❒ Calcium chloride IVP augments cardiac output and blood pressure, whereas calcium-channel blockers decrease inotropic effect.
- ❒ The current CCRN format requires a good understanding of the electrical system of the heart and the ability to interpret dysrhythmias and 12-lead ECGs. Whereas specific sections are provided on dysrhythmias and 12-lead analysis, it is important to understand the basic anatomy and physiology of the electrical conduction system.
- ❒ When patients experiencing shock are in Trendelenburg position, the increased flow to the baroreceptors in the carotid and aortic bodies sends a "false message" to the vasomotor center that compensatory vasoconstriction is responding better than it actually is. This is why Trendelenburg in shock resuscitation is no longer considered evidence-based.

Review Questions:

1. Which of the following is the outermost lining of the heart?
   a. endocardium
   b. myocardium
   c. transcardium
   d. pericardium

Answer: D. Rationale: "Endo," meaning "within" is associated with the innermost lining of the heart, so eliminate A. The myocardium is associated with the heart's middle layer, so eliminate option B. The "-transcardium" is somewhat of a contrived term, eliminate C as well. The prefix in pericardium, "peri," means "outside." Option D is the best answer.

2. Which of the following are atrioventricular (AV) valves?
   a. mitral and tricuspid
   b. pulmonic and aortic
   c. mitral and aortic
   d. tricuspid and pulmonic

Answer: A. Rationale: This is a straight knowledge question. The mitral and tricuspid valves (Choice A) are called the AV valves because they separate the atriums and the ventricles. An easy way to remember these is to remember that L (left) and M (mitral) are close to one another in the alphabet and are on the left side of the heart. R (right) and T (tricuspid) are also close in the alphabet and are on the right side of the heart. The aortic and pulmonic valves (all mentioned in B, C, and D) are called the semilunar valves. Choose A.

3. Which electrolyte is responsible for initial depolarization?
   a. sodium
   b. potassium
   c. chloride
   d. calcium

Answer: A. Rationale: The electrolyte responsible is sodium (option A), which rushes into the cell to depolarize it. An easy way to remember this is to remember that sodium is the cation (positively charged) that is available in the highest extracellular quantities (reference range 135–145 mEq/L), just waiting to rush into the cell. Potassium is largely intracellular, so eliminate B. Chloride is an ion of rapid *repolarization* in phase 1, so eliminate C. Calcium, option D, is more involved in the slow calcium channels of phase 2, the plateau phase of repolarization. Choose A.

2

Diagnosis and Treatment of Cardiovascular Disorders

CHAPTER OVERVIEW AND OBJECTIVES

There is no section specifically on testing in the CCRN exam. However, several questions, either directly or indirectly, address cardiovascular assessment via diagnostic tests. In this short section, cardiac diagnostic tests are categorized according to what they do and when they are indicated. Depending on the importance of the test, they will also be covered in chapters on specific cardiac conditions later in this book. This section should help you familiarize yourself with the tests that may be on the exam.

2.1 INVASIVE AND NONINVASIVE DIAGNOSTIC TESTS

Cardiac Isoenzyme and Protein Level

Following trauma or hypoxia, enzymes and proteins leak from damaged cells. These isoenzymes and proteins are used in the identification of myocardial injury, most commonly myocardial infarction (MI). Any myocardial injury, however—including that due to cardiopulmonary resuscitation, cardiac contusion, and cardiac surgery—will elevate cardiac enzymes and proteins. Some tests are better than others at avoiding confounding factors. The most common cardiac enzymes and proteins are listed in **Table 2-1**.

Electrocardiography

The electrocardiogram (ECG) is the most commonly used noninvasive diagnostic test for patients with known or suspected cardiac disease. The ECG is a graphic tracing of the *electrical* forces produced by the heart. A bedside monitor is primarily used to assess heart rate, rhythm, and life-threatening dysrhythmias. The 12-lead ECG provides more detailed information than a bedside monitor including:

- Myocardial injury and ischemia
- Conduction disturbances
- Axis orientation
- Heart size such as when there is atrial or ventricular enlargement

It is important to note that although the ECG's simplicity makes it very useful, it is of limited accuracy and should be used in conjunction with other information, such as physical assessment and laboratory tests. The ECG is not simple to interpret despite its simplicity of use. Many factors alter the ECG's appearance and many of these factors are not clinically significant. However, it is essential for the intensive care unit (ICU) nurse to be able to identify important changes on the ECG, since many times it is the bedside nurse who is responsible for interpreting the ECG.

Echocardiography

Echocardiography (echo) is excellent at identifying structural changes in the heart. Echo uses pulses of reflected ultrasound to evaluate cardiac structure and function. There are different types of echo, including two-dimensional and transesophageal techniques. Transesophageal echo is more specific but requires the patient to swallow a device resembling a thick nasogastric tube and requires sedation to perform.

Echo can detect:

- Valve disturbances
- Septal defects
- Presence of pericardial fluid
- Abnormalities of ventricular muscle movement
- Evaluation of ejection fraction (EF)

TABLE 2-1. COMMON CARDIAC ENZYME AND PROTEIN DETERMINATIONS USED IN DIAGNOSING CARDIAC INJURY

Cardiac Test	*Purpose*
CPK	Nonspecific muscle enzyme, found in muscle and heart tissue. Some studies have indicated that the greater the rise in the CPK, the greater the damage to the heart. This test is less useful when muscle damage is also present.
CPK-MB	A more specific cardiac muscle enzyme. Among the most common tests used in diagnosing myocardial injury. Highly specific for cardiac injury, although it can also rise with muscle damage.
LDH	A nonspecific muscle enzyme whose chief value in cardiac diagnostics is its slow rise and persistent elevation. It is used to detect MIs that may be >24-h old.
Subforms of CPK-MB	Cardiac isoenzyme subforms (CPK-MB_1 and -MB_2) may be the fastest changing of myocardial enzymes. Evidence exists that MIs can be identified within 2 h of occurrence if these forms are measured and (CPK-MB_2 > CPK-MB_1) the short-lived CPK-MB_2 is found to exceed CPK-MB_1.
Troponin I	A very specific cardiac muscle protein, one of the first of a new generation of diagnostic tests for cardiac assessment. It rises rapidly, like CPK-MB, but stays elevated for about 8 days.
Myoglobin	A very specific cardiac muscle protein which elevates and returns to normal rapidly. May be useful in rapid detection, with a higher precision than before, of myocardial injury.

CPK, creatine phosphokinase; LDH, lactic dehydrogenase; MI, myocardial infarction.

In conditions such as MI and cardiac contusion, it can detect what part of the heart is damaged by noting dysfunctional movement in the muscle of the heart. It is an essential aspect of identifying disturbances in physical properties of the heart. Since it is noninvasive, many cardiologists consider it one of the diagnostic tests of choice.

Radionuclide Myocardial Perfusion Imaging

Myocardial perfusion imaging (MPI) detects pathologic cardiac conditions through the external detection of photons emitted from the body after the administration of radioisotopes. These pictures are taken both at rest and after stress to the heart. These scans are useful in detecting abnormalities in:

- Cell function
- Blood flow
- Left ventricular wall motion as well as ventricular size
- Left ventricular volume
- Ejection fraction

MPIs are commonly known as nuclear stress tests. One form of a nuclear stress is called a thallium scan that is used to evaluate regional myocardial perfusion and viability. Thallium scans can be performed with the patient at rest or during exercise. For those patients unable to exercise, dobutamine and dipyridamole thallium scanning is used to increase coronary blood flow in place of exercise. Vasodilators such as adenosine may also be used in place of dobutamine. Other radioisotopes such as technetium-99m (Cardiolite) or regadenoson (Lexiscan) may be used in place of thallium.

Positron emission tomography (PET) is a sophisticated imaging technique that measures specific radioisotopes injected into the body via the blood. PET scans may be used to determine the exact part of the heart that is threatened by a loss of oxygen. It is capable of distinguishing dysfunctional but viable myocardium from areas of infarction.

Cardiac Catheterization

Cardiac catheterization involves the insertion of catheters into cardiac chambers and blood vessels to measure intracardiac pressures, oxygen saturation, and coronary blood flow. Angiography, a part of the cardiac catheterization procedure, is used specifically to examine the blood vessels by injecting measurable contrast material. Coronary angiography generally involves the injection of a radiopaque contrast medium into the chambers of the heart, coronary arteries, and great vessels. The passage of the contrast dye is followed and filmed as the heart beats spontaneously.

Cardiac catheterization is usually performed to evaluate the presence and severity of coronary artery atherosclerosis. **In anticipation of cardiac surgery, virtually all patients undergo cardiac catheterization (the gold standard test for confirmation of coronary occlusions)**. Cardiac catheterization may also involve placement of coronary stents during procedures known as percutaneous coronary intervention (PCI).

Electrophysiology Studies

Electrophysiology studies (EPSs) are used to assess the conduction of electricity through the heart, which it can do with much more specificity than the surface ECG. EPSs provide definitive diagnostic information on cardiac dysrhythmias, such as premature ventricular contractions (PVCs), and help direct proper therapies. The results of EPSs are similar to those of cardiac catheterization. Intracardiac catheters placed under fluoroscopic guidance are used to record intracardiac electrical activity. They are often used to provoke cardiac dysrhythmias in a controlled, treatment-ready setting. Treatment plans for various dysrhythmias often emerge from the results of EPSs. Many hospitals are not equipped to perform EPSs; therefore, those patients needing such studies must be referred to more specialized settings.

2.2 PHARMACOLOGICAL TREATMENT

Treatment of abnormal hemodynamics centers on improving either cardiac output or systemic vascular resistance (SVR). In the treatment of inadequate cardiac output, the components of stroke volume *(preload, afterload, and contractility) are the most commonly manipulated parameters.* A large number of cardiac therapies are available to treat hemodynamic abnormalities.

Treatment of Low Cardiac Output States

Treatment of conditions that cause low stroke volume and low cardiac output usually centers on the left ventricle. Normally, low cardiac output is caused by weakening of the left ventricle (due, for example, to heart failure [HF], MI, or cardiomyopathy) or inadequate blood volume (hypovolemia). *If the problem is a weak left ventricle, therapies that might be used include (1) reducing preload; (2) reducing afterload; and (3) increasing contractility.* There are also a few physical interventions, such as allowing the patient to sit up or attempting to reduce his or her anxiety, as well as mechanical support of the heart with intra-aortic balloon pumps and ventricular assist devices. Most therapies, however, focus on pharmacologic support. It is this treatment modality that is most important for the bedside clinician to understand.

Improving the Strength of the Heart

In the patient presenting with symptoms of left ventricular dysfunction, relief is obtained by improving the strength of the heart. This is also referred to as inotropic therapy. *Inotropic therapy* increases the strength of cardiac contraction. As a consequence of the improved strength, an increase in ejection fraction, stroke volume, cardiac output, and, ideally, tissue oxygenation (eg, improved SvO_2 and lactate) occur.

Several inotropes are available (**Table 2-2**). These include **dobutamine (Dobutrex), dopamine, amrinone, milrinone, epinephrine, and digoxin**. The inotrope most commonly used is **dobutamine**. Dobutamine acts by stimulating *beta cells of the sympathetic nervous system,* which in turn strengthens contraction (positive *inotropic* response) and makes the heart beat faster (positive *chronotropic* response). Since beta stimulation also causes smooth muscle relaxation, blood vessels dilate. This results in a drop in preload (pulmonary capillary wedge pressure and central venous pressure) and afterload (SVR).

Better contractility agents, like levosimendan (Simdax), are still being investigated in the United States. However, the disadvantage to inotropes are the lack of evidence to support their effect on long-term survival. In addition, they increase myocardial oxygen consumption at a time when the heart may be starved for oxygen. Owing to these concerns, inotropes are likely more limited in their application.

Dopamine is also used, particularly in moderate dosages (2–10 μg/kg/min). However, dopamine *stimulates alpha cells of the sympathetic nervous system, causing vasoconstriction (increased SVR).* This vasoconstriction might increase the blood pressure, but it also causes an increase in myocardial work.

There are times when sympathetic stimulation cannot provide any more improvement in contractility. At this time, drugs having different mechanisms of action, such as the phosphodiesterase inhibitors amrinone and **milrinone**, might be used. These drugs increase the availability of intracellular calcium and the strength of the heart.

Digitalis preparations such as digoxin are not used in acute situations. These drugs might be used in chronic ventricular dysfunction but not in acute failure.

Improving Cardiac Strength through Preload Reduction

The strength of the heart might be improved if overstretched myocardial muscle fibers can be allowed to shrink back to normal. *Preload reduction can accomplish this goal. Preload reduction is done through vasodilation or with diuretics.*

Diuretics are commonly used for preload reduction, mainly because they help reduce the excess fluid in the circulatory system that results from renal compensation for decreased blood flow through the kidneys. Many types of diuretics are available (**Table 2-3**). All diuretics work by blocking reabsorption of sodium and water. They usually produce a rapid increase in urine output. The efficacy of the diuretic is measured by improvement in cardiac performance.

Preload reduction can also occur with *vasodilation*. Drugs such as **nitroglycerin, diltiazem,** and **morphine** can reduce preload through vasodilation (**Table 2-4**). Vasodilation causes an "internal phlebotomy" by reducing the amount of blood returning to the heart.

TABLE 2-2. COMMON INOTROPIC (CONTRACTILITY) DRUGS

	Dose	*Onset*	*Route*	*Drip Conc.*
Dobutamine (Dobutrex) beta-adrenergic	2–10 μg/kg/min, Max of 20 μg/kg/min	1–2 min, peak ~10 min	IV	250 mg/250 mL D_5W or NS
Dopamine (Intropin) beta adrenergic and alpha adrenergic at high doses	2–10 μg/kg/min, Max of 20 μg/kg/min	<5 min	IV	400 mg/250 mL D_5W or NS
Milrinone (Primacor)	Usual dose of 0.375–0.75 μg/kg/min	2–5 min	IV	20 mg/100 mL
Digoxin (IV) (Lanoxin)—note digoxin is mainly used for rate control in arrhythmias rather than its inotropic effects	For the treatment of heart failure, loading 8–12 μg/kg in divided doses over 12–24 h q 6–8 h. Maintenance dosing of 2.4–3.6 μg/kg/min once daily	5–30 min	IV	NA
Digoxin (PO) (Lanoxin)	Loading 0.5 mg × 1 then 0.25 mg q 6 h until desired effect or total digitalizing dosage is achieved—note that loading dose is generally not recommended Maintenance 0.125–0.25 mg/day	1–2 h	PO	NA

D_5W, 5% dextrose in water; NA, not applicable; NS, normal saline.

TABLE 2-3. DIURETICS

	Dose	Onset	Route	Drip Conc.
Mild				
Mannitol (osmotic diuretic)—not a first-line drug for diuresis	12.5–200 g/day	1-3 h	IVP (filter) or IV drip	50 g in NS or D_5W to 250 mL final volume
Spironolactone (Aldactone) (K^+ sparing class)	25–200 mg/day	24–48 h	PO	NA
Moderate				
Chlorothiazide (Diuril) (thiazide class)—usually used as adjunctive to loop diuretic therapy	500–1000 mg/day, max daily dose 2000 mg/day	PO: 1–2 h IV: 15 min	PO/IV	NA
Hydrochlorothiazide (Hydrodiuril) (thiazide class)	25–100 mg/day, max daily dose 200 mg/day	2 h	PO	NA
Metolazone (Zaroxolyn, Microx) (nonthiazide)—typically adjunct to loop diuretic therapy	2.5–20 mg/day	1 h	PO	NA
Strong				
Furosemide (PO) (Lasix) (loop diuretic)	Initial 20–40 once and titrate every 6–8 h to effective dose. Max dose of 600 mg/day	1 h	PO	NA
Furosemide (IV) (Lasix) (loop diuretic)	Initial 20–40 once and titrate every 6–8 h to effective dose. If continuous infusion, 10–40 mg/h	5 min	IV	1 g in NS or D_5W to 250 mL final volume
Ethacrynic acid (PO) (Edecrin) (loop diuretic)—used as an alternative agent	25–50 mg/day, max dose of 400 mg/day in two divided doses	30 min	PO	NA
Ethacrynic acid (IV) (Edecrin) (loop diuretic)—used as an alternative agent	50 mg/day as a single dose. Max single dose of 100 mg.	5 min	IV	No standard drip
Bumetanide (PO) (Bumex) (loop diuretic)	0.5–1 mg/day, max of 10 mg/day	30 min–1 h	PO	NA
Bumetanide (IV) (Bumex) (loop diuretic)	0.5–1 mg/day, max of 10 mg/day. If continuous infusion, initial rate of 0.5 mg/h	Within 30-60 minutes	IV	No standard drip
Torsemide (Demadex) (loop diuretic)	Initial 10–20 mg/day. Max dose of 200 mg/day.	Within 1 h	PO	NA

NA, not applicable.

Increasing Cardiac Strength through Afterload Reduction

One of the best methods for improving cardiac performance is to reduce the work that the heart must do to eject blood. This can be accomplished by afterload reduction, which can be achieved with many different drugs (**Table 2-5**). However, only a few of these drugs are commonly used in critical care.

The use of afterload reducers is common in two situations: during hypertensive episodes and when the cardiac output is low and the SVR is high. The principles of their use are similar in both situations.

While potentially dangerous, a commonly used drug to reduce resistance is **nitroprusside. Nitroprusside** acts quickly and is effective only with continuous administration. Once stopped, its effect will wear off in minutes. It is very effective at reducing resistance and is frequently used in ICUs. **Nitroprusside** use has two disadvantages. First, it breaks down into cyanide. Cyanide levels therefore need to be monitored daily in patients on nitroprusside and **sodium thiosulfate may be added to the solution to decrease the risk of toxicity**. The medication needs to be protected from light. Second, it acts as a nonselective arterial dilator. This dilation can open flow into areas that do not need more oxygen. However, as more flow enters these areas, some areas that need more oxygen (ischemic myocardium) might have flow diverted from them. This is called the *"coronary steal" phenomenon.*

KEY CLINICAL CONCEPT

The addition of sodium thiosulfate to the IV bag of nitroprusside to decrease risk of cyanide toxicity commonly appears on the exam.

In order to avoid the problems with **nitroprusside**, other afterload reducers, such as calcium channel blockers, beta-blocking agents, IV **nitroglycerin**, and natriuretic peptides

TABLE 2-4. VASODILATORS

	Dose	*Onset (min)*	*Route*	*Drip Conc.*
Nitroglycerin (IV) (Tridil, Nitrostat IV) (nitrate vasodilator)	Initial 5–10 µg/min, max of 400 µg/min. Titrate to desired effect; at high dose becomes afterload-reducing agent	1–2	IV	50 mg in D_5W or NS to a final volume of 250 mL
Nitroglycerin (SL) (Nitrostat)	Initial 0.3–0.4 mg at onset; repeat every 5 min if angina persists; may administer up to 3 tablets in a 15-min period. For patients with refractory angina, up to 0.6 mg as a single dose may be considered	1–3	SL	NA
Diltiazem (IV) (Cardizem) (calcium channel blocker)	20 mg (average) bolus over 2 min. May repeat with 25-mg bolus then start drip	1–2	IV	125 mg in D_5W or NS to a final volume of 125 mL
Diltiazem (PO) (Cardizem) (calcium channel blocker)	Tablets: Extended-release 120–180 mg once daily; increase as needed at 7–14 day intervals; usual effective dose 240–360 mg/day Immediate-release 30 mg 4 times daily; increase as needed at 1–2 day intervals; usual effective dose 240–360 mg/day in 3–4 divided doses	30–60	PO	NA
Nifedipine (PO) (Procardia, Procardia XL, Adalat) (calcium channel blocker)	Immediate-release Capsules: 30 mg total daily dose in 3–4 divided doses, max of 180 mg/day Sustained release: 30–60 mg/day in once-daily dosing, max of 120 mg/day; increase the dose every 7–14 days until desired response is achieved	Capsules: 5–10 Sustained release: 20	PO	NA

NA, not applicable.

TABLE 2-5. AFTERLOAD REDUCERS

Direct Arterial Dilator	*Dose*	*Onset*	*Route*	*Drip Conc.*
Sodium nitroprusside (Nipride, Nitropress)	For hypertensive emergency, initial 0.25–0.5 µg/kg/min; titrate as needed by 0.5 µg/kg/min every 5 min to achieve target blood pressure To avoid toxicity, limit dose to ≤2 µg/kg/min if possible Max dose of 10 µg/kg/min	Within 2 min	IV	50 g in D_5W to a final volume of 250 mL
Hydralazine (IV) (Apresoline)	For hypertensive emergency, 10–20 mg every 4–6 h as needed; may increase dose to a max of 40 mg/dose if necessary	10–80 min	IV, IM	NA
Nitroglycerin (IV) (Tridil, Nitrostat IV) (nitrate vasodilator)	Initial: 5–10 µg/min; titrate as needed based on response and tolerability in increments of 5–10 µg/min every 3–5 min up to 200 µg/min	1–2 min	IV	50 mg in D_5W or NS to a final volume of 250 mL
Nitroglycerin (SL) (Nitrostat)	Initial 0.3–0.4 mg at onset; repeat every 5 min if angina persists; may administer up to 3 tablets in a 15-min period. For patients with refractory angina, up to 0.6 mg as a single dose may be considered	1–3 min	SL	NA
Alpha inhibitors				
Prazosin (Minipress)	1–20 mg total daily dose in 2–3 divided doses	30 min–3 h	PO	NA
Phentolamine (Regitine) - Generally used in the setting of catecholamine excess (eg, pheochromocytoma)	IV: 1–5 mg bolus; maximum single dose: 15 mg. A continuous infusion may be administered after initial bolus dosing (eg, 1 mg/h titrated to blood pressure response) to a maximum infusion rate of 40 mg/h	1–2 min	IV	No standard drip
Clonidine (Catapres)	0.1 mg PO twice daily, initially. May increase dose by 0.1 mg/day every 7 days if further control is needed Usual dosage range: 0.1–0.8 mg/day	30–60 min	PO	NA

(*Continued*)

TABLE 2-5. AFTERLOAD REDUCERS (*CONTINUED*)

Direct Arterial Dilator	***Dose***	***Onset***	***Route***	***Drip Conc.***
Methyldopa (PO) (Aldomet) (loop diuretic)	Initial: 250 mg 2–3 times daily; titrate daily dose at least every 2 days based on response; usual dose range: 250 mg–1 g daily in 2–4 divided doses; maximum dose: 3 g/day in divided doses	3–6 h	PO	NA
Methyldopa (IV) (Aldomet) (loop diuretic)	250 mg–1 g every 6–8 h; maximum dose: 1 g every 6 h	2 h	IV	NA
Calcium channel blockers				
Diltiazem (IV) (Cardizem)	20-mg (average) bolus over 2 min; may repeat with 25-mg bolus then start drip	1–2 min	IV	125 mg in D_5W or NS to a final volume of 125 mL
Diltiazem (PO) (Cardizem)	Tablets: Extended-release 120–180 once daily; increase as needed at 7–14 day intervals; usual effective dose 240–360 mg/day Immediate-release 30 mg 4 times daily; increase as needed at 1–2 day intervals; usual effective dose 240–360 mg/day in 3–4 divided doses	30–60 min	PO	NA
Nifedipine (PO) (Procardia, Procardia XL, Adalat)	Immediate-release Capsules: 30 mg total daily dose in 3–4 divided doses, max of 180 mg/day Sustained release: 30–60 mg/day in once-daily dosing, max of 120 mg/day; increase the dose every 7–14 days until desired response is achieved	Capsules: 5–10 min	PO	NA
Nicardipine (IV) (Cardene)	For hypertensive emergency initial dose of 5 mg/h; titrate by 2.5 mg/h at 5–15-min intervals to achieve target blood pressure; max dose of 15 mg/h	1–5 min	IV	25 mg/250 mL D_5W or NS
Nicardipine (PO) (Cardene)	Initial: 20 mg 3 times daily; usual dosage: 20–40 mg 3 times daily (allow ≥3 days between dose increases)	1–2 h	PO	
Ace inhibitors (most common agents in use)				
Captopril (PO) (Capoten)—not used as commonly anymore	Initial dose of 6.25–25 mg 2–3 times daily; for patients in an acute care setting, may titrate as frequently as every 8 h (based on pharmacokinetic properties), as needed, up to 50 mg 3 times daily	15–30 min	PO	NA
Enalapril (PO) (Vasotec)	Initial dose of 5–10 mg once daily; evaluate response after ~2–4 weeks and titrate dose (eg, increase the daily dose by doubling), as needed, up to 40 mg/day in 1 or 2 divided doses	1 h	PO	NA
Enalapril (IV) (Enalaprilat)	1.25 mg/dose, given over 5 min every 6 h; may titrate as needed to a maximum dose of 5 mg/dose every 6 h	Within 15 min	IVP	NA
Lisinopril (Zestril/ Prinivil)—most common ACE-inhibitor	Initial dose of 5–10 mg once daily; evaluate response after ~2–4 weeks and titrate dose (eg, increase the daily dose by doubling) as needed, up to 40 mg once daily	1 h	PO	NA
Benazepril (Lotensin)	Initial: 10 mg once daily; evaluate response after ~2–4 weeks and titrate dose (eg, increase the daily dose by doubling), as needed, up to 40 mg daily in 1 or 2 divided doses	1–2 h	PO	NA
Beta blockers				
Atenolol (PO) (Tenormin) (beta-1 selective)	Initial dose of 25 mg once or twice daily; titrate at ≥1 week intervals as needed based on response and tolerability up to 100 mg/day in 1 or 2 divided doses	Within 1 h	PO	NA

(*Continued*)

TABLE 2-5. AFTERLOAD REDUCERS (CONTINUED)

Direct Arterial Dilator	*Dose*	*Onset*	*Route*	*Drip Conc.*
Metoprolol (PO) (Lopressor = immediate-release, Toprol-XL = extended-release) (beta-1 selective)	Immediate-release (metoprolol tartrate) = initial dose of 50 mg twice daily; titrate at weekly (or longer) intervals as needed based on patient response; maximum dose: 400 mg/day; usual dosage range: 100–200 mg/day in 2 divided doses Extended-release (metoprolol succinate) = initial dose of 25–100 mg once daily; titrate at weekly (or longer) intervals as needed based on patient response; maximum dose: 400 mg/day; usual dosage range: 50–200 mg once daily	Within 1 h	PO	NA
Metoprolol (IV) (Lopressor)	For acute ventricular rate control use 2.5–5 mg over 2 min; repeat dose every 5 min as needed; maximum total dose: 15 mg	Within 20 min	IV	NA
Propranolol (PO) (Inderal) (beta-non selective)	For hypertension use an initial dose of 80 mg/day in 1–4 divided doses based on chosen formulation (may choose an IR or ER formulation); titrate at ≥1-week intervals as needed based on patient response; usual dosage range: 80–160 mg/day in 1–4 divided doses based on chosen formulation	1–2 h	PO	NA
Esmolol (Brevibloc) (beta-1 selective)	For hypertensive emergency, use an initial loading dose of 250–500 μg/kg over 1 min, followed by a continuous infusion of 25–50 μg/kg/min. Titrate infusion by 25–50 μg/kg/min every 5 min as needed to achieve target blood pressure while maintaining adequate heart rate	2–10 min	IV	NA
Labetalol (PO) (Normodyne or Trandate) (beta-blocker with alpha-blocking activity)	Initial dose of 100 mg twice daily; may increase as needed every 2–3 days by 100 mg twice daily (titration increments not to exceed 200 mg twice daily) until desired response is obtained; usual dosage range: 200–800 mg/day in 2 divided doses	2–4 h	PO	NA
Labetalol (IV) (Normodyne or Trandate)	For hypertensive emergency, intermittent IV dosing includes the use an initial dose of 10–20 mg over 1–2 min followed by 20–80 mg every 10 min until target blood pressure is reached Continuous IV infusion, use an initial loading dose of 10–20 mg over 2 min (optional if intermittent dosing is used), followed by 0.5–2 mg/min; some patients may require titration up to 10 mg/min	Within 5 min	IV	200 mg in D_5W or NS to a final volume of 200 mL

ACE, angiotensin-converting enzyme; D_5W, dextrose 5% in water; NA, not applicable; NS, normal saline.

(eg, **Nesiritide**) are used. The advantage of agents like natriuretic peptides is that they do not directly reduce cardiac contractility. Calcium channel blockers and beta blockers reduce afterload, but they unfortunately also tend to weaken the heart. If calcium channel blockers (eg, **nicardipine**) or beta blockers (eg, **metoprolol, labetalol**) are used, their effect on both SVR and cardiac output must be monitored.

There are other afterload reducers, most notably the **angiotensin-converting enzyme (ACE) inhibitors**. ACE inhibitors are most often used in the management of nonacute forms of cardiac failure because they do not activate compensating neurohumoral responses as do other afterload reducers. This makes them attractive for long-term use in such situations as HF. *They tend to reduce SVR without increasing cardiac output. The net effect is a substantial reduction in myocardial oxygen consumption.*

Management of Hypovolemia

When hypovolemia is present, the circulating blood volume must be replenished by one of three therapies: blood (eg, whole blood, packed cells), crystalloids (normal saline, lactated Ringer's solution), and colloids (**albumin**). The choice of therapy depends on the clinical situation. General guidelines for fluid replacement are as follows:

1. **Blood** is used when the patient is actively bleeding and the *hemoglobin levels are in the range of less than or equal to 7 g/dL or when acute coronary syndrome exists.* Blood is the only fluid replacement that actually carries oxygen.
2. **Crystalloids** are used when volume depletion does not have to be corrected rapidly, when depletion of more than vascular volume is suspected, or when hypovolemia is suspected but is not a clear diagnosis.

TABLE 2-6. VOLUME EXPANDERS

	Dose	*Onset*	*Route*	*Drip Conc.*
Hetastarch (Hydroxyethyl starch; Hespan, Hextend) (plasma volume expander) BLACK BOX WARNING due to risk of kidney injury, coagulopathy, and increased mortality	500–1000 mL once; may repeat as needed based on assessment of intravascular volume status. Doses >1500 mL/day are usually not required	30 min	IV	NA
Albumin	Initial 12.5–25 g (250–500 mL); repeat after 15–30 min as needed	Varies	IV	Comes as a 5%, 20%, or 25% solution
Crystalloids (see the following)	100–1000 mL/5–30 min	30 min	IV	Titrate to effect
Normal saline	NA	NA	IV	NA
Lactated Ringer's solution	NA	NA	IV	NA

NA, not applicable.

3. **Colloids** are used when rapid volume expansion is necessary, but the use of blood is not indicated or blood is not available.

Considerable controversy exists regarding the proper fluid replacement therapy. *Generally, crystalloids are the first agent used in suspected hypovolemia* (**Table 2-6**). They are inexpensive and do not cause any allergic reactions. However, they take longer to expand the vascular volume than either colloids or blood.

Treatment of Low Systemic Vascular Resistance

Many hemodynamic problems are a result of disturbances of blood flow. In **sepsis**, one of the most common of these disturbances, *SVR is abnormally low.* Other conditions can cause this situation as well, including hepatic disease and **neurogenic shock**. The key to all treatment is reversal of the underlying problem. For example, in sepsis, antibiotics might be the primary treatment, and hemodynamic interventions are viewed primarily as supportive therapies.

The primary hemodynamic therapies are aimed at achieving three goals: (1) maintaining circulating blood volume with volume expansion; (2) increasing blood flow with inotropic therapy; and (3) maintaining blood flow with agents to increase the SVR. These three components may also be thought of as, *"The tank, the pump, and the pipes."*

Maintaining blood flow with volume expansion and inotropic therapy has already been discussed. Maintaining blood flow with agents to increase the SVR is done with one of four agents (**Table 2-7**). All of these agents work by stimulating the *alpha*$_1$ *cells of the sympathetic nervous system.* These drugs produce *vasoconstriction*, and some also increase the cardiac output. These are potent drugs that should elevate blood pressure and blood flow. However, they must be used with caution because they might elevate the SVR and blood pressure but not increase tissue oxygenation.

Alpha stimulants cause marked vasoconstriction. These drugs are so potent that they are given centrally to avoid the tissue damage that would result in the event of infiltration during peripheral intravenous administration.

TABLE 2-7. COMMON VASOPRESSORS

	Dose	*Onset*	*Route*	*Drip Conc.*
Dopamine (Intropin) alpha adrenergic	2–5 μg/kg/min continuous IV infusion, initially. Titrate by 5–10 μg/kg/min until desired hemodynamic and/or renal response is attained. Usual dosage of 2–20 μg/kg/min	<5 min	IV	400 mg/250 mL D_5W or NS
Epinephrine (Adrenaline)—the initial vasopressor of choice in anaphylactic shock; typically an add-on agent to levophed in septic shock	Initial dose of 1–15 μg/min (0.01–0. μg/kg/min) Usual dose range of 1–40 μg/min (0.01–0.5 μg/kg/min)	<5 min	IV	5 mg/500 mL or 4 mg/100 mL D_5W or NS
Norepinephrine (Levophed)—initial vasopressor of choice in septic, cardiogenic, and hypovolemic shock	Initial dose 5–15 μg/min (0.05–0.15 μg/kg/min) For cardiogenic shock, initial 0.05 μg/kg/min Usual maintenance dose range of 2–80 μg/min (0.025–1 μg/kg/min)	1–2 min	IV	8 mg/500 D_5W
Phenylephrine (Neosynephrine) (pure alpha-adrenergic vasoconstrictor)	Initial dose of 40–160 μg/min until stabilized (alternatively, 0.5–2 μg/kg/min) Usual dose range of 20–400 μg/min (0.25–5 μg/kg/min)	1–2 min	IV	10 mg/250 mL D_5W or NS

D_5W, dextrose 5% in water; NS, normal saline.

TABLE 2-8. LEFT VENTRICULAR DYSFUNCTION: HEMODYNAMIC AND SYSTEMIC EFFECTS

Increased preload	Reduced subendocardial perfusion Decreased renal perfusion Antidiuretic and aldosterone released, causing sodium and fluid retention Increased blood volume Fluid overload Increased beta natriuretic peptide (BNP)
Increased afterload	Catecholamines and angiotensin II released, causing vasoconstriction via the renin-angiotensin-aldosterone compensatory mechanism Impaired vascular smooth muscle relaxation Increased systemic vascular resistance
Impaired contractility	Decreased cardiac output due to reduced left ventricular reserve Decreased skeletal muscle blood flow Decreased exercise capacity Poor forward blood flow Increased backward pressure into the pulmonary vasculature

Specific Cardiovascular Drugs

Drugs specific to clinical conditions are discussed in the chapters about those conditions. For example, thrombolytics are presented in the chapter on acute coronary syndrome and antidysrhythmics are covered in chapters on dysrhythmias. This section is designed as a general review of treatment of hemodynamic disturbances. For more information on specific drug therapy, locate the specific condition of interest.

KEY CLINICAL CONCEPT

You can expect several questions, perhaps as many as 10, that directly or indirectly address pharmacologic treatments for abnormal hemodynamics or dysrhythmias. It is not necessary or desirable to review all therapies while preparing for the CCRN exam. However, it is critical to understand the most common therapies and how they work. If you have a good understanding of this section, you should be well prepared for the CCRN exam questions on this content.

2.3 IMPLICATIONS OF CARDIOVASCULAR DYSFUNCTION ON OTHER ORGAN SYSTEMS

In assessing the effect of cardiovascular dysfunction on other organs, it is helpful to understand the blood flow from each ventricle, since the effects of dysfunction are different in each ventricle. For example, **left ventricular dysfunction** results in a failure to move blood to the tissues adequately. This threatens every organ's ability to maintain its normal metabolic activity. Since any threat to circulation threatens oxygen delivery, all tissues are at risk when left ventricular function is disturbed. In addition, a *backup of blood into the lungs will eventually occur, causing pulmonary symptoms such as orthopnea* (**Table 2-8**).

Right ventricular dysfunction results in a loss of blood flow through the lungs and a *backup of blood into the venous system, causing symptoms such as venous engorgement* (**Table 2-9**).

Since any organ can be affected, symptoms of dysfunction may be found in any organ. **Table 2-10** shows the effects of ventricular dysfunction on each organ.

KEY CLINICAL CONCEPT

As it fails, the cardiovascular system will affect every other organ system. Most of these effects are covered in the following chapters on specific organ systems. It is not likely that the CCRN exam will address the specific effects of cardiovascular dysfunction on other organs directly. More likely, the exam will include a few questions that integrate the cardiovascular system into the dysfunction of other systems. This short section is a review of the general effects of the cardiovascular system on other organs.

TABLE 2-9. RIGHT VENTRICULAR DYSFUNCTION: HEMODYNAMIC AND SYSTEMIC EFFECTS

Increased preload	Passive organ congestion Hepatic engorgement Hepatojugular reflux Coagulopathies Elevated liver enzymes Gastric congestion Dependent, peripheral edema Distended neck veins Decreased cardiac output due to the reduced forward flow from the right ventricle (see Table 2-8)

TABLE 2-10. END-ORGAN EFFECTS OF VENTRICULAR DYSFUNCTION

Left Ventricular Failure	*Right Ventricular Failure*	*Organ System*	*Effect*	*Clinical Presentation*
+	+	Central nervous system	Reduced cerebral perfusion due to decreased cardiac output	Altered level of consciousness Disorientation Confusion Lethargy Anxiety
			Deceased skeletal muscle perfusion	Insomnia Dizziness/syncope Fatigue Deceased exercise capacity
+	+	Renal system	Reduced renal perfusion, causing Na^+ retention and fluid accumulation	Fluid overload Increased SVR Oliguria during day Nocturia Metabolic acidosis Weight gain Peripheral edema Hyponatremia Hypokalemia due to diuretic therapy Dark, concentrated urine
	+	Hepatic system	Passive congestion and reduced perfusion of liver due to elevated systemic venous pressure cause liver damage and dysfunction and deficiencies in coagulation factors	Hepatomegaly Abdominal distention Hepatojugular reflex Elevated liver enzymes (AST, ALT, LDH, GGT, lipase, etc) Elevated PT, PTT, INR
	+	Gastrointestinal system	Passive congestion of gut slows due to visceral edema	Nausea/vomiting Anorexia Ascites Nutritional deficiencies Poor oral medication absorption Cachexia
+		Pulmonary system	Backward pressure due to poor left ventricular systolic function, causing pulmonary edema	Gravity-dependent crackles Wheezes Orthopnea Dyspnea on exertion Paroxysmal nocturnal dyspnea Low Pao_2/Sao_2/pH Use of accessory muscles Cheyne–Stokes respirations Productive cough of blood-tinged, frothy sputum
+		Cardiovascular system	Fluid overload of left ventricular	S_3 and/or S_4 Systolic murmur of mitral regurgitation Stretching of myocardium and valvular radius PMI shifts to the left
			Poor left ventricular contractility	Pulsus alternans Deceased pulse pressure Cold/discolored extremities Cool, clammy skin Deceased capillary refill Diaphoresis

(Continued)

TABLE 2-10. END-ORGAN EFFECTS OF VENTRICULAR DYSFUNCTION (*CONTINUED*)

Left Ventricular Failure	*Right Ventricular Failure*	*Organ System*	*Effect*	*Clinical Presentation*
+	+		Reduced subendocardial perfusion	Ischemic symptoms Dysrhythmias Atrial or ventricular bundle branch block
	+		Fluid overload	Jugular vein distention Pulsus paradoxus Pedal edema

Pao_2, arterial oxygen pressure; PMI, point of maximal impulse; PT, prothrombin time; PTT, partial thromboplastin time; Sao_2, arterial oxygen saturation.

KEY CLINICAL CONTENT CHECKLIST

- ❒ The addition of sodium thiosulfate to the IV bag of nitroprusside to decrease risk of cyanide toxicity commonly appears on the exam.
- ❒ You can expect several questions, perhaps as many as 10, that directly or indirectly address pharmacologic treatments for abnormal hemodynamics or dysrhythmias.
- ❒ As it fails, the cardiovascular system will affect every other organ system. It is not likely that the CCRN exam will address the specific effects of cardiovascular dysfunction on other organs directly. More likely, the exam will include a few questions that integrate the cardiovascular system into the dysfunction of other systems.

Review Questions:

1. **A patient with stage D, HFrEF has been admitted to the intensive care unit for 2 days for acute heart failure exacerbation. The patient is on guideline directed medical therapy but experiencing continued fatigue, poor perfusion, and continued edema. The patient's systolic blood pressure has consistently been around 90/54. The heart rate is 60. Which medication would most likely be indicated to improve cardiac output?**
   a. Digoxin
   b. Nitroprusside
   c. Nitroglycerin
   d. Dobutamine

Answer: D. Rationale: The patient is in end-stage heart failure and showing signs of poor perfusion and decreased cardiac output that are signs of a need for improved contractility of the heart. While digoxin may help improve contractility, this patient is in acute heart failure and experiencing a low heart rate and blood pressure. Therefore, digoxin would not be the best choice. Nitroprusside is an afterload reducer and would not be indicated in this patient as their blood pressure is 90/54. Nitroglycerin is also not indicated in this patient as they do not need preload reduction. The best choice would be dobutamine to improve contractility and cardiac output, thereby improving the patient's symptoms.

2. **Vasodilators, such as nitroglycerin, will have all of the following effects except:**
   a. Decreased preload
   b. Increased contractility
   c. Decreased SVR
   d. Decreased afterload

Answer: B. Rationale: Vasodilators such as nitroglycerin will open the vessels, therefore decreasing SVR (a measurement used to determine afterload) and decreasing preload. They do not have an effect on contractility of the heart.

3

The Normal ECG

CHAPTER OVERVIEW AND OBJECTIVES

Generally, the CCRN exam requires interpretation of fewer than three rhythm strips (if any), but it may also have a few questions regarding 12-lead electrocardiogram (ECG) analysis. However, there may or may not be rhythm strips or 12-lead ECGs to actually interpret (eg, ischemia, injury, and effects of major electrolytes like potassium). If you understand the major dysrhythmias and key concepts of 12-lead ECGs, you will be fine. **The CCRN is not a test on ECGs or 12 leads, but more on how they relate to given clinical conditions. 12 leads are more likely to be described in scenarios than actually shown or displayed.**

In this chapter, a review of normal and preferred electrocardiogram (ECG) leads, as well as the normal components of ECG waves, is provided. Review this chapter carefully if ECG monitoring is not one of your strengths. However, if you have a basic understanding of dysrhythmias, lead placement, and identifying injury and ischemia **(especially the acute changes)**, this chapter will not add much to your CCRN preparation.

- Understand changes occurring on a 12-lead ECG for various clinical situations, including myocardial infarction and abnormal waveforms that signify potential cardiac abnormalities.
- Describe a systematic approach when analyzing ECGs.

3.1 COMPONENTS OF THE NORMAL ECG

The electrocardiograph is a machine that records the electrical activity of the heart on special paper. The result is an electrocardiogram (ECG or EKG). The electrical activity measured by the ECG is the electrical potential between two points on the body: a positive pole and a negative pole. When one is monitoring patients in critical care, all monitoring leads have one negative and one positive pole. For example, in lead I, the right arm is negative and the left arm is positive. Electrical activity in the heart is monitored by these two poles. Electrical activity that is directed toward the positive pole results in an upright deflection. Activity heading toward the negative pole is upside down. The sum of all cardiac electrical activity (referred to as cardiac vectors) is generally in a direction that is inferior and to the left. The leftward direction of cardiac electrical activity is primarily due to the size and therefore electrical activity of the left ventricle.

The 12-lead ECG is the graphic recording of the electrical output of the heart from 12 different positions. A 12-lead ECG can be diagnostic in drug toxicity, conduction disturbances, electrolyte imbalances, ischemia, and infarction, and can aid in determining the size of the heart chambers and axis orientation of the heart.

Cardiac monitoring uses rhythm strips to assess heart rate, rhythm, and dysrhythmias. Rhythm strips may be run on any one of the 12 leads used in a 12-lead ECG and several other special leads.

The most common leads used to monitor patients are leads II and V_1. Lead II is a common lead, although it is highly limited in the information it can reveal to the clinician. Lead II has a negative pole attached to an electrode placed on the upper chest near the right arm and a positive pole attached to an electrode placed on the lower left side of the chest. Lead II normally sees electrical activity in the heart in an upright ECG pattern, since its positive electrode is on the left side of the body. *Lead II is especially useful in assessing P waves* and QRS complexes that have a small amplitude. It is not, however, the ideal monitoring lead. *V_1 is a better routine monitoring lead.* MCL_1 is modified chest lead 1. It is the bipolar equivalent of V_1 on the 12-lead ECG.

V_1 is an excellent monitoring lead, perhaps the best of the six common chest leads of the 12-lead ECG. In V_1, the positive electrode is attached to an electrode placed to the right of the sternum at the fourth intercostal space (**Fig. 3-1**). Since the V_1 positive electrode is placed to the right of the sternum, it views

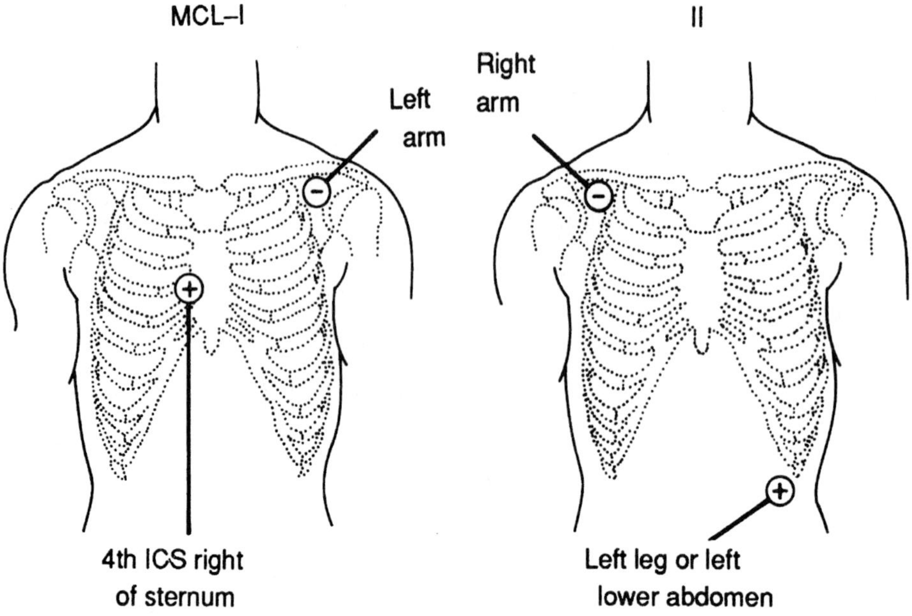

Figure 3-1. Normal placement for leads V_1 and II.

the cardiac electrical activity as heading away from it and therefore sees the QRS complex as primarily upside down. The V (vector) leads are technically called unipolar leads, since the negative pole is the computer-calculated center of all the ECG leads and only the positive electrode is physically visible.

V_1 gives more information on conduction defects, such as right and left bundle branch blocks, than do other routine monitoring leads. As such, it is the routine lead employed to identify most dysrhythmias, particularly aberrant atrial premature contractions, from premature ventricular contractions. The one situation for which V_1 is not as useful is with newer monitoring systems that employ ST-segment analysis. ST-segment analysis operates better when large R waves are sensed. If large R waves are desired, lead II, V_5, or V_6 are employed.

In monitoring dysrhythmias, develop the practice of using multiple leads. Use of a single lead for all situations limits your ability to interpret complex dysrhythmias.

A key ingredient to accurate dysrhythmia analysis is the correct application of lead placement. *Although the CCRN exam generally does not ask specific questions on lead placement,* such questions are possible. More importantly, accurate lead placement has an effect on correct rhythm and 12-lead analysis. Studies have indicated significant changes in QRS morphology with incorrect lead placement.

ECG Paper

The CCRN exam will not ask questions about the ECG paper. However, you must know the time grids within the ECG paper to make interpretations of dysrhythmias and 12-lead analysis.

The ECG paper has a series of horizontal lines exactly 1 mm apart (**Fig. 3-2**). The horizontal lines represent voltage (or amplitude). ECG paper also has vertical lines that represent time. Each vertical line is 0.04 s apart. To help in measuring waveforms, every fifth line is darker than the other lines, both horizontally and vertically. The intersection of these lines produces both small boxes (the lighter lines) and large boxes (the darker, bolder lines). Horizontally, each small box represents 1 mm (0.1 mV) and each large box represents 5 mm (0.5 mV). (Note that each large box is made up of five small boxes.) Vertically, each small box represents 0.04 s and each large box represents 0.20 s with a printer paper speed of 25 mm/s. Because of the design of ECG paper, one can measure the duration of impulses (wavelengths) and the amplitude (height) of impulses. All waves will be either isoelectric (no net electrical activity, or flat),

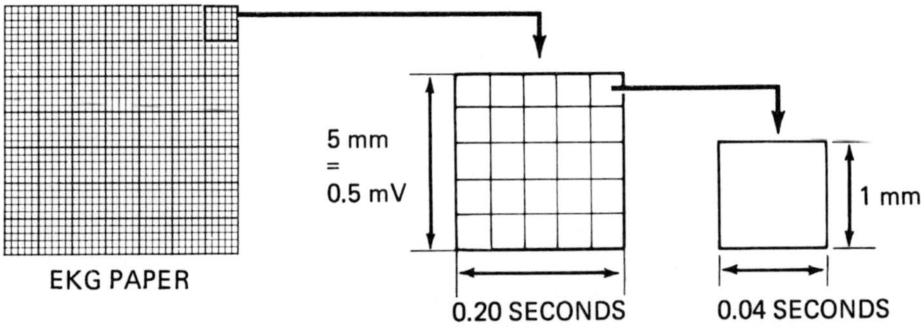

Figure 3-2. ECG paper.

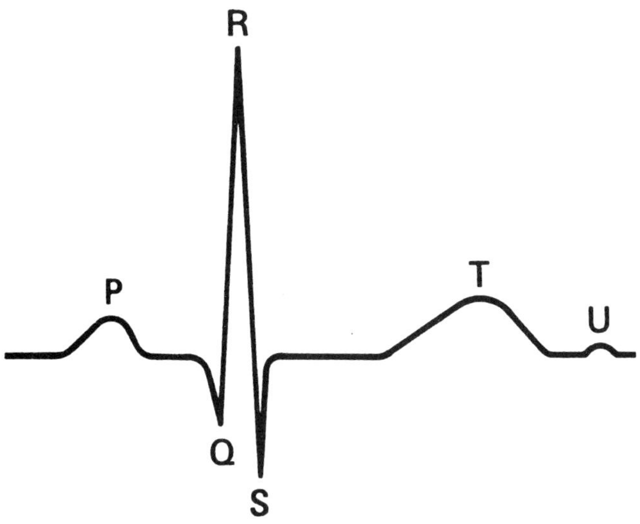

Figure 3-3. The normal PQRST deflections, lead II.

positively deflected (upright, toward the positive pole), or negatively deflected (downward, toward the negative pole).

3.2 COMPONENTS OF A CARDIAC CYCLE

Before a rhythm strip can be labeled, a systematic analysis of each portion of the strip and the relation of each wave to the electrical activity in the cardiac cycle is made. The interpretations will be made using lead II or V_1 in this text. It is conventional to label the components of the cardiac cycle P, QRS, and T. (There is no reason why these specific letters were chosen.)

There are three prominent deflections in the ECG: the P wave, the QRS complex, and the T wave (**Fig. 3-3**).

P Wave

This represents the generation of an electrical impulse and depolarization of the atria (**Fig. 3-4**). The P wave is important in determining whether the impulse started in the sinoatrial (SA) node or elsewhere in the atrium.

KEY CLINICAL CONCEPT

P-mitrale is evidenced by an enlarged, sometimes notched P-wave. This is suggestive of atrial enlargement and often appears on the exam.

QRS Complex

The QRS complex is composed of three separate waveforms, which represent ventricular depolarization (**Fig. 3-5**). Multiple variations exist in the shape of the QRS complex. A Q wave is the first negative deflection and may or may not be present. **A large Q wave may be indicative of myocardial death.** *To be clinically significant, the Q wave should be greater than 0.04 s and the depth should be greater than one-third the height of the R wave.*

The R wave is the first positive deflection in the complex. The R wave is usually large in leads where the positive electrode is on the left (I, II, III, aVL, aVF, V_5, V_6) and small in leads where the positive electrode is on the right (V_1, V_1, V_2, aVR).

The S wave is the negative deflection following the R wave. The S wave can be useful in interpreting terminal electrical activity in the heart. The S wave is large in leads where the positive electrode is on the right and small in leads where the positive electrode is on the left.

T Wave

The T wave is the third major deflection in the ECG (**Fig. 3-6**). It represents repolarization of the ventricles. In most lead II of a healthy heart, the T wave is positively deflected. **In ischemia or infarction, the T wave may be inverted.**

Intervals and Segments

There are four other intervals and segments of a rhythm strip and an ECG that must be identified.

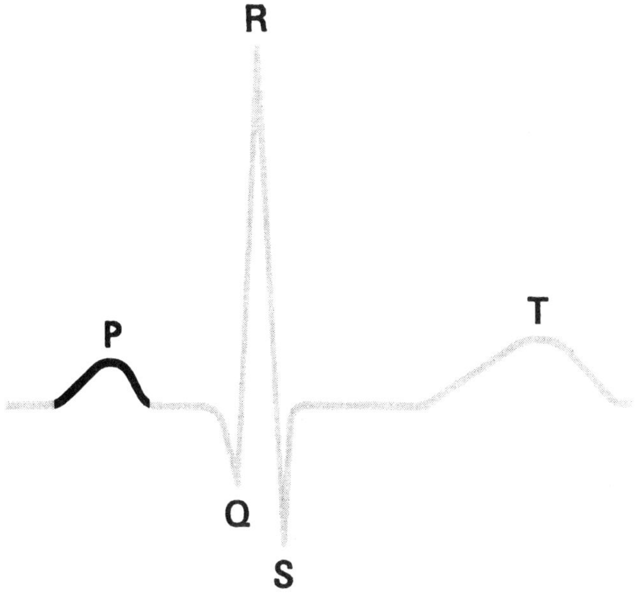

Figure 3-4. The P wave.

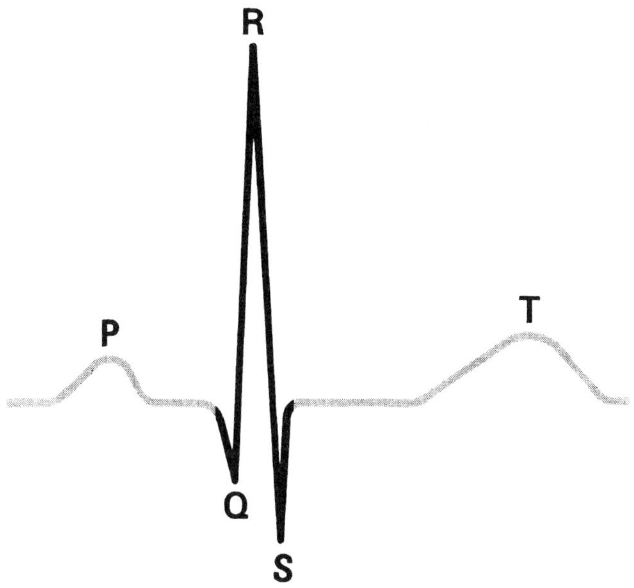

Figure 3-5. The QRS complex.

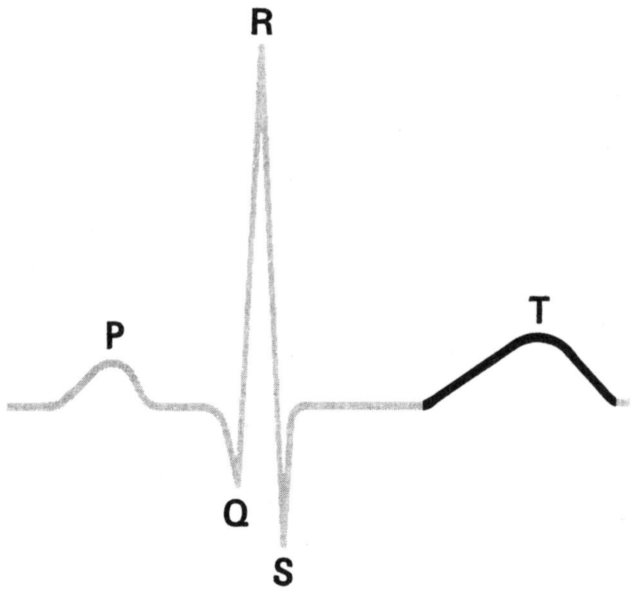

Figure 3-6. The T wave.

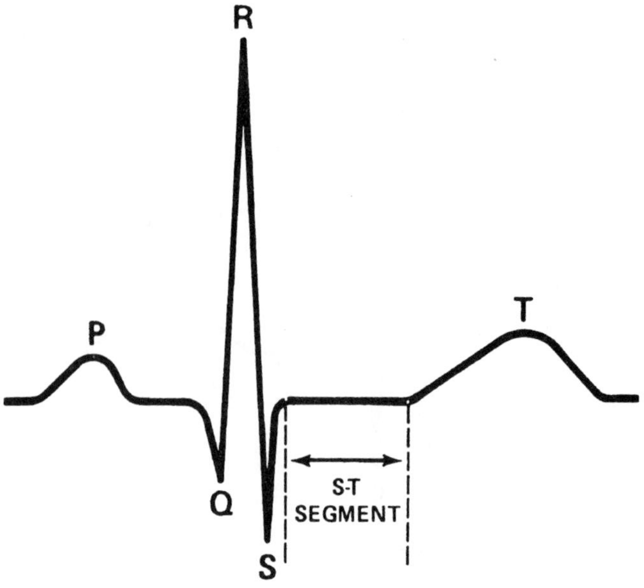

Figure 3-8. The ST segment.

PR Interval. The PR interval (**Fig. 3-7**) represents the time for the electrical impulse to spread from the atrium to the atrioventricular (AV) node and His bundle. It is measured from the beginning of the P wave to the beginning of the QRS complex. Normally, this interval is 0.12 to 0.20 s.

ST Segment. The ST segment (**Fig. 3-8**) represents the time from complete depolarization of the ventricles to the beginning of repolarization (recovery) of the ventricles. In the healthy heart, the ST segment is flat or isoelectric. Since no net electrical activity is present during the recovery phase of the cardiac cycle, the wave is not deflected in either direction. **In myocardial injury, the segment may be elevated. In ischemia, the ST segment is depressed.**

PR Segment. This segment (**Fig. 3-9**) represents the normal delay in the conduction of the electrical impulse in the AV node. It is normally isoelectric and is measured from the end of the P wave to the beginning of the R wave. Duration of the PR segment varies. Clinically, the PR segment is not usually addressed.

QT Interval. This interval (**Fig. 3-10**) represents the total time required for depolarization and repolarization (recovery) of the ventricles. It is measured from the beginning of the QRS complex to the end of the T wave. It is normally less than 0.40 s but is dependent on heart rate, sex, age, and other factors. **Antidysrhythmics such as amiodarone may also prolong the QT interval to more than 0.40.** A QT interval that is corrected for heart rate is called the QTc. **A QTc more than 450 ms is considered elevated and is associated with a higher risk of developing lethal arrhythmia such as torsade de pointes.**

Occasionally another wave is seen after the T wave and before the next P wave. This is called a **U wave** (**Fig. 3-11**).

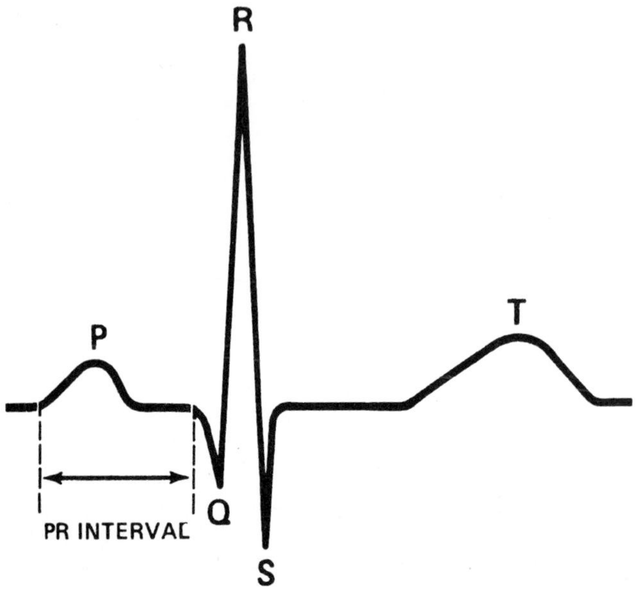

Figure 3-7. The PR interval.

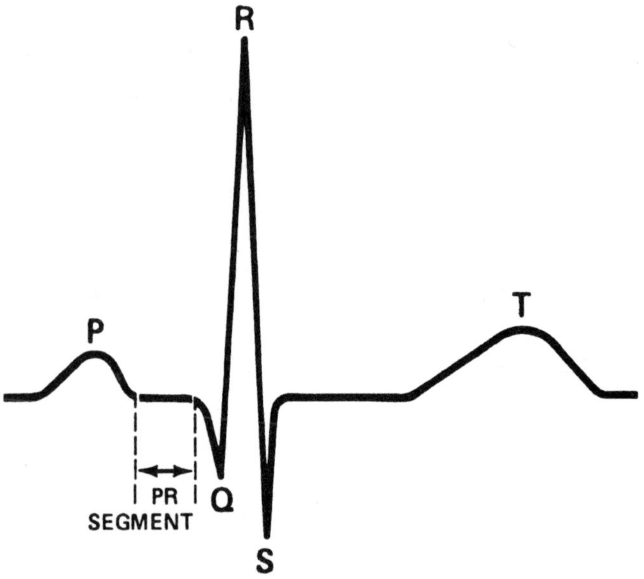

Figure 3-9. The PR segment.

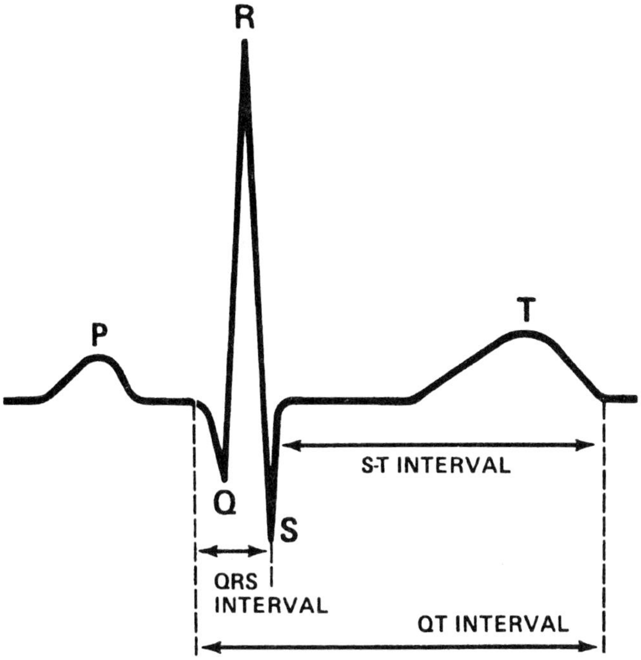

Figure 3-10. The QRS, ST, and QT intervals.

*The U wave may represent repolarization of the Purkinje fibers or **hypokalemia.*** It may or may not be seen.

3.3 INTERPRETATION OF A RHYTHM STRIP

Five basic steps are followed in analyzing a rhythm strip (or an ECG) to aid in the interpretation and identification of a rhythm. Each step should be followed in sequence. Eventually this will become a habit and will enable the clinician to identify a strip correctly, accurately, and quickly.

Step 1

Determine the rates at which the atria and the ventricles are depolarizing. These rates may not be the same. *To count the rate of the atria, count the number of P waves present in the 6-s*

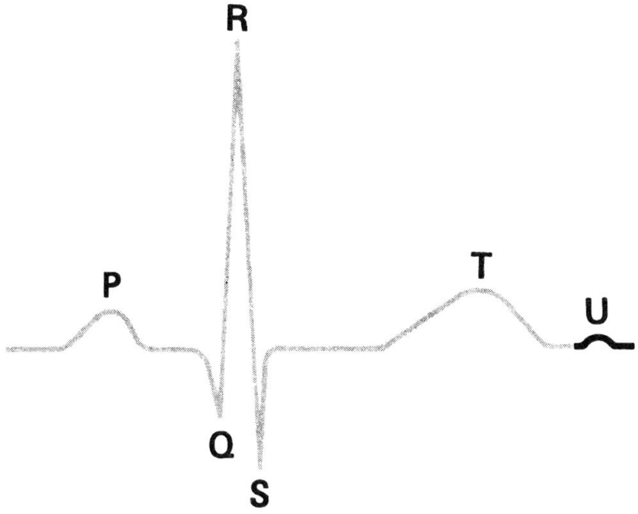

Figure 3-11. The U wave.

rhythm strip and multiply by 10. (Each mark at the top edge of the ECG paper represents 3 s, and each inch of the ECG paper equals 1 s.) This gives the atrial rate per minute.

Count the number of QRS complexes in a 6-s strip and multiply by 10. This gives the ventricular rate per minute. **For the CCRN exam, this is all that is needed.**

For regular rhythms, another method may be used. Find the peak of one QRS complex that lands on a heavy dark line. Then find the next QRS complex. The rate is as follows: If the QRS complexes are separated by one large block (five small blocks), the rate is 300. If there are two blocks, the rate is 150; three blocks, 100; four blocks, 75; five blocks, 60. The rate becomes less accurate after this.

Step 2

Determine whether the rhythm is regular or irregular **(for the purposes of the exam, the degree of regularity will be obvious, and calipers are not needed)**. The most accurate method is to measure the interval from one R wave to the next. (Set one point of the cardiac calipers on the tip of the first R wave and the other point on the tip of the next R wave.) Then move the cardiac calipers from R to R. If the measurement is the same (or varies <0.04 s between beats), the rhythm is regular. If the intervals vary by more than 0.04 s, the rhythm is irregular. Often, one can tell by simply looking at the strip that the rhythm is irregular. However, if it looks regular, it is best to measure the R-to-R intervals to be certain.

Step 3

Analyze the P waves. A P wave should precede every QRS complex. All of the P waves should be identical in shape. The normal P wave is fairly sharply curved, less than 3 mm in height, and less than 0.1 s in width in lead II. If the P wave is abnormally shaped or varies in shape from wave to wave, the stimulus may have arisen from somewhere in the atrium other than in the SA node. Almost all impulses that originate in the SA node will meet the "normal" shape and size previously stated if heart function is normal. **A biphasic P (a single P wave moves above and below the baseline) may indicate *left atrial enlargement*; a peaked P may indicate right atrial enlargement**, and both these P waves originate in the SA node. If there is no P wave or if the P wave does not precede the QRS complex, the impulse did not originate in the SA node.

Step 4

Measure the PR interval. This is done from the beginning of the P wave to the beginning of the QRS complex. It should be between 0.12 and 0.20 s. Intervals outside this range indicate a conduction disturbance between the atria and the ventricles.

KEY CLINICAL CONCEPT

Wolff-Parkinson-White (WPW) syndrome is identified with two key characteristics on an ECG: a short PR interval less than 0.12 and the appearance of a delta wave. The short PR interval is due to accessory pathways that allow for abnormal conduction through the atria to the ventricles at a faster rate than if they moved through the AV node.

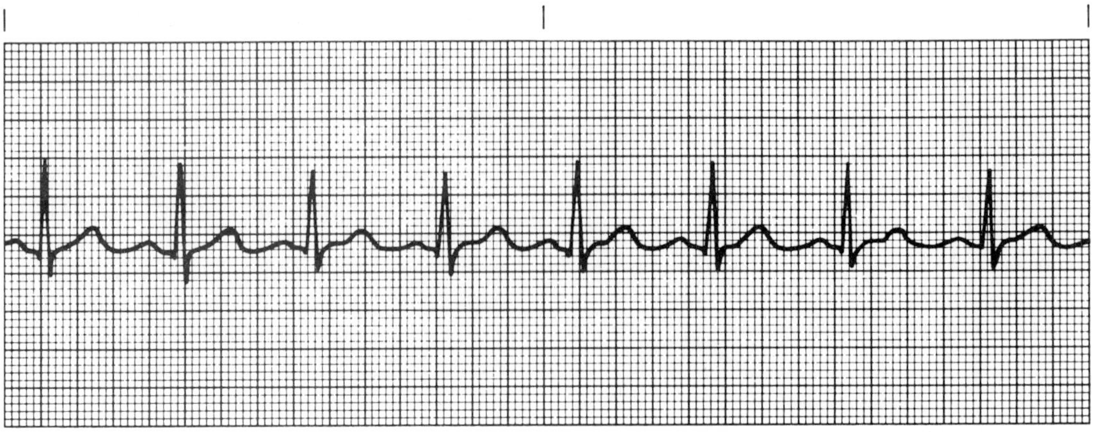

Figure 3-12. Lead II normal sinus rhythm.

QUICK TIP! On the exam you will not likely be directly asked if you know a PR >0.20 is abnormal. The exam will assume you already know that. Instead, you would be expected to know clinical conditions to suspect why it may be >0.20, such as due to beta-blockers, calcium-channel blockers, or ischemia.

Step 5

Measure the width of the QRS complex. This is done from the beginning of the Q (if present, otherwise the R) to the end of the S wave. The normal duration is 0.06 to 0.12 s. A QRS measurement of greater than 0.12 s indicates an intraventricular conduction abnormality *(such as due to heart failure or to drugs such as amiodarone).*

Figure 3-12 is a 6-s lead II rhythm strip. Let us analyze this rhythm strip by applying the five steps just mentioned.

- Step 1: The atrial rate is 80 (eight P waves in 6 s). The ventricular rate is 80 (eight R waves in 6 s). The heart rate is 80.
- Step 2: There is less than a 0.04-s variation from R wave to R wave, so the rhythm is regular.
- Step 3: The P waves are all the same shape, size (in height), and duration. Each P wave appears immediately before a QRS complex. These factors indicate that the impulse starts in the SA node.
- Step 4: The PR interval is about 0.16 s. This is within the normal duration range, indicating normal conduction of the impulse from the SA node to the AV node.
- Step 5: Each QRS complex is less than 0.10 s in duration, which is normal.
- Interpretation of the strip: Normal sinus rhythm.

KEY CONTENT CHECKLIST

- ❒ Lead II is useful for assessing P waves and QRS complexes; however, V_1 is a better lead for routine monitoring and diagnostic purposes.
- ❒ ECG paper has horizontal lines that represent amplitude and are 1 mm apart. The vertical lines represent time, and each line is 0.04 seconds apart.
- ❒ P wave represents depolarization of the atria.
- ❒ A notched P wave, somewhat resembling an M shape, may represent atrial enlargement (also known as P-MITRALE). A peaked P wave may represent right atrial enlargement.
- ❒ A large, significant Q wave should be greater than 0.04 seconds and at least one-third the height of the R wave. A large Q wave may represent myocardial death.
- ❒ Understand how ECG changes relate to clinical concepts. For example, understand that T wave inversion may demonstrate ischemia or infarction.
- ❒ ST segment is elevated in myocardial injury and depressed in ischemia.
- ❒ QT intervals may be prolonged by antidysrhythmic such as amiodarone. Prolonged QTs can increase the risk of lethal dysrhythmias.
- ❒ U waves may represent repolarization of the Purkinje fibers or hypokalemia.
- ❒ Follow a systematic approach for interpreting rhythm strips.
- ❒ WPW syndrome is identified with two key characteristics on an ECG: a short PR interval less than 0.12 and the appearance of a delta wave. The short PR interval is due to accessory pathways that allow for abnormal conduction through the atria to the ventricles at a faster rate than if they moved through the AV node.

Review Questions:

1. A patient is admitted with acute cholecystitis and is experiencing fever as well as nausea/vomiting. Your patient complains of chest discomfort, so a 12-lead ECG is completed. There are no signs of acute ischemia; however, upon review of the ECG, it is noted your patient is in sinus rhythm with a heart rate of 86 and the QTc is 526. All of the following medications may be contributing to the increased QTc except which one?

a. Ciprofloxacin
b. Ondansetron
c. Sotalol
d. Morphine

Answer D. Rationale: All of the other medications are in drug classes that may cause QT prolongation. Ciprofloxacin is a fluoroquinolone, which is a drug class that is known to cause QT prolongation. While ciprofloxacin is one of the less likely of this drug class to cause QT interval prolongation it is still possible. Ondansetron is known to cause QT prolongation, especially when used with other medications that cause prolongation. ECGs should be monitored when using in patients at higher risk. Sotalol is part of an antiarrhythmic class and is a non-selective beta blocker. Due to this mechanism of action, they are known to cause QT prolongation and ECGs should be monitored. Choose D.

Questions 2 and 3 refer to the following scenario:

A 65-year-old man is admitted to your unit with chest pain. The chest pain developed 2 hours ago at his home. The pain went away while he rested but then returned. Currently, he has substernal chest pain radiating to the left arm and chin. The pain is the same regardless of position. No change in the pain occurs during inspiration. Vital signs are as follows: blood pressure 132/86 mm Hg, pulse 96 bpm, respiratory rate 25 breaths/min. The patient's 12-lead ECG shows depressed ST segments in the inferior leads. Small Q waves, less than one-third the height of the R wave, are present in the inferior leads.

2. Based on the preceding information, which condition is likely to be developing?

a. Angina
b. Acute MI
c. Pericarditis
d. Pericardial tamponade

Answer: A. Rationale: Based on the case information, the patient in this question is likely suffering from unstable angina, option A. The absence of ST elevation makes acute MI less likely, eliminating B. ST elevation is also often seen in pericarditis, ruling out option C as well. Pericarditis chest pain also tends to improve when sitting forward, however, the pain persists regardless of patient's position in this case. Signs of pericardial tamponade are also absent such as hypotension, tachycardia, and pulsus paradoxus, so eliminate D as well. Choose A.

3. What would be the most likely treatment for the condition?

a. Nitrates and beta blockers
b. Thrombolytic therapy
c. Pericardiocentesis
d. Nonsteroidal anti-inflammatory drugs (NSAIDs) and consider steroids

Answer A. Rationale: This patient is suffering from acute coronary syndrome (ACS), and central to the care of patients with ACS is the reduction of afterload and myocardial oxygen demand with nitrates and beta blockers, option A. Thrombolytic therapy would not be appropriate because this patient is not having an acute MI, so eliminate B. Pericardiocentesis would also not be appropriate since signs of pericardial tamponade are not present (see rationale for question 72), so eliminate option C as well. Option D is more appropriate for pericarditis treatment. Choose A.

4

The 12-Lead ECG

CHAPTER OVERVIEW AND OBJECTIVES

The CCRN exam can include questions that require an understanding of the 12-lead electrocardiogram (ECG). The most important questions to answer relate to the acute coronary syndrome, where ischemia or injury may be present. **This should be the most important part of preparing for the CCRN exam in regards to 12-lead interpretation**. Other less common questions involving the 12-lead ECG usually focus on conditions such as left and right ventricular (RV) hypertrophy, left and right bundle branch blocks, differentiating aberrant atrial premature contractions from premature ventricular contractions (PVCs), and identifying myocardial infarction (MI) patterns. This chapter provides the information necessary to interpret these conditions. However, keep in mind the number of questions regarding a 12-lead ECG will be limited. **Often, it is not the interpretation of the 12-lead ECG, which is key to a question, but what does an abnormal component of the 12-lead ECG indicate? For example, you may be told that the ST segment is elevated in certain leads, and you need to apply that information to a scenario.**

- Identify key characteristics of acute myocardial infarction and injury on a 12-lead ECG and the associated area of injury.
- Understand basic characteristics of bundle branch blocks.

4.1 IDENTIFYING MYOCARDIAL INFARCTION AND ISCHEMIA

In reviewing the 12-lead ECG for infarction and ischemic injury patterns, keep in mind that the ECG is not foolproof (**Table 4-1**). In a small but substantial percentage of patients who have an MI, the ECG will show no evidence of damage. Changes in serum cardiac biomarkers are more accurate, but they take longer to determine. The speed with which an ECG can be obtained is the primary reason why it still has clinical value.

The first step in identifying an MI is to look at the ST segment. It is one of the first parts of the ECG to change with MI. **Typically, if an MI is occurring, the ST segment will be elevated** (**Fig. 4-1**). Elevation of the ST segment is a strong warning sign of cardiac injury. *The ST segment may be* **depressed if only ischemia** *of the heart exists* (**Fig. 4-2**). To identify changes in the ST segment, examine where the ST segment is 0.08 s (two small blocks) from the end of the QRS (**Fig. 4-3**).

The ST segment in the area opposite the MI might show depression, a concept referred to as reciprocal change (**Fig. 4-4**).

The T wave may also indicate cardiac ischemia and may change before the ST segment does. It usually becomes inverted with cardiac ischemia (**Fig. 4-5**) but may also be tall and peaked.

Significant Q-wave formation is the primary indication that a patient has had an MI. Q waves are negative deflections in front of R waves and are small in size (**Fig. 4-6**). *They are considered significant (also known as pathologic) if they are wide (>0.04 s) and large (greater than one-third the height of the R wave).* **Q waves indicate cardiac muscle death when present in contiguous leads.**

TABLE 4-1. 12-LEAD ECG LEADS

Lead	*View of the Heart*
I	Lateral wall
II	Inferior wall
III	Inferior wall
aVR (augmented vector of the right)	
aVL (augmented vector of the left)	Lateral wall
aVF (augmented vector of the foot)	Inferior wall
V_1	Ventricular septum
V_2	Anterior wall
V_3	Anterior wall
V_4	Anterior wall
V_5	Lateral wall
V_6	Lateral wall

Because they take about 24 hours to form, if a Q wave is present, one can estimate that the MI occurred at least 1 day earlier. From a nursing perspective, we would want to determine whether cardiac damage was occurring before the muscle actually died, which may indicate an opportunity to mitigate further ischemic damage. To do this, we look for ST-segment changes before the formation of a Q wave. *If the Q wave is present, you know that the MI is too old for some treatments, such as thrombolysis.*

In reading a 12-lead ECG, it is necessary to identify the location of any injury. The heart is normally divided into four parts, each identified with different ECG leads.

KEY CLINICAL CONCEPT

Consider committing to memory the groups of contiguous leads that are associated with the parts of the heart, especially: Anterior/septal, lateral, and inferior.

Part of the Heart	*Leads*
Anterior/septal MI	V_1–V_4
Lateral MI	I, aVL, V_5, V_6
Inferior MI	II, III, aVF
Posterior MI	V_1, V_2
Right ventricular MI	V_3R, V_4R, V_5R, V_6R

Anterior MIs are usually the most dangerous because of the amount of muscle damaged and the *injury to the ventricular conduction system.* This usually represents obstruction of the **left anterior descending (LAD) artery**. Lateral MIs might

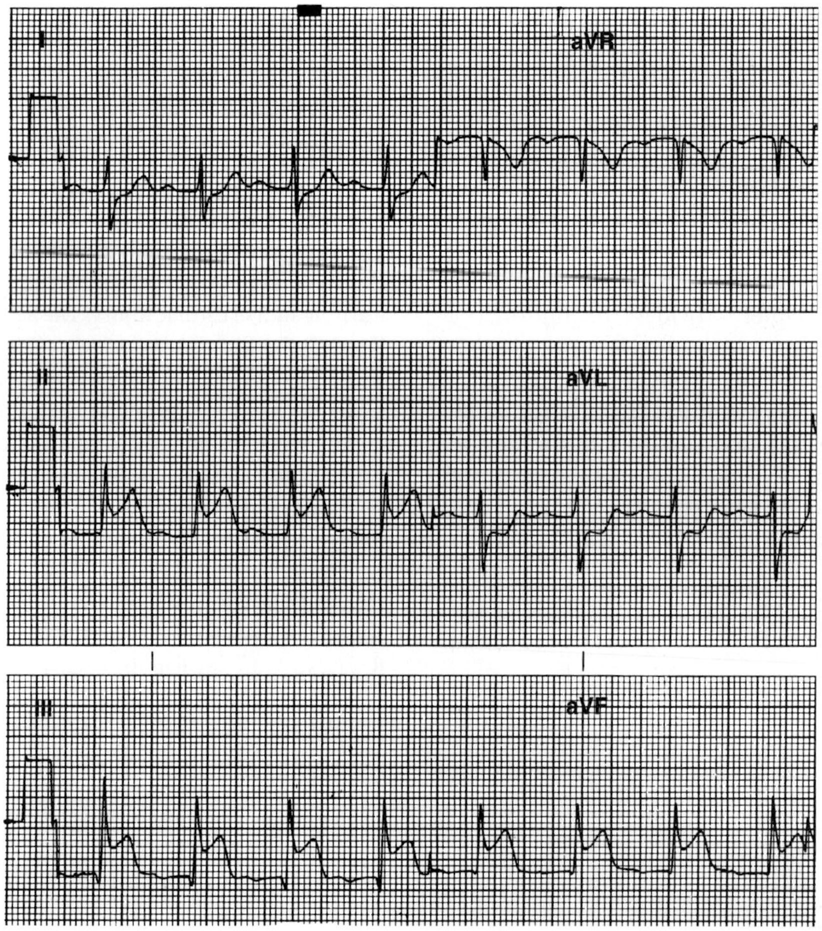

Figure 4-1. ST-segment elevation during MI.

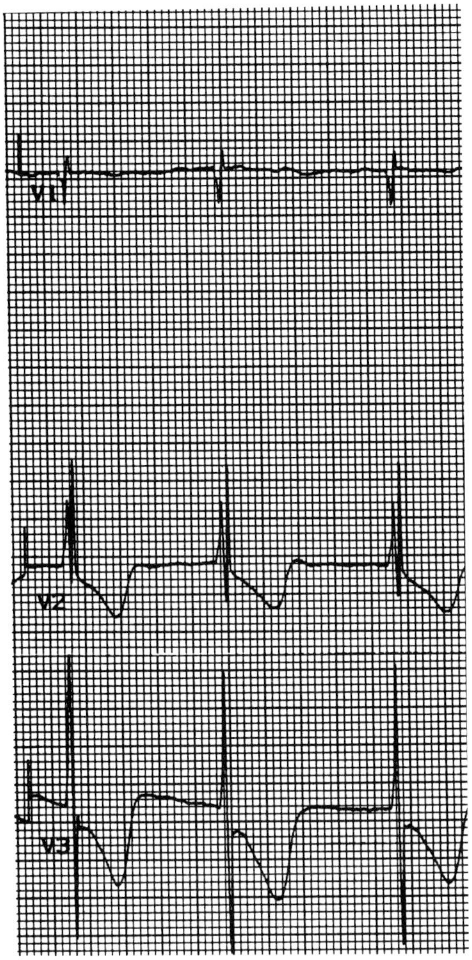

Figure 4-2. ST-segment depression during myocardial ischemia.

accompany anterior MIs or occur alone. **Lateral MIs** usually occur with obstruction of the **circumflex artery**. **Inferior MIs** are the second most dangerous type. *They frequently produce dysrhythmias, such as second-degree heart block.* **Inferior MIs** are most associated with obstruction of the **right coronary artery.** ***Inferior MIs are also commonly associated with RV MIs***. RV MIs are identified by using right-sided precordial chest leads, specifically V_3R to V_6R. Posterior MIs are difficult to see with the normal ECG. When the V_1 and V_2 leads are used to examine the back of the heart, the criteria for cardiac death are usually reversed. Instead of having a Q wave indicate an MI, the presence of a large R wave in V_1 and V_2 (the mirror test) might indicate a posterior MI. A posterior MI can be the result of obstruction of either the circumflex or the right coronary artery.

Injury Patterns

The more areas of the heart that are damaged, the more dangerous the MI becomes. For example, an anterior/lateral MI is more dangerous than either one individually. Common patterns include anterior/lateral, inferior/posterior, and anterior/septal.

KEY CLINICAL CONCEPT

The most important aspects of the ECG to understand have to do with identifying myocardial ischemia and injury. Your understanding of how to identify evidence of infarction or ischemia on an ECG will be tested on the CCRN exam.

4.2 AXIS DEVIATION

Axis calculation refers to identifying the source of major electrical activity in the heart. This is done by using vectors. A vector is a quantity that has magnitude and direction. Cardiac vectors represent electrical activity and force and are identified by arrows. If a cardiac vector is headed toward a positive lead on an ECG, it is represented by an upright arrow. If it is headed away from the positive electrode, it is viewed as negative. Normally, the mean cardiac vector is directed inferiorly and to the left (**Fig. 4-7**). If all the electrical activity in the heart were averaged, the net direction of electrical impulses would be toward the area of largest muscle concentration—that is, the left ventricle.

Vectors are usually represented on a circular diagram known as the hexaxial (six axes) reference system (**Fig. 4-8**). As Fig. 4-8 shows, the circle is divided into 30-degree segments. Each lead is represented, separated by 30-degree increments. The axis is

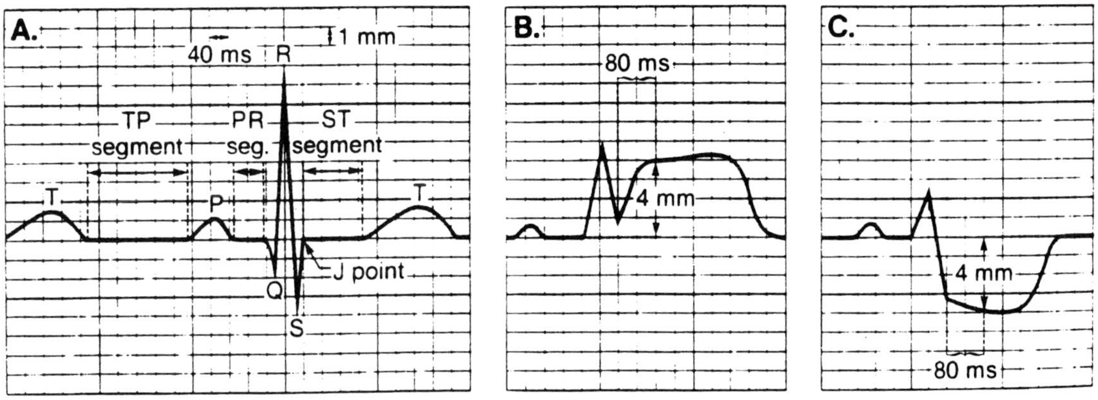

Figure 4-3. Correct location for measuring ST-segment changes.

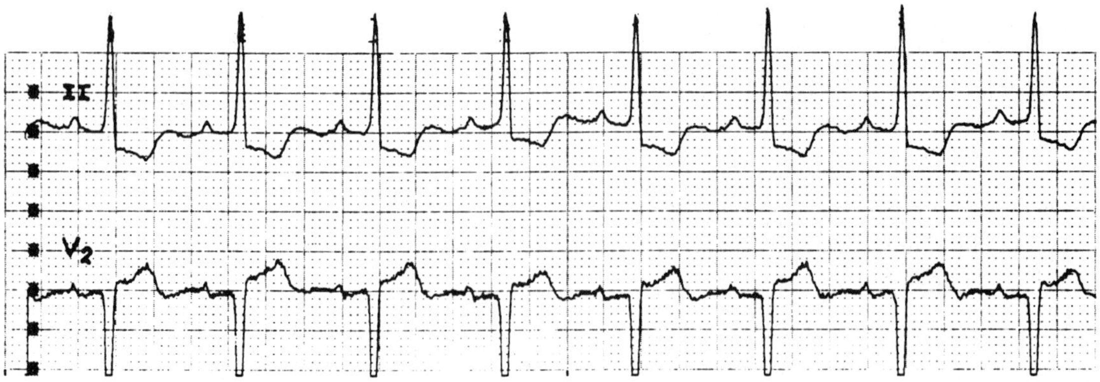

Figure 4-4. Reciprocal changes in the ECG during MI.

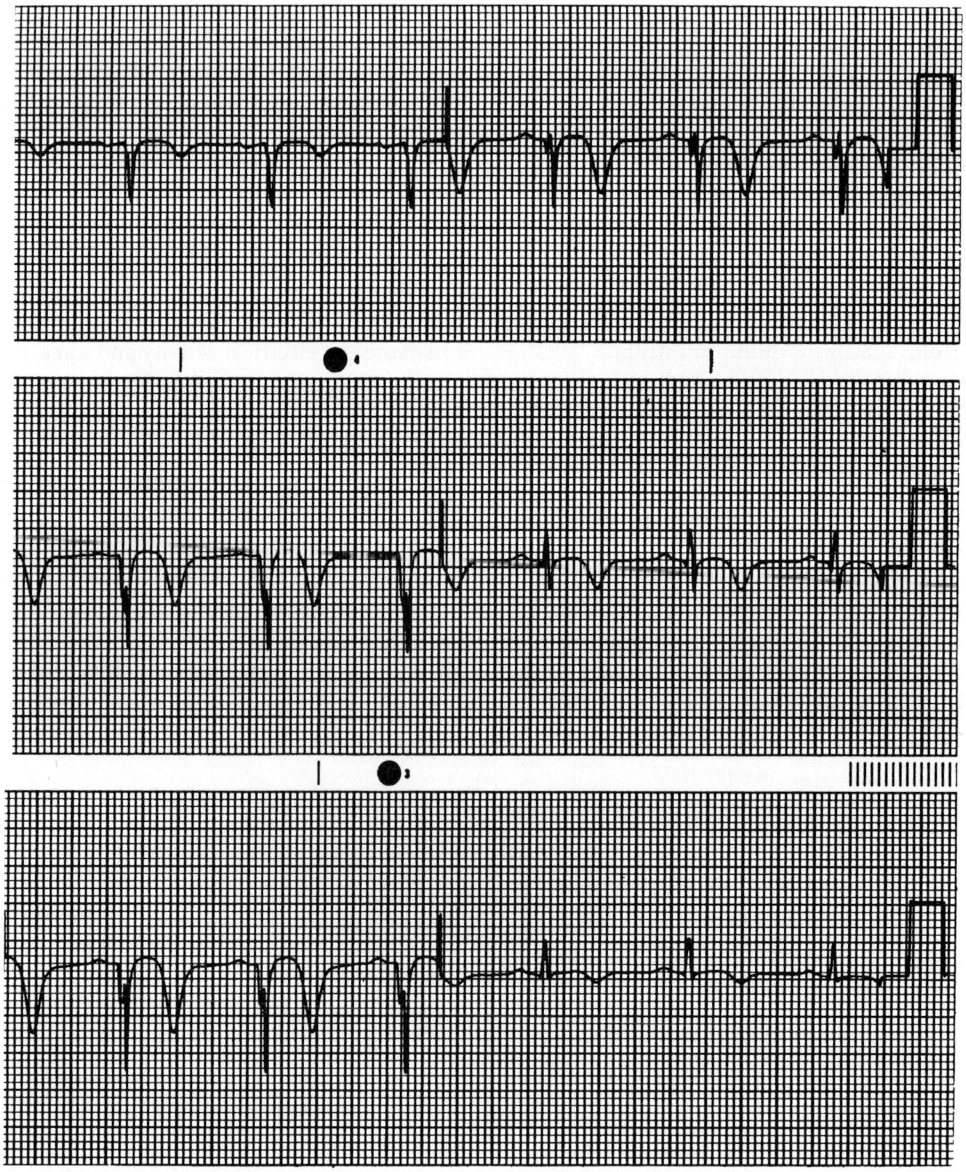

Figure 4-5. T-wave inversion with myocardial ischemia.

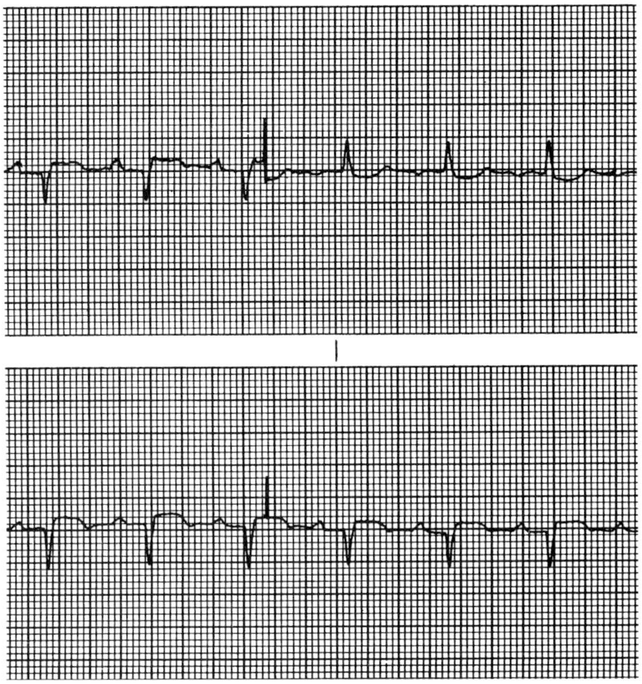

Figure 4-6. Q waves indicating myocardial death.

indicated by the number to which the major cardiac vector is pointing.

The axis can deviate. Typically, these deviations are classified as right axis deviation, left axis deviation, extreme right axis deviation, or indeterminate (**Fig. 4-9**). Causes for these changes are listed in **Table 4-2**.

Determining if an axis is normal or abnormal can be done by examining the largest QRS complex in the frontal plane

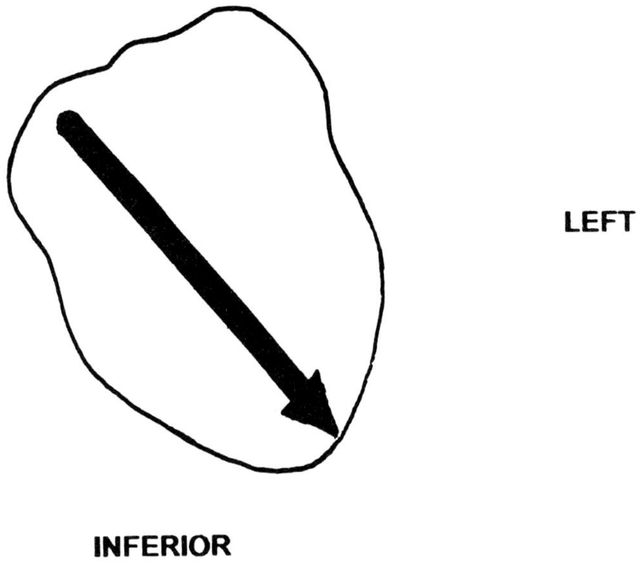

Figure 4-7. Representation of the mean cardiac vector.

leads—that is, I, II, III, aVR, aVL, and aVF. The largest QRS complex results when the cardiac vector heads directly toward or away from the positive electrode.

Using **Fig. 4-10** as an example, we can calculate the axis as follows: Note the locations of the positive and negative electrodes in each lead. Then observe the QRS complex in the 12-lead ECG. Note that, lead III has the largest deflection. This means the vector is 120 degrees. In **Fig. 4-11**, aVL has the largest QRS. This means the vector is −30 degrees (330 degrees).

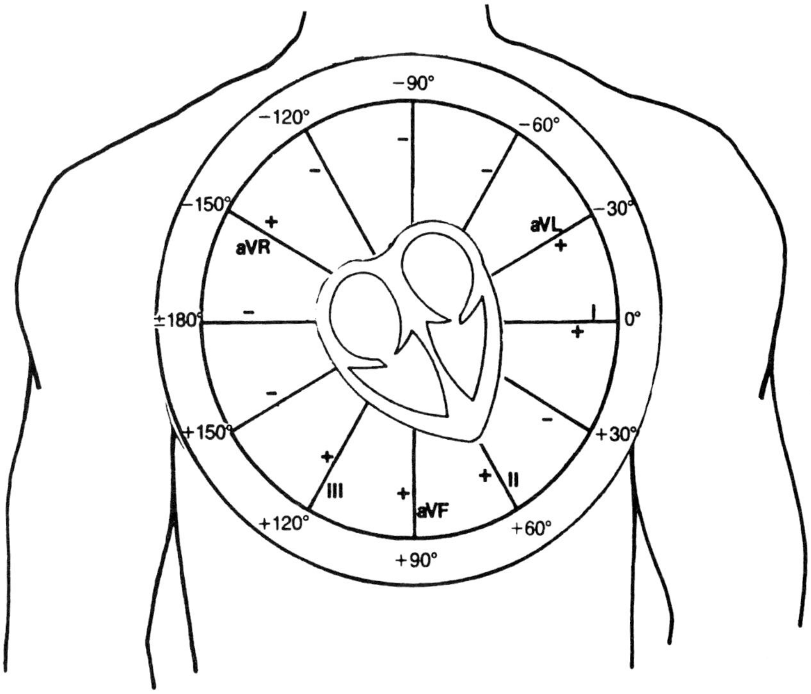

Figure 4-8. Geometric circle for vector measurement.

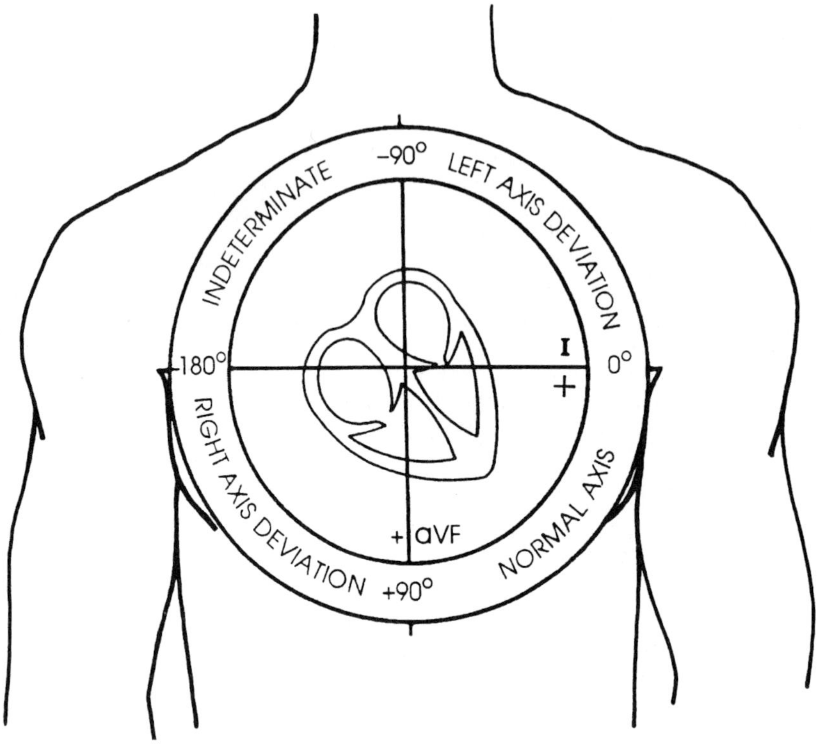

Figure 4-9. Normal and abnormal axes.

> **KEY CLINICAL CONCEPT**
>
> It is necessary to understand the axis of the heart in order to interpret a 12-lead ECG. However, it is unlikely that the CCRN exam will have a question regarding axis deviation.

4.3 BUNDLE BRANCH BLOCKS

Interpreting bundle branch blocks focuses on identifying changes in the QRS complex. Normally, the QRS complexes in the frontal plane (I, II, III, aVL, aVF) have small Q and S waves. V_1 has a small r wave and a large S wave. Conduction blocks can change this appearance. Bundle branch blocks are usually preceded by normal P waves and PR intervals. The primary difference is seen in the QRS complexes. However, these changes may only occur in certain ECG leads. Therefore, it is important to monitor leads correctly.

To understand conduction blocks, it is important to understand how the ventricles depolarize. Normally, the ventricles depolarize in the following manner: As the impulse spreads from the bundle of His, the left bundle depolarizes slightly ahead of the right. This causes the ventricular septum to be depolarized in a left-to-right direction. Leads with a positive electrode on the right side of the heart view this depolarization wave (vector) as coming toward it, creating an R wave (**Fig. 4-12**). Leads with a positive electrode on the left side of the heart view this wave as heading away from it, creating a Q wave.

TABLE 4-2. COMMON CAUSES FOR AXIS DEVIATIONS	
Left axis deviation	Left anterior fascicular block Left ventricular hypertrophy PVCs
Right axis deviation	Left posterior fascicular block Right ventricular hypertrophy
Extreme right axis deviation	PVCs
PVC, premature ventricular contraction.	

As the impulse spreads to the rest of the heart, the main depolarization wave is directed inferiorly and to the left (**Fig. 4-13**). This is due to the influence of the large left ventricle related to the size of the right ventricle. Depolarization in this manner creates an S wave for right-sided leads and an R wave for left-sided leads.

With conduction disturbances, these normal depolarization waves can be altered. Understanding the changes in depolarization waves is the key to interpreting conduction defects.

Right Bundle Branch Block

A right bundle branch block (RBBB) has two common characteristics, a triphasic pattern (rSR′) in lead V_1 or V_2 and a deep S wave in lead I (**Fig. 4-14**). Since the right bundle is blocked, a delayed rightward vector is created. This causes a third wave heading toward the positive electrode in V_1, resulting in a triphasic pattern. It simultaneously produces a wave headed away from the positive electrode in lead I. This causes a deep S wave in lead I. It will also cause a deep S wave in other lateral leads, such as V_6.

A RBBB might have a widening of the QRS but usually by no more than 0.14 s. P waves are usually visible in front of the rSR′

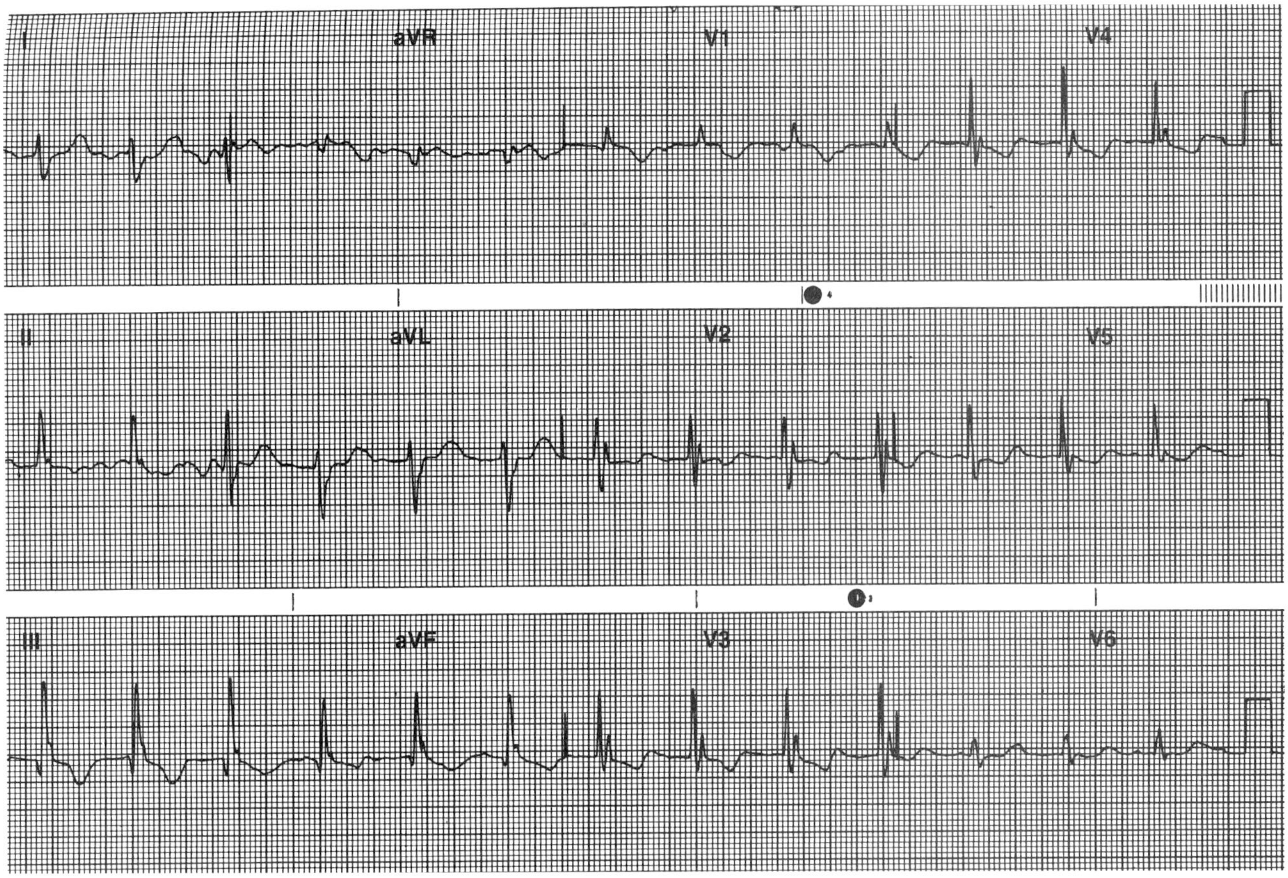

Figure 4-10. Sample lead III axis calculation.

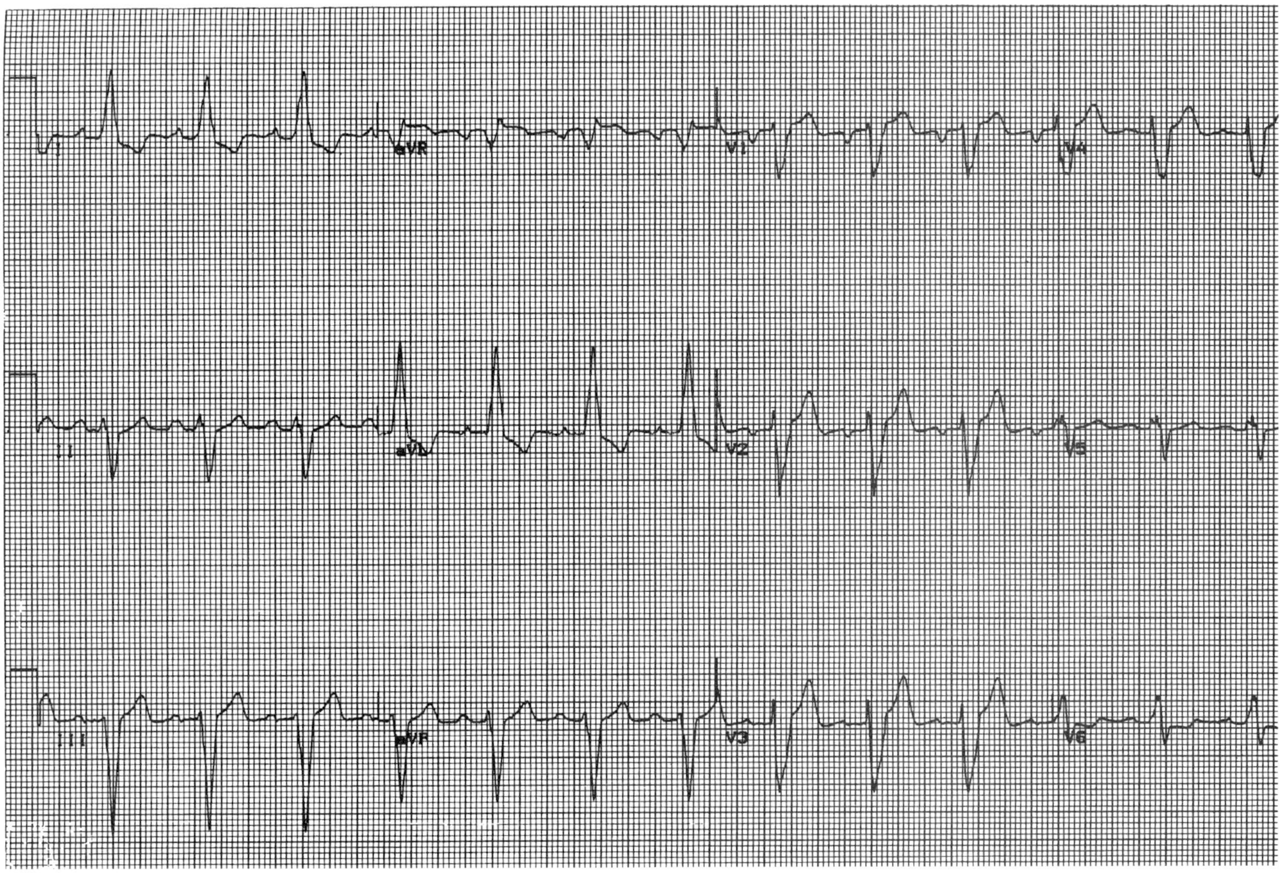

Figure 4-11. Sample aVL axis calculation.

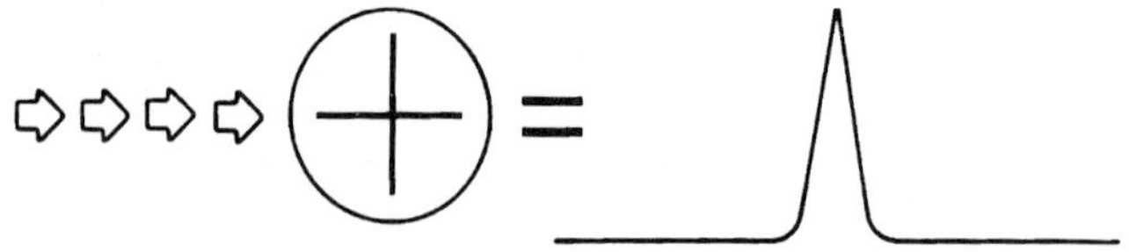

Figure 4-12. Depolarization occurring toward the positive electrode.

pattern, although they might be lost in the preceding T wave. Variations of the rSR′ pattern are occasionally found; however, the CCRN exam is not likely to cover complex variations from these common conduction patterns.

Left Bundle Branch Block

A left bundle branch block (LBBB) also has two common characteristics, a QS wave in lead V_1 and a wide, notched R wave in leads I and V_6 (**Fig. 4-15**). With a LBBB, the normal initial septal depolarization is altered. The first vector created is from the right bundle, creating a rightward-directed depolarization wave. This is seen by right-sided chest leads (like V_1) as headed away from it, creating a Q wave. Left-sided chest leads see this as an R wave (lead I).

LBBBs are almost always wide (>0.12 s) and frequently notched. P waves are usually visible but can be lost in the preceding T wave. As with RBBBs, there are some variations from these patterns, but they are not as common.

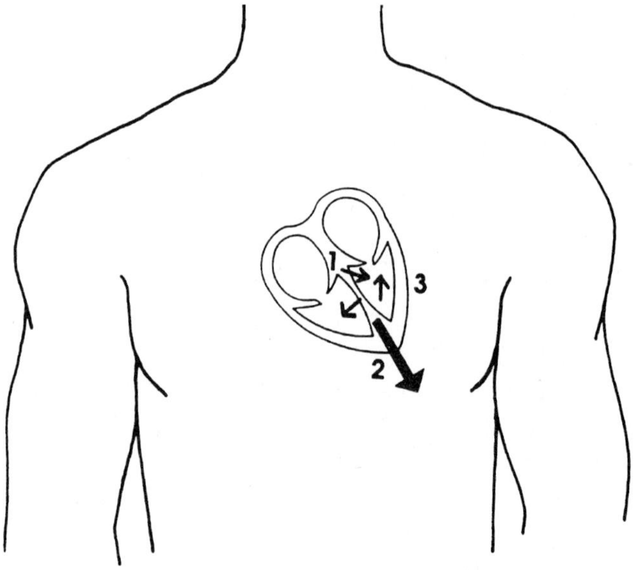

Figure 4-13. Ventricular depolarization vectors.

Left Anterior Fascicular Blocks (Anterior Hemiblock)

A left anterior fascicular block (anterior hemiblock) occurs when the anterior portion of the left bundle is obstructed (**Fig. 4-16**). The result is a shift in axis forces to the left (usually greater than −60 degrees). This left axis deviation also causes leads II, III, and aVF to become inverted.

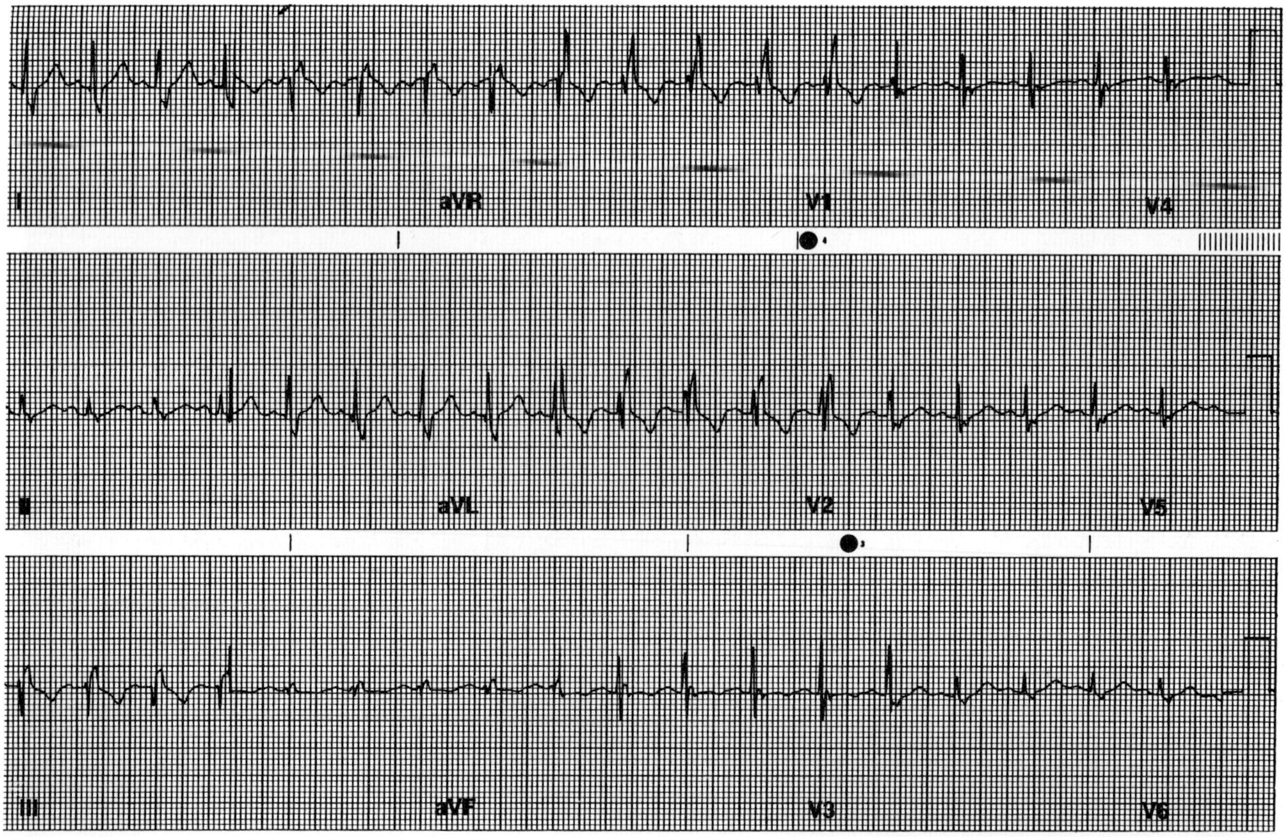

Figure 4-14. RBBB characteristics.

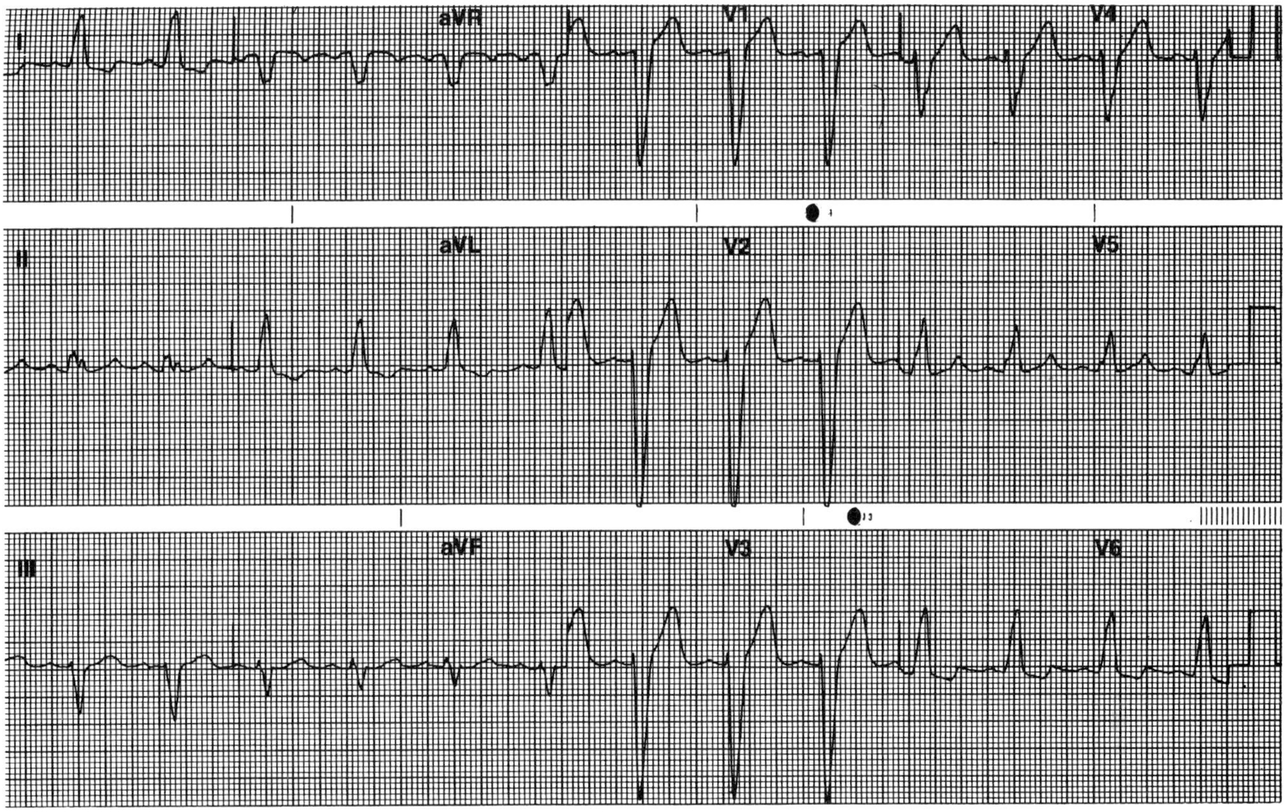

Figure 4-15. LBBB characteristics.

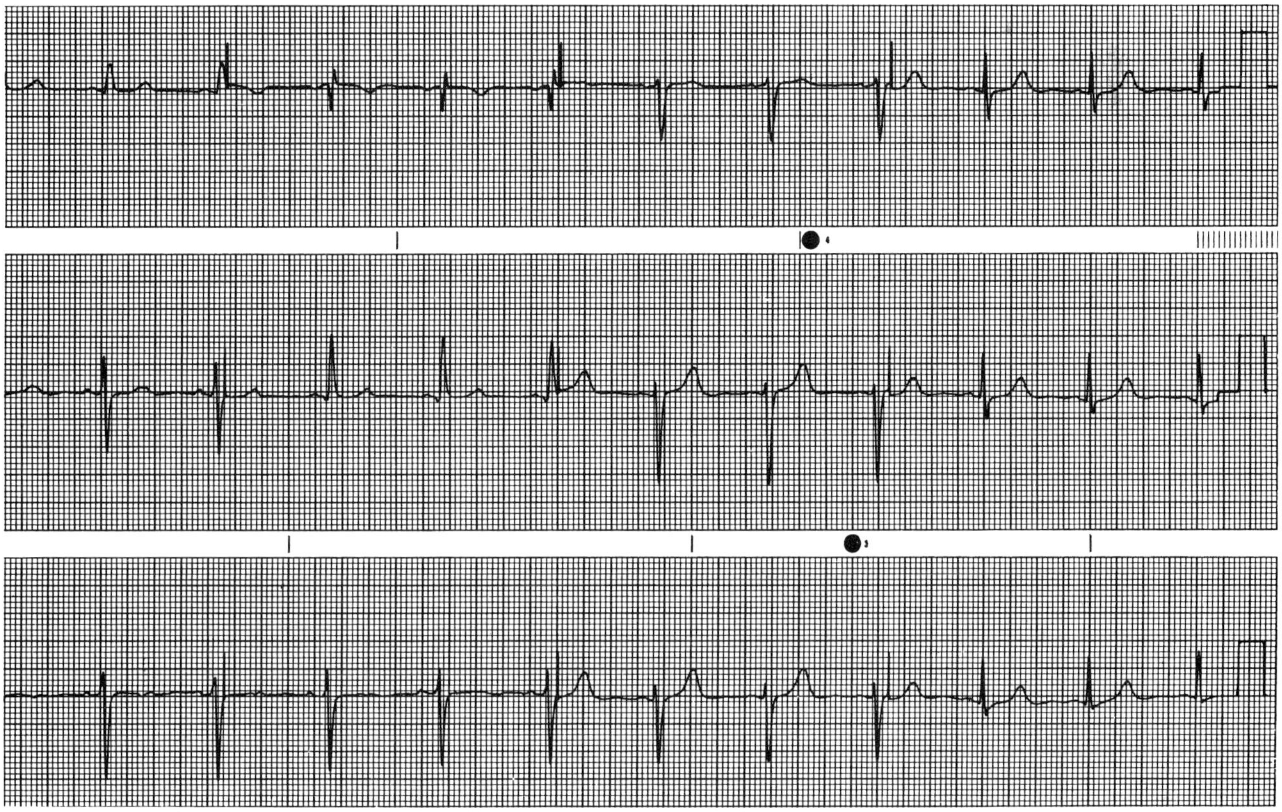

Figure 4-16. **Left** Anterior fascicular block characteristics.

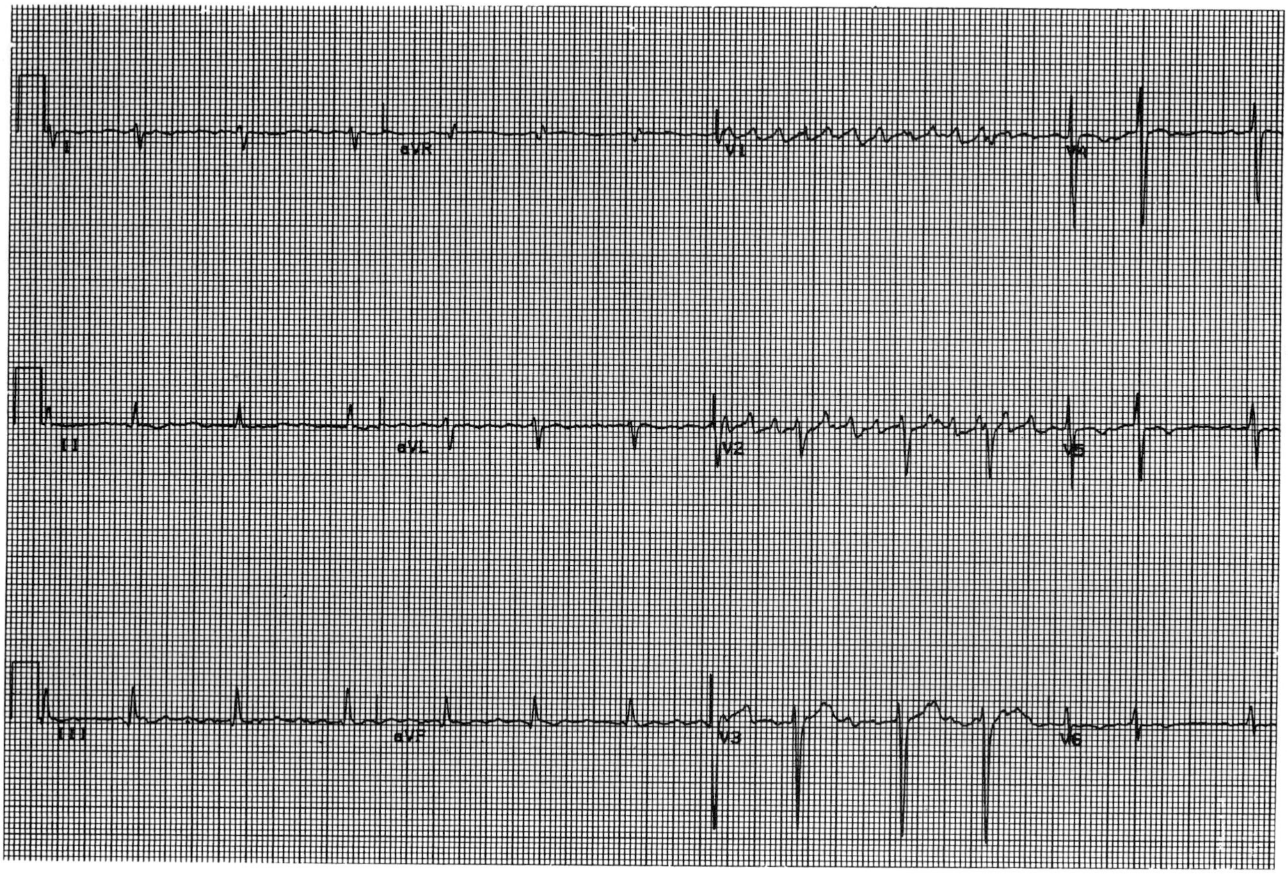

Figure 4-17. **Left** Posterior fascicular block characteristics.

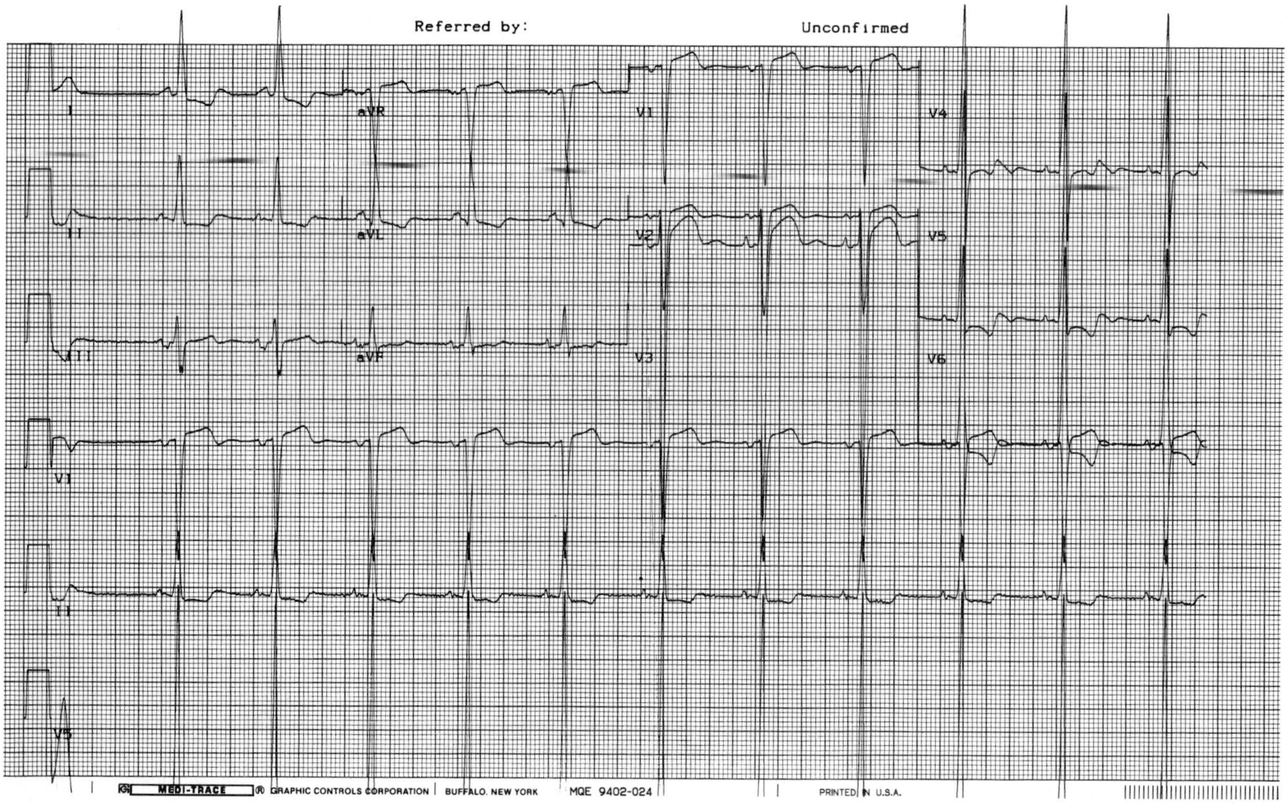

Figure 4-18. Left ventricular hypertrophy.

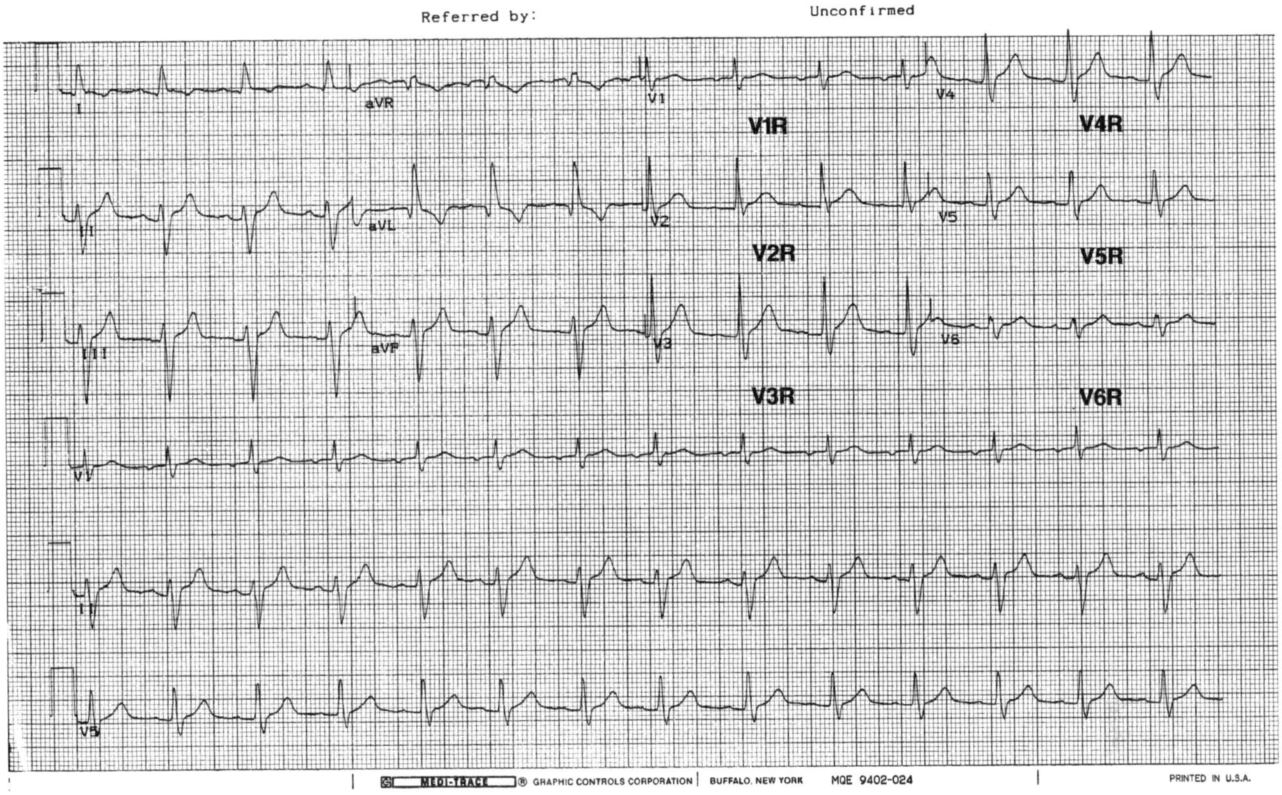

Figure 4-19. Right precordial leads.

Small Q waves may be noted in leads I and aVL. There may or may not be a prolongation of the QRS complex.

Left Posterior Fascicular Block (Posterior Hemiblock)

A left posterior fascicular block (posterior hemiblock) occurs when the posterior portion of the left bundle is obstructed. The result is a shift in the axis to the right. The vector in this direction causes large R waves in II, III, and aVF (**Fig. 4-17**). Small r waves with deep S waves are present in I and aVL. There may or may not be a prolongation of the QRS.

QUICK TIP! Bundle branch blocks may be on the CCRN exam. It is possible that at least two questions addressing this area might be included. It is helpful to have a basic understanding of this topic.

4.4 LEFT AND RIGHT VENTRICULAR HYPERTROPHY

Left ventricular hypertrophy (LVH) causes more electrical forces to be generated on the left side of the heart. This can understandably lead to left axis deviation. The leads viewing the heart on the left side (such as V_5 and V_6) will reflect the increased electrical activity by having large R waves. Leads on the right side show large S waves, the opposite of large R waves. The most common criterion for diagnosing LVH is a combination of right and left precordial chest leads that demonstrate tall R waves and deep S waves. For example, if the height of the R wave in V_5 combined with the depth of the S wave in V_1 exceeds 35 mm, the voltage criterion for LVH is present (**Fig. 4-18**).

Right ventricular hypertrophy (RVH) is better noted from right precordial leads. Leads V_3R and V_4R are better able to pick out changes in RV size through the presence of large R waves (R:S ratio >1). Figure 4-19 illustrates right precordial leads. In addition to possible right axis deviation, the best criteria for RVH include a large R wave in V_1 and V_2 and a deep S in V_5 and V_6. **Table 4-3** lists criteria for LVH and RVH.

TABLE 4-3. CRITERIA FOR LEFT AND RIGHT VENTRICULAR HYPERTROPHY

Condition	*Leads and Criteria*	
Left ventricular hypertrophy	S wave in V_1 + R wave in V_5 or V_6 >35 mm	
	$R_1 + S_3$	>26 mm
Right ventricular hypertrophy	V_3R and V_1 and V_2, R > S V_4R, R:S ratio >1:1	

KEY CONTENT CHECKLIST

- ❒ If you understand the concepts briefly presented in this chapter, you should do well on the CCRN 12-lead questions. It is more likely that questions will be oriented toward infarction and ischemia, although an occasional question on other areas may appear.
- ❒ Consider committing to memory the groups of contiguous leads that are associated with the parts of the heart, especially: Anterior/septal, lateral, and inferior
- ❒ The most important aspects of the ECG to understand have to do with identifying myocardial ischemia and injury. Your understanding of how to identify evidence of infarction or ischemia on an ECG will be tested on the CCRN exam.
- ❒ It is necessary to understand the axis of the heart in order to interpret a 12-lead ECG. However, it is unlikely that the CCRN exam will have a question regarding axis deviation.
- ❒ Bundle branch blocks may be on the CCRN exam. It is possible that at least two questions addressing this area might be included. It is helpful to have a basic understanding of this topic

Review Questions:

1. Left posterior fascicular block is seen when which conduction defect occurs?

a. Obstruction of the left main bundle branch
b. Obstruction of the right main bundle branch
c. Blockage of the posterior portion of the right bundle
d. Blockage of the posterior portion of the left bundle

Answer: D. Rationale: The left main is a coronary artery, but option A is not specific enough to address anterior or posterior blocks, so eliminate this option. Options B and C can also be eliminated because the right bundle branch only has one fascicle and the question refers to fascicular block (hemiblock), so eliminate B and C as well. The left bundle involves two fascicles and could be responsible for a hemiblock. Posterior fascicular blocks (hemiblocks) involve the posterior portion, so choose D.

2. An atrial premature beat with aberrant conduction usually has which of the following characteristics? (See Chapter 11 if need more information on aberrant conduction.)

a. Left bundle branch block
b. Left anterior fascicular block
c. Right bundle branch block
d. Left posterior fascicular block

Answer: C. Rationale: The rSR′ in V_1 is a common feature between the right bundle branch block and an atrial premature beat with aberrant conduction, making option the C the best answer. A 12-lead ECG is often needed to differentiate between the two.

3. Which of the following leads are used in the diagnosis of an inferior MI?

a. V_1, V_2, V_3, V_4
b. I, aVL
c. V_5, V_6
d. II, III, aVF

Answer: D. Rationale: V_1 to V_4 are anteroseptal leads, so eliminate option A. I and aVL are high lateral leads, so eliminate option B as well. Option C can also be ruled out because V_5 and V_6 are left lateral leads. The only inferior leads listed are II, III, and aVF—choose D. Picture where the electrodes are placed to perform a 12-lead ECG in order to provide yourself with a "mental roadmap" to locate where these affected areas may be.

5

Hemodynamic Monitoring

CHAPTER OVERVIEW AND OBJECTIVES

The purpose of this chapter is to review the concepts associated with hemodynamic monitoring, discuss the technology utilized in hemodynamic monitoring, and present methods for interpreting hemodynamic parameters. It is essential that nurses who are planning to take the CCRN exam understand the content of this chapter. There will be several questions taken directly from material covered here. Normally, the questions focus on interpreting and applying hemodynamic data in clinical scenarios. There will be few if any questions on hemodynamic technology, and no questions will be manufacturer-specific. However, to be safe, key concepts in hemodynamic monitoring, in terms of both interpretation and technology, are presented.

After reading this chapter, the reader will understand:

- Starling's law and how increasing or decreasing preload affects myocardial contractility, stroke volume, and cardiac output.
- The effect of increasing or decreasing afterload on cardiac output.
- The role of tissue oxygenation monitoring in early detection of shock and evaluating the patient's response to treatments.

5.1 MONITORING HEMODYNAMIC DATA

Hemodynamic data are produced by noninvasive, less invasive, and invasive technologies. Noninvasive monitoring of heart rate (HR), blood pressure (BP), respiratory rate (RR), and oxygen saturation (SaO_2) is ubiquitous in acute care. Critically ill patients often require additional hemodynamic data for appropriate diagnosis and treatment. Over the past two decades, the proliferation of less invasive monitoring has significantly reduced the use of invasive, flow-directed pulmonary artery (PA) catheters, which are also called Swan–Ganz catheters. These less invasive technologies include, but are not limited to, esophageal Doppler, bioreactance, pulse contour analysis, capnography, and cardiac ultrasound. Central venous line oximetry is also increasingly popular.

Cardiac Output, Stroke Volume, and Tissue Oxygenation

Depending on the technologies selected, less invasive hemodynamic monitoring may include assessment of tissue oxygenation, cardiac output (CO), stroke volume (SV), and/or stroke volume variation (SVV). Invasive hemodynamic monitoring measures the same variables except for SVV, in addition to right and left heart preload and afterload. In unstable patients, SvO_2 or $ScvO_2$ data help clinicians determine if oxygen delivery (DO_2) to the tissues is adequate relative to tissues' oxygen consumption (VO_2). However, **stroke volume** changes before other parameters, even tissue oxygenation (such as SvO_2 and lactate).

KEY CLINICAL CONCEPT

SV is the most important "macrocirculatory" parameter to optimize. SvO_2 levels (or serum lactate) are the most important "microcirculatory" (tissue oxygenation) parameters to optimize

Tissue Oxygen Delivery, Consumption, and Monitoring

The circulatory system's primary function is delivering oxygenated blood to body tissues. Disease processes that cause hypoxemia or impair tissue perfusion negatively affect tissue oxygenation. Several parameters reflect tissue oxygenation (**Table 5-1**). However, the most helpful in terms of real-time monitoring is the mixed venous oxygen saturation (SvO_2) measurement. SvO_2 values are obtained from the fiberoptic oximetry in the PA. Central venous oxygen saturation ($ScvO_2$) values are measured in the superior vena cava (SVC) via a central line with a fiberoptic oximeter. SvO_2 is a more accurate

TABLE 5-1. MEASURES OF TISSUE OXYGENATION

Parameter	Normal Level	Consider Intervention
SvO_2	60–75%	<60% or >75%
$ScvO_2$	70–80%	<70% or >85%
Sto_2	75–85%	<70% or >90%
Lactate	<2 mmol/L	>2 mmol + pH <7.25 >4 mmol indicates shock

measure of tissue oxygenation than $ScvO_2$ as it reflects the oxygen content of blood from the coronary sinus, inferior vena cava (IVC), and SVC. $ScvO_2$ only measures blood oxygen content in the SVC, which may not correlate to actual DO_2 or VO_2 in the lower body. There are two ways to measure venous oxyhemoglobin:

1. Sampled directly from the distal port of the PA catheter or right atrium. When measuring the SvO_2 in the PA, draw the sample slowly so as not to aspirate pulmonary capillary blood, which is similar to an arterial blood gas (ABG) sample.
2. Once either device is calibrated, fiberoptics produce continuous SvO_2 or $ScvO_2$ data displayed on a monitor (**Fig. 5-1**). This allows for earlier correction of hemodynamic variables contributing to alterations in DO_2 and VO_2. Another benefit is avoiding the excessive blood draws needed for intermittent SVO_2 or $ScvO_2$ monitoring.

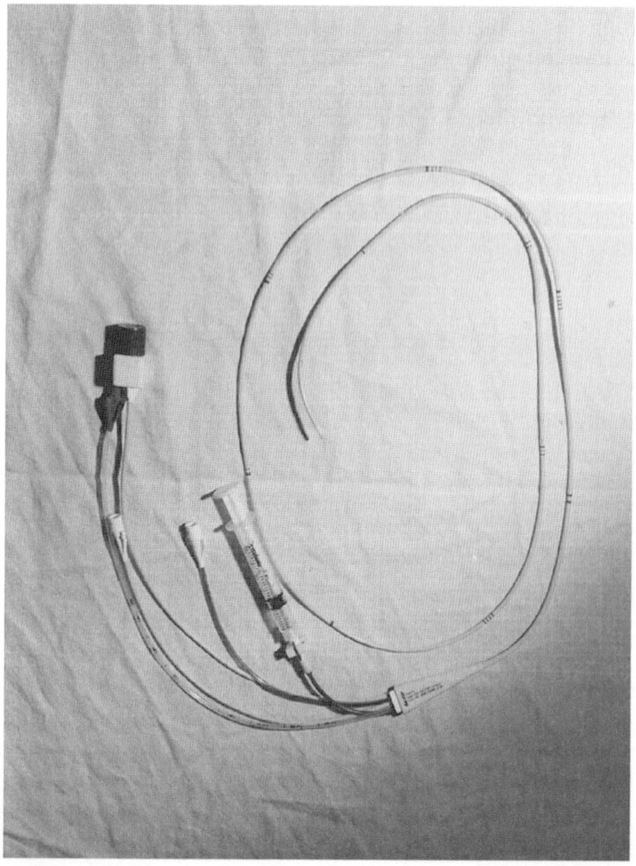

Figure 5-1. Flow-directed pulmonary artery catheter and triple-lumen oximeter.

Tissue oxygenation monitoring (SvO_2) reveals the **amount of oxygenated blood returning from the venous system into the right heart traveling to the PA. SvO_2 reflects a patient's global oxygen supply and demand.** Oxygen bound to hemoglobin molecules is referred to as oxyhemoglobin. **Under normal physiologic conditions, 25% of oxygen is removed from hemoglobin as it passes through capillary beds. This means 75% of the blood returning to the PA should be oxygenated. In theory, a normal SvO_2 is 75%.**

Delivering more oxygen (DO_2) than the tissues need may create an oxygen reserve for use during times of physiologic stress. If the tissues are deprived of oxygen, either by too little delivery of oxygen (oxygen delivery, DO_2), **physiologic decreases (hypotension, hypoxia, anemia), or if there is an increase in tissue demand (fever, pain, anxiety, increased work of breathing), higher than normal amounts of oxygen are released from hemoglobin (oxyhemoglobin dissociation) to improve tissue oxygen concentrations.** This is referred to as a right shift of the *oxyhemoglobin dissociation curve.* When tissues extract more oxygen, less oxygenated blood (oxyhemoglobin) returns to the PA, leading to lower SvO_2 levels. **An SvO_2 less than 60% signals either impaired DO_2 or increased VO_2, and requires investigation**. Without intervention, inadequate DO_2 leads to anaerobic metabolism and subsequent metabolic acidosis.

In clinical situations such as hypothermia, tissues are unable to utilize the delivered oxygen due to increased binding of O_2 to hemoglobin, which increases the amount of oxygenated blood returned to the PA. This is referred to as a **left shift of the oxyhemoglobin dissociation curve.** As a result, SvO_2 increases. *SvO_2 values more than 75% are abnormal and require investigating the underlying cause(s). Other increases in oxygen supply or decreases in demand cause elevated values, such as anesthesia, neuromuscular blockade, or 100% Fio_2 delivery.*

Determining the potential causes of clinically significant hemodynamic changes is often a daunting task. Fortunately, SvO_2 monitoring facilitates this.

KEY CLINICAL CONCEPT

- Under normal physiologic conditions, 25% of oxygen is removed from hemoglobin as it passes through capillary beds. This means 75% of the blood returning to the PA should be oxygenated. In theory, a normal SvO_2 is 75%.
- SvO_2 values less than 60% signal either impaired DO_2 or increased VO_2, and require investigation. Without intervention, inadequate DO_2 leads to anaerobic metabolism and subsequent metabolic acidosis.
- SvO_2 values more than 75% are abnormal and require an investigation of the underlying cause(s).
- Expect at least 1 or 2 questions regarding the oxyhemoglobin dissociation curve on the test

Thenar Tissue Oxygen Saturation Monitoring

Thenar skeletal muscle oxygen saturation (StO_2) monitoring is a noninvasive method estimating regional oxygen supply and demand. The sensor placed on the thenar aspect of the thumb detects oxyhemoglobin in the microcirculation via near-infrared spectroscopy. The theory behind this technology is that decreasing DO_2 shifts blood flow to vital organs and away from skeletal muscle, causing the skeletal muscle to extract more oxygen from the blood to prevent local tissue hypoxia. **StO_2 (%) = Oxyhemoglobin/Total Hemoglobin × 100.** Normal StO_2 levels are more than 75%. Values less than 75% are associated with increased oxygen extraction. There are numerous studies in the literature regarding the utility of StO_2 monitoring. The data are heterogeneous with some studies showing types of patients (eg, trauma) with higher StO_2 levels having better outcomes, while others found no evidence for routine StO_2 monitoring in cardiac surgery or septic shock.

Lactate Values

Lactate (also referred to as lactic acid) levels are used as a laboratory biomarker of tissue oxygenation. **Normal levels are less than 2 mmol/L. If a lactate level is more than 2.0, the patient may be developing** *anaerobic metabolism.* If lactate levels are increasing, an ABG or venous blood gas (VBG) may reveal metabolic acidosis (pH < 7.40, $HCO_3^- < 22$). Since lactate levels can increase without producing hypoxia if metabolic acidosis is not present, it is important to monitor both lactate and parameters such as bicarbonate, pH, and base excess. For example, a patient with a lactate level of 4.4 mmol/L, a pH of 7.30, and a bicarbonate (HCO_3^-) level of 18 (which is low), would be suspected to have Type A metabolic acidosis (hypoperfusion) and tissue hypoxia.

Lactate levels are used as an indicator of shock and marker of shock resuscitation. Lactate levels do not change as rapidly as SvO_2 or $ScvO_2$ levels, making drug titration a little more difficult if lactate levels are used. Normally, lactate levels are drawn (either arterial or venous samples) every 2 to 4 hours until they return to normal. Trending SvO_2 or $ScvO_2$ allows more frequent assessment of the patient's response to treatment, with confirmation of a positive response as lactate levels normalize.

KEY CLINICAL CONCEPT

- Lactate levels more than 2 mmol/L indicate impaired tissue oxygenation and may require intervention. Lactates should be assessed every 2 to 4 hours until they are less than 2 mmol/L.
- Trending SvO_2 or $ScvO_2$ allows more frequent assessment of the response to treatment, with lactate levels confirming the improvement.

Cardiac Output and Cardiac Index

Normal hemodynamic parameters are given in **Table 5-2.** *Normal CO is usually in the range of 4 to 8 L/min.* The cardiac index (CI), an adjustment of CO based on the body surface area (BSA) (size of the person), is more accurate than CO. **A normal cardiac index (CI) is 2.5 to 4 L/min/m². Levels below 2.2 L/min/m² indicate threats to tissue oxygenation and may require intervention.**

Generally, the CI is a better parameter to use than the CO. Some patients tolerate a low CI without clinical problems. *It is more useful to track trends* in the CI than to monitor single data points, since temporary changes in values may not be clinically significant. Monitoring both CI and tissue oxygenation (SvO_2) increase the early identification of hemodynamic alterations.

CO is determined by two factors: HR and stroke volume. It is essential to understand how abnormal HRs and low stroke volume affect CO. Abnormal CO is most commonly related to a problem with stroke volume.

TABLE 5-2. NORMAL HEMODYNAMIC PARAMETERS

Parameter	*Normal Level*	*Consider Intervention*
Stroke volume	50–100 mL/beat	<50 mL
Stroke volume index	25–45 mL/m²	<25 mL
Cardiac output	4–8 L/min	<4 L/min
Cardiac index	2.5–4 L/min/m²	<2.2 L/min/m²
Cardiac power index	0.5–0.7 W/m²	<0.4 W/m²
Ejection fraction	>50%	<40%
Wedge pressure (PCWP or PAOP)	8–12 mm Hg	<8 (hypovolemia)[a] >12 (hypervolemia) >15 (LV dysfunction)[a]
Central venous pressure	2–6 mm Hg	<2 (hypovolemia)[a] >10 (hypervolemia, RV dysfunction)
Pulmonary artery systolic pressure	15–35 mm Hg	>35 mm Hg
Pulmonary artery diastolic pressure	8–15 mm Hg	<8 or >15 mm Hg
Pulmonary mean arterial pressure	10–20 mm Hg	>20 mm Hg at rest
Right ventricular end-diastolic volume	100–160	<100 mL (hypovolemia)

[a]If stroke volume is also low.
PAOP, pulmonary artery occlusive pressure; PCWP, pulmonary capillary wedge pressure.

KEY CLINICAL CONCEPT

Hemodynamic values that are "indexed" are more accurate than standard values since they take into account a patient's body surface area (BSA).

Esophageal and Surface Doppler Cardiac Output Monitoring

Esophageal and surface Doppler, give indications of cardiac strength though **peak velocity (PV) measurements (normal 50–120 cm/s).** These technologies also give indications of volume status through **flow time (FTc), with normal levels of 330 to 360 mm/s.** If a patient has a low PV, then LV contractility is weakened. If the flow time is low, then hypovolemia is suspected. Although esophageal Doppler monitoring (EDM) is available for ICU use, it is best likely suited for use in the OR as patients must be intubated and sedated during EDM, and the ultrasound probes dislodge easily.

Stroke Volume, Stroke Volume Index, and Ejection Fraction

Stroke volume (SV) and stroke volume index (SVI) are dynamic indicators of preload responsiveness. A large meta-analysis demonstrated reduced mortality when using dynamic measures of preload responsiveness such as stroke volume (SV) or stroke volume (index), compared to static preload measurements such as CVP, when administering goal-directed fluid resuscitation.

SV is the amount of blood ejected with each heartbeat. Normal **SV is 60 to 100 mL per beat.** The SVI, like CI, is a more useful measure that individualizes the stroke volume based on the patient's BSA. **Normal SVI is 33 to 47 mL/m²/beat.**

Multiple cardiac abnormalities such as ischemia, valvular disease, and myocarditis are associated with lower SV/SVI. The LV ejection fraction (EF) is defined as the amount of blood pumped per beat (SV) in relation to the amount of blood available to be pumped (end-diastolic volume).

$$\mathbf{EF = (SV/EDV) \times 100}$$

For example, assume the LV end-diastolic volume (LVEDV), (the amount of blood remaining in the LV just before systolic contraction), is 100 mL and the stroke volume is 65 mL. Since 65 mL of the possible 100 mL in the ventricle is ejected, the ejection fraction is 65%. A normal EF is 50% to 75%. A "borderline" EF is 41% to 49%. An EF less than 40% represents cardiomyopathy or heart failure.

In any condition in which the heart begins to malfunction, the stroke volume/index will decline; however, in certain circumstances, such as LV failure and sepsis, the stroke volume may not initially decline because of the heart's compensatory mechanisms. If a patient with coronary artery disease begins to have LV dysfunction, the left ventricle will dilate, causing the LVEDV to increase. Although the increase in LVEDV might prevent a drop in stroke volume, dysfunction can still be detected by observing a drop in the ejection fraction. For example, a patient with severe coronary artery disease may develop ischemic cardiomyopathy. The LV is mildly dilated. Although the heart muscle begins to weaken, the increase in LVEDV allows the SV to stay within the normal range:

LVEDV	125 mL
Stroke volume	65 mL
Ejection fraction	42% = (65/125) × 100/125

Regulation of Cardiac Output

Three factors regulate CO: preload, afterload, and contractility. Definitions of preload, afterload, and contractility are presented in **Table 5-3**. Preload is affected by myocardial muscle stretching as a result of the amount of blood in the ventricle, as well as the ventricle's ability to relax (lusitropy).

According to **Starling's law**, the more the heart muscle (myocardium) stretches, the more forceful its contraction, unless it stretches beyond the point of maximal contractility. If the myocardium stretches too much, its contraction weakens. The amount of ventricular stretch depends on **preload**, which is the amount of blood volume in the ventricle at the end of diastole. In standard PA catheters, RV preload is measured by evaluating RA pressure (RAP), commonly referred to as central venous pressure (CVP) since the SVC and IVC deliver blood into the RA. CVP reflects RV filling pressures and function. **Normal CVP is 2 to 6 mm Hg.** Some PA catheter models are capable of measuring right ventricular end-diastolic volume (RVEDV) which may more precisely evaluate RV preload than CVP. Normal RVEDV is 100 to 160 mL. The PA catheter's location in the RA, RV, and PA, allows accurate evaluation of right heart function, but only allows *estimation* of left heart function.

PAOP or PAD pressures are used to evaluate left heart filling pressures. By occluding the PA, the PAOP estimates left atrial pressure (LAP). As with the right heart, the LAP is used as a surrogate for LV preload. **The normal PAOP range is 8 to 12 mm Hg.** *A PAOP less than 8 mm Hg may indicate hypovolemia. An elevated PAOP (>15 mm Hg) along with elevated CVP (>8 mm Hg) may*

TABLE 5-3. DETERMINANTS OF STROKE VOLUME

Preload	Amount of stretch in a muscle just before contraction	CVP estimates RV preload. PAOP estimates LV preload. Also estimated by SV, SVI, FTc, and SVV.
Afterload	Resistance a muscle faces as it attempts to contract	PVR/PVRI represents resistance to RV blood ejection. SVR/SVRI represents resistance to LV blood ejection.
Contractility	Strength of the muscle contraction	Estimated by SV and PAOP or CVP. If the stroke volume is low and the PAOP or CVP is high, then the heart is assumed to be weakened Can also be estimated by ejection fraction and peak velocity

CVP, central venous pressure; FTc, flow time; PAOP, pulmonary artery occlusive pressure; PVR, pulmonary vascular resistance; SV, stroke volume; SVR, systemic vascular resistance; SVV, stroke volume variation.

indicate fluid volume overload or biventricular failure (the point where the muscle is stretching excessively). Cardiogenic shock is associated with PAOP more than 15 mm Hg. Pulmonary edema occurs when PAOP is more than 18 mm Hg. Conversely, when the ventricular filling pressure is too low (< 8 mm Hg), it is assumed that the blood volume is low (hypovolemia).

QUICK TIP! If a hemodynamic value is particularly relevant to an exam question, the value in the scenario will typically be very low, normal, or very high to facilitate interpretation "Borderline" values and hemodynamic values are rarely on the test.

It is important to understand that volumes such as RVEDV are more precise estimates of preload than pressures since a variety of factors such as chamber size and intrathoracic pressures can produce higher pressures, even if the amount of volume in the ventricle is unchanged. *Compare changes in filling pressures with SV/SVI to obtain a more accurate hemodynamic picture and to avoid misinterpreting filling pressures.* If the filling pressures elevate, they should decrease the stroke index if they are clinically significant. In cases of hypovolemia, the filling pressures and SV/SVI will be low. **In other words, filling pressures are guides for how to best optimize the SV/SVI. An SV increase *more than or equal to* 10% after a fluid challenge demonstrates fluid responsiveness, even if the BP does not change.**

KEY CLINICAL CONCEPTS

- It is essential to assess SV/SVI along with the filling pressures, as assessment of filling pressures alone can be misleading.
- A SV increase more than and equal to 10% after a fluid challenge demonstrates fluid responsiveness, even if the BP does not change.

Stroke Volume Variation

Controlled mechanical ventilator modes, such as assist control, continuous mandatory ventilation, and pressure-regulated volume control, deliver consistent tidal volumes, regardless of whether the patient initiates the breath or if the ventilator generates the preset tidal volume. In patients on controlled modes, who are not breathing above the set RR, fluctuations in SV, called stroke volume variation (SVV) may reflect intravascular volume status. SVV is unreliable in spontaneously breathing patients, including those on pressure support ventilation (PSV) or synchronized intermittent mandatory ventilator modes (SIMV) due to insufficient intrathoracic pressures to detect fluid-responsive states. A recent study demonstrated that SVV is less reliable in patients receiving tidal volumes of 6 mL/kg of predicted body weight (PBW) compared to those receiving tidal volumes of 8 mL/kg of PBW. In patients who meet these criteria, SVV may be used to guide fluid administration. **Normal SVV is 10% to 15%.** SVV more than 15% is associated with hypovolemia. In those with elevated SVV, fluid resuscitation is given until a SVV less than 13% is achieved.

Heart Rate

The heart rate (HR) must be evaluated to detect early changes in hemodynamics. *Since CO is a product of stroke volume multiplied by HR*, any change in SV will normally produce a change in the HR. If the SV is high, the HR may decrease (as seen in adaptation to exercise). The exception to this guideline is during an increase in metabolic rate, in which both the stroke volume and the HR increase.

If the SV falls, HR normally increases to maintain CO. Sinus tachycardia should prompt assessment of CO and SV. *Generally, bradycardia and tachycardia are significant because they may reflect a potentially dangerous shift in CO. Bradycardia that develops suddenly almost always impairs CO.* Tachycardia, a more common clinical situation, may also indicate a threat to CO.

Common causes of sinus tachycardia:

1. Increase in metabolic rate (fever, hyperthyroidism, exercise)
2. Sympathetic nervous system activation (anxiety, fear, pain, substance withdrawal, shock, drugs that mimic the SNS response such as dopamine)
3. Hypoxia (pulmonary embolus, pulmonary edema, pneumonia)
4. Decreased SV
   a. Reduced myocardial contractility (MI, heart failure, cardiogenic shock, myocarditis)
   b. Low preload (hypovolemia, hemorrhage, and drugs or disease states that decrease venous return to the heart such as sepsis)

Sinus tachycardia requires an investigation of the cause. It may be easily identified as a result of anxiety or pain, but it is important to consider other causative factors. Anxiety may be an early sign of mental status change. Pain may occur from ischemia. Assessing the patient for changes such as tachypnea, hypotension, hypoxia, diminished urine output, and physical exam findings (eg, dry oral mucus membranes or poor skin turgor) will help determine if the sinus tachycardia is the result of a pathologic process (eg, anemia, hypovolemia, MI, sepsis) requiring immediate intervention. All factors need to be considered in evaluating a rapid HR. For example, a clinician must rule out other factors before assuming that the HR is increased due to a reduced stroke volume.

KEY CLINICAL CONCEPT

Sinus tachycardia may signal the presence of an underlying disease process such as sepsis. It is important to relate the increased HR to other vital signs and physical exam findings to identify possible causes.

A number of pathologies can cause sinus tachycardia If the HR is increased and a raised metabolic rate or a psychological factor does not appear to be the cause, then a **lower stroke volume is suspected and an investigation into its cause is necessary.** *The two most common reasons for a low SV are* (1) *hypovolemia and* (2) *LV dysfunction*. Both of these increase HR, provided the patient is able to increase HR to compensate for low SV or increased metabolic oxygen demand. Patients who may not develop tachycardia include those on medications which slow HR such as metoprolol (Lopressor) or diltiazem (Cardizem), those with heart block, autonomic nervous system dysfunction (eg, due to drugs), or neurogenic shock. Without intervention, HR will continue to increase.

An increased HR can compensate for a decrease in stroke volume, although this compensation is limited. *As the HR increases, there is less time for ventricular filling.* Because an increased HR reduces diastolic filling time, this can lead to reduced SV. There is no specific HR at which diastolic filling is reduced so severely that stroke volume decreases. However, it should be remembered that as the HR increases, stroke volumes can be negatively affected.

Another important concept regarding HR is the effect it has on myocardial oxygen consumption (MVO_2). The higher the HR, the more oxygen the heart demands. Typically, the MVO_2 can only be estimated, due to the difficulty of direct measurements. Increased contractility and vascular resistance also affect MVO_2. Keeping HR and MVO_2 as low as possible, particularly in patients with myocardial ischemia, protects myocardial function.

Hemodynamic Pressures

The most common invasive hemodynamic pressures are central venous pressure (CVP), pulmonary artery systolic pressure (PAS), pulmonary artery diastolic pressure (PAD), and pulmonary artery occlusive pressure (PAOP). PAOP is also referred to as pulmonary capillary wedge pressure (PCWP) and is sometimes monitored in critically ill patients. The advent of newer, less invasive technologies are increasing and replacing the use of intracardiac pressures.

Interpreting Arterial Pressures

Both noninvasive (cuff) and arterial blood pressures (ABP) are frequently used to assess the adequacy of blood flow to the tissues. Although the BP is often misleading, it is still one of the most commonly used parameters in hemodynamic monitoring. Whereas the role of BP in patient assessment needs serious review based on its inaccuracy, the measurement of BP is still a standard of care. BP is determined by two factors: CO and systemic vascular resistance (SVR).

This relationship can be illustrated by the formula:

Blood Pressure = Cardiac Output × Systemic Vascular Resistance

The sympathetic nervous system (SNS) and renin-angiotensin-aldosterone system (RAAS) activation compensates for hypovolemia and vasodilation. These compensatory mechanisms affect both CO and SVR, maintaining BP for some time after a pathophysiologic change. This relationship is illustrated as **CO = HR × SV.** This fact is critical to the interpretation of BP. BP will not reflect early clinical changes in hemodynamics because of a compensatory mechanism by which CO and SVR interact to maintain adequate BP. CO is maintained by HR and SV. If SV decreases, HR increases to maintain the CO near normal levels. Although this interaction is not always predictable, it works as follows: If CO decreases, the SVR increases just enough to overcome the fall in CO and maintain BP at near-normal levels (**Table 5-4**). Conversely, if SVR falls, CO rises to maintain BP. As a result, **hypotension is a later sign of shock as a result of failing CO and/or SVR.**

The key point to these interactions is that the BP cannot signal early clinical changes. If a patient begins to bleed postoperatively, the BP will generally not reflect this event until it becomes so severe that an increase in the HR and SVR no longer compensates. This is also the case for patients who have heart failure or myocardial infarction.

TABLE 5-4. REGULATION OF BLOOD PRESSURE

Cardiac Output	*Systemic Vascular Resistance*	*Effects on Blood Pressure*
Normal	Normal	Normal
Decreased	Increased	Remains near normal
Increased	Decreased	Remains near normal
Increased	Increased	Rapidly elevates
Decreased	Decreased	Rapidly falls

Normotension is present when the systolic pressure (SBP) is 90 to 130 mm Hg, the diastolic pressure (DBP) is 60 to 80 mm Hg, and mean arterial pressure (MAP) is 65 to 105 mm Hg. A lower BP is considered normal for the patient if there are no signs of hypoperfusion. Hypoperfusion and/or tissue hypoxia are likely present if the SvO_2 or $ScvO_2$ are low, along with clinical signs such as mental status change, tachypnea, and/or urine output less than 30 mL/kg/h. It is important to consider tissue oxygenation data in the context of BP. **Stage I HTN is defined as an SBP more than 130 mm Hg or DBP more than 80 mm Hg. Stage II HTN is present if SBP** is **more than 140 mm Hg or SBP** is **more than 90 mm Hg.** It is also important to consider a patient's usual BP. For example, a patient with HTN and an SBP that ranges from 160 to 170 mm Hg can have significant hypoperfusion. For example, tissue hypoxia can result even though such BPs are within a "normal" range. In patients with HTN, SBPs more than 40 mm Hg below baseline may reflect hypoperfusion.

KEY CLINICAL CONCEPT

- Do not assume that a BP within a normal range represents adequate tissue perfusion. This is especially important in patients with HTN, since their BP may appear "normal" when it is actually much lower than their baseline. In patients with HTN, SBPs more than 40 mm Hg below their baseline may reflect hypoperfusion.
- If tissue hypoxia is suspected when a BP is "normal," consider checking SvO_2 or a lactate level to verify.

Interpreting Pulmonary Artery Pressures

PA and intracardiac pressures are typically obtained from a flow-directed catheter inserted into a major vein and directed into the right atrium, through the right ventricle (RV) and into the PA (**Figs. 5-2** and **5-3**). Since the pulmonary vasculature is normally a low-resistance system, the PA pressures are significantly lower than systemic pressures.

Normal Pulmonary Artery Pressure Ranges:

- **Pulmonary Artery Systolic Pressure (PASP): 15 to 35 mm Hg**
- **Pulmonary Artery Diastolic Pressure (PADP): 8 to 15 mm Hg**
- **Pulmonary Mean Arterial Pressure (PMAP): 10 to 20 mm Hg**

If the pressure in the pulmonary vasculature rises, the capillary hydrostatic pressure exceeds capillary osmotic pressure and fluid is forced out of the vessels. Interstitial and alveolar flooding can occur, impairing oxygen and carbon dioxide exchange, such as in pulmonary edema (or other example here).

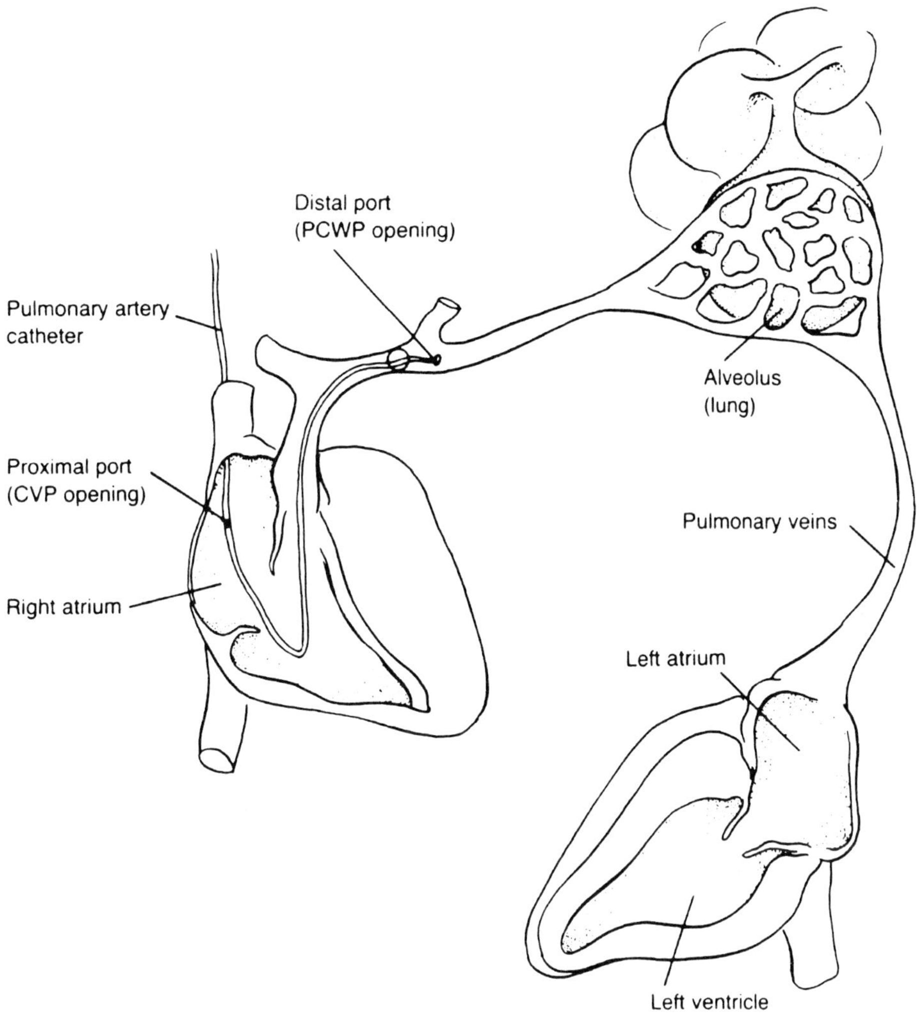

Figure 5-2. Pulmonary artery catheter in place within the pulmonary artery. (Reproduced with permission from Ahrens TS. *Hemodynamic Waveform Recognition*. Philadelphia: Saunders, 1993.)

The PA pressures can be helpful in diagnosing many clinical conditions. For example, **mean pressure more than 25 mm Hg at rest is considered pulmonary hypertension (PH).**

Interpreting Central Venous Pressure

As previously mentioned, **CVP measures right atrial pressure (RAP). CVP is a surrogate for RVEDP** (RV preload) (**Fig. 5-4**). **LAP is referred to as the PCWP or PAOP.**

The guidelines for interpreting the CVP have traditionally been relatively simple. **Normal CVP is 2 to 6 mm Hg. CVP goals may vary depending on disease state and the presence of positive pressure ventilation**. For example, in mechanically ventilated patients with high intrathoracic pressures, a CVP of 12 mm Hg may be needed to maintain adequate preload. **Generally speaking, low CVPs indicate hypovolemia or decreased venous blood return to the right heart (venodilatation). A high CVP can occur in hypervolemia, RV dysfunction, or pulmonary hypertension.**

When evaluating hemodynamics, it is important to trend the data and compare different values to get a complete picture of the patient's physiology. Left ventricular stroke volume (SV) or SVI evaluate how the LV is responding to preload. Measuring baseline SV/SVI and observing how it changes with IV fluid challenges is a more accurate assessment of preload responsiveness than assessing changes in CVP.

- Hypovolemia is typically present if both the CVP and the SV/SVI index are low.
- A low CVP in the presence of a normal SV/SVI, maybe the result of right atrial dilation, which makes the CVP appear low. Therefore, hypovolemia may not be present. A high CVP with a normal SV/SVI can indicate increased intravascular volume or RV dysfunction.
- A high CVP and a low SV/SVI usually indicates RV failure. Perhaps the most difficult part of interpreting pressures is that normal pressures do not indicate normal cardiac functioning.

Interpreting the Pulmonary Capillary Wedge Pressure

LV preload data are commonly obtained by pulmonary artery occlusion pressure (PAOP), which is also referred to as the pulmonary capillary wedge pressure (PCWP) or wedge pressure. The use of the PAOP to estimate LVEDP is based on the assumption that a measurement from an obstructed pulmonary capillary will reflect an uninterrupted flow of blood to the left atrium and LAP, since there are no valves in the pulmonary arterial system. A second

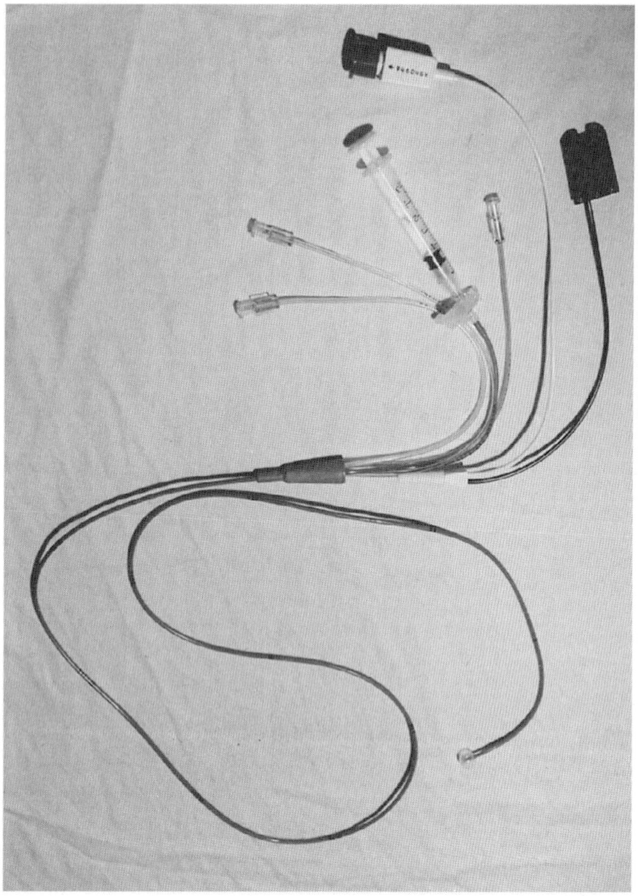

Figure 5-3. Fiberoptic pulmonary artery catheter and triple-lumen oximeter.

assumption is that when the mitral valve is open, LAP reflects LVEDP. As long as these assumptions are accurate, it is acceptable to use the PAOP to estimate LVEDP. The rules for interpreting the PAOP are relatively simple and similar to those of CVP interpretation. **Normal PAOP is 8 to 12 mm Hg.** *If the PAOP is low, hypovolemia is likely. If the PAOP is normal, normovolemia is present. If the PAOP is high, LV dysfunction or fluid volume overload is present.* However, PAOP interpretation has the same limitations as CVP interpretation, plus a few more. As with the CVP, the PAOP should not be interpreted in isolation. In analyzing the PAOP, always use the SV or SVI to put the PAOP in context. If the PAOP and the SV/SVI are low, hypovolemia is probable. If the PAOP is low and the SV/SVI is normal, hypovolemia is unlikely. The low PAOP may result from LV dilatation. If the PAOP is high and the SV/SVI is low, LV dysfunction or failure is likely. However, if the PAOP is high and the SV/SVI is normal, LV dysfunction may not be present (or clinically significant).

Effects of Elevated Pulmonary Artery Occlusion and Left Ventricular End-Diastolic Pressures

- LVEDP 15: Pulmonary hypertension (PH), RV dysfunction, and peripheral edema can occur.
- *LVEDP 18: Pulmonary interstitial edema occurs.*
- *LVEDP 25: Pulmonary alveolar edema occurs.*

Derived Parameters

Several hemodynamic measurements are derived or calculated from other variables. These calculated parameters have more clinical value in some patients than others. Their utility depends on the patient's diagnosis and comorbidities. Some common derived hemodynamic parameters are listed in **Table 5-5**. Even though most bedside monitors will perform the calculations automatically, it is essential for the critical care nurse to know the variables in the calculations to better understand how hemodynamic values interact and to interpret the data.

Systemic and Pulmonary Vascular Resistance

One of the most common derived parameters is vascular resistance. *Vascular resistance is frequently assumed to represent afterload, or the resistance the ventricles face during the ejection of blood.* It is important to keep in mind that afterload is not measured by vascular resistance alone. Afterload is also influenced

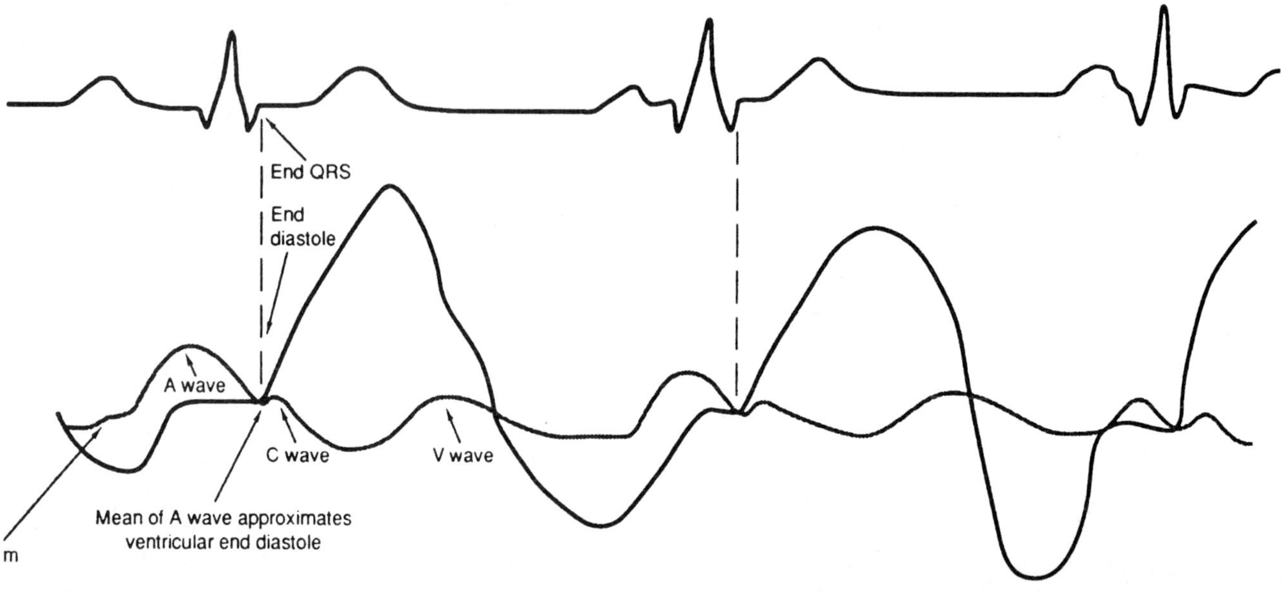

Figure 5-4. Correlation of ventricular end-diastole pressure with atrial pressure. (Reproduced with permission from Ahrens TS. *Hemodynamic Waveform Recognition*. Philadelphia: Saunders, 1993.)

TABLE 5-5. NORMAL DERIVED HEMODYNAMIC PARAMETERS

Parameter	*Normal Level*	*Consider Intervention*
Mean arterial pressure (MAP)	70–110 mm Hg	<65 mm Hg
Mean pulmonary arterial pressure (MPAP)	15–25 mm Hg	>25 mm Hg
Systemic vascular resistance (SVR)	900–1300 dynes/s/cm^5	<800 dynes/s/cm^5 >1500 dynes/s/cm^5
Pulmonary vascular resistance (PVR)[a]	40–150 dynes/s/cm^5	>200 dynes/s/cm^5

[a]where MAP = [(2 × DBP) + SBP]/3; MPAP = [(2 × DPAP) + SPAP]/3; SVR = [MAP – CVP × 80]/CO; PVR = [MPAP – PAOP × 80]/CO.
CO, cardiac output; DBP/SBP, diastolic/systolic blood pressure; DPAP/SPAP, diastolic/systolic pulmonary artery pressure.

by blood viscosity and valvular resistance. While these values can change, vascular resistance can be used to estimate afterload since viscosity and valvular resistance tend to change less often than blood vessel resistance. **Two types of vascular resistance are commonly measured, systemic and pulmonary.**

Systemic vascular resistance (SVR) represents LV afterload. Normal SVR is 800 to 1200 dynes-sec/cm^{-5}. In clinical practice, this formula is:

$$\text{SVR} = \frac{\text{Mean Arterial Pressure} - \text{Right Atrial Pressure}}{\text{Cardiac Output}}$$

As with other hemodynamic parameters, **the index derived from a patient's BSA is more accurate than the unindexed parameter. The normal systemic vascular resistance index (SVRI) is 1970 to 2390 dynes-sec/cm^{-5}/m^2.**

$$\text{SVRI} = \frac{80 \times (\text{Mean Arterial Pressure} - \text{Right Atrial Pressure})}{\text{Cardiac Index}}$$

SVR/SVRI increases due to myriad issues including, pain, agitation, hypertension, hypovolemia, hemorrhage, low cardiac output, and cardiogenic shock. *The higher the SVR/SVRI, the more resistance the LV faces during systole. High SVR/SVRI can decrease LV SV/SVI and subsequently CO/CI.* Hypertension directly increases SVR/SVRI. Vasoconstriction raises SVR/SVI to compensate for a low CO/CI. *It is important for the clinician to determine why the SVR is elevated.* Since SVR/SVRI increase to maintain BP to compensate for low CO/SI, it is essential to evaluate preload and preload responsiveness and intervene before adding afterload reducing agents. If CO/CI are adequate and the patient is hypertensive, afterload-reducing (vasodilator) agents, such as nicardipine (Cardene), are indicated.

SVR/SVRI decreases when a disease state, such as sepsis, or vasodilator medications are administered. The SVR/SVRI can also be reduced in hepatic disease (because of increased collateral circulation) or neurogenic-induced central vasodilation. If the SVR/SVRI is low, the LV encounters less resistance to the ejection of blood. CO/CI usually increases as a result. If the SVR/SVRI is reduced, vasodilatation is present. In hypotensive patients, vasopressors are indicated to raise SVR/SVRI. In addition to adding vasoconstrictors to increase BP and SVR/SVRI, **address treatment of the underlying disease process is paramount. Failure to treat the causative condition will result in patient deterioration. Utilizing only vasopressors without treating the underlying cause will provide only short-term success.**

PVR reflects the resistance the RV faces as it contracts and ejects blood into the PA. The PVR is normally less than 250 dynes/s/cm^5. **Normal pulmonary vascular resistance index (PVRI) is 255 to 285 dynes-second/cm^{-5}/m^2.** PVR/PVRI increases from hypoxia, lung disease, left-sided heart disease (left HF, mitral regurgitation or stenosis, aortic regurgitation or stenosis), acute or chronic pulmonary emboli, and RV failure. (See Chapter 17 for more detailed discussion on PVR elevation.) Patients with acutely high PVR/PVRI may benefit from the beta-1 and beta-2 dobutamine or the phosphodiesterase type III inhibitor milrinone. Both dobutamine and milrinone work to improve contractility and decrease PVR/PVRI through vasodilatation. For patients with hypoxia, improving blood oxygen levels should help decrease hypoxia-induced pulmonary vasoconstriction and lower PVR/PVRI. For those with other causes of high PVR/PVRI, the pressures should improve by treating the underlying condition, for example, mitral valve repair or replacement for mitral regurgitation. Patients with pulmonary arterial hypertension (PAH) have markedly elevated PVR/PVRI. No known cure exists for this condition, although use of prostacyclins (epoprostenol, iloprost), endothelin receptor antagonists (bosentan), and vasodilators such as oral phosphodiesterase type V inhibitors (sildenafil, tadalafil) may help alleviate symptoms and prolong life. Patients with PAH may require lung transplants or combined heart/lung transplants.

KEY CLINICAL CONCEPT

- If CO/CI are low, it is important to assess preload first, and intervene for low SV/SVI.
- Deciding when a hemodynamic parameter, such as CO or BP, has changed in a clinically significant manner is one of the most important responsibilities facing the bedside clinician.
- Although this traditional interpretation of hemodynamics is somewhat simplistic, it is adequate for CCRN qualification.

5.2 INTERPRETING HEMODYNAMIC WAVEFORMS

Reading CVP and PAOP (Wedge) Waveforms

One critical point to remember when reading CVP and PAOP (or PCWP) tracings is that they are used to estimate ventricular end-diastolic pressures. Therefore, only one part of the PAOP and CVP tracing correlates with ventricular end-diastolic pressure. That part occurs just before closure of the mitral and tricuspid valves prior to ventricular systole. To identify this point, the electrocardiogram (ECG) is used as the reference point. Since the mitral and tricuspid valves close just

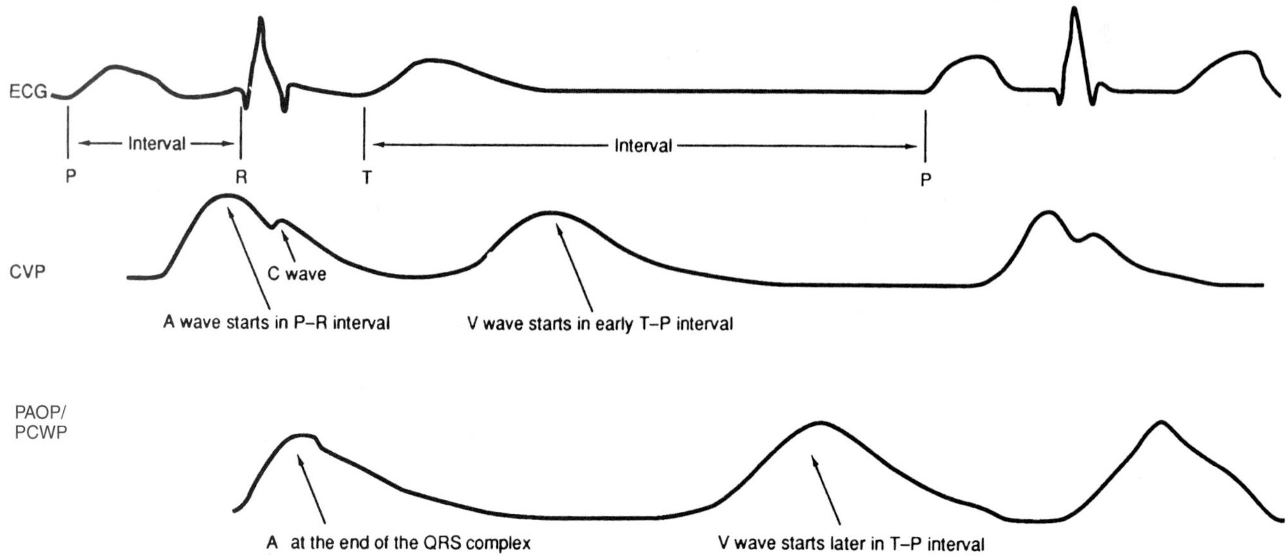

Figure 5-5. Reading CVP and PAOP waveforms. (Reproduced with permission from Ahrens TS. *Hemodynamic Waveform Recognition*. Philadelphia: Saunders, 1993.)

before ventricular contraction, the valves must still be open during the QRS complex (**Fig. 5-5**). For the CVP waveform, identify the point near the end of the QRS and draw a line straight down. The point at which this line intersects with the wave is the CVP value. For the PAOP waveform, the line is drawn about 0.08 seconds after the QRS complex (**Fig. 5-6**). This difference from the CVP reflects the time needed for the wave to travel from the left atrium back to the PA catheter.

Abnormal CVP and PAOP Waveforms

Abnormal waveforms can make reading pressure values difficult. Fortunately, abnormal waveforms are easy to avoid by using the techniques outlined above for obtaining CVP and PAOP values. *Probably the two most common abnormal waves are large A and V waves.* Large A waves occur when the atrium and ventricles contract simultaneously (as in third-degree heart block or premature ventricular contractions). Large V waves are seen in conditions such as mitral or tricuspid regurgitation and ventricular failure (Fig. 5-6).

Arterial Waveforms

An arterial waveform has three common characteristics: (1) a rapid upstroke, (2) a dicrotic notch, and (3) a progressive diastolic runoff (**Fig. 5-7**).

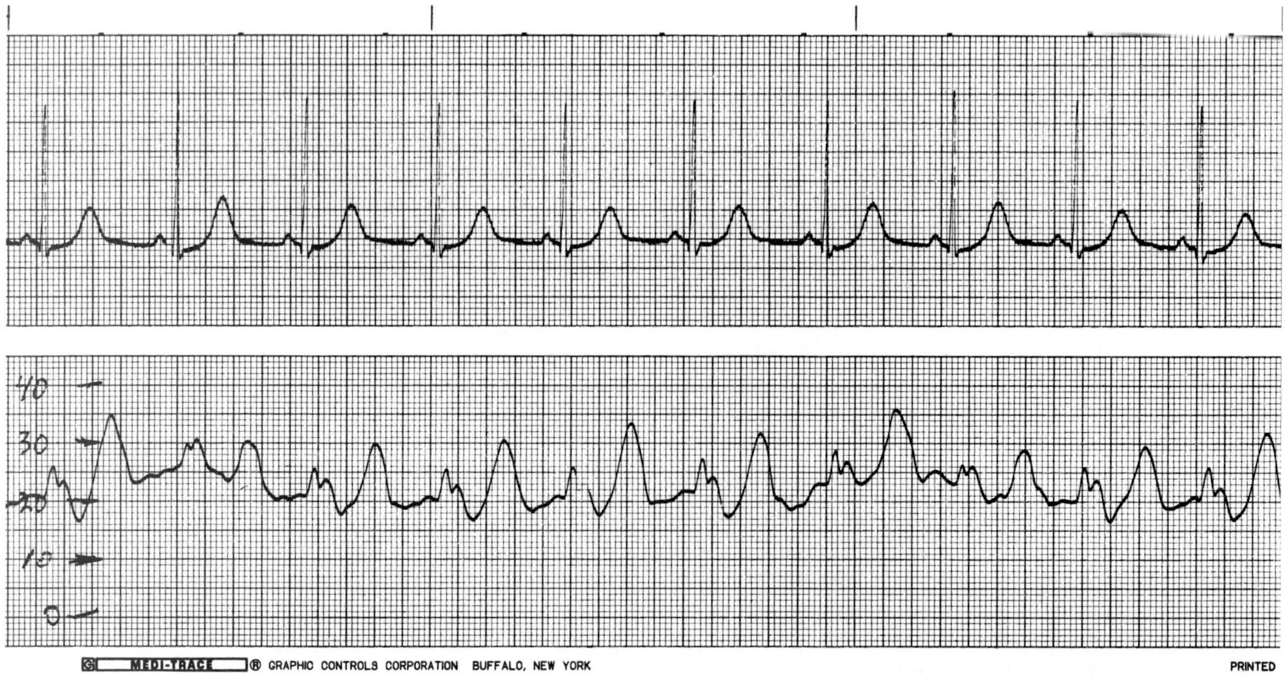

Figure 5-6. Abnormal V waves in a PAOP waveform.

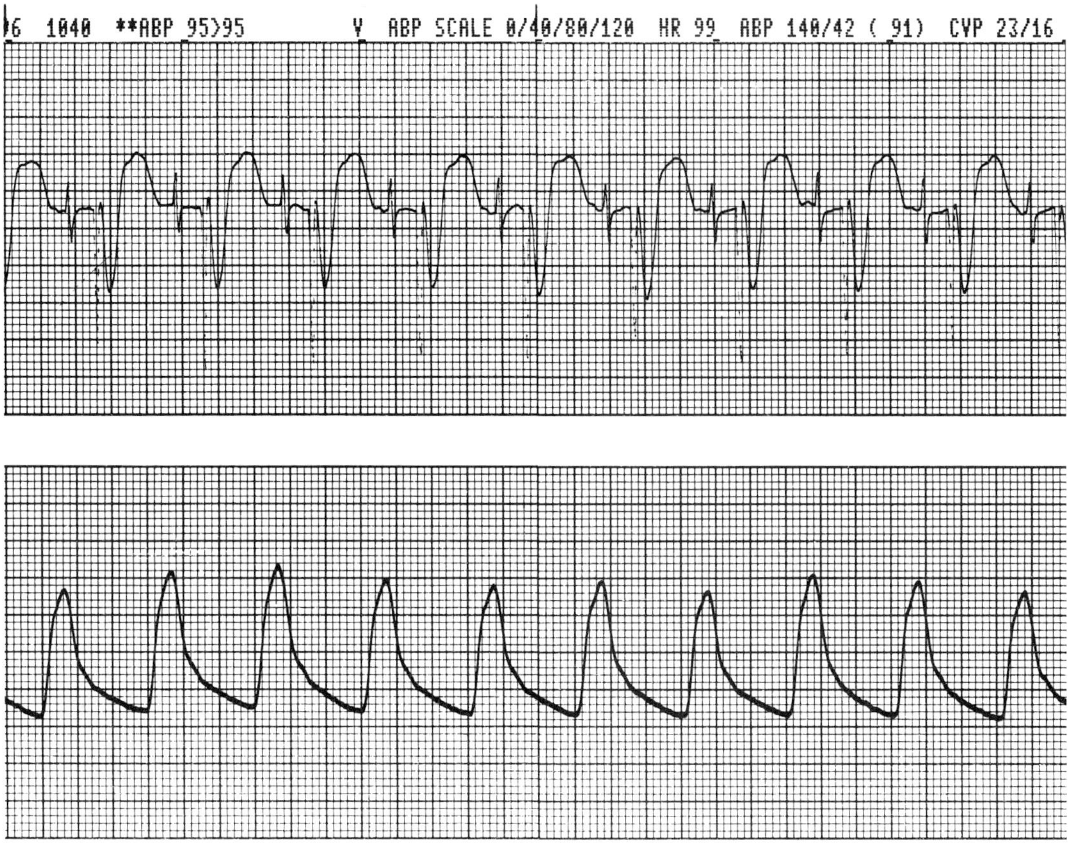

Figure 5-7. Normal arterial waveform.

A ventricular waveform is similar to an arterial wave in that it also has three common characteristics (eg, a rapid upstroke, a rapid diastolic drop, and an end-diastolic pressure rise) (**Fig. 5-8**). Systole and diastole are read in the same manner as on an arterial waveform. Normally a ventricular waveform is not monitored. **If a ventricular waveform is present on the monitor, it is important to verify the correct location of the catheter. A catheter that is floating freely in the ventricle tends to cause premature**

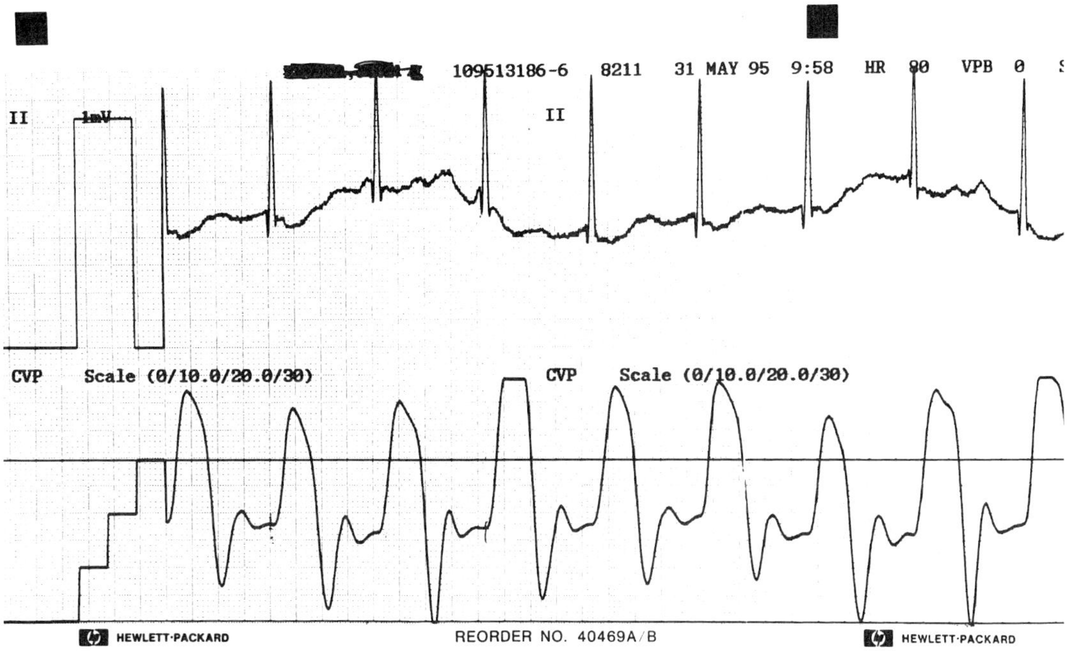

Figure 5-8. Normal ventricular waveform.

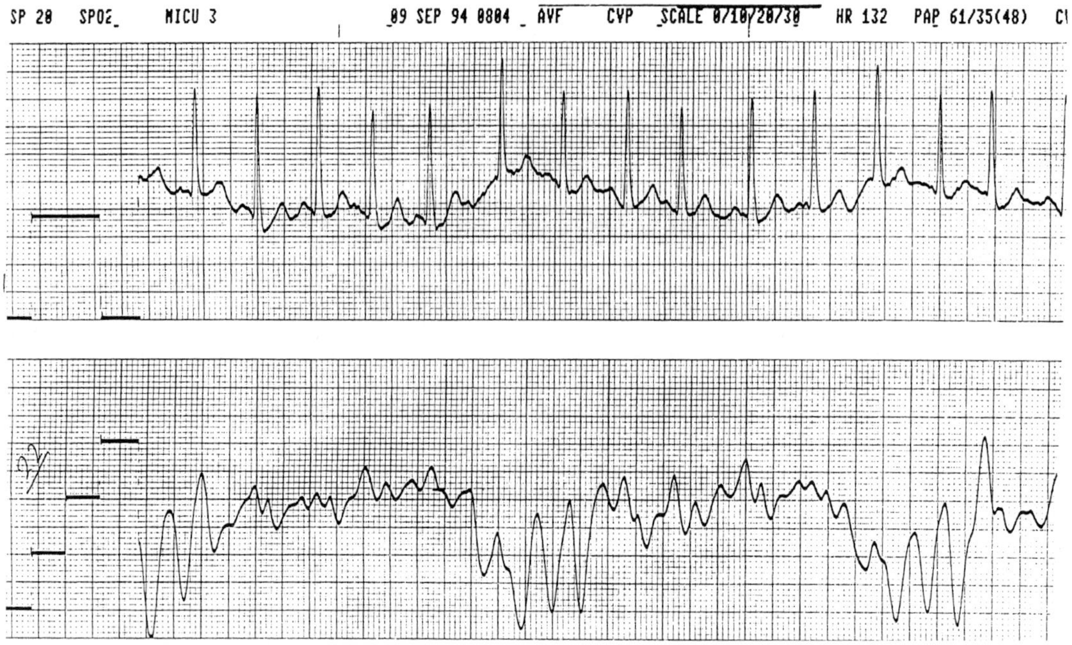

Figure 5-9. Spontaneous inspiratory artifact.

ventricular contractions, ventricular tachycardia, or ventricular fibrillation.

Respiratory Artifact

Waveforms obtained from blood vessels in the chest are subject to artifact. This artifact occurs because the transducer is referenced to atmospheric pressure, not pleural pressure. **To avoid this artifact, read respiratory waveforms at end-expiration.** End-expiration is the point at which atmospheric and pleural pressures are relatively close.

> **KEY CLINICAL CONCEPT**
>
> All hemodynamic measurements should be taken at end expiration. *A spontaneous inspiration or a patient-triggered ventilator inspiration produces a decrease in the waveform due to a fall in pleural pressure (**Fig. 5-9**). A ventilator inspiration will produce a positive deflection due to an increase in unmeasured pleural pressure (**Fig. 5-10**). To avoid artifact, find the point just before the inspiration* (spontaneous, triggered ventilator, or unassisted ventilator) occurs (eg, "end expiration"). This will avoid most artifacts (**Fig. 5-11**).

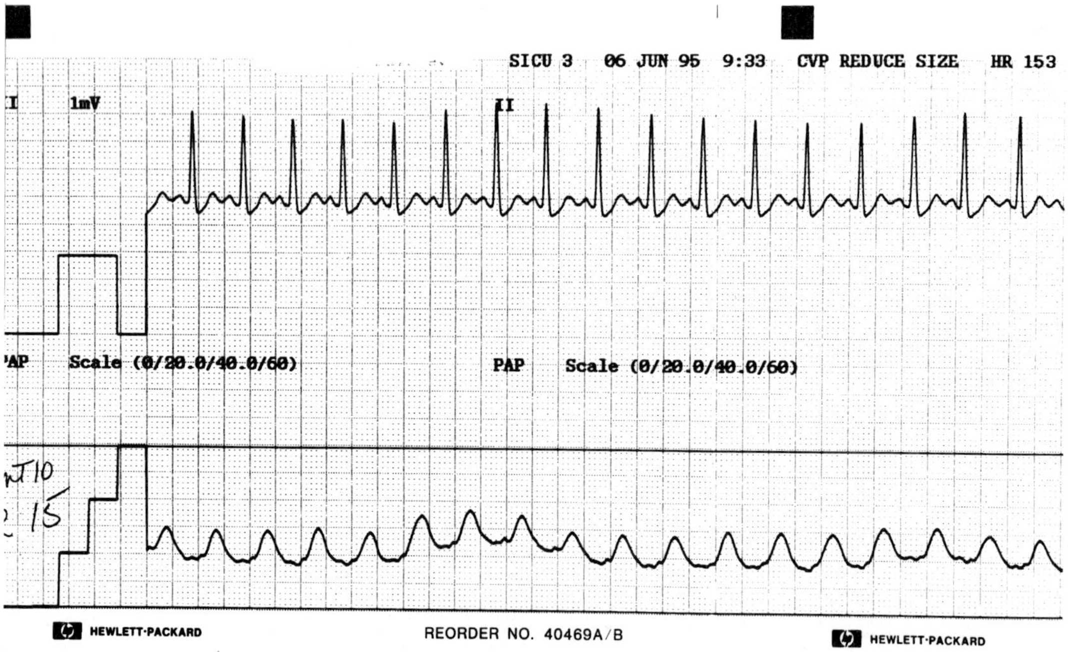

Figure 5-10. Respiratory artifact from mechanical ventilation.

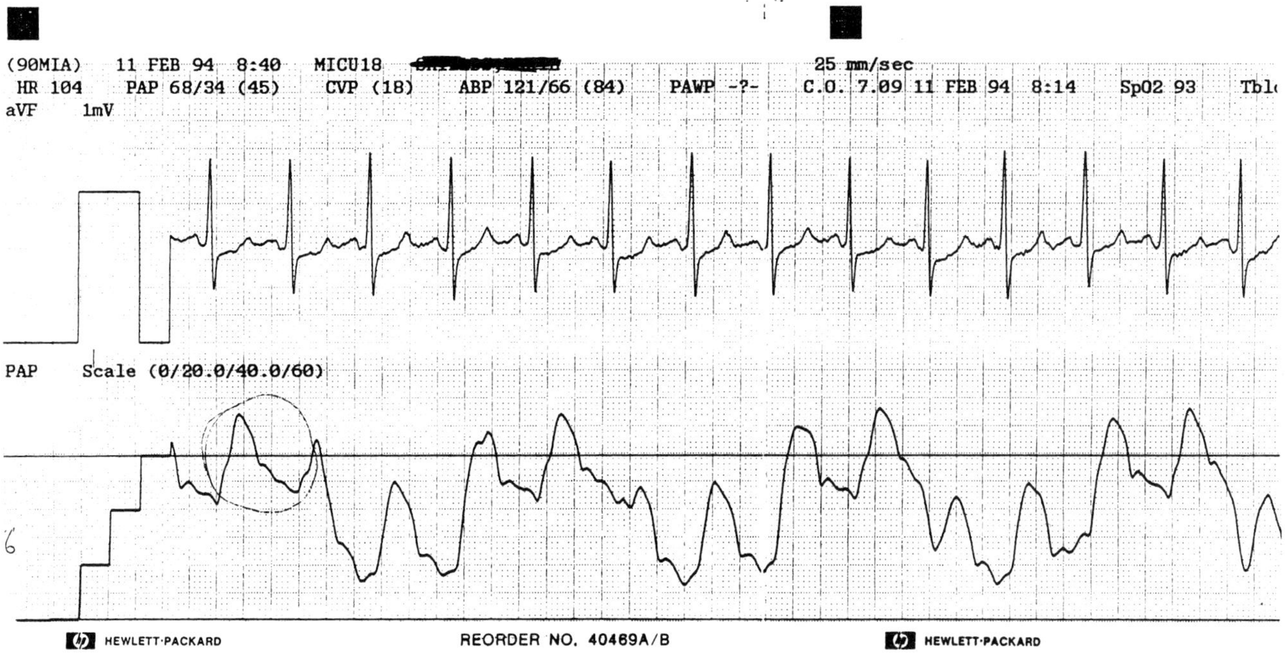

Figure 5-11. Avoiding inspiratory artifact in a patient with a respiratory rate greater than the ventilator rate.

QUICK TIP! Reading hemodynamic waveforms is the key to obtaining the pressures used in hemodynamic monitoring. Learning how to read waveforms for the CCRN exam is very easy, as there are very few questions that address this content. It is unlikely that you will actually have to read waveforms on the exam.

5.3 OBTAINING ACCURATE HEMODYNAMIC VALUES

Ensuring Accuracy

To obtain accurate values, five steps are necessary:

1. Set the transducer to zero.
2. Ensure that the transducer is leveled. *(This should be done whenever the patient or transducer moves from the original level position.)*
3. Read the waveform accurately.
4. For arterial catheters, perform a **square-wave test** to verify data accuracy.
5. Calibrate the transducer, if indicated. (If necessary at all, this is required only once.)

"Zeroing" the Transducer and Leveling the Transducer to the Phlebostatic Axis

Zero referencing eliminates the effects of hydrostatic and atmospheric pressures. "Zeroing" is done by exposing the transducer to air and pushing or activating a zero button (**Fig. 5-12**).

Leveling is the process of aligning the **phlebostatic axis** (usually 5 cm below the sternal angle) with a zero point, usually the transducer attached to the pressure tubing. For example, leveling a PA or any vascular catheter is done by opening a stopcock at the level of the midaxillary line (**Fig. 5-13**). Level the transducer with a carpenter's level or a laser level, prior to obtaining the first set of hemodynamic data and any time the patient or transducer has moved from their original positions. After this initial combined effort, only leveling is required and then only if the patient or transducer has moved from the original position.

KEY CLINICAL CONCEPT

Transducers must be leveled and zeroed at the phlebostatic axis to provide accurate hemodynamic data.

Arterial Catheter Square-Wave Test

The **square-wave test** ensures the pressure tubing system used to flush the arterial catheter does not interfere with transmitting waveforms to the transducer. Obstructions such as air or blood decreases the arterial waveform amplitude. This type of waveform is referred to as *"overdamped"* (**Fig. 5-14**). Overdamping

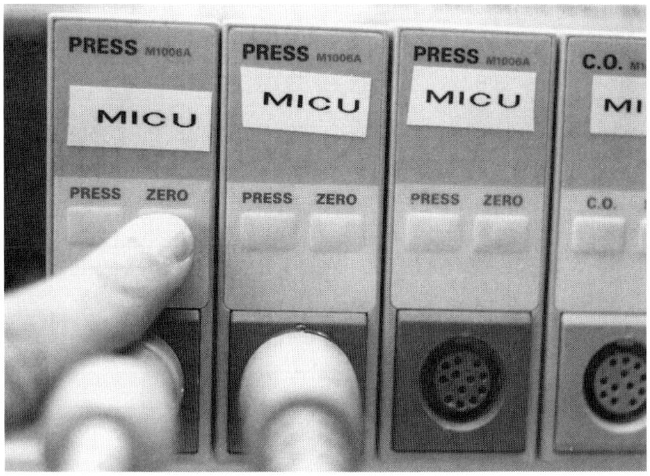

Figure 5-12. "Zeroing" a transducer.

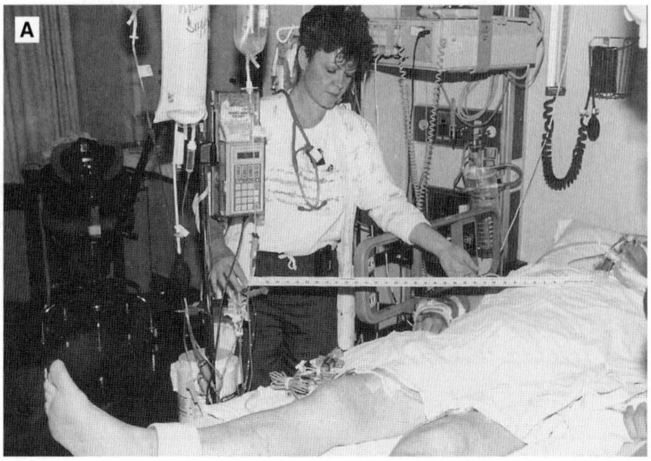

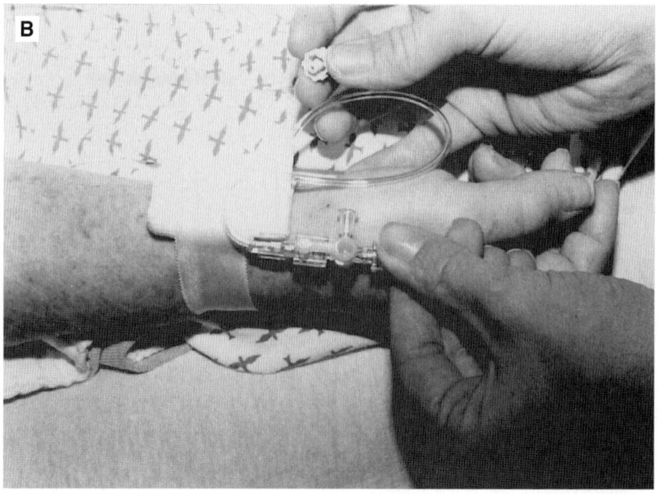

Figure 5-13. a. Leveling a transducer to the catheter tip. b. Leveling a radial artery catheter.

decreases systolic blood pressure (SBP) and increase diastolic blood pressure (DBP). If something, such as excessive tubing length, increases the waveform amplitude, it becomes *"underdamped"* (**Fig. 5-15**). Underdamping increases SBP and decreases DBP.

The ideal square-wave test is called an *"optimally damped"* test (**Fig. 5-16**). It is important to remember that the square-wave test is the best method available for checking the accuracy of systolic and diastolic arterial pressure readings. **The MAP may be more reliable whether or not an over or underdamped waveform is present and is more accurate than comparing an arterial pressure to a cuff pressure.**

QUICK TIP! All disposable hemodynamic transducers are precalibrated. Periodically, a calibration check may be indicated. It is unlikely that calibration questions will appear on the CCRN exam.

Factors to Consider During Hemodynamic Monitoring

Patient position during hemodynamic monitoring can be anywhere from flat to about 40 degrees of upper-body elevation. In this range, hemodynamic readings should be consistent. *It is not necessary that patients lie flat for hemodynamic values to be obtained.* However, there is little evidence to support accurate readings when a patient is turned to either side or is prone.

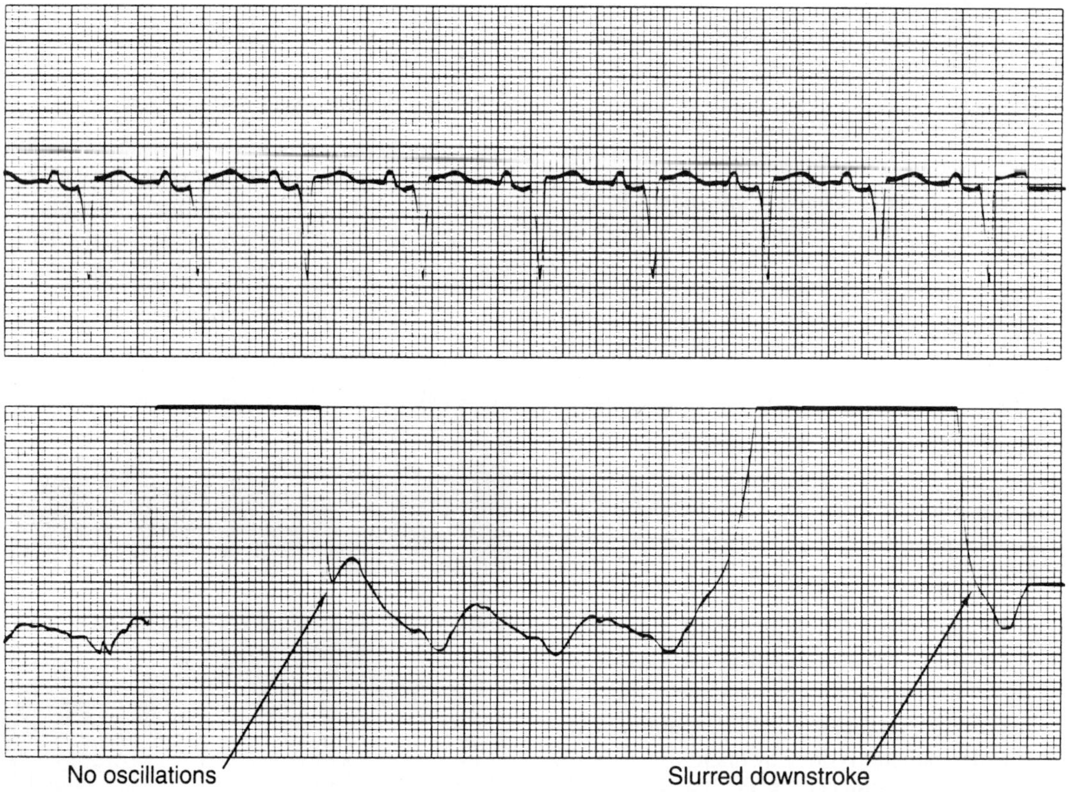

Figure 5-14. Overdamped square-wave test. (Reproduced with permission from Ahrens TS. *Hemodynamic Waveform Recognition*. Philadelphia: Saunders, 1993.)

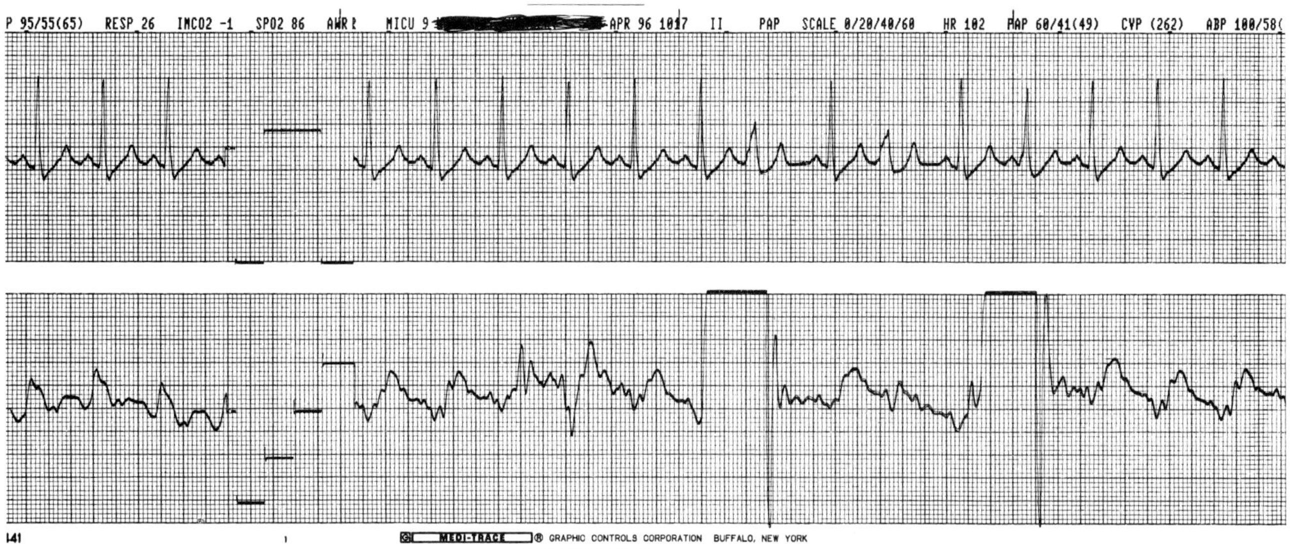

Figure 5-15. Underdamped square-wave test.

Measuring Cardiac Output and Cardiac Index

PA catheters employ thermodilution to assess CO and cardiac index (CI). Thermodilution measures cardiac output based on temperature changes as blood passes by sensors within the catheter. Depending on the type of PA catheter used, CO output data may be obtained manually or automatically. Manual thermodilution requires the clinician to inject crystalloid fluid into the PA catheter to intermittently assess CO (CO_{int}). Newer PA

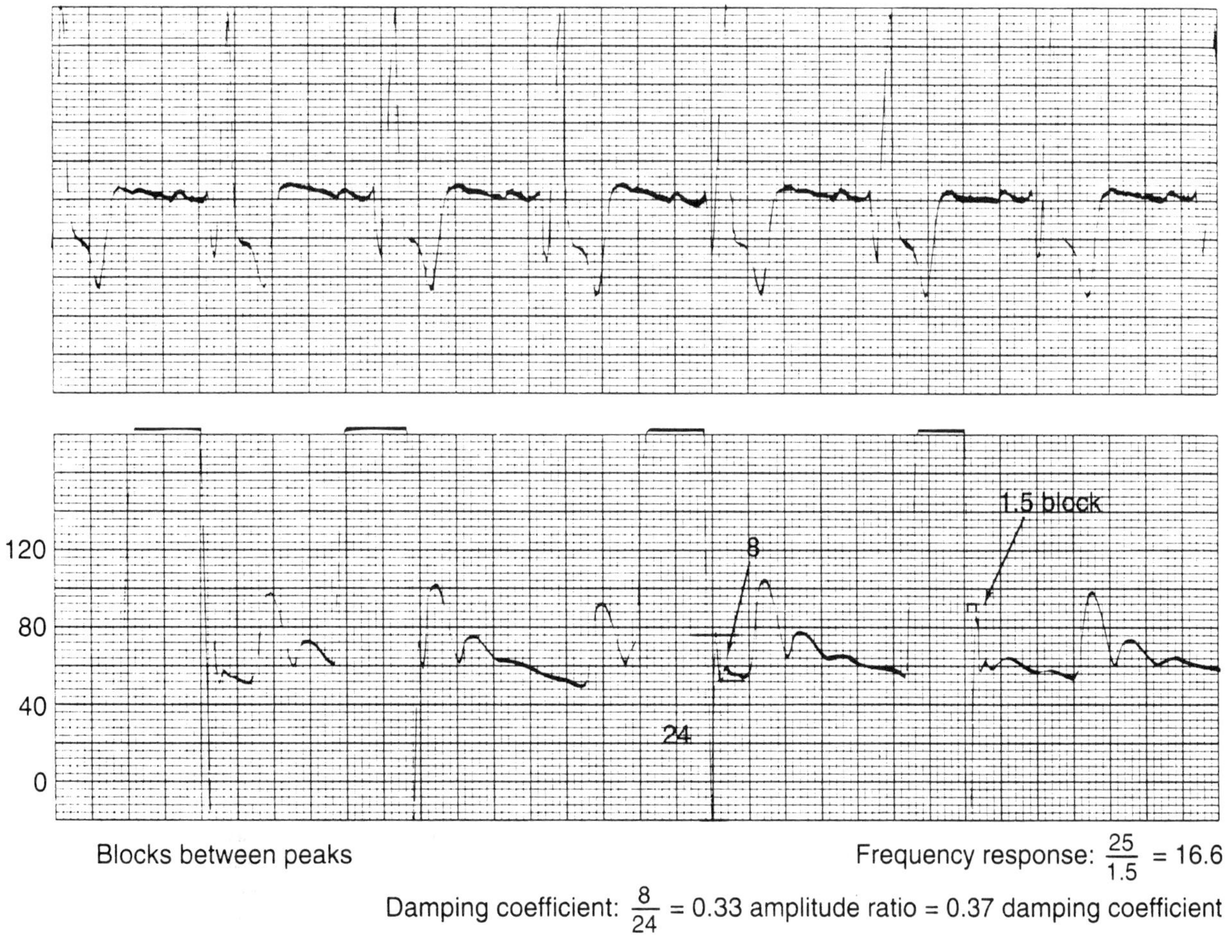

Figure 5-16. Optimally damped square-wave test. (Reproduced with permission from Ahrens TS. *Hemodynamic Waveform Recognition*. Philadelphia: Saunders, 1993.)

catheters allow for continuous cardiac output (CO_{cont}) monitoring. CO_{cont} devices change blood temperature via heaters which turn on and off automatically, inducing thermodilution to generate CO data. According to a recent meta-analysis, traditional intermittent manual CO (CO_{int}) measurements are the most accurate. However, CO_{cont} catheters are more widely used for their convenience and potential to prevent contamination compared to CO_{int}. Over the last two decades, the invasive nature and risk of myriad complications associated with PA catheters have decreased their use. Currently, there are multiple noninvasive and less invasive methods for measuring CO and SV, such as pulse contour analysis and bioreactance. The Fick method is used to measure CO during heart catheterization procedures. *The exam is less likely to focus on a particular technology*, like the PA catheter.

QUICK TIP! Although it is unlikely that the Fick equation itself will be on the CCRN exam, it is important to understand how CO, Hgb, and arterial oxygen content affect oxygen delivery to the tissues (DO_2).

The Fick Method

$$\text{Cardiac output} = \frac{Vo_2/10}{1.34 \times \text{Hgb} \times (Sao_2 - SvO_2)}$$

Cardiac Index

$$\text{Cardiac Index} = \frac{\text{Cardiac Output}}{\text{Body Surface Area}}$$

A few key points to be mindful of when measuring CO:

- The presence of the following limit the accuracy of thermodilution measurements: ventricular or atrial septal defect, tricuspid regurgitation, or dysrhythmias. They have less, or no, effect on technologies outside the heart, such as esophageal Doppler.
- Injecting at a consistent point in the respiratory cycle will help reduce variability in readings (only necessary for manual thermodilution techniques). (All outputs should be within 10% of each other.)
- If the CO measurements are inconsistent, use the Fick equation to measure CO.

KEY CLINICAL CONCEPT

If CO/CI has changed more than 10%, suspect the patient's clinical condition has changed.

Cardiac Power Index

The cardiac power index (CPI) is a newer data point that reflects LV stroke work (LVSW). It is derived from CI and MAP. Normal CPI is 0.5 to 0.7 w/m^2. Low CPIs during rest are seen in HF and cardiogenic shock. Although CPI is not yet widely used, it can determine response to inotropic agents and predict prognosis.

$$\frac{\text{Cardiac Power Index} = \text{Cardiac Index} \times \text{Mean Arterial Pressure}}{451}$$

QUICK TIP! The information obtained from hemodynamic monitoring technology must be verified for accuracy by the bedside clinician. However, the CCRN exam is unlikely to include many specific questions in this area. Only the steps necessary to obtain accurate values are provided. You might want to review this content for your own clinical practice and just to be safe for the exam.

KEY CONTENT CHECKLIST

- ❒ Sinus tachycardia may signal the presence of an underlying disease process such as sepsis. It is important to relate the increased HR to other vital signs and physical exam findings to identify possible causes.
- ❒ Under normal physiologic conditions, 25% of oxygen is removed from hemoglobin as it passes through capillary beds. This means 75% of the blood returning to the PA should be oxygenated. In theory, a normal SVO_2 is 75%.
- ❒ SvO_2 values less than 60% signal either impaired DO_2 or increased VO_2, and require investigation. Without intervention, inadequate DO_2 leads to anaerobic metabolism and subsequent metabolic acidosis.
- ❒ SvO_2 values more than 75% are abnormal and require investigating the underlying cause(s).
- ❒ Lactate levels more than 2 mmol/L indicate impaired tissue oxygenation and may require intervention. Lactates should be assessed every 2 to 4 hours until they are less than 2 mmol/L.
- ❒ Trending SvO_2 or $ScvO_2$ allows more frequent assessment of the response to treatment, with lactate levels confirming the improvement.
- ❒ Hemodynamic values that are "indexed" are more accurate than standard values since they take into account a patient's body surface area (BSA).
- ❒ It is essential to assess SV/SVI along with the filling pressures to avoid misinterpreting the filling pressure.
- ❒ A SV increase *more than or equal to* 10% after a fluid challenge demonstrates fluid responsiveness, even if the BP does not change.
- ❒ In patients with sinus tachycardia it is important to assess SV, since optimizing SV is the first step in improving hemodynamics.
- ❒ Deciding when hemodynamic changes, such as CO/CI or BP, are clinically significant is one of the

most important responsibilities facing the bedside clinician.

- Do not assume that a BP within a normal range represents adequate tissue perfusion. This is especially important in patients with HTN, since their BP may appear "normal" when it is actually much lower than their baseline. In patients with HTN, SBPs more than 40 mm Hg below baseline may reflect hypoperfusion. If hypoperfusion is suspected, consider checking an SvO_2 or lactate level.
- You will not have to know how to operate hemodynamic monitoring devices on the exam. Instead, you will need to know what the hemodynamic values mean for that patient, how to treat them, and what response to treatment to expect.
- Although this traditional interpretation of hemodynamics is somewhat simplistic, it is adequate for CCRN qualification.
- Learning how to read waveforms for the CCRN exam is very easy as there are very few questions that address this content. It is unlikely that you will actually have to read waveforms on the exam.
- The information obtained from hemodynamic monitoring technology must be verified for accuracy by the bedside clinician. However, the CCRN exam is unlikely to include many specific questions in this area.
- Transducers must be leveled and zeroed at the phlebostatic axis to provide accurate hemodynamic data.
- All hemodynamic measurements should be taken at end expiration.
- Although systolic and diastolic arterial BPs are altered if the waveform is overdamped or underdamped, MAPs may be more reliable.
- Suspect the patient's clinical condition has changed if CO has changed more than 10%.

Review Questions:

1. Which of the following parameters does not assess left ventricular (LV) preload?

a. Central venous pressure (CVP)
b. Pulmonary artery occlusion pressure (PAOP)
c. Left atrial pressure (LAP)
d. Left ventricular end-diastolic pressure (LVEDP)

Answer: A. Rationale: The correct answer is A. CVP is a measure of RV preload. LAP, PAOP, and LVEDP assess LV preload.

2. The (PAOP) is used to estimate which of the following pressures?

a. Left atrial pressure and LV end-diastolic pressure
b. Right atrial pressure and RV end-diastolic pressure
c. Central venous and pulmonary arterial pressures
d. Mean pulmonary artery and RV peak pressures

Answer: A. Rationale: The correct answer is A. Occluding the PA reflects pressures within the left atrium and left ventricle. All three are measurements of LV preload. Both parameters in answer B assess RV preload. The parameter in answers C and D are not related to PAOP.

3. Which of the following is the most common reason for both the PAOP and CVP to increase?

a. Left ventricular failure
b. Excess blood volume
c. Right ventricular failure
d. Pulmonary hypertension

Answer: B. Rationale: The correct answer is excess blood volume (hypervolemia) since it would raise both RV and LV filling pressures. LV failure (answer A) would cause PAOP to increase initially, and if not corrected RV failure could occur. RV failure (answer C) would cause CVP to increase. Pulmonary hypertension (answer D) initially affects RV function.

REFERENCES

Bednarczyk JM, Fridfinnson JA, Kumar A, et al. Incorporating dynamic assessment of fluid responsiveness into goal-directed therapy: a systematic review and meta-analysis. *Crit Care Med.* 2017;45(9):538–1545. doi: 10.1097/CCM.0000000000002554.

Bojar RM. *Manual of perioperative care in adult cardiac surgery,* 6th ed. John Wiley & Sons, Inc. Hoboken, New Jersey.

Brien LD, Oermann MH, Molloy M, and Tierney C. Implementing goal directed therapy for fluid resuscitation in the cardiovascular intensive care unit. *AACN Adv Crit Care.* 2021;31(4):364–370.

Edwards Clinical Education. *Quick guide to cardiopulmonary care,* 4th ed. Irving, CA: Edwards Lifesciences, 2018. Available at: https://edwardsprod.blob.core.windows.net/media/Gb/devices/monitoring/hemodynamic%20monitoring/quick-guide-to-pulmonary-care-4th-edition.pdf

Edwards Lifesciences. *Swan-Ganz flow-directed monitoring catheters product guide.* 2018b. Available at: https://eifu.edwards.com/eifu/pages/viewers/pdf?projectKey=5970f1b346e0fb00015e5f4d&itemKey=5c92c68246e0fb0001b4552f.

Edwards Lifesciences. (n.d.). *How you manage volume matters: using advanced hemodynamic parameters for perfusion management.* Available at: https://www.edwards.com/healthcare-professionals/conditions-procedures/fluid-management.

Johnson A, Stevenson J, Gu H, Huml J. Stroke volume optimization: utilization of the newest cardiac vital sign: considerations in recovery from cardiac surgery. *Crit Care Nurs Clin North Am.* 2019;31(3):329–348. doi: 10.1016/j.cnc.2019.05.004.

Johnson AP, Fallon T, Thorgesen D. Dynamic and static cardiac function measurements during sepsis. *Crit Care Nurse.* 2022;42(2):76–78. doi: 10.4037/ccn2022643.

Kaufmann T, van der Horst ICC, Scheeren TW. This is your toolkit in hemodynamic monitoring. *Curr Opin Crit Care.* 2020;26(3):303–312. doi: 10.1097/MCC.0000000000000727.

Kouz K, Michard F, Bergholz A, et al. Agreement between continuous and intermittent pulmonary artery thermodilution for cardiac output measurement in perioperative and intensive care medicine: a systematic review and meta-analysis. *Crit Care.* 2021;25(1):125. doi: 10.1186/s13054-021-03523-7.

Monnet X, Teboul JL. Prediction of fluid responsiveness in spontaneously breathing patients. *Ann Transl Med.* 2020;8(12):790. doi: 10.21037/atm-2020-hdm-18.

Morimoto R, Mizutani T, Araki T, et al. Prognostic value of resting cardiac power index depends on mean arterial pressure in dilated cardiomyopathy. *ESC Heart Failure.* 2021;8(4): 3206–3213. doi: 10.1002/ehf2.13446.

Myatra SN, Prabu NR, Divatia JV, Monnet X, Kulkarni AP, Teboul JL. The changes in pulse pressure variation or stroke volume variation after a "tidal volume challenge" reliably predict fluid responsiveness during low tidal volume ventilation. *Crit Care Med.* 2017;45(3):415–421. doi: 10.1097/CCM.0000000000002183.

Nardi O, Zavala E, Martin C, et al. Targeting skeletal muscle tissue oxygenation (StO_2) in adults with severe sepsis and septic shock: a randomised controlled trial (OTO-StS Study). *BMJ Open.* 2018;8(3):e017581. doi: 10.1136/bmjopen-2017-017581.

Pinksy MR. Combining functional hemodynamic measures to increase precision in defining volume responsiveness. *Crit Care Med.* 2017;45(3):558–559. doi: 10.1097/CCM.0000000000002242.

Rong LQ, Rahouma M, Neuburger PJ, et al. Use of pulmonary artery pulsatility index in cardiac surgery. *J Cardiothorac Vasc Anesth.* 2020;34(5):1220–1225. doi: 10.1053/j.jvca.2019.09.023.

Rosenkranz S, Howard LS, Gomberg-Maitland M, Hoeper MM. Systemic consequences of pulmonary hypertension and right-sided heart failure. *Circulation.* 2020;141(8):678–693. doi: 10.1161/CIRCULATIONAHA.116.022362.

VanDyck TJ, Pinsky MR. Hemodynamic monitoring in cardiogenic shock. *Curr Opin Crit Care.* 2021;27(4):454–459. doi: 10.1097/MCC.0000000000000838.

Vincent JL, Joosten A, Saugel B. Hemodynamic monitoring and support. *Crit Care Med.* 2021;49(10):1638–1650. doi: 10.1097/CCM.0000000000005213.

6

Acute Coronary Syndrome (Angina Pectoris and Myocardial Infarction)

CHAPTER OVERVIEW AND OBJECTIVES

This chapter emphasizes the key features of the origin, symptomatology, and medical and nursing interventions associated with acute coronary syndrome (ACS). Angina (including coronary artery vasospasm and unstable angina [UA]) and myocardial infarction (MI) are common test items on the CCRN exam. **The ability to differentiate them as well as the different treatments to anticipate will be key for the exam.**

Expect the CCRN exam to contain many questions on assessing and treating coronary artery disease (CAD). This chapter provides brief but key concepts in the area of CAD. Expect several questions in the CCRN exam on the assessment, diagnosis, and treatment of angina and MI.

After studying this chapter, you should be able to:

- Differentiate the various forms of ACS including their associated symptoms and treatments.
- Identify the treatments for STEMI and NSTEMI including medical management.
- Understand the ECG lead changes associated with the different locations of MI.

6.1 ACUTE CORONARY SYNDROME

Acute coronary syndrome (ACS) is described as a continuum of coronary artery disease (CAD) where there is a sudden decrease in blood flow to the heart. ACS includes diseases in which there is narrowing of the blood vessel (angina) all the way to a complete occlusion of the coronary artery, which can result in MI. MIs are subdivided into ST-segment elevation myocardial infarctions (STEMIs) and non–ST-segment elevation myocardial infarctions (NSTEMIs).

6.2 PATHOPHYSIOLOGY OF ACS

Plaque (atheroma) rupture with the precipitation of vasospasm and clot formation is the likely precipitating event in myocardial ischemia and ACS. A combination of chronic lipid accumulation and acute endothelial injury with subsequent thrombosis formation probably forms the basis for plaque formation and eventual obstruction of blood flow.

Plaque and clot formation are well-studied causes for MI and ACS, yet there is increasing evidence for the role of inflammation in the generation of the obstruction. The inflammation may be subclinical and initially unrelated to the plaque. Markers of inflammation, such as C-reactive protein, are increasingly being seen as suggestive of CAD. A normal level of C-reactive protein is 0.03 to 10 mg/dL. If CRP is elevated and there are no other inflammatory processes known, inflammation is likely in the coronary artery rather than from any ischemic area.

Over time, atherosclerotic lesions (atheromata) form. These lesions are asymmetrical, isolated thickenings in the coronary arteries (as well as other arteries throughout the body). They form in the intima, the innermost lining of the blood vessels of the heart. The atheroma consists of several different types of cells, including endothelial, smooth muscle, and inflammatory cells. The atheroma is preceded by a fatty deposit, which is composed of lipid cells beneath the endothelium. Why such an atheroma develops is still under investigation but is believed to be caused by continued injury within the endothelial wall. In the past, it was thought that the atheroma caused severe narrowing of the coronary artery, which caused the symptoms of ACS. Such narrowing is likely not the only cause, owing to the development of collateral circulation as the plaque extends. Recent research suggests that it is not always the degree of narrowing as much as it is the degree to which the atheroma or plaque is activated, resulting in plaque rupture or endothelial rupture.

Activation of an atheroma or plaque may be initiated by the rupture of a thin plaque or by an inflammatory response. The activation may be the result of hemodynamic flow or shear factors. This process takes place over time, but for unclear reasons, the plaque will elicit an inflammatory response. That is, the inflammatory macrophages, T cells, and mast cells will help cause a clot to form at the site of the plaque.

After an MI, ventricular remodeling occurs. This includes changes in the size, shape, and thickness of the ventricle, which can occur in both the infarcted and noninfarcted areas.

Risk Factors

There are some relatively well-known risk factors for the development of ACS. These can be divided into modifiable and nonmodifiable risk factors.

Unalterable Risk Factors

1. A hereditary predisposition to the development of atherosclerosis.
2. Age, since ACS is more prevalent in older persons than in younger persons.
3. Gender appears to be a factor in the development of atherosclerosis, since the condition develops earlier in men than in women. However, recent evidence suggests incidence of myocardial disease in postmenopausal women begins to approach that in men.

Medically Alterable Risk Factors

1. Hypertension has been shown to be related to the development of atherosclerosis. Close medical treatment of hypertension may slow the development of atherosclerosis.
2. Diabetics develop atherosclerosis more often than nondiabetics. Close medical treatment and control of diabetes may reduce the atherosclerotic process.
3. Hyperlipidemia may have an important bearing on the development and/or progression of atherosclerosis. The presence of low-density lipoproteins appears to be a precursor to the development of atherosclerosis. Medical treatment of hyperlipidemia will help slow the atherosclerotic process.

Personal Alterable Risk Factors. The following can be altered by the individual to decrease the possibility or progression of atherosclerosis:

1. Weight control can be beneficial in reducing the risk of CAD.
2. Cigarette smokers have a higher incidence of heart disease than do nonsmokers. Elimination of smoking will reduce the risk of MI.
3. Sedentary lifestyles predispose to the development of atherosclerosis. Exercising three to four times per week for 30 minutes or activity that pushes the heart rate into the target zone or aerobic exercise will reduce the rate of CAD.
4. Moderate alcohol intake may reduce the risk of CAD. However, the limitation to moderate intake is difficult for many people, and the risk of alcoholism may outweigh the benefit.

If an individual is sufficiently motivated, these last four risk factors can be incorporated into a personal lifestyle.

Prognosis

One cannot change unalterable risk factors; however, a focus on addressing modifiable personal risk factors, combined with medical treatment, can reduce one's overall risk for CAD. If risk factors are not modified, atherosclerosis may progress from the development of angina and ischemia to MI, heart failure, or sudden death. Despite the prognosis with alterable risk factors, coronary atherosclerosis is still one of the leading causes of death in the United States.

Identification and Treatment of ACS. In this section, an easy-to-follow guideline for the treatment of ACS is presented (**Figs. 6-1** and **6-2**). The guideline walks through the diagnosis and treatment of a patient with symptoms of cardiac disease.

The following sections provide a brief overview of MI and angina. **The guidelines presented in Figs. 6-1 and 6-2 contain much of what the CCRN will likely expect you to know, including patient characteristics to expect and treatments to anticipate.** These next sections provide additional background information that should help strengthen your overall knowledge of ACS.

KEY CLINICAL CONCEPT

The CCRN will not ask many questions on the pathophysiology of ACS. However, it is important to understand a few key concepts. These should prepare you for the exam as well as clinical practice.

6.3 ANGINA PECTORIS

Angina can result from a reduced blood flow, low-oxygen content, or myocardial oxygen demand in excess of supply. Most types of angina result in minimal injury to no injury to the myocardial muscle. Autopsy results of patients with angina have demonstrated frequent total occlusion of coronary vessels with subsequent development of extensive collateral circulation. The development of collateral circulation can allow maintenance of coronary perfusion and no permanent injury to the myocardium even when cardiac catheterization results indicate total occlusion. Differing types of lesions are noted during cardiac catheterization (**Fig. 6-3**).

Causes of reduced blood flow to the myocardium include atherosclerosis, valvular dysfunction, hypotension, and coronary vasospasm. Low-oxygen content can also precipitate anginal episodes. Causes of low-oxygen content include reduced hemoglobin and low oxygen pressure/saturation (Pao_2/Sao_2) levels. Causes of excessive oxygen demand relative to perfusion include hypertension, exercise, and increased metabolic rate. Many predisposing

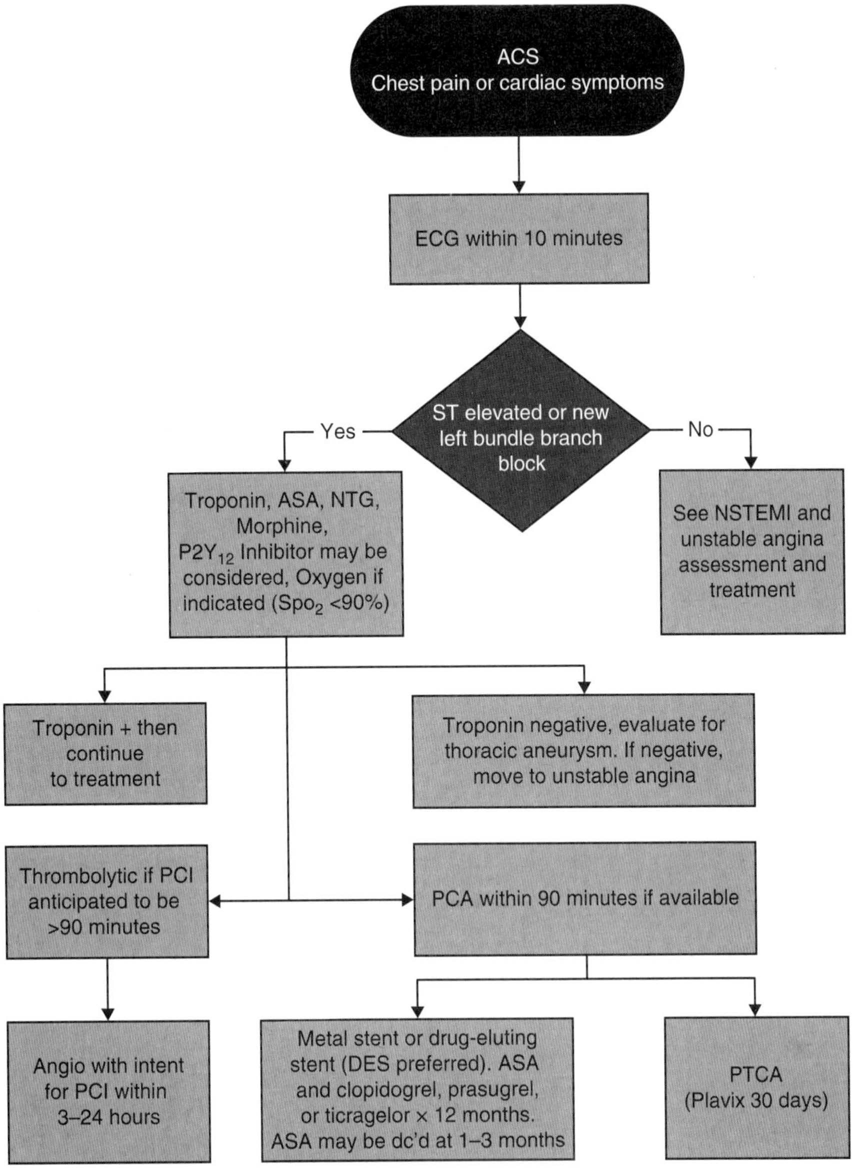

Figure 6-1. Algorithm to assess and treat ST-elevation MI (STEMI).

factors can precipitate reduced blood flow, decreased oxygen content, or increased myocardial oxygen demand.

The occurrence of angina is variable, depending substantially on the degree of collateral circulation that has developed. Angina can be suddenly precipitated by any event that increases oxygen demand (such as anxiety, stress, eating, or exercise) or reduces blood flow (smoking).

Clinical Presentation

The typical clinical presentation of angina presents with pain is the primary symptom. This pain may be described as burning, squeezing in a tight band, or as extreme heaviness or pressure on the lower sternum, and may radiate to the neck, jaws, shoulders, arms, and stomach. **Atypical symptoms often found in African Americans and women are fatigue, shortness of breath, indigestion-type symptoms, and shoulder/back discomfort.** Characteristically, the pain begins after eating or physical activity and subsides with rest. The pain usually lasts 1 to 4 minutes, but it may require as long as 10 minutes to subside completely. Anginal pain should always last less than 30 minutes. Pain for more than 30 minutes suggests MI and the need for immediate treatment. Not all CAD will present with anginal symptoms. Some patients can have evidence of ischemia without symptoms. *This possibility of ischemia without pain serves as a reminder to educate patients with angina and MI, especially diabetic patients who often have vague symptoms of angina.* Frequent evaluation of cardiac status, as with exercise testing, can enable the clinician to detect symptoms early, rather than waiting for an anginal episode to indicate ischemia.

Diagnosis

Diagnosis of angina is based on history and electrocardiogram (ECG) findings. Cardiac markers are usually normal. **The 12-lead ECG usually has depressed ST segments over the affected area.** ST-segment elevation **(Prinzmetal's angina)** can occur but is less common.

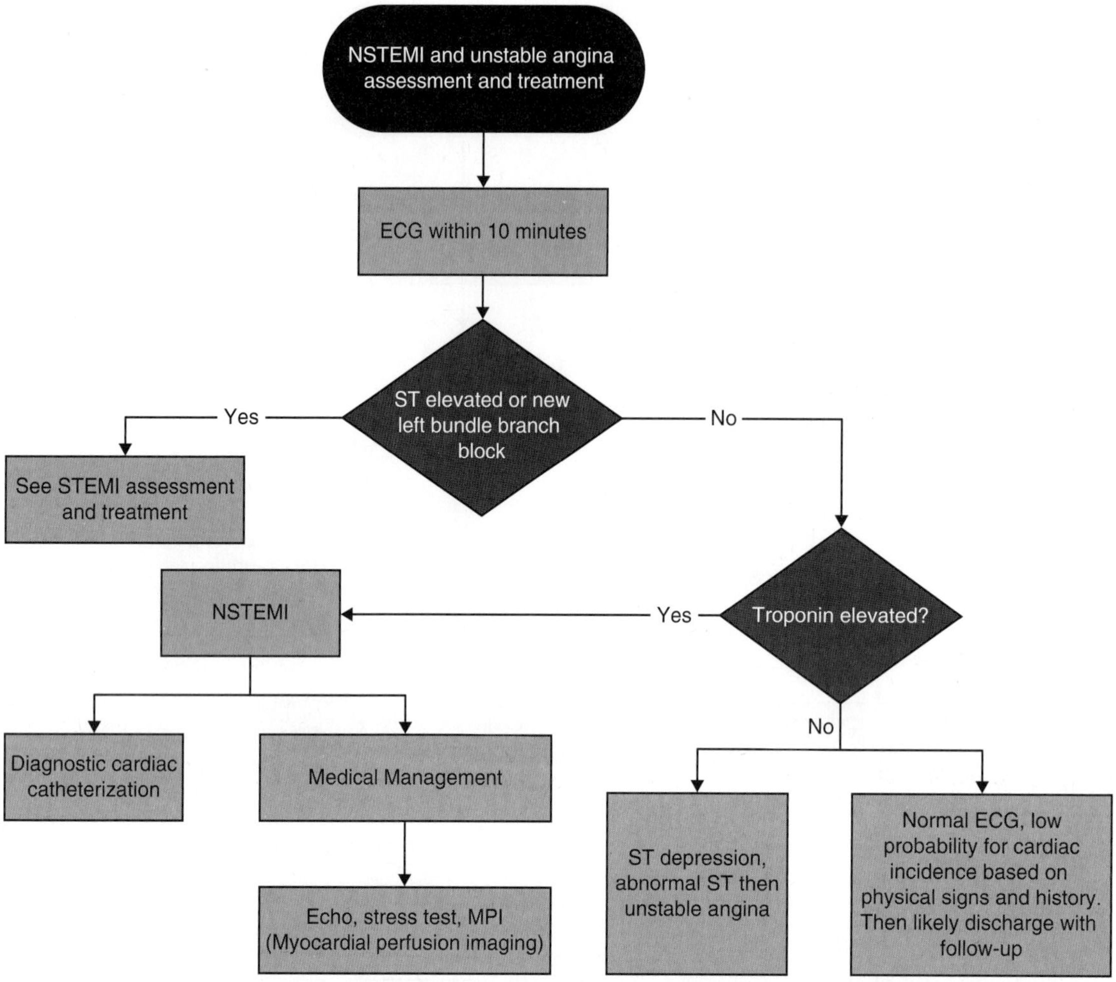

Figure 6-2. Algorithm to assess and treat non–ST-elevation MI (NSTEMI) and unstable angina.

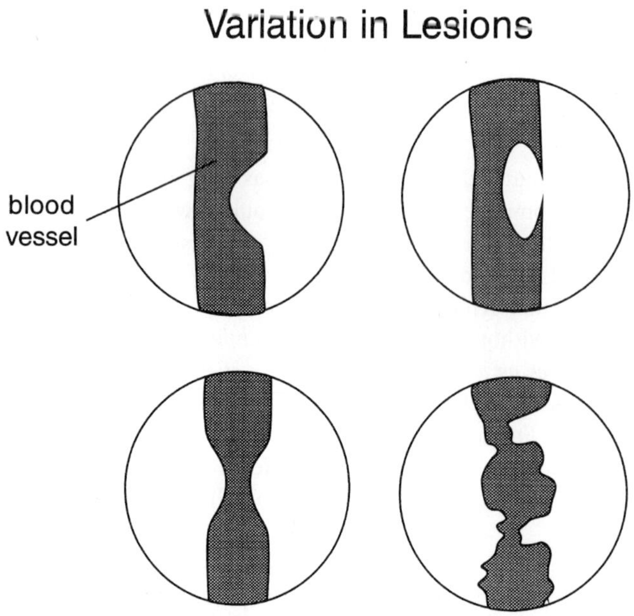

Figure 6-3. Different types of lesions noted during cardiac catheterization.

KEY CLINICAL CONCEPT

Prinzmetal's angina is also termed, "variant angina" and Is angina due to coronary spasm and NOT CAD. Treatment may include calcium channel blockers.

Treatment

The pathology of angina is plaque formation without rupture, leading to narrowing of the coronary artery and diminished blood flow. The goal is to dilate the vessels so as to increase the size of the arterial lumen, decrease oxygen demand, and increase oxygen availability. Vasodilators, such as sublingual **nitroglycerin**, usually relieve the angina within ½ minute. **Nitroglycerin** taken before an activity may prevent an attack. Changing one's lifestyle to eliminate the alterable risk factors may help to decrease the severity and frequency of attacks. If the anginal attacks increase in frequency or intensity (crescendo angina), stress testing and/or cardiac catheterization to determine the extent of the disease is indicated. **Nitrates** and **beta blockers** may be used alone or in combination to resolve anginal episodes. The patient may be a candidate for angioplasty or coronary artery bypass surgery, which will stop the angina and decrease the risk of MI. The patient is advised to exercise within the limits of pain and obtain adequate rest while awaiting surgery or intervention. Coronary artery bypass grafting (CABG) is the treatment for failure of medical intervention. CABG has demonstrated the potential for alleviating symptoms of angina although may or may not necessarily prolong life.

Unstable Angina

The pathology of UA includes plaque formation with rupture and platelet activation, hence varying degrees of blood supply and unpredictable discomfort. There are several variations of angina, the most prevalent being UA. It differs from stable angina in that it is more easily triggered. UA may involve crescendo angina, may occur at rest, and is characterized by increasing severity and frequency. Clinically, the patient may complain that it takes less activity to stimulate an anginal episode and that the severity of symptoms is increasing.

Treatment of UA usually requires additional medical therapy. Beta blockers **(eg, metoprolol)** are helpful in reducing myocardial oxygen consumption. Nondihydropyridine calcium channel blockers **(eg, verapamil, diltiazem)** may be useful in reducing afterload and myocardial oxygen use if beta blockers are contraindicated and the patient does not have other contraindications (eg, decreased left ventricle [LV] function).

Another type of angina is **Prinzmetal's variant angina,** or PVA. The origin of PVA is thought to be both coronary vasospasm and stenosis. The patient presents with symptoms most often including pain at rest and other symptoms of angina. Patients tend to be younger women who do not have the usual cardiac risk factors (except for smoking). The attacks can be triggered by drinking iced liquids, alcohol, cocaine, nicotine, and other factors. The attacks tend to fall into a circadian rhythm, often occurring early in the morning and during the menstrual cycle. *Calcium channel blockers* have a potential benefit due to their ability to relieve or prevent vasospasm.

The ECG shows reversible ST-segment elevation rather than depression. Dysrhythmias may occur with this form of angina, often with marked ST-segment elevation (>4 mm). Sudden cardiac death is markedly more likely with dysrhythmias caused by PVA.

The pathogenesis of PVA is not well understood. Activation of the autonomic nervous system (alpha-adrenergic receptors) seems to be a major factor. Precipitating events are those that stimulate alpha-adrenergic receptors (eg, acetylcholine) and blocked by alpha-receptor blockers *(eg, atropine, prazosin, and clonidine).* Autonomic nervous system involvement is supported by the fact that surgical sympathetic denervation has worked on patients unresponsive to medical therapy.

PVA is diagnosed by 24-hour Holter monitoring (to find episodes of symptoms associated with ST-segment elevation) and sympathetic stimulation with ergonovine. Exercise testing and coronary angiography are of little value in the diagnosis of PVA.

Calcium channel blockers have a positive effect in reducing the anginal episode, as do nitrates. **Diltiazem and nifedipine** are effective in reducing episodes of PVA.

Beta blockers and high-dose aspirin may aggravate PVA. If medical therapy fails, both UA and PVA may require CABG, angioplasty, or stent placement. With treatment and smoking cessation, prognosis with PVA is usually good.

Coronary Artery Vasospasm

Coronary artery vasospasm, a form of variant angina, is a transient narrowing of a large coronary artery. The origins are unclear but could include sympathetic stimulation, prostaglandin mediation, or pharmacologic stimulation. Treatment is similar to that for angina, with more emphasis on calcium channel blockers as well as nitroglycerin.

6.4 ACUTE MYOCARDIAL INFARCTION (STEMI AND NSTEMI)

MI is the actual necrosis, or death, of myocardial tissue because of reduced blood supply (loss of oxygen) to a specific area of the heart (**Fig. 6-4**).

Etiology

In most MIs, atherosclerotic heart disease is present. The remaining cases of MI are likely due to coronary artery spasm in which the artery constricts enough to prevent blood from reaching the myocardium.

Most MIs have been demonstrated to be the result of the formation of a coronary thrombus on top of an atherosclerotic plaque. The rapid identification of MI is crucial to treatment. **If onset of symptoms to the time of treatment is ≥12 hours, myocardial muscle generally becomes irreversibly damaged.** Although this time period can vary and some tissue can

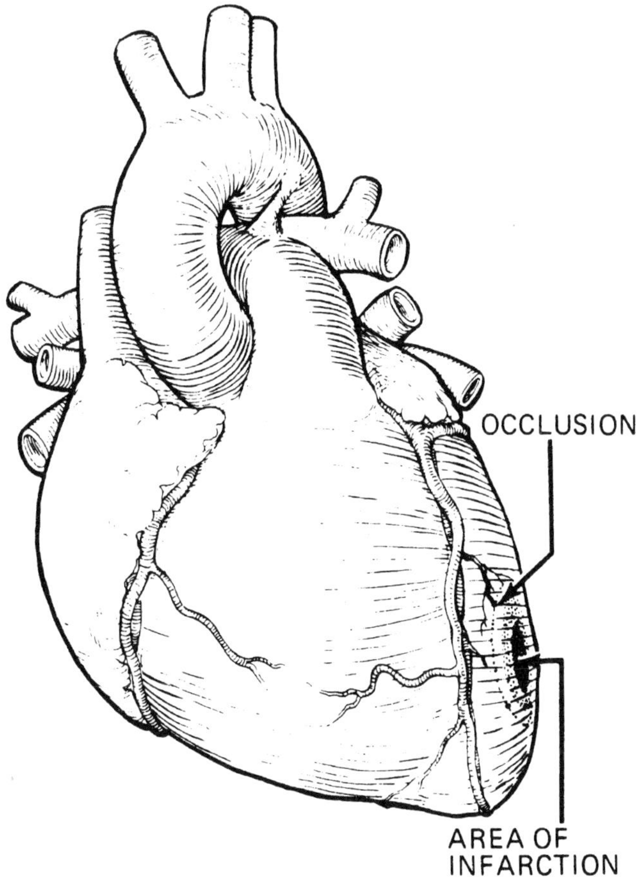

Figure 6-4. Myocardial infarction.

be salvaged later, the earlier the treatment, the more likely the recovery.

KEY CLINICAL CONCEPT

Clinical goals for ischemic chest pain include obtaining a 12-lead ECG within 10 minutes of the onset of symptoms. In the event of STEMI, the goal from onset of symptoms to stent deployment is less than 90 minutes (within acute care). However, research has shown the faster the stent is deployed the better outcomes for the patient.

Diagnosis and Clinical Presentation

Chest pain—with nausea (and maybe vomiting), diaphoresis, and weakness—is the most common symptom of an MI. The pain of an infarct differs from angina pain. With an MI, the chest pain is constant, severe, and not relieved by nitroglycerin. The location of the pain is similar to that of anginal pain. It is, however, not relieved with rest or lying down. The duration of pain exceeds 30 minutes, without relief. In fact, it often occurs at rest without a clear precipitating event. As the pain, nausea, weakness, and diaphoresis continue, the patient becomes dyspneic and often becomes extremely apprehensive, often developing a sense of impending doom.

QUICK TIP! Generally, if symptoms in a patient scenario are relevant to an answer on the exam, they will often appear as, "classic" symptoms as described here. However, for ischemic chest pain questions, be mindful of the "silent" or atypical symptoms that may be present in pre-menopausal women, diabetics, and the elderly.

However, MIs may present without any symptoms or with only mild signs, such as indigestion. These "silent" MIs are extremely difficult to treat, since the signs are not severe enough to prompt a visit to the hospital or physician.

TABLE 6-1. AREAS OF THE HEART AND THEIR CORRESPONDING ECG LEADS FOR INTERPRETATION OF MYOCARDIAL INFARCTION

Location	*ECG Location*	*ECG Changes*
Anterior	V_2–V_4	Q waves, ST-segment elevation
Inferior	II, III, aVF	Q waves, ST-segment elevation
Lateral	I, aVL, V_5, V_6	Q waves, ST-segment elevation
Right ventricular	V_3R–V_6R	ST-segment elevation
Posterior	V_1, V_2	Large R wave
Septal	V_1	Q waves, ST-segment elevation

The 12-lead ECG reveals initial T-wave inversion, followed quickly by ST-segment elevation in the affected area. Q-wave formation, indicating cellular death, occurs after 24 h and is considered more diagnostic of past MI. **Areas of the heart and their corresponding ECG leads for MI interpretation are presented in Table 6-1. Fig. 6-5** gives an example of MI of the anterior septal region; **Fig. 6-6** gives an example of an inferior MI.

Abnormalities in serum cardiac markers are the best diagnostic criteria for MI, specifically **high sensitivity troponin (hs-cTn)**. The troponin complex consists of three subunits: TnT, TnI, and TnC and Both TnT and TnI can be performed using a high sensitivity assay. High-sensitivity troponins are now considered the preferred method of measurement for troponin in the evaluation of chest pain when available as they will detect lower levels of the troponin protein. This faster identification of myocardial injury may result in faster treatment and better patient outcomes in ACS. However, high-sensitivity

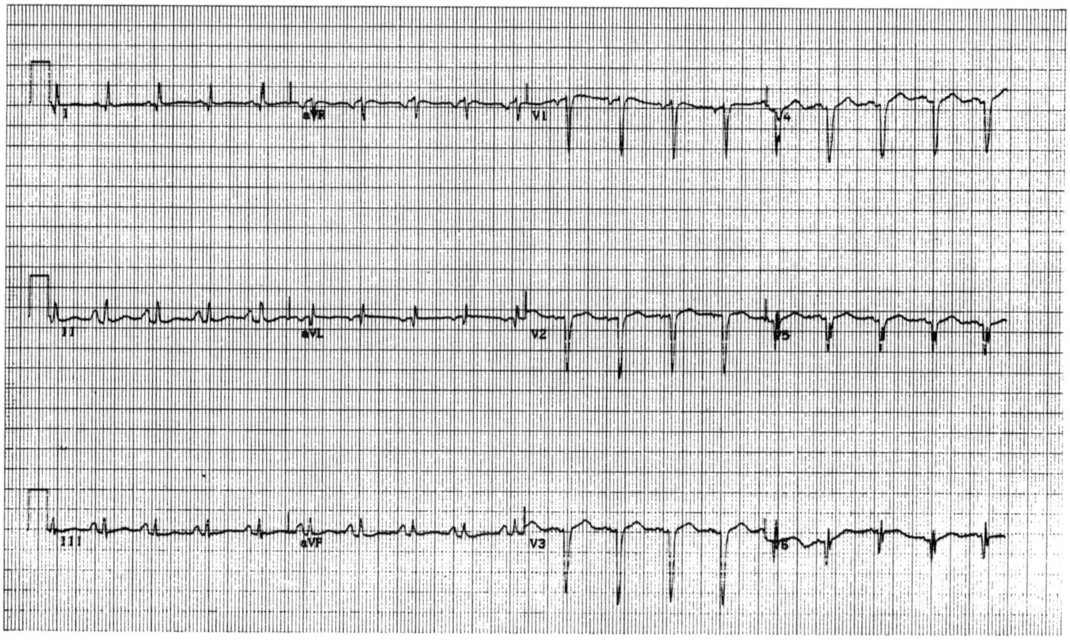

Figure 6-5. Anterior septal myocardial infarction.

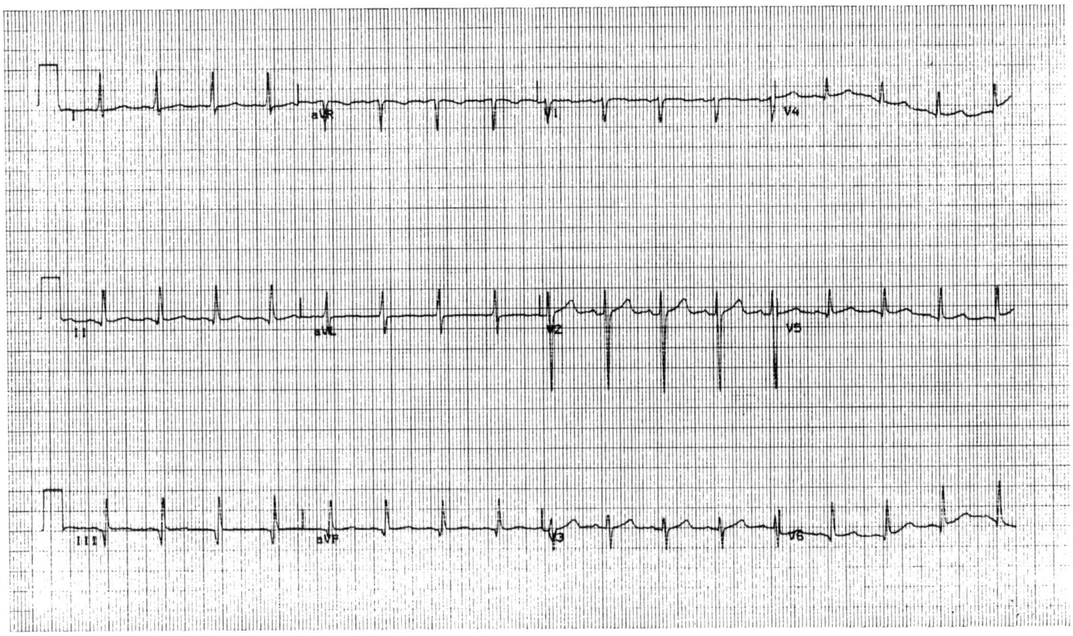

Figure 6-6. Inferior myocardial infarction.

troponin may be elevated for nonacute causes; therefore, the clinical presentation of the patient must be considered. Serial values are important in evaluating the significance of the hs-cTn as nonacute causes will rarely show an increase within a couple hours.

If high-sensitivity assays are not available troponin I (cTnI) is considered the best evaluation method. Normally, traditional troponin levels are not detectable in blood assays. cTnI levels above greater than 0.4 ng/mL may be considered diagnostic of MI, although even lower levels are now being identified as consistent with MIs. cTnI levels have replaced creatine phosphokinase (CPK) isoenzymes as the main biomarkers for MIs.

Troponin levels may remain elevated for more than 8 days or even longer with decreased renal excretion. If a patient has had a recent MI, the troponin level will not indicate how recent the event was. This is why some centers still use CPK isoenzymes, including the subset of MB bands. The CPK-MB band is specific for cardiac muscle. If the CPK-MB band rises above 12 IU, MI can be diagnosed (**Table 6-2**). CPK isoenzymes rise within hours of injury, peaking within 24 hours and returning to normal within a few days.

Other diagnostic tests include the use of echocardiography and radionuclide imaging. Echocardiography reveals MIs by identifying defects in regional wall motion. Negative results also help rule out MIs.

Location of Infarction

Occlusions of the ***right coronary artery result in an inferior MI.*** Inferior MIs have a lower mortality rate than anterior MIs. Symptoms associated with an inferior MI include more mild *AV node dysrhythmias, such as first- and second-degree type I blocks.* Approximately 30% of inferior MIs include right ventricular (RV) infarction. **Symptoms of RV infarction include hypotension from a decrease in the preload available to the LV because of decreased RV emptying.**

> **KEY CLINICAL CONCEPT!**
>
> Patients with RV infarction are preload dependent; therefore, caution is advised with administration of nitroglycerin or other medications that will decrease preload (diuretics, beta blockers, morphine). RV infarctions are best treated with fluids to increase preload and inotrope support to increase contractility.

Occlusion of the left anterior descending coronary artery results in an anterior MI. Anterior MIs have a higher mortality rate and are associated with more serious dysrhythmias. Rhythm disturbances are more likely to include second- and third-degree blocks. *Anterior MIs are also most likely responsible for diminished ejection fraction and symptoms of heart failure.*

Less serious MIs are lateral and posterior, each with lower mortality rates than inferior or anterior MIs. More dangerous

TABLE 6-2. SERUM CARDIAC MARKERS AND PROTEINS USED IN THE DIAGNOSIS OF MYOCARDIAL INFARCTION

CPK	30–200 IU	Not specific by itself for MI; the size of MI is referenced to the degree of total CPK elevation (ie, the higher the CPK, the greater the size of the MI)
CPK-MB	<5 ng/mL	>8 ng/mL suggests MI
Troponin I	<0.15, normal; >0.4–1.4, cardiac injury likely; >1.4 ng/mL suggests MI; elevates within 4 h of MI and remains elevated for up to 5–10 days	
hs-cTn	<99th percentile of the upper reference limit is considered normal (varies based on assay used in each lab). Available as Hs- cTnI or Hs-cTnT. All results need to be evaluated based on the value trend and the clinical picture.	

MIs are those that affect multiple regions, such as anterolateral MIs. When more than 40% of the LV is acutely damaged, mortality is extremely high.

RV MIs are less common but are associated with obstruction of the right coronary or left circumflex artery. Mortality is lower with RV MIs. Diagnosis is made from the ECG, indicating a posterior MI pattern (large R waves in V_1 and V_2) and ST-segment elevation in the right precordial leads (eg, V_2R to V_4R).

Symptoms include elevated central venous pressure (CVP) despite normal pulmonary artery occlusive pressure (PAOP). Venous congestion, the result of the high CVP from RV failure, is the primary symptom. Treatment centers on maintaining CVP values higher than normal, up to 25 mm Hg, in order to improve blood flow through the right ventricle. In severe RV failure, less blood is pumped into the lungs, and a drop in PAOP results.

Treatment and Complications

Figs. 6-1 and 6-2 provide a simple overview of treatment for STEMI and NSTEMI, respectively. Immediate reperfusion is the main goal in treating an MI. **Table 6-3** is a summary of key treatments in ACS. Reperfusion can be either in the cardiac catheterization lab or via a thrombolytic drug. In the cath lab, a stent will be placed (perhaps a drug-eluting stent [DES], which reduces the rate of reocclusion) to reestablish reperfusion.

Pain relief is a prime objective and is usually accomplished with intravenous analgesics such as **morphine sulfate**. Vasodilators such as **nitroglycerin** may be used but may also produce unwanted hypotension and may not relieve pain.

TABLE 6-3. THROMBOLYTIC AND OTHER THERAPIES USED IN TREATING ACS

Drug Class	*Examples of Drugs*	*Dose and Route*
Antiplatelet	Clopidogrel (Plavix)	Loading Dose of 600 mg followed by maintenance dose of 75 mg daily. A lower dose of 300 mg should be considered in patients after fibrinolytic therapy.
	Aspirin	160–325 mg PO chewable. Maintenance dose of 75–100 mg orally daily.
	Prasugrel	Loading Dose of 60 mg orally; followed by maintenance dose of 10 mg. In patients with body weight <60 kg, a maintenance dose of 5 mg orally daily is recommended.
	Ticagrelor	In patients ≥7 5 years of age, a dose of 5 mg orally daily can be used if deemed necessary. Loading dose of 180 mg orally, MD of 90 mg orally twice daily. Maybe chewed for faster action.
Antithrombin	Direct thrombin inhibitors	For pts who receive UFH, repeat activated clotting time (ACT). If ACT is not in therapeutic range, then give 0.75 mg/kg IV bolus then 1.75 mg/kg/h IV infusion.
	Bivalirudin	For patients who have not received previous anticoagulant therapy; 0.75 mg/kg bolus, 1.75 mg/kg/h IV infusion.
	Argatroban	200 µg/kg/min IV; Then 15 µg/kg/min IV Infusion. For patients who have not received previous anticoagulant therapy; 350 µg/kg/min IV; Then 15 µg/kg/min IV Infusion.
Anticoagulants	Unfractionated heparin	Weight-based IV bolus (approx. 2000–5000 U) to achieve an ACT of 250–300 s.
	Enoxaparin (Lovenox)	0.5–0.75 mg/kg IV bolus.
	Warfarin (Coumadin)	PO dose to maintain INR of 2.5–3.5.
Thrombolytics	Alteplase	Weight > 67 kg: 15-mg IV bolus followed by 50-mg infusion over 30 min, then 35-mg infusion over the following 60 min for a total of 100 mg over 120 min.
	Reteplase	
	Tenecteplase (TNKase)	Weight < 67 kg: 15-mg IV bolus followed by 0.75-mg/kg infusion over 30 min (not to exceed 50 mg), then 0.5-mg/kg infusion over the following 60 min (not to exceed 35 mg).
		10 U IV over 2 min followed in 30 min by a second injection of 10 U IV over 2 min.
		Weight-based IV injection: range of 30–50 mg. Do not exceed 50 mg.
GP IIb/IIIa inhibitors: all have reduced dosages with renal impairment	Abciximab (ReoPro)	0.25-mg/kg IV bolus followed by 0.125 µg/kg/min for 12 h. Max of 10 g/min infusion for 12 h.
	Eptifibatide (Integrilin)	180-mg IV bolus (repeat 180-mg IV bolus after 10 min for PCI patients) followed by 2 µg/kg/min for 18 h.
	Tirofiban (Aggrastat)	Bolus of 25 µg/kg over 3 min. Maintenance infusion of 0.15 µg/kg/min for up to 18 h.
	Cangrelor	Bolus of 30 µg/kg. Maintenance infusion of 4 µg/kg/min for at least 2 h or duration of procedure whichever is longer.
Beta blocker	Atenolol	5–10 mg IV, 100 mg PO daily.
	Metoprolol	15 mg IV, then 50–100 mg daily.

Thrombolytic Therapy. If the patient cannot get to a cath lab for a primary percutaneous coronary intervention (PCI) within 120 minutes (from first medical contact), thrombolysis is the treatment of choice. Thrombolytics require clear evidence of MI before they are administered. Usually at least ST-segment elevation or a new left bundle branch block is required for treatment.

Nursing care of the patient with thrombolytic therapy centers on reducing potential episodes of bleeding. Only those arterial punctures and venipunctures that are absolutely necessary should be performed. Finger oximetry should be employed, for example, rather than drawing blood gases to obtain a Pao_2 level. If venipuncture must be performed, extra time must be spent holding the site to achieve hemostasis. Avoidance of automated blood pressure cuffs is encouraged, owing to severe bruising from the high cuff pressures associated with automated systems.

It is important to assess the patient for signs of bleeding. Hypotension, tachycardia, or specific organ changes (ie, reduced level of consciousness) are indicators of possible bleeding.

Reperfusion dysrhythmias are common. Bradycardias are frequently seen after infusion of thrombolytic agents. Ventricular tachycardias are also common.

Cardiac catheterization is performed as soon as possible, perhaps even during the acute MI episode. Percutaneous coronary intervention (PCI) is indicated for patients who present with symptom onset of less than 12 hours, evidence of cardiogenic shock, or hemodynamic or electrical instability. Stent placement, angioplasty, atherectomy, thrombectomy, or surgery (CABG) may be performed at this time. For patients who are not candidates for PCI may need revascularization with CABG (**Table 6-4**).

KEY CLINICAL CONCEPT

Generally speaking, "notifying the provider" is not the correct answer on the exam. However, in cases where nursing management is maximized and definitive treatment requires provider, procedural, or surgical management, consider choosing, "notify provider..." For example, in a situation involving ST elevation and ischemic chest pain refractory to morphine and nitroglycerin.

TABLE 6-4. CRITERIA FOR PCI IN MI PATIENTS

Clear Criteria
PCI should be performed in new onset LBBB or ST elevation if symptom onset <12 h earlier
Other indications: Cardiogenic shock Persistent ischemia Electrical instability Patient is not a candidate for thrombolytic therapy
Uncertain Criteria
Clinical appearance of MI but not clear based on ECG
Ongoing ischemia, heart failure, or electrical instability in patients with symptoms >12 h.
Prior CABG—dependent on which artery needs revascularization

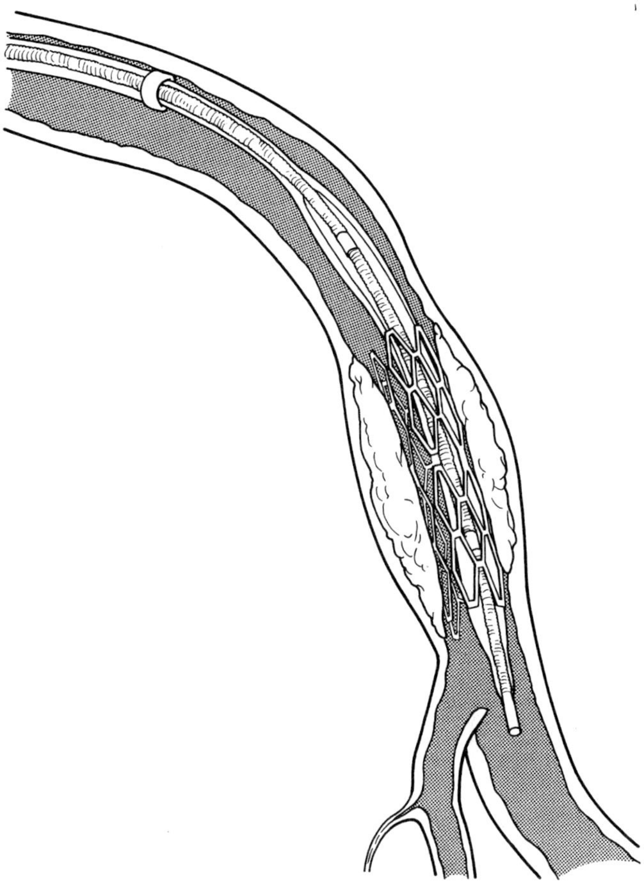

Figure 6-7. Stent inflated by a balloon.

Intracoronary Stent Placement. Stent placement has become the treatment of choice in reperfusion. A stent is a device that holds open the coronary artery where narrowing has occurred. The design of stents is continuing to evolve. A balloon is used to open the stainless-steel stent, which remains in place after the balloon is deflated (**Fig. 6-7**).

The most common problem following stent placement is the development of reocclusion due to endothelial overgrowth. This complication has been markedly reduced by the DES, which decreases and/or prevents endothelial overgrowth. This has made the DES the preferred stent. Reocclusion due to platelet activation and aggregation also results in reocclusion of the stented vessel; therefore, antiplatelet therapy is necessary following stent placement. Clopidogrel, an antiplatelet agent, is used for up to 12 months following stent placement. The DES requires antiplatelet therapy for 12 months, while bare metal stents require therapy with clopidogrel for a shorter time. The patient's ability to use clopidogrel for an extended period of time can be a determining factor for the use of angioplasty, bare metal stents, or DES.

Angioplasty. Angioplasty is the dilatation of a stenotic coronary artery through the insertion of a catheter into the artery. This technique has markedly declined in use since the development of the DES. Once the catheter is inserted, the stenotic area (identified by cardiac catheterization) is compressed by expanding a balloon at the end of the catheter. Angioplasty has the benefit of avoiding CABG while maintaining good results in expanding the stenotic area.

Nursing care of the patient treated with a stent or angioplasty includes care of the cardiac catheterization insertion site rest, immobility of the puncture site, arterial compression at the site in the event of rebleeding, distal pulse checks, and observation for signs of reocclusion (dysrhythmias). If the stenosis recurs, chest pain or symptoms of decreased cardiac output may occur.

Atherectomy and Thrombectomy. Atherectomy is removal of the atherosclerotic plaque by excision. It is not routinely performed but may be used to improve success of a PCI in patients with fibrotic or heavily calcified lesions. Thrombectomy is aspiration of the clot. In patients with diagnosis of STEMI routine thrombectomy before PCI is no longer recommended. The primary objective in these patients should be treatment with PCI.

Medical Therapy. If cardiac support is necessary, **dobutamine and milrinone** are positive inotropic (strengthening) therapies that may be used in states of low cardiac output. **Dopamine** is reserved for episodes of hypotension or at low doses (<5 μg/kg/min). If medical support is not adequate, **intra-aortic balloon pumping** has been demonstrated to effectively increase hemodynamic performance.

Vasodilators, such as **nitroglycerin or nitroprusside**, may be cautiously employed in an attempt to reduce preload and afterload. Continuous hemodynamic monitoring is necessary to accurately manipulate many of the cardiac medications. It is critical to reduce myocardial work in order to avoid episodes of congestive heart failure. The use of angiotensin-converting enzyme **(ACE) inhibitors (enalapril)** has become a key aspect of post-MI treatment because of their ability to reduce afterload (systemic vascular resistance) without increasing cardiac output. Other therapies, such as beta blockers **(labetalol)**, may also be used. However, beta blockers should be used with caution in patients who already have heart failure. Beta blockers have negative inotropic (weakening) effects on the heart. However, their effect in reducing myocardial oxygen consumption usually offsets the negative effects on the heart; therefore, they are commonly used in treating an MI.

Outpatient therapy is centered on the use of statins. These drugs have given strong indications that they can restrict the development of atherosclerosis. Statins are HMG-CoA reductase inhibitors. By blocking the conversion of HMG-CoA mevalonate kinase, they inhibit hepatic cholesterol synthesis, thus decreasing the amount of low-density lipoprotein. In addition to their impact of lipid synthesis, statins have been shown to have anti-inflammatory effects as well. This dual effect has made statins almost a required part of ongoing preventive therapy.

Continuous cardiac monitoring is used to provide for the early identification of and intervention in dysrhythmias. Dysrhythmias can be a common cause of early sudden death. If the patient survives the initial infarction and subsequently dies, death is usually due to a shock syndrome. Dysrhythmias of all types, including conduction disturbances, occur.

Oxygen therapy is indicated when Spo_2 is less than 90% or patient is experiencing dyspnea to ensure that the myocardium receives enough oxygen for its needs. An intravenous line is started for use in emergency situations. Food, usually low in sodium, is given as tolerated.

Hemodynamic monitoring must be continuous for early intervention in heart failure, ventricular failure with pulmonary edema, and cardiogenic shock. Bed rest and emotional support are necessary to help heal the injured myocardium. Use of platelet inhibitors to decrease clotting is part of standard therapy. Currently, low-dose **aspirin** (325 mg) appears adequate to avoid early reocclusion.

Long-term immobility may result in venous pooling, with an increased risk of thromboembolism. Passive and active range-of-motion exercises and sequential compression devices help reduce this risk.

Less common but equally lethal complications of an MI include pericarditis, papillary muscle rupture, ventricular aneurysm, and ventricular rupture. These complications are generally seen 5 to 10 days following the acute infarction event. Sudden death commonly occurs with the last three of these complications.

Papillary muscle ruptures are commonly associated with anterior or inferior wall MIs. Symptoms include a new loud murmur, hemodynamic instability, and acute mitral regurgitation. Diagnosis is made by echo.

Ventricular septal ruptures are more common in patients who have experienced anterior/septal wall MIs. Symptoms of this complication include acute shortness of breath, S_3 heart tone, and crackles.

Recovery

Recovery begins as soon as myocardial injury and necrosis stop. Scar tissue develops (**Fig. 6-8**) at the necrotic area. This process takes 6 to 8 weeks to complete.

Emotional support of the patient and family is a key factor in recovery. Cardiac patients often feel that their active and productive lives are over. It is not uncommon to see the patient and family members going through the stages of grief following an MI. Symptoms of *depression* must therefore be identified early in the course and the patient referred for treatment. Recent data point to chronic illness from ACS or the recurrence of a CV event with associated depression. The nurse plays an essential role in educating the patient and family as to lifestyle changes and the elimination of alterable risk factors, thus helping both the patient and family to work through this difficult process.

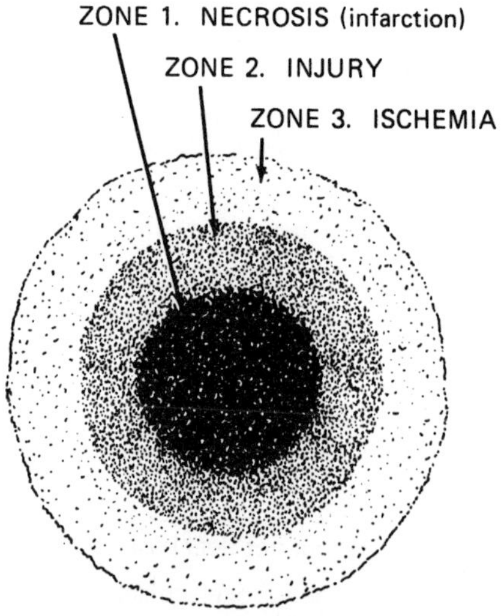

Figure 6-8. The development of scar tissue following myocardial infarction.

KEY CONTENT CHECKLIST

- ❒ The CCRN exam will not ask many questions on the pathophysiology of ACS; however, understanding the general principles for what is occurring during ACS is important.
- ❒ Prinzmetal's angina is also termed, "variant angina," and is angina due to coronary spasm and NOT CAD. Treatment may include calcium channel blockers.
- ❒ Atypical symptoms often found in African Americans and women are fatigue, shortness of breath, indigestion-type symptoms, and shoulder/back discomfort.
- ❒ Scenarios in the exam will most certainly ask you which areas of the heart are associated with specific changes on the 12-lead ECG and the signs and symptoms of each. It is important to have a good understanding of areas of the heart and the associated ECG leads for interpreting an MI.
- ❒ Understand the difference between RV MIs in comparison to LV MIs. RV MIs are typically treated with inotropes and fluids whereas LV MIs has conservative fluid administration.
- ❒ Typically, notify the provider is not the correct answer on the exam unless nursing management has been exhausted and a provider is needed for medical, surgical, or procedural intervention.

Review Questions:

1. **Inferior MIs produce conduction defects different from those seen in anterior MIs. Which type of dysrhythmia is more likely to occur in *inferior* as opposed to anterior MIs?**
   a. Second-degree type I
   b. Second-degree type II
   c. Multiform PVCs
   d. Third-degree heart block

Answer: A. Rationale: Inferior MIs are associated with dysfunction of the SA node, making option A the best answer. Options B, C, and D all impact the conduction pathway farther down as compared to option A. Option A suggests a defect on the uppermost portion of the conduction pathway compared to the other options, choose A.

2. **Which ECG change indicates an increased chance of sudden death following an MI?**
   a. Left bundle branch block (LBBB)
   b. Right bundle branch block (RBBB)
   c. Sinus tachycardia
   d. Second-degree type II heart block

Answer: A. Rationale: New-onset left bundle branch block is considered a STEMI-equivalent finding in the setting of suspected acute MI. Right bundle branch blocks are not at serious in comparison, eliminating option B. Sinus tachycardia is too vague and nonspecific of a finding, eliminating option C as well. Second-degree type II heart block may require urgent attention, however, is not as emergent as a STEMI-equivalent finding, which mandates PCI within 90 minutes unless proven otherwise. Choose A.

3. **Unstable angina (UA) is characterized by all the following features but one. Which feature does NOT characterize UA?**
   a. Increasing frequency of chest pain
   b. Chest pain at rest
   c. Increasing severity of symptoms
   d. Q-wave formation

Answer: D. Rationale: The presence of pathologic Q waves (deep and wide) indicates irreversible myocardial ischemia. All the other symptoms listed are associated with UA.

7

Conduction Blocks

CHAPTER OVERVIEW AND OBJECTIVES

Conduction blocks can be expected to be tested with one to four questions. **Often, the CCRN exam will not ask directly about conduction blocks but will put them in a clinical situation.** If you have an actual electrocardiogram (ECG) strip with a conduction block, there is likely to be only one test item.

After studying this chapter, you should understand the following:

- Differentiate the various conduction blocks and their clinical significance.
- Examine the clinical implications of bundle branch blocks (BBBs).
- Understand key pacemaker nomenclature and indications for pacing.

7.1 FIRST-DEGREE HEART BLOCK

Etiology

First-degree atrioventricular (AV) junctional block may be caused by heart disease (coronary artery disease [CAD]), acute myocardial infarction (MI), AV node ischemia, and drugs that act at the AV node (eg, digitalis). In first-degree block the AV node delays the progression of the impulse from the sinoatrial (SA) node for an abnormal length of time, but all impulses are conducted (**Fig. 7-1**).

Identifying Characteristics

The rate is normal; the rhythm is regular; P waves are normal; and the PR interval is prolonged beyond 0.20 seconds. The QRS complex is normal, and conduction is normal except for the prolonged delay at the AV node.

Risk

First-degree block is not a serious dysrhythmia in itself. It may progress to a second-degree type I block and, less commonly, to a second-degree type II or third-degree block; however, this is not common.

Treatment

If the PR interval is less than 0.25 seconds and it does not increase, no treatment may be required. The length of the PR interval is not as significant as the effect on stroke volume and heart rate. No treatment is indicated unless a bradycardia results.

Nursing Intervention

Document the dysrhythmia with a rhythm strip. Monitor the patient closely for progression to a slower heart rate or a worsening block. If progression develops, document with a rhythm strip and notify the physician immediately.

7.2 SECOND-DEGREE BLOCK TYPES I AND II

The terms Mobitz I and Wenckebach (named after cardiac physiologists of the early twentieth century) are sometimes used instead of type I. Mobitz II is also used in place of type II. These terms are not used in this section, although it is helpful to remember that you may see them on the exam or in clinical practice.

Both types I and II are AV junctional blocks. The AV node delays the progression of the SA node impulse for longer than normal and the AV node halts progression of some SA node

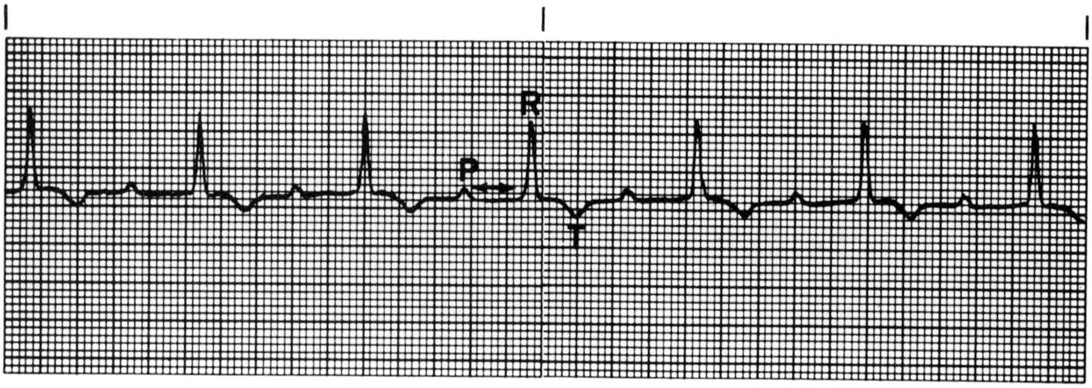

Figure 7-1. First-degree AV heart block.

impulses, which never reach the ventricular conduction system. The characteristics, treatment, and prognosis for these two forms of second-degree AV block differ. The type I form of second-degree block is considered first.

Second-Degree Type I

Etiology. Conduction arises normally from the SA node and progresses to the AV node. With each succeeding impulse, it becomes more difficult for the AV node to conduct the impulse. Eventually, one impulse is not conducted and a QRS complex does not occur. The progression then begins again. Ischemia or injury to the AV node is the cause of this progression (**Fig. 7-2**).

Identifying Characteristics. The following are the key components of second-degree type I heart block:

1. A progressive prolongation of the PR interval
2. A progressive shortening of the R to R interval before each pause
3. A pause in the ventricular rhythm that is less than twice the PP interval or sinus cycle length
4. The cycle repeats itself and the length of the PR interval following the dropped QRS should match the first PR interval in the cycle.

Risk. *Second-degree type I is often a temporary block following an acute MI.* It may, however, progress to a complete (third-degree) block. For this reason, second-degree type I is considered a potentially dangerous dysrhythmia, although by itself it usually does not produce a clinical problem.

Treatment. Frequently no treatment is indicated. If the ventricular rate is slow, **atropine** may increase AV conduction. Epinephrine may be used to increase the rate of the SA node and thus the overall rate. On occasion, an external pacemaker or temporary transvenous pacemaker may be inserted.

Nursing Intervention. Document the dysrhythmia with a rhythm strip. Monitor the patient, although this dysrhythmia is normally not clinically significant. If the ventricular rate slows enough to produce symptoms, notify the physician.

> QUICK TIP! Generally speaking, bradycardia does not require treatment in exam scenarios unless it is symptomatic (causing dizziness, diaphoresis, chest pain, hypotension, etc).

Second-Degree Type II

Etiology. An impulse originates in SA node and progresses normally to the AV node. Below the AV node in the common bundle or bundle branches, impulses are blocked on a regular basis, with every second, third, or fourth impulse not being conducted. In this block, a QRS complex is regularly missing. This dysrhythmia is due to disease of the AV node, the AV junctional tissue, or the His–Purkinje system (**Fig. 7-3**).

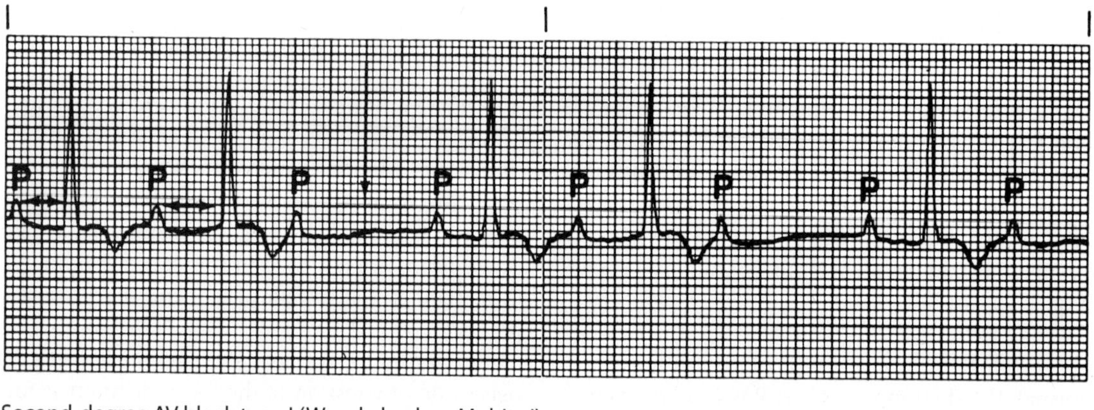

Figure 7-2. Second-degree AV block type I (Wenckebach or Mobitz I).

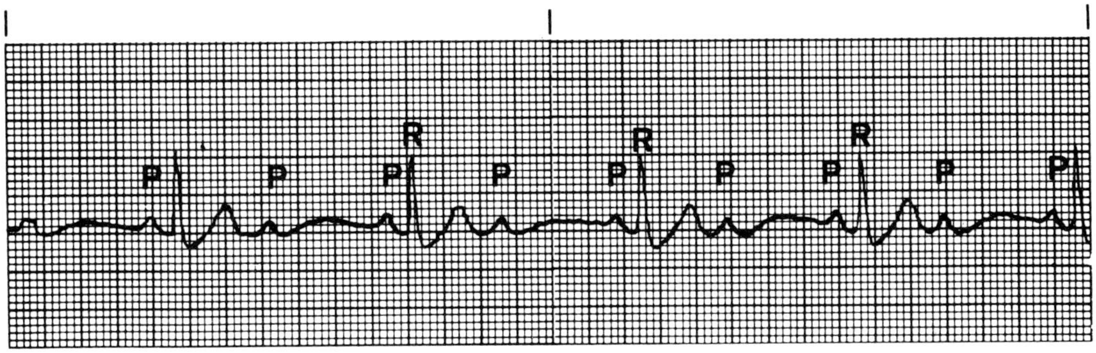

Figure 7-3. Second-degree AV block type II.

Identifying Characteristics. The atrial rate may be normal. The ventricular rate is usually one-half or one-third of the atrial rate (referred to as 2:1 or 3:1 block). At times, the block rate may be even greater than 3:1. The ventricular rate depends on the frequency of the block. (In 4:1 block, there are four atrial beats to every one QRS complex.)

- The atrial rhythm is regular.
- Ventricular rhythm is regular if the frequency of the block remains consistent or it may be irregular if the frequency of the block is inconsistent.
- P waves are normal and will look the same even when the QRS complex is dropped.
- The PR interval is constant whenever it can be measured.
- The QRS complex may be normal or widened.
- Conduction is normal in the atria and may be abnormal in the ventricles.

Risk. Type II block is unpredictable and may suddenly advance to complete heart block or ventricular standstill; *this is especially common after inferior infarction* and is a dangerous warning dysrhythmia.

Treatment. If the ventricular response is slow, **atropine or epinephrine** may be tried. Because the condition is so unpredictable, a temporary pacemaker is often the treatment of choice. A permanent pacemaker is frequently necessary.

Nursing Intervention. Document the dysrhythmia with a rhythm strip. Determine the width of the QRS complex. Monitor the patient closely for a widening of the QRS complex. The width of the QRS complex indicates the location in the conduction system of the block. The wider the complex, the lower in the bundle branch system the block will be. Document the widening, if it occurs, with a rhythm strip, notify the physician immediately, and prepare for the insertion of a transvenous pacemaker or use of an external pacemaker. Assess the patient frequently for hemodynamic compromise if the ventricular response is slow (3:1 and 4:1 block).

Although types I and II heart blocks are differentiated by the changes in the PR interval, another feature is important to bear in mind with these two types of dysrhythmias. Consider that the *right coronary artery* is responsible for feeding the AV node in most of the population. In addition, the *right coronary artery* supplies the inferior region of the left ventricle. Therefore, in **inferior MIs,** a common dysrhythmia is AV block, specifically second-degree type I block. Clinically this is relevant, since type I blocks may appear like type II blocks (ie, in 2:1 patterns). These 2:1 blocks are generally less dangerous, though, because the bundle branches remain intact. If a pacemaker is required, a temporary one will usually suffice.

Anterior MIs are different, however, in their effect of producing type II blocks. An **anterior MI** is usually the result of obstruction of the *left anterior descending (LAD) artery.* This artery also feeds the left and right bundle branches. In the presence of an **anterior MI,** a type II block may also appear in a 2:1 pattern. This pattern is more dangerous with an **anterior MI,** since the block is due to loss of ventricular conduction system, that is, the left and/or right bundle system. Type II blocks, especially in the presence of an **anterior MI,** may require more attention as they can rapidly progress to third-degree heart block. Pacemakers for this dysrhythmia are usually permanent.

KEY CLINICAL CONCEPT

Inferior MIs are generally caused by a blockage of the right coronary artery and may result in AV blocks, specifically a second-degree type I block. An anterior MI is generally caused by blockage of the LAD and may result in a second-degree type II block that may progress to a third-degree block.

7.3 THIRD-DEGREE BLOCK—COMPLETE HEART BLOCK

Etiology

Ischemia or injury to the AV node, junctional tissue, or His–Purkinje tissue is the cause of complete heart block. The ischemia may be secondary to CAD, acute MI, drug use (eg, digitalis toxicity, cocaine), systemic disease, or electrolyte imbalances (especially in renal patients) (**Fig. 7-4**).

Identifying Characteristics

Atrial rates are faster than ventricular rates. P waves are not conducted through the AV node. The ventricular rate is 30 to 40 (unless there is a junctional escape mechanism). The rhythm is regular for both the atria and the ventricles; therefore, your

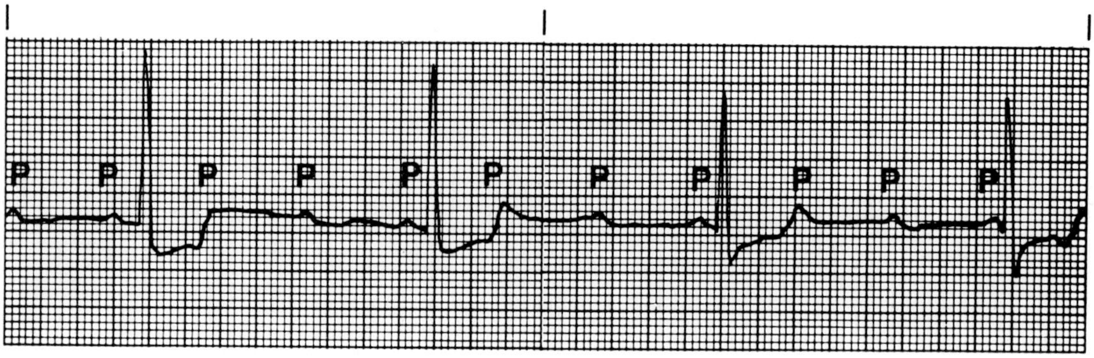

Figure 7-4. Third-degree (complete) AV block.

P-P intervals and R-R intervals will march out even though they are depolarizing completely independently of one another. P waves are normal and not associated with a QRS complex so they may appear all throughout the cardiac cycle. The PR interval is not constant. QRS complexes are close to normal if they arise near the AV node. The QRS complex may be wide and bizarre if the impulse arises from the ventricles. There is no AV conduction. The atrial pacemaker controls the atria, and the ventricular pacemaker controls the ventricles, this is known as an AV dissociation (see Figure 7-4).

Risk

The main danger of third-degree heart block is the possibility that bradycardia will produce a decrease in cardiac output, leading to hypotension and myocardial ischemia. The loss of AV synchrony in third-degree block is a key reason for the decrease in cardiac output. *Third-degree heart block is a potentially lethal dysrhythmia. Additionally, there is a risk of ventricular standstill if there is no escape mechanism from the junction or ventricles.*

Treatment

Immediate pacemaker insertion is the treatment of choice. A temporary or transcutaneous pacing may be tried initially until the presence of the block has been determined to be permanent. *Complete heart block may be temporary after MI,* and pacing should be available for several days after the return of a normal sinus rhythm.

Nursing Intervention

Document the dysrhythmia with a rhythm strip and notify the physician immediately. Monitor the patient for signs of ventricular failure and hypotension. Hemodynamic status is compromised by the slow ventricular rate, and circulatory collapse is not uncommon.

7.4 ATRIOVENTRICULAR DISSOCIATION

Many conditions can be termed AV dissociation. Ventricular tachycardia and conduction defects where the atrial and ventricular rhythms do not match can all be examples of AV dissociation. Some clinicians make the mistake of using the term "third-degree block" synonymously with "AV dissociation"; however, third-degree block is only one form of AV dissociation.

Etiology

The many causes of AV dissociation include anesthesia, medications, infections, acute MI, and ischemic heart disease (**Fig. 7-5**).

Identifying Characteristics

The PR interval is inconsistent, since the atrial and ventricular pacemakers are independent of one another. The P wave, usually normal in form, may vary slightly in measurements. The P wave may fall immediately before, during, or after a QRS complex during the absolute refractory period of the ventricles

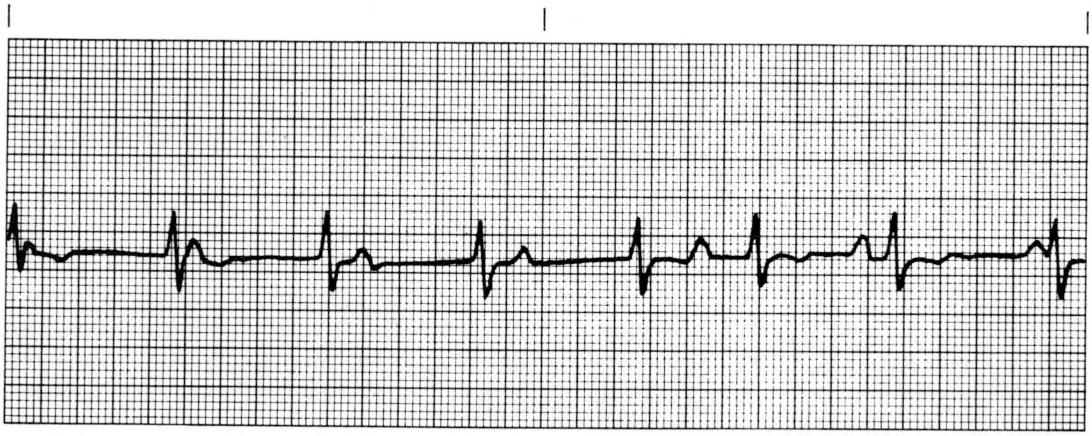

Figure 7-5. One type of AV dissociation.

(the period in which they cannot depolarize). The QRS complex may be normal or abnormal, depending on whether the ventricular pacemaker is at or below the bundle of His.

Risk

AV dissociation by itself is significant, since atrial and ventricular contractions are not in synchrony. The loss of synchrony can produce a substantial reduction in cardiac output. However, rather than treat AV dissociation, the underlying rhythm producing AV dissociation should be addressed.

Treatment

Treatment is dependent on the underlying rhythm and the effect on hemodynamics. Treatments range from pacemakers for bradycardias to antidysrhythmics for ventricular tachycardia.

Nursing Intervention

Monitor the patient closely for signs of cardiac decompensation and progression of the dysrhythmia. Document the dysrhythmia with a rhythm strip and notify the physician.

TABLE 7-1. CRITERIA FOR VENTRICULAR CONDUCTION DEFECTS

Condition	*Lead*	*QRS Appearance*
Right bundle branch block	V_1 or V_2	rSR′, rsr′, rsR′
	I and V_6	Deep S wave
Left bundle branch block	I and V_6	Wide QRS (>0.12)
	I and V_6	Notched QRS
	V_1	QS wave
Left Anterior fascicular block	I, aVF	Left axis > 30 degrees
	I, aVL	Initial Q wave
	II, III, aVF	Small R wave, deep S wave
Left Posterior fascicular block	I, aVL	Deep S wave
		Right axis
	I, aVL	Initial R wave
	III, aVF	Large R wave

7.5 BUNDLE BRANCH BLOCKS

BBBs are also termed intraventricular conduction defects. There may be a right or left BBB. In addition, the left bundle has two divisions, referred to as fascicles. These fascicles may also become blocked. Obstructions of the fascicles are termed hemiblocks. There may be a left anterior hemiblock of the anterior fascicle of the left bundle branch or there may be a left posterior hemiblock of the posterior fascicle of the left bundle branch. Trifascicular blocks involve both left bundle fascicles and the right bundle branch. Bifascicular blocks usually involve the right bundle branch and one fascicle of the left bundle branch or both fascicles of the left branch. BBBs may be suspected by observing a rhythm strip (due to a wide QRS or abnormal QRS configuration) but *cannot* be diagnosed by a rhythm strip. A 12-lead ECG is necessary to diagnose a BBB.

Criteria for diagnosing conduction defects are listed in **Table 7-1**. It is useful to identify conduction defects for several reasons, ranging from identifying areas of disease in the heart to assessing the significance of injury patterns. In addition, it is helpful to interpret conduction defects, particularly right BBBs, in differentiating atrial premature contractions with aberrant conduction from PVCs.

> QUICK TIP! The need to distinguish between an RBBB versus an LBBB on an ECG tracing rarely, if ever, appears on the exam. However, be aware of the clinical significance. For example, new-onset LBBB is considered MI-equivalent until proven otherwise.

Etiology

Several different factors may cause a BBB. For example, an acute MI may cause ischemia in the intraventricular conduction system. This is probably the most common cause. However, other factors, such as chronic degeneration with fibrous scarring, may permanently block the bundle branches, or such blocks may be congenital or rate-dependent (ie, they appear only at certain heart rates).

Identifying Characteristics

Rate is usually normal, although it may vary if the BBB varies. Rhythm is regular. P waves may be normal. The PR interval is normal. The QRS complex is wide (>0.12 s) and may be notched, depending on the lead viewed.

Risk

The development of BBBs indicates marked ischemia of the intraventricular conduction system, and BBBs are potentially more dangerous than AV blocks, since these blocks are subjunctional. The involvement of more than one fascicle often progresses to complete heart block. In these instances, the prognosis is poor.

Treatment

It is not uncommon for the BBB to cause no symptoms. Because of the lack of symptoms, most BBBs require no direct treatment. Many patients tolerate conduction defects such as BBBs for long periods of time without developing any problems. The potential danger of the BBB, however, is that it can deteriorate into a more severe obstruction, such as complete heart block. In this case, the treatment is focused on improving the heart rate, as with atropine or a pacemaker. Chronic BBB associated with systolic failure (*ejection fraction* [EF] < 40%) can lead to ventricular dyssynchrony and symptoms of *heart failure* (HF). Biventricular pacemakers can be implanted in HF patients already on maximal medical HF treatment in order to improve ventricular synchrony and symptoms. However, questions about biventricular pacemakers are not likely to appear on the exam.

Nursing Intervention

The primary consideration is to identify the conduction defect and document the type of block. Notify the physician if the block is new. Monitor the rhythm and be aware of the potential for a bradycardia, such as complete heart block, to develop.

QUICK TIP!

- The CCRN exam can have one to four questions on cardiac conduction defects. This section provides an overview of how these conduction problems identified and treated.
- For more information on BBBs, see the complete review in Chapter 4.

7.6 PACEMAKERS

There are many pathologic states that may be most efficiently treated by the use of an artificial pacemaker. Pacemakers may be particularly useful in the treatment of symptomatic bradycardias that have not responded to **atropine or epinephrine**.

KEY CLINICAL CONCEPT

- For the purposes of the CCRN, pacemakers do not have to be understood in great depth. There have been remarkable advances in pacemakers, ranging from very simple ones to complex pacemaker/defibrillators. This section focuses on what you need to know for the exam and most critical care situations.
- The three primary abnormal pacemaker rhythms to be familiar with are **(1) failure to fire** (no spike when there should be one), **(2) failure to sense** (spikes appearing in inappropriate places), and **(3) failure to capture** (a spike with no R wave after it)

Definition

A pacemaker is a system consisting of a lead and a pulse generator. The generator is capable of producing repeated, timed bursts of electrical current for a prolonged period of time. The bursts of electrical current are of sufficient magnitude to initiate depolarization of the heart.

Modes of Pacing

There are two modes of pacing. Temporary pacing is the mode used mainly to manage emergencies such as acute heart block and cardiac arrest. There are two types of temporary pacemakers: transvenous and transcutaneous (external). In the transvenous or mode, the lead is inserted into the right atrium or ventricle. The pulse generator is external. Insertion routes include the transvenous (brachial via cutdown), subclavian, femoral, or jugular (via percutaneous entry), and postsurgical (endocardial). The power supply for temporary pacing is an external battery (the pulse generator). For a specific insertion procedure, the nurse is referred to their institution's policy.

Transcutaneous cardiac pacing has gained increasing acceptance and works by sending direct current transcutaneously between electrodes placed on the skin. The advantages of transcutaneous pacing is the ease of use (it can be applied in a matter of minutes) and the fact that no invasive equipment is necessary, such as the difficulty associated with inserting the transvenous wire.

In the transcutaneous mode of pacing, the nurse must be aware of the *potential for some discomfort* to the patient because of the electrical stimulation, which will cause superficial as well as cardiac muscle contraction. Some conscious patients may complain of pain on stimulation, particularly if the milliampere (mA) setting (energy delivered) is high. *Sedatives or analgesics may be required.*

Permanent pacing with a fully implantable system is a second mode of pacing the heart. The pulse generator, which is implanted into the patient, contains the circuit for the specific pacing mode selected and a battery that provides energy to the circuit. The components are encased in a nonconductive plastic material that does not react with body tissue.

Indications for Pacing

The major indication for pacing is the development of second-degree type II or third-degree heart block. *Pacemakers can be used for any bradycardia that is producing hypotension or signs of reduced cardiac output.*

Chronic heart block of varied degrees may be treated by pacing if the patient has syncopal episodes, HF, convulsions, or evidence of cerebral dysfunction.

Intermittent complete heart block (third degree) is often treated with a pacemaker. Usually there is evidence of block in one or two of the three bundle branches (fascicles). Thus, these patients rely solely on the third fascicle, which may become dysfunctional at any time.

Complete heart block that develops in conjunction with an acute MI may be an indication for pacing. If the infarction is **anterior, the involved artery is usually the LAD.** This results in ischemia or necrosis of part of the ventricular septum with damage to the intraventricular conduction system below the His bundle. These patients may die despite the insertion of a pacemaker because of the extent of myocardial damage. If the infarction is **posterior or inferior**, the artery involved is usually the **right coronary** (90% of the time) or the **circumflex** (10% of the time). The area of damage is the AV node area. Types I and II may be indications for pacing. Type I may progress into a type II (2:1) or higher block. Type II, because it occurs below the AV node, often progresses into third-degree heart block. A block that develops after infarction is usually transient and responds to atropine or a brief period of time with a temporary pacemaker.

Conduction defects may occur after a cardiac surgical procedure. For this reason, most cardiac surgeries (eg, coronary artery bypass grafting) include the use of pacing wires attached to the epicardium for postoperative management. Some centers also use a pacing port through a pulmonary artery catheter.

Pacemakers may be used in other rhythm disturbances if bradycardia is a component of the dysrhythmia. Sick sinus syndrome indicates dysfunction of the SA node. This may occur as sinus bradycardia, sinus arrest, and/or brady–tachy syndromes.

Pacemakers may also be used to treat tachydysrhythmias, such as atrial or ventricular tachycardia. In these rhythms, the pacemaker rate is increased to a level higher than the tachycardia. Once the pacemaker is controlling the rate, the rate is slowed to a more acceptable level. This is known as overdrive pacing.

A pacemaker may be used as a diagnostic aid to evaluate SA node and AV node function. They may be used to eliminate multiple ectopic foci by overriding the rate of the foci, or they

TABLE 7-2. FIVE-POSITION PACEMAKER CODE

I. Chamber Paced	*II. Chamber Sensed*	*III. Mode of Response*	*IV. Rate Modulation*	*V. Multisite Pacing*
V = ventricle	V = ventricle	I = inhibited	R = Rate modulation	O = None
A = atrium	A = atrium	T = triggered		A = Atrium
D = atrium and ventricle (dual)	D = atrium and ventricle (dual)	D = atrial triggered and ventricular inhibited		V = Ventricle
	O = none	O = none	O = none	external = Dual (A + V)

may be used to abolish reentry phenomena by delivering a premature stimulus that breaks the reentry pattern.

Types of Pacing Modes

There are several types of pacing modes. These are categorized according to the Inter-Society Commission on Heart Disease (ICHD) nomenclature, given in **Table 7-2**. There are two codes: a simplified three-letter one and more comprehensive five-letter code. Table 7-2 contains the five-letter code. In the CCRN exam, only a few pacing modes may be addressed. *As a rule, the CCRN exam requires you to remember only the simpler three-letter code.*

The major concept to remember is that the pacemaker electrically paces a cardiac chamber (*the first letter*), senses an electrical impulse in a cardiac chamber (*the second letter*), and discharges the impulse in either a triggered or inhibited manner (*the third letter*). In critical care, the inhibited manner is almost always used.

If a patient had a transvenous pacemaker inserted that would pace and sense only in the ventricle, the ICHD description would be a VVI. If the pacemaker paced both atrium and ventricle but sensed only in the ventricle, the pacemaker would be a DVI (AV sequential) pacemaker.

QUICK TIP! For the purposes of the exam, the main three-letter modes to know are VVI, AAI, DDD, DOO, and to a lesser-extent DVI

Nursing Care

The patient with a temporary pacemaker will need documentation as to the effectiveness of rhythm capture and sensing. The electrical signal indicating that a pacemaker impulse has occurred should be evident only immediately prior to capturing a paced beat (**Fig. 7-6**). If a pacemaker signal is present and the heart is not in a refractory mode, a captured beat should follow. If no beat occurs, this would be called **failure to capture** (**Fig. 7-7**). Causes of failure to capture include loose or inadequate connections, low/dead batteries, low voltage (mA), or improper positioning of the leads. **Failure to sense** would be a paced beat or pacemaker artifact occurring too soon after a spontaneous beat. The spontaneous beat should inhibit the next paced impulse; if it does not, **failure to sense** is present (**Fig. 7-8**). Causes of failure to sense can be the position of the lead but most commonly is due to incorrect sensitivity settings. If no pacemaker spikes occur at all or do not appear where they should, **"failure to fire"** (also called, **"failure to pace"**) is present. Causes of failure to fire may include dead batteries, loose connections, incorrect settings and lead dislodgment. Notify the physician if either of these conditions occurs more than once.

Care of the pacemaker insertion site is the same as for any central intravenous catheter. It is important to explain the purpose and duration of the pacemaker carefully in order to avoid causing the patient unnecessary anxiety.

KEY CLINICAL CONCEPT

The major concept to remember is that the pacemaker electrically paces a cardiac chamber (the first letter), senses an electrical impulse in a cardiac chamber (the second letter), and discharges the impulse in either a triggered or inhibited manner (the third letter)

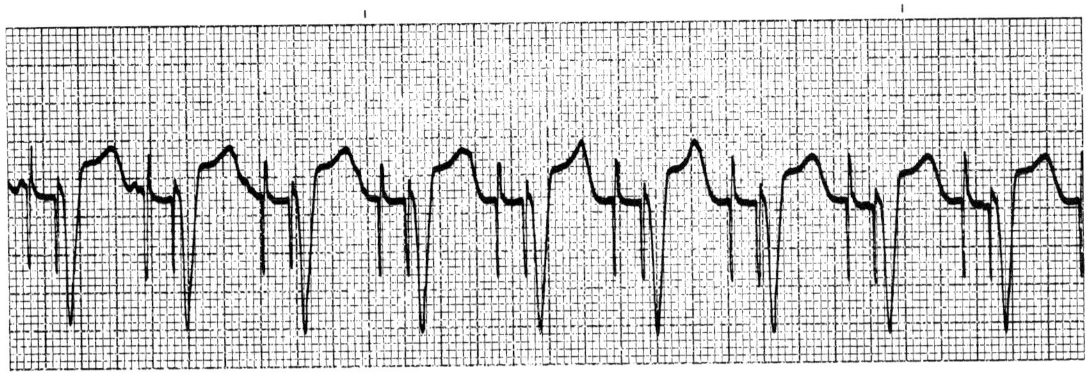

Figure 7-6. Normal pacemaker (DVI) electrical pattern.

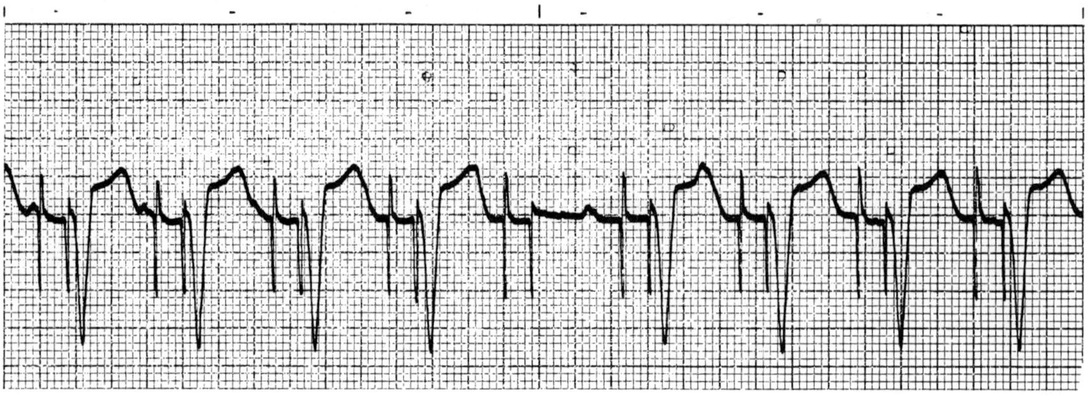

Figure 7-7. Failure of pacemaker to capture.

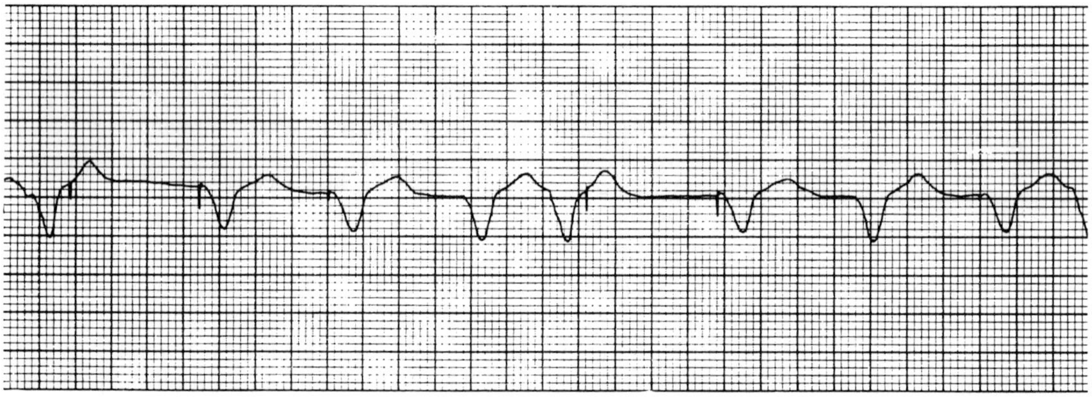

Figure 7-8. Failure of pacemaker to sense.

KEY CONTENT CHECKLIST

- Often, the CCRN exam will not ask directly about conduction blocks but will put them in a clinical situation.
- The CCRN exam can have one to four questions on cardiac conduction defects. For more information on BBBs, see the complete review in Chapter 4.
- Generally speaking, bradycardia does not require treatment in exam scenarios unless it is symptomatic (causing dizziness, diaphoresis, chest pain, hypotension, etc).
- The need to distinguish between an RBBB versus an LBBB on an ECG tracing rarely, if ever, appears on the exam. However, be aware of the clinical significance. For example, new-onset LBBB is considered MI-equivalent until proven otherwise.
- Inferior MIs are generally caused by a blockage of the right coronary artery and may result in AV blocks, specifically a second-degree type I block. An anterior MI is generally caused by blockage of the LAD and may result in a second-degree type II block that may progress to a third-degree block.
- Third-degree heart block is a potentially lethal dysrhythmia. Additionally, there is a risk of ventricular standstill if there is no escape mechanism from the junction or ventricles.
- For the purposes of the CCRN, pacemakers do not have to be understood in great depth.
- Pacemakers can be used for any bradycardia that is producing hypotension or signs of reduced cardiac output.
- The three primary abnormal pacemaker rhythms to be familiar with are **(1) failure to fire** (no spike when there should be one), **(2) failure to sense** (spikes appearing in inappropriate places), and **(3) failure to capture** (a spike with no R wave after it).
- The major concept to remember is that the pacemaker electrically paces a cardiac chamber (the first letter), senses an electrical impulse in a cardiac chamber (the second letter), and discharges the impulse in either a triggered or inhibited manner (the third letter).
- For the purposes of the exam, the main three-letter modes to know are VVI, AAI, DDD, DOO, and to a lesser-extent DVI.

Review Questions:

1. **Which of the following is NOT an example of AV dissociation?**
   a. Ventricular tachycardia
   b. Third-degree heart block
   c. First-degree heart block
   d. Atrial tachycardia with 2:1 block

Answer: C. Rationale: In this negatively stated question, it is asking, "AV dissociation is present in each of these options EXCEPT..." Options B and D can be eliminated quickly because third-degree block is complete A–V dissociation and atrial tachycardia with 2:1 block suggest AV block every other beat. VT can also be ruled out as P waves in VT are either not present or unable to assess, so eliminate A as well. Be careful not to be misled by the name "first-degree block," even though it is a part of the heart block continuum, no AV dissociation exists with this rhythm. Choose C.

2. **Which type of medication is common in the treatment of unstable angina?**
   a. Diuretics
   b. Inotropic agents
   c. Beta blockers
   d. Sympathetic stimulants

Answer: C. Rationale: Beta blockers are considered antianginal medications since they decrease heart rate, thereby lowering myocardial oxygen demands. Option A is used to decrease preload in patients with heart failure but does not affect angina. Options B and D are both sympathetic stimulants would likely worsen the angina.

3. **A patient is admitted with presyncope and chest pain. Which one of the symptoms below would make the RN suspect the patient may have aortic stenosis?**
   a. Fatigue
   b. Palpitations
   c. Shortness of breath
   d. Unexplained weight loss

Answer: C. Rationale: The triad of symptoms in severe aortic stenosis is syncope or presyncope, chest pain (angina), and shortness of breath (due to reduction in LV cardiac output). Fatigue and palpitations can happen in a number of disease processes including aortic stenosis, but they are not major symptoms of aortic stenosis, eliminating options A and B. Unexplained weight loss is not typically seen in aortic stenosis (however, perhaps in TB or oncology), eliminating option D.

8

(Congestive) Heart Failure, Pulmonary Edema, and Hypertensive Crisis

CHAPTER OVERVIEW AND OBJECTIVES

The assessment of abnormal hemodynamics, particularly regarding left ventricular (LV) and right ventricular (RV) failure, is a common topic for questions in the CCRN exam. **However, the focus of the exam is on acute heart failure (HF) rather than the management of chronic HF.** This chapter reviews the major concepts normally employed in the assessment of acute ventricular failure as well as its diagnosis and associated interventions. Expect several questions on the CCRN exam from this content area.

After studying this chapter, you should be able to:

- Understand the two main types of HF including the associated symptoms, common assessment findings, and treatments.
- Differentiate signs and symptoms of RV HF and LV HF.
- Identify the clinical symptoms and management of hypertensive crisis.

It is important to understand advances HF research in the course of studying conditions such as HF, pulmonary edema, and hypertensive crisis. The management of these conditions begins long before intensive care unit (ICU) admission. However, in order to understand hospital treatment of HF (formerly referred to as "congestive heart failure" [CHF]), pulmonary edema, and hypertensive crisis, it is helpful to understand the disease process of HF in general. An overview of HF, along with contributing factors such as hypertension, will provide a better understanding of the assessment and treatment of HF overall.

Before discussing the specific clinical conditions of HF, pulmonary edema, and hypertension, the factors that regulate cardiac output (ie, *preload, afterload, and contractility*) will be reviewed. Ventricular failure can be assessed and treated by regulating these three components. Although ventricular failure can be assessed by noting each component of cardiac output, each ventricle is assessed slightly differently. For example, *preload of the left ventricle* is partially assessed by the **pulmonary artery occlusive (or wedge) pressure (PAOP)**, while *preload of the right ventricle* is assessed by the **central venous pressure (CVP)**. Other factors used to differentiate LV and RV influences are listed in **Table 8-1**.

The specific pressures frequently used in the assessment of ventricular preload are listed in **Table 8-2**.

QUICK TIP! Although the pressures in Table 8-2 are general examples, the CCRN exam is likely to utilize values such as these when clinical scenarios are provided in situations describing ventricular failure. The CCRN will not expect you to act on "borderline" hemodynamic pressures.

More sophisticated measures to estimate cardiac performance, such as echocardiography, are available. However, the basic guidelines listed in Tables 8-1 and 8-2 are useful in assessing cardiac performance in most clinical practice settings. Because of the common application of these concepts, it is helpful to understand their role in clinical assessment.

QUICK TIP! Table 8-2 lists reference ranges for hemodynamic pressures. On the exam, these values will appear extreme (ie, very high or very low) if they are relevant to the question. For example, a CVP of 1 to 2 or a PAOP of >20.

8.1 HEART FAILURE

HF is the inability of the heart to pump blood through the systemic circulation in an amount sufficient to meet the body's needs. HF normally refers to biventricular failure, although it is important

TABLE 8-1. METHODS TO ASSESS LEFT AND RIGHT VENTRICULAR PERFORMANCE

Parameter	*Right Ventricle*	*Left Ventricle*
Preload	CVP	PAOP
Afterload	PVR	SVR
Contractility	Ejection fraction, peak velocity	Ejection fraction, peak velocity

CVP, central venous pressure; PAOP, pulmonary artery occlusive (wedge) pressure; PVR, pulmonary vascular resistance; SVR, systemic vascular resistance.

TABLE 8-2. USE OF THE PULMONARY ARTERY OCCLUSIVE (WEDGE) PRESSURE (PAOP) AND CENTRAL VENOUS PRESSURE (CVP)

Value	*Stroke Index*	*Condition Indicated*
PAOP		
<8	<25	Hypovolemia
8–12	25–45	Normal
12–18	<35	Beginning failure or fluid overload
>18	<25	LV failure
CVP		
0–5	<25–45	Normal or hypovolemia
5–10	25–45	Beginning failure or fluid overload
>10	<25	RV failure

to understand that each ventricle can fail independently of the other. LV failure is a common precursor to RV failure and can precede RV dysfunction. RV failure is frequently associated with lung disease or dysfunction, or it may be the result of ischemia of the right-sided coronary circulation. **RV failure will produce LV hypovolemia by failing to move blood through the lungs.**

HF is categorized in stages, that is, A through D (**Table 8-3**). Management of HF is summarized in **Table 8-4**. Management with guideline-directed medical therapy (GDMT) is imperative in keeping patients out of the hospital and controlling their symptoms. HF is the gradual inability of the heart to pump sufficient blood to meet the body's demands. HF can become acute without an obvious cause or may be precipitated by an acute ischemic cardiac event. The presence of RV failure in the face of LV failure usually indicates a more advanced disease state and worse prognosis.

Etiology

Unless specified otherwise, assume that the term "heart failure" implies biventricular failure. Signs and symptoms of HF result from the failure of both ventricles. However, even though signs and symptoms of HF are biventricular in nature, the origin of the failure is usually the left ventricle. Factors commonly influencing the development of LV dysfunction and eventually causing HF are listed in **Table 8-5**.

LV pump failure usually occurs before RV pump failure. The LV myocardium weakens to the extent that it cannot eject blood in the normal amount. This reduces the cardiac output secondary to a reduction in stroke volume (SV). Before SV decreases, however, two changes in myocardial function may take place. First, if the failure is slow, the left ventricle enlarges in both capacity (measured by end-diastolic volume [EDV]) and muscle size. This is called ventricular remodeling. The ventricle changes in shape as well, becoming more spherical. This change in shape makes it less effective at pumping blood and leads to worsening cardiac function. As the remodeling continues, the second problem develops, that is, the ability of the heart to eject blood (measured by SV and ejection fraction [EF]) is reduced. This reduction is initially offset by factors such as increased EDV (ventricular stretch), but it is just a temporary solution.

The factors that produce the change in the shape of the heart are partially modifiable. Neurohumoral factors that contribute to this change include the release of sympathetic stimulants, activation of the renin–angiotensin–aldosterone system, and secretion of vasopressin. Although these neurohumoral factors initially are designed to help the injured or failing heart, they eventually contribute to the development of HF. For example, the sympathetic stimulants (eg, **norepinephrine, dopamine**) help to increase cardiac output by their positive inotropic effects. They also produce vasoconstriction, as will angiotensin II and vasopressin. Aldosterone increases sodium and water

TABLE 8-3. STAGES OF THE EVOLUTION AND PROGRESSION OF CHF

	Definition	*Examples*
Stage A At risk for HF	High risk of heart failure but without symptoms, no structural heart disease or cardiac biomarkers of stretch or injury, signs of failure	Hypertension, coronary artery disease, diabetes, family history of cardiomyopathy
Stage B Pre-HF	Structural heart disease but no signs of failure, evidence of increased filling pressures, Patients with risk factors and increased levels on BNPs or persistent elevated cardiac troponin in the absence of other diagnosis.	Prior MI, systolic dysfunction, valvular heart disease, left ventricular hypertrophy
Stage C Symptomatic HF	Structural heart disease and signs of failure (either in the past or currently)	Symptoms include dyspnea, fatigue, exercise intolerance, orthopnea
Stage D Advanced HF	Refractory heart failure despite maximal medical therapy.	Symptoms that interfere with activities of daily living and with recurrent hospitalizations

2022 AHA/ACC/HFSA Guideline for the Management of Heart Failure: A Report of the American College of Cardiology/American Heart Association Joint Committee on Clinical Practice Guidelines. Circulation (ahajournals.org)

TABLE 8-4. COMMON TREATMENTS OF CHF

Category	*Dose*	*Action*	*Comments*
Acute and Chronic Management			
ACE inhibitors:			
Lisinopril	Initial dose, 2.5–5 mg PO once daily; target dose, 20–40 mg PO qd	Afterload reducer, blocks RAAS	Observe for hypotension, renal dysfunction
Enalapril	Initial dose, 2.5 mg PO bid; target dose, 10–20 mg PO bid		
Captopril	Initial dose, 6.25 mg PO tid; target dose, 50 mg PO tid		
Fosinopril	5–10 mg once daily, target dose, 40 mg once daily		
Perindopril	2 mg once daily target dose, 8–16 mg once daily		
Quinapril	5 mg twice daily, target dose 20 mg twice daily		
Ramipril	1.25–2.5 mg once daily, target dose 10 mg once daily		
Trandolapril	1 mg once daily, target dose 4 mg once daily		
ARB		ARB, angiotensin receptor blocker	
Candesartan	4–8 mg once daily, target 32 mg once daily		
Losartan	25–50 mg once daily, target 50–150 mg once daily		
Valsartan	20–40 mg once daily, target 160 mg twice daily		
ARNi			
Sacubitril/valsartan	49 mg sacubitril and 51 mg valsartan twice daily (therapy may be started at 24 mg sacubitril and 26 mg valsartan twice daily); target dose: 97 mg sacubitril and 103 mg valsartan twice daily		
Beta blockers:			
Metoprolol succinate extended release (metoprolol CR/XL)	Initial dose, 12.5–25 mg PO qd; target dose 200 mg PO qd	Beta blockade (and with third generation, alpha blockade)	
Carvedilol	Initial dose, 3.125 mg PO bid; target dose 25–50 mg PO bid	The result is vasodilation (reducing work of the ventricle) and reduced myocardial work (slows the heart and weakens contractility)	
Bisoprolol	Initial dose, 1.25 mg PO daily; target dose, 10 mg PO qd		
Nitrates:			
Isosorbide dinitrate and hydralazine Fixed dose combination	20 mg isosorbide dinitrate and 37.5 mg hydralazine 3 times daily; Target dose 40 mg isosorbide dinitrate and 75 mg hydralazine 3 times daily		Hypotension. Recommended for all patients self-identifying as African American
Isosorbide dinitrate and hydralazine	20–30 mg isosorbide dinitrate and 25–50 mg hydralazine 3–4 times daily Target dose, 120 mg isosorbide dinitrate total daily in divided doses and 300 mg hydralazine total daily in divided doses	Promote venous dilation, producing a drop in venous return and CVP	Hypotension.

(*Continued*)

TABLE 8-4. COMMON TREATMENTS OF CHF (*CONTINUED*)

Category	*Dose*	*Action*	*Comments*
Diuretics:			
Aldosterone antagonists, Spironolactone	12.5–25 mg PO qd, target 25–50 mg once daily	Inhibit aldosterone release, promoting diuresis	Monitor K, may need to be discontinued in patients whose K >5.5
Eplerenone	25 mg once daily, target 50 mg once daily		
Furosemide	20–40 mg PO once or twice up to 600 mg daily	Inhibit Na reabsorption, promoting diuresis	
Torsemide	10–20 mg once, Max total daily dose 200 mg		
Bumetanide	0.5-1 mg PO qd once or twice, max totally daily dose 10 mg		
Metolazone	2.5 mg once, Max 20 mg daily		
Digoxin	0.125 mg PO qd, 0.25 mg PO qd	Acts as a positive inotrope, increasing contractility	Individualized variable dose to achieve serum digoxin concentration 0.5–<0.9 ng/mL
SGLT2i		sodium glucose cotransporter 2 inhibitor	
Dapagliflozin	10 mg once daily, target 10 mg once daily		Recommended regardless of presence of type 2 diabetes
Empagliflozin	10 mg once daily, target 10 mg once daily		
Primarily Acute Management			
Inotropes:			
Dobutamine	2.5–20 µg/kg/min	Sympathetic stimulant (beta); increases contractility and stroke volume, cardiac output	Caution: MAO-I; CI: sulfite allergy
Milrinone	New guidelines- Bolus Not recommended 0.125–0.75 µg/kg/min	Phosphodiesterase inhibitor, acts by increasing intracellular calcium; result is improved contractility, stroke volume, and cardiac output	Accumulation may occur in setting of renal failure; monitor kidney function and LFTs
Afterload reducers:			
Nitroprusside	10–400 µg/min or 0.5–10 µg/kg/min	All will reduce afterload (SVR) through differing mechanisms	Recommended PO for all patients self-identifying as African American
Hydralazine Fixed dose combination	20 mg isosorbide dinitrate and 37.5 mg hydralazine 3 times daily		

retention in an attempt to maintain cardiac output. However, all these factors will eventually contribute to worsening cardiac performance.

The body will try to compensate for these effects by releasing substances like natriuretic peptides (NPs). These peptides are naturally occurring proteins that produce vasodilation and increase urine output. There are several types of NPs, including atrial (ANP), brain (BNP), and C type. ANP is localized in atrial storage granules, while BNP is located in both the atria and ventricles (despite the term "brain natriuretic peptide").

TABLE 8-5. CONDITIONS THAT CONTRIBUTE TO DEVELOPMENT OF HEART FAILURE

Systemic hypertension	Atrial and ventricular tachydysrhythmias	Ischemic heart disease, eg, MI, angina
Infiltrative cardiac disease (eg, sarcoidosis, amyloid)	Cardiomyopathy (Genetic, familial, stress induced, peripartum)	Valvular heart disease (eg, aortic stenosis, mitral regurgitation)
Myocarditis	Endocrine/Metabolic disorders (eg, hyperthyroidism, obesity)	Autoimmune/rheumatologic disorders
Cardiotoxicities (chemotherapies, substance abuse)		

The NPs are elevated in HF. Serum BNP levels are useful as a clinical tool in the diagnosis of HF. Although there are different testing methods to measure BNP, one common method used at the point of care has demonstrated that a value of >100 pg/mL is strongly suggestive that a patient has HF. Some authors have suggested that an elevated BNP is among the most accurate methods of identifying HF.

As this process progresses, HF develops. A weakened LV is signaled by a decrease in strength, for example, in EF. Normally, about 70% of the EDV is ejected with each beat. The amount of blood thus ejected is the SV. The amount of blood ejected (SV) in comparison with the EDV is termed the EF (SV/EDV = EF). As the contractile ability of the heart worsens, the EF falls. **As the EF decreases to less than 40%, exercise limitations become evident** and progress to interfere with activities of daily living. Newer technologies, like esophageal Dopplers, measure contractility by different techniques (eg, peak velocity).

QUICK TIP! The CCRN exam is unlikely to include newer technologies that measure contractility on the exam.

If the left ventricle cannot pump all the blood it receives from the atrium, a buildup of blood and pressure occurs in the left atrium. As the pressure in the left atrium increases, it becomes more difficult for blood to enter the atrium from the pulmonary veins. As the blood in the pulmonary veins becomes unable to flow into the left atrium, it backs up in the lung vessels. **When pressure in the pulmonary capillaries (PAOP) exceeds 18 to 25 mm Hg, fluid from the capillaries leaks into the interstitial spaces.** Once this leakage of fluid into the pulmonary interstitial space exceeds the ability of the pulmonary lymphatics to drain the fluid, pulmonary edema begins to develop.

HF can be categorized into two main types: heart failure with preserved ejection fraction (HFpEF) and heart failure with reduced ejection fraction (HFrEF). Patients whose ejection fraction is between 40% and 50% are known to have heart failure with mildly reduced ejection fraction (HFmrEF). HFpEF was previously known as diastolic dysfunction and HFrEF was previously known as systolic dysfunction. Symptoms differentiating the two main types of HF are listed in **Table 8-6** and summarized below.

TABLE 8-6. SYMPTOMS OF SYSTOLIC AND DIASTOLIC HEART FAILURE

	HFrEF (Systolic Failure)	*HFpEF (Diastolic Failure)*
Stroke volume	Reduced	Reduced
Ejection fraction	Reduced (<40%)	Normal (≥50%)
Age	all ages, 50–70 years common	More common in age >60 years
Sex	More common in men	More common in women
Heart sounds	S_3	S_4
Heart cavity size	Enlarged	Often normal

QUICK TIP! Regarding Table 8-6: The exam does not contain much information regarding heart sounds. However, awareness of S_3 and S_4 sounds will be important. An S_3 is suggestive of pulmonary edema or fluid overload. An S_4 indicative of a stiff, less compliant ventricle, resulting in sub-optimal filling (eg, post-acute MI)

HFrEF

HFrEF is characterized by a decrease in muscle strength. Forward blood flow falls, producing systemic hypoperfusion. SV and EF also fall. This also causes pulmonary congestion, but it is more dangerous because of the potential to decrease forward blood flow.

HFpEF

HFpEF is the inability of the ventricle to fully relax. The result is increasing pressure and volume in the ventricle. This produces pulmonary congestion as pressures "back up" the pulmonary veins. In diastolic dysfunction, the strength of the heart is often normal (eg, EF and peak velocity are within normal levels). SV is gradually reduced owing to the limitation in ventricular chamber size.

In both types of HF, pulmonary compliance can compensate for some increases in pressure as the heart becomes dysfunctional. Since the lung vasculature is distensible, it can accept a moderate amount of increased pressure and volume. However, without intervention, the pressure in the pulmonary capillaries increases to the point that the right ventricle cannot eject its blood into the lungs for oxygenation. As the backflow pressure increases, the **right ventricle fails and the CVP increases**. Then blood from the right atrium cannot drain completely, and consequently the right atrium cannot accommodate all of the blood entering from the venae cavae. *Since venous blood flow to the heart is impeded, venous pooling and eventual organ congestion with venous blood occurs.*

Left Versus Right Heart Failure

Right HF is most commonly caused by left HF and then by all the factors that cause left HF. Right HF may also be caused by isolated right coronary ischemia, pulmonary emboli, pulmonary hypertension, and chronic obstructive pulmonary disease.

Left HF alone can occur from the same factors that cause HF. Since left HF occurs before right HF in these cases, initial symptoms of left HF differ from those of HF. Because of the potential for left heart before right HF, measures that formerly were used to estimate left heart function by right-sided measures (such as CVP) have been demonstrated to be inaccurate.

Clinical Presentation

Symptoms of LV and RV failure are presented in **Table 8-7**.

QUICK TIP! Prepare to see symptoms of LV and RV failure on the exam as they commonly appear on the test in multiple questions.

Complications

The major complications of HF are the progression of failure and loss of cardiac output and oxygen delivery. In addition, progression of cardiac failure can lead to the development of lethal dysrhythmias. It is also important to keep in mind that therapies to treat HF may cause drug toxicity (including oxygen toxicity) and fluid and electrolyte imbalances.

TABLE 8-7. SYMPTOMS OF LEFT AND RIGHT VENTRICULAR FAILURE

Left Ventricle	*Right Ventricle*
Orthopnea	Distended neck veins
Dyspnea of exertion	Dependent edema
Crackles	Hepatic engorgement
Low Pao_2/Sao_2/Spo_2	Hepatojugular reflux
S_3, S_4	Anorexia or nausea/vomiting
Cough	

Treatment and Nursing Intervention

The goal of treating HF is to improve ventricular function and prevent the progression to right HF. There are three methods of treatment, which are based on the factors regulating SV.

Inotropes

The first method of treatment is to improve the contractility of the ventricle. Depending on the severity of the problem, different agents may be attempted. For example, in mild HF, preload and afterload reducers would be initiated. In severe HF, inotropes would be added. Improving contractility can occur with positive inotropic agents such as **dobutamine** and **milrinone**. New agents are being considered (eg, levosimendan [Simdex]) but have not been shown to improve outcomes. Within the limits of Starling's law and balancing the good (improved cardiac output, SV) against the bad (increased myocardial oxygen consumption), this method of treatment can be useful in the short term. However, long-term use has been shown to worsen mortality and is considered palliative. Indications for the use of these inotropes are centered around low cardiac indices (SI < 25 mL/m^2 and a CI < 2.2 L/min/m^2) and high PAOP (>18 mm Hg).

In theory, these agents are good treatments because of their ability to directly improve SV, EF, and cardiac output. However, inotropes come with a cost—that is, increased myocardial oxygen consumption at a time when oxygenation of the heart is threatened. Digitalis preparations, such as **digoxin**, have been used in the chronic control of HF. Their role in acute HF is less clear.

Part of the less than optimal effectiveness of inotropes (especially **dobutamine**) may involve "downregulation," which refers to the lack of responsiveness of cardiac muscle to sympathetic stimulation. In HF, sympathetic stimulation has been occurring for a long time. This chronic stimulation leads eventually to failure of the cardiac muscle to respond to further stimulation. Because of the failure of long-term oral inotropes in the presence of HF, the current therapy emphasizes manipulation of preload and afterload to improve contractility.

Biventricular Pacing. Downregulation and the increased oxygen demand of inotropes has made biventricular pacing a more common treatment for poor contractility. *One* required indication for biventricular pacing is evidence of a bundle branch block (BBB) and HFrEF of <36%. The dyssynchrony of RV and LV contraction in a BBB compounds the pump failure. When the right and left ventricles contract at the same time, the septum is stable. When the right and left ventricles contract one after the other in a BBB, the septum moves back and forth, causing less efficient ejection of blood from the ventricles. Biventricular pacing restores synchronized ventricular contraction, thus maximizing the efficiency of ventricular contraction and increasing cardiac output.

Reduction of Afterload. Afterload is the resistance of the blood, valves, and blood vessels that the left ventricle must overcome to eject blood. A decrease in any of these factors will decrease afterload. *Reduction in afterload (estimated by the SVR) eases the work of the left ventricle.* Reduced work may allow for improved contractility, thereby increasing SV and cardiac output. Afterload agents include vasodilators of several different pharmacologic types, including **nitroprusside**, angiotensin-converting enzyme (ACE) inhibitors (**captopril** and **enalapril**) **OR** angiotensin-receptor blockers (ARB), and many other agents. *Angiotensin receptor-neprilysin inhibitor (ARNi) is preferred in place of an ACE/ARB when it is tolerated and feasible for patients.* Patients can only be on either an ACE, ARB or ARNi as the ARNi is a combination medication consisting of sacubitril/valsartan (Entresto). Common agents used to reduce afterload in HF are included in **Table 8-8**. *The intra-aortic balloon pump* **(IABP)** *is a nonpharmacologic afterload reducer.*

TABLE 8-8. AFTERLOAD REDUCERS—CATEGORIES OF AGENTS

Calcium Channel Blockers (Not Commonly Used in CHF)	*Beta Blockers*	*Angiotensin-Converting Enzyme Inhibitors*	*Direct Arterial and Venous Dilators*	*SGLT2i*
Amlodipine (Lotrel, Norvasc) Nimodipine (Nimotop) Felodipine (Plendil)	First generation: Second-generation: metoprolol, bisoprolol, Third generation:, carvedilol,	Captopril (Capoten) Enalapril (Vasotec) Fosinopril (Monopril) Lisinopril (Prinivil) Quinapril (Accupril) Perindopril (Aceon) Ramipril (Altace) Trandolapril (Mavik)	Nitroprusside nipride) Nitroglycerin	Dapagliflozin Empagliflozin

Notes: Per the 2022 guidelines (Table 13)—nondihydropyridine calcium channel blockers—diltiazem and verapamil—are myocardial depressants and generally not well tolerated in HF. Verapamil had no impact of survival or major cardiac events post-MI, including in those patients with HFrEF after acute MI. In patients with nonischemic cardiomyopathy, diltiazem had no impact on mortality but, in HFrEF after acute MI, diltiazem was associated with a higher risk of recurrent HF.

Second-generation dihydropyridine calcium channel blockers, including amlodipine and felodipine, have greater selectivity for calcium channels in vascular smooth muscle cells and less myocardial depressant activity. By reducing peripheral vasoconstriction and LV afterload, calcium channel blockers were thought to have a potential role in the management of chronic HF. The PRAISE-1 (Prospective Randomized Amlodipine Survival Evaluation-1) study showed a reduction in mortality in the subgroup of patients with nonischemic cardiomyopathy who received amlodipine

TABLE 8-9. PRELOAD REDUCERS

Diuretics			
Loop	***Thiazides***	***Potassium-Sparing***	***Vasodilators***
Bumetanide (eg, Bumex)	Chlorothiazide (eg, Diuril) Chlorthalidone (eg, Hygroton)	Spironolactone (eg, Aldactone) and eplerenone	Nitroglycerin
Torsemide	Hydrochlorothiazide (eg, Hydrodiuril)		
Furosemide (eg, Lasix)	Metolazone (eg, Zaroxolyn) Indapamide		

Reduction of Preload. If the volume of blood entering the left atrium can be lowered, stress on the left ventricle is reduced. Diuretic therapy (as with **furosemide** and **thiazides**), and *fluid and sodium restriction are examples of treatment of preload.* Examples of diuretics used in the treatment of HF are listed in **Table 8-9**.

Other Treatment. A new drug class, sodium-glucose cotransporter-2 inhibitor (SGLT2i) is now recommended for all patients with HF. While its benefits are not fully understood it has shown to decrease hospitalizations and reduce risk of cardiovascular mortality. This class of medication has a mild diuretic effect and reduces sodium reabsorption as well as increases delivery of sodium to the distal tubule. Additionally, this class has been shown to improve smooth muscle relaxation. Overall, it helps to reduce preload and afterload.

Close monitoring of the patient and his or her response to these treatments is very important in the early detection of a deteriorating state requiring more aggressive therapy.

High-Output Failure

Some conditions are associated with high cardiac output. When associated with symptoms of HF, these conditions are called high-output failure. **Table 8-10** lists conditions commonly associated with high-output failure. Treatment of high-output failure is based on relieving the underlying condition, such as excess catecholamines and thyroid dysfunction.

8.2 PULMONARY EDEMA

Pulmonary edema is the most serious progression of HF. *It may occur when pressure in the pulmonary vasculature (PAOP) exceeds 18 to 25 mm Hg.* This results in the extravasation of fluid from pulmonary capillaries into interstitial tissue and intra-alveolar spaces. The intrapulmonary shunt worsens, as is evident by the need for high oxygen requirements (increased FIO_2) and worsening intrapulmonary shunts (eg, *PaO_2/FIO_2 ratios worsen*).

Etiology

Acute pulmonary edema is usually the result of LV failure, although noncardiac forms of pulmonary edema (eg, adult respiratory distress syndrome) exist. Symptoms of HF are exacerbated in pulmonary edema. Dyspnea and orthopnea become markedly pronounced; crackles may be heard throughout the lungs and may be accompanied by blood-tinged, frothy sputum. Hypoxemia will worsen as lung function deteriorates from the increased fluid. Restlessness and anxiety precede a changing level of consciousness as cerebral oxygenation falls.

TABLE 8-10. CAUSES OF HIGH-CARDIAC-OUTPUT FAILURE

Hyperthyroidism Severe anemia Arteriovenous fistula	Thiamine deficiency Paget's disease

Radiographic Changes

Changes due to pulmonary edema occur on chest x-ray s in stages equal to the progression and/or severity of the pulmonary edema. The first change is an enlargement of the pulmonary veins. As interstitial edema occurs, the vessels become poorly outlined and foggy. This is frequently referred to as hilar haze. As intra-alveolar edema develops, the chest x-ray shows a density in the inner middle zone. This gives the appearance of a "bat wing" or "butterfly" at the hilum.

Treatment and Nursing Intervention

The treatment for pulmonary edema is the same as for HF, with a few exceptions. The goal of therapy is to resolve the pulmonary edema by improving cardiac function, which will improve renal function while supporting respiratory needs. *The goal is to decrease preload, decrease afterload, and increase contractility.*

Preload is reduced by diuretic therapy. For example, **furosemide (Lasix)** has been a mainstay in the management of pulmonary edema for decades. Pulmonary edema responds well to **furosemide**, possibly because of its vasodilatory effect as much as its diuretic action. Anxiety is best treated by improving cardiac function and providing constant reassurance to the patient that treatments are being given. Some clinicians still use analgesics such as **morphine sulfate**, which is given intravenously to both relieve anxiety and cause vasodilation, resulting in a reduced afterload. At times, patients with a history of long-standing use of diuretics are refractory to the diuretic effects, and it becomes difficult to decrease the preload. Ultrafiltration via dialysis or renal replacement therapy can be considered for fluid removal. Newer modalities of mechanical fluid removal are also being developed.

Cardiac function can be immediately supported with inotropes (eg, **dobutamine**). If no response from **dobutamine** is seen, **milrinone** can be given. It is important to monitor the patient's response to make sure that the benefit of inotropes is worth the cost. If hypotension exists, mid-dose vasopressors (eg, **dopamine, norepinephrine**) may be given. However, it is advisable to use as minimal a dose as possible and titrate to tissue oxygenation endpoints (eg, SvO_2 or $ScvO_2$).

Normally, hypoxemia is treated, but not in isolation. Improving arterial oxygenation is important, but not at the expense of tissue oxygenation (a danger in using any positive-pressure therapy, such as mechanical ventilation or positive end-expiratory pressure [PEEP]). Hypoxemia can be treated by increasing the fraction of inspired oxygen (FIO_2). Oxygen therapy is usually administered by a high-flow face mask system, with oxygen concentrations over 50% being required. *The addition of continuous positive airway pressure (CPAP) or intubation and implementation of PEEP may be necessary for patients whose hypoxemia (PaO_2 levels < 60 mm Hg) does not respond to oxygen therapy.*

KEY CLINICAL CONCEPT

PEEP can decrease preload by compressing the inferior vena cava. However, when positive pressure is applied, care must be taken to avoid a decrease in cardiac output.

Nursing intervention focuses on monitoring significant changes in preload, afterload, and contractility. If the preload (PAOP) changes, the nurse must observe whether other parameters (eg, SV, cardiac output, and SvO_2) have changed. Trends in data analysis are more important than a single set of numbers. It is very important to monitor treatments over several readings as opposed to a single point-in-time to ensure the accurate assessment of clinical conditions.

Emotional support of the patient with pulmonary edema is made difficult by the patient's fear of shortness of breath. It is important to decrease this fear concurrently while providing treatment.

8.3 HYPERTENSION AND HYPERTENSIVE CRISIS

Hypertension is not a disease but rather the symptom of a disease. Guidelines from AHA/ACC define hypertension parameters as the following: normal, <120/<80 mm Hg; elevated blood pressure, 120 to 129/<80 mm Hg; stage 1 hypertension, 130 to 139/80 to 89 mm Hg; stage 2 hypertension, ≥140/≥90 mm Hg. Primary hypertension (idiopathic, or of unknown cause) is common in the general population, with up to 30% of the population being affected. Hypertensive crises, however, occur only in a small percentage of the hypertensive population.

Mean arterial pressure (MAP) is routinely lower in normal populations (MAP of between 60 and 90 mm Hg) than in chronic hypertensive patients (MAP commonly between 120 and 160). The fact that hypertensive patients have higher mean pressures is important when therapeutic endpoints are identified. The patient with chronic hypertension may tolerate a higher MAP, and rapid reduction to normal levels is generally not necessary.

The severity of the hypertensive disturbance can be identified according to the guidelines of the Joint National Committee on Detection, Evaluation and Treatment of High Blood Pressure, published periodically to identify best practices in treating hypertension. *Emergencies* are blood pressure levels that need treatment within 1 hour; *urgencies* are blood pressure levels that need treatment within 1 day. The characteristics of emergencies are listed in **Table 8-11**.

TABLE 8-11. CHARACTERISTICS OF EMERGENCY HYPERTENSION
Diastolic blood pressure >120 mm Hg
Presence of one of the following:
Acute aortic dissection
LV failure with or without pulmonary edema
Myocardial ischemia
Acute renal failure
Cerebrovascular or subarachnoid bleed
Hypertensive encephalopathy
Head injuries
Grade 3–4 Keith–Wagener–Barker retinopathy
Eclampsia and toxemia of pregnancy
Burns
Medication interaction
Pheochromocytoma crisis or sympathetic crisis

Etiology

Hypertension may be classified by etiology.

1. Unknown origin accounts for 90% of all cases of hypertension identified. This is termed essential hypertension.
2. Adrenal origin results from a tumor (**pheochromocytoma**) secreting epinephrine and norepinephrine, Cushing's disease, or a brain tumor.
3. Renal origin is due either to an interruption of blood supply or to a disease state of the kidney itself (eg, pyelonephritis).
4. Cardiovascular hypertension can be in response to either HF or myocardial ischemia or it may act as their cause. Postoperative hypertension is common, particularly early in CABG recovery. The postoperative hypertension is probably due to excess catecholamine release.
5. The origin of obstetric hypertension is unclear, but the condition usually presents in the second trimester of pregnancy.
6. Medications that cause vasoconstriction.
7. Lack of compliance with medical therapy in "known" hypertension or inadequate treatment of such hypertension. Also, certain drugs may cause hypertension.

KEY CLINICAL CONCEPT

Suspicion of pheochromocytoma may be confirmed by a 24-hour urine test for catecholamines. However, a more definitive diagnostic test would be an abdominal CT. If confirmed, definitive management is surgery.

Clinical Presentation of Hypertensive Crisis

The most common symptom is severe headache accompanied by nausea, vomiting, restlessness, and mental confusion, which may rapidly advance to coma and/or convulsions. Signs of a specific organ injury may be present. For example, myocardial ischemia, cerebral vascular accident, hematuria, or retinopathy may become evident. Sudden elevations in blood pressure are more likely to present with symptoms than are gradual elevations.

Treatment

Treatment of hypertensive crisis centers around the reduction of blood pressure to safe levels without producing a subsequent hypotension. Remember, hypotensive symptoms can appear at higher than expected pressures in the patient with chronic hypertension. **Gradual reduction of the MAP to 110 to 115 mm Hg is acceptable. Then, if the patient is showing no symptoms of hypotensive effects, further reductions to about 85 mm Hg are generally safe.** There are certain exceptions to these guidelines such as patients with aortic dissection would require rapid reduction of blood pressure. Therapeutic modalities to achieve the MAP reduction generally involve a rapidly acting agent initially, with conversion to an oral agent as soon as possible. A diuretic is frequently added to counter potential water and sodium disturbances resulting from normal renal mechanisms to compensate for the hypertension. Examples of rapidly acting and oral maintenance agents are listed in **Table 8-12**.

TABLE 8-12. MEDICATIONS TO TREAT HYPERTENSIVE EMERGENCIES

Intravenous Medications			
Agent	***Dose***	***Onset of Action***	***Actions and Precautions***
Sodium nitroprusside (Nipride)	0.25–10 µg/kg/min as IV infusion	Immediate/1–10 min after infusion	Action: Direct arterial dilator Side effects: Nausea, vomiting; may cause thiocyanate toxicity, methemoglobinemia, acidosis, cyanide poisoning. Keep IV and delivery set shielded from light.
Nitroglycerin	5–100 µg/min as IV infusion	2–5 min/5–10 min	Action: Venodilation Side effects: Headache, tachycardia, vomiting, flushing, methemoglobinemia; requires special delivery system due to due to drug binding to IV tubing.
Nicardipine (Cardene)	5–15 mg/h IV infusion	1–5 min/15–30 min, but may exceed 12 h after prolonged infusion	Action: Calcium channel blockade Side effects: Tachycardia, nausea, vomiting, headache, increased intracranial pressure; hypotension may be protracted after prolonged infusion.
Hydralazine (Apresoline)	5–20 mg as IV bolus or 10–40 mg IM; repeat every 4–6 h	10 min IV/>1 h (IV) 20–30 min IM/4–6 h (IM)	Action: Direct vascular smooth muscle relaxation Side effects: Tachycardia, headache, vomiting, aggravation of angina pectoris, sodium and water retention and increased intracranial pressure.
Fenoldopam mesylate	0.1–0.3 µg/kg/min IV infusion	<5 min/30 min	Action: Peripheral dopamine$_1$-receptor antagonism Side effects: Headache, tachycardia, flushing, local phlebitis, dizziness.
Esmolol (Brevibloc)	500 µg/kg is typical loading dose given over 1 min; then initiate IV infusion at 25–0 µg/kg/min; titrate incrementally up to maximum of 300 µg/kg/min. May consider repeating a loading dose (eg, ≤500 µg/kg) prior to each up-titration step.	1–5 min/15–30 min	Action: Beta blockade Side effects: First-degree heart block, congestive heart failure, asthma.
Labetalol (Normodyne, Trandate)	Initial bolus of 20 mg IV followed by 20–80 mg IV bolus every 10 min (maximum 300 mg) or 0.5–2 mg/min as IV loading infusion following an initial 20 mg IV bolus (maximum 300 mg)	5–10 min/2–6 h	Action: Beta blockade Side effects: Bronchoconstriction, heart block, orthostatic hypotension, bradycardia.
Enalaprilat (Vasotec)	0.625–1.25 mg every 6 h IV	Within 30 min/12–24 h	Action: ACE inhibition Side effects: Renal failure in patients with bilateral renal artery stenosis, hypotension.

(Continued)

TABLE 8-12. MEDICATIONS TO TREAT HYPERTENSIVE EMERGENCIES (*CONTINUED*)

Intravenous Medications			
Agent	***Dose***	***Onset of Action***	***Actions and Precautions***
Phentolamine	5–10 mg as IV bolus	1–2 min/10–30 min	Action: Alpha-adrenergic blockade. Used primarily in pheochromocytoma Side effects: Tachycardia, orthostatic hypotension.
Oral Agents			
Captopril	6.25–25 mg PO, repeat as needed; SL, 25 mg	15–30 min/6–8 h SL 10–20 min/2–6 h	Action: ACE inhibition Side effects: Hypotension, coughing, renal failure in patients with high-grade bilateral renal artery stenosis, angioedema.
Clonidine	0.1–0.2 mg PO, repeat hourly as required to total dose of 0.6 mg	30–60 min/8–16 h	Action: Alpha-adrenergic antagonism Side effects: Hypotension, drowsiness, light-headedness, dry mouth.
Labetalol	200–400 mg PO, repeat every 2–3 h	1–2 h/2–12 h	Action: Beta blockade Side effects: Bronchoconstriction, heart block, orthostatic hypotension.
Prazosin	1–2 mg PO, repeat hourly as needed	1–2 h/8–12 h	Action: Alpha-adrenergic blockade Side effects: Syncope (first dose), palpitations, tachycardia, orthostatic hypotension.

KEY CONTENT CHECKLIST

- ❐ HFrEF is caused by decreased strength of the ventricle (systolic HF). HFpEF is caused by the ventricles inability to relax (diastolic HF).
- ❐ An S_3 is suggestive of pulmonary edema or fluid overload. An S_4 indicative of a stiff, less compliant ventricle, resulting in suboptimal filling (eg, postacute MI)
- ❐ PEEP can decrease preload by compressing the inferior vena cava. Take caution when increasing PEEP to monitor cardiac output.
- ❐ Know the difference symptoms for RV and LV failure as they commonly appear on the exam.
- ❐ Suspicion of pheochromocytoma may be confirmed by a 24-hour urine test for catecholamines. However, a more definitive diagnostic test would be an abdominal CT. If confirmed, definitive management is surgery.
- ❐ Gradual reduction of blood pressure of about 10% to 20% in the first hour followed by another 5% to 15% over the next 23 hours is generally indicated in hypertensive urgency to prevent ischemic damage.

Review Questions:

1. RV failure is manifest by which of the following signs?
a. Increased CVP
b. Increased PAOP
c. Decreased pulmonary artery pressure
d. Increased systemic arterial pressure

Answer: A. Rationale: Option A, increased CVP, is the most closely associated option with RV failure and is the chamber directly behind the affected area. Option B, increased PAOP, is more closely associated with LV failure. Option C may be seen but is in front of (ie, "downstream") from the affected area and is not the best answer. Option D, increased systemic arterial pressure may be seen in acute decompensated LVF but is a secondary sign. Choose A.

2. Which stage of HF poses a high risk of HF but is not associated with structural disease or symptoms?
a. Stage A
b. Stage B
c. Stage C
d. Stage D

Answer: A. Rationale: This is a straight knowledge question. Stage A HF is an early class of HF common in hypertensives, diabetics, patients with substance abuse, or certain comorbid conditions that place a patient at increased risk for developing structural signs of HF. Stages B, C, and D indicate more advanced stages of HF, respectively (with stage D representing end-stage HF). Choose A. When in doubt in a staged question such as this with options that indicate a continuum, consider using the "cluster technique" and eliminate the middle options (options B and C) initially to narrow it down.

3. Which of the following would not be an expected treatment in decompensated acute HF?
a. Inotrope (eg, milrinone or dobutamine)
b. Diltiazem
c. Beta NP (eg, nesiritide)
d. Diuretic (eg, furosemide)

Answer: B. Rationale: Diltiazem is a nondihydropyridine calcium channel blocker. Besides lowering blood pressure, it lowers heart rate and can decrease myocardial contractility. Inotropes and diuretics (A and D) are the mainstay of treatment in decompensated CHF. Although its use is declining, nesiritide (Natrecor) (option C) is a synthetic b-type NP for the treatment of decompensated CHF.

9

Cardiogenic Shock

CHAPTER OVERVIEW AND OBJECTIVES

Expect a few questions addressing the assessment and treatment of cardiogenic shock (CS). An understanding of hemodynamic monitoring will substantially assist in answering these questions. Many of the principles of treating CS are covered in the earlier discussion of the treatment of heart failure.

After studying this chapter, you should understand the following:

- Major causes, pathophysiology, and stages of CS.
- Hemodynamic changes associated with worsening CS.
- Indications for inotrope, vasopressor, and mechanical circulatory support (MCS) in CS.

9.1 ETIOLOGY

Cardiogenic shock (CS) is caused by cardiac dysfunction, and like other forms of shock, it. leads to tissue hypoperfusion and cellular hypoxia. Acute myocardial infarction (AMI) is the leading cause of CS, occurring in approximately 10% of AMIs. It can occur immediately or later in the course of both ST-segment elevation myocardial infarction (STEMI) and non–ST-segment elevation myocardial infarction (NSTEMI). *CS is the leading cause of in-hospital deaths after AMI.* In addition to AMI, there are numerous other etiologies of CS (**Table 9-1**).

9.2 PATHOPHYSIOLOGY

Regardless of the etiology of CS, ventricular function decreases, triggering compensatory neurohormonal mechanisms to improve cardiac output (CO), blood pressure (BP), and tissue perfusion. Two of these key mechanisms are as follows:

1. *Sympathetic nervous system (SNS) stimulation.* Release of sympathetic neurotransmitters as **epinephrine, norepinephrine, and dopamine** (also known as catecholamines), which act to increase heart rate, as well as improve contractility, and vasoconstriction to increase BP. The resulting tachycardia decreases the amount of time blood can flow into the coronary arteries and increases myocardial oxygen demand (MVO_2) and potentially worsens myocardial ischemia.
   - **Epinephrine** is a beta-1 agonist that improves contractility and increases heart rate, resulting in improved CO and increased BP.
   - **Norepinephrine** is primarily an alpha agonist and potent vasoconstrictor. It also has some effect on beta-1 receptors, increasing contractility and HR. The increased contractility and heart rate subsequently raise CO. Vasoconstriction maintains BP, perfusion pressures, and improves vital organ blood flow.
2. *Activation of the renin–angiotensin–aldosterone system (RAAS).* RASS activation promotes vasoconstriction along with sodium and water retention. This mechanism acts to increase an already normal or elevated total vascular volume compartment. This mechanism, like SNS stimulation, is designed to help maintain blood flow, but can actually make the situation worse. The increased vasoconstriction caused by angiotensin II raises systemic vascular resistance (SVR) and leads to decreased CO.

9.3 IDENTIFYING CHARACTERISTICS

CS occurs along a continuum that ranges from patients who are at risk for CS to those in extremis. The Society for Coronary Angiography and Intervention (SCAI) developed criteria to help clinicians with earlier identification and treatment of CS. There are six SCAI classes. **At-risk** patients have risk factors for CS but do not have any symptoms. Patients in

TABLE 9-1. COMMON ETIOLOGIES OF CARDIOGENIC SHOCK

Acute Myocardial Infarction	Mechanical	Impaired Contractility	Vascular
• STEMI • NSTEMI	• Acute mitral or aortic valve reguriguation • Intraventricular septal rupture • Left ventricular free wall rupture • Aortic stenosis, hyperobstructive cardiomyopathy (HCOM), or other left ventricular outflow tract (LVOT) obstruction • Poor LV inflow (left atrial myxoma, mitral stenosis)	• Ischemic cardiomyopathy (ICM) • Nonischemic cardiomyopathy (NICM) • Myocarditis • Arrhythmias • Right ventricular (RV) failure • Pulmonary embolus leading to RV failure	• Thoracic aortic dissection

the **beginning** stage of CS have vital sign changes such as hypotension and/or tachycardia, which may require fluid administration. Patients in the **classic** stage have evidence of hypoperfusion and require vasoactive medications or mechanical circulatory support (MCS) to maintain cardiac index (CI) and BP.

Deteriorating patients having worsening vitals and hypoperfusion, requiring increasing doses or additional medications or MCS to maintain CI and BP. Patients in **extremis** are typically unresponsive and highly unstable despite multiple interventions, these patients are close to or have cardiovascular collapse, and are at high risk of dying. The final class consists of patients who are postcardiac arrest. Patients with CS will present with the physical exam findings, vital signs, hemodynamic alterations, and lab abnormalities, as listed in **Table 9-2**.

TABLE 9-2. SCAI CLASSIFICATION OF CARDIOGENIC SHOCK

A At Risk	B Beginning	C Classic	D Deteriorating	E Extremis
Normal physical exam findings	JVD Rales	Volume Overload Evidence of hypoperfusion. ("cold, clammy")	Signs of ongoing or worsening hypoperfusion	May be unconscious Weak, thready pulses May have undergone several defibrillations
Normal vital signs	SBP < 90 mm Hg or MAP < 60 mm Hg or >30 points below baseline HR > 100	Hypotension Tachycardia	Hypotension Tachycardia	Hypotension Tachycardia
Normal hemodynamics	Elevated CVP	CI < 2.2 PAOP > 15 mm Hg	Same as stage C, but requiring higher doses or additional vasoactive agents or MCS	Severe hypotension despite maximal hemodynamic support and/or CPR in progress
Normal lactate Normal kidney function	Normal lactate Renal function mildly abnormal Elevated BNP	Lactate > 2 mmol/L. Elevated BNP AKI Abnormal LFTs	Rising BNP Worsening BNP, Cr, eGFR, & LFTs	Acidosis (pH < 7.2) Lactate > 8 mmol/L

AKI, acute kidney injury; BNP, brain natriuretic peptide; CI, cardiac index; Cr, creatinine; eGFR, estimated glomerular filtration rate; JVD, jugular venous distention; LFTs, liver function tests; MAP, mean arterial pressure; MCS, mechanical circulatory support; PAOP, pulmonary artery occlusion pressure; SBP, systolic blood pressure.

Data from references Naidu et al., 2022; SCAI, 2022; VanDyck & Pinsky, 2021; Baran et al., 2019.

KEY CLINICAL CONCEPT

"Classic" CS is diagnosed when cardiac dysfunction resulting in SBP <90 mm Hg for >30 minutes or requiring pharmacology support to maintain SBP >90 mm Hg due to a CI <2.2 L/min/m^2, and PAOP >15 mm Hg.

QUICK TIP! The CCRN exam will not ask specific questions about the SCAI Classification; however, the information in Table 9-2 will help you prepare to answer exam questions about CS.

9.4 TREATMENT

In patients with CS, rapid intervention to improve myocardial function is paramount to preventing hypoperfusion, multiorgan failure, and death. Much of the current treatment centers on pharmacologic or MCS of the heart. If CS is caused by an AMI, urgent percutaneous coronary intervention (PCI) with stenting is indicated. The CULPRIT-SHOCK trial showed decreased 30-day mortality in AMI patients with CS who underwent PCI of the blocked artery responsible for the AMI. If the patient's coronary artery disease (CAD) is not amenable to PCI, an intra-aortic balloon pump (IABP) may be inserted by the cardiologist prior to transferring the patient to the operating room (OR) for emergent coronary artery bypass graft (CABG) surgery.

Pharmacologic Treatment

Improving Cardiac Output by Using Diuretics to Reduce Preload. Unless contraindicated by hypotension, preload reduction is typically the first intervention ordered to improve CO. Intravenous (IV) loop diuretics, such as **furosemide** or **bumetanide**, lower the circulating blood volume. Less blood returned to the heart decreases the myocardial stretch in the ventricles, resulting in improved myocardial contractility and pulmonary congestion. Vasodilatory agents such as nitroglycerin that also decrease preload are contraindicated in CS (SBP < 90 mm Hg or >30 points lower than baseline).

Improving Cardiac Output by Using Inotropes to Increase Contractility. Although the use of pulmonary artery catheters has declined over the years, patients may benefit from invasive hemodynamic monitoring to facilitate inotropic and/or vasoactive drug selection and accurate assessing its effects. Inotropic agents such as **dobutamine, milrinone, and dopamine** are commonly used to raise CO. **Epinephrine** is used primarily after cardiac surgery, but it can also be used to treat CS. *Improving contractility with these agents increases the risk of tachyarrhythmias and increases myocardial oxygen consumption (MvO_2).*

KEY CLINICAL CONCEPT

- Heart rate (HR) × stroke volume (SV) = cardiac output (CO).
- Increasing either or both HR and SV will increase CO.
- Improving CO will improve oxygen delivery to the tissues (DO2) and may improve SVO_2.

Improving Cardiac Output/Preload Reduction. Diuretics and vasodilators (**nitroglycerin**) may be employed. The use of a pulmonary artery catheter may facilitate assessment of the effectiveness of these agents. The goal of preload reduction is to reduce the stretch of ventricular muscle and improve myocardial contractility while reducing pulmonary congestion.

Improving Blood Pressure. Catecholamine infusions, such as **norepinephrine** and **dopamine**, are frequently used to raise SBP and MAP. **Norepinephrine** is the vasopressor of choice in severe hypotension (SBP < 70 mm Hg), since it stimulates not only alpha-1 receptors causing vasoconstriction but also beta-1 receptors to increase myocardial contractility and CO. Although, **norepinephrine** raises HR (positive chronotropy), it has less of a tachycardic effect than **dopamine**. **Dopamine** is often avoided in patients with tachyarrhythmias, as it may induce atrial fibrillation and/or lead to severe tachycardia, both of which lower CO. *Use of these drugs is not without risk because of the increased Mvo_2 associated with their vasoconstrictive properties.* Vasopressin acts on the V1a receptors in the vasculature to cause vasoconstriction. Providers may opt for a fixed-rate **vasopressin** infusion to support BP and reduce the risk of tachyarrhythmias. **Phenylephrine** is an alpha agonist that raises BP and SVR (LV afterload) but has no inotropic properties. It is not commonly used for BP support in CS patients due to the risk of increasing SVR, which in turn can lead to decreased stroke volume (SV) and CO. **Phenylephrine** should be avoided in patients with low heart rates, since it can induce reflex bradycardia. However, an improved BP does not always improve blood flow. Use of oxygenation parameters, such as venous oxygen saturation (SvO_2) values and lactate levels, will help determine whether an improvement in BP has improved blood flow.

KEY CLINICAL CONCEPT

- Cardiac output (CO) × systemic vascular resistance (SVR) = mean arterial pressure (MAP)
- Increasing CO or SVR increases MAP.
- Increasing MAP may increase tissue perfusion.

Adjuncts to Pharmacologic Support. As previously discussed, AMI patients with CS benefit from rapid revascularization. If PCI is not available and there are no contraindications, a fibrinolytic agent such as tissue plasminogen activator (tPA) may be ordered to restore coronary artery blood flow. MCS devices are frequently used in CS patients. Such support ranges from IABPs, right, left, or biventricular assist devices (VADs), or venoarterial (VA) extracorporeal life support (ECMO).

Ensuring Adequate Oxygenation and Ventilation. Patients with CS often develop pulmonary edema (resulting in **shunt**), resulting in hypoxia. It's important to monitor hemodynamics in patients receiving positive pressure ventilation, as increasing **positive end-expiratory pressure (PEEP) may increase CVP and decrease CO.**

Treating Lactic Acidosis

Lactic acidosis is a frequent cause of metabolic acidosis. As acidosis worsens electrolyte imbalances occur, the arrhythmia threshold decreases, and the cardiovascular system becomes less responsive to vasopressor infusions. Although lactate and pH will normalize as perfusion is reestablished, patients with severe systemic pH (<7.20) may benefit from sodium bicarbonate ($NaHCO_3^-$) boluses or continuous infusions to improve the physiologic vasopressor therapy and allow other interventions to improve tissue perfusion. ***It is important to remember, however, that sodium bicarbonate may provide a temporary solution but does not fix the underlying issue of hypoperfusion.***

Intra-Aortic Balloon Pump

IABP pumps **reduce left ventricular afterload and increase coronary artery perfusion pressure (CPP), which improves blood flow into the coronary arteries.** IABPs augment coronary artery blood flow in patients with angina refractory to PCI and those who need emergent cardiac surgery (eg, severe left main coronary artery [LMCA] stenosis or AMI with multivessel CAD). IABPs are also used as adjunctive to inotropes and other vasoactive meds in CS and in patients with decompensated acute on chronic systolic heart failure (HF). **Contraindications to the use of the IABP include the presence of aortic aneurysms, suspected aortic dissection, significant aortic regurgitation, severe untreated (eg, no prior stent placement) peripheral arterial disease (PAD), uncontrolled bleeding, and sepsis.**

> **KEY CLINICAL CONCEPT**
>
> IABPs (1) increase coronary artery perfusion pressure during diastole, and (2) lower LV afterload (SVR) during systole.

Insertion of the IABP. The IABP is most commonly inserted in the femoral artery, although the axial or brachial arteries or surgical transthoracic placement may be used in cases of significant arterial disease in the abdominal aorta. Using echocardiographic or fluoroscopic guidance, the IABP is advanced into the descending thoracic aorta until the radiopaque marker at the tip is 2 to 3 cm below the takeoff of the left subclavian artery (**Fig. 9-1**). Patients with femoral IABPs are on strict bedrest and must avoid bending the affected extremity. Most patients will be systemically heparinized to prevent thrombosis during IABP therapy. Cardiac surgery patients are not anticoagulated in the early post-operative period due to the risk of bleeding.

> **QUICK TIP!** The CCRN will not include technical questions about the IABP and are more theoretical in nature. Questions on the CCRN regarding the IABP tend to address counterpulsation triggers, who would benefit and why. There may be one or two IABP questions on the exam.

IABP Counterpulsation. Current IABP models have automatic timing mechanisms to prevent inappropriate counterpulsation. Semiautomatic timing should be selected in specific instances where it may improve hemodynamics. IABP counterpulsation (inflation and deflation) is triggered by either an electrocardiogram (ECG trigger) or an arterial pressure (pressure trigger). Electrocardiogram (ECG) triggers are used unless a patient has significant dysrhythmias or pacemaker misfiring. In those cases, pressure triggering is indicated. Both triggers synchronize IABP counterpulsation to occur at the appropriate intervals to prevent worsening hemodynamic compromise.

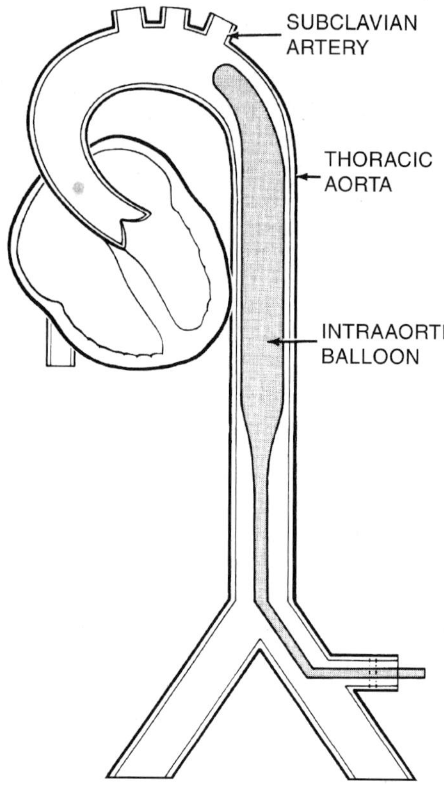

Figure 9-1. The intra-aortic balloon pump (IABP) in the thoracic aorta.

Balloon **inflation occurs during diastole**, after the closure of the aortic valve (identified by the *"dicrotic notch"* on the arterial line) closure, **increasing diastolic aortic root pressure and coronary artery perfusion pressure, improving coronary artery and cerebral blood flow** (**Fig. 9-2**). If the IABP is set to ECG trigger, **balloon inflation will occur at the midpoint of the T wave.** If the arterial pressure trigger is selected, **balloon inflation will occur at the dicrotic notch.**

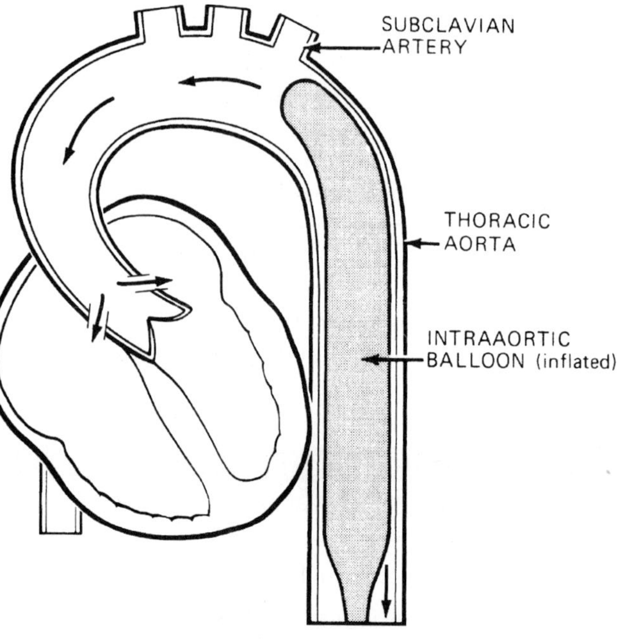

Figure 9-2. The IABP inflated during ventricular diastole.

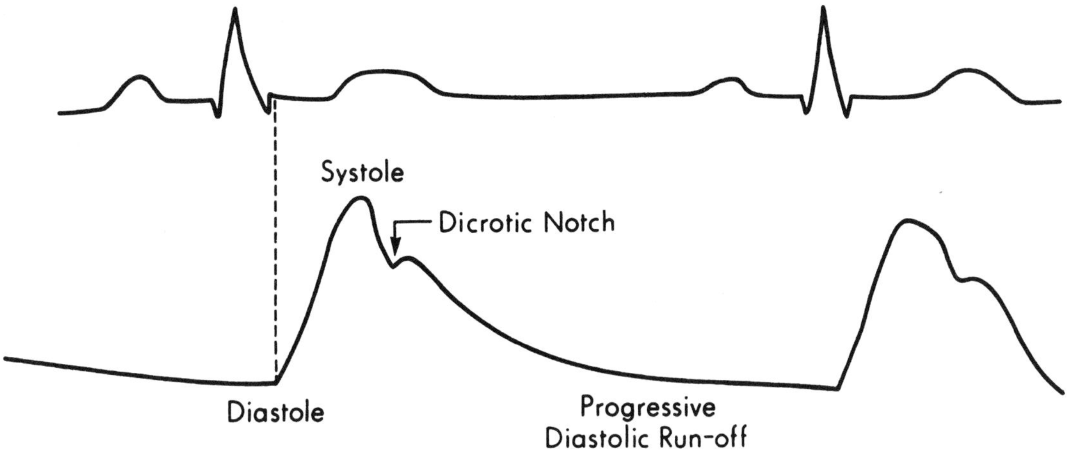

Figure 9-3. Normal arterial waveform.

Balloon **deflation occurs at the end of diastole, just prior to systole**. Deflation of the standard 40-mL balloon displaces 40 mL of blood away from the aortic valve, **reducing LV afterload**, raising SV, and increasing CO by to 0.5–1 L/min. Patients with significantly reduced LV function achieve the most CO augmentation. If the ECG trigger is chosen, **deflation will occur at the R wave in the QRS (Figs. 9-3 and 9-4)**.

QUICK TIP! The two key timing errors to avoid with IABP therapy are **(1) early inflation and (2) late deflation.** The CCRN exam may include questions regarding the ECG and pressure triggers indicating systole and diastole.

Assessing for IABP Complications. Patients with IABPs are at risk for limb ischemia due to the large diameter of intra-aortic balloon catheters, circulation to the leg (or arm) inferior to the insertion site is compromised to varying degrees. It is extremely important to monitor pulses, as well as the temperature and appearance of the leg (or arm) below the insertion site, and compare the findings with those of the extremity on the opposite side, and document appropriately.

Daily chest-radiographs (CXR) are indicated to verify IABP placement. Nurses should check for IABP dislodgement by documenting the depth in centimeters at the time of insertion and during physical assessments. Frequently evaluate pulses to rapidly identify and intervene for suddenly diminished or absent pulses that result from IABP migration. Monitor hourly vital signs and urine output. Abrupt oliguria or anuria may result from IABP occlusion of the renal arteries.

QUICK TIP! IABPs have the potential for numerous complications, including thrombosis, embolic stroke, bleeding, hematoma, infection, and balloon rupture. Critical limb ischemia and IABP dislodgement are the most likely to appear on the CCRN exam.

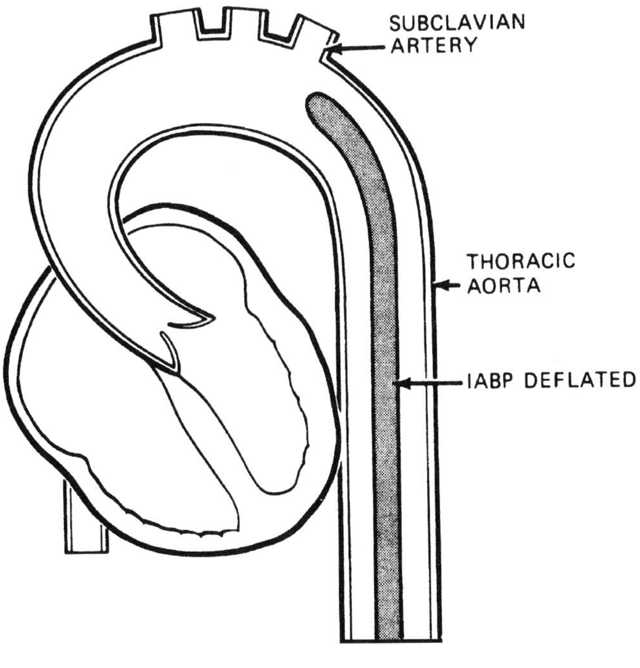

Figure 9-4. The IABP deflated prior to ventricular systole.

IABP Weaning and Removal. The patient is weaned off the IABP usually by lowering the frequency of counter pulsation. At the time of insertion, counterpulsation is normally 1:1 (1 counterpulsation for every heartbeat). When weaning is initiated, the ratio is decreased to 2:1 (1 counterpulsation for every 2 heartbeats), then 3:1 (1 counterpulsation for every 3 heartbeats), according to the patient's tolerance. Weaning may also be achieved by decreasing the balloon inflation volume (augmentation), depending on the IABP model and provider preference.

A complication of IABP therapy is balloon rupture. For this reason, the balloons are inflated a rapid-exchanging gas (eg, helium) to prevent air embolism.

QUICK TIP!

- Although percutaneous MCS (pMCS) device insertion is increasing, at this time, MCS is not a testable item on the updated 2020 CCRN exam blueprint.
- The CCRN will not include technical questions about the IABP. Questions on the CCRN regarding the IABP tend to address who would benefit and why. There may be one or two questions about the IABP on the exam.

KEY CONTENT CHECKLIST

- ❒ "Classic" CS is diagnosed when cardiac dysfunction resulting in SBP <90 mm Hg for >30 minutes or requiring pharmacology support to maintain SBP >90 mm Hg due to a CI <2.2 L/min/m^2, and PAOP >15 mm Hg.
- ❒ Heart rate (HR) × stroke volume (SV) = cardiac output (CO).
- ❒ Increasing either or both HR and SV will increase CO.
- ❒ Improving CO will improve oxygen delivery to the tissues (DO_2) and may improve SVO_2.
- ❒ Cardiac output (CO) × systemic vascular resistance (SVR) = mean arterial pressure (MAP)
- ❒ Increasing CO or SVR increases MAP.
- ❒ Increasing MAP may increase tissue perfusion.
- ❒ IABPs increase coronary artery perfusion pressure (CPP) during diastole, and lower LV afterload (SVR) during systole.

Review Questions:

1. **A patient with CS has a heart rate of 110, BP 69/49, RR 28, oxygen saturation of 90% on 100% NRBM. Which of the following vasoactive agents would the nurse most likely administer?**
   a. Dobutamine (Dobutrex)
   b. Dopamine (Intropin)
   c. Norepinephrine (Norepinephrine)
   d. Phenylephrine (Neosynephrine)

Answer: A. Rationale: The correct answer is C. Norepinephrine is the agent of choice to treat severe hypotension. Answer A is not correct since dobutamine may cause hypotension. Answer C is not correct as dopamine may significantly increase tachycardia. Answer D is incorrect as phenylephrine is a potent vasoconstrictor without the inotropic effects needed to treat CS

2. **A patient is in CS after a blunt cardiac injury (BCI) sustained in a motor vehicle collision (MVC). Which of the following would prompt the RN to prepare to administer packed red blood cells (PRBCs)?**
   a. CVP 1 mm Hg, PAOP 7 mm Hg, SvO_2 40%
   b. Hemoglobin 8.5 mg/dL, CI 2.4 L/min/m^2
   c. SVR 800 dynes/s/m^2, CI 5.0 L/min/m^2
   d. CVP 8 mm Hg, PAOP 12 mm Hg, SvO_2 65%

Answer: A. Rationale: A is the correct answer since the low CVP and PAOP indicate hypovolemia, and the low SvO_2 indicates either poor oxygen delivery or increased tissue extraction of oxygen, all which would be improved by a PRBC transfusion. Answer B is not correct as transfusion is not indicated for a hemoglobin of 8.5 g/dL in a patient with a normal cardiac index (CI). Answer C is incorrect as the low SVR and the high CI are more consistent with distributive shock (eg, sepsis) and not cardiogenic or hypovolemic shock. Answer D is not correct as the CVP, PAOP, and SVO_2 are within normal parameters, suggesting euvolemia and adequate oxygen delivery to the tissues.

REFERENCES

Asber SR, Shanahan KP, Lussier L, et al. Nursing management of patients requiring acute mechanical circulatory support devices. *Crit Care Nurse.* 2020;40(1):e1–e11. doi: 10.4037/ccn2020764.

Baran DA, Grines CL, Bailey S, Burkhoff D, et al. SCAI clinical expert consensus statement on the classification of cardiogenic shock. *Catheter Cardiovasc Interv.* 2019;94(1):29–37.

Bojar RM. *Manual of perioperative care in adult cardiac surgery.* 6th ed. John Wiley & Sons, 2021.

Brien LD, Oermann MH, Molloy M, Tierney C. Implementing goal directed therapy for fluid resuscitation in the cardiovascular intensive care unit. *AACN Adv Crit Care.* 2020;31(4):364–370.

Gordon D, Spiegel R. Fluid resuscitation: history, physiology, and modern fluid resuscitation strategies. *Emerg Med Clin North Am.* 2020;38(4):783–793. doi: 10.1016/j.emc.2020.06.004.

Holcomb B. Intra-aortic balloon pump securement. *Crit Care Nurse.* 2022;42(6):79–81. doi: 10.4037/ccn2022985.

Samsky MD, Morow DA, Proudfoot AG, Hockman JS, Theile H, Rao SV. Cardiogenic shock after acute myocardial infarction: A review. *JAMA.* 2021;326(18):1840–1850. doi: 10.1001/jama.2021.18323.

Society for Coronary Angiography and Intervention. SCAI shock classification checklist. 2022. Retrieved from: https://scai.org/clinical-practice/quality-improvement/scai-shock-resource-center

Thiele H, Akin I, Sandri M. PCI strategies in patients with acute myocardial infarction and cardiogenic shock. *N Engl J Med.* 2017;377(25):2419–2432. doi: 10.1056/NEJMoa1710261.

VanDyck TJ, Pinsky MR. Hemodynamic monitoring in cardiogenic shock. *Curr Opin Crit Care.* 2021;27(4):454–459. doi: 10.1097/MCC.0000000000000838.

10

Hemorrhagic (Hypovolemic) Shock

CHAPTER OVERVIEW AND OBJECTIVES

The CCRN exam is likely to include several questions that test your knowledge of treatment of the major forms of shock. In this chapter, a simple approach to understanding hypovolemic shock is presented. This approach should provide you with the information necessary to successfully answer questions on the concept of hypovolemic shock. **Table 10-1** presents a simple guide to identifying hypovolemia. If you follow it, you will be able to recognize any case of hypovolemia on the CCRN.

After studying this chapter, you should be able to understand:

- Early versus late signs of hypovolemic shock.
- Indications for crystalloid, colloid, and blood/blood product transfusions to restore intravascular volume.
- Markers of shock and endpoints of resuscitation.

This section presents a brief review of the physiology of microcirculatory compensation in shock. This compensation is not restricted to hypovolemia but occurs in all forms of shock.

10.1 PATHOPHYSIOLOGY OF HYPOVOLEMIC SHOCK

Hypovolemic shock is caused by a *loss of circulating blood volume* that decreases tissue perfusion. *Although this loss of blood volume is commonly associated with bleeding, it also is commonly accompanied by early sepsis.* Sepsis presents in a phasic manner, with early phases presenting with low cardiac outputs (COs) while the later phase presents with a hyperdynamic state with high COs. This chapter emphasizes early identification and treatment of hypovolemia. The hemodynamic changes associated with sepsis are discussed in Chapter 5.

Hypovolemic shock occurs when there is a threat to tissue oxygenation secondary to a loss of **CO and stroke volume**. The threat to tissue oxygenation is accompanied by several clinical factors, including:

- A low SvO_2 (<60%) or low $ScvO_2$ (<70%)
- High lactate (>4 mmol)
- Low mean arterial pressure (MAP) (<60 mm Hg).
- **Perhaps most importantly, hypovolemia is accompanied by a low stroke volume (normal varies, but <50 mL is usually abnormally low).**

Stroke volume (SV) can also be interpreted with Doppler values (a low flow time [FTc] of <330 m/s) or pulse contour devices showing a stroke volume variation of >10%. *An easier way to assess if a patient is hypovolemic is to give fluids and see if the stroke volume increases by >10%.* If it does, an additional fluid bolus should be given. Fluid should be administered until no further increase in stroke volume is seen.

Loss of circulating intravascular volume can occur due to myriad reasons including major bleeding, coagulopathy, vomiting, high nasogastric tube output, diarrhea, insensible fluid losses, or capillary leakage. Specific causes of hypovolemic shock are listed in **Table 10-2**. When a patient is admitted with hypotension of unknown origin, hypovolemia must be suspected and treated before other forms of therapy are instituted.

QUICK TIP! The CCRN exam contains shock questions on each type of shock (cardiogenic, hypovolemic, anaphylactic, neurogenic, and septic). The review presented here is designed to build on previous chapters and improve your ability to recognize and differentiate etiologies, signs and symptoms of hypovolemic shock from those of cardiogenic, obstructive, and distributive shock.

TABLE 10-1. HYPOVOLEMIA: EASY REVIEW AND APPLICATION
Presents with a threat to tissue oxygenation
SvO_2 or $ScvO_2$ is low (<60% or <70%, respectively)
Lactate is elevated (>4 mmol)
Cardiac output is low
Heart pumps <4 L/min
Cardiac index is low (<2.5 mL/m²)
Stroke volume is low (<50 mL)
Stroke index is low (<25 mL/m²)
Cardiac filling pressures are low or normal
CVP is <6
PAOP is <8

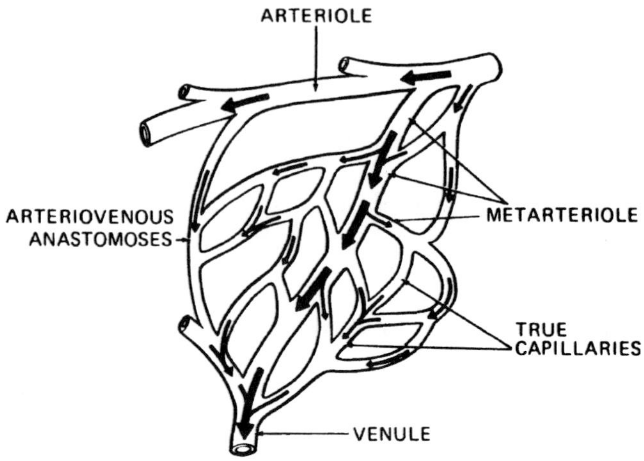

Figure 10-1. Components of the microcirculation.

10.2 PATHOPHYSIOLOGY

The loss of circulating blood volume leads to a **reduction in preload** (stretch of the ventricular muscle) and *eventually a reduction in* ***SV*** *and* ***CO****. Heart rate (HR) increases to compensate for loss of SV in order to maintain adequate CO.* In the early stages of hypovolemic shock, this HR *increase is* substantial enough to prevent a hypotension.

Sympathetic nervous system (SNS) stimulation raises circulating catecholamine (eg, **epinephrine, norepinephrine, dopamine**) levels causing vasoconstriction. The renin–angiotensin–aldosterone system (RAAS) activation induces fluid retention and vasoconstriction. By working together, the SNS and RAAS increase systemic vascular resistance (*SVR*) *and BP* as a second compensatory mechanism. Again, the BP does not change markedly until the SVR can no longer regulate the BP. Simultaneously, at the same time that HR and SVR are compensating for loss of stroke volume, microcirculatory changes are also occurring to maintain blood flow to vital organs.

Microcirculation Physiology

> QUICK TIP! It is unlikely that this content will be directly addressed on the exam. However, this information is good background material for understanding how blood flow is regulated at the tissue level.
>
> *These mechanisms occur in all forms of initial compensation to loss of blood flow—for example, all initial stages of shock.*

The microcirculation of blood vessels regulates blood supply to the tissues (**Fig. 10-1**). The microcirculatory system consists of capillaries, arterioles, and venules. Capillaries form the vascular system between arterioles and venules. The arterioles bifurcate at points called metarterioles or precapillary arterioles.

Muscle sphincters are located where metarterioles bifurcate into true capillaries. This precapillary sphincter acts as an *autoregulatory system*. The precapillary sphincter constricts in cases of shock and SNS stimulation to maintain perfusion of the vital organs. *This constriction directs available blood from nonessential tissues, such as the stomach, to vital organs, especially the heart and brain.* The release of *catecholamines* in early shock results in vasoconstriction of the microcirculatory vessels at the precapillary sphincter level. The precapillary sphincter *constricts in an attempt to increase venous return to the heart* (by preventing blood flow in unnecessary tissues), which in turn improves CO and tissue perfusion (**Table 10-3**). *This is the first major compensatory mechanism to be activated with the onset of shock.*

Many chemical and neurohormonal factors alter the regulation of the microcirculatory system. Neurochemical controls provide

TABLE 10-2. CAUSES OF HYPOVOLEMIC AND CARDIOGENIC SHOCK

Hypovolemic	*Cardiogenic*
Trauma	Myocardial infarction
Postoperative bleeding	Atrial tachydysrhythmias (atrial tachycardia, flutter, fibrillation)
Gastrointestinal bleeding	Ventricular tachycardia, fibrillation
Burns	Congestive heart failure
Capillary leak syndromes	Papillary muscle rupture Septal or ventricular wall rupture Tension pneumothorax Pericardial tamponade

TABLE 10-3. REGULATION OF THE MICROCIRCULATORY SYSTEM

Chemical	*C*	*D*	*Humoral*	*C*	*D*
Hypoxemia		+	Catecholamines		
Hydrogen		+	Epinephrine	+	+
Potassium		+	Norepinephrine	+	
Hypercapnia	+		Dopamine	+	+
Hyperosmolarity	+		Amines		
			Serotonin	+	+
			Acetylcholine		+
			Histamine		+
			Polypeptides		
			Angiotensin	+	
			Kinins	+	
			Vasopressin	+	

C, vasoconstriction; D, vasodilatation.

a negative feedback response that results in adaptive responses to maintain cellular oxygenation. This may slow the rate of hemodynamic changes if the hypovolemia is mild or has a slower onset. If the shock is severe or develops rapidly, this negative feedback of the microcirculatory system can't continue to compensate. Without immediate intervention, **preload and SV continue to drop,** significant tachycardia and hypotension ensue. As shock progresses, tissue perfusion, cellular hypoxia, and metabolic acidosis worsen, and may cause cardiac arrest.

Movement of fluid from the interstitial space into the vasculature, increases plasma volume and helps compensate for hypovolemia. Hydrostatic pressure changes in the capillaries alter fluid exchange across the capillary membrane. Over time, plasma oncotic pressure decreases, and fluid moves into capillary beds. After hemorrhage, the liver synthesizes albumin. Albumin raises the intravascular oncotic pressure, reversing the fluid shift and raising intravascular volume.

The *renin–angiotensin–aldosterone cascade* is activated by decreased renal blood flow. **Renin** is released. Renin loses two amino acids, converting it to the vasoconstrictor **angiotensin I** (AT I). The **angiotensin converting enzyme (ACE)**, cleaves AT I into **angiotensin II** (AT II). **Angiotensin II** is one of the most potent vasoconstrictors known. In combination with catecholamines, AT II raises SVR and BP. The adrenal glands release **aldosterone in response to AT II. Aldosterone** increases renal sodium retention and water reabsorption in the nephrons leading to higher intravascular fluid volume.

A low CO, secondary to hypovolemia stimulates the posterior pituitary gland to increase the release of **antidiuretic hormone (ADH),** which is also called arginine **vasopressin** since it acts on vasopressin (V) receptors. At lower levels, ADH acts on the (V2) receptors in the kidney to reabsorb water from the convoluted tubules and collecting ducts. At higher levels, ADH acts on the V1a receptors in the vasculature, inducing vasoconstriction and increasing arterial pressure.

Presentation of Acute Hypovolemia

Hypovolemic patients may report lightheadedness or dizziness when changing positions to sitting or standing. (Specific symptoms of hypovolemic shock are listed in Table 10-1.) This phenomenon is called **orthostasis**, and it may indicate hypovolemia. Orthostatic vital signs are measured after changing the patient's position from supine to sitting and from sitting to standing. Orthostasis is present if the systolic blood pressure (SBP) decreases >20 mm Hg and the diastolic blood pressure (DBP) decreases >10 mm Hg. HR normally increases 10 to 15 BPM above baseline with position change. Critically ill patients may not report lightheadedness or dizziness if they are bedbound, intubated, sedated, or have other barriers to communication As a result, acute hypovolemia may go unnoticed until hypotension and compensatory tachycardia occur. Fortunately, there are more subtle clinical changes that can help nurses recognize shock and intervene sooner.

The earliest sign of shock is mental status change. Elevated respiratory rates (>20 breaths/min) and **reduction in urine output (<0.5 mL/kg/h)** occur before HR increases and BP drops. *A gradually increasing HR coupled with a downtrending BP may be a clue to impending hypovolemic shock.* In hypovolemia, pulse pressure (SBP – DBP) narrows as shock progresses, indicating a drop in CO. Measurements of **preload** decrease. In patients with central lines, **CVP is normal to low**. Patients with pulmonary artery catheters will have **normal to low CVP, pulmonary artery diastolic pressures (PAD) or pulmonary artery occlusion pressures (PAOP). These findings help differentiate hypovolemic from cardiogenic or obstructive shock.**

KEY CLINICAL CONCEPT!

- Altered mental status is the earliest sign of tissue hypoperfusion, followed by tachypnea and oliguria. Significant sinus tachycardia (HR > 120) and hypotension (SBP <90 or >40-point drop from baseline) are late findings.
- Pulse pressure is narrowed in hypovolemic shock.
- Normal to low filling pressures (CVP, PAD, PAOP) may indicate hypovolemia.

QUICK TIP! Hypovolemic is a common cause of pulseless electrical activity (PEA) cardiac arrests.

10.3 COMPLICATIONS

Ongoing hypoperfusion decreases oxygen delivery to the tissues (DO_2). Cellular metabolism changes from aerobic to anaerobic, generating lactic acid, and inducing metabolic acidosis. Lactate levels >4 mmol indicate shock and correspond with low SvO_2 (or $ScvO_2$).

Acidosis lowers the arrhythmia threshold and impairs the coagulation cascade. As shock progresses, patients may be obtunded, anuric, have cool clammy or mottled skin, weak peripheral pulses, and sluggish cap refill, in addition to worsening tachypnea, hypotension, and tachycardia (HR > 140). Severe hypovolemia leads to cerebral anoxia and cardiac arrest (eg, PEA).

Sustained hypoperfusion due to hypovolemia will lead to impaired organ function and eventually cell death. It is possible that apoptosis (preprogrammed cell death) may be stimulated by hypoperfusion. Hypovolemia requires rapid treatment to avoid a potentially harmful or even fatal outcome.

10.4 TREATMENT

Treatment of hypovolemic shock focuses on restoring intravascular volume, reversing systemic anticoagulants (eg, heparin, apixaban, rivaroxaban, warfarin, etc), and stopping any ongoing blood loss. The initial treatment of hypovolemia is administration of isotonic crystalloid fluids, such as 0.9% saline or lactated ringers. The amount of fluid ordered depends on degree of hypovolemia, cause of the bleeding (eg, trauma vs. GI bleed), and patient-specific factors. Many providers and treatment guidelines recommend using lactated ringers since it has a lower level of chloride than 0.9% saline and may help prevent the hyperchloremic metabolic acidosis that accompanies large-volume 0.9% saline resuscitation. Alternatively, some providers are opting for balanced fluids such as Plasma-Lyte and sodium acetate to prevent acid-base and electrolyte imbalances. In theory, these fluids have desired benefits, but there are currently no data to support their use over standard crystalloids. Administering warmed fluids, if possible, will help decrease the risk of coagulopathy. Large volumes of room-temperature fluids can cause hypothermia and coagulopathy that increases the risk of ongoing blood loss. Current literature recommends mindfulness of the total amount of crystalloid volume administered in the first 24 hours due to the risks of coagulopathy, respiratory failure, and abdominal/extremity compartment syndrome.

Administration of whole blood or a combination of packed red cells (PRBCs) along with **platelets**, **plasma**, and/or **cryoprecipitate** (alone or as part of mass transfusion protocol) may be required to replaced lost blood, platelets, and plasma clotting factors including fibrinogen.

Viscoelastic tests such as thromboelastography (TEG) or rotational thromboelastography (ROTEM) have been shown to reduce the amount of products administered by identifying specific coagulation deficiencies, allowing for targeted transfusion instead of indiscriminately using multiple products. Blood administration increases vascular volume, osmotic pressure, and oxygen-carrying capacity. Intravenous **calcium**, **prothrombin concentrates**, **recombinant factor VII**, **DDAVP**, and the administration of antifibrinolytic agents, such as **tranexamic acid (TXA)**, may be indicated.

In addition to blood, providers may order other types of colloids to expand the circulating blood volume. Colloids, such as albumin, contain high-molecular-weight solutes and are available in different concentrations (eg, 12.5% vs 25% albumin). The colloidal agents increase plasma oncotic pressure, shifting fluid from the interstitial spaces into the blood stream. Recent research suggests that albumin has no benefit over crystalloid resuscitation.

In addition, the optimal method to administer the saline is to have a goal (the concept of goal-directed therapy). The best criterion to use in determining how much fluid to give is the SvO_2 level. Although normal saline can be administered at an estimated volume (eg, 20 mL/kg), the exact amount that should be given is not known. That is why it is best to administer fluids until the SvO_2 level returns to normal (eg, 70%).

Blood and Blood Product Transfusions

Blood and blood production transfusion is associated with risks such as immune system modulation and is an independent risk factor for hospital acquired infections such ventilator associated pneumonia, as well as transfusion associated acute lung injury (TRALI), and transfusion-associated circulatory overload (TACO). *Blood transfusion is not indicated unless the patient is actively bleeding, has signs of acute coronary syndrome (ACS), is symptomatic (eg, dizzy, light-headed, hypotensive), or hemoglobin <7 g/d. Blood should be given with caution.* After 1 unit of PRBCs, hemoglobin should rise by 1 g/dL and hematocrit should rise by 3%. Ongoing blood loss should be considered when hemoglobin and hematocrit don't increment as expected.

KEY CLINICAL CONCEPT

Blood transfusion is not indicated unless the patient is actively bleeding, has signs of acute coronary syndrome (ACS), is symptomatic (eg, dizzy, lightheaded, hypotensive), or hemoglobin <7 g/d. Blood should be given with caution.

If blood is given, a better endpoint is tissue oxygenation (eg, SvO_2) rather than an arbitrary hemoglobin value.

Endpoints of Resuscitation

There are several methods available for determining the completion of volume resuscitation. These are the most commonly used by providers:

- Restoration of mental status.
- Urine output ≥ 0.5 mL/kg/h (or 30 mL/h).
- Mean arterial pressure (MAP) ≥ 60 mm Hg.
- Resolution of tachycardia.
- Hemoglobin above target, eg, >7.0 g/dL.
- Lactate <2 mEq/L × 2 consecutive measurements. (Also, the higher a patient's lactate (when associated with a decrease in pH), the higher the morbidity and mortality.)
- Normalization of base deficit (>−5 is considered shock).
- Stroke volume variation (SVV) <13.
- Normalization of SvO_2 occurs when tissue oxygen delivery (DO_2) improves.

10.5 NURSING INTERVENTION

Hemodynamic monitoring of hypovolemic shock usually commonly involves arterial blood pressure. CVP and $ScvO_2$ may be used in selected patients. In patients with pulmonary artery catheters, resuscitation should increase CVP, PAD, PAOP, and SvO_2. Newer research is moving away from using static measures such as filling pressures and towards assessing vascular structures or dynamic variables to assess fluid responsiveness. Some examples include point-of-care ultrasound (POCUS) to assess the inferior vena cava (IVC) and passive leg raise (PLR). Nondilated IVC and BPs that increase are predict that the patient's BP will be responsive to fluid administration. Patients who have dilated IVCs or whose BP don't change with PLR will likely not respond to fluid administration. Other dynamic variables include less invasive technologies, such as esophageal Dopplers, bioimpedance and pulse contour analysis with the ability to measure SV, SVI, or SVV.

The Trendelenburg position is no longer recommended to raise BP in shock patients. It is associated with risk of aspiration, facial/laryngeal edema, hypoventilation, cardiac arrhythmias, and decreased lower extremity arterial blood flow. *In cases of severe shock, a supine position with legs elevated 20 to 30 degrees by pillows may increase venous return.* Whether this helps improve survival is not known.

Cardiovascular status, in addition to hemodynamic status, is continuously monitored for signs of dysrhythmias. Dysrhythmias due to acidosis and electrolyte disturbances are common hypovolemia and large volume transfusion.

Vasomotor tone is normally controlled by constriction secondary to sympathetic and catecholamine agents. Vasoactive infusions, such as **norepinephrine (Levophed), dopamine, or phenylephrine (Neosynephrine)** may be administered to maintain BP in conjunction with volume resuscitation.

Acid–base disturbances may be severe. Metabolic acidosis with respiratory alkalosis compensating to normalize an acidotic pH is common. Respiratory acidosis is corrected by adequate ventilation. Metabolic acidosis may be corrected by increasing blood flow to the organs. If the pH is severely acidotic (<7.20), sodium bicarbonate ($NaHCO_3$) may be used to raise the pH (>7.20). An initial loading dose for sodium bicarbonate is 1 mEq/kg of body weight. Additional doses or $NaHCO_3$ infusions may be indicated depending on the ABG values. *The use of sodium bicarbonate remains controversial, as it may not be helpful in correcting the underlying cause of the acidosis. However, it may help raise pH in order to "buy time" for other treatments to be work.* However, changes in the guidelines for its application may alter the above recommendations.

Urine output is monitored hourly, usually via an indwelling Foley catheter, or external urinary drainage devices. Lab monitoring of blood urea nitrogen (BUN) and creatinine may show acute kidney injury (AKI) due to prerenal azotemia is the first renal response. **The BUN may rise disproportionately to the creatinine, creating an increased BUN/creatinine ratio (>20:1).** Severe or sustained hypovolemia may result in acute tubular necrosis (ATN).

QUICK TIP! The CCRN exam may include a question regarding the suspected etiology of oliguria. It is important to note that prerenal AKI is associated with an increased BUN/creatinine ratio (>20:1).

Nutritional support is essential, since a shock state rapidly depletes glucose storage with a resulting negative nitrogen balance, and protein catabolism increases acidotic states. Enteral feeding is preferred.

Emotional support of the patient and families is paramount and includes reassurance and explanation of procedures. Families may be provided with information by way of brochures or websites that will help explain medical conditions in an easy-to-understand manner. Brief explanations in lay terms about the patient's condition, and the use of monitoring equipment will decrease anxiety and promote family-centered care.

KEY CONTENT CHECKLIST

- ❒ Altered mental status is the earliest sign of tissue hypoperfusion, followed by tachypnea and oliguria. Significant sinus tachycardia (HR > 120) and hypotension (SBP <90 or >40-point drop from baseline) are late findings.
- ❒ Pulse pressure (SBP – DBP = PP) is narrowed in hypovolemic shock and suggests low SV.
- ❒ Normal to low filling pressures (CVP, PAD, PAOP) may indicate hypovolemia.
- ❒ Blood transfusion is not indicated unless the patient is actively bleeding, has signs of acute coronary syndrome (ACS), is symptomatic (eg, dizzy, lightheaded, hypotensive), or hemoglobin <7 g/d. Blood should be given with caution.

Review Questions:

1. A patient reports dizziness when moving from sitting to standing. Vital signs are HR 82, BP 105/60, RR 14, oxygen saturation 98% on 3 L NC. Hemoglobin is 9.2 g/dL. Which of the following are most consistent with orthostatic hypotension?

a. BP 101/57 and HR 92
b. BP 98/60 and HR 104
c. BP 90/48 and HR 95
d. BP 103/53 and HR 90

Answer: C. Rationale: The correct answer is C since the SBP has decreased >20 points and the DBP >10 points from baseline. HR is normally expected to increase 10 to 15 bpm during position changes. Answers A, B, and D do not meet the SBP or DBP change criteria.

2. An 80-kg patient with admitted from the emergency department (ED) with acute pancreatitis is increasingly anxious and urine output has decreased to 25 mL/h for the last 2 hours, despite 2 L of crystalloid fluid. Vital signs are T 101.0, HR 105, RR 20, and BP 110/50. Which of the following findings indicates the patient may benefit from additional IV fluid resuscitation?

a. Distended inferior vena cava
b. Flat neck veins
c. BP increases to 122/60 with PLR
d. BP increases to 130/62 with the Trendelenburg positioning

Answer: C. Rationale: The correct answer is C. Increased BP with PLR indicates fluid responsiveness. Answer A is incorrect as a distended inferior vena cava can indicate obstructive shock or fluid volume overload. Answer B, all though it seems like the patient could benefit from IV fluid, is not an indicator of fluid responsiveness. Answer D is incorrect since the Trendelenburg position has been associated with myriad undesired physiologic responses.

REFERENCES

Cannon JW. Hemorrhagic shock. *N Engl J Med.* 2018;378(4):370–379. doi: 10.1056/NEJMra1705649.

Casey DD, Brown RM, Semler MW. Resuscitation fluids. *Curr Opin Crit Care.* 2018;24(6): 512–518. doi: 10.1097/MCC.0000000000000551.

Gordon D, Spiegel R. Fluid resuscitation: history, physiology, and modern fluid resuscitation strategies. *Emerg Med Clin North Am.* 2020;38(4):783–793. doi: 10.1016/j.emc.2020.06.004.

Semple JW, Rebetz J, Kapur R. Transfusion-associated circulatory overload and transfusion-related acute lung injury. *Blood.* 2019;133(17):1840–1853. doi: 10.1182/blood-2018-10-860809.

11

Interpreting Dysrhythmias

CHAPTER OVERVIEW AND OBJECTIVES

The CCRN exam can be expected to directly address either the interpretation or treatment of sinus and atrial dysrhythmias. There are only a few questions on the CCRN that will ask you to interpret dysrhythmias. The most likely dysrhythmias are atrial tachycardia, flutter, and fibrillation. The most important concepts in this area are the correct interpretation of dysrhythmias and the treatment each would require. Most of this information is included in a basic ECG course. However, if the interpretation of dysrhythmia is not a strength for you, review this chapter carefully.

After studying this chapter, you should be able to:

- Identify key characteristics in distinguishing sinus, atrial, atrioventricular nodal, and ventricular dysrhythmias.
- Describe appropriate treatments for the various dysthymias within the chapter.

QUICK TIP! There may be several questions where dysrhythmias are a part of the test question or scenario on the CCRN Exam.

All dysrhythmias are caused by a disturbance in the formation of the cardiac impulse or a disturbance in its conduction. The classification of dysrhythmias is shown in **Table 11-1**.

Every dysrhythmia has specific identifying characteristics. The first four dysrhythmias discussed in this chapter originate in the sinoatrial (SA) node. The next six dysrhythmias originate in the atrium but not in the SA node. The final eight dysrhythmias originate from electrical impulses initiated in the junctional tissue around the atrioventricular (AV) node. (*Note:* All rhythm strips are 6 s, lead II.)

11.1 SINOATRIAL NODE DYSRHYTHMIAS

Sinus Arrhythmia (or Sinus Dysrhythmia)

Etiology. Variations of impulse formation in the SA node are caused by the vagus nerve and changes in venous return to the heart. This results in an irregular rhythm with alternating fast and slow rates (**Fig. 11-1**).

Identifying Characteristics. The rate varies, generally between 60 and 100 bpm. The rate increases with inspiration and decreases with expiration. Both atrial and ventricular rhythms are regularly irregular if the variation is due to a regular breathing pattern. The P waves are normal and the PR interval is within normal limits. The QRS complex is normal. The difference between normal sinus rhythm and sinus arrhythmia is seen in the variation in the R-R intervals. In sinus arrhythmia, the variation is at least 0.04 s between the shortest and longest R-R intervals. The variation in normal sinus rhythm is less than 0.04 s.

Risk. There is no risk for the patient because this dysrhythmia is generally a normal variant and causes no hemodynamic compromise.

Treatment. Generally, no treatment is needed.

Nursing Intervention. Document the dysrhythmia with a rhythm strip. This interpretation can be substantiated if the patient holds his or her breath and the rate stabilizes.

Sinus Bradycardia

Etiology. **Parasympathetic (vagal)** control over the SA node due to ischemia, vagal nerve stimulation, pain, drugs, sleep, hypoxia, electrolyte imbalances, or athletic conditioning decreases the formation of electrical impulses (**Fig. 11-2**).

Identifying Characteristics. The rate is less than 60 bpm but typically more than 40 bpm. Both atrial and ventricular rhythms are usually regular. P waves are normal and there is a P wave for each QRS. The PR interval is within normal typically near the upper limit of the range. The QRS complex is normal. Conduction is normal.

Risk. This dysrhythmia may lead to syncopal attacks, angina, premature beats, ventricular tachycardia, heart failure (HF), and cardiac arrest. It is a serious warning dysrhythmia if the rate is low (about 40) and accompanied by hypotension

TABLE 11-1. CLASSIFICATION OF DYSRHYTHMIAS

Dysrhythmias Due to Disorders in Impulse Foundation or Accessory Pathway	*Dysrhythmias Due to Conduction Disturbances*
SA node dysrhythmias	SA block
Sinus tachycardia	AV blocks
Sinus bradycardia	First-degree AV block
Sinus arrhythmia	Second-degree type I AV block
Wandering pacemaker	Second-degree type II AV block
SA arrest	Third-degree (complete) AV block
Atrial dysrhythmias	Intraventricular blocks
Premature atrial contractions	Left bundle branch blocks
Paroxysmal atrial tachycardia	Right bundle branch blocks
Atrial flutter	Bilateral bundle branch blocks
Atrial fibrillation	
AV nodal area (junctional) dysrhythmias	
Premature junctional contractions	
Junctional escape rhythm	
Paroxysmal junctional tachycardia	
Junctional tachycardia	
Ventricular dysrhythmias	
Premature ventricular contractions	
Ventricular tachycardia	
Ventricular fibrillation	
Ventricular asystole	

(blood pressure below 90/60 mm Hg). Sinus bradycardia is generally benign but should be assessed for its effect on hemodynamics especially in older, sedentary people.

Treatment. No treatment may be necessary if the rate is close to 60 bpm or if the patient is asymptomatic. If the patient is symptomatic, first try to find out whether there is a reversible cause, such as hypoxemia.

KEY CLINICAL CONCEPT!

Treatment of bradycardia is usually only indicated when the patient is symptomatic or hemodynamically unstable.

Lack of patient tolerance of bradycardia may be evident with symptoms such as shortness of breath, dizziness, signs of poor peripheral perfusion, and fatigue.

Treat the symptom to resolve the bradycardia. For example, give supplemental oxygen if the oxygen saturation is low. If more severe symptoms are present (eg, hypotension or signs of HF), intravenous **atropine** is the drug of choice to increase the heart rate. **Dopamine** or **epinephrine** infusions may also be attempted if **atropine** is not effective. *An external or temporary pacemaker may be required if pharmacologic management is unsuccessful.*

Nursing Intervention. Document the dysrhythmia with a rhythm strip and assess whether the patient is symptomatic. Monitor and document the effectiveness of drug therapy. *Do not administer drugs, such as digitalis or beta blockers,* that may further slow the heart rate. Be especially alert for premature ventricular contractions (PVCs). If PVCs occur, obtain a rhythm strip and notify the physician; *do not treat with lidocaine* or other agents that may eliminate the PVCs. PVCs associated with a bradycardia are generally treated with **atropine** or another therapy to remove the cause of the bradycardia. As the heart rate increases, the PVCs usually disappear.

Sinus Tachycardia

Etiology. Sinus tachycardia may be caused by many factors and identifying the etiology is key to successful treatment of the dysrhythmia. Common etiologies include hypoxia, hypovolemia, anemia, pulmonary embolism, acute myocardial infarction (MI), and stimulation of the sympathetic nervous system (anxiety, physical exertion, and fever). Cardiac decompensation is the most serious cause of sinus tachycardia. The increase in heart rate during HF is a compensatory response due to a reduced stroke volume. (**Fig. 11-3**).

Identifying Characteristics. The rate is greater than 100 and is usually between 100 and 160 bpm. Both atrial and ventricular rhythms are regular. The P wave is normal but may be difficult to identify because of the rapid rate. (*Note:* Look for the P wave superimposed on the T wave with fast rates). The PR interval is usually at the lower limits of normal.

Risk. Regardless of the etiology, prolonged sinus tachycardia may precipitate HF in patients with borderline cardiac function. When the body is requiring increased cardiac output, the heart rate will increase to increase the blood flow to the end organs and tissues. The ability to tolerate a prolonged sinus tachycardia is dependent on the patient's underlying cardiac function as this increased heart rate increases the amount of oxygen the heart requires (MvO_2).

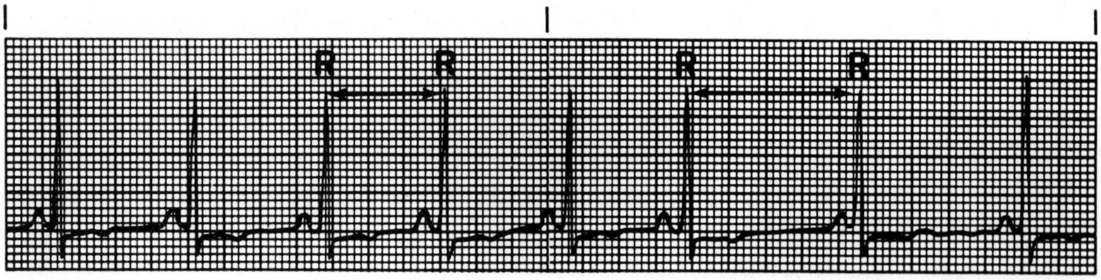

Figure 11-1. Sinus arrhythmia.

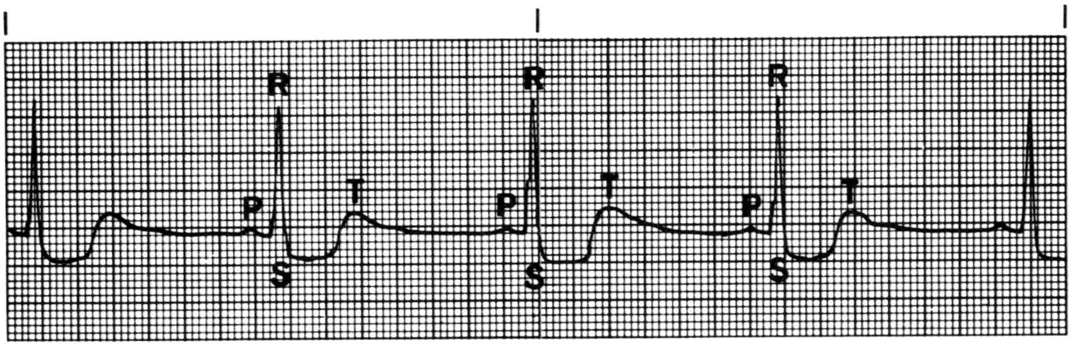

Figure 11-2. Sinus bradycardia.

Treatment. Effective treatment depends on controlling the underlying cause. Normally sinus tachycardia does not in itself require treatment. In case of a persistent sinus tachycardia that is compromising cardiac output, pharmacologic treatment may be required, with drugs such as calcium channel blockers (eg, **verapamil**), beta blockers (eg, **esmolol, diltiazem**), or **adenosine** or digitalis preparations (eg, **digoxin**).

QUICK TIP! Generally speaking, revolving the underlying physiologic cause is the focus of treatment for sinus tachycardia (eg, pain, fear, anxiety, fever, volume depletion).

Nursing Intervention. Document the dysrhythmia with a rhythm strip. Monitor the patient for signs of left ventricular (LV) failure (restlessness, orthopnea, cough, shortness of breath). Attempts to calm the patient and decrease the patient's stress may be helpful.

Sinus Pause/Arrest, Sinoatrial Block

Etiology. These more complex atrial dysrhythmias will rarely be on the CCRN exam. Therefore, this information is more supplemental than essential. Ischemic injury to the SA node is the most common and important cause of SA block. There is a technical but not a clinical difference between sinus pause/arrest and SA block. In the pause/arrest, the SA node does not form an electrical impulse. In SA block, the SA node initiates an impulse, but it is prevented from leaving the node and thus cannot be visualized. Regardless of this difference, the end result is that no impulse stimulates the atria or the ventricles. The terms "pause" and "block" are often used interchangeably. Sinus disease, vagal effect, hypoxia, digitalis toxicity, and parasympathetic stimulation may be causes of SA block (**Fig. 11-4**).

QUICK TIP! The appearance of obscure dysrhythmias, such as, "wandering atrial pacemaker" on the exam is less likely.

Identifying Characteristics. The rate is usually slower than normal. Rhythm (both atrial and ventricular) is generally regular except for the arrest/block complex. P waves are absent in arrest and block for a specific time. Otherwise, P waves are normal. The PR interval is absent in the arrest/block complex. The QRS complex may be normal or abnormal in arrest, depending on the escape site. No QRS complexes are seen during the block. Conduction depends on the escape site in arrest and is absent in sinus block for that specific interval.

Risk. The greatest risk is that both sinus pause/arrest and sinus block may proceed to a reduced cardiac output if the arrest or block is frequent. If the arrest or block is infrequent and self-limiting, it is not dangerous.

Treatment. If the arrest or block is rare, it does not require treatment. *If the arrest is frequent, treatment is essential.* If drugs are the underlying cause, they should be evaluated and stopped. **Atropine** and **epinephrine** may be effective at increasing the heart rate. If these are not effective and the patient is symptomatic, an **external pacemaker** could be applied initially, but long-term treatment will require a permanent pacemaker.

Nursing Intervention. Document the dysrhythmia with a rhythm strip. If a drug is the possible underlying cause, withhold the drug until it is reordered. Monitor the patient closely

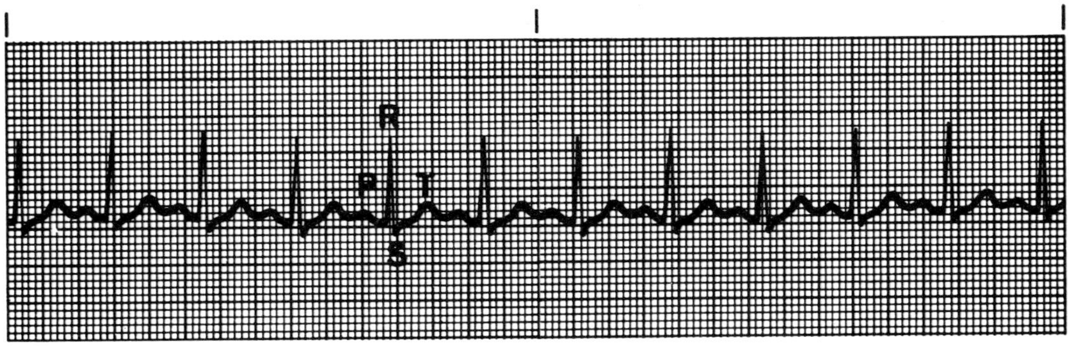

Figure 11-3. Sinus tachycardia.

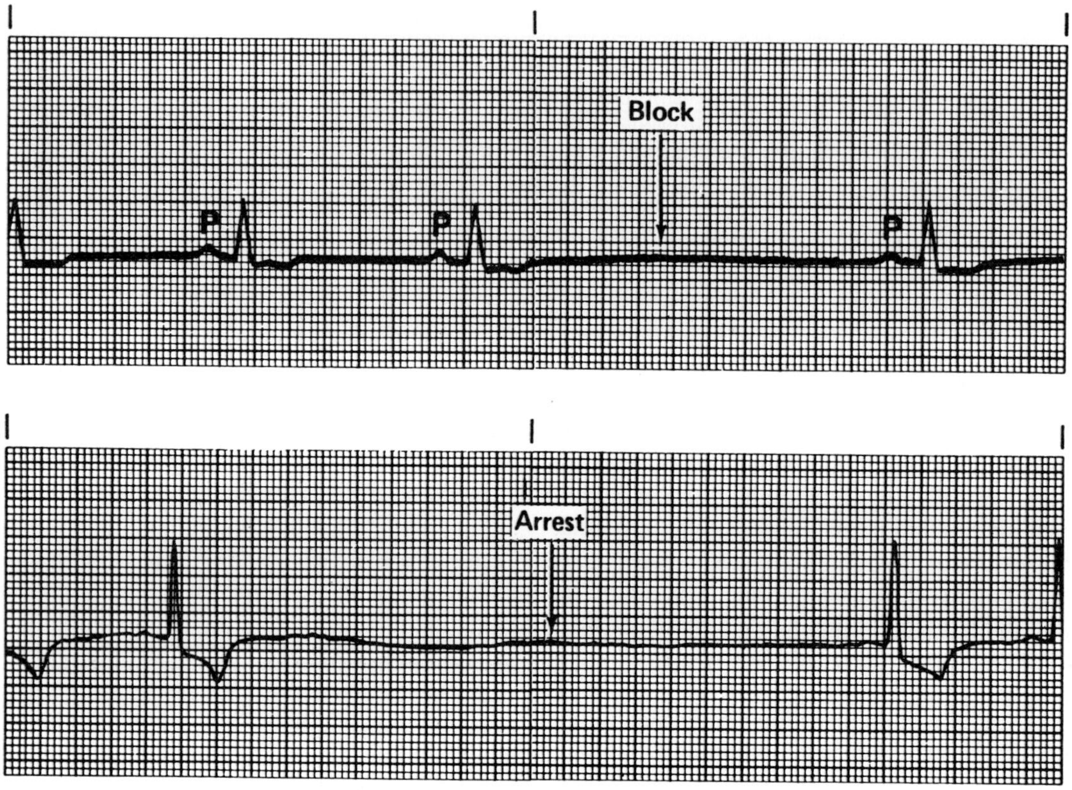

Figure 11-4. SA arrest or block.

to determine whether the frequency of arrest or block is increasing. If it is, document with rhythm strips and notify the physician; a pacemaker may be indicated.

11.2 ATRIAL DYSRHYTHMIAS

Paroxysmal Atrial Tachycardia

Etiology. The term paroxysmal atrial tachycardia (PAT) describes several causes for a rapid atrial heart rate (**Fig. 11-5**). Another term, paroxysmal supraventricular tachycardia (PSVT or just SVT), is also used to describe this rhythm. In PAT, excessive sympathetic stimulation or abnormal conduction situations are present. Abnormal conduction situations include AV nodal reentry problems or the presence of accessory pathways.

Identifying Characteristics. Three characteristics are associated with PAT:

1. It starts suddenly.
2. Ends abruptly.
3. The ventricles respond either to every impulse created by the focus (1:1 conduction) or to most impulses, creating a rapid ventricular response.

Both atrial and ventricular rates are usually between 150 and 250. The rhythm is regular. P waves are present but may be very difficult to identify. The P wave will not have the normal, smooth, rounded shape of a sinus P wave, since this impulse originates in the atrium tissue, not in the SA node. The PR interval varies. It may be within normal limits and is frequently greater than might be expected for the rate. However, in some

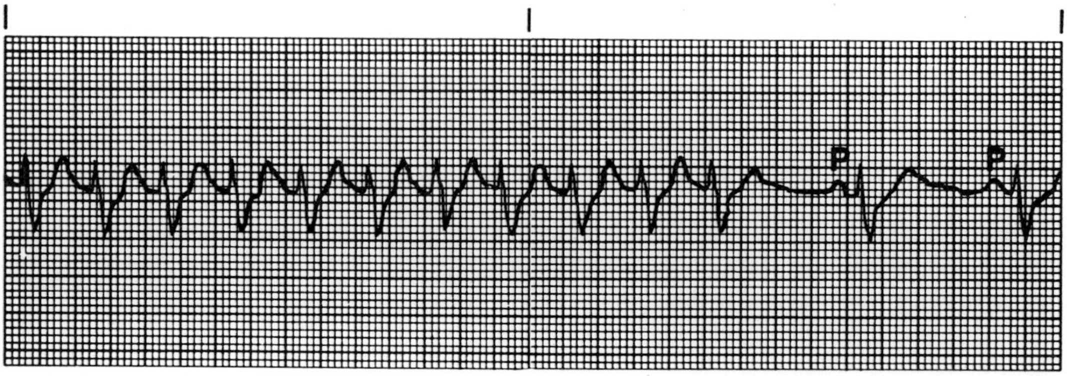

Figure 11-5. Paroxysmal atrial tachycardia.

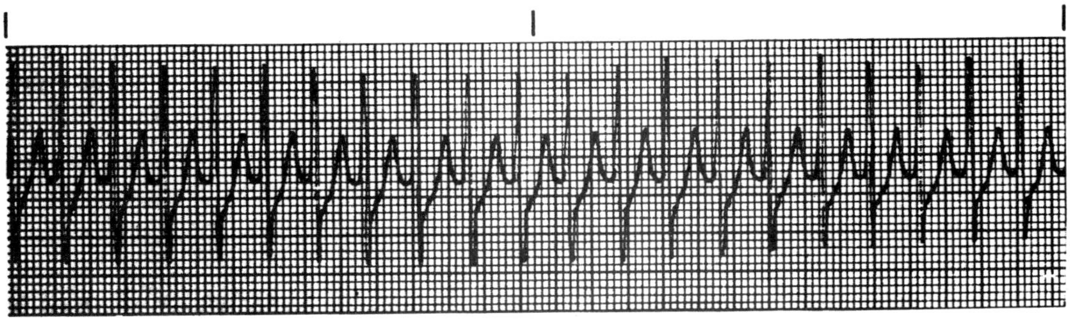

Figure 11-6. Atrial tachycardia.

accessory pathway situations, the PR interval may be shortened. The QRS complex is usually normal. Once again, however, if the problem is due to an accessory pathway, an initial distortion in the QRS complex may be present. This distortion is sometimes seen as a delta wave, causing a slurring of the upstroke on the R wave of the QRS complex.

Risk. PAT frequently stops spontaneously. If it does not, the rapid rate may lead to myocardial ischemia and eventually cardiac decompensation. If PAT occurs after a MI or in a patient with limited cardiac function, it may lead to increased myocardial ischemia, injury, and LV failure.

Treatment. *Vagal stimulation and other vagal maneuvers, such as coughing and pressure on the eyes, may terminate the dysrhythmia.* Having the patient perform a **valsalva maneuver stimulates the vagus nerve**. If this fails to terminate the rhythm, carotid massage by the doctor (or nurse if allowed) often terminates PAT. *If this fails and the patient is asymptomatic, drug therapy may be tried.* Beta blockers such as **esmolol, digoxin,** nondihydropyridine calcium channel blockers (**verapamil or diltiazem**), or **adenosine** given intravenously may terminate PAT. If the patient is symptomatic (complains of angina and becomes diaphoretic, short of breath, and hypotensive), **synchronized cardioversion** may be used immediately. Cardioversion usually terminates PAT.

KEY CLINICAL CONCEPT

When treating SVT, medications are usually indicated if the patient is symptomatic but hemodynamically stable. However, if the patient is unstable (chest pain, short of breath, hypotensive), cardioversion is usually indicated.

Surgical interventions and radiofrequency ablation are increasingly seen as options for the patient with PAT. To cut the accessory pathway surgically (or eliminate the path with radiofrequency ablation), extensive electrical mapping of the heart in an electrophysiology lab to locate the origin of the abnormal pathway is required.

Nursing Intervention. Document the dysrhythmia with a rhythm strip. Assess and monitor the patient for signs of ischemia and decompensation. Medicate as ordered by the physician. Be prepared for synchronized cardioversion.

Atrial Tachycardia

The impulse of atrial tachycardia originates in the atrium. The rate of atrial tachycardia is constant. The difference between PAT and atrial tachycardia is only that PAT starts and stops suddenly. Atrial tachycardia is a constant regular rhythm, not irregular. All other parameters of PAT apply to atrial tachycardia (**Fig. 11-6**).

Premature Atrial Contractions

Note: Premature atrial contractions (PACs) are also called atrial premature beats.

Etiology. On occasion, an irritable focus within the atrium or an impulse through an accessory pathway causes an unexpected, early complex initiating depolarization. The irritable focus does not become the heart's pacemaker except for this single beat (**Fig. 11-7**). Causes of PACs include increased sympathetic nervous system activity, stimulants, drugs such as inotropes, albuterol, and epinephrine, hypoxia, electrolyte imbalances, myocardial ischemia, and digoxin toxicity.

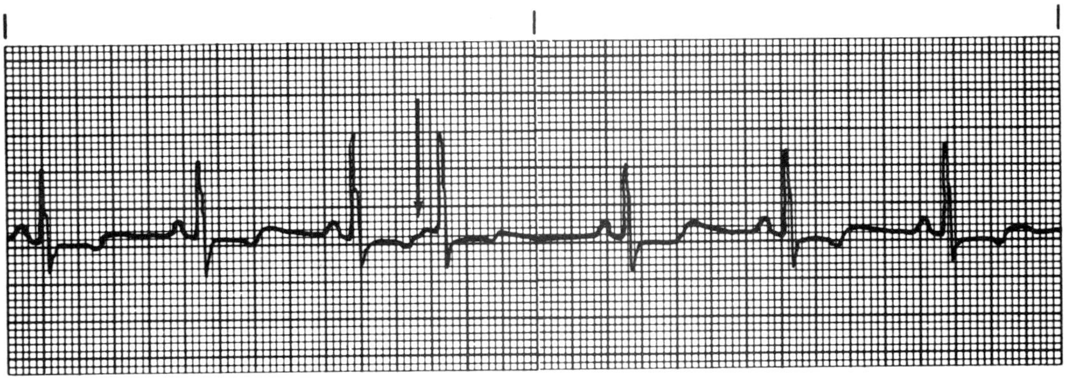

Figure 11-7. Premature atrial contraction.

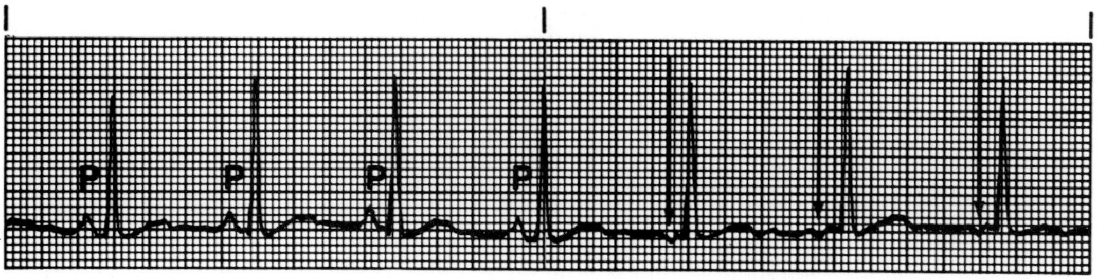

Figure 11-8. Wandering atrial pacemaker.

Identifying Characteristics. The underlying rate is usually normal. The rhythm has an occasional irregularity due to the premature nature of the beat and a brief pause after the premature beat. The P wave is abnormally shaped for the premature beat only. The PR interval is usually prolonged but may be normal or shortened. The QRS complex is normal. PACs may be blocked or may have an aberrant (abnormal or wide QRS) conduction. Conduction below the atria (junctional and ventricular) is usually normal.

QUICK TIP! A biphasic, or "double-humped" P-wave may also be called, "P mitrale." This may suggest atrial enlargement and often comes up on the exam.

Risk. If PACs occur infrequently, there is no risk. The greater the number of PACs the higher the risk of the patient converting to a more dangerous dysrhythmia such as atrial flutter, atrial fibrillation, or atrial tachycardia

Treatment. Those PACs that require treatment are more likely those causing symptoms that disrupt normal activities. Common treatments for PACs include correcting the underlying cause such as correcting hypoxia, repleting electrolytes for hypokalemia or hypomagnesemia, and decreasing or discontinuing causative medications. Pharmacologic therapy includes nondihydropyridine calcium channel blockers and beta blockers.

Nursing Intervention. Document the dysrhythmia with a rhythm strip. Monitor the patient for increasing frequency of PACs. More frequent PACs may cause anxiety, some hemodynamic compromise, hypotension, and dyspnea. Document an increase in frequency with rhythm strips and notify the physician of the increase.

Wandering Atrial Pacemaker

Etiology. Various foci within the atrium or from the AV node supersede the SA node as the pacemaker for a variable number of beats (**Fig. 11-8**). It is commonly seen in the very young, athletes, and the elderly.

Identifying Characteristics. Rate is usually normal but may be slow. Rhythm is frequently regular but can be irregular due to varied conduction pathways. P waves are abnormal, and they change in size, shape, and deflection. There should be three or more P waves with differing morphology representing the various foci firing within the atrium. The PR interval may vary or may be constant. The QRS complex is normal. Conduction is abnormal in the atrium and sometimes in the AV node. Below the AV node, conduction is normal.

Risk. Generally, there is no risk. The presence of a wandering atrial pacemaker is normally insignificant, although it may indicate the presence of SA disease.

Treatment. Usually no treatment is necessary. If the rhythm produced symptoms, the symptoms would be treated. For example, a bradycardia could be treated with **atropine.** If it is drug-induced medications should be stopped and re-evaluated.

Nursing Intervention. Document the dysrhythmia with a rhythm strip. Monitor for an unacceptably low ventricular rate (<50 bpm) and treat as necessary.

Atrial Flutter

Etiology. An irritable atrial focus or accessory pathway may supersede the SA node and produce atrial flutter. This is a fairly common dysrhythmia in atherosclerotic heart disease and valvular heart disease (**Fig. 11-9**). Other common causes include HF, inflammatory heart diseases, cardiomyopathy, excessive alcohol use, hypoxia, and thyrotoxicosis.

Identifying Characteristics. The atrial rate is rapid, usually 250 to 350 bpm. Atrial rhythm is regular, and ventricular rhythm varies with the number of impulses transmitted through the AV node. The P wave is replaced by a flutter wave (F wave). Flutter waves have no isoelectric interval between the waves

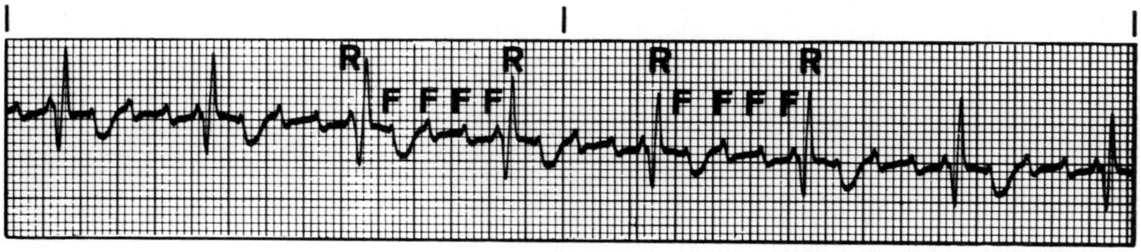

Figure 11-9. Atrial flutter.

and appear sawtooth. The PR interval is not measurable. The QRS complex is usually normal. Conduction is abnormal in the atria, and the AV node normally blocks many of the F waves.

Risk. Pulmonary vascular congestion may occur quickly if the patient has limited cardiac function and the AV node conducts almost all of the F waves. There is the possibility of severe hemodynamic compromise. *If the ventricular response is rapid, there is insufficient filling time for the ventricle. The rapid rate can cause a reduction in cardiac output and hypotension.* Rapid response of the ventricle increases myocardial oxygen demand, which cannot be met due to the decreased cardiac output.

Treatment. Antiarrhythmics such as **amiodarone** are frequently used to treat the condition. Treatment may involve *beta blockers* or non-dihydropyridine *calcium channel blockers* to slow the rate. **If the ventricular response is rapid and the patient is hemodynamically compromised, synchronized cardioversion with low voltage is the preferred treatment.** If the rhythm is unclear, adenosine can be given in an attempt to slow the rhythm so that a better diagnosis can be made.

Nursing Intervention. Document the dysrhythmia with a rhythm strip. Monitor the patient closely for signs of hemodynamic compromise. The physician should be notified when this dysrhythmia develops. If **adenosine** is used, the patient should be warned about a potentially temporary negative feeling as the drug is administered.

Atrial Fibrillation

Etiology. Many irritable foci develop in the atrium to such a degree that normal atrial contraction becomes impossible. This condition may be caused by rheumatic heart disease (particularly mitral stenosis), HF, cardiomyopathy, coronary disease, hypertension, valvular disease, thyrotoxicosis, and congenital heart disease. It is also commonly seen acutely after open heart surgery or in patients with pulmonary embolism (**Fig. 11-10**).

Identifying Characteristics. The atrial rate is not measurable but is probably greater than 300 bpm. At such a high atrial rate, the AV node cannot accept all the stimuli it receives. Consequently, the atrial and ventricular rates are markedly different. The atrial and ventricular rhythms are irregular. P waves are nonexistent and are replaced by fibrillatory waves (f waves). There is no true PR interval. The QRS complex may be normal or abnormal. Ventricular response may be slow, normal, or very rapid. Conduction is abnormal in both the atria and the AV node. The number of impulses that the AV node transmits determines the degree of AV block.

Risk. There may be a rapid development of pulmonary vascular congestion. *In atrial fibrillation lasting more than 24 hours, thrombi may form in the left atrial appendage. This can lead to embolization and stroke.* Marked hemodynamic disturbance is common if the rhythm is of recent onset. Angina and increased myocardial ischemia may occur due to the increase in myocardial oxygen demand (MvO_2).

Treatment. If the dysrhythmia is not causing hemodynamic compromise, medications such as *beta blockers*, nondihydropyridine *calcium channel blockers* (**diltiazem**), **amiodarone**, or less commonly *digitalis preparations* (**digoxin**) may be employed to control the ventricular rate. If hemodynamic compromise develops, synchronized cardioversion is essential to reduce and control the ventricular response. The longer presence of atrial fibrillation without appropriate anticoagulation increases the risk of atrial thrombus. Ideally, an anticoagulant is administered for at least 3 weeks prior to cardioversion in patients who have experienced atrial fibrillation for more than 48 hours or an unknown duration. However, when this is not feasible, anticoagulation should be initiated as soon as possible.

Atrial fibrillation patients who have a high risk of stroke require long-term anticoagulation for stroke prophylaxis. Systemic anticoagulants such as warfarin, and nonvitamin-K anticoagulants (apixaban, dabigatran, edoxaban, rivaroxaban) are used in patients with higher stroke risk. Ablation is also an option for people with symptomatic atrial fibrillation who do not respond to antiarrhythmic therapy.

Nursing Intervention. Document the dysrhythmia with a rhythm strip. Notify the physician if atrial fibrillation develops suddenly. Monitor the patient carefully for hemodynamic compromise and embolization. Contact the physician if a rapid ventricular response develops or if an unacceptably low ventricular response develops (<50 bpm).

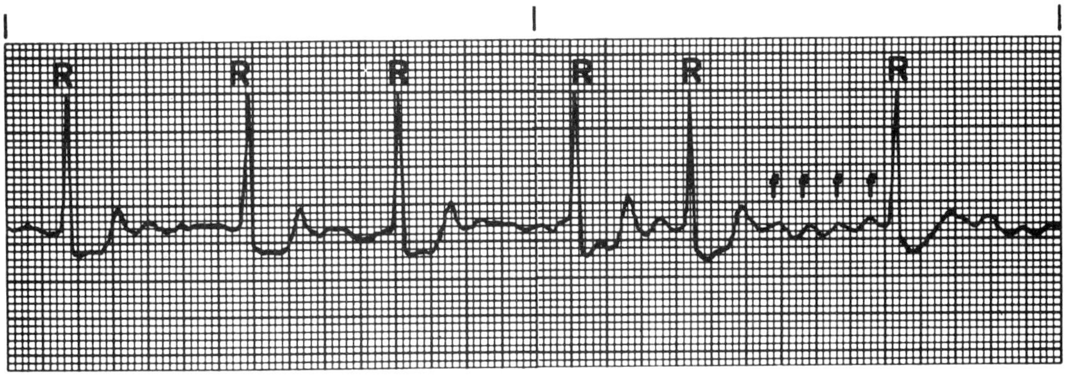

Figure 11-10. Atrial fibrillation.

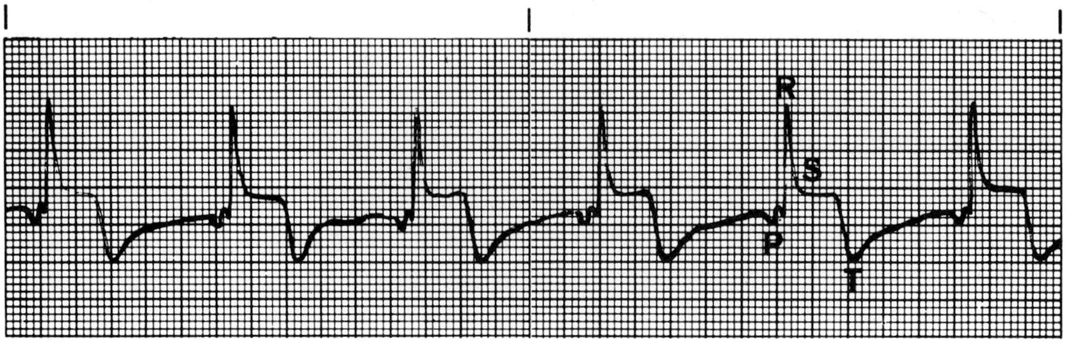

Figure 11-11. Junctional rhythm.

11.3 ATRIOVENTRICULAR NODE AND VENTRICULAR DYSRHYTHMIAS

Junctional Rhythm

Etiology. This dysrhythmia is often due to an acute MI, a SA block, digitalis toxicity, or treatment with drugs that slow the atrial rate (eg, **digitalis** and **procainamide**) (**Fig. 11-11**).

Identifying Characteristics. The rate is usually 40 to 60 bpm. The rhythm is usually regular. If seen, the P wave is usually inverted (negatively deflected) and may precede or follow the QRS complex or be buried within it. This inverted P wave is caused by the electrical impulse originating in junctional tissue and moving both down into the ventricles (a normal path) and back up into the atrium (retrograde movement, an abnormal path). The PR interval, if present, is less than 0.12 seconds and often is not measurable. The QRS complex is normal unless a P wave is buried in it. Conduction to the atria is abnormal owing to its retrograde depolarization of the atria.

Risk. The junctional impulse formation is slow. The junctional rhythm is normally a protective rhythm, taking over as the pacemaker of the heart when the SA node slows to rates below 40 to 60 bpm. Hemodynamic balance may be compromised by a slow ventricular rate, leading to poor cardiac output and perhaps ventricular failure.

Treatment. Medications that increase the heart rate, such as **atropine, dopamine, or epinephrine**, *are considered if the bradycardia were associated with hemodynamic compromise.* If medications fail to work, *pacemakers* can be used to override the slow rate. If drug toxicity is the underlying cause, the drug should be stopped immediately.

Nursing Intervention. Document the dysrhythmia with a rhythm strip. Monitor the patient closely. *PVCs may occur and do not respond well to lidocaine or other ventricular antidysrhythmic agents, since the PVCs are usually a result of decreased cardiac output.* Increasing the heart rate is a more effective method of eliminating the PVCs. Monitor for signs of hemodynamic compromise. Notify the physician immediately if compromise occurs.

Premature Junctional Contraction

Etiology. An irritable focus in the junctional tissue initiates an early impulse. The impulse depolarizes the ventricles normally and the atria in a retrograde fashion. Coronary artery disease (CAD), acute MI, and digitalis toxicity are frequent causes. Any factor that increases junctional ischemia may produce a premature junctional contraction (PJC) (**Fig. 11-12**).

Identifying Characteristics. The underlying rate may be normal or slow. The rhythm is regular except for the premature (early) beat. P waves are abnormal, inverted, and may precede, follow, or be buried in the QRS complex of the PJC. The PR interval varies with the position of the pacemaker and is frequently not measurable. The QRS complex is normal unless the P wave is buried in it or aberration occurs. Conduction is normal through the ventricles and retrograde through the atria.

Risk. PJCs may lead to a SVT if frequent. If rare, PJCs do not pose a threat for the patient.

Treatment. Generally, no treatment is necessary for PJCs. If drug toxicity is the underlying cause, the offending medication should be stopped immediately.

Nursing Intervention. Document the dysrhythmia with a rhythm strip (to justify junctional origin rather than ventricular origin).

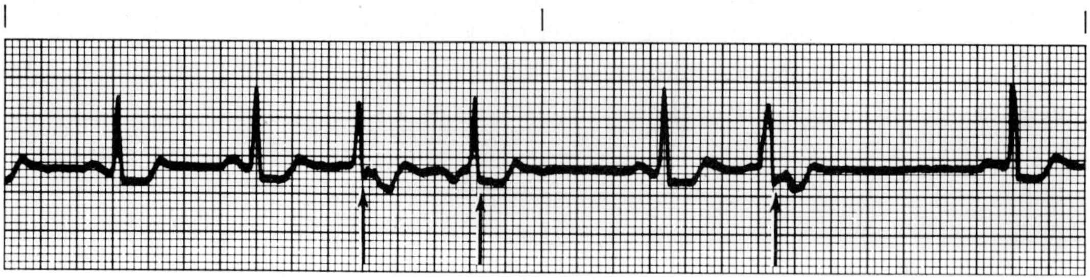

Figure 11-12. Premature junctional contraction.

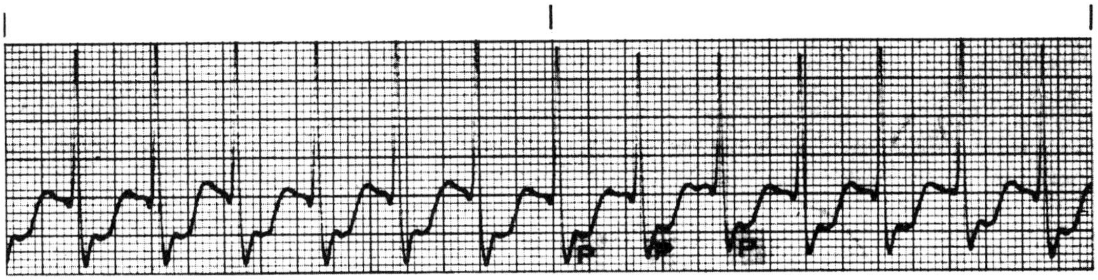

Figure 11-13. Paroxysmal junctional tachycardia.

Monitor the patient for increasing frequency of PJCs and notify the physician if the frequency does increase.

Accelerated Junctional and Junctional Tachycardia

Etiology. Accelerated junctional rhythm and junctional tachycardia are generally caused by cardiac ischemia, inflammatory heart disease, or digitalis toxicity. (**Fig. 11-13**).

Identifying Characteristics. *Accelerated junctional* and *junctional Tachycardia* rhythms have the same characteristics as junctional rhythm except the heart rates differ. Accelerated junctional rhythms range from 60 to 100 bpm and junctional tachycardia is generally 100 to 180 bpm. The rhythm is typically regular. P waves are abnormal and inverted (when visible), and they may precede, follow, or be buried in the QRS complex. If present, the PR interval is shortened (<0.12) or not measurable. The QRS complex is normal unless the P wave is buried in it or it is aberrantly conducted. Conduction of the QRS may be normal. Atrial conduction is retrograde. Junctional tachycardia may be *paroxysmal* (PJT) with the distinguishing criteria being an abrupt start and stop to the rhythm. PJT may be difficult to distinguish from PAT and therefore these rhythms are often called SVT.

Risk. The faster the rate, the greater the likelihood of a decreased cardiac output.

Treatment. Treatment of accelerated junctional rhythms may include treating the underlying cause or utilizing medications such as **beta blockers, diltiazem, verapamil, or flecainide** to slow the heart rate and potentially reestablish a sinus rhythm. Additional options may include ablation.

Nursing Intervention. Document the dysrhythmia with a rhythm strip. Assess the patient for hemodynamic compromise. If compromise occurs, notify the physician and medicate as the situation dictates.

Idioventricular Rhythm

Etiology. In this rhythm, there is no functioning pacemaker above the ventricles. The ventricles initiate an impulse to generate a heart rate. Normally, a ventricular pacemaker is very slow, generally less than 40 bpm. The terms *"idioventricular pacemaker"* (which means unknown ventricular pacemaker) and *"ventricular escape rhythm"* both apply to this dysrhythmia. All diseases and injuries that cause loss of function from the SA node down are etiologic factors (**Fig. 11-14**).

Identifying Characteristics. The ventricles initiate a rate at their inherent ability, usually 20 to 40 bpm. The rhythm is regular but may slow as a *"dying heart syndrome"* progresses. There is no P wave. There is no PR interval. The QRS complex is wide and bizarre, measuring 0.12 seconds or more.

Risk. The imminent danger is *ventricular standstill.* It is possible that the electrical event is not leading to an effective contraction, which means that electrical mechanical dissociation (PEA) has developed. This rhythm is normally a protective or compensatory response and is known as the rhythm of last resort, therefore *treatment becomes urgent.*

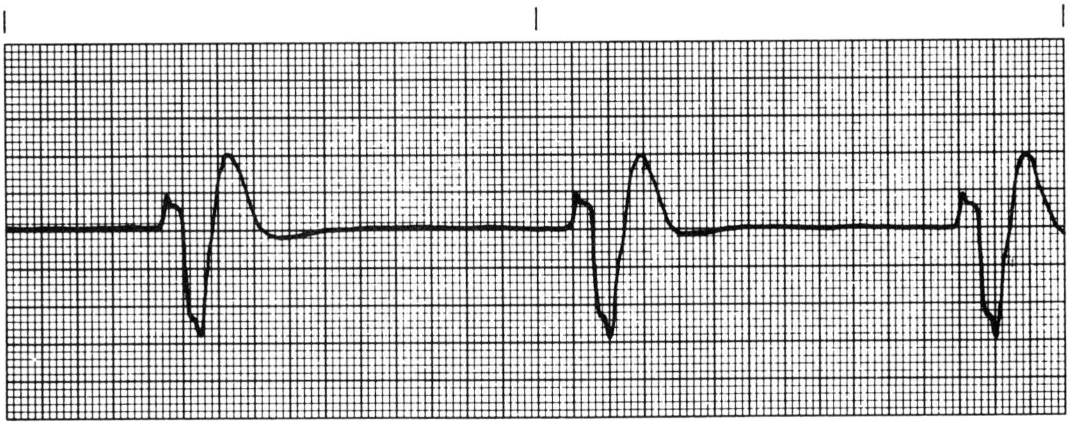

Figure 11-14. Idioventricular rhythm.

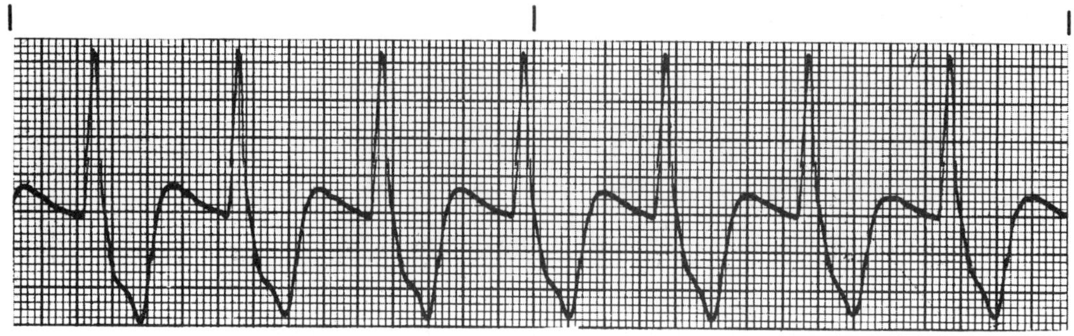

Figure 11-15. Accelerated idioventricular rhythm.

Treatment. A pacemaker is the only reliable and totally effective form of treatment. In a crisis, until a transvenous or external pacemaker can be applied, **atropine** or isoproterenol hydrochloride **(Isuprel)** may accelerate the heart rate.

Nursing Intervention. Document the dysrhythmia with a rhythm strip. Notify the physician immediately. Assess and treat the patient continuously for hypotension and other signs of hemodynamic compromise. *Prepare an external pacemaker for use or be prepared to assist in the insertion of a transvenous pacemaker.*

Accelerated Idioventricular Rhythm

Etiology. The etiology is the same as for idioventricular rhythm (**Fig. 11-15**).

Identifying Characteristics. These are the same as for an idioventricular rhythm with the exception that the rate is usually greater than 40 bpm.

Risk. The immediate risk is that the accelerated focus may cease and the dysrhythmia may convert to an idioventricular rate or cardiac standstill. The accelerated idioventricular rhythm generally poses no danger by itself.

Treatment. No treatment is indicated unless the patient demonstrates signs of hemodynamic compromise in which treatment is the same as idioventricular rhythm. Since the rate is normal, this dysrhythmia may generate an adequate cardiac output.

Nursing Intervention. Monitor the patient for signs of hypotension or HF. Document the rhythm strip and monitor patient closely for hemodynamic compromise.

Premature Ventricular Contraction or Complex

PVCs are also termed premature ventricular beats (PVBs) or ventricular premature contractions (VPCs). PVC can also be called a premature ventricular complex as not all PVCs result in a contraction of the ventricle or produce a palpable pulse.

Etiology. An irritable focus in the ventricle initiates a contraction before the normally expected beat. The irritability may be due to acute MI, CAD, HF, drug toxicity, hypoxia, electrolytes (hypokalemia and hypomagnesemia), acidosis, increased *sympathetic* nervous system activity, or infusions of inotropic medications (**Fig. 11-16**).

Identifying Characteristics. The rate is variable. Rhythm is irregular because of the premature beat. P waves are not visible and therefore there is no PR interval. The QRS complex is wide and bizarre, exceeding 0.12 seconds and frequently being greater than 0.14 seconds. It usually has a compensatory pause that is equal to two P-P distances following the PVC.

Risk. The danger of a PVC is the possibility of increasing myocardial irritability, leading to an increasing frequency of PVCs. With an increased occurrence of PVCs, ventricular tachycardia and/or ventricular fibrillation may occur. There is an increased potential for problems when any of the following occur:

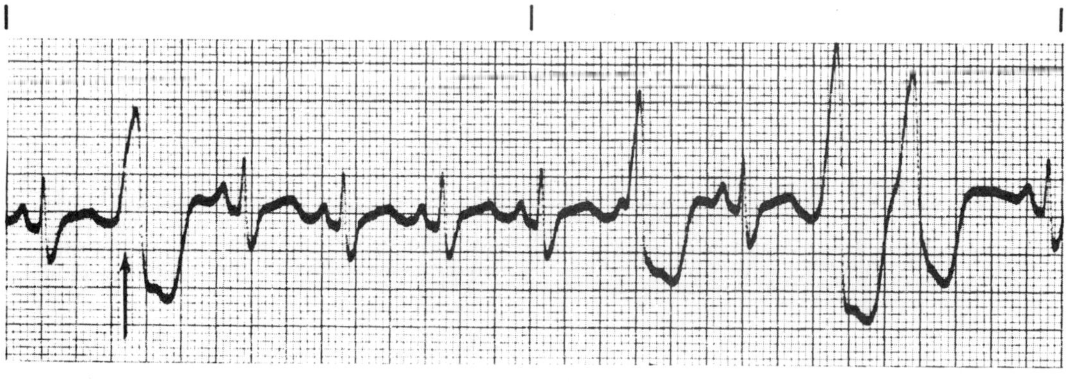

Figure 11-16. Premature ventricular contraction (PVC, PVB, or VPC).

1. PVCs occur from more than one focus (multifocal PVCs).
2. PVCs occur more often than 6 per min, including rhythms such as bigeminy (every other beat is a PVC); or short runs of PVCs occur frequently (two to three sequential PVCs) every few beats.
3. There are variable coupling intervals (the period between the beginning of a normal QRS and the beginning of the QRS of the PVC).
4. The PVC occurs on the T wave of the preceding complex **(described as the R-on-T phenomenon). If the PVC occurs on the T wave, it may precipitate lethal arrhythmias such as ventricular tachycardia or ventricular fibrillation.**

Treatment. Treatment of PVCs depends on their clinical significance. Acute development of PVCs might indicate myocardial ischemia, acidosis, hypoxia, hypokalemia, or hypomagnesemia. *Correcting the underlying cause prevents PVCs.* For example, if hypokalemia is present, potassium may terminate the PVCs. If the PVCs are asymptomatic, observation might be the best clinical treatment. If elimination of PVCs is desired, agents such as **beta blockers, lidocaine,** and **amiodarone** can be used. If **lidocaine** or **amiodarone** treatment is unsuccessful, **procainamide** or **bretylium** may be tried.

QUICK TIP! Just as treatment of PVCs should center around the underlying cause, treating the underlying cause is a key theme and focus of questions throughout the CCRN exam.

Chronic PVC control is usually managed with oral medications such as beta blockers and nondihydropyridine calcium channel blockers. If PVCs are not controlled by conventional therapies, class IC antiarrhythmics **(flecainide or propafenone)** or class III antiarrhythmics **(amiodarone or sotalol)** may be indicated.

Nursing Intervention. Document the dysrhythmia with a rhythm strip. Monitor the patient closely for increasing frequency of PVCs or the development of multifocal PVCs. Notify the physician. Treat the patient with medications as ordered. Observe the patient and monitor closely for ventricular tachycardia and ventricular fibrillation.

Differentiating APCs with Aberrant Conduction from PVCs

APCs with abnormal (aberrant) conduction can mimic PVCs. Criteria that help differentiate APCs with aberrant conduction from PVCs have been described in both medical and nursing research articles. **Table 11-2** provides the criteria necessary to aid differentiation. The key to identifying an aberrantly conducted APC centers around two features. First, identify any characteristics of an APC that are different from those of a PVC. For example, in **Fig. 11-17**, note the P wave on the downstroke of the T wave. This is suggestive of an APC. Second, note the shape of the QRS complex. The morphology or appearance of the QRS complex is a key factor in differentiating APCs with aberrancy from PVCs.

TABLE 11-2. DIFFERENTIATING APCs WITH ABERRANT CONDUCTION FROM PVCs

Criteria for PVCs	*Criteria for APCs*
Extreme right axis Rr′ in V_1 rS in V_6 Precordial concordancy (all V leads show same axis pattern, ie, upright or inverted) Initial R wave >0.03 s Beginning of R to nadir (lowest point) of S wave >0.10 s	rSR′ in V_1 Bi- or triphasic QRS Normal axis

QUICK TIP! The CCRN exam rarely has a question regarding a rhythm strip, or on differentiating between APCs and PVCs with aberrant conduction.

Monomorphic Ventricular Tachycardia

Etiology. Advanced irritability of the ventricles allows a ventricular focus to become the heart's pacemaker. The myocardial irritability may be due to arteriosclerotic heart disease (ASHD), HF, acute MI, cardiomyopathy, electrolyte imbalance, hypoxia, acidosis, or occasionally drugs (**Fig. 11-18**).

Identifying Characteristics. The rate is greater than 100 up to 180 bpm. The rhythm is regular or only slightly irregular. P waves are not present and therefore there is no measurable PR interval. The QRS complex is wide and bizarre, resembling essentially a salvo (or burst) of PVCs. A ventricular focus initiates ventricular depolarization. In monomorphic vtach the complexes are very similar in shape and size.

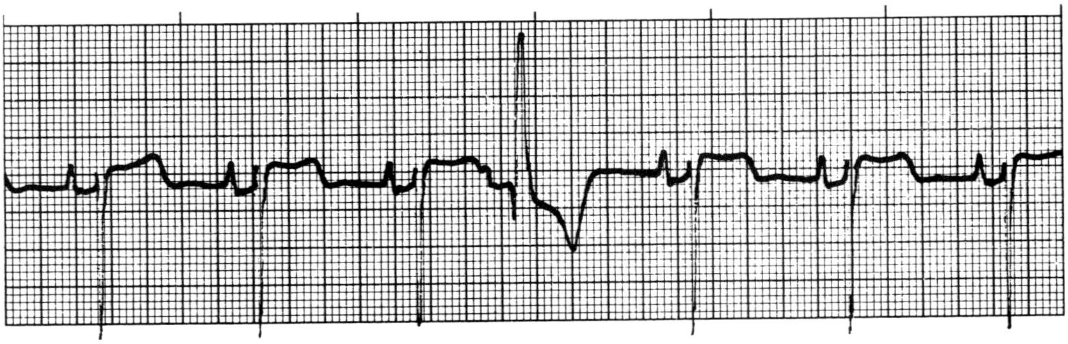

Figure 11-17. Aberrantly conducted APC.

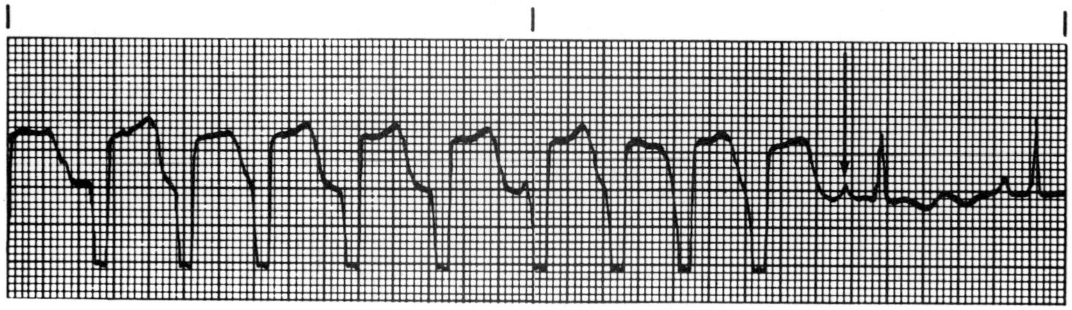

Figure 11-18. Ventricular tachycardia terminating spontaneously.

Risk. The risk with ventricular tachycardia is the potential to develop dangerous or lethal reductions in cardiac output and loss of pulse.

Treatment. Nonsustained ventricular tachycardia (NSVT) is defined as lasting less than 30 seconds before spontaneously converting out of the rhythm. NSVT can indicate an increased likelihood of developing sustained ventricular tachycardia. Treatment should focus on correcting potential contributing factors such as electrolyte imbalances or hypoxia. For sustained ventricular tachycardia the patient should be assessed and promptly treated with electrical **cardioversion** or antiarrhythmic drugs such as **lidocaine** or **amiodarone**. If the patient loses a pulse, CPR should be initiated immediately with prompt **defibrillation.**

Nursing Intervention. Document this dysrhythmia with a rhythm strip and alert the provider. Medications such as **amiodarone, beta blockers, verapamil, or procainamide** may be employed to treat ventricular tachycardia. *If the patient is without a pulse, immediate defibrillation* and institution of cardiac arrest procedures are essential.

Torsades de Point (Polymorphic Ventricular Tachycardia)

Etiology. Torsades can be provoked due to myocardial ischemia or prolonged QT intervals. If the QT is not prolonged the rhythm is typically identified solely as *polymorphic ventricular tachycardia.*

Identifying Characteristics. Torsades de pointe is a form of polymorphic ventricular tachycardia. It has a varying morphology of QRS complexes that appear to twist or rotate along a point. The rhythm is irregular. There are no P waves and therefore no PR interval. The rate is difficult to count due to the irregularity in shape and size of the QRS complexes. QRS complexes are difficult to measure.

Risk. Patients are generally hemodynamically unstable and prompt treatment is required. Torsades may decompensate to ventricular fibrillation if not treated promptly.

Treatment. Patients generally do not have a pulse and therefore initiation of CPR with prompt **defibrillation** would be necessary. IV **magnesium** should also be considered in the treatment of torsades with defibrillation. Correction of any underlying causes is necessary such as discontinuing medications that may be prolonging the QT.

Nursing Intervention. Monitor QT intervals and alert the provider if QT intervals are prolonged, especially when initiating new medications that may further prolong the QT.

Ventricular Fibrillation

Etiology. Owing to extensive ventricular irritability, ventricular fibers fail to depolarize in sequence; instead, they depolarize individually, creating an uncoordinated series of muscle depolarizations. No substantial cardiac output is generated. Ventricular fibrillation may occur after an acute MI. It may, however, occur as a result of ASHD, HF, digitalis or another drug toxicity, and electrolyte imbalance (**Fig. 11-19**).

Identifying Characteristics. There is no identifiable rate. The rhythm is irregular and not measurable. P waves are replaced by undulating waves as the baseline. The PR interval is nonexistent or not measurable. The QRS complex is an undulating asymmetrical line.

Risk. The development of hemodynamic collapse may occur within seconds, followed by death within 4 to 8 min.

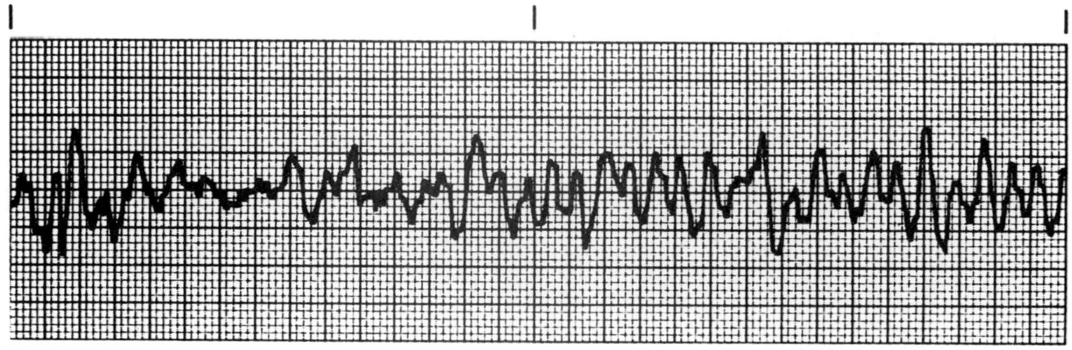

Figure 11-19. Ventricular fibrillation.

Treatment. *Immediate defibrillation* is the only possible means of establishing a viable cardiac rhythm.

If initial defibrillations are unsuccessful, begin cardiopulmonary resuscitation (CPR) and establish an artificial airway and venous access. Repeat defibrillations after medical therapies (eg, with **amiodarone**). **The key is successful defibrillation.** Without a return to spontaneous circulation within minutes, survival is unlikely. End-tidal CO_2 levels ($PETCO_2$), which are indicators of cardiac output, have been shown to aid in identifying which patients will survive. A persistently low $PETCO_2$ level (<10) is highly correlated with increased mortality.

Evaluation of patient symptoms and tolerance of the dysrhythmia is a key factor in determining appropriate treatments. Always assess your patient first when evaluating dysrhythmias.

KEY CONTENT CHECKLIST

- ❐ There may be several questions where dysrhythmias are a part of the test question or scenario on the CCRN exam.
- ❐ The most common dysrhythmias likely to be addressed on the CCRN exam involve disturbances of the AV node (junctional rhythms, atrial fibrillation, and conduction blocks) and ventricular ectopy (PVCs, ventricular tachycardia, and fibrillation).
- ❐ Treating the cause of the elevated heart rate is generally the focus of managing sinus tachycardia.
- ❐ When treating SVT, medications are usually indicated if the patient is symptomatic but hemodynamically stable. However, if the patient is unstable (chest pain, short of breath, hypotensive), cardioversion is usually indicated.
- ❐ A biphasic, or "double-humped" P wave may also be called, "P mitrale." This may suggest atrial enlargement and often comes up on the exam.
- ❐ Treating the underlying cause is a key theme and focus of questions throughout the CCRN exam.

Review Questions:

1. **Interpret the following ECG rhythm strip.** ***See art below.***
   a. Sinus tachycardia
   b. Paroxysmal atrial tachycardia
   c. Atrial flutter
   d. Atrial fibrillation

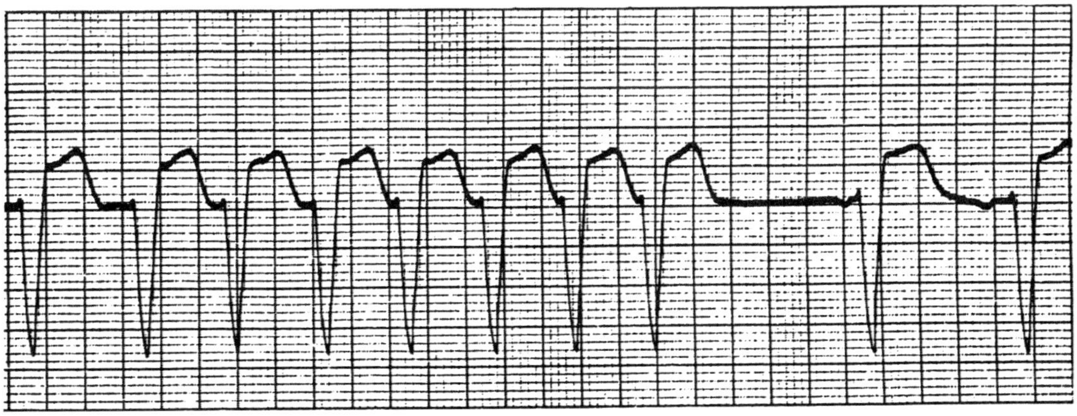

Answer: B. Rationale: Since this tracing presents with irregularity, option A can be eliminated quickly. Options C and D may also be eliminated due to the fact that neither the sawtooth nor the chaotic baselines of atrial flutter or atrial fibrillation are observed. Paroxysmal atrial tachycardia (PAT) however is characterized by a rapid rate (>100) and abrupt onset or cessation back into an organized rhythm with controlled rate (<100) as illustrated toward the end of this tracing. Choose B.

2. **What is the inherent rate of the AV nodal area?**
   a. 20 to 40.
   b. 40 to 60.
   c. 60 to 80.
   d. The AV nodal area has no inherent rate.

Answer: B. Rationale: This is a straight knowledge question. The inherent rate of the AV nodal area is 40 to 60, option B. 20 to 40 is the inherent rate of the His–Purkinje system, eliminating option A. 60 to 80 is within the normal sinus node range, eliminating option C as well. Option D is not true. Choose B.

3. **Interpret the following ECG rhythm strip.** ***See art below.***
   a. Multiform PVCs
   b. Ventricular tachycardia
   c. Ventricular fibrillation
   d. Torsade de pointes

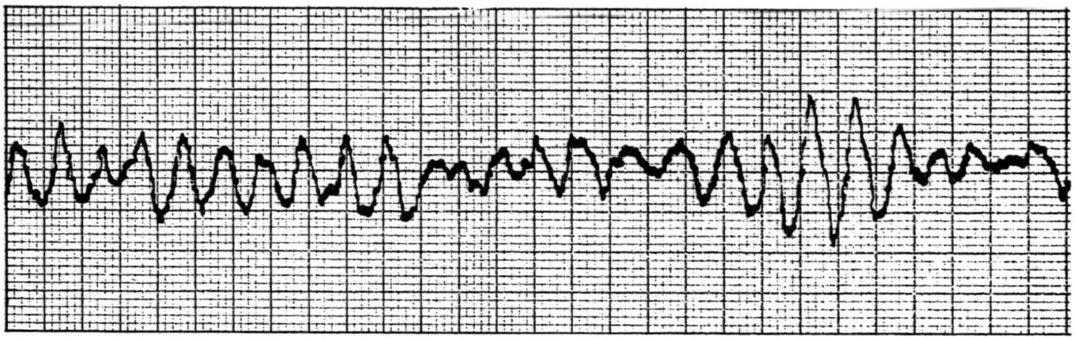

Answer: C. Rationale: In this tracing there is no clear organized underlying rhythm, which helps to eliminate option A quickly. The presence of R or S waves is also not clear enough, which helps to eliminate VT, option B. Torsade de pointes by definition is polymorphic VT, with QRSs that vary in shape, amplitude, and duration. This tracing illustrates waves that are smaller, monomorphic, and consistent in nature, making option C the best answer.

REFERENCES

2015 ACC/AHA/HRS guideline for the management of adult patients with supraventricular tachycardia Executive summary (heartrhythmjournal.com)

2019 AHA/ACC/HRS Focused Update of the 2014 AHA/ACC/HRS Guideline for the Management of Patients with Atrial Fibrillation: A Report of the American College of Cardiology/American Heart Association Task Force on Clinical Practice Guidelines and the Heart Rhythm Society in Collaboration with the Society of Thoracic Surgeons (ahajournals.org)

12

Cardiomyopathies and Pericarditis

CHAPTER OVERVIEW AND OBJECTIVES

It would be disproportionate to devote many pages to cardiomyopathies when the CCRN exam will have no more than a few questions on this topic. Pericarditis has been removed from the current CCRN exam. Therefore, this chapter is intentionally short, with an emphasis on practical information that will be seen both in practice and on the exam. Much of the information in this chapter is also found in the discussion of (formerly "congestive") heart failure (HF) (Chapter 8).

After studying this chapter, you should be able to:

- Describe the various types of cardiomyopathies and their associated clinical symptoms.
- Understand the effects of various cardiomyopathies on cardiac function and the associated treatments.
- Understand the clinical presentation of pericarditis and appropriate nursing actions and considerations.

12.1 CARDIOMYOPATHIES

Clinical Presentation

In the past, cardiomyopathy was roughly defined as heart muscle disease of unknown etiology. However, that is not true, because the origins of some types, such as ischemic cardiomyopathy, are known. Possible origins of cardiomyopathy are listed in **Table 12-1**. Regardless of the origin, the disease tends to involve most of the muscles of the heart both structurally and functionally, although some parts of the heart may be more affected than others. This presents a clinical picture whereby cardiomyopathy can appear very differently in different patients. *One patient might exhibit more left-sided dysfunction while another might exhibit right-sided dysfunction.* Some patients might have systolic ventricular failure, others might have diastolic dysfunction. The most common presentation appears to be a combination of the above. All cardiomyopathies will involve increased ventricular pressures by the time such patients present with symptoms.

There are three most common presentations of cardiomyopathy included in the CCRN exam **dilated, hypertrophic,** and **restrictive** and will be discussed in further detail below (**Fig. 12-1**).

Dilated Cardiomyopathy. The most common type of cardiomyopathy is dilated, in which the heart muscle begins to stretch and dilate, causing the walls to become thin; thereby, resulting in weakened contractility. Due to the weakened contractility the symptoms tend to resemble those of heart failure (HF) (formerly referred to as congestive heart failure [CHF]). The patient will have a decreased stroke volume and ejection fraction as well as symptoms of pulmonary congestion. Left ventricular (LV) volumes are increased. Eventually, hypotension will occur, with death resulting from severe LV failure. Dilated cardiomyopathy presents with a highly compliant ventricle. This usually means that *higher ventricular filling pressures (a pulmonary artery occlusive pressure, or PAOP, of 20 mm Hg)* can be tolerated relatively easily. Fluid administration in the presence of this PAOP can be employed without a major increase in extravascular lung water. However, the key parameter to monitor is **stroke volume** (and ideally ejection fraction).

Dilated cardiomyopathy is usually treated similarly to HF. Inotropic agents (**dobutamine** or **milrinone** in acute cases, **digoxin** in chronic cases), diuretics, vasodilators (eg, **ACE inhibitors**, **angiotensin II antagonists**), and **beta blockers** are commonly used. Aggressive measures such as cardiomyoplasty and mechanical support devices may be used until heart transplantation is possible.

Hypertrophic Cardiomyopathy. Hypertrophic cardiomyopathy is more of a *diastolic dysfunction* as a result of the *inability of the heart to relax* during diastole due to the thickened, stiff ventricular walls. Often hypertrophic cardiomyopathy is due to genetic mutations of genes found in the heart muscle. Clinical symptoms include pulmonary congestion but close to normal stroke volume and ejection fraction, at least until end stages.

In hypertrophic cardiomyopathy, the focus is on reducing afterload, particularly with beta blockers. A new medication,

TABLE 12-1. POSSIBLE CAUSES OF CARDIOMYOPATHY	
Dilated	Idiopathic (unknown) Inflammatory/infectious Autoimmune disease Toxic (drugs, alcohol) Hereditary Ischemic (eg, coronary artery disease) Metabolic (uremia, vitamin deficiency) Endocrine (thyroid) Heart valve disorders
Restrictive	Idiopathic Interstitial disease (sarcoidosis) Eosinophilic heart disease Radiation Drug toxicity
Hypertrophic	Genetic/Hereditary Systemic hypertension

mavacamten, was recently approved specifically for patients with symptomatic, obstructive hypertrophic cardiomyopathy. This medication is a myosin inhibitor which helps the heart to relax. Diuretics and other afterload reducers, such as calcium channel blockers, might be used. If atrial dysrhythmias (such as atrial fibrillation) develop, electrotherapy (cardioversion) or drugs for supraventricular tachycardia would be employed. Inotropes should be avoided in patients with hypertrophic cardiomyopathy.

Restrictive Cardiomyopathy. Restrictive cardiomyopathy presents with a very noncompliant ventricular muscle, leading to presentations of HF. Ventricular volumes are decreased, although stroke volume and ejection fraction can be maintained at near-normal levels.

Treatment of restrictive cardiomyopathy is difficult. The focus is generally on diuretics and afterload reducers in an attempt to improve diastolic function. Although this might help temporarily, eventually systemic hypotension results, with a worsening of clinical symptoms. Treatments tend to be supportive, although if a specific condition is present, such as eosinophilic cardiomyopathy, cytotoxic agents (hydroxyurea), or steroids might be used.

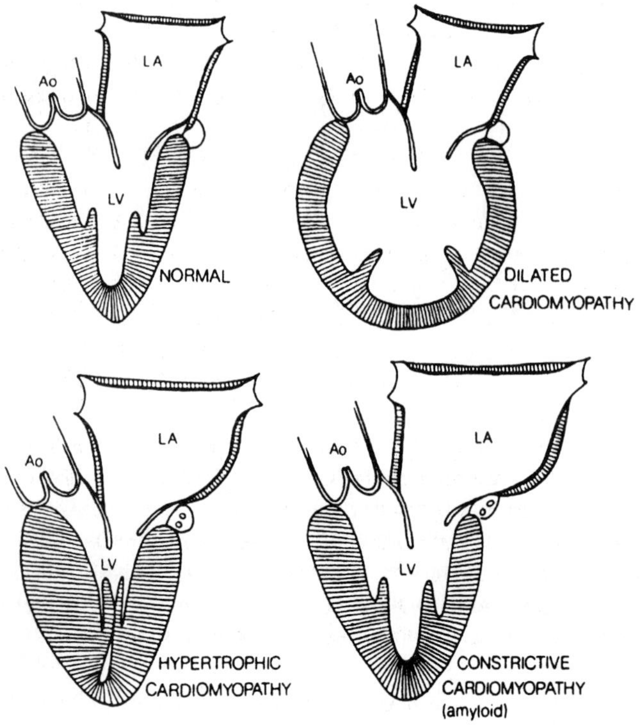

Figure 12-1. Types of cardiomyopathies.

Diagnosis

Echocardiograms (ECG) cardiac magnetic resonance imaging (MRI), genetic testing, exercise stress tests, and cardiac catheterization may be useful in assessing cardiac function and determining the type of cardiomyopathy. An endomyocardial biopsy is generally recommended if prior testing is inconclusive on the etiology of cardiomyopathy. No curative measures currently exist.

> **KEY CLINICAL CONCEPT**
>
> A subtype of hypertrophic cardiomyopathy is "IHSS," or "idiopathic hypertrophic subaortic stenosis." It basically consists of an enlarged, hypertrophic ventricular septum. Enhanced contraction actually worsens cardiac output, therefore drugs such as digoxin are contraindicated. Treatment instead includes beta blockers to reduce the LV outlet obstruction.

12.2 PERICARDITIS

Etiology

Pericarditis may be present or may develop in essentially any disease process. It may be viral or bacterial in etiology (most common); have a metabolic cause, as in uremia; or have an unknown cause. It may be secondary to systemic disease or myocardial trauma, or it may follow acute myocardial infarction (MI).

Clinical Presentation

Symptoms vary with the etiology of the pericarditis. Most commonly, pain is present. The pain may mimic an acute MI, angina, or pleurisy. **Pain usually increases with deep respiration and when the patient is lying supine. Sitting up and leaning forward usually diminishes the pain.**

Other symptoms that may be present:

- *Fever due to* the infectious or inflammatory process.
- *Pericardial friction rub, a scratchy, superficial sound,* may be present for only a few days (post-MI) or prolonged for many days (uremia).
- **ST-segment elevation on all leads except aVR on an ECG is a classic finding.**

Complications

Complications of pericarditis include dysrhythmias, tamponade, and restriction of ventricular contraction.

Signs of Tamponade

- **Equalization of pressures in the heart, particularly the central venous pressure (CVP) and PAOP, may signal the presence of tamponade.**
- Muffled heart sounds during auscultation

KEY CLINICAL CONCEPT

Increased and equalizing PA catheter pressures is a classic sign of pericardial tamponade. The increased pressures in this case however are "falsely elevated," not due to increased volume, but to the increased mediastinal pressures external to the heart.

Treatment

Pain relief is essential to promote normal and adequate ventilation. **Anti-inflammatory and steroid therapies** may be tried. Treatment of the underlying cause is imperative. **Antipyretic** agents will control the fever if the patient is uncomfortable. Pericardiocentesis or a pericardial window may be performed if there is a possibility of tamponade developing. Anticoagulants are contraindicated to avoid an increase in pericardial fluid.

Nursing Intervention

Perform continuous ECG monitoring for signs of dysrhythmias that may indicate the early development of cardiac tamponade. The most dangerous dysrhythmia is electromechanical dissociation (an ECG pattern is present but there is no pulse, ie, "PEA"). Monitoring with a noninvasive Doppler is more sensitive to early changes. The nurse should be prepared to assist with an emergency pericardiocentesis if it becomes warranted. Especially close auscultation of cardiac sounds is imperative for early intervention. Medications to relieve pain and fever are administered as ordered.

Arterial blood gases or pulse oximetry should be monitored at regular intervals to determine ventilatory status and allow early intervention if hypoxemia develops. Emotional support and explanations of the reasons for the close monitoring will help to alleviate some of the patient's anxiety.

Cardiac Tamponade

If fluid accumulates in the pericardial sac, there is a potential for the development of cardiac tamponade. Cardiac tamponade will have a constrictive effect on the heart, producing a condition initially like diastolic dysfunction (the heart cannot relax and fill with blood). This is particularly aggravated on inspiration, where increased right ventricular (RV) volume (due to inspiration) increases the pericardial pressure, thus limiting LV expansion and producing a drop in blood pressure during inspiration. The term **"pulsus paradoxus,"** where the systolic blood pressure decreases by about 20 mm Hg during inspiration, describes a condition that is commonly seen with cardiac tamponade. Other clinical features include **equalization of left and right filling pressures (the CVP and PAOP are about the same)** pulmonary and venous engorgement (leading to **widened mediastinum** on chest X-ray), or a **decreased EKG amplitude**.

Treatment involves treating the underlying cause of the fluid or blood in the pericardial sac. Emergent treatment might involve pericardiocentesis. **Decreasing PEEP may also be a consideration if the PEEP is believed to potentially decrease venous return.**

KEY CONTENT CHECKLIST

- ❒ The three most common types of cardiomyopathy are dilated, hypertrophic, and restrictive. Understanding the physiology associated with each helps to understand why certain treatments are recommended for some but contraindicated in others.
- ❒ A subtype of hypertrophic cardiomyopathy is "IHSS," or "idiopathic hypertrophic subaortic stenosis." It basically consists of an enlarged, hypertrophic ventricular septum. Enhanced contraction actually worsens cardiac output, therefore drugs such as digoxin are contraindicated. Treatment instead includes beta blockers to reduce the LV outlet obstruction.
- ❒ Increased and equalizing PA catheter pressures is a classic sign of pericardial tamponade.
- ❒ The increased pressures in pericarditis are "falsely elevated," not due to increased volume, but to the increased mediastinal pressures external to the heart.
- ❒ Pulsus paradoxus is an exaggerated decrease in the systolic blood pressure by 10 to 20 mm Hg during inspiration.
- ❒ High PEEP pressures can decrease venous return.

REFERENCE

Ommen SR, Mital S, Burke MA, et al. 2020 AHA/ACC guideline for the diagnosis and treatment of patients with hypertrophic cardiomyopathy: a report of the American College of Cardiology/American Heart Association Joint Committee on Clinical Practice Guidelines. *Circulation.* 2020;142:e558–e631. doi: 10.1161/CIR.0000000000000937

13

Treatment of Cardiac, Valvular, Vascular Insufficiency, and Trauma

CHAPTER OVERVIEW AND OBJECTIVES

Cardiovascular surgery has assumed a greater role in critical care over the past decade, and the CCRN exam reflects this trend. Do not be surprised by questions on cardiovascular surgery (extensive cardiac surgical experience is not required as long as the key principles/concepts are understood). Use this section in conjunction with the preceding chapters to apply hemodynamic analysis to the concept of cardiovascular surgery. This will help in understanding the assessment of and need for the surgical treatment of cardiovascular disorders.

After studying this chapter, you should understand the following:

- Common issues after cardiac surgery, including identification and nursing interventions for bleeding and hemodynamic instability.
- Signs and symptoms of mitral regurgitation and aortic stenosis.
- Signs and symptoms of cardiac tamponade.
- Presentation of and nursing interventions for thoracic aortic dissection

13.1 CARDIAC, VALVULAR, AND VASCULAR SURGERY

Cardiovascular surgery in the critical care environment can include many procedures, although the key surgical interventions involve the cardiac or vascular circulation. The cardiac disturbances that require emergency surgery include acute coronary artery obstruction, ventricular septal rupture, pericardial tamponade, and papillary muscle rupture. Other than acute coronary artery obstruction, the problems present with symptoms similar to those of cardiogenic shock and are not discussed here (see Chapter 5).

Knowledge of these common problems and the associated nursing care will prepare you for most CCRN questions in this area, including emergent surgical procedures. With the greater emphasis on the cardiovascular component of the CCRN exam, an understanding of cardiovascular surgical concepts has increased in importance.

Coronary Artery Bypass Grafting

Coronary artery bypass grafting (CABG) is the technique of using blood vessels obtained from another part of the body to route blood flow around coronary artery blockages. The left internal mammary artery (LIMA) is generally used because of its long-term patency. The greater saphenous vein is generally harvested because most patients requiring surgical revascularization need three or more bypass grafts. Radial arteries are increasingly used as bypass conduits due to their longevity compared to vein grafts. Gastroepiploic arteries require laparoscopic harvesting and are only used in rare cases when no other conduit is available.

Determination of the Need for CABG

Indications for surgical revascularization continue to be revised as the roles of less invasive forms of treatment are refined. Percutaneous coronary intervention (PCI) with coronary stent placement with or without percutaneous transluminal coronary angioplasty (PTCA), and CABG are the most common revascularization therapies. General criteria for invasive revascularization are presented in **Table 13-1**.

Surgical revascularization remains the treatment of choice in patients with left main coronary artery (LMCA) disease, multivessel disease, or complex lesions. CABG is indicated if LMCA stenosis is >50% and in non-LMCA coronary arteries with >70% stenosis. Recent studies have demonstrated improved long-term morbidity and mortality in patients with diabetes, LV dysfunction (ejection fraction [EF] <45%), and ischemic mitral regurgitation who undergo CABG compared to PCI. Other considerations

TABLE 13-1. INDICATIONS FOR CORONARY ARTERY BYPASS GRAFTING

• Acute STEMI in patients with anatomy not suited to PCI or those with mechanical complications (ventricular septal defect, acute mitral regurgitation due to papillary muscle rupture). • PCI failure. High complexity left main coronary artery stenosis (> 50%). • Intermediate to high complexity two-vessel CAD (> 70% stenosis). • Three-vessel CAD.
CAD, coronary artery disease; PCI, Percutaneous coronary intervention.

include age, general health status, frailty, associated cardiac disease, and comorbid conditions.

Advances in minimally invasive cardiac surgery have changed traditional surgery methods and require advanced surgical training. Minimally invasive direct coronary artery bypass (MIDCAB) can be performed on patients who need bypass grafting of the left anterior descending (LAD) artery. Hybrid procedures consisting of robotic surgery to bypass the LAD are done in conjunction with percutaneous interventions for other vessels (right coronary artery, circumflex artery, or both), in which the major sternal incision is eliminated in favor of a small incision. Off pump, or "beating heart" CABG, allows the heart to beat during surgery, eliminating the need for the cardiopulmonary bypass (CPB) machine.

Pain relief from bypass surgery is individualized and usually focuses on management of surgical pain since such surgery is effective primarily if blood flow to viable cardiac muscle is reestablished.

Indications for emergency operation are as follows:

1. Highly complex coronary anatomy not suitable for PCI
2. Complications of PCI (eg, arterial dissection)
3. Ischemia that is uncontrolled by medical therapy and PCI
4. Hemodynamic instability or LV dysfunction with coronary anatomy not suited for PCI

Patients with hemodynamic instability (hypotension), unremitting chest pain despite maximal medical treatment and/or intra-aortic balloon pump (IABP) placement require emergent CABG. Elective surgeries are utilized for those patients with hemodynamic stability and symptoms partially controlled through medical therapy. Unfortunately, surgical revascularization is not curative. Some patients require reoperation because of the progression of coronary artery disease (CAD) or loss of graft patency. Patients undergoing reoperation have at least double the operative risk because their average age is higher and the atherosclerotic disease is more advanced. They tend to have longer surgeries due to the presence of adhesions and scar tissue. They are more likely to receive blood and blood products during the procedure. Patients undergoing reoperation tend to be more challenging to care for postoperatively.

Surgical Procedure

The surgical techniques utilized during CABG are unlikely to be covered on the CCRN exam. (However, a "post-CABG patient" may appear in a scenario. If it does, do not worry, as key information to answer the question will not be specific to CABG patient care).

During CABG, several surgical techniques are employed to improve success rates. The patient is typically cooled to near 28°C to 30°C (to reduce oxygen demand) and is placed on CPB. CPB is a technique for diverting blood from the heart during surgery while simultaneously oxygenating the blood and removing carbon dioxide. During CPB, three maneuvers help achieve safe and successful extracorporeal oxygenation: hemodilution, hypothermia, and anticoagulation. While these techniques help reduce complications, they also form the basis for many of the postoperative observations by the critical care nurse. In addition, autotransfusion is typically employed to aid in the replacement of normal blood loss during surgery. Autotransfusion is the reinfusion of shed mediastinal blood. In most centers, all mediastinal bloodshed is filtered and returned to the patient to decrease the need for blood transfusions.

Physiologic consequences of CPB include the following:

1. Damage to blood elements (eg, platelets, red blood cells, white blood cells, and plasma proteins)
2. Incorporation of abnormal substances into the blood (eg, air, fibrin particles, and platelet aggregates)
3. A systemic inflammatory response, which results in increased capillary permeability and fluid in the interstitial space
4. An initial decrease in systemic vascular resistance (SVR), then a progressive increase as hypothermia is induced
5. An increase in circulating catecholamines
6. Alterations in vascular tone

As fluid leaks from the blood vessels, the nurse should be alert for the need to give volume (either crystalloid or colloid) to maintain fluid status. Patients may gain several pounds following CPB owing to fluid shifting into the interstitial space. Careful observation of urine output to assess intravascular volume is an important part of patient assessment. Impaired gas exchange as manifested by low arterial oxygen pressure/saturation (Pao_2/Sao_2) levels may also indicate excess capillary leaking. Improved blood gases can indicate clearing of third-space volume. Atelectasis is common due to CPB pump run (lungs are deflated during the procedure) and postoperative pain. Pain control, incentive spirometry, and early mobilization decrease atelectasis and improve oxygenation.

Some patients will have a coagulopathy as a result of heparin administration during CPB and loss of platelets and plasma clotting factors. Measurement of the activated partial thromboplastin time (aPTT) detects an excessive heparin effect after CPB. **Protamine sulfate** *is given to reverse heparin-induced anticoagulation.* Protamine sulfate can cause a severe adverse *histamine reaction accompanied by profound vasodilation, systemic hypotension, and elevated pulmonary artery (PA) pressures*, and may require fluid and/or vasoactive medications to maintain adequate tissue perfusion. Patients may require treatment with antifibrinolytic agents such as **aminocaproic acid (Amicar) or tranexamic acid (TXA)**, administration of **vasopressin (DDAVP)**, and/or **platelet, plasma, or cryoprecipitate transfusions.**

KEY CLINICAL CONCEPT

Protamine sulfate *is given to reverse heparin-induced anticoagulation.* Protamine sulfate can cause a severe adverse *histamine reaction accompanied by profound vasodilation and hypotension.*

Postoperative Measures

The primary postoperative assessments following CABG involve hemodynamic monitoring, pain relief, dysrhythmia control, and recovery from surgical techniques such as CPB. Hemodynamic monitoring centers on maintaining adequate blood pressure (BP), cardiac indices **(> 2.2 L/min/m²)**, and tissue oxygenation **(SvO_2 above 60%).** Acceptable BP and cardiac index (CI) are achieved through providing sufficient **preload (assessed via central venous pressure [CVP] and/or pulmonary artery diastolic pressure [PAD]), left ventricular afterload reduction [SVR or SVRI],** and the use of **inotropes** to enhance contractility and maintain normal **stroke volume.** (PAD is used as a surrogate for pulmonary artery occlusion pressure [PAOP] in cardiac surgery patients to avoid potential injury from inflating the PA catheter balloon while obtaining the PAOP.) As the patient warms postoperatively, vasopressors may initially need to be used to maintain BP. A temporary external pacemaker, antidysrhythmic agents, and sedatives may also be employed to optimize hemodynamic status.

More aggressive measures to maintain CI may be required. This would include the use of artificial devices for mechanical circulatory support (MCS). Devices that may be utilized include an IABP, ventricular assist devices (VADs) for right, left, or biventricular support, or venoarterial extracorporeal membrane oxygenator (VA ECMO); however, few if any questions on the CCRN exam cover MCS devices at this time.

Problems encountered in the early postoperative period include the following:

1. Bleeding: either from a surgical site or due to a coagulopathy. This may result in cardiac tamponade. Postoperative blood loss should not exceed 300 mL/h in the first 2 to 3 hours. After this time, bleeding should be less than 100 to 150 mL/h. Persistent bleeding (> 200 mL in 1 hour or > 2 mL/kg × 2 hours) is associated with the need for blood and blood product transfusion. The total average blood loss is 1 L. The surgeon should be notified of excessive postoperative blood loss.
2. Low-cardiac-output syndrome, where the stroke volume (SV)/stroke volume index (SVI) or CI is low. Postoperative causes of low CI include hypovolemia, elevated SVR, myocardial dysfunction, cardiac tamponade, and dysrhythmias.
3. Profound hypotension.
4. Hypertension.
5. Electrolyte imbalances (primarily hypokalemia, hypomagnesemia, and hypocalcemia).
6. Dysrhythmias (primarily bradycardia, premature ventricular contractions [PVCs], atrial fibrillation, atrial flutter).
7. Cardiac arrest (resulting pulseless electrical activity (PEA), ventricular tachycardia (VT), ventricular fibrillation (VT).

Core temperature measurements are obtained by either pulmonary artery catheter or rectal (or bladder) temperature probes. **Shivering is the body's response to combating hypothermia.** *Although this reflex is effective, it increases oxygen consumption, lowering SvO_2.* The nurse can aid in rewarming the patient through external methods (blankets, radiant lights) and internal methods (warmed blood or IV fluid, warmed inspired gases). Avoidance of marked shivering is one key goal of rewarming therapy.

During rewarming, the patient may be hypotensive due to vasodilation. Volume replacement and vasopressors may be required to initially combat the decreased SVR/SVRI. Administering volume will also improve CVP and PAD, CVP since fluid administration will increase **preload.**

The nurse must maintain pain reduction while simultaneously allowing for the recovery of ventilatory function. Aggressive pulmonary toilet may include endotracheal suctioning initially. After extubation encouraging coughing and use of the incentive spirometer will aid in reducing pulmonary complications. The nurse's support in pain reduction and the sensitivity shown for the patient's adjustment to temporary dependence on nursing will help the patient to adapt to the immediate postoperative recovery.

Dysrhythmia control centers on two factors. First, any metabolic disturbance that may precipitate either atrial or ventricular dysrhythmias should be corrected. For example, potassium (K^+) and magnesium (Mg) levels should be monitored when dysrhythmias, particularly ventricular ectopy (PVCs), exist. Second, pharmacologic or electrical therapy can be utilized to control dysrhythmias. Pharmacologic treatments are dictated by the type of dysrhythmia. Beta blockade is started in all patients who do not have contraindications such as bradycardia, heart blocks, hypotension, vasopressor, or inotropic support. **Metoprolol** is the most commonly used. Beta blockers lower myocardial oxygen (MvO_2) demand and help prevent both atrial and ventricular arrhythmias (class II antiarrhythmics). For example, atrial tachycardias are treated with agents such as beta blockers **(metoprolol, esmolol),** non-dihydropyridine calcium channel blockers **(verapamil, diltiazem), amiodarone, adenosine,** or a combination of these agents. Electrical cardioversion may also be used. VTs and PVCs are treated with amiodarone or lidocaine.

Electrical therapy is usually performed through epicardial pacing wires placed on the right atrium and the right or both ventricles near the end of the CABG procedure. These pacing wires can be used postoperatively to manage both supraventricular tachycardias and bradycardias. Postoperative bradycardia is the most common indication for the use of the pacing wires. *Atrial (for bradycardia) or atrioventricular (AV) sequential (for Mobitz II second-degree or third-degree AV block) pacing is preferable to ventricular pacing because* **atrial kick accounts for 15% to 30% of cardiac output.** Certain dysrhythmias (paroxysmal atrial tachycardia, atrial flutter) may be treated with rapid overdrive pacing. A wide variety of external temporary pacemakers are available.

Complications of Cardiac Surgery

Potential complications of cardiac surgery include hemorrhage, cardiac tamponade, myocardial infarction (MI), ventricular dysfunction, dysrhythmias, and death. In addition, patients may be predisposed to problems with other organ systems (eg, neurological, pulmonary, renal).

Cardiac tamponade is among the most challenging complications to manage in the postoperative period. This is a condition in which the *heart is compressed* by blood that has accumulated in the pericardial space or mediastinum. As a result, the heart is unable to fill adequately, causing cardiac output and BP to fall. *The usual signs of tamponade are enlargement of the cardiac silhouette on roentgenography (CXR), sinus tachycardia, orthopnea, pulsus paradoxus, jugular venous distention (JVD), and* *acute hypotension.* Unless the fluid is evacuated, *equalization of right and left heart filling pressures (CVP and PAD) will occur and PEA ensues.* Typically, patients with initially heavy bleeding from *chest tubes suddenly stop bleeding* and become hypotensive. Temporary measures to support cardiac function include volume administration and inotropic support. Emergent treatment involves reopening the sternal incision in the intensive care unit (ICU) and an immediate return to the operating room.

> **QUICK TIP!** Beck's Triad (muffled heart tones, pulsus paradoxus, and JVD) are classic signs of cardiac tamponade that frequently show up on the CCRN exam.

Cardiac Transplantation

Heart transplantation is generally not covered on the CCRN exam. Nonetheless, transplantation may be an option for patients with end-stage cardiomyopathy, and you should be familiar with the procedure.

In patients with end-stage cardiomyopathy, optimizing goal-directed medical therapy (GDMT), insertion of biventricular pacemaker/defibrillators (Bi-V AICD), may require a temporary or permanent VAD (LV, RV, or both). These devices may be used as a bridge to a decision regarding transplant, as a bridge to transplant, or as destination therapy for patients who are not transplant candidates. CABG in this stage often will not improve cardiac performance. It is also indicated in patients with refractory malignant ventricular dysrhythmias and those with pulmonary hypertension and subsequent RV failure. Once identified as a candidate for transplantation an extensive work-up is performed to identify any contraindications for transplant (**Table 13-2**). After the work-up is completed, the patient is categorized as to severity according to the United Network for Organ Sharing (UNOS) status classifications, which were updated to 6 tiers in 2018 to allocate hearts to the most critically ill patients. ICU patients on VA-ECMO, those with biventricular VADs, and those on MCS with life-threatening ventricular arrhythmia (Status 1) are the highest priority on the UNOS waiting list.

Status 2 patients include those requiring MCS support with a total artificial heart (TAH), IABP, LVAD, RVAD, MCS device malfunction/failure. Patients with VT or VF not requiring MCS are also Status 2.

Less priority is given to patients with intractable angina, non-ICU patients who are on inotropic medications or MCS or at home with surgically implanted VADs and/or inotrope infusions such as **dobutamine**. Transplant candidates typically have an expected survival of less than a year without transplantation. The time between being placed on the list and undergoing transplantation is highly variable and can serve as a major source of anxiety to the potential recipient.

The success rate for transplantation is very good, with 1-year survival for heart transplants of 85% to 90%. After that, the yearly mortality is approximately 4% per year over the next 11 years. However, the shortage of donors means that not all patients who might benefit from transplantation actually undergo the procedure.

The surgical procedure has been improved since the time of the first transplantation in 1966, but the prime difference has been in the area of immunosuppression. Suppression of rejection through such agents as cyclosporine, azathioprine, and corticosteroids has been the major factor in improving outcome following transplantation.

TABLE 13-2. ELIGIBILITY CRITERIA FOR CARDIAC TRANSPLANTATION

1. End-stage, ischemic, valvular, or congenital heart disease with maximal medical therapy, not amenable to conventional or high-risk surgery
2. NYHA functional class III–IV congestive heart failure with maximal medical therapy
3. Prognosis for 1-year survival, < 75%
4. Age, generally < 65 years
5. Psychologically stable, compliant, reliable patient able to understand the procedure and risks involved
6. Strong family support system
7. Able to adhere to complex medical regimen
8. Absence of the following contraindicating factors:
   Systemic disease or infection
   Serious, irreversible impairment of hepatic, renal, or pulmonary functions
   Recent cerebrovascular accident or neurologic deficits
   Recent pulmonary embolization or infarction
   Peptic ulcer disease
   Active substance abuse
   Pulmonary vascular resistance > 6 Wood units
   Psychological instability
   Malignancy
9. Relative contraindications:
   Advanced peripheral atherosclerosis
   Diabetes mellitus

Postoperative care is similar to that for CABG surgery with the exception of medications for immunosuppression. *The electrocardiogram (ECG) has two sinus nodes initially (due to the retention of the recipient sinus node), and the recipient sinus node gives P waves unrelated to the QRS complex. Since the transplanted heart has no innervation from the autonomic nervous system, normal cardiac responses to various reflexes do not occur. In addition, the patient will feel no angina-like pain.* Because of the denervation, sympathetic stimulants such as **isoproterenol** may be necessary to increase heart rate (HR) and support cardiac function until the ventricle adjusts to the absence of autonomic innervation. A more long-term issue in these patients is hypertension. Many drugs used to prevent transplant rejection can cause significant hypertension. These patients may be on two or more antihypertensive agents for BP control.

- An ECG with two p waves prior to a QRS. This is an ECG manifestation seen in patients with transplanted hearts.
- Transplanted hearts are denervated. **Isoproterenol (Isuprel)** is used to treat symptomatic sinus bradycardia occurs, since the HR will not respond to **atropine**.

Valvular Heart Disease

The cardiac valves allow unidirectional forward flow of blood through the heart. Dysfunctional cardiac valves are classified as *stenotic or regurgitant (insufficient).* A **stenotic** valve restricts the forward flow of blood during the portion of the cardiac cycle when the valve should be open. A cardiac valve that does not close completely allows backward flow of blood is regurgitant. **Regurgitation** occurs during the portion of the cardiac cycle when the valve should be closed.

Valves that are **stenotic** cause an *elevated afterload*, subsequently resulting in *hypertrophy* of the atrium or ventricle, which is contracting against the *increased pressure load.* As the stenosis worsens, patients become more symptomatic due to the paucity of blood being ejected through the defective valve and the results of blood backing up into other chambers or vasculature.

Valve pathology is caused by a number of disorders such as infective endocarditis (IE), degenerative changes of the tissue, trauma, papillary muscle rupture from MI, systemic diseases, and others. Although it is less common in industrialized countries, *rheumatic fever is a common etiology of valvular stenosis.* The aortic and mitral valves are more commonly affected by acquired valvular heart disease than the tricuspid or pulmonic valves.

Mitral regurgitation (MR) *allows blood to flow back into the left atrium.* The patient presents with dyspnea, orthopnea, paroxysmal nocturnal dyspnea, elevated PAOP, *pulmonary hypertension,* decreased CO, crackles, a holosystolic murmur heard best at the apex, S_3, atrial fibrillation. As it progresses, it can lead to pulmonary hypertension and eventually to *right heart failure.* The progression of mitral insufficiency is slow, and such patients may remain asymptomatic for years. However, if the mitral insufficiency occurs rapidly (endocarditis, ruptured papillary muscle) the presentation will be very acute and patients have more severe symptoms and hemodynamic compromise compared to those with chronic MR. MR is treated either by surgically repairing or replacing the MV. Patients who are at high risk for open surgical mitral valve surgery may meet criteria to undergo a percutaneous mitral valve repair. Postoperative care of patients requiring valvular surgery is similar to the general care of the cardiac surgery patient, with the exception of higher incidences of heart block which require temporary epicardial pacing and possibly permanent pacemaker (PPM) insertion.

KEY CLINICAL CONCEPT

- The signs and symptoms of acute MR are similar to acute left heart failure.
- Acute MR is associated with a holosystolic (throughout systole) murmur heard at the fourth to fifth intercostal space (ICS) and radiates to the left axial.
- Patients who undergo multiple valve repair or replacement surgery are at higher risk of having heart block and requiring temporary epicardial pacing and/or permanent pacemaker insertion.

Mitral stenosis (MS) is most commonly caused by rheumatic fever. The symptoms develop as the size of the opening decreases. As the opening becomes smaller, symptoms include dyspnea on exertion and progressive fatigue. *Atrial fibrillation (AF) is very common in patients with MS due to dilatation of the left atrium.* Later signs include cough, hemoptysis, elevated PAOP, elevated RV pressures, and right heart failure. Medical therapy for MS focuses on treating pulmonary edema and anticoagulation for stroke prophylaxis. However, the definitive treatment for MS is surgical mitral valve replacement (MVR).

QUICK TIP! On the CCRN exam, patients with MS often have atrial fibrillation (AF).

Aortic regurgitation (AR) results in *LV overload, causing dilation and hypertrophy of the left ventricle.* It can be caused chronically by a thoracic aortic aneurysm, which enlarges the annulus (door frame) of the valve and prevents the leaflets from closing appropriately. AR can also occur from endocarditis. The presentation of AR includes *fatigue, dyspnea, paroxysmal nocturnal dyspnea, orthopnea,* angina, widened pulse pressure, S_3 heart sound, diastolic murmur heard best in aortic area and Erb's point, sinus tachycardia, and elevated PAOP. Patients who present with acute AR are typically more symptomatic and hemodynamically unstable than those who have chronic AR. Symptoms of heart failure, HTN, and dysrhythmias are medically managed. Aortic valve replacement (AVR), and much less frequently, aortic valve repair, is the definitive treatment for the disorder.

Aortic stenosis (AS) obstructs the ejection of blood from the LV into the systemic circulation during systole, **raising LV afterload.** It is most commonly seen in elderly patients due to calcium deposition which fuses the valve leaflets. It can also occur in younger patients who have a congenital bicuspid aortic valve (BAV). AS symptoms worsen as the disease progresses. Symptoms of severe AS include *syncope or presyncope, angina, and dyspnea.* Pulmonary congestion and LV failure occur late in the disease process. Surgical AVR is the treatment of choice for patients with low to moderate surgical risk Patients who are intermediate to high risk for open surgical AVR may qualify for transcatheter aortic valve replacement (TAVR).

KEY CLINICAL CONCEPT

The classic symptoms of severe AS are pre-syncope or syncope, angina, and dyspnea/shortness of breath.

Types of Replacement Heart Valves: Biological versus Mechanical

Patients who are referred for surgical valve replacement must consider the type of valve they would prefer to be implanted. There are benefits and risks associated with both biological and mechanical replacement valves. Bioprosthetic heart valves are derived from bovine or porcine pericardial tissue. They do not require life-long anticoagulation. Unfortunately, they have a higher rate of deterioration especially in younger patients, leading to an increased need for future valve replacement procedures. Mechanical valves are more durable, which decreases the risk of needing subsequent valve replacement surgery. However, all mechanical heart valves regardless of position, such as aortic or mitral, require lifelong anticoagulant therapy with warfarin. If oral anticoagulation is held prior to an invasive procedure or surgery, the patient must be bridged with therapeutic low molecular weight heparin (LMWH) subcutaneously or unfractionated heparin to prevent valve thrombosis and/or thromboembolism.

Vascular Surgery

The two most common problems requiring vascular surgery are aneurysms and occlusions. Aneurysms are more problematic when they occur in major arteries. Occlusions are problematic when they occur in major arteries or veins.

Aortic Aneurysms

The two common types of aortic aneurysms are thoracic (TAA) and abdominal (AAA). Approximately 75% of aneurysms occur in the abdominal aorta. For most patients, an aneurysm results from a combination of HTN, atherosclerosis, and hyperlipidemia weakening the vessel. It can increase in size over time, especially if HTN is not adequately controlled. Congenital bicuspid aortic valves (BAV) and inherited connective tissue disorders, such as Marfan's disease are less-common causes of TAA. It is estimated that 5% of individuals over the age of 60 have an AAA.

Ruptured Abdominal Aortic Aneurysms

At least 50% of patients who experience a ruptured AAA die before reaching the hospital. Although the risk of rupture correlates with aneurysm size, even small aortic aneurysms can rupture. The risk of rupture is higher with a AAA diameter of > 5.5 cm for men and > 5.0 cm for women. Symptoms most commonly associated with a ruptured AAA are abdominal and back pain, tender pulsatile abdominal mass, hypotension, and/or shock. These symptoms occur in 50% or less of patients. The location of pain is dependent on the location of the retroperitoneal hematoma.

Mortality with a ruptured AAA ranges from 15% to 88% and is most commonly the result of a delay in operating. The team must be prepared for the massive infusion of fluid and blood products perioperatively. The same complications exist with the ruptured AAA as with elective AAA repair, but they occur with greater frequency. Patients with ruptured AAA repair have a 50% chance of *renal failure* and a 20% chance of an *MI*. The patient usually has a longer ventilator course and is more prone to *colon ischemia* than with elective AAA repair.

Although bowel and spinal cord ischemia are less common complications, they are associated with a high incidence of morbidity and mortality. Respiratory complications may be avoided through routine use of incentive spirometry, early ambulation, and, if necessary, postural drainage and percussion.

Aortic Dissection

Aortic dissections are potentially life-threatening because of the rapid progression of shock, loss of vascular volume, potential bleeding into the pericardial sac (with resultant tamponade), myocardial infarction, and disruption of the aortic valve leading to acute AR and cardiogenic shock. *Dissections are almost always caused by uncontrolled HTN.* Severely high BPs can cause an intimal tear in the aorta. This tear produces a false lumen for blood to pass through. **The presentation is one of hypertension with severe unremitting chest, which is often described as "ripping or tearing" and/or abdominal pain frequently radiating to the back.** Aortic dissections are classified as either Stanford Type A (ascending aorta) or Type B (descending aorta). Type A dissections are surgical emergencies. Type B dissections are often managed medically with BP and HR control. If the dissection is progressing on scan or the patient develops signs of lower blood flow to the internal organs or extremities, transcatheter endovascular aortic repair (TEVAR) using a covered intra-aortic stent may be performed.

The immediate treatment is control of BP and HR to prevent excessive shear stress on the aorta, which can lead to rupture. General management includes keeping the HR less than 70 bpm and keeping the BP less than 120 mm Hg (or lower depending on surgeon preference). **Esmolol**, an IV beta blocker, is the drug of choice since it lowers both HR and BP and is titratable. If the BP target is not met with esmolol alone, an additional agent(s) such as **nicardipine** or **sodium nitroprusside** may be indicated.

KEY CLINICAL CONCEPT

- Medical management of aortic dissections focuses *on* keeping the HR less than 70 bpm and keeping the BP less than 120 mm Hg (or lower depending on surgeon preference).
- **Esmolol,** an IV beta blocker, is the drug of choice since it lowers both HR and BP, and is titratable. **Labetalol,** a combination beta and alpha-blocker may also be used.
- If the BP target is not met with **esmolol** alone, an additional agent(s) such as **nicardipine** or **sodium nitroprusside** may be indicated

Diagnosis of Aneurysms

Angiography remains the gold standard for diagnosis of aortic emergencies due to its specificity and sensitivity; however, it is invasive and not frequently used. The use of **computed tomography angiography (CTA)** and magnetic resonance angiography (MRA) are commonly used to evaluate abdominal and thoracic aortic aneurysms and dissections. Transesophageal echocardiogram may also be useful in evaluating ascending aortic disease processes. Ultrasound may be used to detect and follow the progression of AAA.

Treatment of Aneurysms

Replacement of the aneurysm with a graft is the most common surgical intervention. **Figure 13-1** contains an example of the surgical replacement technique. The closer the aneurysm is to the heart, the more difficult the surgery will be. Thoracic aneurysms of the descending aorta and abdominal aneurysms offer the surgeon a better operative field and reduce postoperative complications.

Endovascular surgical grafting techniques have become more commonplace. If effective, this approach will eliminate the need for cross-clamping of the aorta and therefore decrease most of the complications of major aortic surgery.

Postoperative Considerations

The most serious complication following aortic surgery is MI, accounting for almost half of the postoperative mortality from aortic surgery. Monitoring cardiovascular performance such as CI, stroke index or volume, PAOP, CVP, ST segments, and ECG rhythms is helpful in assessing cardiac performance.

The second most common complication is bleeding, which results from injury or from coagulopathies. The nurse must be aware of symptoms of hypovolemia (see Chapter 10), indicating

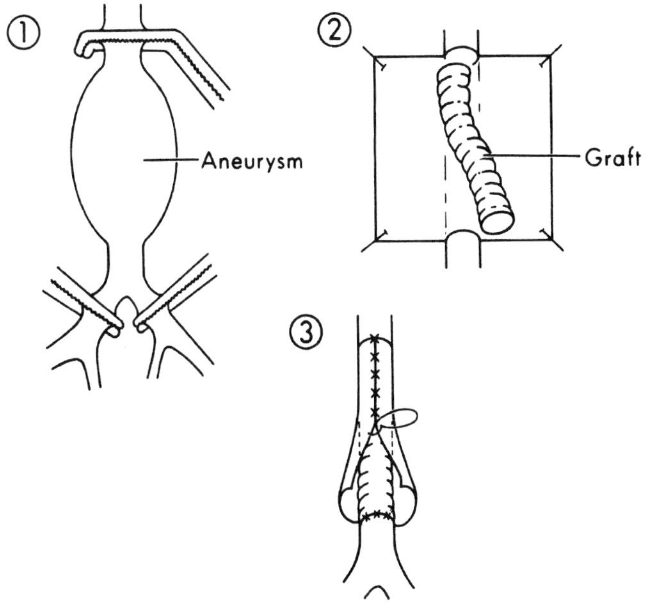

Figure 13-1. Aneurysm graft technique.

a potential bleed. *The presence of a strong pulse on palpation of the femoral artery gives an indication of adequate patency of the aorta.*

Renal failure, the third complication, is especially great in patients with preexisting kidney disease. *Acute renal failure is usually caused by periods of prolonged ischemia either from extended aortic cross-clamping above the renal arteries; hypotensive episodes before, during, or after surgery;* and/or embolization of atherosclerotic plaques (atheroembolism) to the renal arteries. Renal function is assessed through the measurement of urine volume, intake and output, and serum and urine creatinine and electrolytes.

Acute limb ischemia is most commonly the result of atheroembolism and can occur in one or both legs. Significant cutaneous ischemia may occur despite maintenance of palpable pedal pulses (blue-toe syndrome or "trash foot"). Assessment of pulses, skin color, temperature, movement, and sensation should be completed hourly. **Pain in an extremity can be a significant indicator of acute ischemia.**

KEY CLINICAL CONCEPT

- Acute limb ischemia and limb trauma can cause compartment syndrome. The "6 Ps" can be helpful for identifying compartment syndrome. The 6 Ps include pain, pallor, pulselessness, paresthesia, and poikilothermia (limb temperature is the same as the ambient air). The earliest manifestation of limb compartment syndrome is loss of sensation. Pulselessness and poikilothermia are late signs of compartment syndrome and may signal irreversible nerve and muscle damage.
- In contrast, venous occlusions are associated with redness, swelling, maintaining a pulse, and a tendency to be chronic.
- Acute limb ischemia and/or compartment syndrome can cause rhabdomyolysis.

Occlusive Disorders

Obstruction of arterial or venous flow due to atherosclerosis is the most common cardiovascular disturbance. Obstruction can occur anywhere along the major arterial tree; in critical care settings, however, aortofemoral obstructions are most likely to bring the patient to the ICU setting.

Obstruction due to arterial flow usually results in *pain during exercise.* Lower extremity obstruction is more common than upper extremity obstruction. Pain in the legs on activity due to obstruction is called *intermittent claudication.* Arterial obstructions are potentially more dangerous because of the loss of oxygen and substrates necessary for the generation of energy. **Venous obstructions** tend to be more chronic and are less likely to be seen in the critical care setting.

Clinical indications of decreased arterial blood flow include diminished pulses, loss of temperature (cool skin), change in color (pallor suggestive of arterial obstruction) and distal necrosis may be observed as it progresses, as well as diminished sensation. If the obstruction is sudden, severe pain distal to the obstruction is a common symptom. In **chronic arterial obstruction**, arterial ulcers may occur. The skin is typically shiny, has a lack of hair growth, and is not edematous. **Chronic venous insufficiency (CVI)** can lead to venous ulcers, peripheral edema, cyanosis, and brawny (bronze-like) skin discoloration.

Assessment of the need for surgery generally includes Doppler ultrasound studies and possibly abdominal aortic ultrasound and CT examinations. Angiography with or without intervention (stenting) is commonly performed. Surgery is indicated for complex lesions and those that cannot be successfully treated percutaneously.

Surgical Intervention

The optimal surgical method to relieve obstruction to blood flow depends on the location of the obstruction. **Figure 13-2** illustrates the most common types of surgical procedures to bypass obstructions of the aorta and femoral arteries.

Endovascular therapies (balloon angioplasties, atherectomy, and laser angioplasties) can provide effective symptom relief in patients with peripheral vascular disease.

Postoperative Considerations

Assessment of blood flow is an important nursing measure both pre- and postoperatively. *Blood flow assessment includes pulse quality, capillary refill, and sensation.* Pulse presence does not necessarily mean that the graft has good patency. *Doppler assessment is a better parameter to measure flow than palpation.*

Loss of flow following surgery can be due to failure of the bypass graft or obstruction as a result of clot formation. It can also result from **compartment syndrome** (*severe edema caused by tissue reperfusion injury*). In the case of clot formation, there is a danger of potential embolization. **In arterial surgery,** the emboli will obstruct a site beyond the site of surgery and may result in loss of a portion of the extremity involved. If obstruction is on the **venous side,** the emboli will result in *pulmonary embolization.* Symptoms of pulmonary emboli are chest pain,

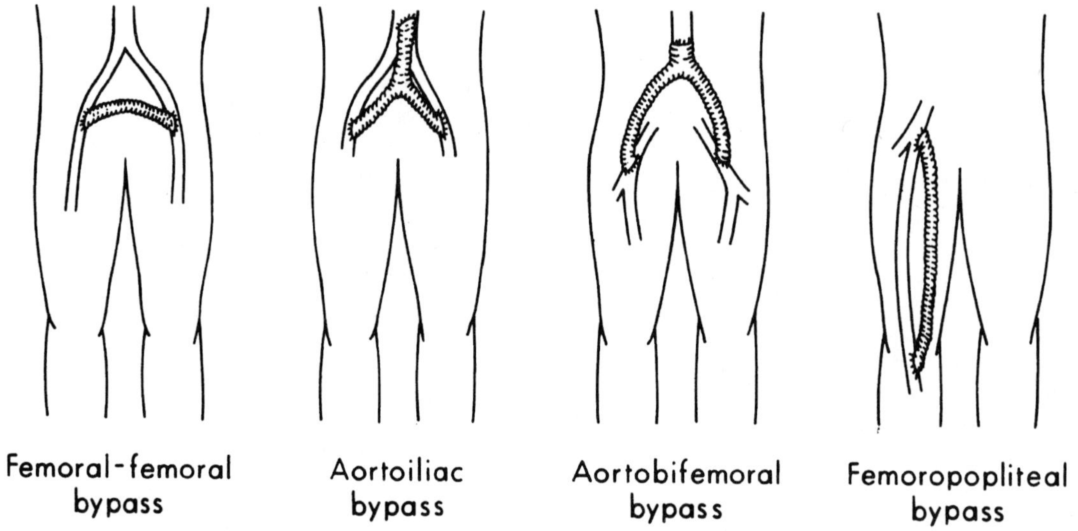

Figure 13-2. Femoral vascular bypass techniques.

shortness of breath, decreased Pao_2/Sao_2, and elevation of pulmonary artery pressures.

13.2 CARDIAC TRAUMA

Cardiac injuries can be among the most life-threatening traumatic injuries and are second in mortality only to neurologic injuries. Most are the result of motor vehicle crashes and are therefore due to blunt trauma. There is an increasing number of chest injuries due to gunshot wounds and stabbings. Injury to the heart and/or great vessels causing disruption of the structures can reduce circulating blood volume and leads to hypovolemia and shock. Direct trauma to the heart muscle, as in myocardial contusion, can lead to a decrease in myocardial contraction, resulting in low cardiac output.

> QUICK TIP! Expect about two questions on the exam covering cardiac trauma. This section, in conjunction with the previous sections, will enable the clinician to understand the hemodynamic effects of cardiovascular trauma.

Blunt Cardiac Injury

Blunt cardiac injury (BCI) is a common term used to describe any traumatic injury to the heart. It spans from cardiac or valve rupture and coronary arterial injury to stunning or contusion of the myocardium. Cardiac contusion is the most common blunt injury to the heart. It is rarely fatal. Suspect BCI if the patient has anterior chest wall trauma and/or fractures of the sternum or ribs. The most commonly seen ECG changes are sinus tachycardia (not specific in trauma patients) and the development of premature atrial contractions (PACs) or PVCs. In patients with suspected BCI, monitor telemetry for 24 to 48 hours. Troponin I (cTnI) or troponin T (cTnT), are the most accurate indicators of BCI. *Unlike in MI, positive troponin levels do not affect BCI treatment.* Treatment is based on the patient's symptoms. Two-dimensional echocardiography and/or multigated angiography may be useful in determining abnormalities in ventricular wall movement and EF. Severe visceral injury may result in delayed cardiac rupture, ventricular septal defect, ventricular aneurysm, and/or cardiogenic shock. All of which require conventional treatment.

Although uncommon, BCI can result in **cardiac tamponade** from tearing of either coronary arteries or veins. Even though it is caused by a small amount of blood (as little as 50 mL), clinical deterioration occurs more rapidly in these cases since the pericardium has not had time to stretch to accommodate the fluid volume (as seen with chronic pericardial effusions).

> **KEY CLINICAL CONCEPT**
> The most commonly seen ECG changes in BCI are sinus tachycardia (not specific in trauma patients) and the development of premature atrial contractions (PACs) or PVCs.

Cardiac Rupture

This is a blunt trauma injury and is the most common cause of death. Chamber rupture most commonly occurs in the right ventricle, followed by the left ventricle, right atrium, and left atrium. There is no treatment for cardiac rupture other than emergent surgical intervention.

Valvular Injury

This is a blunt trauma injury. The aortic valve is the most commonly injured valve. Signs and symptoms are valve regurgitation and heart failure. Specific treatment could include valve repair or replacement in conjunction with medical heart failure therapy.

Cardiac Tamponade

This may result from blunt or penetrating trauma to the pericardium and/or heart. Blood enters the pericardial sac. As more blood enters the sac, *more pressure is placed against the heart,*

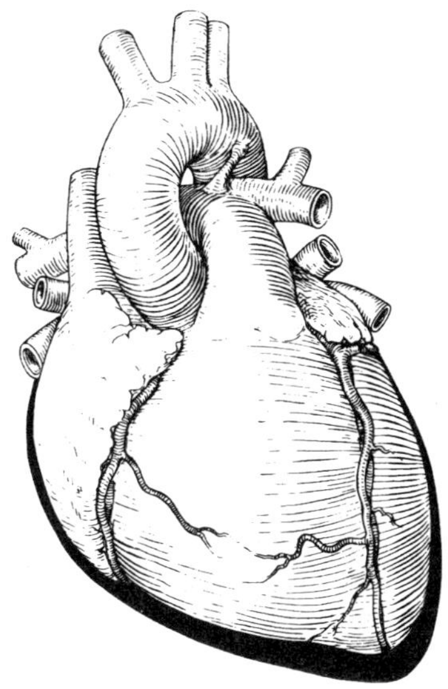

Figure 13-3. Cardiac tamponade.

thus inhibiting or compromising ventricular filling (**Fig. 13-3**). A subsequent decrease in SV and narrow pulse pressure leads to a decrease in CO.

Cardiac tamponade *presents with hypotension, muffled or distant heart sounds, and distended neck veins. Additional clues are a falling systolic blood pressure (SBP), narrow pulse pressure (due to low cardiac output), pulsus paradoxus (a drop of >10 mm Hg in SBP during inspiration), elevated CVP, and various degrees of shock.* In a trauma patient, the classic symptoms may be obscured by hypovolemic shock.

QUICK TIP! On the CCRN exam, pulsus paradoxus (which is also called a paradoxical pulse is present if there is a drop of >10 mm Hg in SBP during inspiration) is a key indicator of cardiac tamponade.

Treatment and Nursing Intervention

The objective of treatment is to confirm the diagnosis and relieve the tamponade. *Pericardiocentesis* is not recommended in blunt trauma patients due to the small amount of blood that causes the tamponade and the risk of RV injury during the procedure. *Pericardial exploration (pericardial window) is the diagnostic and treatment procedure of choice* in blunt cardiac trauma (**Fig. 13-4**). The underlying cause of the tamponade must be determined. If the cause of the tamponade is not readily apparent or readily controlled, a thoracotomy may be indicated for direct diagnosis and repair of the underlying problem.

Blunt Aortic Injury

Blunt aortic injury (BAI) is the result of a blunt trauma deceleration injury causing a shearing of the fixed and mobile portions of the aorta. The aorta is tethered at three points: the

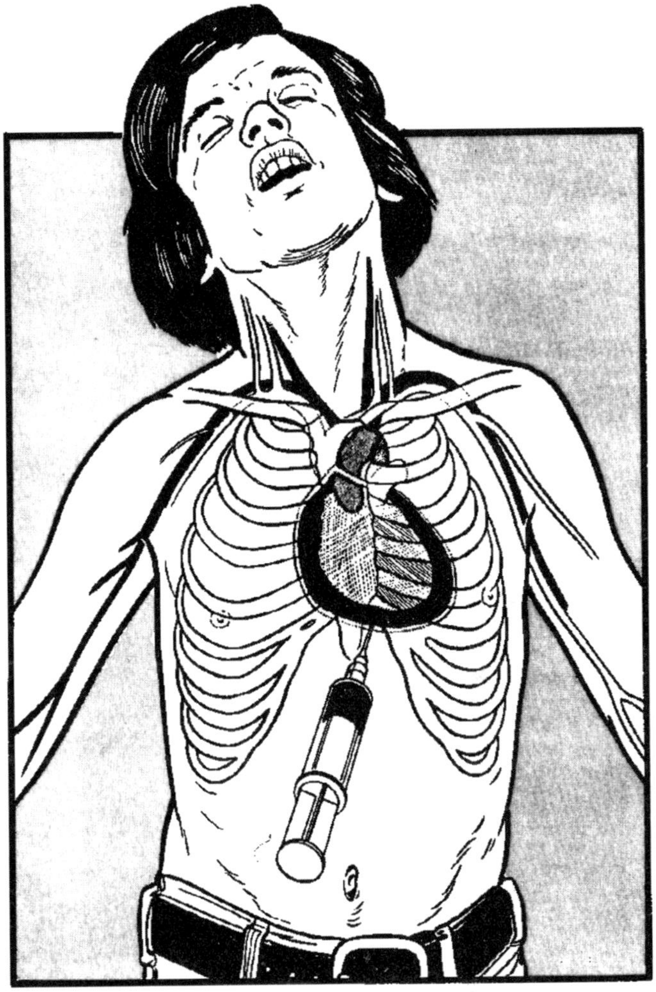

Figure 13-4. Paraxiphoid approach to pericardiocentesis.

aortic valve, the ligamentum arteriosum (located near the take-off of the left subclavian artery), and the hiatus of the diaphragm. **Figure 13-5** identifies the most common sites of aortic rupture. Eighty-nine percent of BAI occur at the isthmus as a result of the ligamentum arteriosum's tethering of the aorta. **Patients who have a complete aortic transection die immediately.** Those who survive the initial injury have a high risk of death: 30% mortality in 6 hours, 50% mortality in 24 hours, and 70% mortality in 1 week if the injury is not definitively repaired.

Chest roentgenography (CXR) may reveal a widened mediastinum (> 8 cm in diameter), which is suggestive of aortic injury; however, 7% of patients with BAI have negative chest radiographs. As with thoracic aortic aneurysms, the *aortogram is still the gold standard for identifying the area of rupture. However, CTA and MRA are more commonly used due to the ease of performing the tests and their less invasive natures. Symptoms may include a lower BP and pulse alterations* in the upper extremities **(decreased left brachial and radial pulses if the left subclavian artery is affected)**, and pulse alterations in the lower extremities. Shortness of breath, weakness, *chest or back pain* may be present depending on the presence of other thoracic injuries.

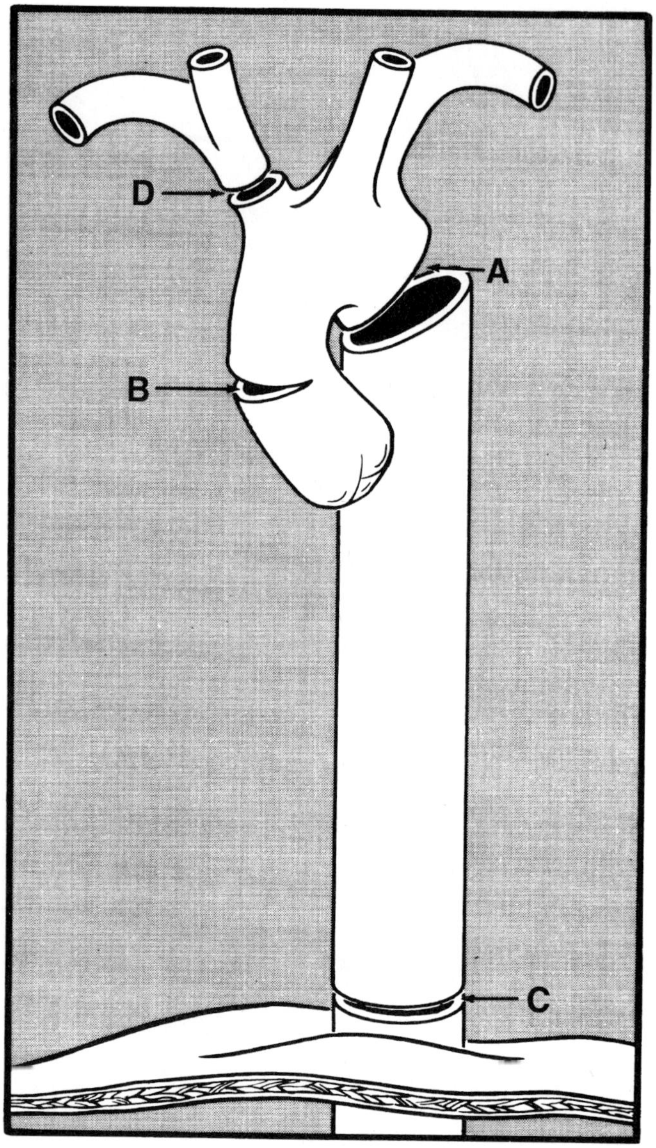

Figure 13-5. Sites of aortic rupture: (**A**) arch of aorta; (**B**) area just above aortic valve; (**C**) end of thoracic aorta; (**D**) subclavian vein. The aortic arch is the most common site; the subclavian vein is the least common.

QUICK TIP! On the CCRN exam, if a CXR report reveals a "widened mediastinum" the patient in the scenario likely has a thoracic aortic dissection or increased mediastinal bleeding that may suggest cardiac tampondade.

Treatment and Nursing Intervention

As with thoracic aneurysms and dissections, the *initial treatment focuses on keeping the HR less than 70 and the SBP less than 120 (or lower) to prevent aortic rupture.* Definitive treatment is either surgical or endovascular aortic repair.

Nursing interventions include monitoring the respiratory, cardiovascular, neurologic, and renal systems. Nursing care of the patient on ventilatory support and in need of close monitoring before and after surgery applies to the patient with a BAI.

KEY CONTENT CHECKLIST

- ❒ **Cardiac tamponade** *presents with hypotension, muffled or distant heart sounds, and distended neck veins. Additional clues are a falling systolic blood pressure (SBP), narrow pulse pressure (due to low cardiac output), pulsus paradoxus (a drop of >10 mm Hg in SBP during inspiration), elevated CVP, and various degrees of shock.*
- ❒ **Protamine sulfate** is given to reverse heparin-induced anticoagulation. Protamine sulfate can cause a severe adverse histamine reaction accompanied by profound vasodilation, systemic hypotension, *and elevated pulmonary artery (PA) pressures. Protamine reactions* may require fluid and/or vasoactive medications to maintain adequate tissue perfusion.
- ❒ Transplanted hearts are denervated. **Isoproterenol** is used to treat symptomatic sinus bradycardia that occurs since the HR is unresponsive to **atropine.**
- ❒ The signs and symptoms of acute MR are similar to acute left heart failure.
- ❒ Acute MR is associated with a holosystolic (throughout systole) murmur heard at the fourth to fifth ICS and radiates to the left axial.
- ❒ Patients who undergo multiple valve repair or replacement surgery are at higher risk of having heart block and requiring temporary epicardial pacing and/or permanent pacemaker insertion.
- ❒ The classic symptoms of severe AS are pre-syncope or syncope, angina, and dyspnea/shortness of breath.
- ❒ Medical management of aortic dissections focuses *on* keeping the HR less than 70 bpm and keeping the BP less than 120 mm Hg (or lower depending on surgeon preference).
- ❒ **Esmolol**, an IV beta blocker, is the drug of choice since it lowers both HR and BP and is titratable. **Labetalol,** a combination beta and alpha-blocker may also be used.
- ❒ If the BP target is not met with esmolol alone, an additional agent(s) such as **nicardipine** or **sodium nitroprusside** may be indicated
- ❒ Acute limb ischemia and limb trauma can cause compartment syndrome. The "6 Ps" can be helpful for identifying compartment syndrome. The 6 Ps include pain, pallor, pulselessness, paresthesia, and poikilothermia (limb temperature is the same as the ambient air). The earliest manifestation of limb compartment syndrome is loss of sensation. Pulselessness and poikilothermia are late signs of compartment syndrome and may signal irreversible nerve and muscle damage.
- ❒ In contrast, venous occlusions are associated with redness, swelling, maintaining a pulse, and a tendency to be chronic.
- ❒ Acute limb ischemia and/or compartment syndrome can cause rhabdomyolysis.
- ❒ The most commonly seen ECG changes in BCI are sinus tachycardia (not specific in trauma patients) and the development of premature atrial contractions (PACs) or PVCs.

Review Questions:

1. **A patient who was recently admitted from the emergency department with hypertensive crisis reports "ripping" chest pain that radiates to the back. On exam, the patient has a loud diastolic murmur heard best at right sternal border, second intercostal space, and diminished pedal pulses. After notifying the medical team, which intervention would the nurse anticipate?**
   a. CT angiography of the chest, abdomen, and pelvis for suspected aortic dissection
   b. Emergent cardiac catheterization for acute coronary syndrome
   c. Echocardiogram and medical management of aortic regurgitation
   d. Adding an additional medication for BP control

Answer: A. Rationale: The patient in this scenario has classic signs and symptoms of an aortic dissection. In addition to heart rate and blood pressure control, the patient needs emergent CTA or MRA of the chest, abdomen, and pelvis to confirm the diagnosis and aid in surgical planning. Answer B is not correct as the physical exam findings are not consistent with an acute coronary syndrome. Answer C is incorrect as it does not address finding the cause of the new aortic regurgitation murmur. Answer D is incorrect. Although the patient in this scenario may need additional medications added for BP control, this answer does not investigate potential causes of the new symptoms and exam findings.

2. **A patient who was admitted to the cardiothoracic intensive care unit (CTICU) after coronary artery bypass grafting three times and a bioprosthetic aortic valve replacement is being treated with protamine sulfate and aminocaproic acid infusions due to excessive chest tube output. The patient is also receiving IV magnesium sulfate and perioperative cefazolin (Ancef). The patient develops severe vasodilation, resulting in systemic hypotension and pulmonary hypertension. The nurse suspects the patient is experiencing:**
   a. Anaphylaxis from cefazolin (Ancef)
   b. Vasodilation due to magnesium sulfate
   c. An allergic reaction to aminocaproic acid
   d. A reaction to protamine sulfate

Answer: D. Rationale: The patient in this scenario is experiencing a classic reaction to protamine sulfate. Answer A is not correct as there are no signs of anaphylaxis other than hypotension. Answer B is not correct, although magnesium sulfate can cause vasodilatation and lower blood pressure, pulmonary hypertension would not be expected. Answer C is not correct as there are no other signs of an allergic reaction besides hypotension.

REFERENCES

Adler Y, Charron P, Imazio M, et al. The 2015 European Society of Cardiology Guidelines on the diagnosis and management of pericardial diseases. *Eur Heart J*. 2015;36(42): 2921–2962. doi: 10.1093/eurheartj/ehv318.

Appleton C, Gillam L, Koulogiannis K. Cardiac tamponade. *Cardiol Clin*. 2017;35(4):525–537. doi: 10.1016/j.ccl.2017.07.006.

Bastopcu M, Sargin M, Kuplay H, Erdoğan SB, Yapici N, Aka SA. Risk factors for vasoplegia after coronary artery bypass and valve surgery. *J Card Surg*. 2021;36(8), 2729–2734. doi: 10.1111/jocs.15663.

Batra G, Ahlsson A, Lindahl B, Lindhagen L, Wickbom A, Oldgren J. Atrial fibrillation in patients undergoing coronary artery surgery is associated with adverse outcomes. *Upsala J Med*, 2019;124(1):70–77.

Baumgartner H, Falk V, Bax JJ, et al. 2017 ESC/EACTS Guidelines for the management of valvular heart disease. *Eur Heart J*. 2017;38:2739–2791.

Bojar RM. *Manual of Perioperative Care in Adult Cardiac Surgery*. 6th ed. John Wiley & Sons, Inc. 2021.

Bollinger D, Tanaka KA. Coagulation management strategies in cardiac surgery. *Curr Anesthesiol Rep*. 2017;7:265–272.

Brien LD, Oermann MH, Molloy M, Tierney C. Implementing goal directed therapy for fluid resuscitation in the cardiovascular intensive care unit. *AACN Adv Crit Care*. 2020;31(4):364–370.

Davidson LJ, Davidson CJ. Transcatheter treatment of valvular heart disease: a review. *JAMA*. 2021;325(24), 2480–2494. doi: 10.1001/jama.2021.2133.

Demirci C, Zeman F, Schmid C, Bernhard F. Early postoperative blood pressure and blood loss after cardiac surgery: a retrospective analysis. *Intensive Crit Care Nurs*. 2017;42: 122–126.

Engelman DT, Ali WB, Williams JB, et al. Guidelines for perioperative care in cardiac surgery: enhanced recovery after surgery society recommendations. *JAMA Surgery*. 2019;154(8): 755–766.

Faroux L, Guimaraes L, Wintzer-Wehekind J. Coronary artery disease and transcatheter aortic valve replacement: JACC state-of-the-art review. *J Am Coll Cardiol*. 2019;74(3):362–372. doi: 10.1016/j.jacc.2019.06.012.

Flint N, Wunderlich NC, Shmueli H, Ben-Zekry S, Siegel RJ, Beigel R. Aortic regurgitation. *Curr Cardiol Rep*. 2019;21(7):65. doi: 10.1007/s11886-019-1144-6.

Geng J, Qian J, Cheng H, Ji F, Liu H. The influence of perioperative dexmedetomidine on patients undergoing cardiac surgery: a meta-analysis. *PLoS One*. 2016;11(4):e0152829.

Gillinov AM, Bagiella E, Moskowitz AJ, et al. Rate control versus rhythm control for atrial fibrillation after cardiac surgery. *NEJM*. 2016;374, 1911–1921.

Hillis LD, Smith PK, Anderson JL, et al. 2011 ACCF/AHA guideline for coronary artery bypass graft surgery: a report of the American College of Cardiology Foundation/American Heart Association Task Force on Practice Guidelines developed in collaboration with the American Association for Thoracic Surgery, Society of Cardiovascular Anesthesiologists, and Society of Thoracic Surgeons. *J Am Coll Cardiol*. 2011;58(24):e123–e210.

Honasoge AP, Dubbs SB. Rapid fire: pericardial effusion and tamponade. *Emerg Med Clin North Am*. 2018;36(3):557–565. doi: 10.1016/j.emc.2018.04.004.

Horr SE, Mentias A, Houghtaling PL,et al. Comparison of outcomes of pericardiocentesis versus surgical pericardial window in patients requiring drainage of pericardial effusions. *Am J Cardiol*. 2017;120(5):883–890. doi: 10.1016/j.amjcard.2017.06.003.

Lawton JS, Tamis-Holland JE, Bangalore S, et al. 2021 ACC/AHA/SCAI Guideline for Coronary Artery Revascularization: a report of the American College of Cardiology/American Heart Association joint committee on clinical practice guidelines. *J Am Coll Cardiol*. 2021;S0735-1097(21):06158-1. doi: 10.1016/j.jacc.2021.09.006.

Liu J, Yang BQ, Itoh A, Masood MF, Hartupee JC, Schilling JD. Impact of new UNOS allocation criteria on heart transplant practices and outcomes. *Transplant Direct*. 2021;7(1): e642. doi: 10.1097/TXD.0000000000001088.

Li P, Qu L, Qi D, et al. Significance of perioperative goal-directed hemodynamic approach in preventing postoperative complications in patients after cardiac surgery: a meta-analysis and systematic review. *Ann Med*. 2017;49(4):343–351.

Marra A, Ely EW, Pandharipande PP, Patel MB. The ABCDEF bundle in critical care. *Crit Care Clin*. 2017;33(2):225–243.

Myles PS, Smith JA, Forbes A, et al. Tranexamic acid in patients undergoing coronary-artery surgery. *N Engl J*. 2017;376(2):136–148. doi: 10.1056/MEJMoa1606424.

Osawa EA, Rhodes A, Landoni G, et al. Effect of perioperative goal-directed hemodynamic resuscitation therapy on outcomes following cardiac surgery: a randomized clinical trial and systematic review. *Crit Care Med.* 2016;44(4):724–733. doi: 10.1097/CCM.0000000000001479.

Otto CM, Nishimura RA, Nishimura RA, et al. 2020 ACC/AHA guideline for the management of patients with valvular heart disease: a report of the American College of Cardiology/American Heart Association Joint Committee on Clinical Practice Guidelines. *Circulation.* 2020;72–227.

Parrino PE. Cardiopulmonary bypass: An introduction. *CTS Net.* 2018. doi:10.25373/ctsnet.7364945.

Pereira KM, De Asis CS, Cintra HL, et al. Factors associated with the increased bleeding in the postoperative period of cardiac surgery. *J Clin Nurs.* 2018;28(5-6):850–861.

Richards JE, Samet RE, Koerner AK, Grissom TE. Tranexamic acid in the perioperative period. *Adv Anesth.* 2019;37:87–110. doi: 10.1016/j.aan.2019.08.009.

Shaefi S, Mittel A, Loberman D, Ramakrishna H. Off-pump versus on-pump coronary artery bypass grafting: a systematic review and analysis of clinical outcomes. *J Cardiothorac Vasc Anesth.* 2019;33(1):232–244. doi: 10.1053/j.jvca.2018.04.012.

Thompson-Brazill KA. Pain control in the cardiothoracic surgery patient. *Crit Care Nurs Clin North Am.* 2019;31(3):389–405. Doi: 10.1016/j.cnc.2019.05.007.

Thompson-Brazill KA, Tierney CC, Brien L, Wininger JW, Williams JB. Enhancing family-centered care in cardiothoracic surgery. *Crit Care Nurs Clin North Am.* 2020;32(2):295–311. doi: 10.1016/j.cnc.2020.02.010.

Tierney CC, Oermann MH, Molloy MA, Brien L, Neisler C. Implementing a weaning protocol for cardiac surgery patients using simulation: a quality improvement project. *Dimens Crit Care Nurs.* 2019;38(5):248–255.

Venuta F, Diso D, Anile M, Rendina EA, Onorati I. Chest tubes: generalities. *Thorac Surg Clin.* 2017;27(1):1–5.

York NL, Kane C, Smith CS. Identification and management of acute cardiac tamponade. *Dimens Crit Care Nurs.* 2018;37(3):130–134. doi: 10.1097/DCC.0000000000000295.

PART I
Cardiovascular Practice Exam

Questions 1 and 2 are based on the following scenario:
A 72-year-old man is admitted to the unit with the diagnosis of acute inferior wall myocardial infarction (MI). He has a history of peripheral vascular disease and chronic obstructive pulmonary disease (COPD). During your shift, he begins to complain of shortness of breath. His 12-lead electrocardiogram (ECG) shows ST-segment depression in leads V_1 to V_4. He has dependent crackles in his posterior lobes along with expiratory wheezing. His pulse oximeter reading is 0.95 on 2 L/min per nasal cannula. He has the following laboratory data:

pH	7.37
$Paco_2$	52
Pao_2	69
HCO_3	33
CPK-MB	4
Troponin I	0.1

He has an S_3 (gallop) and a III/VI systolic murmur. The following hemodynamic information is available:

Blood pressure	104/60
Pulse	101
Stroke index	20
Cardiac index	2.0
Pulmonary arterial pressure	40/24
Pulmonary artery occlusive pressure (PAOP)	22
Central venous pressure (CVP)	11

1. **Based on this information, what is probably happening?**
   (A) exacerbation of the COPD
   (B) development of heart failure
   (C) development of inferior MI
   (D) development of pericardial tamponade
2. **Based on the above information, what would be the best treatment to improve the symptoms?**
   (A) oxygen therapy and thrombolytic
   (B) vasopressin (increasing afterload)
   (C) nitroprusside (afterload reducer) and fluids (preload increaser)
   (D) dobutamine (inotrope) and/or Lasix (preload reducer)
3. **A 76-year-old woman in your unit has the diagnosis of heart failure (HF). The physician inserts a pulmonary artery catheter to help assess therapeutic interventions. One of the therapies she selects is dobutamine. With the addition of dobutamine to the treatment regimen, which parameters would you expect to see change if the therapy is successful?**
   (A) increase in stroke volume
   (B) increase in wedge pressure
   (C) increase in systemic vascular resistance (SVR)
   (D) decrease in mean arterial pressure

Questions 4 and 5 are based on the following scenario:
A 71-year-old man is admitted to your unit with shortness of breath, orthopnea, and progressive reduction in exercise tolerance. He states he has "not ever been to a doctor." His lung sounds demonstrate crackles in most of his posterior lobes. A pulse oximeter indicates a value of 0.89. A pulmonary artery catheter is placed to help identify the origin of the shortness of breath. The following data are available:

Blood pressure	118/70
Pulse	110
Respiratory rate	28
Temperature	37.1
Cardiac index	2.2
Stroke index	20
Pulmonary arterial pressure	36/22
PAOP	20
CVP	6

4. **Based on the above information, what condition is likely developing?**
   (A) noncardiogenic pulmonary edema
   (B) primary pulmonary hypertension
   (C) sepsis
   (D) left ventricular (LV) failure
5. **What therapy would most likely improve his symptoms?**
   (A) oxygen therapy
   (B) phenylephrine
   (C) furosemide
   (D) carvedilol
6. **What is the approximate normal right atrial CVP value?**
   (A) 2 to 6 mm Hg
   (B) 5 to 10 mm Hg
   (C) 8 to 12 mm Hg
   (D) 12 to 18 mm Hg
7. **Which of the following statements regarding the coronary sinus is correct?**
   (A) It provides arterial blood flow to the lateral LV wall.
   (B) It provides arterial blood flow to the sinus node.
   (C) It is the main venous drainage vessel of the heart.
   (D) It stimulates secretion of the atrial natriuretic factor.
8. **Left atrial pressure approximates which pressure?**
   (A) pulmonary mean pressure (PMAP)
   (B) LV end-diastolic pressure (LVEDP)
   (C) right atrial pressure
   (D) CVP (or superior to the right atrium)

9. **Of the following four factors, three determine stroke volume. Identify the factor that does NOT affect stroke volume.**
   (A) preload
   (B) afterload
   (C) contractility
   (D) capillary permeability

10. **The A wave on the CVP and PAOP tracing represents which physical event?**
    (A) ventricular filling
    (B) atrial contraction
    (C) atrial filling
    (D) tricuspid and mitral valve movement

11. **The C wave on the CVP and PAOP tracing occurs due to which anatomic event?**
    (A) pulmonic and tricuspid valve closure
    (B) aortic and mitral valve opening
    (C) mitral and tricuspid valve closure
    (D) mitral and tricuspid valve opening

12. **What is the normal right ventricular (RV) end-diastolic pressure?**
    (A) 2 to 6 mm Hg
    (B) 5 to 10 mm Hg
    (C) 10 to 15 mm Hg
    (D) greater than 20 mm Hg

13. **Which of the following is an estimate of right ventricular preload?**
    (A) PAOP
    (B) CVP
    (C) pulmonary artery mean pressure
    (D) coronary sinus pressure

14. **Afterload is estimated by which parameter?**
    (A) CVP
    (B) PAOP
    (C) stroke volume
    (D) SVR

15. **Which hemodynamic waves are produced and found on the atrial pressure waveform?**
    (A) A, C, and V waves
    (B) arterial systolic waves
    (C) augmented diastolic waves
    (D) X, Y, and Z waves

16. **LV failure alone presents with all but one of the following signs. Select the INCORRECT sign.**
    (A) increased CVP
    (B) increased PAOP
    (C) increased LVEDP
    (D) increased pulmonary mean arterial pressure

17. **Two circumstances may produce a systolic murmur. One exists when backward flow of blood (regurgitant flow) occurs through a valve that is normally closed during systole. The second exists when blood has difficulty getting past a valve (stenosis) that is normally easily opened. Which two situations may produce a systolic murmur?**
    (A) aortic stenosis and mitral regurgitation
    (B) pulmonic regurgitation and tricuspid stenosis
    (C) aortic and tricuspid stenosis
    (D) pulmonic and mitral regurgitation

18. **All of the following but one are considered key treatments in the management of HF. Which one is NOT a key treatment in HF?**
    (A) angiotensin-converting enzyme (ACE) inhibitors
    (B) beta blockers
    (C) diuretics
    (D) nitroprusside

19. **The PAOP is used to estimate which of the following pressures?**
    (A) left atrial pressure and LVEDP
    (B) right atrial pressure and RV end-diastolic pressure (RVEDP)
    (C) central venous and pulmonary arterial pressures
    (D) mean pulmonary artery and RV peak pressures

20. **Pericardial tamponade presents with all but one of the following symptoms. Identify the symptom NOT associated with pericardial tamponade.**
    (A) equalization of left and right atrial pressures (CVP and PAOP)
    (B) LV failure without RV involvement
    (C) hypotension
    (D) distended neck veins

21. **LV preload is estimated from all of the following pressures but one. Identify the one pressure that does NOT permit one to estimate LV preload.**
    (A) CVP
    (B) PAOP
    (C) left atrial pressure
    (D) LVEDP

22. **RV failure is manifest by which of the following signs?**
    (A) increased CVP
    (B) increased PAOP
    (C) decreased pulmonary artery pressure
    (D) increased systemic arterial pressure

Questions 23 and 24 refer to the following scenario:
A 62-year-old man is admitted to your unit with the diagnosis of acute subendocardial infarction. At present he has no chest pain and his vital signs are normal. As you talk with him, he complains of sudden severe shortness of breath. His blood pressure is 80/50 mm Hg, pulse 118, respiratory rate 34. Heart sounds are easily heard but he has a new systolic murmur, grade V/VI. Hemodynamic data indicate the following:

Pulmonary artery pressure	38/25
PAOP	24
CVP	7
Cardiac output	3.2
Cardiac index	1.7

23. **Based on the preceding information, which condition is likely to be developing?**
    (A) pericardial tamponade
    (B) mitral valve rupture
    (C) ventricular wall rupture
    (D) aortic valve rupture

24. **Which treatment would be indicated for this condition?**
(A) immediate surgery
(B) dopamine nitroprusside
(C) fluid challenges
(D) thrombolytic therapy

25. **Dysfunction of the papillary muscle producing mitral regurgitation would be seen in which part of the left atrial PAOP tracing?**
(A) giant A waves
(B) absent A waves
(C) giant C waves
(D) giant V waves

26. **Phase 0 of cellular impulse transmission refers to which phase of electrical action?**
(A) depolarization
(B) early repolarization
(C) end repolarization
(D) myocardial relaxation

27. **Spontaneous diastolic repolarization occurs during which phase of the cardiac action potential?**
(A) phase 0
(B) phase 1
(C) phase 3
(D) phase 4

28. **Which cation activates the second (slow channel) inward flow of ions during cardiac depolarization?**
(A) sodium
(B) potassium
(C) chloride
(D) calcium

29. **Which ion leaves the cell during depolarization to counter the inward flow of sodium?**
(A) phosphate
(B) potassium
(C) chloride
(D) calcium

30. **Which of the following cardiac chambers contains deoxygenated blood?**
(A) right ventricle
(B) left ventricle
(C) pulmonary veins
(D) left atrium

31. **Where is the sinoatrial (SA) node located?**
(A) right atrium
(B) left atrium
(C) right ventricle
(D) superior vena cava

32. **Which component of blood pressure regulation has the strongest effect on controlling the blood pressure?**
(A) stroke volume
(B) cardiac output
(C) SVR
(D) mean arterial pressure

33. **Which of the following corresponds most closely to the normal ejection fraction?**
(A) 10% to 20%
(B) 25% to 35%
(C) 40% to 50%
(D) greater than 60%

34. **Starling's law involves which of the following relationships?**
(A) As fluid fills the lungs, gas exchange decreases.
(B) As coronary blood flow increases, preload falls.
(C) As afterload increases, stroke volume improves.
(D) As muscle stretches, contraction strength initially increases.

35. **Which of the following would normally cause a patient with chest pain to be transferred to the cardiac catheterization lab as quickly as possible?**
(A) lactate level of 1.8
(B) Troponin I (cTnI) of less than 1
(C) ST-segment elevation in leads V_1 to V_4
(D) CVP of 8 mm Hg

36. **Which of the following is the most common reason for the PAOP and CVP to increase?**
(A) left and right ventricular failure
(B) excess blood volume
(C) RV failure
(D) pulmonary hypertension

37. **Reduction of myocardial oxygen consumption is best achieved through which of the following changes?**
(A) reducing afterload
(B) reducing preload
(C) increasing contractility
(D) increasing preload

38. **Which neurologic structure or system has the strongest effect on regulating the heart rate?**
(A) sympathetic nervous system
(B) parasympathetic nervous system
(C) adrenergic system
(D) cerebellum

39. **Which of the following could produce giant A waves?**
(A) aortic stenosis
(B) mitral regurgitation
(C) mitral stenosis
(D) hypovolemia

40. **What is the preferred first treatment for ventricular fibrillation?**
(A) nifedipine
(B) lidocaine 1 mg/kg
(C) synchronized cardioversion, 50 to 100 J
(D) defibrillation, 200 to 300 J monophasic or 120 to 180 biphasic

41. **Which of the following leads are used in the diagnosis of a lateral MI?**
(A) V_1, V_2, V_3, V_4
(B) I, aVL, V_5, V_6
(C) V_2R, V_3R, V_4R
(D) II, III, aVF

42. Which of the following leads are used in the diagnosis of a RV MI?

(A) V_1, V_2, V_3, V_4
(B) I, aVL, V_5, V_6
(C) aVR, aVL, aVF
(D) V_1, V_2, V_4R, V_6R

43. Interpret the following ECG rhythm strip. Sinus rhythm with. . . . ***See waveform below.***

(A) LV premature ventricular contraction (PVC)
(B) atrial premature contractions (APCs) with aberrant conduction
(C) RV PVC
(D) interpolated PVC

44. Interpret the following ECG rhythm strip. ***See waveform below.***

(A) sinus tachycardia
(B) atrial tachycardia
(C) atrial flutter
(D) atrial fibrillation

45. Interpret the following ECG rhythm strip. ***See art below.***

(A) sinus tachycardia
(B) paroxysmal atrial tachycardia
(C) atrial flutter
(D) atrial fibrillation

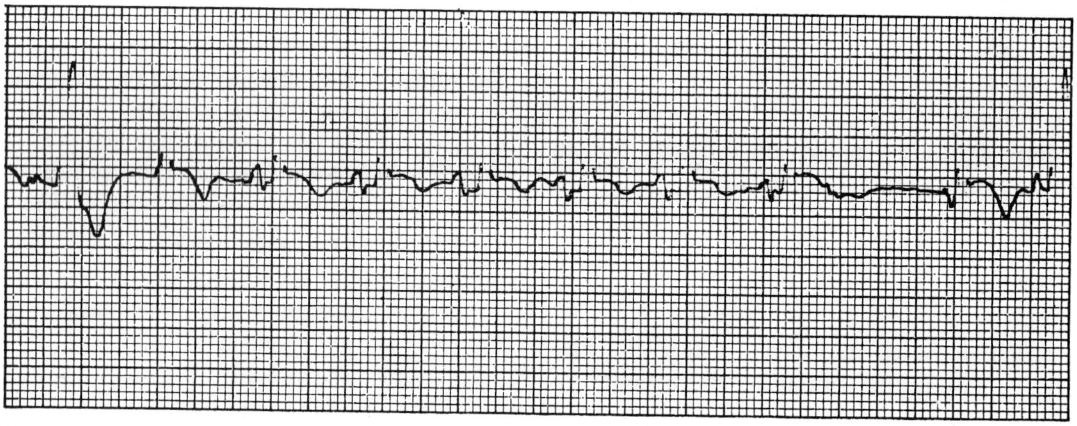

Question 43.

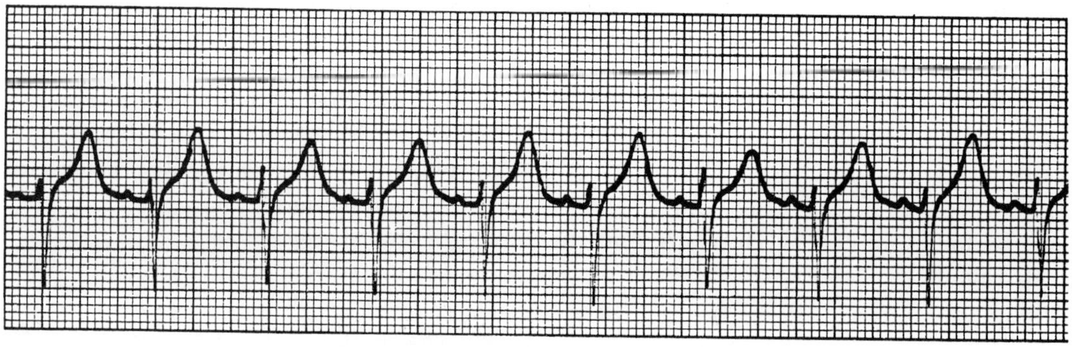

Question 44.

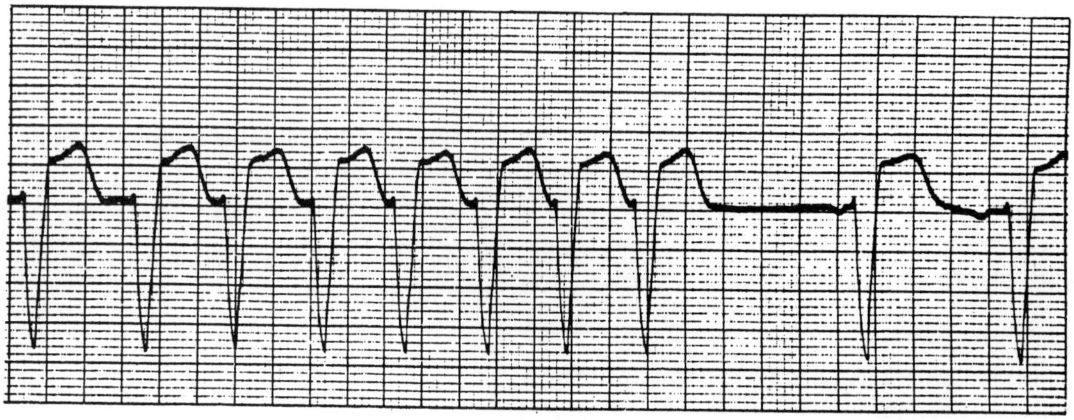

Question 45.

46. **Interpret the following ECG rhythm strip.** ***See art below.***
    (A) sinus tachycardia
    (B) atrial tachycardia
    (C) atrial flutter
    (D) atrial fibrillation

47. **Interpret the following ECG rhythm strip.** ***See art below.***
    (A) sinus tachycardia
    (B) atrial tachycardia
    (C) atrial flutter
    (D) atrial fibrillation

48. **Interpret the following ECG rhythm strip.** ***See art below.***
    (A) first-degree block
    (B) second-degree block type I
    (C) second-degree block type II
    (D) third-degree block

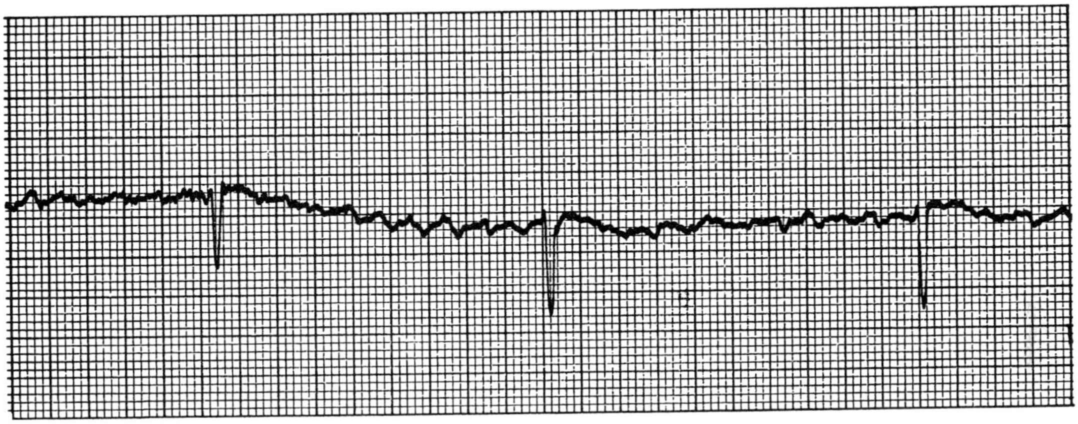

Question 46.

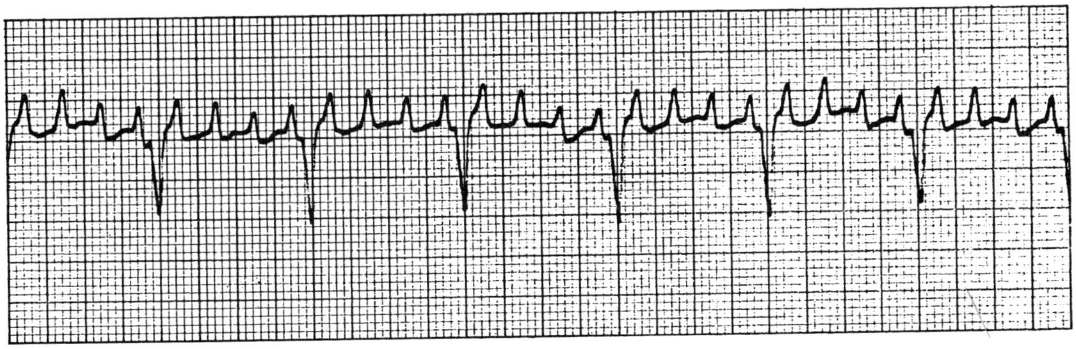

Question 47.

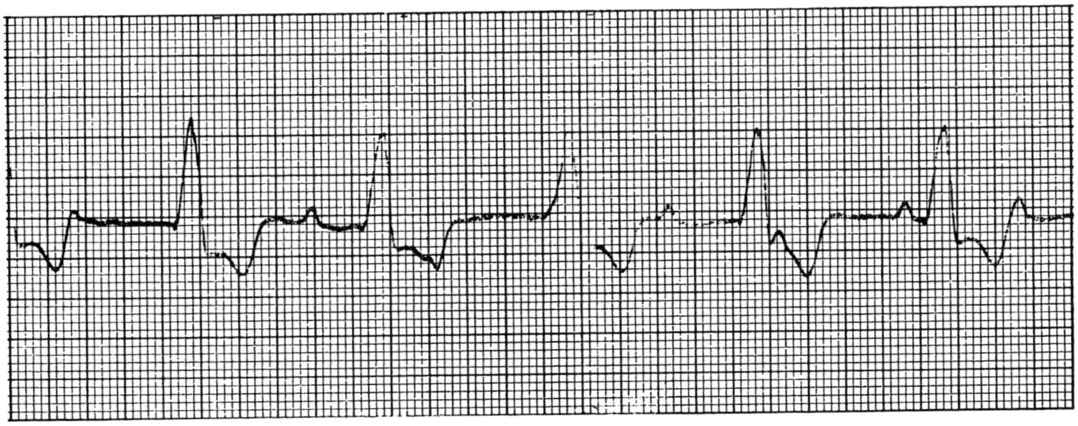

Question 48.

49. Interpret the following ECG rhythm strip. ***See art below.***

(A) first-degree block
(B) second-degree block, type I
(C) second-degree block, type II
(D) third-degree block

50. Interpret the following ECG rhythm strip. ***See art below.***

(A) first-degree block
(B) second-degree block, type I
(C) second-degree block, type II
(D) third-degree block

51. Interpret the following ECG rhythm strip. ***See art below.***

(A) first-degree block
(B) second-degree block, type I
(C) second-degree block, type II
(D) third-degree block

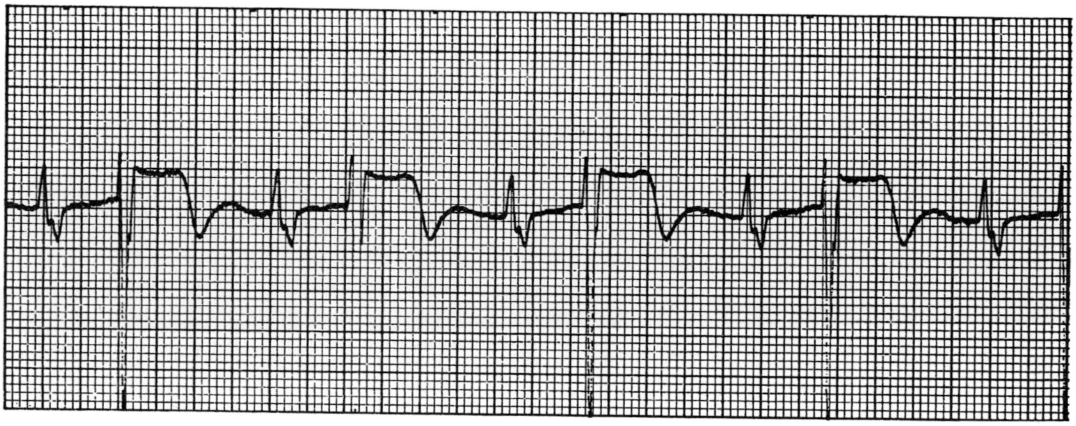

Question 49.

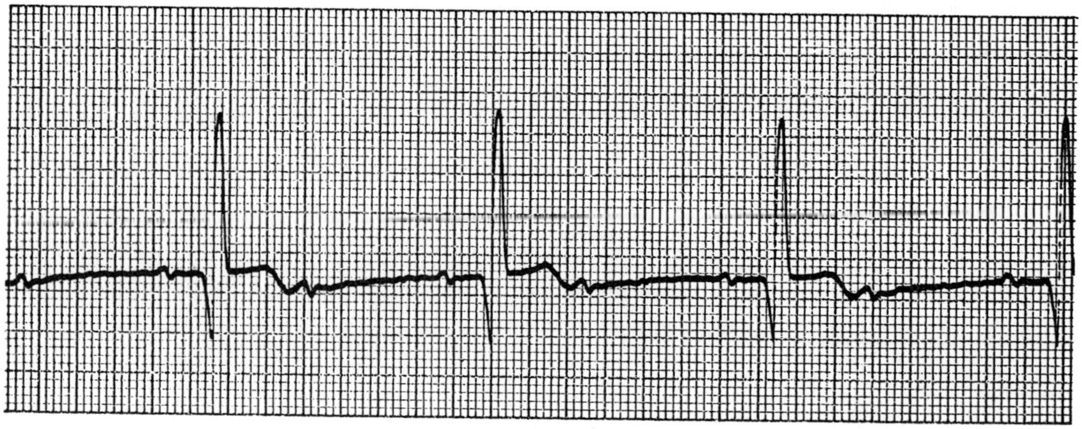

Question 50.

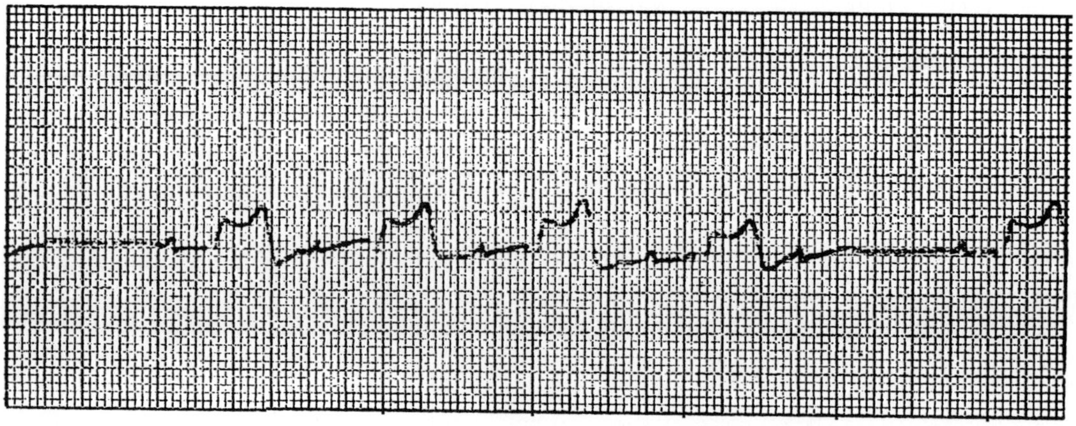

Question 51.

52. Interpret the following ECG rhythm strip. ***See art below.***
(A) multiform PVCs
(B) ventricular tachycardia
(C) ventricular fibrillation
(D) SVT with aberrancy

53. Interpret the following ECG rhythm strip. Atrial fibrillation with. . . . ***See art below.***
(A) multiform PVCs
(B) ventricular tachycardia
(C) ventricular fibrillation
(D) torsade de pointes

54. Interpret the following ECG rhythm strip. ***See art below.***
(A) multiform PVCs
(B) ventricular tachycardia
(C) ventricular fibrillation
(D) torsade de pointes

55. APCs with aberrant conduction can be differentiated from PVCs by noting ECG changes. All of the following but one are associated with PVCs rather than APCs. Identify the one associated with APCs.
(A) taller left peak (Rr’) in V_1
(B) right bundle branch block
(C) marked left axis deviation
(D) rS pattern in V_6

56. Which of the following corresponds most closely to the definition of precordial concordancy?
(A) rsR’ in V_1 to V_4
(B) all QRS complexes have the same axis in V_1 to V_6
(C) all T waves are inverted in V_1 to V_6
(D) left axis deviation in I and aVF

57. Inferior MIs produce conduction defects different from those seen in anterior MIs. Which type of dysrhythmia is more likely to occur in ***inferior*** **as opposed to anterior MIs?**
(A) second-degree type I
(B) second-degree type II
(C) multiform PVCs
(D) third-degree heart block

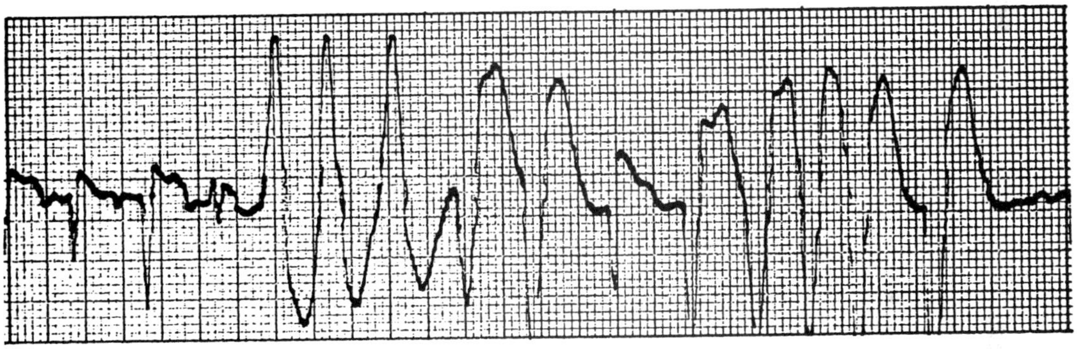

Question 52.

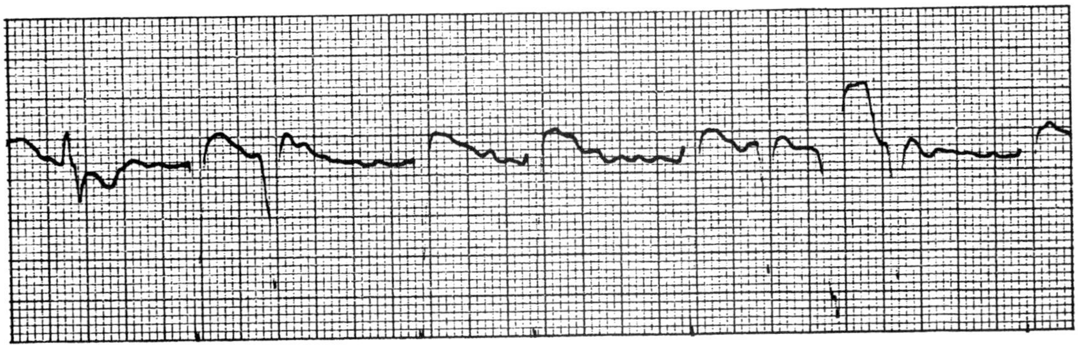

Question 53.

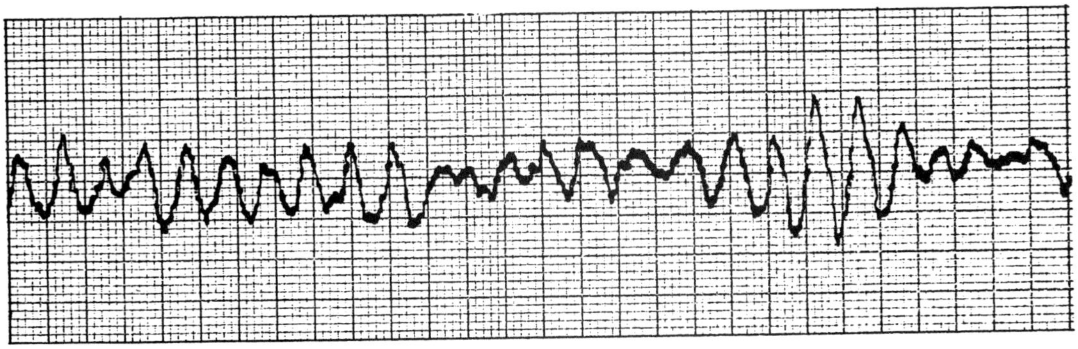

Question 54.

58. Left anterior fascicular block is manifest by which of the following 12-lead ECG patterns?

(A) left axis deviation greater than −30 degrees
(B) right axis deviation greater than +90 degrees
(C) Q wave in V_1 to V_3
(D) large R wave in I and aVL

59. Left posterior fascicular block is manifest by which of the following 12-lead ECG patterns?

(A) left axis deviation greater than −30 degrees
(B) right axis deviation greater than +90 degrees
(C) Q wave in V_1 to V_3
(D) large R wave in I and aVL

60. LV hypertrophy is manifest by which of the following ECG changes?

(A) left anterior fascicular block patterns
(B) left bundle branch block patterns
(C) S wave in V_1 and R wave in V_5 totaling greater than 35 mm
(D) R wave in III and S wave in aVL totaling greater than 30 mm

61. RV hypertrophy is manifest by which of the following ECG changes?

(A) right anterior fascicular block patterns
(B) right bundle branch block patterns
(C) S wave in V_1 and R wave in V_5 totaling greater than 35 mm
(D) R:S ratio greater than 1:1 in V_1

62. Which of the following is NOT an example of AV dissociation?

(A) ventricular tachycardia
(B) third-degree heart block
(C) first-degree heart block
(D) atrial tachycardia with 2:1 block

63. What is the initial treatment of sinus tachycardia?

(A) verapamil
(B) initially carotid massage, then digoxin
(C) esmolol or propranolol
(D) there is no primary treatment; the source of the tachycardia must be found

64. Which of the physical treatments listed below is NOT a form of parasympathetic stimulation for atrial tachycardia?

(A) carotid massage
(B) pressure on the eyeball
(C) Valsalva maneuver
(D) hepatojugular reflux

Questions 65 and 66 refer to the following scenario:

A 72-year-old man is admitted to your unit with the diagnosis of anterior MI. During your shift, you note that he has developed a 2:1 heart block and a constant PR interval, with a ventricular response rate of 42. His blood pressure is 84/50 mm Hg.

65. Based on the preceding information and considering the type of MI, which type of heart block is likely?

(A) first-degree
(B) second-degree type I
(C) second-degree type II
(D) third-degree

66. Which treatment is likely to be most effective in stabilizing this rhythm?

(A) pacemaker
(B) nicardipine
(C) dopamine IV drip
(D) epinephrine IV drip

67. For what does the first letter in VVI stand?

(A) ventricular paced
(B) ventricular sensed
(C) ventricular inhibited
(D) ventricular programmed

68. For what does the second letter in VVI stand?

(A) ventricular paced
(B) ventricular sensed
(C) ventricular inhibited
(D) ventricular programmed

69. In the following rhythm strip, identify the pacemaker operational state for this patient who has a VVI pacemaker. *See art below.*

(A) capturing properly at 1:1
(B) failing to sense
(C) failing to capture
(D) producing pacemaker-generated ventricular ectopic beats

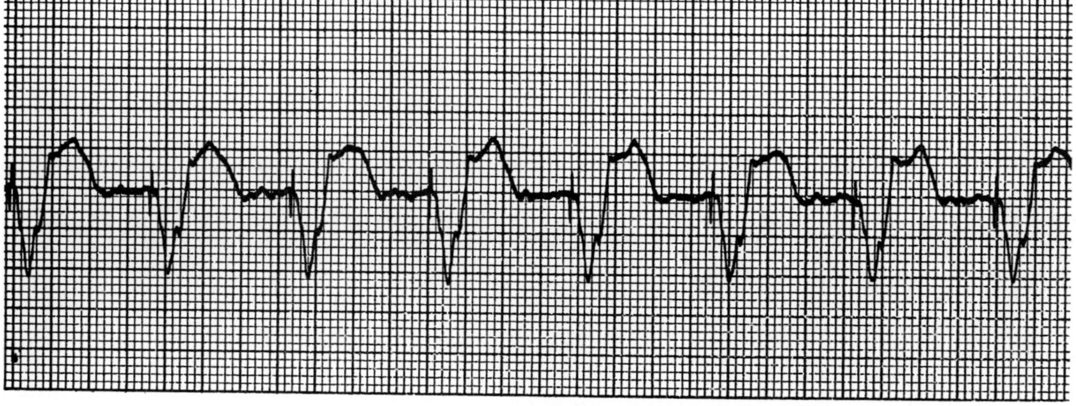

Question 69.

70. Which of the following is an advantage of a transcutaneous pacemaker?
(A) It is easy to apply.
(B) It requires lower electrical stimulation to capture the heart rate.
(C) It requires peripheral intravenous access.
(D) Electrical stimulation is not perceived by the patient.

Questions 71 and 72 refer to the following scenario:
A 45-year-old man is admitted to the unit with the diagnosis of inferior MI. Currently, he has no chest pain or shortness of breath. Two hours after admission, he develops a bradycardia of 50 bpm with a blood pressure of 86/54 mm Hg. He also develops uniform PVCs at the rate of 10/min.

71. Based on the diagnosis of inferior MI, how long will the bradycardia last?
(A) It will usually be permanent and symptomatic.
(B) It will usually be transient and possibly symptomatic.
(C) Bradycardias are so uncommon with inferior MIs that the congestive heart failure (CHF) will exist until the failure is resolved.
(D) It will usually be permanent but asymptomatic.

72. Treatment for this dysrhythmia would most likely include which medication in the event of symptomatic bradycardia?
(A) lidocaine
(B) dopamine
(C) atropine
(D) diltiazem

73. What is the inherent rate of the AV nodal area?
(A) 20 to 40.
(B) 40 to 60.
(C) 60 to 80.
(D) The AV nodal area has no inherent rate.

74. Anterior MIs produce conduction defects different from those seen in inferior MIs. Which type of dysrhythmia is *more likely* to occur in anterior than inferior MIs?
(A) APCs with aberrancy
(B) second-degree type I
(C) second-degree type II
(D) multiform PVCs

75. Passage of the electrical impulse through the AV node is represented by which ECG complex?
(A) PR interval
(B) QRS complex
(C) ST segment
(D) T wave

76. Atrial tachycardia is initially treated with which pharmacological agent?
(A) atropine or isoproterenol
(B) diltiazem or adenosine
(C) digitalis or pronestyl
(D) carvedilol or metoprolol

Questions 77 and 78 refer to the following scenario:
A 66-year-old woman is admitted to your unit with the diagnosis of anterolateral MI. She has no complaints of chest pain or discomfort. While you are interviewing her, she goes into the rhythm displayed below. You ask her how she feels and she replies "I feel fine. You look worried though. Is something wrong?" Her blood pressure is 118/78 mm Hg.

77. What is your interpretation of the dysrhythmia? *See art below.*
(A) accelerated idioventricular rhythm
(B) aberrantly conducted APCs
(C) artifact
(D) ventricular tachycardia

78. What would be the treatment for this rhythm?
(A) observation; no treatment necessary
(B) amiodarone
(C) synchronized defibrillation at 50 J
(D) unsynchronized defibrillation at 200 J

79. A junctional rhythm has all of the following characteristics but one. Which of the following characteristics is NOT indicative of a junctional rhythm?
(A) normal QRS complex
(B) wide QRS complex
(C) heart rate between 40 and 60 bpm
(D) absent P waves

80. Which lead is most likely to detect aberrantly conducted APCs?
(A) lead II
(B) lead III
(C) lead aVF
(D) V_1 lead

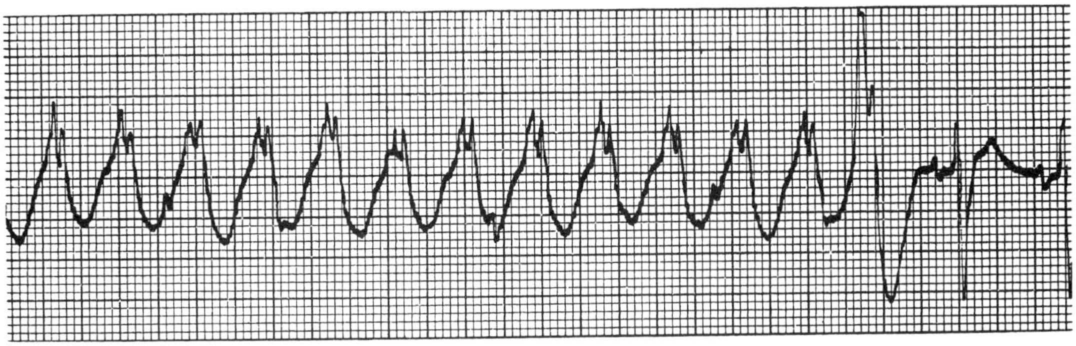

Question 77.

81. Which ECG change indicates an increased chance of sudden death following a MI?
(A) left bundle branch block (LBBB)
(B) right bundle branch block (RBBB)
(C) sinus tachycardia
(D) second-degree type II heart block

82. APCs with aberrant conduction can be differentiated from PVCs by noting ECG changes. All of the following findings but one are associated with APCs rather than PVCs. Identify the one associated with PVCs.
(A) second R wave larger than the first in V_1
(B) RBBB
(C) right axis deviation
(D) AV dissociation

83. Which of the following isoenzymes is most diagnostic in identifying MI?
(A) Troponin I (cTnI)
(B) CPK-MB band
(C) Troponin K (cTnK)
(D) CPK-BB band

Questions 84 and 85 refer to the following scenario:
A 51-year-old man is admitted to your unit with the symptoms of crushing chest pain that is unrelieved by nitrates or rest. He has elevated ST segments elevated 3 mm in V_1 through V_4 with ST-segment depression in II, III, and aVF. His blood pressure is 94/64 mm Hg, pulse 110, and respiratory rate 32.

84. Based on the preceding information, which type of MI would most likely be represented by the ECG changes?
(A) anterior
(B) inferior
(C) lateral
(D) posterior

85. Is ECG confirmation of an MI with irreversible ischemia present in this patient?
(A) no, due to the absence of Q waves
(B) no, due to ST-segment depression in the inferior leads
(C) yes, due to ST-segment elevation in V_1 through V_4
(D) yes, due to the absence of lateral ECG changes

86. Which stage of HF poses a high risk of heart failure but is not associated with structural disease or symptoms?
(A) Stage A
(B) Stage B
(C) Stage C
(D) Stage D

87. Unstable angina is characterized by all of the following features but one. Which feature does NOT characterize unstable angina?
(A) increasing frequency of chest pain
(B) chest pain at rest
(C) increasing severity of symptoms
(D) Q-wave formation

88. Troponin I (cTnI) levels stay elevated for how long following an MI?
(A) up to 8 to 10 days
(B) about 3 h
(C) peaks immediately and stays elevated for 14 days
(D) about 3 days

89. Sympathetic stimulants, such as dopamine, are not indicated in hypovolemia until the blood volume has been corrected. Which of the following is the best explanation for this approach?
(A) Massive sympathetic stimulation is already present and cannot reach effectiveness without adequate fluid volume.
(B) Sympathetic stimulation works only when vasodilation is the primary problem.
(C) Sympathetic stimulation cannot occur until vascular baroreceptors have been inactivated.
(D) Dopamine is indicated in hypovolemia before fluid replacement.

90. Which type of medication is common in the treatment of unstable angina?
(A) diuretics
(B) inotropic agents
(C) beta blockers
(D) sympathetic stimulants

91. Thrombolytic therapy is commonly associated with complications. Which of the following is NOT a complication of thrombolytic therapy?
(A) intracranial hemorrhage
(B) bleeding from venipuncture sites
(C) ventricular ectopy due to reperfusion
(D) extension of the MI due to embolic phenomena

92. Which of the following is an indication for angioplasty or stent placement?
(A) 80% proximal stenosis of a coronary artery
(B) 100% distal occlusion of a coronary artery
(C) 75% in three or more coronary arteries
(D) vasospasm

93. Which of the following are treatments for Prinzmetal's variant angina?
(A) beta blockers, ACE inhibitors
(B) aspirin, nitrates
(C) beta blockers, angiotensin receptor blockers
(D) nitrates, calcium channel blockers

94. Indications for thrombolytic therapy include the following *except:*
(A) new left bundle branch block
(B) onset of pain less than 2 h prior to the initiation of therapy
(C) history of stroke within the previous 3 months
(D) ST-segment elevation in the anterior leads

95. Dopamine is used with caution in patients with MI for which reason?
(A) its potential for increasing myocardial oxygen consumption
(B) because it has no inotropic component
(C) because it may cause reflex bradycardia
(D) due to decreasing the risk of atrial fibrillation development

96. Pulsus paradoxus is utilized to identify which of the following conditions?
(A) cardiac tamponade
(B) MI
(C) respiratory failure
(D) ruptured papillary muscle

97. Nitroglycerin primarily affects which component of stroke volume?
(A) preload
(B) afterload
(C) contractility
(D) stroke volume variation

Questions 98 and 99 refer to the following scenario:
A 65-year-old woman is admitted to the unit with chest pain. Physically, she has no shortness of breath or orthopnea, some noticeable jugular venous distention, and clear breath sounds. Her ECG shows large R waves in V_1 and V_2. Hemodynamic studies reveal the following:

Blood pressure	102/72 mm Hg
Pulse	105
Pulmonary arterial pressure	30/16
PAOP	13
CVP	16
Cardiac output	4.6
Cardiac index	2.4

98. Which condition is likely to be present based on the preceding information?
(A) LV hypertrophy
(B) RV infarction
(C) LV infarction
(D) pericardial tamponade

99. What other leads may be useful in establishing a diagnosis in this patient?
(A) V_2, V_3, V_4
(B) V_5, V_6
(C) aVF, aVR
(D) V_4R, V_5R, V_6R

100. Hemodynamic support would most likely include which of the following strategies?
(A) fluids to keep the CVP elevated
(B) diuretics to reduce the CVP
(C) dopamine to increase the blood pressure
(D) nitroglycerin to reduce the preload

101. Which of the following is NOT a symptom of pericarditis?
(A) sudden, sharp pain and possible fever
(B) increased pain in the left lateral position
(C) pericardial friction rub
(D) chest pain unchanged with deep breathing

Questions 102 and 103 refer to the following scenario:
A 59-year-old man is admitted to your unit with the diagnosis "rule out myocardial infarction." He states that at work, 1 h ago, he felt severe chest pain, became cool and clammy, and felt nauseated. He came immediately to the hospital. The ECG indicates ST-segment elevation in leads II, III, and aVF. ST-segment depression exists in I, aVL, V_5 and V_6. His vital signs are as follows:

Blood pressure	98/68 mm Hg
Pulse	107
Respiratory rate	32

102. Which type of MI is represented by the ECG?
(A) anterior
(B) inferior
(C) lateral
(D) posterior

103. Based on the preceding description, which initial treatment is indicated?
(A) percutaneous coronary interventions (cardiac catheterization) for stent placement
(B) thrombolytic therapy
(C) coronary artery bypass grafting (CABG)
(D) supplemental oxygen

104. The use of furosemide (Lasix) in pulmonary edema due to acute systolic heart failure is designed to improve myocardial function by:
(A) reducing preload and improving myocardial contractility
(B) reducing afterload and decreasing myocardial oxygen consumption
(C) increasing preload and improving contractility
(D) improving contractility while increasing afterload

105. Which of the following medications is NOT a positive inotrope?
(A) epinephrine
(B) dobutamine
(C) milrinone
(D) nitroprusside

106. A patient presents with acute shortness of breath. Vital signs are: T 102.3°F, HR 126, RR 32, oxygen saturations 85% on room air. On exam, the patient is using accessory muscles to breathe, there are crackles 2/3 of the way up bilaterally, and a IV/VI diastolic murmur at the right sternal border, second intercostal space. Based on these findings, the RN suspects the patient has developed:
(A) tricuspid insufficiency (regurgitation) due to endocarditis
(B) mitral stenosis from rheumatic heart disease
(C) aortic insufficiency (regurgitation) due to endocarditis
(D) respiratory distress from pneumonia

107. Which of the following is not a sign of right heart failure?
(A) hypoxia
(B) dependent edema
(C) jugular venous distention
(D) dependent edema

108. Pericarditis presents on the 12-lead ECG with which of the following changes?
(A) Q waves in precordial leads
(B) left axis deviation
(C) generalized elevation of ST segments
(D) depression of ST segments

109. Which of the following are characteristics of PVA?
(A) unprovoked chest pain with ST-segment elevation
(B) chest pain during exertion with ST-segment depression
(C) absence of chest pain with Q-wave formation
(D) abdominal pain with referred pain in left arm

110. The physician orders nitroprusside and dobutamine in a cardiac surgery patient with clear lung sounds, no JVD or dyspnea, no dependent edema, a cardiac index of 1.9 L/min/m^2, ABP of 183/99, and SVR of 1659 dynes. The goal of this regimen would likely be to
(A) reduce preload and improve contractility
(B) increase preload and reduce afterload
(C) reduce afterload and reduce contractility
(D) reduce afterload and improve contractility

111. Orthostatic hypotension results from which of the following conditions?
(A) LV failure
(B) pulmonary hypertension
(C) hypovolemia
(D) portal hypertension

112. Orthostatic hypotension is manifest by which of the following clinical symptoms following a change from lying down to sitting up?
(A) a fall in systolic blood pressure of more than 25 mm Hg and a decrease in diastolic blood pressure of more than 10 mm Hg
(B) systolic blood pressure is unchanged while a decrease in diastolic blood pressure of more than 10 mm Hg occurs
(C) a decrease in systolic blood pressure while diastolic blood pressure increases slightly
(D) an increase in systolic blood pressure while diastolic blood pressure falls

113. Which of the following inflammatory markers is suggestive of coronary artery inflammation?
(A) increased white blood cell count (WBC)
(B) decreased interleukin 6 (IL-6)
(C) increased high-sensitivity C-reactive protein (CRP)
(D) increased procalcitonin

114. Which medication has the strongest effect (assuming normovolemia) in elevating the blood pressure?
(A) dobutamine (Dobutrex)
(B) isoproterenol (Isuprel)
(C) esmolol (Brevibloc)
(D) dopamine (Intropin)

115. In a patient admitted with the diagnosis of blunt cardiac injury (BCI), which physical sign would correlate best with this diagnosis?
(A) distended neck veins
(B) sinus tachycardia with premature atrial and ventricular contraction
(C) shortness of breath
(D) ecchymotic area over the entire sternum

116. Furosemide (Lasix) is considered to affect primarily which component of stroke volume?
(A) preload
(B) afterload
(C) contractility
(D) aortic distensibility

117. A 69-year-old woman with a history of coronary artery disease (CAD) is admitted with substernal chest pain that is unrelieved by rest or sublingual nitroglycerin. The pain started at rest. While in the unit, her chest discomfort resolves. Two years earlier, she had a coronary angiogram that showed more than 75% narrowing of her left anterior descending artery. Medical treatment since then had been successful until this episode. Her 12-lead ECG shows ST-segment depression in anterior leads. Her troponin I is 0.02. Based on this information, what is the likely diagnosis?
(A) stable angina
(B) RV infarction
(C) anterior MI
(D) unstable angina

118. The statin category of drugs exerts its beneficial effect by which of the following mechanisms?
(A) inhibiting thrombin formation
(B) increasing triglycerides
(C) decreasing high-density lipoprotein levels
(D) reducing LDL levels and anti-inflammatory properties

119. Physical signs associated with decompensated LV failure include all of the following but one. Identify the one sign that is NOT associated with decompensated LV failure.
(A) dependent crackles in the lungs
(B) S_3 heart sound
(C) dependent edema and hepatomegaly
(D) hypoxia

Questions 120 and 121 refer to the following scenario:
A 72-year-old man is admitted with the diagnosis of congestive heart failure. He complains of shortness of breath but not of chest pain. He has bibasilar crackles and distended neck veins. His vital signs are as follows: blood pressure 112/82 mm Hg, pulse 110, respiratory rate 29. Pulmonary artery catheter readings reveal the following:

PA pressures	38/23
PAOP	22
CVP	15
Cardiac output	3.6
Cardiac index	2.1

120. Based on the preceding data, which condition does this patient exhibit?
(A) LV failure alone
(B) RV failure alone
(C) biventricular failure
(D) COPD

121. All of the following medications but one would be used to treat the condition. Identify the medication that would NOT be used for this patient.
(A) dobutamine
(B) nitroglycerin
(C) furosemide
(D) high-dose dopamine

Questions 122 and 123 refer to the following scenario:
A 68-year-old woman is admitted to your unit complaining of fatigue, shortness of breath, and "swollen feet." She has the following vital signs: blood pressure 188/106 mm Hg, pulse 108, respiratory rate 30. Pulmonary artery catheter readings reveal the following:

PA pressures	42/25
PAOP	21
CVP	17
Cardiac output	3.3
Cardiac index	1.9

122. If a vasoactive medication were to be used in this patient, which of the following would be the optimal agent to employ?
(A) milrinone (Primacor)
(B) phenylephrine (Neo-Synephrine)
(C) nicardipine (Cardene)
(D) norepinephrine (Levophed)

123. Why would she be having shortness of breath and fatigue?
(A) biventricular failure
(B) underlying chronic lung disease
(C) RV failure
(D) pulmonary hypertension

Questions 124 and 125 refer to the following scenario:
A 75-year-old woman is admitted to your unit from the emergency department with severe shortness of breath and orthopnea. She is very anxious and restless. She has a history of congestive heart failure and was fine until this morning, when the respiratory difficulties started and became progressively worse. Her ECG shows nonspecific ST-segment changes. Breath sounds reveal crackles throughout her lungs. Her blood pressure is 102/56 mm Hg, pulse 118, respiratory rate 38. Her pulse oximetry is 0.83 on a 50% high-humidity face mask.

124. Based on these symptoms, which condition is probably developing?
(A) RV failure
(B) pulmonary edema
(C) MI
(D) pulmonary emboli

125. Which of the following would probably NOT be used in the treatment of this patient?
(A) morphine
(B) nifedipine
(C) dobutamine
(D) furosemide

126. A patient with pneumonia is admitted to a rural hospital without a cardiac catheterization lab. On hospital day 1, the patient developed ST-segment elevation in leads II, III, and aVF, in addition to ST depression in leads I, aVL, V_5, and V_6. Which of the following is an absolute contraindication for administering a thrombolytic to this patient?
(A) BP 178/90
(B) ischemic stroke 2 months ago
(C) recent cardiopulmonary resuscitation (CPR)
(D) ankle fracture 3 months ago

127. A patient is admitted with presyncope and chest pain. Which one of the symptoms below would make the RN suspect the patient may have aortic stenosis?
(A) fatigue
(B) palpitations
(C) shortness of breath
(D) unexplained weight loss

128. The use of furosemide (Lasix) and morphine in pulmonary edema is designed to improve myocardial function by
(A) reducing preload and myocardial oxygen consumption
(B) reducing afterload and myocardial oxygen consumption
(C) increasing preload and improving contractility
(D) improving contractility while increasing afterload

129. Which of the following medications is a beta-blocker?
(A) clonidine
(B) nifedipine
(C) carvedilol
(D) captopril

130. A patient presents with an anterior wall ST-elevation myocardial infarction (STEMI). The patient continues to have angina despite percutaneous intervention and stent placement. The cardiologist is planning to insert an intra-aortic balloon pump (IABP) to improve coronary artery perfusion. Which of the following physical findings is a contraindication to IABP placement?
(A) + 1 dorsalis pedis and posterior tibial pulses in both lower extremities
(B) aortic regurgitation/insufficiency
(C) pulmonic regurgitation/insufficiency
(D) crackles 2/3 of the way up during bilateral lung field auscultation

131. Which of the following is NOT a calcium channel blocker?
(A) nifedipine
(B) diltiazem
(C) verapamil
(D) metoprolol

132. Pericarditis presents on the 12-lead ECG with which of the following changes?
(A) Q waves in precordial leads
(B) left axis deviation
(C) generalized elevation of ST segments
(D) depression of ST segments

133. A patient is status post a thoracotomy for right ventricle repair after a gunshot wound to the chest. The patient is becoming tachycardic and hypotensive. Which of the following would prompt the RN to administer packed red blood cells (PRBCs)?
(A) CVP 1 mm Hg, pulmonary artery diastolic (PAD) 9 mm Hg, SvO_2 40%
(B) Hemoglobin 8.5 mg/dL, cardiac index 2.4 L/min/m^2
(C) SVR 800 dynes/s/m^2, cardiac index of 5.0 L/min/m^2
(D) CVP 10 mm Hg, PAD 22 mm Hg, SvO_2 60%

134. A patient presented to the emergency department with a headache and blurred vision. Initial blood pressure was 210/105. A sodium nitroprusside infusion is started prior to transfer to the ICU. Upon arrival, the patient is complaining of lightheadedness and dizziness. Which of the following is the highest priority for the RN to assess?
(A) perform a neurologic exam
(B) draw blood for thiocyanate monitoring
(C) assess blood pressure
(D) assess urine output

135. Early stages of hypovolemic or cardiogenic shock may exhibit normal blood pressure due to which of the following compensatory mechanisms?
(A) increased SVR and tachycardia
(B) increased preload
(C) decreased afterload
(D) increased stroke volume

136. Where should inflation of the balloon in an IABP occur?
(A) near the R wave on the ECG
(B) during end-diastole
(C) during end-systole
(D) at the dicrotic notch

137. Which of the following is one danger of open abdominal aortic aneurysm (AAA) repair?
(A) obstruction of renal blood flow
(B) interference with coronary diastolic filling
(C) creation of pulmonary emboli
(D) pericardial tamponade

138. Deflation of the balloon in an IABP should occur at what point?
(A) near the T wave on the ECG
(B) before the R wave
(C) at end-systole
(D) near the dicrotic notch

139. Hypovolemic shock differs from cardiogenic shock by exhibiting which one of the following hemodynamic changes?
(A) high preload
(B) low preload
(C) high SVR
(D) low stroke volume

140. Which of the following agents would most reliably raise the blood pressure in cardiogenic shock?
(A) dopamine
(B) dobutamine
(C) milrinone
(D) nitroprusside

141. Which of the following are two benefits of an IABP assist?
(A) decreased preload and increased afterload
(B) increased contractility and decreased afterload
(C) decreased afterload and increased coronary artery perfusion pressure
(D) increased coronary artery perfusion pressure and increased preload

142. A 71-year-old man is admitted with a history of CAD and CHF. He is on the following medications. Which of these medications are not consistent with long-term management of CHF?
(A) diuretics
(B) beta blockers
(C) ACE inhibitors
(D) alpha agonists

143. A 41-year-old woman is admitted to the unit following a motor vehicle collision that resulted in the need for exploratory laparotomy with subsequent splenectomy. When she returns from surgery, she has heart rate of 124, respiratory rate 28, blood pressure 88/50, stroke volume of 25 mL, and a $ScvO_2$ level of 0.43. What course of action would be appropriate at this time?
(A) observation only
(B) administration of a normal saline fluid bolus
(C) antibiotic administration
(D) blood transfusion

144. Cardiogenic shock is characterized by which of the following parameters?
I. cardiac index less than 2.2 L/min/m^2
II. PAOP greater than 22 mm Hg
III. CVP between 5 and 10 mm Hg
(A) I only
(B) I and II
(C) II and III
(D) III only

Questions 145 and 146 refer to the following scenario:
A 67-year-old woman with hypotension is admitted to your unit from the emergency department. Her husband states that she had complained of shortness of breath earlier in the day, and since noon he has not been able to wake her. She is currently unresponsive except to painful stimuli. Her blood pressure is 78/50 mm Hg, pulse 118. A pulmonary artery catheter is inserted and gives the following information:

PA pressures	44/26
PAOP	25
CVP	15
Cardiac output	3.7
Cardiac index	1.6
SvO_2	0.40

145. Based on the preceding information, which condition is developing?
(A) cardiogenic shock
(B) hypovolemic shock
(C) pulmonary embolus
(D) sepsis with a low SVR

146. Which treatment should be initiated for this patient?
(A) fluid bolus
(B) dobutamine and dopamine
(C) furosemide and nitroprusside
(D) epinephrine and furosemide

Questions 147 and 148 refer to the following scenario:
A 58-year-old man is admitted to your unit with hypotension and the diagnosis "rule out myocardial infarction." He has a blood pressure of 82/52 mm Hg, pulse 122. During physical assessment, he exhibits marked orthopnea, extreme anxiety, and crackles throughout his lungs that are more prominent posteriorly. He is to have a pulmonary artery catheter inserted in the next hour.

147. Based on these symptoms, what would you expect the hemodynamic data from the pulmonary artery catheter to reveal?
(A) PAOP less than 10, SI more than 25 mL/m^2, CI (cardiac index) less than 2 L/m^2
(B) PAOP more than 22, SI less than 25 mL/m^2, CI less than 2 L/m^2
(C) CVP more than 15, CI more than 4 L/m^2
(D) SVR more than 2000 dynes/s/cm, CI more than 4 L/m^2

148. What treatment would be most effective initially for this patient?
(A) high-dose dopamine and nitroprusside
(B) furosemide and dobutamine
(C) dobutamine and epinephrine
(D) digitalis and furosemide

149. You receive a phone call from the radiologist about a patient involved in a high-speed motor vehicle crash just admitted to your unit. The radiologist is concerned about the patient's widened mediastinum. Which of the following injuries does the RN suspect?
(A) blunt aortic injury or cardiac tamponade
(B) pericarditis
(C) mitral valve rupture
(D) myocardial contusion

Questions 150 and 151 refer to the following scenario:
A 57-year-old man is admitted to your unit postoperatively for repair of a fractured femur and a splenectomy after a motor vehicle accident. Four hours postoperatively, his level of consciousness begins to decrease. Vital signs are as follows: blood pressure 88/58 mm Hg, pulse 113, respiratory rate 28. His skin is cool and clammy. He has no complaints of shortness of breath; breath sounds are clear. His pulmonary artery catheter provides the following data:

Pulmonary arterial pressure	21/7
PAOP	4
CVP	2
Cardiac output	3.6
Cardiac index	1.7

150. Based on the preceding information, which condition appears to be developing?
(A) LV failure
(B) RV failure
(C) cardiogenic shock
(D) hypovolemic shock

151. Which of the following would least reliably increase the vascular volume?
(A) 0.9% normal saline (NS)
(B) lactated Ringer's (LR)
(C) 5% dextrose in water (D_5W)
(D) albumin

152. A patient is admitted to your unit with a descending aortic dissection (Type B). The surgeon wants to manage the patient medically. Target systolic blood pressure is less than 120 mm Hg. Which of the following antihypertensives will decrease blood pressure without raising heart rate?
(A) nitroglycerin
(B) hydralazine
(C) sodium nitroprusside (Nipride)
(D) esmolol (Brevibloc)

Questions 153 and 154 refer to the following scenario:
A 71-year-old woman is in your unit following colon resection. Because of an episode of hypotension in the operating room, a pulmonary artery catheter was inserted. On postoperative day 1, her morning hematocrit was 35, hemoglobin 11.5. Her afternoon hematocrit is 27, hemoglobin 9. She has no complaints of pain that differ from those reported in the morning. The following are the pulmonary artery catheter readings from the morning and afternoon. She has received 1 L of normal saline over the past 12 h. The house officer is not concerned over the change, attributing it to dilutional factors.

	Morning	Afternoon
Blood pressure	98/58 mm Hg	94/56 mm Hg
Pulse	102	115
PAP	24/12	20/8
PAOP	10	5
CVP	4	2
Cardiac output	3.9	3.7
Cardiac index	2.5	2.4

153. Based on the preceding information, which condition is developing?
(A) the data support dilutional reasons for the drop in hematocrit and hemoglobin
(B) hypovolemia
(C) LV failure
(D) pericardial tamponade

154. Which parameters best separate dilutional from actual decreases in the hematocrit and hemoglobin?
(A) heart rate, cardiac output
(B) stroke volume, heart rate, and PAOP
(C) PAOP and PA pressures
(D) PA pressures and SVR

155. Why would the cardiac output not change substantially if the patient were developing hypovolemia?
(A) The stroke volume increased to offset the loss of blood volume.
(B) The PAOP decrease reduced myocardial oxygen consumption and improved contractility.
(C) The heart rate increased to offset the loss of blood volume.
(D) The mean arterial pressure increased to offset the loss of blood volume.

156. Which of the following is NOT an indication for a CABG?
(A) 75% narrowing of the left main coronary artery
(B) 90% narrowing of the left anterior descending (LAD) coronary artery not amenable to stenting
(C) 80% narrowing of the right coronary artery amenable to stenting
(D) multiple-vessel disease

157. Which of the following is a common sign in cardiac tamponade?
(A) decreased PAOP
(B) increased diastolic blood pressure
(C) decreased systolic blood pressure more than 10 mm Hg upon inspiration (pulsus paradoxus)
(D) ejection fraction more than 75%

158. Which blood vessel is commonly used as the graft vessel in a CABG?
(A) femoral vein
(B) axillary artery
(C) a coronary artery that is unobstructed
(D) internal mammary artery

159. Nursing care of the patient following cardiopulmonary bypass surgery includes observation of all of the following measures but one. Which of the following is NOT routinely assessed postoperatively?
(A) cardiac index
(B) pulmonary gas exchange
(C) urinary bladder pressures
(D) PAOP and CVP

160. Which of the following best defines pulse pressure?
(A) highest heart rate minus lowest heart rate in a 24-h period
(B) systolic BP – diastolic BP
(C) systolic BP + 2 (diastolic BP)/3
(D) ratio of the BP of the ankle (dorsalis pedis) to the BP of the upper arm (systolic brachial BP)

161. Which of the following is the best method to treat cardiomyopathy?
(A) heart transplantation since there is no "cure" for cardiomyopathy
(B) CABG
(C) IABP assist
(D) coronary angioplasty

162. What is the most common type of aortic aneurysm?
(A) ascending thoracic
(B) descending thoracic
(C) abdominal
(D) aortic arch

163. Dissecting aneurysms present with several symptoms. Which of the following is NOT a symptom of a dissecting AAA?
(A) gastrointestinal bleeding
(B) severe abdominal pain
(C) pain radiating to the back
(D) palpable abdominal mass

164. Dissection of an artery occurs because of which type of injury to the blood vessel?
(A) intimal tear
(B) weakness of the entire vessel wall
(C) transects the arterial wall
(D) bleeding into an already formed aneurysm

165. Which of the following is the most common complication following open surgery to repair a ruptured AAA?
(A) acute renal failure
(B) mesenteric ischemia
(C) paralysis
(D) compartment syndrome

166. A patient with chronic atrial fibrillation is admitted with nausea, visual changes, and syncope. An ECG demonstrates second-degree Mobitz II (classic) heart block. Which one of the patient's medications is likely the cause of these symptoms?
(A) verapamil (Calan)
(B) digoxin (Lanoxin)
(C) losartan (Cozaar)
(D) warfarin (Coumadin)

167. All of the following but one are symptoms of obstructed arterial flow. Select the one that represents venous, NOT arterial, obstruction.
(A) pallor of the skin
(B) cyanosis of the skin
(C) intermittent claudication
(D) decreased pulses

168. Which of the following is a common sign of acute arterial obstruction?
(A) pain distal to the obstruction
(B) edema distal to the obstruction
(C) cyanosis distal to the obstruction
(D) warm skin distal to the obstruction

169. Deep venous thrombosis can potentially dislodge from the original location and the clot(s) can travel to distant locations. Which of the following could result from the emboli of a deep venous thrombosis located in the femoral vein?
(A) loss of the dorsalis pedis pulse
(B) loss of pulses in the femoral artery
(C) superior vena cava syndrome
(D) pulmonary emboli

170. Which of the following is NOT a routine nursing care monitoring parameter commonly measured in a patient after open heart surgery?
(A) temperature
(B) PAOP
(C) cardiac output
(D) ejection fraction

Questions 171 and 172 refer to the following scenario:
A 57-year-old man is admitted to your unit following a CABG. At 0400 he is alert and oriented and is extubated without difficulty. At 0500, he is lethargic, although he has not received analgesics. He has a mediastinal chest tube that has drained 500 mL in the last hour. Pulmonary artery catheter and blood gas information is listed below:

	0400	0500
Blood pressure	100/70 mm Hg	95/66 mm Hg
Pulse	100	115
PAD	15	12
CVP	10	6
Cardiac output	4.3	3.9
Cardiac index	2.5	2.3
PaO_2	82	80
SaO_2	0.96	0.95
FiO_2	0.40	0.40
$PaCO_2$	37	39
pH	7.37	7.35
HCO_3^-	24	23

171. Based on the preceding information, the patient is probably developing which of the following?
(A) tension pneumothorax
(B) mediastinal bleeding
(C) acute respiratory distress syndrome
(D) congestive heart failure

172. Which interventions are a priority for the patient?
(A) draw stat hemoglobin, hematocrit, aPTT, PT-INR, platelet, and fibrinogen level
(B) initiation of dobutamine
(C) placing the patient supine to decrease chest tube output
(D) added pleural and mediastinal chest tubes

Questions 173 and 174 refer to the following scenario:
A 62-year-old man is admitted to your unit postoperatively following AAA repair. Four hours after returning from the operating room, he begins to complain of chest pain and shortness of breath. Breath sounds are equal with inspiratory crackles noted posteriorly. Heart sounds indicate a clear S_1, S_2, and S_3.

173. On the basis of this information, the patient is most likely developing which of the following?
(A) pulmonary edema
(B) pulmonary emboli
(C) tension pneumothorax
(D) dissecting thoracic aneurysm

Before answering questions 174 and 175, please read the following additional information:

Based on the development of chest pain, cardiac enzymes and a transthoracic echocardiogram have been done, but the results are pending. An EKG shows sinus tachycardia with nonspecific ST changes. A pulmonary artery catheter is inserted and blood gases are obtained. Analysis of this formation discloses the following:

Blood pressure	106/64 mm Hg
Pulse	112
PAOP	20
CVP	11
Cardiac output	3.4
Cardiac index	1.8
PaO_2	68
SaO_2	0.92
FiO_2	0.40
$PaCO_2$	37
pH7	40
HCO_3^-	25

174. Based on the preceding information, which condition is most likely to be developing?
(A) myocardial infarction
(B) pulmonary emboli
(C) tension pneumothorax
(D) dissecting thoracic aneurysm

175. Treatment to support hemodynamics would most likely include which of the following?
(A) diltiazem
(B) dobutamine
(C) dopamine
(D) nitroprusside

Questions 176 and 177 refer to the following scenario:
A 68-year-old woman is admitted to your unit after a CABG. Eight hours following surgery, she is extubated and experiencing only mild chest discomfort. Over the next hour, she begins to complain of vaguely increasing discomfort. Her pleural tube is bubbling in the water seal chamber. No drainage is present from the mediastinal tube. Her blood pressure fluctuates with respiration, decreasing by 20 mm Hg during inspiration. Her lung sounds are clear; heart sounds are normal but distant.

176. Based on the preceding information, which condition is most likely to be developing?
(A) tension pneumothorax
(B) pneumomediastinum
(C) left ventricular failure
(D) pericardial tamponade

Before answering question 177, please read the following additional information:

A pulmonary artery catheter reveals the following information:

Blood pressure	92/58 mm Hg
Pulse	115
PAOP	18
CVP	18
Cardiac output	3.2
Cardiac index	1.9

177. Which of these parameters would you suspect in a patient developing the above condition?
(A) hypotension and tachycardia
(B) equalization of ventricular filling pressures
(C) decreased cardiac index and cardiac output
(D) all of the above

178. Which treatment would be considered definitive in this patient?
(A) inserting tissue plasminogen activator into the existing mediastinal tube
(B) insertion of a new mediastinal tube at the bedside
(C) return to the operating room for mediastinal exploration
(D) reintubation and placing the patient on positive-pressure ventilation

179. Interpret the following 12-lead ECG. *See art below.*
(A) left anterior fascicular block
(B) left posterior fascicular block
(C) RBBB
(D) LBBB

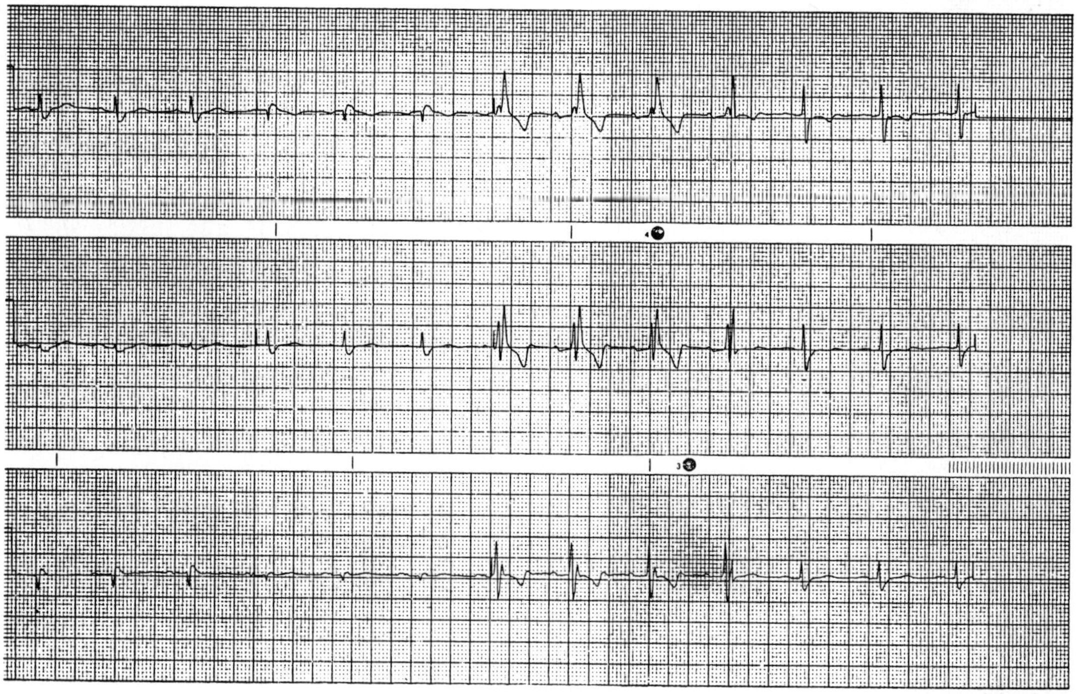

Question 179.

180. Interpret the following 12-lead ECG. ***See art below.***

(A) anterior MI
(B) inferior MI
(C) posterior MI
(D) lateral MI

181. Interpret the following 12-lead ECG. ***See art below.***

(A) anterior MI
(B) inferolateral MI
(C) posterior MI
(D) lateral MI

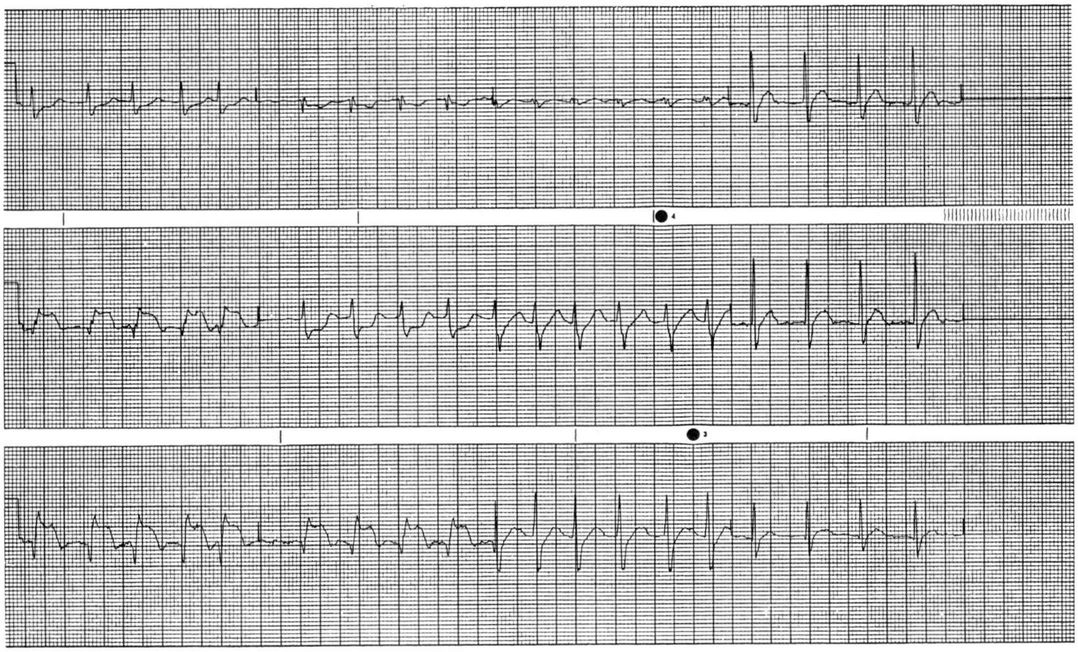

Question 180.

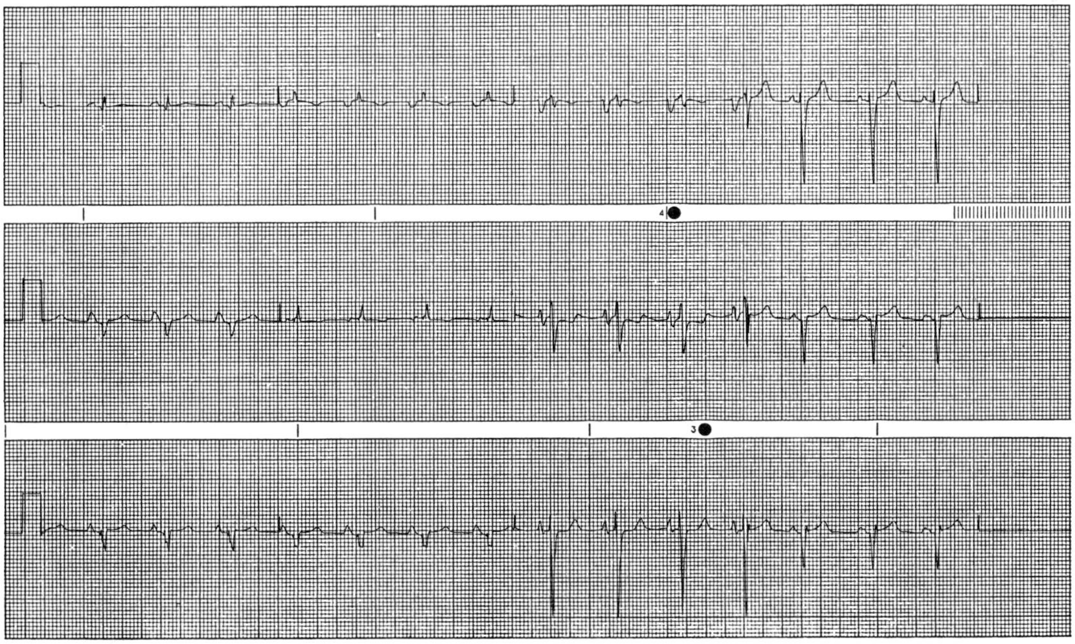

Question 181.

182. In the following ECG, identify the major ECG abnormality. ***See art below.***

(A) inferior ischemia
(B) LV hypertrophy
(C) RV hypertrophy
(D) anterior ischemia

183. Interpret the following 12-lead ECG. ***See art below.***

(A) anterior MI
(B) new inferior MI
(C) posterior MI
(D) anterior and old inferior MI

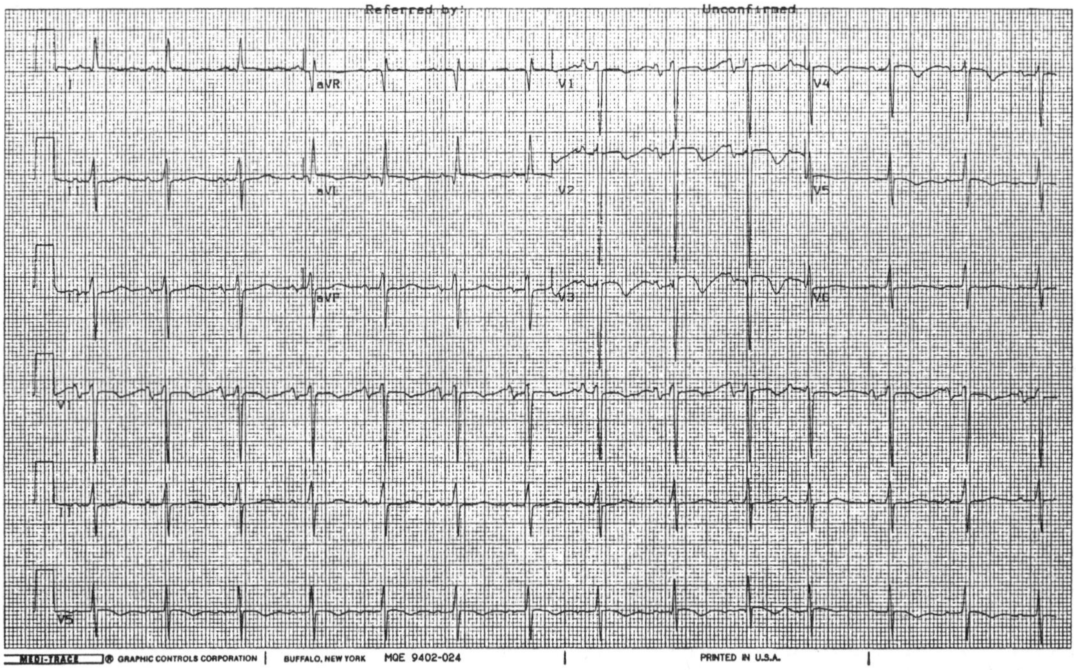

Question 182.

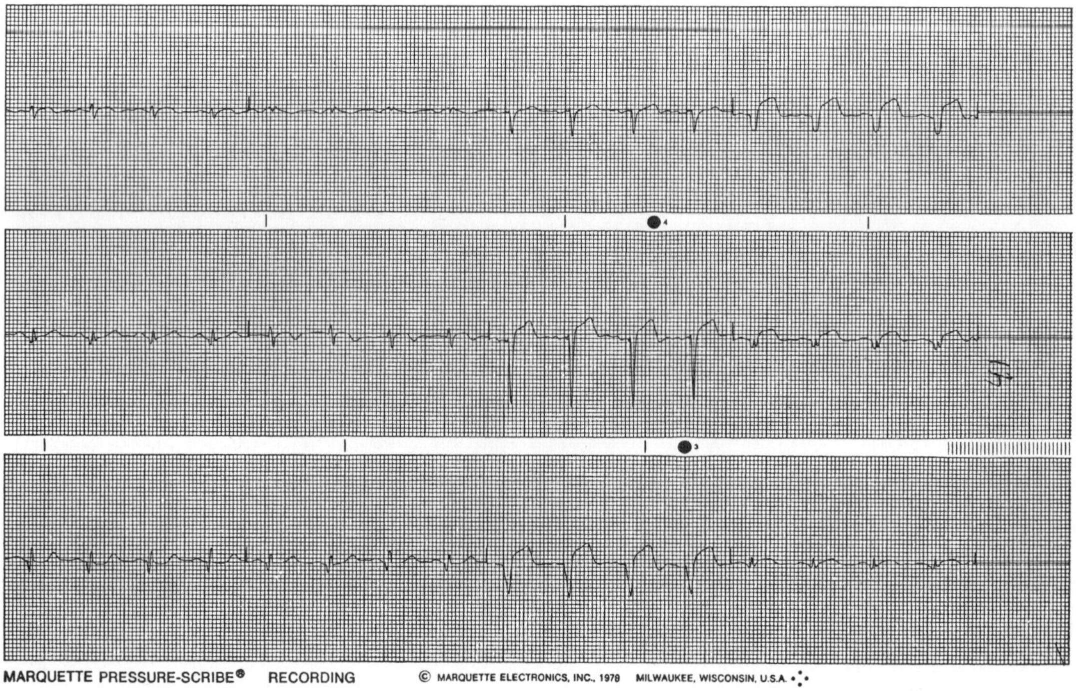

Question 183.

184. In the following ECG, identify the major ECG abnormality. ***See art below.***

(A) inferior ischemia
(B) lateral ischemia and LV hypertrophy
(C) RV hypertrophy
(D) anterior ischemia

185. Interpret the following 12-lead ECG. ***See art below.***

(A) Left anterior fascicular block
(B) Left posterior fascicular block
(C) RBBB
(D) LBBB

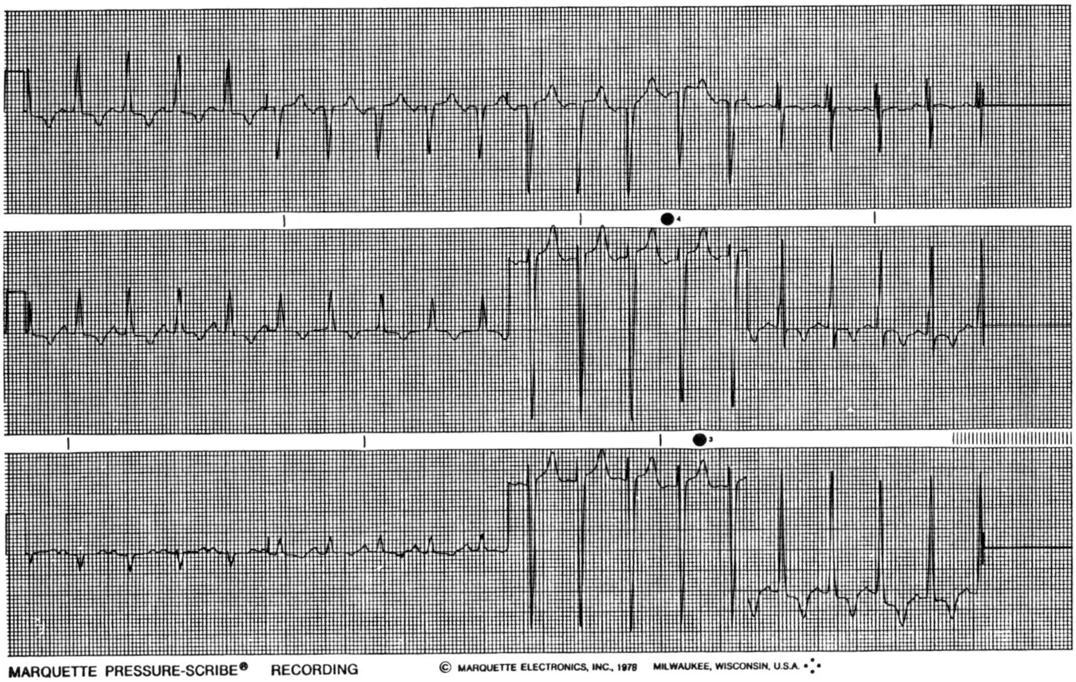

Question 184.

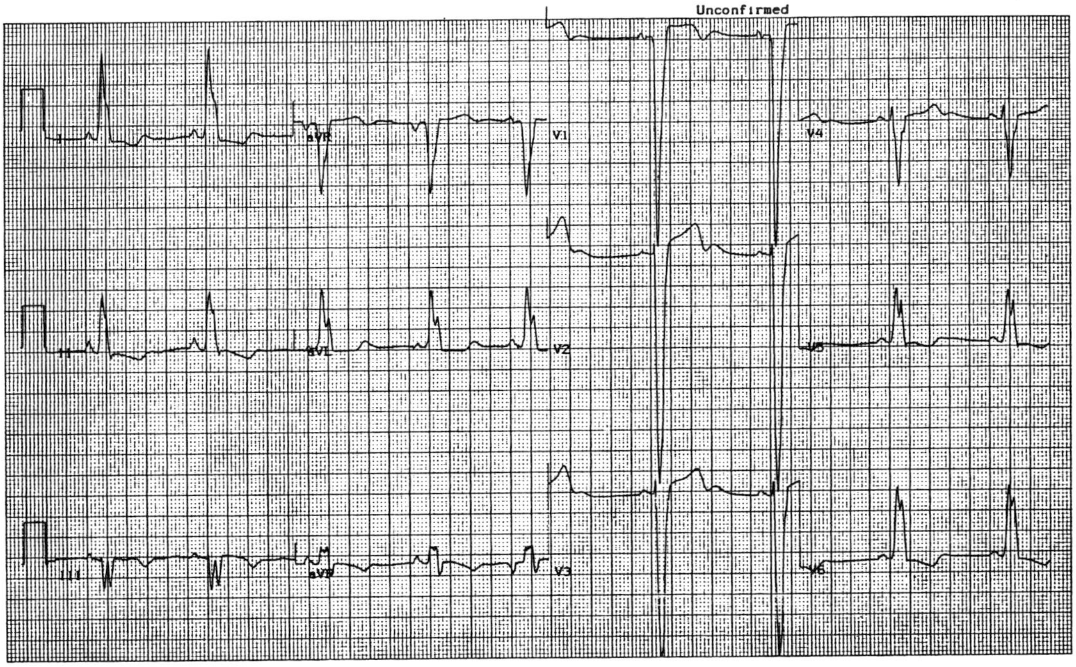

Question 185.

186. Interpret the following 12-lead ECG. ***See art below.***

(A) anterior fascicular block
(B) posterior fascicular block
(C) RBBB
(D) LBBB

187. Which abnormality is present in the following ECG? ***See art below.***

(A) left ventricular ectopy
(B) pericarditis
(C) left axis deviation
(D) right axis deviation

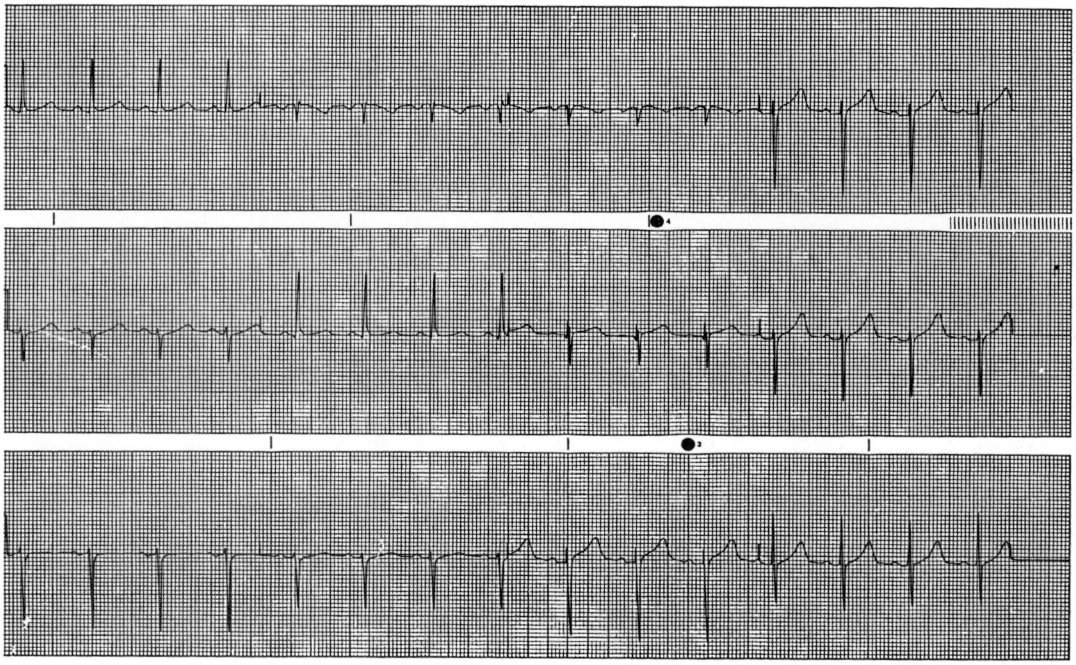

Question 186.

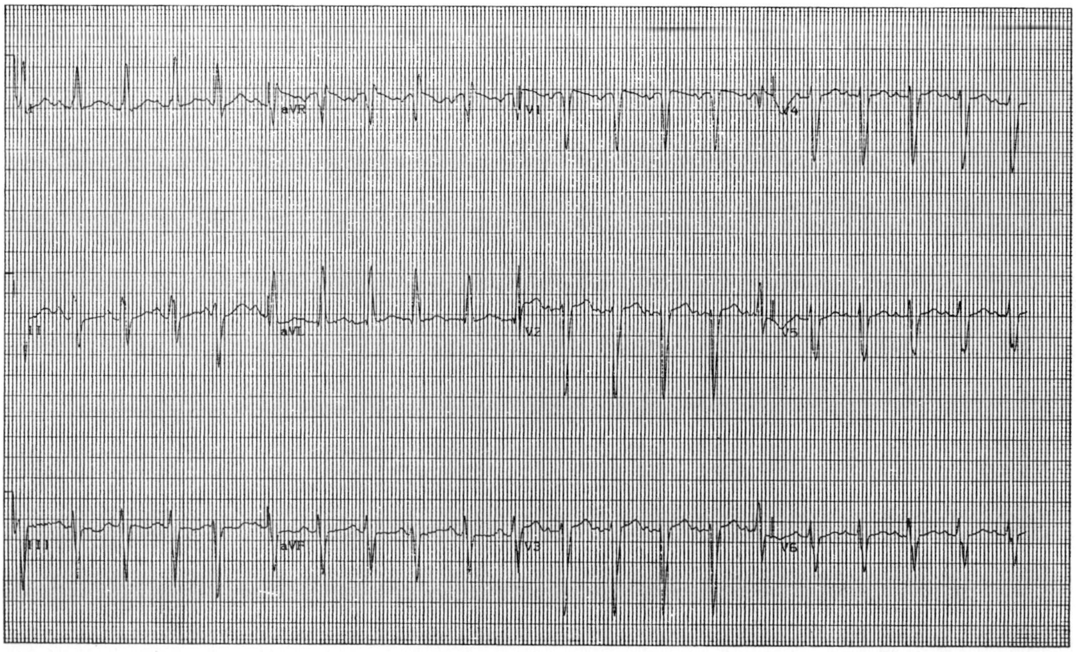

Question 187.

188. In the following ECG, identify the major ECG abnormality. ***See art below.***
(A) inferior ischemia
(B) LV hypertrophy
(C) RV hypertrophy
(D) anteroseptal lateral ischemia with RBBB

189. Interpret the following 12-lead ECG. ***See art below.***
(A) anterior fascicular block
(B) atrial tachycardia with aberrancy
(C) ventricular tachycardia
(D) LBBB

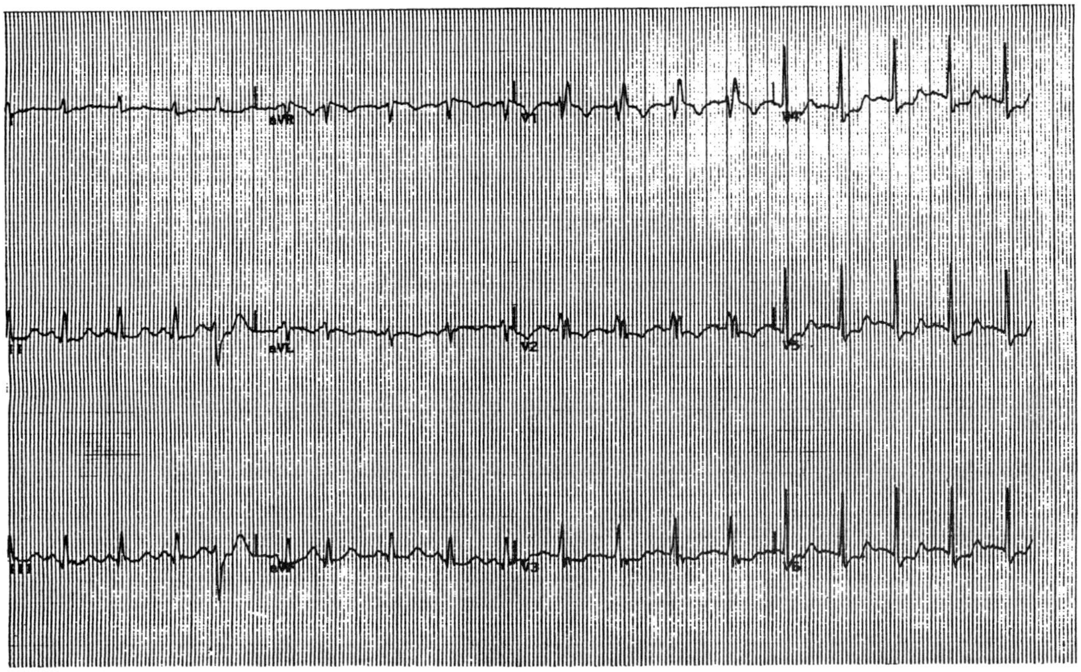

Question 188.

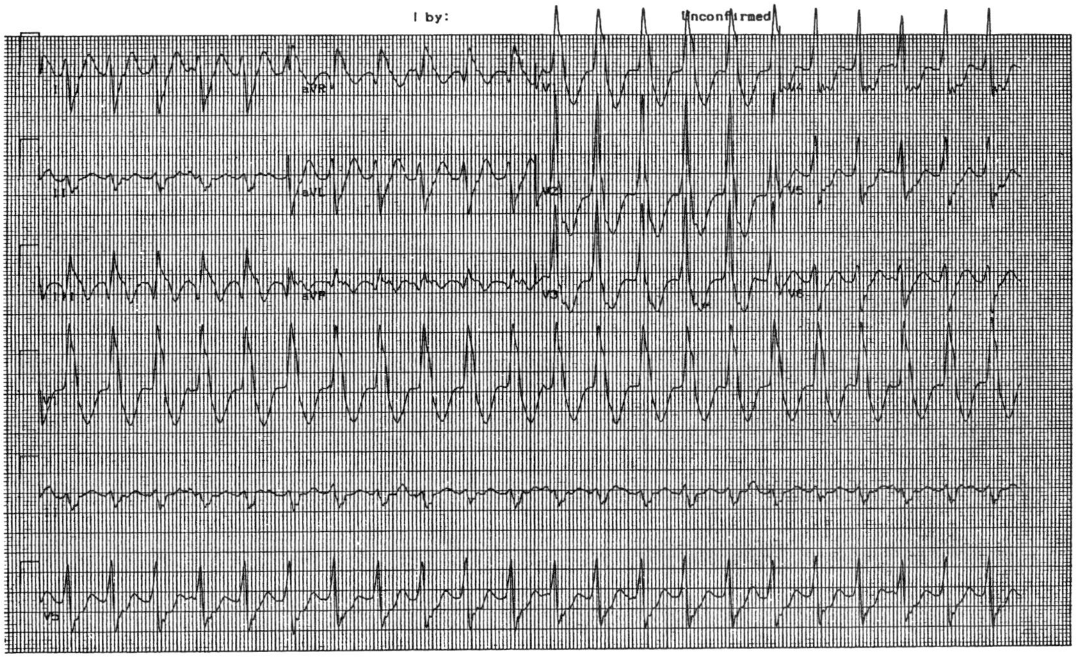

Question 189.

PART I
Cardiovascular Practice Exam

Practice Fill-Ins

1. ______
2. ______
3. ______
4. ______
5. ______
6. ______
7. ______
8. ______
9. ______
10. ______
11. ______
12. ______
13. ______
14. ______
15. ______
16. ______
17. ______
18. ______
19. ______
20. ______
21. ______
22. ______
23. ______
24. ______
25. ______
26. ______
27. ______
28. ______
29. ______
30. ______
31. ______
32. ______
33. ______
34. ______
35. ______
36. ______
37. ______
38. ______
39. ______
40. ______
41. ______
42. ______
43. ______
44. ______
45. ______
46. ______
47. ______
48. ______
49. ______
50. ______
51. ______
52. ______
53. ______
54. ______
55. ______
56. ______
57. ______
58. ______
59. ______
60. ______
61. ______
62. ______
63. ______
64. ______
65. ______
66. ______
67. ______
68. ______
69. ______
70. ______
71. ______
72. ______
73. ______
74. ______
75. ______
76. ______
77. ______
78. ______
79. ______
80. ______
81. ______
82. ______
83. ______
84. ______
85. ______

86. ____
87. ____
88. ____
89. ____
90. ____
91. ____
92. ____
93. ____
94. ____
95. ____
96. ____
97. ____
98. ____
99. ____
100. ____
101. ____
102. ____
103. ____
104. ____
105. ____
106. ____
107. ____
108. ____
109. ____
110. ____
111. ____
112. ____
113. ____
114. ____
115. ____
116. ____
117. ____
118. ____
119. ____
120. ____
121. ____
122. ____
123. ____
124. ____
125. ____
126. ____
127. ____
128. ____
129. ____
130. ____
131. ____
132. ____
133. ____
134. ____
135. ____
136. ____
137. ____
138. ____
139. ____
140. ____
141. ____
142. ____
143. ____
144. ____
145. ____
146. ____
147. ____
148. ____
149. ____
150. ____
151. ____
152. ____
153. ____
154. ____
155. ____
156. ____
157. ____
158. ____
159. ____
160. ____
161. ____
162. ____
163. ____
164. ____
165. ____
166. ____
167. ____
168. ____
169. ____
170. ____
171. ____
172. ____
173. ____
174. ____
175. ____
176. ____
177. ____
178. ____
179. ____
180. ____
181. ____

182. ______________________________
183. ______________________________
184. ______________________________
185. ______________________________
186. ______________________________
187. ______________________________
188. ______________________________
189. ______________________________

PART I
Answers

1. **B** Rationale: The key to answering this question is identification of the underlying cause in the context of the acute change (the ST depression). Although shortness of breath and wheezing may be associated with an exacerbation of COPD, dependent crackles, elevated PAOP, and S3 suggest fluid overload, so eliminate option A. These findings are also not primarily associated with inferior MIs, so eliminate option C. Pericardial tamponade is associated with increasing and equalizing filling pressures; however, the CVP is normal, so eliminate option D. Since the acute findings are associated with new-onset left ventricular (LV) failure, option B is the best answer.
2. **D** Rationale: Since oxygen therapy is less likely to correct the underlying cause of fluid overload and since no ST-elevation is identified, eliminate option A. Option B can also be eliminated because vasopressin would increase afterload on an already failing left ventricle. The PAOP of 22 also makes fluids and incorrect choice, so eliminate C. Dobutamine would improve the contractility of the failing LV causing pulmonary edema, and Lasix would also aid in reducing preload, so choose option D.
3. **A** Rationale: The overall purpose of hemodynamic monitoring is to help optimize blood flow and tissue oxygenation. Stroke volume is the purest, most sensitive and evidence-based macrocirculatory parameter that allows clinicians to do this, option A. Initiating dobutamine in this patient may improve this patient's pulmonary edema by decreasing wedge pressure, so eliminate B. Dobutamine also does not increase SVR and may actually decrease it, so eliminate C. Dobutamine may decrease the mean arterial pressure (MAP); however, this would not necessarily indicate successful treatment, so eliminate D as well.
4. **D** Rationale: The shortness of breath, orthopnea, exercise intolerance, and crackles in the scenario are all suggestive of HF. Noncardiogenic pulmonary edema is associated with a normal PAOP, and since the PAOP of 20 is elevated in this scenario, eliminate A. Although the pulmonary artery systolic pressure is greater than 30, this is likely caused by the patient's cardiac failure (which would be secondary pulmonary hypertension), so eliminate B. Sepsis is also unlikely given that no temperature or WBC are offered and no source of infection is identified, so eliminate C. The symptoms of HF coupled with the PAOP in the setting of a low cardiac index make LV failure, D, the best answer.
5. **C** Rationale: The fluid volume overload at this patient's alveolar–capillary interface creates shunt, which by definition is not corrected with increasing oxygen therapy, so eliminate option A. Eliminate B as well since this patient's BP is normal and phenylephrine would increase afterload on an already failing LV. Carvedilol can be part of the standard of care for HF, but a beta blocker such as this would not be the best answer in the phase of acute LV failure, so eliminate D. Furosemide would help correct the underlying problem, helping to reduce the preload of the LV, so choose C.
6. **A** Rationale: This is a straight knowledge question—the most widely used reference range for the CVP is answer A, 2 to 6 mm Hg. 5 to 10 mm Hg may be used as a target during a resuscitation but is too high for the normal reference range, so eliminate B. Option C is a PAOP reference range and option D would be an elevated PAOP, so eliminate C and D.
7. **C** Rationale: The lateral LV wall is supplied by the circumflex and the sinus node is supplied by the RCA, so eliminate options A and B. It is atrial distension that stimulates the secretion of atrial natriuretic factor, so eliminate D as well. The coronary sinus is best known as the main venous drainage vessel of the heart, so C is the best answer.
8. **B** Rationale: Options C and D essentially refer to the same thing, which can help rule out these two options quickly. In addition, options A, C, and D all refer to the lower pressure, right-sided circulation. B is the only available option referring to the left-sided circulation. The LVEDP is obtained from the PAOP, which is reflective of the column of fluid that extends from the PAOP balloon (through the left atrium) to the LV. Choose B.
9. **D** Rationale: Options A, B, and C all influence stroke volume (ie, the mLs of blood the LV ejects with each beat). Preload reflects the filling of the LV, afterload is associated with the resistance to LV ejection, and contractility impacts the strength of which that volume is ejected. Secondarily, capillary permeability may ultimately affect the mLs pumped by the LV with each beat, but the impact will be indirect. Choose D.
10. **B** Rationale: The A wave represents atrial contraction, so the best answer here is B. Just remember that "A = Atrial contraction." Ventricular filling is more likely to be identified on the PAOP tracing rather than the CVP, so eliminate option A. Atrial filling is more likely to be identified with the V wave, so eliminate C as well. D has contrived irrelevant answers. Choose B.

11. **C** Rationale: The correct answer to this questions is C—mitral and tricuspid valve closure. When examining this list of potential answers, options A and B can be eliminated quickly because they contain both a semilunar and an AV valve in their answers. This narrows down the options to two. Option D, mitral and tricuspid valve opening, occur at the beginning of atrial systole and will be associated with the upstroke of the A wave. So, choose C.

12. **A** Rationale: When approaching this question, remember that the venous, right-sided circulation is a lower-pressure system when compared to the arterial side. Therefore, options C and D can be eliminated quickly, since they may be considered higher pressures. 5 to 10 mm Hg may be considered a target reference range during resuscitation (or may be associated with RV failure), but is too high for what may be considered normal, so eliminate B as well. The correct answer to this question is A—think of the normal RVEDP as being similar to the normal CVP reference range, 2 to 6 mm Hg.

13. **B** Rationale: The PAOP is associated with LV, not RV, preload, so eliminate A. The pulmonary artery diastolic (PAD) pressure may also be associated with LV preload; however, option C asks about pulmonary artery mean pressure, so eliminate C as well. Coronary sinus pressure is also not commonly measured, so eliminate D. However, the CVP is a commonly measured, right-sided filling pressure, so B is the best answer here.

14. **D** Rationale: The approach to this question could include eliminating options A and B quickly, since the CVP and PAOP are both filling pressures that measure preload. Stroke volume is the most sensitive and evidence-based indication of preload responsiveness, and although afterload influences stroke volume, SV is more a measure of flow, so eliminate C. SVR is the isolated parameter intended to measure the resistance (afterload) to LV ejection. Choose D.

15. **A** Rationale: A, C, and V waves are all produced by the CVP, making answer A the best answer. Arterial systolic waves refer more to an arterial line and are more closely associated with LV function, so eliminate B. Augmented diastolic waves are associated with IABP tracings, so eliminate C as well. Waveforms can have an X descent, a Y descent, and a Z point; however, option D is a distractor option. Choose A.

16. **A** Rationale: In the approach to this question, note that both B and C are closely associated with LV failure. However, even if you do not recall this in the moment, B and C can still be eliminated due to the fact that they measure the same thing. Option D, increased pulmonary mean arterial pressure, may secondarily increase due to bloodflow backup into the pulmonary circuit from LV failure. This makes A, increased CVP, the best choice. When bloodflow is traced backward from the LV, the CVP is the furthest "upstream" from all options presented. Choose A.

17. **A** Rationale: During ventricular systole, the semilunar valves (aortic and pulmonic) should be open and the AV (mitral and tricuspid) valves should be closed. Option A provides the only scenario where this should be occurring. A quick test-taking strategy would be to identify that both options C and D identify situations where both types of valves are in stenosis or regurgitation at the same time, allowing you to quickly rule out C and D as options.

18. **D** Rationale: Remember, in these negatively stated questions, the question is essentially asking, "These are all key treatments EXCEPT…" ACE inhibitors and beta blockers (such as carvedilol) are standards of care in HF, so options A and B can be eliminated quickly. Although diuretics are not associated with mortality benefit in HF, they are frequently administered in HF and key to preload reduction and symptom relief in acute HF, so eliminate C. Although afterload reducers are often adjunctive treatment in HF, nitroprusside is less commonly administered compared to the other options and is not considered a standard of care in HF. Choose D.

19. **A** Rationale: The PAOP measures the column of fluid that extends from the tip of the PA catheter in the distal pulmonary artery, through the lung vasculature, through the left atrium, to the left ventricle. Thus, the correct answer is option A. The PAOP primarily takes into account only left-sided cardiac pressures. Options B, C, and D all take into account right-sided cardiac pressures.

20. **B** Rationale: This negatively stated question suggests that all options are characteristics of pericardial tamponade EXCEPT one option. An equalization of all cardiac filling pressures, option A, is a classic finding due to circumferential external pressure on the myocardium. Due to the fact that the pressure distribution is circumferential, both ventricles WOULD BE involved, making, option B the best answer. Hypotension (option C) is a classic finding due to decreased LV filling, and distended neck veins (option D) is a classic finding due to the decreased venous drainage to the heart due to a compressed RA. Choose B.

21. **A** Rationale: This negatively stated question suggests that all options are associated with LV preload EXCEPT one option. Option B (PAOP) and option D (LVEDP) are both indicative of LV preload and are essentially the same thing, so can be eliminated quickly. The left atrial pressure, option C, can indirectly reflect LV preload as this cardiac chamber is in the line of the column of fluid for measuring PAOP, so eliminate option C. Option A, the CVP, is the only option that does not help estimate LV preload and is the only right-sided cardiac chamber of the options listed. Choose A.

22. **A** Rationale: Option A, increased CVP, is the most closely associated option with RV failure and is the chamber directly behind the affected area. Option B, increased PAOP, is more closely associated with LV failure. Option C may be seen but is in front of (ie, "downstream" from) the affected area and is not the best answer.

Option D, increased systemic arterial pressure, may be seen in acute decompensated LVF, but is a secondary sign. Choose A.

23. **B** Rationale: This is a classic picture of a s/p MI mitral valve rupture and the abrupt onset *without chest pain* illustrated here suggests a structural problem has occurred. Option A is unlikely because classic pericardial tamponade involves elevation of all cardiac pressures, and the CVP in this case is low. Also eliminate option C, as ventricular wall ruptures are more likely with full thickness, transmyocardial MIs. Aortic valve ruptures are very rare s/p MI, so eliminate D. Choose B.

24. **A** Rationale: A is the best answer here since immediate surgery is the only definitive management for this structural problem of MV rupture. None of the other options will address the underlying problem. Eliminate option B since nitroprusside will only decrease the SBP further. Fluid challenges (option C) are also inappropriate since the PAOP is already 24. Thrombolytic therapy (option D) is more appropriate in early MI settings and would not address the structural problem of MV rupture. Choose A.

25. **D** Rationale: Eliminate option A as A waves are associated with atrial contraction, which is not associated with the underlying problem in this case. Absent A waves, option B, would be associated with noncontracting atria, which are also not associated with this case, so eliminate B as well. Giant C waves (option C) are associated with closure of the mitral and tricuspid valves; however, an incompetent mitral valve exists in this case, so eliminate C. Giant V waves are associated with poorly compliant atria and the backward flow of blood from mitral regurgitation, choose D.

26. **A** Rationale: Even if you were unsure of the correct choice initially, note that options B, C, and D all relate to repolarization and rest. Option A is the only option that refers to depolarization as suggested by phase 0. Choose A.

27. **D** Rationale: Even if you were unsure of which phase of cardiac potential and ion movement were associated with each option, option D (phase 4) is the only option indicating the complete resting interval between action potentials. Think of the action potential wave as "steps," with the lowest, "bottom" step (-90 mV, electronegativity) suggesting diastole and repolarization.

28. **D** Rationale: The sodium–potassium pumps are associated with rapid channel movement, so A and B can be eliminated initially. Chloride is an anion, so eliminate C as well. Calcium is the "slow channel" cation of phase 2 (the plateau phase). It is by working on this phase that calcium chloride IVP administration can increase contractility and protect the myocardium. Choose D.

29. **B** Rationale: The cell membrane will always favor exchanging a "positive for a positive" or a "negative for a negative." Since sodium is positive and phosphate (option A) and chloride (option C) are negative, they can be eliminated quickly. The "sodium–potassium pump" suggests that sodium largely exchanges with potassium, making option B the best answer. Calcium is more associated with the slow channel phase 2, so eliminate D.

30. **A** Rationale: Left-sided cardiac chambers carry oxygenated blood, so options B and D can be eliminated quickly. The only right-sided chamber mentioned here is A, making option A the best answer. Even though the word "veins" is mentioned in option C, the pulmonary veins carry oxygenated blood to the right atrium from the lungs, thus eliminating option C as well.

31. **A** Rationale: The conduction pathway begins in the right atrium, travels through the bundle of His in the septum, then the apex of the LV and throughout the His–Purkinje system. The conduction impulse also begins with the sinoatrial (SA) node, so choose A. The superior vena cava, option D, is not even a cardiac chamber and can be eliminated quickly. Options B and C refer to either the incorrect side or cardiac chamber in order to confuse the reader.

32. **C** Rationale: Cardiac output and stroke volume relate more to blood flow than blood pressure, so options A and B can be eliminated quickly. Mean arterial pressure is just another way to measure blood pressure, so D can be eliminated as well. Consider the formula MAP = CO × SVR. SVR measures the degree of afterload that compensates for changes in cardiac output (CO). SVR is also one of the primary parameters targeted for treatment of primary systemic hypertension (HTN). Choose C.

33. **D** Rationale: 10% to 20% is associated with severe systolic HF, so eliminate A (also, be careful not to confuse with atrial "kick," which is approximately 10%–15%). A 25% to 35% ejection fraction would suggest advanced HF and 40% to 50% would suggest a depressed EF, so eliminate options B and C as well. A normal ejection fraction is 60% to 65%. Choose D.

34. **D** Rationale: Option A is a true statement but reflects pulmonary shunt and not Starling's law, so eliminate A. Options B and C are not necessarily always true, and neither are they Starling's law, so can be eliminated as well. Option D describes Starling's law, or the "rubber band theory," which suggests that when the cardiac muscle is stretched, the strength of contraction increases. Choose D.

35. **C** Rationale: Acute ST elevation suggesting a STEMI is the primary criteria indicating a transfer to the cardiac catheterization lab as quickly as possible. The lactate level in option A is a normal finding, plus it is only a global indicator of tissue hypoxia and nonspecific with regard to MI, so eliminate A. A troponin I of less than 1 may be present during a STEMI, however does not alone suggest prompt transfer for potential angioplasty, so eliminate B. A CVP of 8 mm Hg, for the purposes of the exam, is a normal finding, thus eliminating D. Therefore, choose C.

36. **A** Rationale: Options C and D only relate to right-sided cardiac failure and therefore can be eliminated quickly. Option A is more specific to the **underlying cause** of PAOP and CVP elevation (as opposed to option B, which is more generally stated), therefore choose A.

37. **A** Rationale: Options C and D actually increase myocardial oxygen consumption (MvO_2) and can be ruled out initially. Then when deciding between options A and B, consider what nitroglycerin does for ischemic chest pain—it vasodilates and lowers the resistance to LV ejection, thus making option A the best remaining answer.

38. **B** Rationale: Options A and C essentially refer to the same "fight or flight" component of the autonomic nervous system and can be eliminated quickly. The parasympathetic nervous system includes the vagus nerve, which is more closely associated with HR control. Consider how vagal maneuvers lower the HR or how atropine (a "parasympatholytic") blocks the parasympathetic (ie, the "rest and digest") side of the nervous system so that sympathetic (ie, "adrenergic") stimulation can take over and accelerate the HR. The cerebellum supports functions such as balance, so eliminate D also and choose B.

39. **C** Rationale: The A waves reflect the intra-atrial chamber pressure during atrial contraction. So, think, "What could cause resistance to atrial contraction?" (which would increase A wave size). Mitral stenosis would help generate enough left atrial pressure to produce giant A waves, so choose C. The aortic valve is further from the tip of the PA catheter than the mitral valve, so eliminate A. Mitral regurgitation creates giant V waves, so eliminate B as well. Hypovolemia is more likely to decrease A wave size than increase it, eliminating D.

40. **D** Rationale: First-line therapy for ventricular fibrillation is defibrillation, so choose D. Since options A and B both refer to drug therapy, they can be ruled out as answers quickly. Option C refers to synchronized cardioversion, which is more appropriate for unstable tachydysrhythmias with a pulse present, such as SVT or atrial fibrillation, usually exceeding a HR rate of 160—so eliminate C as well.

41. **B** Rationale: V_1 to V_4 are anteroseptal leads, so eliminate option A. I and aVL are high lateral leads and V_5 and V_6 are left lateral leads, making option B the best answer. Option C refers to right-sided leads intended to specifically look for right ventricular and/or inferior ischemia or injury, so eliminate C. II, III, and aVF are inferior leads, so eliminate D as well.

42. **D** Rationale: V_1 to V_4 are anteroseptal leads, so eliminate option A. I and aVL are high lateral leads and V_5 and V_6 are left lateral leads, so eliminate option B as well. Option C can be eliminated quickly, since the leads in option C are not contiguous leads (they are all limb leads) and aVR is an indeterminate lead. Option D is the only option that includes right-sided leads to specifically look for right ventricular and/or inferior ischemia or injury, making option D the best answer.

43. **B** Rationale: This ectopic beat occurs early in the tracing and appears similar to the right bundle branch block pattern. An rSR' pattern is seen with a deep S wave, characteristic of atrial premature contractions (APCs) with aberrant conduction. Choose option B. One ECG tracing may be present on the exam to interpret. However, questions this advanced may be less likely to appear.

44. **A** Rationale: This tracing has a P wave for every QRS, is regular, and has a rate between 100 and 150 bpm, which suggests sinus tachycardia, so choose option A. Options C and D can be eliminated quickly because both atrial flutter and atrial fibrillation have irregular R to R intervals, and the tracing presented possesses a regular R to R interval. Atrial tachycardia, option B, is more of a general term which involves the pathway originating within the atria, but outside the sinus node. Since this tracing is sinus in nature (normal P wave morphology and consistent PR intervals), eliminate B as well.

45. **B** Rationale: Since this tracing presents with irregularity, option A can be eliminated quickly. Options C and D may also be eliminated due to the fact that neither the sawtooth nor the chaotic baselines of atrial flutter or atrial fibrillation are observed. Paroxysmal atrial tachycardia (PAT), however, is characterized by a rapid rate (>100) and abrupt onset or cessation back into an organized rhythm with controlled rate (<100) as illustrated toward the end of this tracing. Choose B.

46. **D** Rationale: Sinus tachycardia can be eliminated quickly for this tracing since no consistent P wave is observed and the rate is not greater than 100, so eliminate A. Atrial tachycardia, option B, can also be eliminated since the rate is less than 60. Atrial flutter is an interesting option; however the consistent, symmetrical "sawtooth" baseline of atrial flutter is not present, eliminating C. The chaotic baseline of atrial fibrillation with no discernable P waves is observed here, making option D the best answer.

47. **C** Rationale: The rate for this tracing is approximately 75. Therefore, options A and B can be eliminated quickly since the rate is not greater than 100 (a criteria for any tachycardic rhythm). This tracing does however possess the symmetrical, "sawtooth" baseline of classic atrial flutter, making C the best answer.

48. **D** Rationale: In this tracing option A can be eliminated quickly because first-degree block requires there to be a consistent PR interval, which is absent in this case. Options B and C may also be eliminated as both types of second-degree block require "dropped" QRSs (ie, when the atrial rate exceeds the ventricular rate), and "dropped" QRSs are not observed here. This tracing illustrates complete A–V dissociation, where a regular atrial rate and a regular ventricular rate fire completely independently of one another. So choose third-degree block—option D.

49. **A** Rationale: In this tracing option A, first-degree block is the correct answer because a consistent PR interval and R to R interval is observed throughout. The PR interval is also consistently greater than 0.20. Options B and C can be eliminated as both types of second-degree block require "dropped" QRSs (ie, when the atrial rate exceeds the ventricular rate) and "dropped" QRSs are not observed here. No complete A–V dissociation is observed in the tracing either, where a regular atrial rate and a regular ventricular rate fire completely independent of one another, so option D can be eliminated as well.

50. **C** Rationale: In this tracing, option A can be eliminated quickly because first-degree block requires there to be a consistent PR interval, which is absent in this case. Second-degree block requires progressive prolongation of the PR interval until a QRS is "dropped" (ie, nonconducted). The progressive prolongation is not observed here, so eliminate B. However, the tracing does possess nonconducted QRSs every other beat, resulting in 2:1 A–V conduction, making option C the best answer. No complete A–V dissociation is observed in the tracing either, where a regular atrial rate and a regular ventricular rate fire completely independently of one another, so option D can be eliminated as well. Choose C.

51. **B** Rationale: In this tracing option A can be eliminated quickly because first-degree block requires there to be a consistent PR interval, which is absent in this case. Second-degree block requires progressive prolongation of the PR interval until a QRS is "dropped" (ie, nonconducted). The progressive prolongation ***is*** observed here, making option B the best answer over option C. No complete A–V dissociation is observed in the tracing either, where a regular atrial rate and a regular ventricular rate fire completely independently of one another, so option D can be eliminated as well. Choose B.

52. **B** Rationale: After 2 to 3 normal R wave complexes at the beginning of this tracing, there is a run of R waves that are wide and bizarre and polymorphic in nature at a rate greater than 150. The sustained rate helps eliminate the suspicion that only multiform PVCs are being observed, so eliminate option A. Since clear R waves are seen, ventricular fibrillation, option C, can be ruled out as well. The absence of any right or left bundle branch block-type morphology also helps eliminate SVT with aberrancy, option D. Choose B.

53. **A** Rationale: In this tracing, there is essentially only 1 to 2 nonsustained, wide, bizarre S waves appearing in the underlying rhythm, making option A the best answer. The nonsustained nature of the ectopics make ventricular tachycardia (VT) and torsade de pointes less likely, so options B and D can be eliminated quickly. The presence of QRS complexes also helps eliminate ventricular fibrillation, so option C can be ruled out as well. Choose A.

54. **C** Rationale: In this tracing there is no clear organized underlying rhythm, which helps to eliminate option A quickly. The presence of R or S waves is also not clear enough, which helps to eliminate VT, option B. Torsade de pointes by definition is polymorphic VT, with QRSs that vary in shape, amplitude, and duration. This tracing illustrates waves that are smaller, monomorphic, and consistent in nature, making option C the best answer.

55. **B** Rationale: Right bundle branch block patterns most closely resemble APCs with aberrant conduction of the options listed, making B the best answer. Option A can be eliminated since the taller left peak (Rr') in V_1 is more closely associated with VT or PVCs, as opposed to right bundle branch block pattern where the right peak ("rabbit ear") is taller. Options C and D can also be eliminated because they are both associated with ventricular and not supraventricular activity. Choose B.

56. **B** Rationale: The precordial leads on the 12-lead ECG are V_1 to V_6, and precordial concordance can be very helpful in differentiating wide complex tachycardias from VT. In these situations, if the precordial leads are either all positive or all negative, a high likelihood of VT exists, making option B the best answer. Option A refers to a bundle branch block pattern, option C refers to potential ischemic changes, and option D refers to conditions such as LV hypertrophy.

57. **A** Rationale: Inferior MIs are associated with dysfunction of the SA node, making option A the best answer. Options B, C, and D all impact the conduction pathway farther down as compared to option A. Option A suggests a defect on the uppermost portion of the conduction pathway compared to the other options, so choose A.

58. **A** Rationale: Anterior fascicular blocks (hemiblocks) are a specific type of left bundle branch block associated with left axis deviation, making option A the best answer. Left bundle branch blocks are also associated with PVCs and LV hypertrophy. Right axis deviation would be associated with a right bundle branch block and/or a posterior fascicular block, eliminating option B. Q waves are simply dead tissue, ruling out option C as well. Option D is just a nonspecific reference to high lateral leads. Choose A.

59. **B** Rationale: Posterior fascicular blocks (hemiblocks) are a specific type of left bundle branch block associated with right axis deviation, making option B the best answer. Posterior fascicular blocks are also associated with an RV hypertrophy pattern. Left axis deviation would be associated with an anterior fascicular block, eliminating option A. Q waves are simply dead tissue, ruling out option C as well. Option D is just a nonspecific reference to high lateral leads. Choose B.

60. **C** Rationale: Option C is the best and most specific definition here. Options A and B may be seen with cardiomyopathy or LV hypertrophy physiology; however, these definitions are more vague. Large R waves may also be seen as mentioned in option D; however, the rest of option D is incorrect. Choose C.

61. **D** Rationale: Option D is the best and most specific definition here. Options A and B may be seen with RV hypertrophy physiology; however, these definitions are more vague. Option C describes criteria for diagnosing LV hypertrophy. Choose D.

62. **C** Rationale: This negatively stated question is asking, "AV dissociation is present in each of these options EXCEPT…" Options B and D can be eliminated quickly because third-degree block is complete A–V dissociation and atrial tachycardia with 2:1 block suggests AV block every other beat. VT can also be ruled out as P waves in VT are either not present or unable to assess, so eliminate A as well. Be careful not to be mislead by the name "first-degree block"; even though it is a part of the heart block continuum, no AV dissociation exists with this rhythm. Choose C.

63. **D** Rationale: Many different causes of sinus tachycardia exist, and treatment should primarily be focused on addressing the underlying cause, making option D the best answer. Note that options A, B, and C are all drug therapy, which helps enable the use of the "cluster technique" to eliminate them. The exam will generally not expect drug therapy to be chosen for a treatment unless necessary.

64. **D** Rationale: This is another negatively stated question, asking, in other words, "All of the following are physical parasympathetic stimulation treatments for atrial tachycardia EXCEPT…" Options A, B, and C would all be potential maneuvers to use. The hepatojugular reflux, however, is used to assess for right-sided HF. Choose D.

65. **C** Rationale: In this case, first-degree block is not likely because first-degree occurs in a 1:1 ratio of P waves to QRSs without any AV dissociation, so eliminate A. A constant PR interval is also described in the case, which is uncharacteristic for second-degree type I and third-degree block, so eliminate B and D as well. A constant PR interval with 2:1 AV conduction is consistent with second-degree type II, choose C.

66. **A** Rationale: Based on the available options, a pacemaker would be most appropriate to generate an increased ventricular rate. A calcium channel blocker such as nicardipine would risk further slowing the heart rate or exacerbating the AV block, so eliminate B. Options C and D may be considered due to their ability to increase HR; however, they are not considered first-line therapy. In addition, consider that dopamine and epinephrine are both catecholamines with many similarities, which may serve as a clue to "cluster" and eliminate them as possibilities. Choose A.

67. **A** Rationale: In the three-letter pacemaker code, the first letter stands for the cardiac chamber ***paced***, the second letter stands for the chamber ***sensed***, and the last letter stands for the programmed response to sensing. Therefore, option A is the correct answer. An easy way to remember the order of the first two letters is to remember that P ***("paced")*** comes before S ***("sensed")*** in the alphabet.

68. **B** Rationale: In the three-letter pacemaker code, the first letter stands for the cardiac chamber ***paced***, the second letter stands for the chamber ***sensed***, and the last letter stands for the programmed response to sensing. Therefore, option B is the correct answer. The sensed cardiac chamber is which chamber is being monitored by the pacemaker for intrinsic cardiac activity. An easy way to remember the order of the first two letters is to remember that P ***("paced")*** comes before S ***("sensed")*** in the alphabet.

69. **A** Rationale: This pacemaker is capturing properly with one QRS coming after every one pacemaker spike (1:1), so the correct answer is option A. Failure to sense is when spikes occur randomly across the tracing without consistent relation to QRSs; this is not present, so eliminate B. Failure to capture is when spikes are observed without QRSs after them; this is not observed, so eliminate C as well. Pacemaker-generated ventricular ectopic beats, which look similar to PVCs, are not observed either, which helps to rule out D. Choose A.

70. **A** Rationale: The most significant advantage of a transcutaneous pacemaker is the ease of application of the pads, option A. The rest of the options are not true. Transcutaneous pacemakers require a higher electrical stimulation to capture the heart rate as compared to a transvenous pacemaker, eliminating option B. This higher stimulation is usually perceived by the patient and analgesia is often required, eliminating option D as well. Peripheral intravenous access is technically not required, ruling out option C. Choose A.

71. **B** Rationale: Since the right coronary artery is often the culprit in inferior MIs and also supplies the SA node, bradycardias are common in these cases, eliminating option C. However, the bradycardias are usually transient, self-limiting, and resolve after reperfusion takes place, which also helps eliminate options A and D. Choose B.

72. **C** Rationale: Since the patient has an acute-onset HR of 50 and a BP of 86/54, this question is asking for the first-line treatment for symptomatic bradycardia, which is atropine, option C. Dopamine, option B, may be considered as a second-line treatment, but is not the best answer. Both options A and D may cause further slowing of the HR, which helps eliminate them as well. In addition, the simple treatment of PVCs with lidocaine is no longer recommended. Choose C.

73. **B** Rationale: This is a straight knowledge question. The inherent rate of the AV nodal area is 40 to 60, option B. 20 to 40 is the inherent rate of the His–Purkinje system, eliminating option A. 60 to 80 is within the normal sinus node range, eliminating option C as well. Option D is not true. Choose B.

74. **C** Rationale: In this question option D can be ruled out quickly because PVCs are equally likely to occur with either type of MI. Next, consider that inferior MIs largely impact the SA node (creating bradydysrhythmias, etc), whereas anterior MIs are more likely to impact the AV

node (creating AV blocks, etc). Option C identifies the location furthest down the conduction pathway of the remaining options. Options A and B may be more closely associated with SA node dysfunction, ruling them out. Choose C.

75. **A** Rationale: The QRS complex represents ventricular depolarization, the ST segment represents the end of ventricular depolarization, and the T wave represents ventricular repolarization, eliminating options B, C, and D. The PR interval represents the impulse of atrial depolarization, through the AV node, and up to the ventricles. Choose A.

76. **B** Rationale: In this question option A can be ruled out quickly because these drugs actually increase the HR. Option C can also be eliminated since pronestyl is not considered a first-line agent due to its poor side effect profile. Carvedilol is considered a drug more appropriate for chronic HF treatment, helping to eliminate option D as well. Diltiazem and adenosine are short-acting agents that help further diagnose the rhythm and stabilize the patient quickly. Choose B.

77. **D** Rationale: The HR in this tracing looks to be approximately 150. Therefore, option A can be ruled out quickly here because it is too fast to be accelerated idioventricular rhythm. Also, clear R waves are present without the electrical fling or chaos often observed with artifact, so eliminate option C as well. A 12-lead ECG may be needed to fully differentiate between the remaining two options. However, in the setting of acute MI, consider the more serious remaining answer, option D (note: also observe that the left "rabbit ear" RSR' wave is higher than the right, a finding that also favors VT).

78. **B** Rationale: The rhythm displayed here is "stable" VT (ie, VT with a pulse and without symptoms). Option A, observation, should be eliminated initially because of the likelihood of decompensation into unstable VT. Electrical therapy would also be recommended in the event of conversation to unstable VT. However, since the patient is hemodynamically stable at this time, eliminate options C and D. Medical therapy is recommended as first-line treatment of "stable VT." Choose B.

79. **B** Rationale: This negatively stated question is stating that "all of the following options are true of junctional rhythms EXCEPT…" It is true that junctional rhythms have normal QRS complexes, heart rates 40 and 60/minute, and have absent P waves, which helps eliminate A, C, and D. Junctional rhythms do not have wide QRS complexes; choose B.

80. **D** Rationale: If uncertain with this question, consider first that options A, B, and C are all inferior leads. This could serve as a clue to "cluster" and eliminate them (a much higher likelihood of success on the exam than guessing). V_1 is the only precordial lead listed, and is a preferred lead for evaluating conduction defects, right and left bundle branch blocks, and differentiating PVCs from aberrantly conducted PACs. Choose D.

81. **A** Rationale: New-onset left bundle branch block is considered a STEMI-equivalent finding in the setting of suspected acute MI. Right bundle branch blocks are not as serious in comparison, eliminating option B. Sinus tachycardia is too vague and nonspecific of a finding, eliminating option C as well. Second-degree type II heart block may require urgent attention; however, is not as emergent as a STEMI-equivalent finding, which mandates PCI within 90 min unless proven otherwise. Choose A.

82. **D** Rationale: If you were unsure with this question, note that options A, B, and C are all associated with right-sided changes so can be clustered together and eliminated. A second R wave larger than the first also suggests an RSR', second "rabbit ear" that is larger than the left R wave "rabbit ear," suggesting right bundle branch block. Choose D.

83. **A** Rationale: The most cardio-specific isoenzyme listed below is option A, troponin I. Options B and D are less specific to the cardiac muscle, ruling these options out. Troponin K (cTnK) does not exist. Choose A.

84. **A** Rationale: ST elevation in V_1 through V_4 suggests an anteroseptal MI, making option A the best answer. The inferior leads are II, III, and aVF, eliminating option B. The lateral leads are V_5 and V_6 and the high lateral leads are I and aVL, eliminating option C as well. For a posterior MI to be visualized, leads V_7 to V_9 would need to be obtained via a right-sided 12 lead ECG. Choose A.

85. **A** Rationale: Q waves suggest that dead myocardial tissue and irreversibility is present. Since Q waves are not present, option A is the best answer. ST depression in the inferior leads only reflects reciprocal changes in this example, so eliminate B. ST-segment elevation suggests active ischemic injury from compromised blood flow is occurring; however, this is still reversible, so eliminate option C as well. Option D is irrelevant. Choose A.

86. **A** Rationale: This is a straight knowledge question. Stage A HF is an early class of HF common in hypertensives, diabetics, patients with substance abuse, or certain comorbid conditions that place a patient at increased risk for developing structural signs of HF. Stages B, C, and D indicate more advanced stages of HF, respectively (with Stage D representing end-stage HF). Choose A. When in doubt in a staged question such as this with options that indicate a continuum, consider using the "cluster technique" and eliminate the middle options (options B and C) initially to narrow it down.

87. **D** Rationale: The presence of pathologic Q waves (deep and wide) indicate irreversible myocardial ischemia. All of the other symptoms listed are associated with unstable angina.

88. **A** Rationale: Troponin I stays elevated for up to 10 days post-MI in patients with normal renal function. It starts to rise in about 3 h after the onset of the MI. CK-MB rises within 4 h and resolves in 48 to 72 h.

89. **A** Rationale: Vasoactive agents are indicated in hemorrhagic shock only after intravascular volume is replaced and there is evidence of ongoing shock. Without adequate preload, stroke volume will continue to be low and heart rate will continue to increase in an attempt to maintain cardiac output. Additionally, Dopamine itself is not the best medication to give to tachycardic patients, since it acts on B1 receptors to increase heart rate.

90. **C** Rationale: Beta blockers are considered antianginal medications since they decrease heart rate, thereby lowering myocardial oxygen demands. Option A is used to decrease preload in patients with heart failure, but does not affect angina. Options B and D are both sympathetic stimulants that would likely worsen the angina.

91. **D** Rationale: All of the above, with the exception of extending the MI due to an embolus, are known complications of thrombolytic therapy.

92. **A** Rationale: Percutaneous intervention (stenting) is only indicated in option A since the stenosis is more than 75% and involves a single vessel. Total (100%) occlusions of coronary arteries are not often stented due to the presence of extensive collateral circulation. Multivessel disease (option C) is incorrect as those patients are better served with coronary artery bypass grafting. Vasospasm is treated in the cath lab with either intracoronary verapamil or nitroglycerin. Long-term it is treated with oral calcium channel blockers.

93. **D** Rationale: Vasospasm is treated in the cath lab with either intracoronary verapamil or nitroglycerin. Long-term it is treated with oral calcium channel blockers. Aspirin, ACE inhibitors, and angiotensin receptor blockers are not used to treat Prinzmetal's angina.

94. **C** Rationale: All of the above are indications except for a history of stroke within the previous 3 months due to the risk of iatrogenic stroke that may occur with thrombolytic administration.

95. **A** Rationale: Whenever adding an inotrope or a positive chronotrope (dopamine is both), there is an increase in myocardial oxygen demand (MVO_2). Dopamine does not cause reflex bradycardia, eliminating options B and C. Dopamine can induce atrial fibrillation, eliminating option D.

96. **A** Rationale: Pulsus paradoxus is defined as a decrease of more than 10 mm Hg drop in blood pressure upon inspiration. It is a classic sign of cardiac tamponade, likely to be observed along with Beck's triad: low arterial blood pressure, distended neck veins, and distant, muffled heart sounds.

97. **A** Rationale: Nitroglycerin is both an arterial and venodilator. However, it is primarily a venodilator. As a result, nitroglycerin infusions increase the likelihood of blood pooling in the abdominal and dependent venous circulation. By decreasing the amount of "relative" intravascular volume, nitroglycerin decreases preload (the amount of blood returned to the heart). Although decreasing preload can affect contractility and may affect stroke volume variation, those are not the primary effects, eliminating options C and D.

98. **B** Rationale: Based on the elevated CVP which is higher than the PAOP, and normal cardiac index/output, the patient has right ventricular dysfunction. Out of all of these options, RV infarction is the only one that would lead to a CVP that is higher than the PAOP. As a test-taking strategy, consider "clustering" and eliminating A and C since both are specific LV issues. Tamponade can also be eliminated since the cardiac filling pressures are not equalizing and the cardiac index is normal. Choose B.

99. **D** Rationale: Ideally, a right-sided ECG is used to diagnose a RV infarct. The leads associated with an RV MI on a right-sided ECG are V_4R, V_5R, and V_6R.

100. **A** Rationale: Fluid administration is paramount in RV infarctions in order to improve RV contractility and improve blood flow in to the pulmonary artery (Starling's law). This should also help improve blood pressure. Anything that decreases preload (ie, diuretics, nitroglycerin) will decrease RV cardiac output and lead to hypotension as RVMI patients are often preload-dependent. *After* the patient is adequately fluid loaded, dopamine may improve heart rate, cardiac output, and blood pressure, eliminating option C.

101. **D** Rationale: Pericarditis pain typically increases with respiration. It is also positional. It is worse when lying and improved when sitting forward. Fever is commonly present as a result of the inflammation involved in pericarditis. Pericardial friction rub is generally present in most cases, but it may not be present in all.

102. **B** Rationale: Inferior MIs have ST changes in leads II, III, and aVF. The ST depression in the lateral leads (I, aVL, V_5, and V_6) are reciprocal changes seen with inferior ST-segment elevation MIs.

103. **A** Rationale: The patient is having a STEMI. This requires emergency intervention. The intervention of choice is percutaneous coronary intervention (cardiac catheterization) when available. Thrombolytic therapy is used in situations where percutaneous coronary intervention is not available and there are no contraindications.

104. **A** Rationale: In systolic heart failure, the affected ventricle (in this scenario it is the left ventricle) is volume overloaded. This leads to "overstretch" of the ventricular muscle fibers, lowering contractility and stroke volume (Starling's law). Using furosemide to decrease the amount of circulating intravascular volume decreases the ventricular preload, leading to less ventricular muscle fiber stretch, thereby improving stroke volume and cardiac output. Ultimately, this will lower heart rate and therefore myocardial oxygen demand/consumption.

105. **D** Rationale: All of the agents except for nitroprusside are positive inotropes. Nitroprusside is a vasodilator that decreases afterload and lowers blood pressure.

106. **C** Rationale: The patient has signs of an infection. The pulmonary symptoms and findings are consistent with left heart failure or an insufficient valve on the left side of the heart (mitral or aortic), excluding option A. We can exclude pneumonia since there is no mention of a cough or sputum production. The presence of the murmur points to endocarditis as the culprit. The murmur is at the right sternal border at the second intercostal space, which is where the aortic valve is auscultated. Aortic insufficiency (regurgitation) is a diastolic murmur.

107. **A** Rationale: Hypoxia is associated with left heart failure. All of the other symptoms are seen in right heart failure.

108. **C** Rationale: Pericarditis typically presents with diffuse ST elevations and sloped PR intervals. Q waves are associated with dead myocardial tissue. Left axis deviation is more associated with left ventricular hypertrophy, and ST depressions are more reflective of ischemic changes. Choose C.

109. **A** Rationale: Unprovoked chest pain with ST-elevation is characteristic of Prinzmetal's Variant Angina (PVA), which can mimic unstable angina. PVA is also associated with exposure to cold temperatures. Chest pain during exertion is more associated with stable angina. Absence of chest pain with Q-wave formation may be more associated with conditions such as diabetic neuropathy. Option D may be more associated with a gallbladder attack, but is a confusing option. Choose A.

110. **D** Rationale: Dobutamine is a positive inotrope and a vasodilator. It is used to improve contractility and decrease afterload, both of which will improve cardiac output. The addition of nitroprusside, an alpha-antagonist-type effect, will further decrease afterload with the goal of improving cardiac output.

111. **C** Rationale: Orthostatic hypotension is commonly seen in hypovolemia. LV failure, pulmonary hypertension, and portal hypertension are not common causes of orthostasis.

112. **A** Rationale: In orthostatic hypotension, when changing position from supine to sitting, the heart rate increases by more than 10 bpm, the systolic BP falls more than 25 mm Hg, and the diastolic BP falls more than 10 mm Hg.

113. **C** Rationale: High-sensitivity C-reactive protein (CRP) is a marker of chronic, low-grade inflammation, which is a risk factor for atherosclerosis. CRP levels help stratify patients as either low, intermediate, or high risk for future cardiovascular events. A high WBC count is seen more generally during times of acute inflammation or stress, eliminating option A. IL-6 is secreted by the immune system in response to trauma, eliminating option B. Procalcitonin is typically increased in bacterial infections, eliminating option D.

114. **D** Rationale: Dopamine is an alpha agonist in addition to a positive chronotrope. At doses of 11 to 20 mcgs/kg/min it produces severe vasoconstriction. Dobutamine causes vasodilatation, eliminating option A. Isoproterenol is a beta-agonist used to increase HR in bradycardia and heart block, eliminating option B. Esmolol is a beta blocker, which decreases HR and BP, eliminating option C.

115. **B** Rationale: Sinus tachycardia is common in many trauma patients, including those with blunt cardiac injury. PACs and PVCs are associated with BCI. Some, but not all, patients with BCI may have sternal ecchymosis, eliminating option D. Distended neck veins would be present if the BCI led to cardiac tamponade, eliminating option A. Shortness of breath is too nonspecific of an option, so eliminate C as well.

116. **A** Rationale: Stroke volume is primarily comprised of three main elements: preload, afterload, and contractility. Furosemide decreases circulating volume and preload, eliminating B and C. D is a more obscure option; choose A.

117. **D** Rationale: The patient is presenting with classic signs of unstable angina. Option C is incorrect because the patient's troponin is negative at this point and no ST-segment elevation is identified. Option A, stable angina, can be eliminated because it is unrelieved by rest. B can be eliminated because there are no Q waves, ST-segment elevation, and no inferior injury described. Choose D.

118. **D** Rationale: Statins decrease total cholesterol and low-density lipoprotein (LDL), while increasing high-density lipoprotein (HDL). They also have anti-inflammatory properties which help decrease the risk of cardiovascular events.

119. **C** Rationale: Options A, B, and D occur when the left ventricle fails and leads to pulmonary vascular congestion. The S_3 heart sound is produced when blood is entering a volume-overloaded ventricle. Option C is the correct choice since dependent edema and hepatomegaly are associated with right ventricular failure.

120. **C** Rationale: The presentation demonstrates signs of both right and left ventricular failure. The patient has a low cardiac output which is associated with left ventricular failure but is also seen in right ventricular failure. The key to determining which ventricle(s) is failing is to look at the filling pressures. Both the CVP (right-sided filling pressure) and PAOP (left-sided filling pressure) are high, suggesting biventricular failure. Physical signs such as crackles (LV failure) and distended neck veins (RV failure) also confirm that biventricular failure exists.

121. **D** Rationale: Dobutamine is a positive inotrope and vasodilator as is indicated in the treatment of acute decompensated heart failure. Nitroglycerin and furosemide decrease preload, which can improve contractility, stroke volume, and cardiac output (Starling's law). High-dose dopamine is not indicated since the patient is not hypotensive.

122. **A** Rationale: Milrinone is the best choice since it will improve myocardial contractility and decrease afterload for both the right (PVR) and left heart (SVR), and lower PA pressures. Nicardipine works well as a vasodilator but does not affect inotropic activity. Phenylephrine and norepinephrine are both alpha agonists, which should not be administered to a hypertensive patient.

123. **A** Rationale: The patient is showing signs of biventricular failure. Dependent edema and elevated CVP are signs of right heart failure. Shortness of breath, tachypnea, elevated PA pressures (pulmonary hypertension), and PAOP are signs of left heart failure. There is nothing in the scenario that indicates the presences of chronic lung disease, which eliminates option B. Options C and D focus only on right-sided issues. Choose A.

124. **B** Rationale: All of the signs point to pulmonary edema, which is likely the result of decompensated left ventricular CHF. RV failure and PE (both right-sided issues) would not cause crackles throughout the lung fields, eliminating A and D. ECG findings are nonspecific and there is no mention of a positive troponin, eliminating option C. Choose B.

125. **B** Rationale: Although nifedipine causes vasodilation and decreases afterload, it is generally reserved for the treatment of hypertension. Dobutamine will increase contractility and decrease afterload. Furosemide and morphine will decrease preload, which is desirable in decompensated CHF.

126. **B** Rationale: Out of all of these factors, only an ischemic stroke within the last 3 months is an absolute contraindication to administering a thrombolytic. Although high, the BP is still within parameters for thrombolytic administration, eliminating option A. Recent CPR and recent trauma are relative contraindications (eliminating C and D as the best answer). Thrombolytic administration is up to the discretion of the attending physician based on the risk–benefit to the patient.

127. **C** Rationale: The triad of symptoms in severe aortic stenosis is syncope or presyncope, chest pain (angina), and shortness of breath. Fatigue and palpitations can happen in a number of disease processes including aortic stenosis, but they are not major symptoms of aortic stenosis, eliminating options A and B. Unexplained weight loss is not typically seen in aortic stenosis (however, perhaps in TB or oncology), eliminating option D.

128. **A** Rationale: Morphine acts as a vasodilator (decreasing preload) and decreases perceived shortness of breath, while furosemide decreases circulating volume, thereby decreasing myocardial oxygen consumption. Although morphine also decreases afterload as well, its preload reducing effect better addresses the underlying problem, eliminating option B. Options C and D directly conflict with the intended effect of furosemide and morphine. Choose A.

129. **C** Rationale: The only medication in this list that is a beta blocker is carvedilol. Clonidine is an alpha-antagonist. Nifedipine is a calcium channel blocker. Captopril is an ACE inhibitor.

130. **B** Rationale: The major contraindications to IABP placement are coagulopathy, suspected aortic dissection, severe peripheral arterial disease, and aortic valve insufficiency. The peripheral arterial disease in this patient is probably not severe since the patient still has palpable lower extremity pulses, eliminating option A. Option D is likely pulmonary edema, which is not a contraindication to IABP insertion, nor is option C. Choose B.

131. **D** Rationale: All of the above medications except for metoprolol are calcium channel blockers. Metoprolol is a beta blocker.

132. **C** Rationale: Classic pericarditis findings represent generalized, diffuse ST elevations in several leads on the 12-lead ECG. Q waves suggest dead myocardial tissue, often post-MI, eliminating A. Left axis deviation suggests that the summation of depolarization vectors are left of the apex, such as in LV hypertrophy, eliminating B. Depression of ST segments suggests myocardial ischemia but not pericarditis, eliminating D. Choose C.

133. **A** Rationale: In option A, the patient is volume depleted (low CVP and PAD) and is unable to deliver enough oxygen to the tissues (low SvO_2). Option B has a patient with a lower hemoglobin, but it is above the typical transfusion threshold. The patient has a normal cardiac index, which may be due to the heart rate increasing to improve stroke volume. We would need either filling pressures or tissue oxygenation data to determine if this patient needed blood, eliminating option B. The hemodynamics in option C are consistent with what is seen in distributive shock states such as sepsis, eliminating option C. Giving the patient additional intravascular volume is not indicated in option D, since the patient has high ventricular filling pressures and normal tissue oxygenation.

134. **C** Rationale: Performing a neuro exam is important, but assessing BP is the priority. The sodium nitroprusside infusion may have decreased the patient's blood pressure too quickly, leading to the onset of lightheadedness and dizziness. Urine output is a good sign of organ perfusion, but it is not the priority in this situation, eliminating option D. It is too early to worry about thiocyanate toxicity since the infusion has just started. Generally, thiocyanate levels are checked after 48 to 72 h of sodium nitroprusside administration.

135. **A** Rationale: Norepinephrine, angiotensin II, vasopressin, and cortisol are released as part of the body's response to compensate for shock. All of these can lead to vasoconstriction, which increases blood pressure. By vasoconstricting, they also increase SVR. Heart rate also rises due to the decrease in stroke volume.

136. **D** Rationale: The dicrotic notch is the dip in the arterial waveform that signals the beginning of diastole.

When the IABP is on pressure-trigger, it senses the dicrotic notch and causes the balloon to inflate. This increases coronary artery perfusion pressure. Option B is incorrect since the balloon needs to inflate at the beginning of diastole for maximum benefit. The R wave represents ventricular systole. If the balloon inflates during any part of systole, it will create an obstruction to blood flow from the left ventricle. This eliminates options A and C.

137. **A** Rationale: Since the aneurysm is abdominal, pericardial tamponade and coronary artery blood flow are unlikely. Pulmonary emboli arise from venous sources, not arterial. This eliminates option C. Decreased renal perfusion due to surgical cross-clamping and perioperative low flow may be issues with any open aortic procedure, making option A the best answer.

138. **B** Rationale: The IABP needs to deflate prior to the beginning of ventricular systole or it will impede blood flow out of the left ventricle. When the IABP is on the EKG trigger, it recognizes the R wave as the beginning of ventricular systole and deflates the balloon. The T wave and the dicrotic notch represent diastole, eliminating options A and D.

139. **B** Rationale: In hypovolemic shock, the filling pressures (CVP and PAOP) are low due to the loss of circulating blood volume. In cardiogenic shock, the filling pressures are high. As a result of blood or fluid loss, the cardiac output decreases. The sympathetic nervous system and renin–angiotensin–aldosterone systems are activated, leading to vasoconstriction and increased SVR. Both forms of shock include an elevated SVR and low stroke volume.

140. **A** Rationale: All of the medications listed above, except for dopamine, cause vasodilation which can lower blood pressure. Dopamine is an alpha agonist which increases blood pressure.

141. **C** Rationale: An IABP deflates during systole to decrease afterload and inflates during diastole to increase coronary artery perfusion pressures. It does not affect preload or contractility.

142. **D** Rationale: Beta blockers and ACE inhibitors are part of the core measures for CHF. Diuretics are used to treat fluid volume overload. Alpha agonists would potentially worsen CHF by vasoconstricting and increasing afterload. The increase in afterload could decrease stroke volume and cardiac output.

143. **B** Rationale: The patient is in class III shock based on the HR and BP. The treatment for class III shock is typically blood products, however there is not enough information available to suggest transfusion is necessary. She has a low $ScvO_2$ level, which reflects poor oxygen delivery to the tissues. A fluid challenge is the easiest, quickest, and most conservative way to improve circulating volume as a first-line approach until more information can be obtained about the patient. Choose B.

144. **B** Rationale: Cardiogenic shock is defined by a cardiac index less than 2.2 L/min/m^2 and is associated with a PAOP greater than 18 mm Hg. CVP evaluates the right ventricle. In cardiogenic shock, the CVP is typically normal but may elevate as the left ventricular failure worsens or if failure becomes biventricular.

145. **A** Rationale: Based on the low cardiac index/output and the PAOP more than 18 mm Hg, we need to consider left ventricular failure and cardiogenic shock as causes. The low SVO_2 indicates poor oxygen delivery to the tissues, which occurs in shock. The filling pressures (CVP and PAOP) are elevated, which eliminates options B and D. Although the CVP is higher than normal, the PAOP is also elevated, which makes option C less likely.

146. **B** Rationale: Dopamine and dobutamine will increase cardiac output, stroke volume, and contractility, and raise blood pressure, both of which the patient needs. Increasing BP will help improve renal perfusion, which may lead to increased urine output. Although dopamine can cause tachycardia and the patient is already tachycardic, B is the best option since a fluid bolus will worsen cardiac output (Starling's law) and respiratory status. Furosemide and nitroprusside will further decrease the BP in this already hypotensive patient, eliminating options C and D.

147. **B** Rationale: The patient in this scenario most likely has pulmonary edema and acute LV heart failure due to his MI. This would be associated with a PAOP more than 18 mm Hg and a low cardiac index less than 2.2 L/m^2. The SVR will likely be high, like in option D, but the high CI eliminates this option as well as option C.

148. **B** Rationale: Since cardiogenic shock is characterized by LV dysfunction, an ideal option for this question would include an inotropic infusion (eg, dobutamine), eliminating options A and D. Although epinephrine would likely improve the patient's blood pressure, it would also increase afterload and myocardial oxygen demand on an already failing left ventricle, eliminating C as well. Furosemide also addresses the underlying problem of the volume-overloaded LV. Choose B.

149. **A** Rationale: A mediastinum is considered widened if it is greater than 8 cm in diameter. Widening of the mediastinum is often associated with blunt aortic injury. A traumatic cardiac tamponade would also enlarge the pericardial silhouette. Pericarditis does not widen the mediastinum on radiograph, eliminating option B. Mitral valve rupture and myocardial contusion should not widen the mediastinum, either eliminating options C and D.

150. **D** Rationale: The extremely low cardiac filling pressures coupled with a low cardiac index suggest hypovolemic shock. Options A, B, and C would all include at least one elevated cardiac filling pressure, which helps to "cluster" them and rule them out. Choose D.

151. **C** Rationale: D_5W is a hypotonic fluid that is used to gradually replace free water in patients with hypernatremia. It does not raise intravascular volume as much as isotonic fluids (0.9% NS and LR) or colloids (albumin).

152. **D** Rationale: Esmolol is a beta blocker. It is the preferred antihypertensive for acute aortic emergencies because it decreases heart rate, which helps decrease sheer stress on the aorta. This may help prevent rupture. The other antihypertensives listed will decrease BP, but they do not prevent increases in HR.

153. **B** Rationale: The patient's cardiac filling pressures and BP are decreasing, and the HR is increasing, all of which point to hypovolemia. If the decreased H/H was purely dilutional, the filling pressures would have either not changed or increased and the tachycardia would not have developed, eliminating option A. In LV failure the PAOP would be more than 18 mm Hg, eliminating option C. In pericardial tamponade, the filling pressures increase and equalize as the tamponade progresses, eliminating option D.

154. **B** Rationale: In hypovolemia, stroke volume would drop as an early sign due to decreased ventricular filling (Starling's law). Heart rate would increase secondarily to maintain cardiac output, therefore just looking at the cardiac output alone would not give you sufficient information about volume status. Option B is the best option because it takes into account stroke volume (which decreases in hypovolemia), heart rate, and LV filling pressure (PAOP). Stroke volume is blood flow based and the most sensitive and evidence-based routine hemodynamic parameter for volume status. Options C and D contain only pressure-based parameters, which allows us to eliminate them quickly.

155. **C** Rationale: In hypovolemia, stroke volume would drop due to decreased ventricular filling (Starling's law). Heart rate would increase to maintain cardiac output, therefore just looking at the cardiac output alone would not give you sufficient information about volume status. Stroke volume actually decreases in hypovolemia, eliminating A, and mean arterial pressure (MAP) is a secondary monitoring parameter, eliminating D. Option B may be true in situations such as acute heart failure, but is not the best answer. Choose C.

156. **C** Rationale: Single-vessel disease that is able to be stented is not an indication for CABG. Single-vessel disease that cannot be stented, significant left main disease, and multi-vessel disease are indications for CABG.

157. **C** Rationale: Pulsus paradoxus (decrease in SBP > 10 mm Hg upon inspiration) is a classic sign of cardiac tamponade. It is part of Beck's triad. The other two components of the triad are hypotension and muffled heart sounds. In cardiac tamponade, PAOP increases. Diastolic blood pressure and cardiac output decrease.

158. **D** Rationale: The internal mammary artery (IMA) is a vessel of choice for CABG and is a gold standard for bypass grafting. It is typically used to bypass the either the left main, left anterior descending, or diagonal branches. The greater saphenous vein is also commonly used. Some surgeons will use the radial artery or right IMA, depending on patient characteristics and surgeon preference.

159. **C** Rationale: Hemodynamics such as CI, PAOP, and CVP are important post-op assessments, as is pulmonary gas exchange (arterial blood gas, oxygen saturations). Bladder pressures are not routinely assessed postheart surgery unless there are signs of intra-abdominal hypertension present.

160. **B** Rationale: Pulse pressure is systolic BP diastolic BP. High pulse pressures are associated with high cardiac output (ie, early sepsis) and low pulse pressures are associated with low cardiac output and low stroke volume (ie, class III hemorrhagic shock). Option C is the formula for MAP. D is the ankle–brachial index (ABI). Option A is a general assessment of HR range, however is not a pressure. Choose B.

161. **A** Rationale: Heart transplantation (or surgical treatment) is the only definitive management for cardiomyopathy (CM). CABG and angioplasty revascularize the myocardium, but do not reverse CM, eliminating B and D. IABP provides temporary afterload reduction and coronary artery reperfusion, but also does not correct CM, eliminating C. Choose A.

162. **C** Rationale: Approximately 65% of aortic aneurysms are located in the abdomen. Options A, B, and D may be more associated with aortic dissection rather than aortic aneurysm. Choose C.

163. **A** Rationale: AAAs may be palpable and cause severe abdominal pain that radiates to the back. Dissecting aortic aneurysms are a surgical emergency and carry a significant risk of mortality. Aortic aneurysms are not associated with GI bleeding. Choose A.

164. **A** Rationale: Dissections begin when there is damage to the intimal lining of the aorta. This intimal "tear" allows for blood to create a false lumen between the aortic intima and the media, which allows the dissection to develop. Option D is attractive since many patients with dissections can also have aneurysms, but that is not the correct pathophysiology of aortic dissection and not all dissections begin from aneurysms. Options B and C are not correct because the entire vessel wall may not be weakened, and transection occurs in blunt aortic injury.

165. **A** Rationale: Approximately 50% of patients undergoing ruptured AAA repair will develop renal failure and 20% will develop as MI. Mesenteric ischemia and paralysis are relatively uncommon after this procedure, eliminating options B and C. Option D is somewhat obscure and not enough information is given regarding it. Choose A.

166. **B** Rationale: The nausea, vomiting, visual field disturbances, and heart block are classic sings on digoxin toxicity. Verapamil is a calcium channel blocker that can affect AV conduction and cause heart block, however it would not cause the same physical symptoms of digtoxicity, eliminating A. Losartan and warfarin do not cause any of the above changes, eliminating C and D. Choose B.

167. **B** Rationale: Remember the "5-P's" of arterial occlusion: pain, pallor, pulselessness, paresthesia, and polar sensation (coldness). Options A, C, and D are all included in the 5-P's. Cyanosis is a bluish discoloration and more closely associated with venous insufficiency. Choose B.

168. **A** Rationale: Remember the "5-P's" of arterial occlusion: pain, pallor, pulselessness, paresthesia, and polar sensation (coldness). Option A is the only one available that is included in the 5-P's. Cyanosis, warmth, and edema are more closely associated with venous insufficiency. Choose A.

169. **D** Rationale: When lower extremity DVTs embolize, they travel through the inferior and superior vena cavae to the right side of the heart. From there, they travel into the pulmonary circulation causing pulmonary emboli. Superior vena cava (SVC) syndrome generally occurs from occlusion of the SVC by something outside of the venous system, that is, lung cancer, lymphoma, etc., eliminating option C. DVTs do not travel to the lower extremity arteries, eliminating options A and B (options A and B are also arterial problems).

170. **D** Rationale: Temperature, PAOP, and cardiac output are commonly monitored parameters via pulmonary artery catheter observed by staff in the ICU postcardiac surgery. Ejection fraction is more commonly measured via echocardiogram or a stress test. Choose D.

171. **B** Rationale: The best answer in this scenario is option B given the 500-mL output from the chest tube in the last hour. The hemodynamic changes listed above support this since the pulse pressure is narrowing, the blood pressure is dropping, the patient is becoming more tachycardic, the cardiac index/output are decreasing, and the ventricular filling pressures are decreasing. In acute respiratory distress syndrome or left ventricular CHF, we would expect worsening pulmonary parameters such as hypoxia and hypercarbia, eliminating options C and D. Option A is incorrect, since the respiratory parameters have not worsened significantly and the ventricular filling pressures are decreased. In obstructive shock, ventricular filling pressures are typically elevated.

172. **A** Rationale: Checking hemoglobin, hematocrit, and coagulation tests are a priority when assessing the severity of blood loss. Evaluating platelet counts and aPTT levels can help determine if the cause of bleeding is correctable without surgical intervention—ie, thrombocytopenia or if the heparin given in the OR was not completely reversed. The patient may ultimately need to go to the OR for emergent re-exploration. C is incorrect because it does not assess the cause of the bleeding and may potentially cause more harm—ie, blood builds up in the pericardium and leads to tamponade. Options B and D do not address the underlying cause of blood loss either.

173. **A** Rationale: The shortness of breath combined with the physical findings of crackles on lung auscultation and the presence of an S_3 heart sound indicate pulmonary edema. Pulmonary emboli would not produce crackles or an S_3. Tension pneumothorax findings would likely include absent breath sounds on the affected side and tracheal deviation, eliminating option C. Dissecting thoracic aneurysm would likely include chest pain; however, the crackles and S_3 make A the best answer.

174. **A** Rationale: The EKG changes could be associated with a non-ST-elevation myocardial infarction (NSTEMI). The hemodynamic parameters are consistent with the development of left heart failure and cardiogenic shock; for example, PAOP more than 18 mm Hg, low cardiac index/cardiac output. The high PAOP in this scenario helps exclude a pulmonary embolus (PE) because a PE would be associated with a high CVP since it is an obstruction of blood flow leaving the right heart. In patients with PE, the $PaCO_2$ is typically low. In this scenario the $PaCO_2$ is normal, helping to exclude option B. Tension pneumothorax findings would likely include absent breath sounds on the affected side, hypotension, JVD, and tracheal deviation, eliminating option C. Dissecting thoracic aneurysms may include chest pain, but A is the best answer.

175. **B** Rationale: The patient has a low cardiac index/output and has LV failure. A positive inotrope would work well in this situation. Because the SBP is more than 100 mm Hg, dobutamine would be a better choice since it will also vasodilate and reduce afterload. Reducing afterload will improve stroke volume and cardiac output. Dopamine would be the agent of choice if the patient had mild hypotension. Diltiazem could cause hypotension and likely further decrease cardiac output, eliminating option A. Nitroprusside will only decrease afterload, eliminating option D.

176. **D** Rationale: The lack of drainage from the mediastinal tube may be due to clot formation causing blockage of the chest tube. If the mediastinal tube is not draining, it can cause the development of tamponade. The patient is experiencing pulsus paradoxus (decrease in SBP > 10 mm Hg upon inspiration), which supports the presence of tamponade. Clear breath sounds help rule out option A and C. Bubbling in the water seal chamber when air leaks exist is a normal finding.

177. **D** Rationale: All of the above parameters are consistent with the presence of cardiac tamponade. Tamponade is a type of obstructive shock. As pressure builds in the pericardial sac, there is decreased venous return to the heart and decreased cardiac index/cardiac output. This leads to hypotension. Tachycardia occurs to persevere cardiac output due to decreased ventricular filling. As tamponade progresses, the right and left ventricular filling pressures equalize.

178. **C** Rationale: Postoperative patients with pericardial tamponade require emergency surgery to evacuate blood and clots from the pericardial space. Chest tubes inserted in the mediastinum are done in the operating room under direct visualization, eliminating option B. Inserting tissue plasminogen activator may unclog the tube, but it does not address other potential causes of tamponade, eliminating option A. Reintubation is required during mediastinal exploration, however, initiating positive-pressure ventilation may be worsening the patient's hemodynamics by exerting more pressure on the heart, making option D incorrect.

179. **C** Rationale: In lead V_1 there is an RSR[1] and in V_6 there is a slurred S-wave consistent with a RBBB.

180. **B** Rationale: The ST-segment elevations in lead II, III, and aVF indicate an inferior MI. The ST depression in I and aVL is an expected reciprocal change.

181. **B** Rationale: Inferolateral MI is the correct choice. The ST elevations in leads II, II, and aVF are consistent with an inferior MI. The ST elevations in leads I, aVL, V_5, and V_6 are consistent with a lateral MI.

182. **D** Rationale: ST elevations in V_2, V_3, and V_4 are consistent with an anterior wall STEMI.

183. **D** Rationale: Out of all these choices, option D is the most correct. There is a pathologic Q wave in lead III, which is consistent with a previous inferior wall MI. The ST elevations in V_2 to V_4 are consistent with an anterior MI.

184. **B** Rationale: There is ST depression and T wave inversion in the lateral leads (I, aVL, V_5, and V_6), suggesting lateral ischemia. The deep S waves in V_1 to V_3 and the tall R waves in V_5 to V_6 also suggest LV hypertrophy.

185. **D** Rationale: The best option available is a left bundle branch block. The patient movement during the tracing skews V_1, V_2, V_3 makes it a little more difficult to interpret. In V_1, there is a negative deflection. In lead V_6, there is an RsR[1] in the lateral leads. There is not left axis deviation, q1, and lead II has a positive deflection, eliminating option A. There is no right axis deviation or r1q3, and lead I has a positive deflection, eliminating option B. We can eliminate option C since there is no RsR[1] in V_1 or V_2, and no "slurred" S wave in V_6.

186. **A** Rationale: There is a left anterior fascicular (hemiblock) present since there is a left axis deviation, positive QRS deflection in lead I, and negative deflections in leads II and III. There is also what maybe a small q1 in addition to R3. We can eliminate a posterior fascicular (hemiblock) since there is no right axis deviation and the QRS deflections in leads I, II, and III do not match the criteria. The complexes are narrow (QRS < 0.12), which rules out both LBBB and RBBB, eliminating options C and D.

187. **C** Rationale: There is a positive QRS deflection in lead I and a negative QRS deflection in aVF which supports the presence of a left axis deviation. There is no evidence of left ventricular ectopy or pericarditis, eliminating options A and B.

188. **D** Rationale: There is T-wave inversion in aVL (lateral lead), V_1 (septal lead), V_2 (anterior lead), and ST depression in I (lateral lead), V_3 to V_4 (anterior leads), and V_5 to V_6 (lateral leads). A RBBB is present based on the RsR[1] in V_1 and V_2, and the slightly "slurred" S wave in V_6.

189. **C** Rationale: This is a wide complex tachycardia with a rate of 150. There is poor/absent R-wave progression in the precordial leads. We can eliminate option B since there are P waves present. We are unable to tell if there are bundle branch blocks due to the rhythm.

PART II

PULMONARY

Donna Schweitzer

14

Pulmonary Anatomy and Physiology

CHAPTER OVERVIEW AND OBJECTIVES

The CCRN exam will have a few questions that are directly related to the anatomy of the pulmonary system. Although much of this chapter is explanatory and somewhat theoretical, it is important to be familiar with most of the concepts presented.

Key points:

- *Try to understand the anatomy as it relates to* **clinical application** *rather than memorizing details of anatomy.*
- *This is a long chapter, and it may be useful to read it in sections to improve your understanding of the key concepts.*

After studying this chapter, you should understand the following:

- Pulmonary normal anatomy and physiology.
- Pulmonary gas exchange involves three processes:
  - Ventilation—Movement of air in and out of the lungs
  - Perfusion—Blood flow through the pulmonary capillaries
  - Diffusion—Oxygen and carbon dioxide exchange between the alveoli and capillaries
- Several factors that affect the ability of oxygen to bind and release from hemoglobin.
- Acid–base balance and how it relates to respiratory function.

The major function of the pulmonary system is the exchange of oxygen and carbon dioxide in the body. The pulmonary anatomy includes the thoracic cage, the muscles of the chest, the upper airway, and the lower airway. A grasp of pulmonary physiology is key to understanding pulmonary disturbances; this topic includes gas exchange principles and the analysis of blood gases.

14.1 THE THORACIC CAGE

The thoracic cage (**Fig. 14-1**) is the bony frame of the chest. The thorax is shaped like an inverted cone with the apex about 2.5 cm above the clavicles. The clavicles and first ribs form the protective barrier of the superior portion of the thoracic cage. The diaphragm is the inferior portion of the thoracic cage.

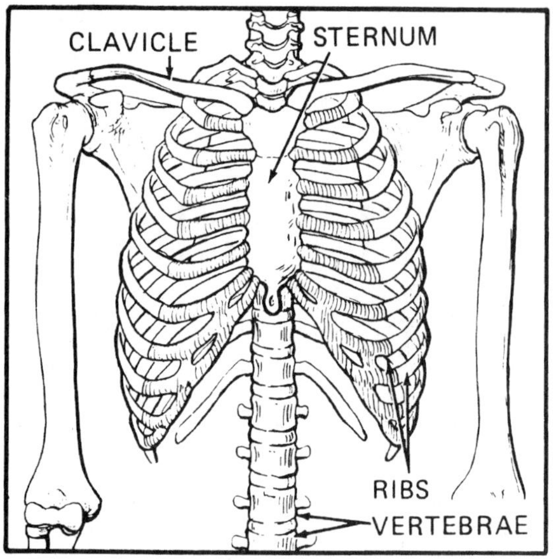

Figure 14-1. The thoracic cage.

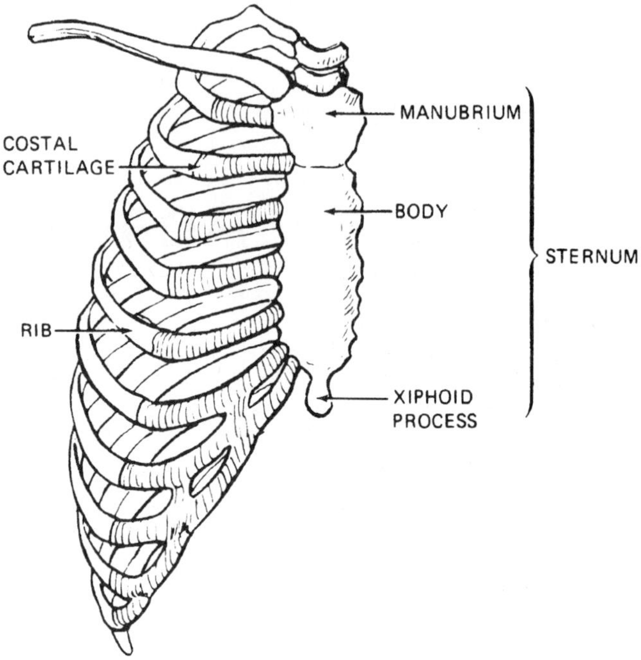

Figure 14-2. The sternum.

The sternum makes up the anterior portion of the thoracic cage and has three connected flat bones: the manubrium, the body, and the xiphoid process. Seven pairs of ribs, called the "true ribs," attach to the sternum. The remaining five ribs form the anterior portion of the thoracic cage. Each rib is attached to the rib above it by intercostal muscles and cartilage. The posterior thoracic cage is formed by the vertebrae and 12 pairs of ribs attached to the vertebrae. The ribs are C-shaped and serve as the bony protective sides of the thoracic cage (**Fig. 14-2**).

Muscles of Respiration

The diaphragm is the major muscle of respiration. On inspiration, the diaphragm contracts (Fig. 14-3), lengthening the chest cavity. The external intercostal muscles contract to raise the ribs, enlarging the diameter of the chest. On expiration, the diaphragm relaxes, becoming dome-shaped and decreasing the size of the thorax (**Fig. 14-3**).

Expiration is passive, accomplished by relaxation of the diaphragm and external intercostal muscles and the lung's normal tendency to collapse. Relaxation of the musculature is the major mechanism for exhalation.

In pulmonary distress and/or disease, *accessory muscles* are used to facilitate inspiration **(which may be an ominous sign).** The accessory muscles of inspiration include the scalene, sternocleidomastoid, trapezius, and pectoralis muscles. The accessory muscles of expiration are made up of the abdominal muscles.

The Lung Parenchyma and Mediastinum. The lung parenchyma and the mediastinum are contained within the bony thoracic cage. The mediastinum is a space midline in the chest and contains the heart, great vessels, trachea, major bronchi, esophagus, thymus gland, lymphatics, and various nerves (**Fig. 14-4**).

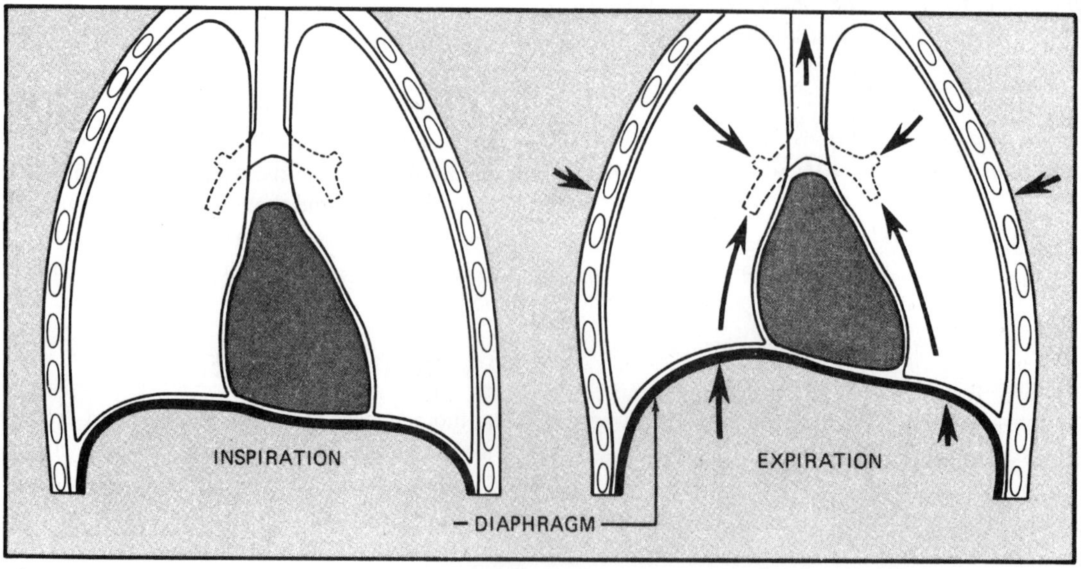

Figure 14-3. The diaphragm on inspiration and expiration.

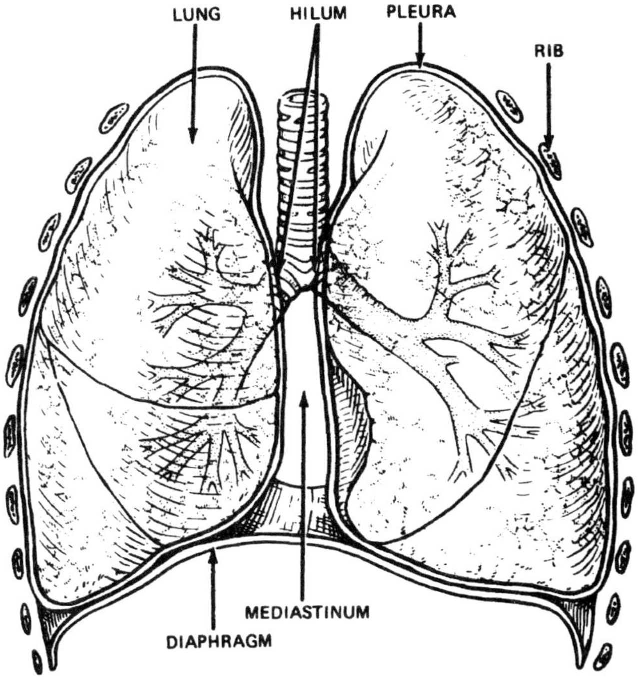

Figure 14-4. The mediastinum and hilum.

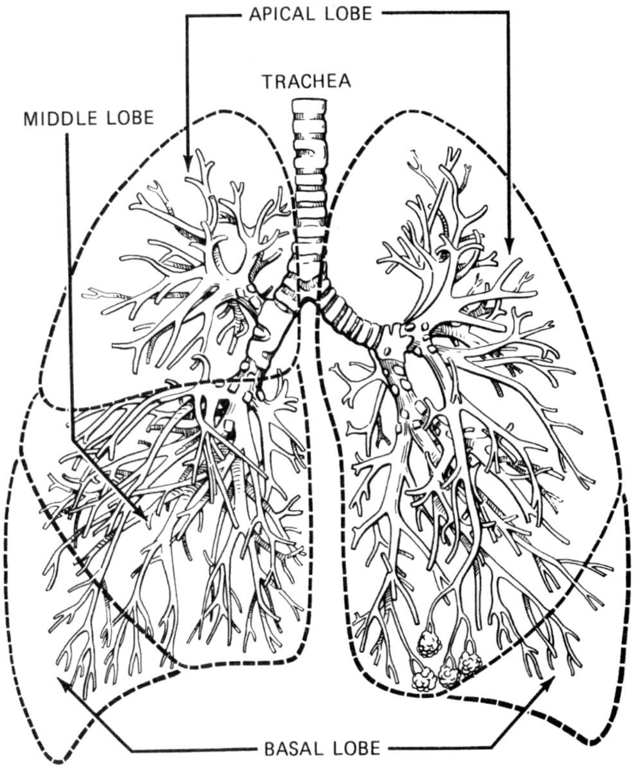

Figure 14-5. Lobes of the lung.

The Pleura. Each lung lies free in its own pleural cavity except at its single point of attachment, the hilum (Fig. 14-4). The pleural covering of each lung is composed of two layers—the visceral and parietal layers. The visceral layer is contiguous with the lung and does not have sensory (pain) nerve fibers. The parietal layer is the outer pleural layer that lines the inside of the thoracic cage and contains sensory nerve fibers. The two pleural layers are separated by a small amount of pleural fluid that allows the two surfaces to slide easily over each other during inspiration and expiration. If the pleura becomes inflamed, movement is restricted and the resulting irritation causes pleuritic pain.

The Lung. Each lung is made up of lobes, with the right lung composed of three lobes and the left lung composed of two lobes. Each lobe of the lung is separated from the adjacent lobe by fissures called lingula. The left lung also has an upper and lower division of its superior lobe, separated by a lingula. The area of the lingula is equal to or smaller than that of the middle lobe of the right lung. Each lobe is further divided into segments: 10 in the right lung and 8 in the left lung (**Fig. 14-5**).

14.2 THE UPPER AIRWAY

The upper airway consists of the mouth, nasopharynx oropharynx, laryngopharynx, and larynx. The purpose of the upper airway is to warm, humidify, and filter the inspired air. This is essential to protect the lower airway and alveoli.

The entire upper airway is lined with a mucous membrane that moisturizes and warms the inspired air by means of the vast blood supply and thick layer of watery mucus produced by serous glands and the thick, tenacious mucus produced by the epithelial goblet cells. The ciliated portions of the upper airway filter pollutants, irritants, and fine particles (1–4 μm in size). Such particles come in contact with the respiratory mucosa and are trapped. They are carried to the pharynx by the mucous blanket, where they are swallowed.

The Nose

Air normally enters the respiratory system through the nose. The nose has skeletal rigidity, which maintains patency during inspiration. The first two-thirds of the nose are cartilaginous and the last third is bony. The nasal septum divides the nose into two fossae; the lateral borders are the alae. The openings between the alae and the nasal septum are the nostrils or nares. The nose has a small inlet and a large outlet, allowing inspired air to have maximum contact with the upper airway mucosa. By sniffing through the nose, inhaled air is directed toward the superior turbinates and olfactory bulb (**Fig. 14-6**).

The first one-third of the nose is lined with nonciliated squamous epithelium. The remaining two-thirds of the nose is lined with ciliated pseudostratified epithelium. Coarse particles larger than 4 μm are entrapped by nasal hairs. The nasopharynx is lined with ciliated pseudostratified epithelium.

The Pharynx

The main function of the pharynx is to collect incoming air from the mouth and nose and project it downward to the trachea. The pharynx is subdivided into the nasopharynx, the oropharynx, and the laryngopharynx (Fig. 14-6).

The nasopharynx is the space behind the oral and nasal cavities and above the soft palate; it contains the orifices of the eustachian tubes. The pharyngeal tonsils (adenoids), an important defense mechanism of the pulmonary system, are in the superior nasopharynx.

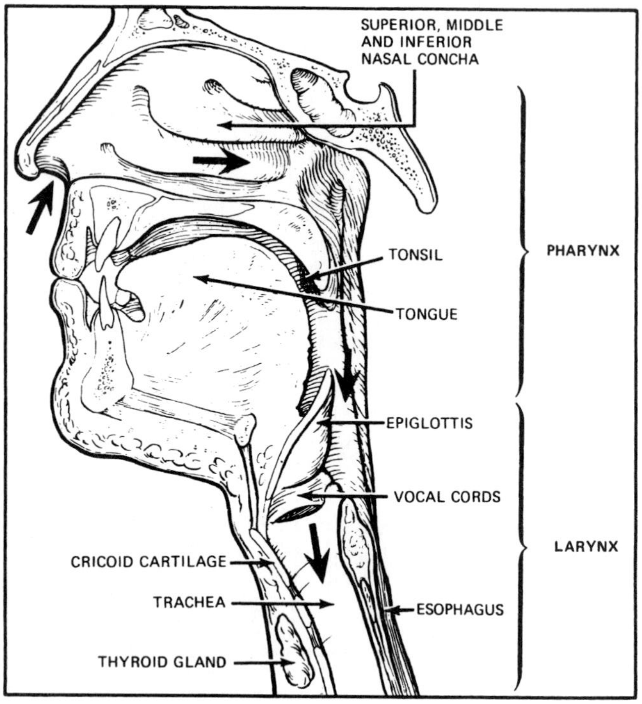

Figure 14-6. The upper airway, pharynx, and larynx.

The oropharynx is the area from the soft palate to the base of the tongue. The function of the oropharynx is to facilitate the passage of air and food. To prevent aspiration into the lungs, the epiglottis secures the airway by closing over the glottis when food is swallowed. The epiglottis is only part of the oropharynx during swallowing, as it lies completely within the larynx during respiration. In addition, the oropharynx contains the Palatine tonsil, which is a large mass of lymphoid tissue that is thought to aid in the prevention of the respiratory and gastrointestinal infections.

The laryngopharynx is the lower portion of the pharynx, extending from the base of the tongue to the opening of the esophagus. The laryngopharynx contains muscles within its wall, the pharyngeal constrictors, that aid in the mechanism of swallowing.

The Larynx

The larynx lies in the anterior portion of the neck, extending from cervical vertebrae C4 to C6 and connecting the upper and lower airway. It aids in speech and is an essential part of the mechanism of coughing. The larynx is composed of cartilage connected by membranes and muscles. The laryngeal mucosa is stratified squamous epithelium above the vocal cords and pseudostratified columnar epithelium below.

The glottis is the opening into the larynx. The epiglottis, a flexible cartilage attached to the thyroid cartilage helps prevent foreign material from entering the airway by covering the glottis during swallowing. In the adult, the thyroid cartilage (**Fig. 14-7**) is the narrowest part of the air passage of the larynx. As muscles in the larynx contract, the vocal cords change shape and vibrate. This vibration of the vocal cords produces sound.

The **cricoid cartilage** is a complete ring located just below the thyroid cartilage, *where the vocal cords are located*. The cricothyroid membrane is an avascular structure that connects

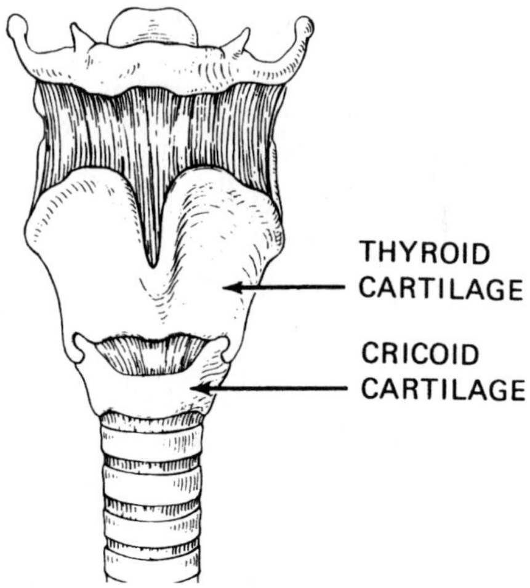

Figure 14-7. The thyroid–cricoid cartilages.

the thyroid and cricoid cartilage s. **It is through this membrane that an airway may be established in an emergency.** Using this anatomical landmark during a cricothyrotomy ensures the posterior wall of the larynx and vocal cords are not injured.

14.3 LUNG DEFENSE MECHANISMS

The mucociliary escalator is the primary protective mechanism for the entire respiratory system. The entire respiratory tree is lined with varying types of epithelial cells as well as cilia, which are fine, hair-like filaments projecting into the airway lumen. Goblet cells in the epithelium produce watery, thick mucus which covers the inner lumen of the airway. The mucous lining is called the mucous blanket. Various mechanisms move the mucous blanket to the pharynx, where it will be swallowed; to the larynx, where coughing will expel it; and to the nose, where it will be expelled by blowing and sneezing. Cilia lining the larger airways help to move the mucous blanket up the respiratory tract by the cilias' continuous undulating movement, referred to as the mucociliary escalator (**Fig. 14-8**).

The sneeze reflex is a reaction to irritation in the nose. The cough reflex is a reaction to irritation in the upper airway distal to the nose. Both processes are complex mechanisms that require the integration of increased intrathoracic pressure, complete and tight closure of the epiglottis and vocal cords, and strong contraction of the abdominal musculature, diaphragm, and intercostal muscles.

14.4 THE LOWER AIRWAY

The lower airway consists of two divisions, the tracheobronchial tree and the lung parenchyma. The tracheobronchial tree is a system of progressively narrower conducting tubes providing air passage to the alveoli. The trachea divides into the right and left mainstem bronchi. Further subdivisions include the bronchi, bronchioles, terminal bronchioles, and alveoli.

Trachea

The trachea extends from approximately C6 to the carina, the point of bifurcation of the right and left mainstem bronchi.

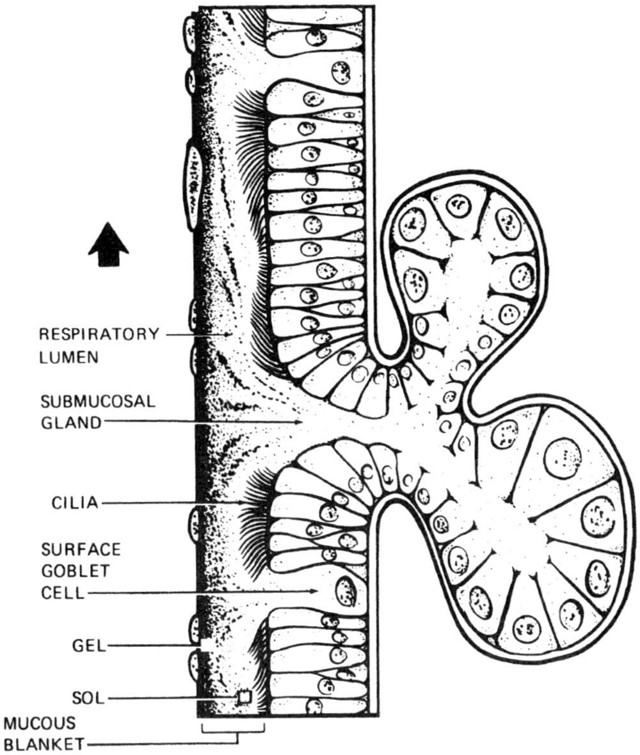

Figure 14-8. The mucociliary escalator.

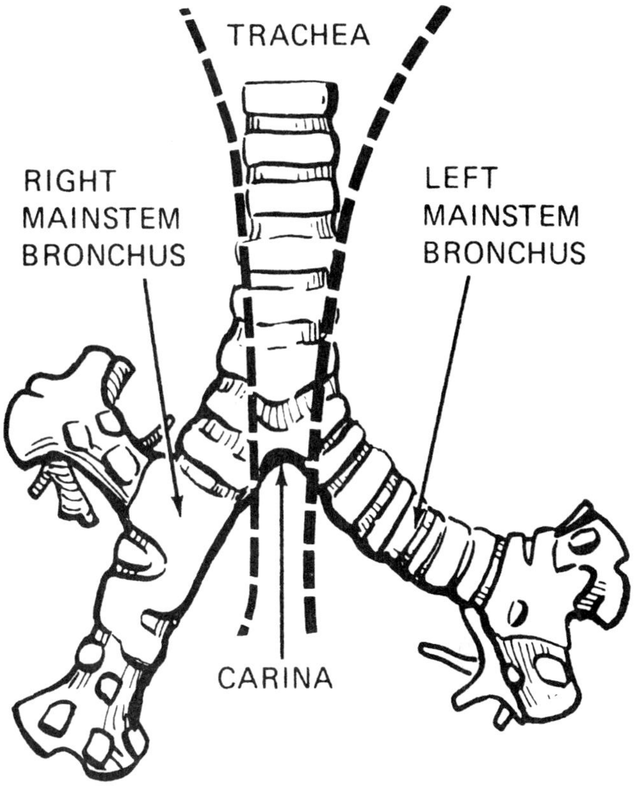

Figure 14-10. Right and left mainstem bronchi.

It is composed of C-shaped cartilaginous rings with a posterior muscle that is membranous and friable. This muscle relaxes on inspiration, increasing the tracheal diameter. On exhalation, the muscle contracts, decreasing the tracheal diameter. Occasionally, the muscle relaxes and bows in on exhalation, decreasing the effectiveness of the mucociliary stream in clearing secretions from the lungs (**Fig. 14-9**).

The trachea divides into the right and left mainstem bronchi at the carina, located at the angle of Louis at the sternomanubrial junction, at about the second intercostal space. The *right mainstem bronchus* comes off the trachea in almost a straight line, while the *left mainstem bronchus* comes off the trachea at an angle of approximately 40 degrees. The right mainstem bronchus is wider in diameter than the left. **Foreign matter tends to lodge in the right mainstem bronchus because of its size and the angle at which it takes off from the trachea** (**Fig. 14-10**).

KEY CLINICAL CONCEPT

Remembering that foreign material is more likely to fall through the right mainstem can be helpful when trying to determine the cause or possibility of aspiration

The right and left mainstem bronchi separate into 22 divisions before the terminal respiratory bronchioles. These divisions are cartilaginous; the terminal respiratory bronchioles are small tubes without cartilage. Only smooth muscle surrounds the respiratory epithelium. Contraction of this smooth muscle results in bronchospasm.

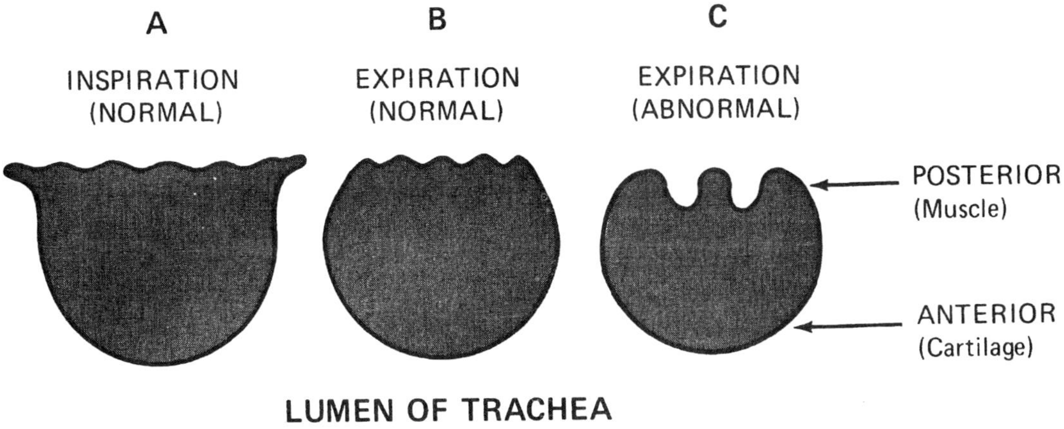

Figure 14-9. Movement of posterior muscles of the trachea.

The respiratory bronchioles branch into alveolar ducts and then into the alveoli, which make up the lung parenchyma. The alveoli and alveolar ducts have common walls, termed septa, which play an important role in the elastic recoil of the lung. The septal wall is composed of smooth muscle that contracts to narrow the lumen of the alveolar duct.

Bronchial Circulation

Bronchi and other lung tissues and structures require their own blood supply for nutrition. There is usually one right bronchial artery that originates from an intercostal artery and two left bronchial arteries that originate from the aorta. The bronchial circulation is not usually involved in alveolar gas exchange. The bronchial veins join the pulmonary veins before arriving at the left atrium, mixing unoxygenated blood with the highly oxygenated pulmonary venous blood.

Alveolar Sacs and Cells

At the terminal end of the tracheobronchial tree are the alveolar sacs. These dead-end structures prevent ambient air from going further. The sacs, made up of 16 or 17 alveoli, each share a common wall with adjacent sacs (**Fig. 14-11**).

The 274 to 790 million alveoli in the normal lung comprise an average total surface area of 40 to 100 m^2, approximately the size of a football field. This surface area is directly related to body length (not weight) and decreases by about 5% per decade.

Alveolar Epithelium

Alveolar sacs are comprised of a single layer of epithelium cells. The alveolar epithelium contains two cell types:

- Type I cells are characterized by cytoplasmic extensions and make up most of the lung. These cells are easily injured or inflamed.
- *Type II alveolar cells* are found where one extension interfaces with another. Type II cells help protect the alveoli by quickly dividing when Type I cells are injured and secreting several antimicrobial products. Type II cells contain organelles that synthesize surfactant.

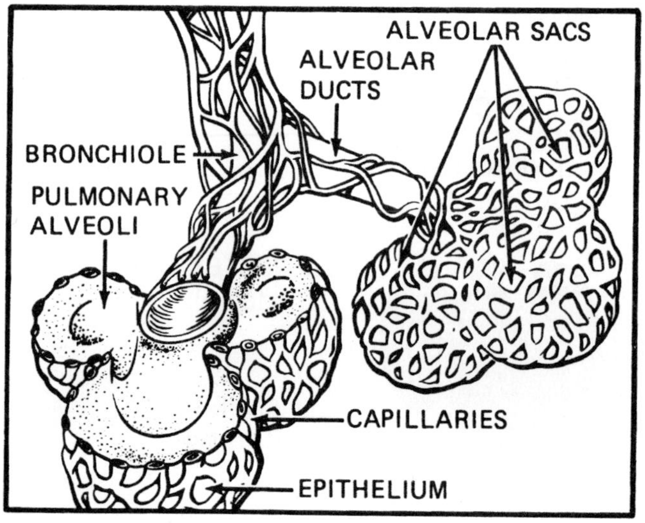

Figure 14-11. Terminal bronchiole and alveolar sac.

QUICK TIP! Damage and dysfunction of the Type II alveolar cells are associated with ARDS pathophysiology.

Pulmonary Surfactant

Alveolar epithelium is lined with a phospholipid protein fluid called *surfactant*. The phospholipid is insoluble but highly permeable to all gases. The function of surfactant is to reduce the surface tension in the alveoli to help keep the alveoli open. Two pathologic states that are complicated by insufficient or absent surfactant are:

1. Infant respiratory distress syndrome (IRDS)—formerly known as hyaline membrane disease
2. Acute respiratory distress syndrome (ARDS)

Surfactant functions by forming a thin, monomolecular layer at the interface of the air and fluid in the alveoli. Without surfactant, an air–fluid interface would produce surface tension that would collapse the small alveoli. By preventing the development of the air–fluid interface, surfactant decreases the surface tension in the alveoli. Surfactant provides stability to smaller alveoli, which have a greater pressure and tend to collapse. Without the proper amount of surfactant, there is a filtration, or movement, of fluid from the alveolar wall capillaries into the alveoli, leading to development of pulmonary edema and/or ARDS. In sum, the effects of the loss of surfactant include stiff, less compliant lungs; atelectasis; and fluid-filled alveoli.

The alveoli are where gas exchange occurs. Oxygen diffuses across the alveolar epithelium, the basement membrane, and the small interstitial space, and through the capillary membrane, the plasma fluid, and the erythrocyte membrane. At this point, the capillary is so small that the erythrocytes must line up in a single column to move through it. Oxygen diffuses rapidly through the erythrocyte membrane and attaches to the hemoglobin molecule of the erythrocyte. Carbon dioxide molecules diffuse across the alveolar-capillary membrane in the opposite direction at a rate 20 times faster than oxygen. The capillary endothelium is very sensitive and is easily damaged by endotoxins, oxygen, and other noxious substances.

14.5 PULMONARY CIRCULATION

The lung receives deoxygenated blood from the right side of the heart via the pulmonary artery. The oxygenated blood is returned to the left side of the heart via the pulmonary vein, where it is pumped from the left ventricle through the cardiovascular system.

The lungs' arterial system follows the bronchial tree, bifurcating at each bronchial division and following close to the bronchus and its subdivisions. As the bronchioles become smaller, some arteries fail to bifurcate and nearby arteries send out branches from their stem to provide oxygenated blood to the central part of the alveolar tissue (**Fig. 14-12**).

The total volume and rate of pulmonary blood circulation is about 5 L/min. Because of gravity, blood flow is greatest to the dependent portions of the lung. Thus, in an erect person, the apex of the lung will have the least circulating blood volume. When the person is lying down, the anterior lung surfaces will have the least circulating blood volume.

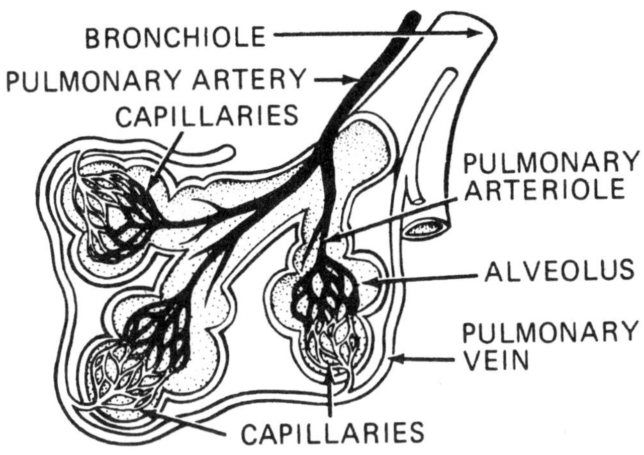

Figure 14-12. Blood flow in the parenchyma.

QUICK TIP! The *"Good Lung Down/Bad Lung Up"* philosophy: Turning the patient with the "good lung down," employs the philosophy that the healthy lung may benefit from improved (dependent) blood flow to well-ventilated alveoli improving the SaO_2, while the diseased lung becomes elevated, thereby improving aeration and ventilation.

The erythrocyte completes the pulmonary circulation very rapidly (within 0.75 seconds at rest). This rapid circulation helps maintain adequate perfusion. The total volume of blood in the pulmonary arteries, veins, and capillaries is about 500 to 750 mL in the average adult male or about 10% to 15% of the total blood volume, serving as a reservoir in times of increased cardiac output.

14.6 CONTROL OF VENTILATION

Three major factors control ventilation: neural, central chemical, and peripheral chemical control mechanisms.

Neural Control

The respiratory center is in the medullary portion of the brain stem. Neurons initiate impulses that result in inspiration. An increase in the rate of impulses results in an increase in respiratory rate; an increase in their strength increases tidal volume.

Normally, chemical factors keep the inspiratory and expiratory centers in balance, resulting in normal ventilatory patterns. The inspiratory center is in the dorsal aspect of the *medulla oblongata*, in close association to the *vagus nerve* and the glossopharyngeal nerves. There appears to be an inherent automaticity in the electrical impulse release for inspiration. The apneustic center, in the pons, acts to prevent the interruption of these inspiratory impulses.

If the apneustic center takes control over the normally balanced ventilation pattern, **apneustic breathing** occurs, which is characterized by gasping deep inhalation with a pause following inhalation and a short expiratory phase. This is typically associated with a critical condition.

Expiration control is in the *pneumotaxic center,* located in the upper pons. The neurons there transmit impulses to limit inspiration. When the **pneumotaxic center** controls ventilation, there is irregular, deep, shallow breathing with randomly spaced periods of varying lengths of apnea.

The walls of the pulmonary bronchi and bronchioles have stretch receptors that interact with the vagus nerve in what is known as the *Hering–Breuer reflex.* When they become overstretched, there is a feedback mechanism to the inspiratory center to prevent hyperinflation of the lungs.

KEY CLINICAL CONCEPT

Central and peripheral chemoreceptors monitor and respond to the chemical composition of blood and fluid around them to alter the respiratory rate and depth in an attempt to correct acidosis or alkalotic states. Acidosis, an increase in hydrogen ions, will stimulate both receptors to increase respiratory rate and depth to correct acidosis. A decrease in PaO_2 will stimulate the peripheral receptors to increase respiration to restore oxygen levels.

Central Chemical Control

Change in cerebral spinal fluid (CSF) pH plays a critical role in the regulation of respirations because PCO_2 is a foundation for cerebral perfusion. Change in CSF pH due to acidosis causes direct relaxation of the smooth muscles and inversely alkalotic CSF causes smooth muscle contraction. Understanding this concept and its application to the critically ill patient is crucial to understanding respiratory pathophysiology.

$Paco_2$ provides the normal neurochemical control of the respiratory cycle because of its effect on the CSF pH. A rise in CSF hydrogen ion concentration will first increase respiratory depth and then the respiratory rate. The central chemical control is less or not sensitive to decreases in PaO_2.

Peripheral Chemical Control

Chemoreceptors are also located at the bifurcation of the internal and external carotid arteries, carotid bodies, and aortic bodies at the aortic arch. These highly vascular neural bodies are stimulated by any decrease in oxygen supply, such as decreased blood flow, decreased hemoglobin, increased pH, or increased $Paco_2$. The most important action of the peripheral chemoreceptors is their quick response to arterial hypoxemia. Stimulation of the carotid and/or aortic bodies will increase cerebral cortical activity, resulting in tachycardia, hypertension, and increased respiratory rate, tidal volume, pulmonary resistance, bronchial smooth muscle tone, and adrenal gland secretions.

KEY CLINICAL CONCEPT

The compensatory vasoconstriction provided by stimulation to the carotid and aortic bodies is why the **Trendelenburg** position is no longer recommended during hypotension. **Trendelenburg** "fools" the receptors into thinking the BP is better when it is not. Best practice instead suggests lying the patient flat with legs elevated if possible (during resuscitation).

Factors Affecting Ventilation

Certain drugs depress the respiratory center by decreasing alveolar ventilation or blocking the central respiratory center.

Decreased alveolar ventilation is characterized by shallow respirations and a respiratory rate of less than 12 breaths per min.

Chronic respiratory disease may alter normal respiratory patterns. Patients with chronic CO_2 retention have a constantly elevated $Paco_2$, thus decreasing the peripheral chemoreceptors' sensitivity to changes in hydrogen ion concentration. A decrease in the level of arterial oxygen pressure (Pao_2) stimulates ventilation. High-flow oxygen therapy may result in apnea, suppressing the hypoxic drive mechanism.

14.7 PROCESS OF RESPIRATION

The process of respiration has four phases. Phase I is ventilation, the movement of ambient air into and out of the lungs. Phase II is the diffusion of oxygen and carbon dioxide in the alveoli. Phase III is the delivery of oxygen and removal of carbon dioxide from the cells. Phase IV is the regulation of ventilation.

Phase I: Ventilation

Normal barometric pressure at sea level is 760 mm Hg. For the average healthy person at rest, the intrapleural pressure is slightly subatmospheric at 755 mm Hg. If the pressures were equal, there would be no flow of air into or out of the lung.

As inspiration begins, the thoracic cage increases in size, producing a negative intrapleural pressure compared to the atmosphere and resulting in airflow into the lungs. If one considers atmospheric pressure to be zero (0), then resting intrapleural pressure is −5 and inspiratory intrapleural pressure is −10. As inspiratory muscle activity ends, the normal elastic recoil of the lung decreases the size of the thoracic cage and gas flows out of the lung.

Lung Pressures

The pulmonary system is a low-pressure system. It allows the capillaries to distend easily to accommodate increased volumes from the systemic circulatory system in times of distress and/or exertion. This distensibility helps regulate resistance to blood flow through the pulmonary system. In the normal disease-free lung, the average pulmonary artery systolic pressure is 25 (±2) mm Hg and the average diastolic pressure is 10 (±2) mm Hg. The pressure necessary to move blood from the right side to left side of the heart is the left atrial pressure, or the pulmonary capillary wedge pressure, or pulmonary artery occlusive pressure (PAOP). **The normal left atrial PAOP is 8 to 12 mm Hg. The mean pulmonary artery pressure must always be higher than the left atrial pressure to move blood from the right heart through the lungs to the left atrium.**

Compliance

Compliance is a measure of the distensibility of the lungs and thorax. Compliance is expressed as change in volume (V) for a change in the intra-alveolar pressure (P). Greater compliance means that there is a larger volume change in the lung for each pressure change. Reduced compliance means that there is less volume change in the lung for each pressure change. *In other words, the more pressure needed to change the volume in the lung, the less compliance.* The standard measure is units of L/cm H_2O. The normal lung plus thorax compliance of an adult is around 0.1 L/cm H_2O.

TABLE 14-1. CAUSES OF DECREASED LUNG COMPLIANCE

Intrathoracic	*Extrathoracic*
Atelectasis	Flail chest
Pneumonia	Barrel chest
Pleural effusion	Pectus excavatum
Empyema	Pectus carinatum
Lung abscess	Kyphosis
Bronchospasm	Scoliosis
Pulmonary edema	Kyphoscoliosis
Bronchitis	Obesity
Asthma	Abdominal compartment syndrome
Emphysema	
Acute respiratory distress syndrome (ARDS)	
Tension pneumothorax	

Any disease that stiffens the lungs will decrease compliance. Diseases that increase congestion in the lungs—such as atelectasis, pneumonia, or pulmonary edema—result in decreased lung compliance and decreased gas exchange. Space-occupying neoplasms, infections, or increased extravascular lung water also decrease lung compliance (**Table 14-1**).

Any condition that limits the ability of the bony thorax to expand will also decrease lung compliance. An example of an extrinsic restrictive cause of decreased compliance is third-trimester *pregnancy.* During the third trimester, the abdominal contents are displaced upward, preventing the diaphragm from descending fully and decreasing the extent of chest wall expansion. *Obesity* and *abdominal distention* also prevent full movement of the diaphragm. The obese patient has decreased lung compliance because of the excess weight on the upper torso. The intercostal muscles cannot function efficiently as they attempt to lift the weight. *Postoperative binders* and *chest splints* decrease lung compliance over large segments of the thorax by limiting its expansion.

There are two types of compliance, static and dynamic. Static compliance (Cst) is the change in lung volume per unit of airway pressure change when the lungs are motionless. Cst can be measured only when there is no flow of gas, at the end of inspiration or expiration. Measurements of Cst provide a reliable index of lung compliance when no airway disease is present, as the presence of airway disease alters the rate of gas flow from the mouth to the alveoli, resulting in inaccurate values. If airway disease is present, most of the resistance to airflow will be in the medium-sized bronchi.

Dynamic compliance (Cdyn) is the measurement of the lungs when in motion, at the end of inspiration and expiration. Dynamic compliance can easily be tested in the clinical area. To get an estimate of the dynamic compliance for the patient on mechanical ventilation, divide the tidal volume (V_T) by the peak airway pressure (PAP). Normal dynamic compliance is about 35 to 55 mL/cm H_2O.

Airway resistance results from the impedance of gas flow by the walls of the airway or obstruction, changing the ratio of alveolar pressure against the rate of airflow. Airway resistance is increased by secretions, artificial airways, endotracheal tubes, bronchospasm, laryngeal or tracheal strictures, edema,

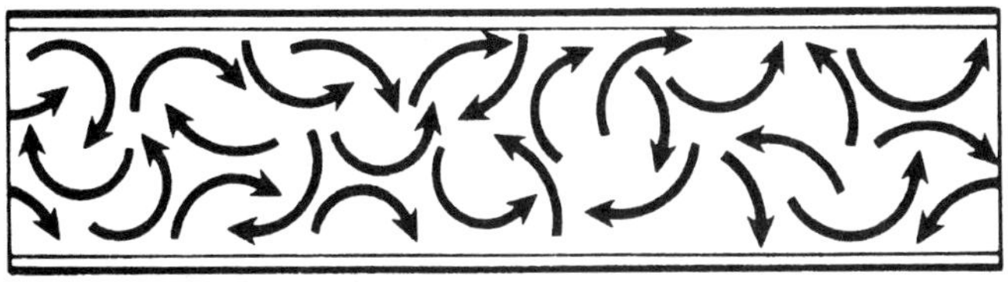

Figure 14-13. Turbulent airflow.

emphysema, or space-occupying lesions. A measure of airway resistance can be made by comparing the Cst and Cdyn.

Elastic Recoil

Intra-alveolar septa are a major factor in the elastic recoil of the interstitial parenchyma. The thorax, pleura, and lung parenchyma have opposing elastic forces. The fluid lining the alveoli and the interstitial parenchyma tends to collapse the lungs, while the thoracic cage and pleura tend to expand them. As long as the thoracic cage and pleura are patent, these elastic forces balance each other. If the integrity of the pleura is compromised, the parenchymal forces become greater and the lung collapses.

Airflow

There are three basic types of airflow within the lung airways, turbulent, transitional, and laminar. Turbulent airflow occurs in large chambers such as the nose and oral pharynx (**Fig. 14-13**). Transitional airflow occurs in large-to-medium airways at points of bifurcation and/or narrowing. As air flows down the tracheobronchial tree, it branches into smaller and smaller tubes, creating transitional airflow (**Fig. 14-14**). Laminar airflow occurs in thin, flat, continuous sheets. The outermost layer of air has minimal contact with the walls of the air passage, providing slight filtering in the small peripheral airways (**Fig. 14-15**).

Lung Volumes

The **total lung capacity (TLC)** is the maximum amount of gas that the lungs can hold (**Fig. 14-16**). The normal amount is about 4000 to 7000 mL. The TLC is composed of four discrete lung volumes measured by spirometry: the **inspiratory reserve volume (IRV)**, the **tidal volume (V_T)**, the **expiratory reserve volume (ERV)**, and the **residual volume (RV)**.

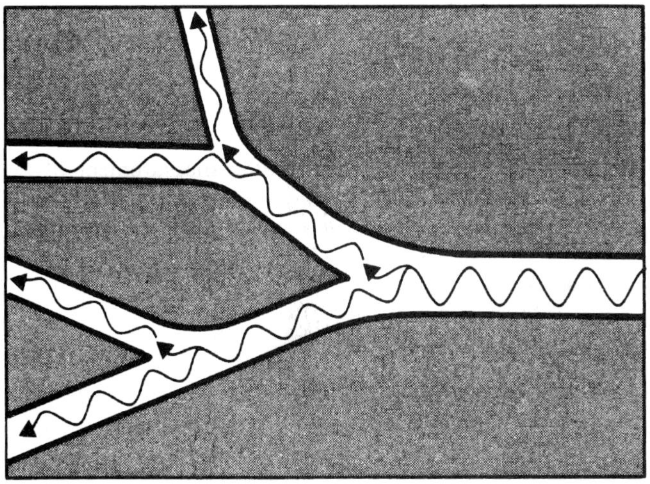

Figure 14-14. Transitional airflow.

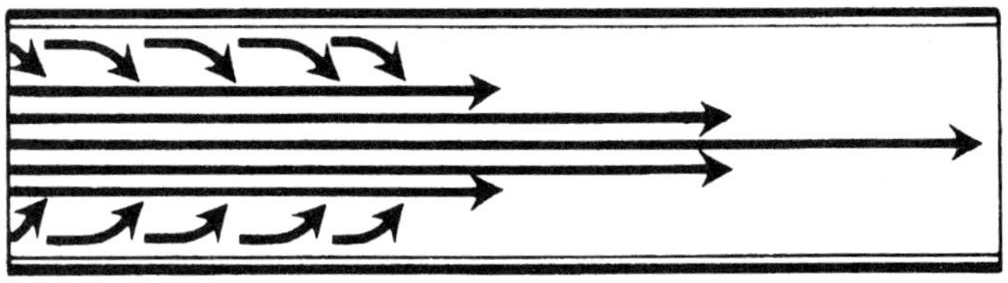

Figure 14-15. Laminar airflow.

This relationship is expressed by the equation TLC = IRV + V_T + ERV + RV.

IRV is the amount of reserve or extra gas that can be inhaled at the end of a normal inspiration. Normal IRV may be as much as 3000 mL.

V_T is the amount of gas that is exhaled or inhaled during normal breathing. Normal V_T is 5 to 10 mL/kg or about 350 to 600 mL in a young adult.

ERV is the amount of gas that can be exhaled after a normal expiration. Normal ERV is about 1000 to 1500 mL.

RV is the amount of gas that always remains in the lungs and cannot be exhaled.

There are four lung capacities, which represent the combination of two or more lung volumes. The values listed for lung capacities are averages and will differ according to body size, weight, and age.

Vital capacity (VC) is the amount of gas that can be forcefully exhaled after a maximum inspiration (VC = V_T + IRV + ERV). Normal is about 4000 to 5000 mL.

The **inspiratory capacity (IC)** is the amount of gas that can be inhaled after a normal exhalation (IC = V_T + IRV). Normal is about 3500 mL.

The **functional residual capacity (FRC)** is the amount of air in the lungs after normal expiration (FRC = ERV + RV). Normal is about 2000 to 3000 mL.

These respiratory volumes and capacities can be used to establish a baseline and monitor the effectiveness of treatment modalities. VC, inspiratory force, and tidal volume are the most frequently measured parameters of respiratory muscle function.

Dead Space

Dead space (V_D) is the amount of inhaled gas that does not take part in gas exchange. Gas exchange occurs only in the terminal bronchioles and alveoli. *There are two types of dead space, anatomic and alveolar.* The conducting airways are ventilated but not perfused by the pulmonary artery and therefore do not participate in gas exchange creating an anatomic dead space. *Anatomic dead space* is estimated to be 1 mL/lb of ideal body weight. For a 150 lb man with each 500-mL tidal volume breath, approximately 350 mL reaches the alveoli. A more accurate measurement can be obtained when a patient is mechanically ventilated. When areas of *alveoli* are not perfused **(such as with a pulmonary emboli)** no gas exchange can occur creating *alveolar dead space.* The total volume of the *anatomic dead space* and *alveolar dead space* is called the physiologic dead space.

The amount of inhaled air that reaches the alveoli and takes part in gas exchange is alveolar ventilation (V_A). In a stable state, the arterial carbon dioxide is inversely related to alveolar ventilation and indicates adequacy of gas exchange. V_A is equal to V_E *(minute ventilation)* minus V_D. *V_E is normally 5 to 10 L/min and is measured by multiplying V_T × respiratory rate.*

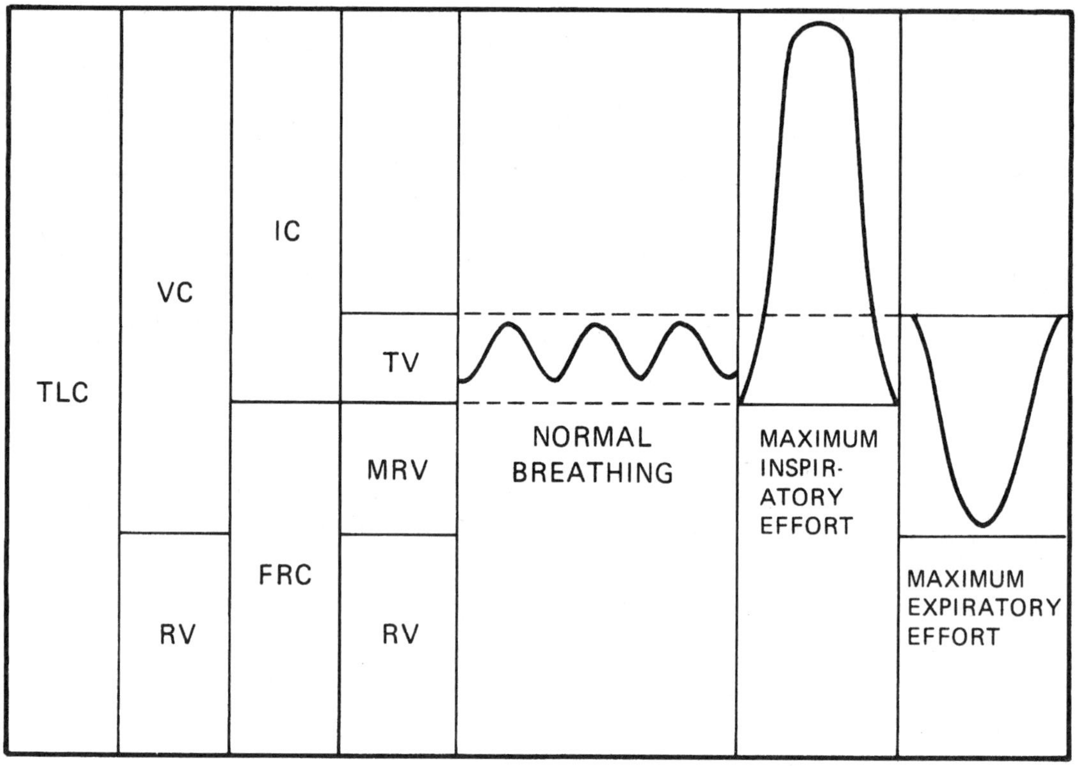

Figure 14-16. Lung volumes and capacities.

Phase II: Gas Diffusion

On inspiration, oxygen concentration or pressure is greater in the alveoli than in the erythrocytes, and the carbon dioxide concentration is greater in the erythrocytes than the alveoli. Therefore, the gas diffuses from the highest level of concentration toward the lower level of concentration.

The actual area of space the gases have to cross to diffuse is very thin, 0.2 to 0.5 μm. The alveoli and capillaries are so small and thin and dense that, under the microscope, they look like a single sheet of blood. Instead, they are made up of six layers: the surfactant, alveolar membrane, interstitial space, capillary endothelial cells, plasma, and erythrocyte membrane. The gases must diffuse through these layers, known as the **alveolar-capillary membrane**, for gas exchange to take place. If the membrane becomes thickened, as in pulmonary edema or interstitial pulmonary fibrosis, the diffusion of gases is slowed. Another factor affecting diffusion through the alveolar-capillary membrane is the available surface area. If an area of the lung is filled with fluid or pus, gas diffusion in that area will be slowed or stopped completely. In emphysema, the alveolar septa collapse, destroying the alveolar structure and decreasing the surface area available for diffusion.

The specific gas composition of the alveolar, arterial, and venous compartments will directly affect the diffusibility of gases (**Table 14-2**).

14.8 OXYGEN TRANSPORT

Once oxygen has penetrated the erythrocyte membrane, it is carried through the systemic circulatory system to all body tissues. Oxygen is transported in only two possible forms in the body, either dissolved in plasma or combined with hemoglobin. The amount of oxygen dissolved in the plasma is very small and amounts to 0.003 mL/100 mL of blood, or 3% of the total body oxygen. Pao_2 measures dissolved oxygen. The remaining 97% of oxygen is transported through the system's circulation in combination with hemoglobin (Hgb); this combination is called oxyhemoglobin. *The transport of oxygen to body tissues is influenced most by cardiac output, hemoglobin concentration, and oxygen–hemoglobin binding and releasing factors.*

TABLE 14-2. COMPOSITION OF PULMONARY GASES

Alveolar	*Arterial*	*Venous*	*Atmospheric*
$P_{H_2O} = 47$	$P_{H_2O} = 47$	$P_{H_2O} = 47$	$P_{H_2O} = 47$
$P_{ACO_2} = 40$	$P_{aCO_2} = 40$	$P_{VCO_2} = 46$	$P_{ICO_2} = 0$
$P_{AO_2} = 100–110$	$P_{aO_2} = 92$	$P_{VO_2} = 40$	$P_{IO_2} = 150$
$P_{AN_2} = 563$	$P_{aN_2} = 563$	$P_{VN_2} = 563$	$P_{IN_2} = 563$
			760 mm Hg

A, alveolar; a, arterial; CO_2, carbon dioxide; H_2O, water; I, inspired; N_2, nitrogen; O_2, oxygen; P, pressure or partial pressure; V, venous.

QUICK TIP! **After oxygen has entered the red blood cell, the blood cells need to be circulated to the peripheral tissues to drop off oxygen. An additional three questions (based on the equations below) can assist in troubleshooting when the patient is displaying signs of poor oxygen delivery (cyanosis, shortness of breath, lactic acidosis):**

1. What is the patient's hemoglobin? Is the patient bleeding? Or anemic?
2. How is the heart function? What is the blood pressure, ejection fraction, or cardiac output?
3. Is there something affecting the hemoglobin's ability to bind or drop off oxygen? Is the patient acidotic, receiving blood products, running a fever?

Cardiac output is usually 4 to 8 L/min. As the cardiac output varies, the quantity of blood oxygenated in the lungs also varies. In normal, healthy lungs, a slight decrease in cardiac output will not greatly alter oxygen content. A markedly decreased cardiac output will alter oxygen content, although the available blood will be maximally oxygenated. *If hemoglobin is low, cardiac output will increase to help compensate and maintain an adequate oxygen content.* The amount of oxygen transported per minute is determined by the cardiac output, even though there are other contributing factors.

Oxygen content (Cao_2) is the maximum potential amount of oxygen the blood can carry. It is expressed as milliliters of oxygen per 100 mL of blood. **Cao_2 = Hgb × 1.34 (cubic centimeters of oxygen) × Sao_2 + (Po_2 × 0.003).** In calculating the oxygen content, the dissolved oxygen in plasma (Pao_2) is usually not included because of its small contribution. Oxygen content is equal to the actual amount of oxygen in both the plasma and the erythrocytes.

QUICK TIP! It would be unlikely that the exam will ask you to calculate the equation for arterial oxygen content. However, the exam will expect you to know that the influence of Hgb and SaO_2 is greater than that of PO_2, according to the equation.

Oxygen saturation (Sao_2) is the ratio comparing the actual amount of oxygen that could be carried with the amount carried, which is expressed as a percentage.

Oxygen Capacity

Hemoglobin has a natural affinity for oxygen. Once the oxygen diffuses through the erythrocyte membrane, it readily attaches to the hemoglobin molecule. With a hemoglobin level of 15 g/100 mL, 100 mL of blood will have enough hemoglobin to carry 20 mL of oxygen. Hemoglobin cannot be oversaturated; 100% is the maximum under human physiologic conditions.

Oxygen Transport

Oxygen transport/oxygen delivery (DO_2) is the amount of oxygen delivered to the cells expressed as milliliters of oxygen per minute. Oxygen transport (DO_2) = Cao_2 × cardiac output × 10, expressed in milliliters per minute. Normal oxygen transport is between 600 and 1000 mL/min or 10 to 12 mL/kg.

The combination of oxygen content and oxygen transport is a more reliable index of oxygenation than the Pao_2 alone because the hemoglobin level and cardiac output are taken into consideration.

Oxygen Consumption (Vo_2)

Oxygen consumption is the amount of oxygen used per minute. Normal Vo_2 is approximately 3.5 mL/kg/min. A 70-kg person would use approximately 245 mL/min of oxygen at rest. Under normal circumstances, only 25% to 30% of the transported oxygen is used by the cells. If oxygen transport is 1000 mL/min and Vo_2 is 250 mL/min, 25% of the oxygen transported was used. The oxygen extraction rate is the difference between the oxygen transported and the oxygen consumed. As the oxygen extraction rate increases, cellular oxygenation is threatened. Rates over 40% require assessment of oxygen transport and consumption components.

QUICK TIP! When a patient is receiving supplemental oxygen, the pulse oximetry does not assess for adequate ventilation. A sedated or medicated patient's respiratory rate or depth may be decreased, causing an increase in $PaCO_2$ while SaO_2 readings are near normal due to supplemental oxygen. Capnography is a better assessment of ventilation when oxygen is in use. Clinical judgment should be utilized regarding the use of capnography, but is a safer assessment of ventilation in the critically ill patient.

Oxyhemoglobin Dissociation

Factors affecting oxygen–hemoglobin binding and releasing include temperature, pH, Pco_2, acidosis or alkalosis, and 2,3-diphosphoglycerate (2,3-DPG). The oxyhemoglobin curve is an S-shaped curve representing the nonlinear relationship of the Pao_2 and the Sao_2 (**Fig. 14-17**).

The amount of oxygen dissolved in the plasma, the Pao_2, provides the driving pressure that forces oxygen to combine with hemoglobin. The driving pressure of dissolved oxygen exists until the alveolar (PAo_2) and arterial (Pao_2) pressures are almost equal. With the oxygen pressure gradient between the alveolus and the erythrocyte at equilibrium, the point of the normal curve is at the upper right. In the healthy person, the oxygen tension is 95 to 97 mm Hg with a hemoglobin saturation (Sao_2) of about 97%.

There is a steep downslope portion to the curve, indicating a move from the lungs into the systemic circulation. The Sao_2 and the Pao_2 are dropping because the hemoglobin is readily giving up oxygen to the tissue capillaries. As the hemoglobin moves through the body, the Pao_2 drops and hemoglobin *loses its affinity for oxygen,* readily releasing it into the tissues. The P50 is a point of reference on the curve when the Sao_2 drops to 50% and the partial pressure of arterial oxygen is about 27 mm Hg. At the P50, the hemoglobin begins to *give up its oxygen much less readily.* The normal curve can be shifted to the right or to the left by many factors. A shift in either direction indicates a change from the normal Sao_2 and Pao_2 relationship.

A shift to the right occurs in acidosis, hypercarbia (increased carbon dioxide), and fever. A shift to the right means that there is less oxygen in the blood. It also means that oxygen is more readily given up to the tissues by the hemoglobin, preventing hypoxia. If shift persists, eventually the decreased oxygen content will not prevent tissue hypoxia. **A shift to the left** occurs in alkalosis, hypocarbia, and hypothermia. In a shift to the left, hemoglobin binds oxygen much more tightly and releases less oxygen to the tissues. The arterial oxygen tension and hemoglobin saturation are only very slightly changed from the normal curve.

2,3-DPG is an important organic phosphate that will shift the normal curve to the right and left. **2,3-DPG** is a phosphate-type enzyme that is present in erythrocytes. An *increase* of **2,3-DPG** in the hemoglobin of erythrocytes *shifts the curve to the right* and facilitates the release of oxygen in the tissues. A *decrease* of **2,3-DPG** in the hemoglobin of erythrocytes *shifts the curve to the left* and hinders the release of oxygen into the tissues.

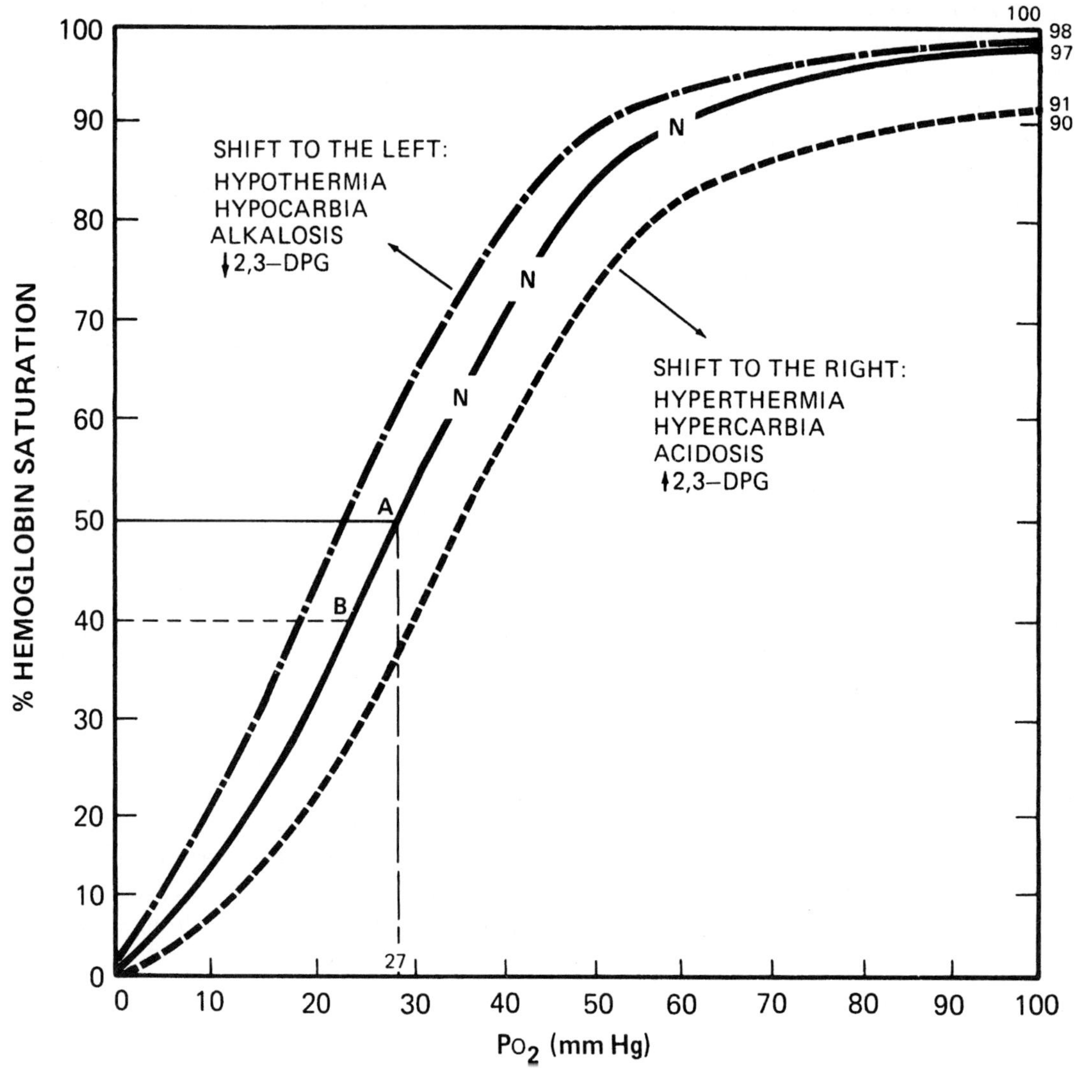

Figure 14-17. Oxyhemoglobin dissociation curve. A, P50, hemoglobin 50% saturated with oxygen; B, hemoglobin binds tightly with oxygen, preventing its release to the tissues, leading to hypoxia; N, normal curve.

QUICK TIP! The oxyhemoglobin dissociation curve will almost certainly appear on the exam. Expect at least one or two questions on this, including factors influencing a shift to the right or left, such as 2,3-DPG. Banked blood, for example, can be low in functional 2,3-DPG, thereby causing a shift to the left. Massive transfusion protocols usually contain an order for calcium chloride or calcium gluconate to increase functional 2,3-DPG and oxygen release to tissues.

Causes of Hypoxemia

Blood volume from the bronchial and cardiac circulation accounts for the 2% to 5% of the blood returning to the left atrium that does not come in contact with inspired air for gas exchange. Anatomic shunt occurs when an alternative pathway allows blood to pass from the right side to the left side of the heart without passing through pulmonary capillaries. Anatomical shunts could be due to an intracardiac shunt (septal defects), pulmonary arteriovenous malformations (AVMs), and hepatopulmonary syndrome (**Fig. 14-18**). The danger of this is that a low Pao_2 (< 60 mm Hg) can produce pulmonary hypertension, increased work of breathing, and low Sao_2 levels.

Decreased alveolar ventilation (VA) results in rising $PACO_2$, causing the displacement of oxygen and lowering of Pao_2. Hypoventilation-induced hypoxemia is easily treated with

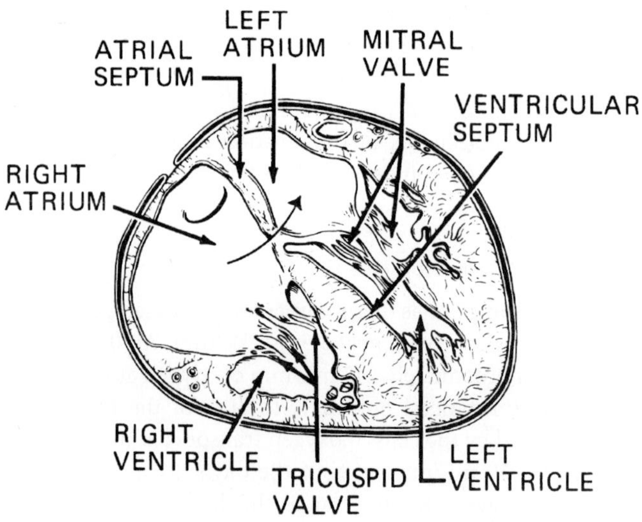

Figure 14-18. Anatomical shunt.

oxygen therapy; however, the decreased VA must be improved or respiratory failure will occur.

Intrapulmonary, or physiologic, shunt occurs when there is adequate pulmonary capillary blood flow but a portion of the alveoli are not being ventilated making them unable to participate in gas exchange (**Fig. 14-19**). Accumulated secretions, atelectasis, pulmonary edema, neoplasms, and foreign objects are only a few of many causes of obstruction.

Intrapulmonary shunts are also referred to as low ventilation/perfusion (V/Q) ratios. When alveolar ventilation is reduced without a subsequent reduction in perfusion, venous blood is not completely oxygenated. Normal venous oxygen levels are low (Pvo_2 35–45 mm Hg and **SvO_2 0.60–0.75**), and more poorly oxygenated blood becomes mixed with oxygenated blood, resulting in hypoxemia (Pao_2 below 60 mm Hg). **Intrapulmonary shunt** is measured by shunt equations or estimated from oxygen tension indices, such as the **Pao_2/Fio_2 ratio or a/A ratio**. *Normal Pao_2/Fio_2 ratio is greater than 286 and* approximately 400 to 500 mm Hg. *The lower it becomes, the worse the intrapulmonary shunt.* The hypoxemia of patients with intrapulmonary shunt will not respond dramatically to oxygen therapy, since the shunted blood will not come in contact with the increased alveolar Po_2. Carbon dioxide elimination will usually not be affected and may be low due to any increase in minute ventilation. *Generally, if the Pao_2/Fio_2 ratio is below 200 the patient will not be able to maintain adequate oxygen levels in their blood without some form of supplemental oxygen therapy.*

14.9 CARBON DIOXIDE TRANSPORT

Carbon dioxide is a by-product of metabolism. It is effectively eliminated only through respiration and is reflected in changes in $Paco_2$ values. Carbon dioxide is transported in the blood in five different states:

- Dissolved in plasma
- As bicarbonate ion
- As carbonic acid
- In combination with hemoglobin
- In an extremely small amount as the carbonate ion

Much like oxygen, only a very small amount of carbon dioxide is transported in the dissolved state, making up about 7% of the total carbon dioxide. The presence of carbon dioxide in a dissolved state creates a pressure gradient or driving force measured as carbon dioxide tension, or $Paco_2$. The pressure gradient of the dissolved carbon dioxide at the tissue level continues until the blood reaches the pulmonary capillaries. Since no carbon dioxide is normally inhaled, the pressure gradient is almost completely one-sided, pushing carbon dioxide from the capillary into the alveoli.

The dissolved carbon dioxide in the blood reacts with water to form carbonic acid. The amount of carbon dioxide that diffuses into the erythrocyte comes into contact with carbonic anhydrase, an enzyme and a strong catalyst, enabling dissolved carbon dioxide to convert to carbonic acid rapidly. About 70% of the body's carbon dioxide waste is handled by the lungs through exhalation. As soon as carbonic acid is formed, it is immediately broken down into hydrogen and bicarbonate ions through the process of dissociation. The hydrogen ions combine with hemoglobin, the bicarbonate ions diffuse into the plasma, and chloride ions diffuse into the erythrocytes to maintain homeostasis. Movement of the bicarbonate ion results in a chloride shift, allowing chloride to move into the erythrocytes. Since this is the body's most important way of transporting carbon dioxide, it is important to review the four steps of the chemical reactions.

1. Carbon dioxide enters the erythrocyte and does the following:
   (A) combines with hemoglobin

   $$CO_2 + Hgb \rightarrow HgbCO_2$$

   (B) combines with water

   $$CO_2 + H_2O$$
   carbon dioxide + water
   $$CA \leftrightarrow H_2CO_3$$

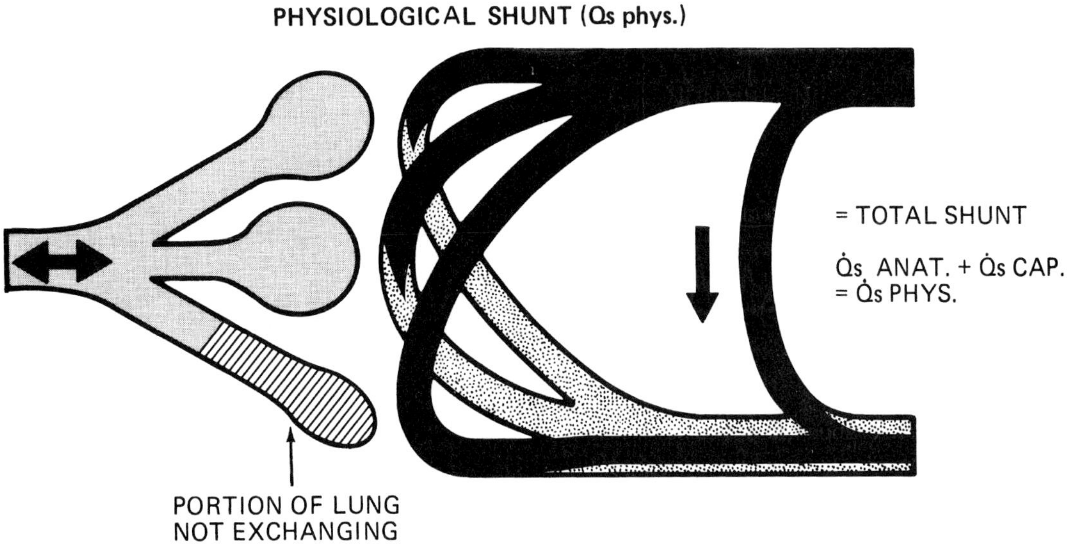

Figure 14-19. Physiological shunt.

2. The carbonic acid of step B dissociates:

$$H_2CO_3 \leftrightarrow HCO_3^- + H^+$$

carbonic acid ↔ bicarbonate ion hydrogen ion

3. Bicarbonate ion leaves the erythrocyte and enters the plasma, allowing the chloride ion to enter the erythrocyte (the chloride shift).
4. The hydrogen ion from step C binds with hemoglobin.

$$H^+ + Hgb \leftrightarrow HHgb$$

14.10 VENTILATION PHYSIOLOGY

The acid–base state in our bodies is kept within a very narrow range. An acid state that is not corrected will eventually result in coma and then death. A base or alkalotic state that is not corrected will eventually result in convulsion, tetany, and eventually death.

An acid is a chemical substance that dissociates into positive or negative electrically charged ions and gives up a hydrogen (H^+) proton to the solution. The positive ion is a cation and the negative ion is an anion. A base is a substance that can and will accept a hydrogen proton while in solution. Water is the most common and abundant base in the body. The pH represents the hydrogen ion concentration and is an expression of the hydrogen ion concentration as a negative logarithm.

Two types of acids are formed in the body: volatile acids and nonvolatile (fixed) acids. These acids are formed by the metabolism of food and by anaerobic glycolysis.

Volatile acids are those that can form a gas; because of an open system, they can be eliminated in their gaseous form. All volatile acids can, therefore, be eliminated by the lungs. The main source of volatile acids is the body's metabolism of glucose and fat. Carbonic acid is the major volatile acid in the body. It is made by the combination of carbon dioxide and water:

$$CO_2 + H_2O \leftrightarrow H_2CO_3$$

The double-direction arrow indicates that the reaction readily moves in either direction.

Acids that cannot be converted into their gaseous form for elimination are termed nonvolatile or fixed acids. Nonvolatile acids are excreted mainly by the kidneys via the urine and in the stool. Nonvolatile acid sources are anaerobic glycolysis, amino acid metabolism, and phosphoprotein/phospholipid metabolism. The kidneys excrete these fixed acids, totaling about 50 mEq/day. Disease can also produce nonvolatile acids.

14.11 ACID–BASE BALANCE

When there is any disruption in the acid–base balance of the arterial blood toward acidosis, the body has three main defense mechanisms: buffering, increasing alveolar ventilation, and/or increasing hydrogen ion elimination as well as increasing bicarbonate reabsorption.

Buffering

Buffering is an immediate response to an acid–base disturbance that prevents changes in hydrogen ion concentration. *Increasing alveolar ventilation begins in 1 to 2 min*utes. As the hydrogen ion concentration builds up, the lungs attempt to reduce their amount by increasing ventilation. The kidneys provide the strongest defense against acid–base disturbances by increasing hydrogen ion elimination and increasing bicarbonate ion reabsorption. *Unfortunately, it takes from several hours to several days for the kidneys to rebalance the hydrogen ion concentration.*

There are three major buffering systems: (1) the bicarbonate buffer system, (2) the phosphate buffer system, and (3) the protein buffer system. The bicarbonate buffer system is the most important system because the end products of the chemical buffer are regulated by both the kidneys and the lungs. The chemical reaction in this system is reversible and occurs extremely rapidly:

$$H^+ + HCO_3^- \leftrightarrow H_2CO_3 3 \leftrightarrow CO_2 + H^+$$

If the buffering moves toward the left, the bicarbonate ion is the end product, regulated by the kidneys. If the buffering moves toward the right, the end product is carbon dioxide, regulated by the lungs. The pH can be shifted up or down by either or both the renal and/or the respiratory system.

The phosphate buffer system is similar to the bicarbonate system in function and buffers best at a slightly different pH than bicarbonate, mainly in the tubular fluids of the kidney. This system buffers strong acids (eg, hydrochloric acid) and strong bases (eg, sodium hydroxide) into weak acids and bases that have little effect on the blood pH.

The protein buffer system is the most inexhaustible buffering system in the body. All the plasma proteins and intracellular proteins, such as hemoglobin, buffer, and the supply of protein is infinite. Proteins buffer carbon dioxide quickly, and it buffers bicarbonate ions over a period of several hours. The importance of this system is that it helps buffer the extracellular fluids through diffusion of carbon dioxide and bicarbonate ion.

Increasing Alveolar Ventilation

If the buffering system has not rectified an acid–base disturbance within minutes, the respiratory system will attempt to compensate. Alveolar hyperventilation increases the rate of carbon dioxide excretion, compensating for a metabolic acidosis. Alveolar hypoventilation does the opposite, compensating for a metabolic alkalosis. As alveolar ventilation increases, the $Paco_2$ decreases. The decreased $Paco_2$ results in a respiratory-induced alkalosis, forcing the hydrogen to combine with HCO_3^-. If alveolar ventilation decreases, the $Paco_2$ level increases, resulting in a respiratory acidosis because of the increased availability of hydrogen.

Increasing Hydrogen Ion Elimination/Bicarbonate Reabsorption

The final mechanism the body can utilize to alter acid–base disturbances is increasing hydrogen ion elimination and bicarbonate ion reabsorption. This defense mechanism involves both the lungs and the kidneys. The kidney function of acid–base disturbances reacts within a few hours of the disturbance; however, it is a slow-acting defense mechanism and may take several days to rebalance the acids and bases. The kidneys can excrete some hydrogen ions in relation to the excretion of nonvolatile acids. This is a very small amount of hydrogen ion elimination since the lungs excrete most of the hydrogen ions. At the same time, the kidneys reabsorb bicarbonate ions in the proximal tubule to equal the excessive number of hydrogen ions. As this reabsorption proceeds, carbon dioxide and water are formed:

$$H^+ + HCO_3^- \leftrightarrow H_2CO_3^- \leftrightarrow CO_2 + H_2O$$

If this reabsorption is not adequate to restore acid–base balance, sodium and hydrogen ions will trade places to maintain electrical neutrality and the sodium bicarbonate return from the kidney tubules to the plasma. If this does not reestablish acid–base balance, the kidneys will conserve still more bicarbonate by substituting ammonium ions (NH_4) for bicarbonate ions. Assuming that the acid–base disturbance continues and all of the possible bicarbonate ions have been retained, hydrogen ions will reach the distal tubules and combine with phosphates. These phosphates will be excreted in the urine. Alterations in potassium and extracellular fluid volume are final efforts of the kidney to restore acid–base balance.

14.12 ACID–BASE DISTURBANCES

The pH expresses the driving pressure of acid–base balance. The pH is a negative logarithm of the blood's hydrogen ion concentration. The smaller the value of the pH, the greater the concentration of hydrogen ions and the more acidic the solution. Conversely, the larger the value of the pH, the smaller the concentration of hydrogen ions and the less acidic the solution. **The normal range of pH for arterial blood is 7.35 to 7.45.**

Acidosis is an acid–base disturbance with a predominant quantity of acid. Acidemia is a state of increased hydrogen ions reflected in an arterial blood pH below 7.35. Alkalosis is an acid–base disturbance in which acids are insufficient in quantity or base is in excess. Acid insufficiency is more commonly a cause than is base excess. Alkalemia is a state of decreased hydrogen ions reflected in an arterial blood pH above 7.45.

There are only two ways by which the pH may be returned toward the normal 7.40 in acid–base disturbances: compensation or correction. Compensation occurs when the body attempts to respond to the acid–base abnormality. If the primary disturbance is respiratory, the kidneys will respond to shift the pH toward normal. If the primary disturbance is metabolic, the respiratory system will attempt to compensate for the alteration.

In **respiratory acidosis,** the lungs are responsible for the altered state. The kidneys will try to compensate by excreting more acid in the urine and increasing reabsorption of the bicarbonate ion. These two concurrent actions will move the pH nearly back to the normal value of 7.40. In **respiratory alkalosis,** the kidneys will try to compensate by increasing the amount of bicarbonate excreted.

In **metabolic acidosis**, the respiratory system is stimulated to increase alveolar ventilation. The hyperventilation increases the excretion of carbon dioxide as an acid waste product of metabolic processes. This is an effective and rapid way to decrease $Paco_2$. The respiratory system can compensate in metabolic acidosis in just a few hours. In **metabolic alkalosis,** the respiratory system will hypoventilate causing carbon dioxide retention and shifting the pH toward normal. The body cannot fully compensate for **metabolic alkalosis**. The hypoventilation necessary for compensation causes a decrease in the Pao_2. When the oxygen level becomes too low, the respiratory system will respond to the decreased oxygen by increasing ventilation. Although this compensatory effort is rapid, it is not a complete compensation. The most significant fact about compensation as a defense mechanism in acid–base disturbance is that *the body never overcompensates and will return the pH to near normal (7.40), but it never "overshoots the mark."*

14.13 RESPIRATORY IMBALANCES

Respiratory Acidosis

The **normal $Paco_2$ is 35 to 45 mm Hg.** *If the $Paco_2$ is elevated above 45 mm Hg and the pH decreased below 7.35, respiratory acidosis is present,* indicating acute or chronic **hypoventilation.** Respiratory acidosis indicates inadequate alveolar ventilation.

Any clinical condition that depresses the respiratory center in the *medulla oblongata* may precipitate hypoventilation and result in respiratory acidosis. These conditions include head trauma, oversedation, and general anesthesia. More rarely, neoplasms in the medulla oblongata or nearby areas with increasing intracranial mass, size, and pressure may cause a respiratory acidosis. Neuromuscular diseases—including myasthenia gravis, Guillain-Barré syndrome, multiple sclerosis, amyotrophic lateral sclerosis, and trauma to the cervical spinal cord—may cause hypoventilation and resultant respiratory acidosis. Inappropriate mechanical ventilation may cause respiratory acidosis. A low respiratory rate or tidal volume and dead space in the tubing may result in respiratory acidosis. Obstructive lung diseases such as COPD may result in a degree of V/Q disturbance, increasing the risk for developing both acute and chronic carbon dioxide retention.

Respiratory acidosis can best be treated by improving ventilation. This includes nursing measures such as protecting the airway through positioning or the use of artificial airways. The key to treatment is to find the cause of the respiratory depression and correct it. A respiratory acidosis requires active treatment if the increase in $Paco_2$ results in a pH of about 7.25. The more alert the patient, the longer intubation and mechanical ventilation can be delayed. For the patient on mechanical ventilation, the respiratory rate is increased to decrease the $Paco_2$ and maintain effective ventilation, or the tidal volume may be increased.

Respiratory Alkalosis

When the $Paco_2$ is decreased below 35 mm Hg and the pH is increased above 7.45, respiratory alkalosis is present, indicating **hyperventilation.** Restrictive lung diseases are common pathologic causes of respiratory alkalosis. Other causes of respiratory alkalosis include anxiety, nervousness, agitation, hyperventilation via mechanical ventilation, and *excessive Ambu-bagging during a cardiopulmonary arrest.*

A respiratory alkalosis is treated by finding the cause of the excessive breathing, such as anxiety, pain, fear, hypoxemic compensation for a metabolic acidosis, or central nervous system (CNS) disturbance. Correcting the causative problem will correct the respiratory alkalosis. If the patient is on mechanical ventilation, decreasing the respiratory rate, decreasing the tidal volume, or adding additional tubing (dead space) may correct the imbalance. If the pH is greater than 7.55, more aggressive measures—such as administration of **acetazolamide (Diamox)**, ammonium chloride, hydrochloric acid, or potassium chloride (KCl)—are used.

14.14 METABOLIC DISTURBANCES

Base Excess

The bicarbonate ion (HCO_3^-) and base excess are the parameters of the arterial blood gas (ABG) used to identify nonrespiratory imbalances. Base excess is an easy guide to use in distinguishing metabolic acidosis from alkalosis. Base excess is the amount of base above the normal level after adjusting the level for hemoglobin. The normal midpoint value is zero. If the base excess is above +2, there is an excess of metabolic base in the body fluids and a metabolic alkalosis exists. If the base excess is below −2, there is not enough metabolic base in the body fluids and a metabolic acidosis exists.

Metabolic Alkalosis

Metabolic alkalosis is a condition with an excess base. *The three most common causes are diuretic therapy, excessive vomiting, and excessive ingestion of alkaline drugs.* Any condition that increases metabolic processes beyond the ability of the body to eliminate or neutralize the waste products results in an increase in bicarbonate ions. These conditions cause a loss of hydrogen ions (diuretics), chloride ions (vomiting), and potassium ions (hyperaldosteronism) through the kidneys. The effect is increased bicarbonate ion reabsorption in the kidneys, which forces excretion of the hydrogen, chloride, and potassium ions in the urine. Loss of gastric secretions from vomiting or through nasogastric suctioning results in metabolic alkalosis. Excessive ingestion of alkaline drugs, such as antacids and soda bicarbonate, may lead to metabolic alkalosis. Less commonly, treatment with corticosteroids, hyperaldosteronism, and Cushing syndrome may result in a metabolic alkalosis.

A metabolic alkalosis is corrected by finding and treating the underlying cause. Most cases of metabolic alkalosis are due to electrolyte disturbances, such as hypokalemia (low potassium) or hyperchloremia (high chloride). In severe disturbances where the pH is greater than 7.60, hydrochloric acid or ammonium chloride may be administered.

QUICK TIP! With respect to the impact of GI losses on the pH, remember that, "If it goes down, then the pH will go down" (eg, diarrhea), and "If it comes up, the pH will go up" (eg, vomiting, excessive NG output, etc.)

Metabolic Acidosis

Metabolic acidosis occurs in the body when there is an increase in endogenous acid production **(lactic acid, ketoacids)**, loss of bicarbonate **(diarrhea, vomiting)**, or accumulation of endogenous acids **(renal failure)**.

Metabolic acidoses are classified in two major groups: those with an increase in unmeasurable anions and those with no increase in unmeasurable anions. To calculate unmeasurable anions, add the serum chloride and the bicarbonate ion values and then subtract this sum from the serum sodium level. Normal anion gap is 4 to 12 mEQ/L plus or minus 2. Any difference over 14, there is an increase in unmeasurable anions known as the **anion gap**. Normally no real anion gap exists, since positive (cations) and negative (anions) ions must always be present in equal numbers. However, it appears as if the anion gap were present, since only the major ions (sodium, chloride, and bicarbonate) are measured.

Common causes of metabolic acidosis with an increase in unmeasurable anions *(anion gap)* include (the specific anion is in parentheses) diabetic or alcoholic ketosis, uremia (phosphates and sulfates), lactic acidosis (lactate), isoniazid or iron overload, substance and salicylate toxicity, methyl poisoning (formic acid), ethylene glycol poisoning (oxalic acid and formic acid), and paraldehyde poisoning.

There are several common causes of metabolic acidosis with no increase in unmeasurable anions *(nonanion gap)*. Diarrhea is probably the most common cause. Large amounts of bicarbonate ion are in the intestines and are washed out in the diarrhea. The more severe the diarrhea, the greater the likelihood of metabolic acidosis. A general guide for the possible development of metabolic acidosis with no increase in unmeasurable anion is the presence below the umbilicus of a drainage tube (except a Foley catheter), such as that for drainage of the pancreas, or an ureterosigmoidostomy and other drainage tubes.

Another cause of nongap metabolic acidosis is uremia. In severe renal failure, the kidneys cannot excrete the acids normally formed daily by the body. As the acids build up, uremia develops, resulting in an increase in unmeasurable anions.

Metabolic acidosis is the most difficult acid–base disturbance to correct. The high hydrogen ion concentration stimulates the body to attempt compensation by increasing both the depth and the rate of respiration **(Kussmaul breathing)**. Compensation is not usually enough by itself. The electrolytes are often quite abnormal and complicate the correction of the acid–base disturbance. **A metabolic acidosis is treated by correcting the cause of the acidosis.** Correction of the underlying cause will reverse the metabolic acidosis. Treatment with an alkali should be reserved for severe metabolic acidosis, pH less than 7.20. **There is controversy over the benefit of using sodium bicarbonate ($NaHCO_3$) in a metabolic acidosis** caused by the accumulation of a metabolized organic acid anion. Sodium bicarbonate may be ordered in a dose of 1 mEq/kg. **If given judiciously, bicarbonate will begin to return the pH to normal while the underlying cause of the imbalance is identified and treated.**

If tissue hypoxia is present, the lactate (normally < 2 mmol) may increase. Lactate values greater than 4, when associated with a decreased pH, are warning signs of tissue hypoxia.

KEY CONTENT CHECKLIST

- ❒ Central and peripheral chemoreceptors monitor and respond to the chemical composition of blood and fluid around them to alter the respiratory rate and depth in an attempt to correct acidosis or alkalotic states. Acidosis, an increase in hydrogen ions, will stimulate both receptors to increase respiratory rate and depth to correct acidosis. A decrease in PaO_2 will stimulate the peripheral receptors to increase respiration to restore oxygen levels.
- ❒ Any disease that stiffens the lungs will decrease compliance. Diseases that increase congestion in the lungs—such as atelectasis, pneumonia, or pulmonary edema—result in decreased lung compliance and decreased gas exchange.
- ❒ The transport of oxygen to body tissues is influenced most by cardiac output, hemoglobin concentration, and oxygen–hemoglobin binding and releasing factors. Assessing each of these factors can also assist in identifying the cause and treatment of hypoxemia.
- ❒ Equation for arterial oxygen content is Cao_2 = Hgb × 1.34 (cubic centimeters of oxygen) × Sao_2 + (Po_2 × 0.003). Given this equation, transfusing PRBCs may have a more significant impact on delivering O_2 to the tissues after a SaO_2 > 90% is achieved.
- ❒ **Shunt** is alveoli are not properly ventilated. Examples: Pulmonary edema, pneumonia, etc.
- ❒ **Deadspace** is when alveoli are not properly perfused. Examples: P.E., fat embolus, etc.
- ❒ Remembering that foreign material is more likely to fall through the right mainstem can be helpful when trying to determine the cause or possibility of aspiration.
- ❒ Damage and dysfunction of the Type II alveolar cells are associated with ARDS pathophysiology.
- ❒ The compensatory vasoconstriction provided by stimulation to the carotid and aortic bodies is why the **Trendelenburg** position is no longer recommended during hypotension. **Trendelenburg** "fools" the receptors into thinking the BP is better when it is not. Best practice instead suggests lying the patient flat with legs elevated if possible (during resuscitation).
- ❒ The oxyhemoglobin dissociation curve will almost certainly appear on the exam. Expect at least one or two questions on this, including factors influencing a shift to the right or left, such as 2,3-DPG. Banked blood, for example, can be low in functional 2,3-DPG, thereby causing a shift to the left. Massive transfusion protocols usually contain an order for calcium chloride or calcium gluconate to increase functional 2,3-DPG and oxygen release to tissues.

Review Questions:

1. The upper airway serves three of the key functions listed below. Select the one function that is NOT served by the upper airway.

a. Humidification of air
b. Removal of particles
c. Warming of inspired air
d. Participation in gas exchange

Answer: D. Rationale: Gas exchange takes place in the lower airways in the alveoli.

2. Right mainstem bronchus intubations are more likely to be performed than left bronchus intubations for which of the following reasons?

a. The right mainstem bronchus has more ciliary clearance of mucus, facilitating passage of the endotracheal tube.
b. The left mainstem bronchus is located several inches lower than the right.
c. The left mainstem bronchus, although wider than the right, sits posterior to the right mainstem bronchus.
d. The right mainstem bronchus is wider and has less angulation than the left.

Answer: D. Rationale: The right mainstem bronchus comes off the trachea in almost a straight line, while the left mainstem bronchus comes off the trachea at an angle of approximately 40 degrees. The right mainstem bronchus is wider in diameter than the left.

3. Normal mixed venous hemoglobin saturation (SvO_2) falls within which of the following ranges?

a. 0.40 to 0.60
b. 0.60 to 0.75
c. 0.80 to 0.90
d. More than 0.95

Answer: B. Rationale: The SvO_2 is the oxygen saturation of "mixed venous" blood that is aspirated from the tip of the pulmonary artery catheter. Remember that a normal SaO_2 (fully oxygenated blood) is more than 95% and in normal circumstances, the body's tissues extract approximately 25% of this via one circuit through the body by the time the blood reaches the pulmonary artery. Thus, 0.25 subtracted from 0.95 = 0.75. Choose B.

15

Diagnosis and Treatment of Pulmonary Disorders

CHAPTER OVERVIEW AND OBJECTIVES

The CCRN exam will include questions that are related to ventilatory and oxygenation failure. This chapter will familiarize you with the diagnostic techniques used to recognize these disorders and the pharmacologic interventions used to treat them.

15.1 INVASIVE AND NONINVASIVE DIAGNOSTIC STUDIES

Diagnostic studies used in identifying respiratory alterations include physical assessment, arterial blood gases (ABGs), pulmonary function tests, and chest radiography.

Physical Assessment

Assessment of the respiratory system includes inspection, palpation, percussion, and auscultation of the lungs.

Inspection

Inspect the patient for respiratory pattern, chest symmetry, clubbing of the fingers, and color.

Five basic terms are used to describe breathing patterns: eupnea, tachypnea, hyperpnea, bradypnea, and apnea.

- **Eupnea:** Regular rhythm and a respiratory rate of 12 to 20 breaths per min (**Fig. 15-1**)
- **Tachypnea:** Increased respiratory rate, above 20 breaths per min, depth of respiration may be normal, shallow, or deep
- **Hyperpnea:** Increased depth of respiration at a normal or increased respiratory rate
- **Bradypnea:** Decreased respiratory rate, less than 12 breaths per min, with normal depth of respiration
- **Apnea:** The absence of breathing (**Fig. 15-2**)

The four common patterns of respiration seen in critical care are:

- **Central neurogenic hyperventilation** (**Fig. 15-3**)—Regular, deep, rapid respirations without periods of apnea caused by neurogenic dysfunction
- **Cheyne–Stokes respiration** (**Fig. 15-4**)—A pattern in which respirations start from apnea, reach a maximum in depth and rate, and then fade back to apnea caused by alterations in acid–base status, an underlying metabolic problem, or neurocerebral insult
- **Kussmaul breathing** (**Fig. 15-5**)—A tachypnea pattern of labored, deep breaths associated with metabolic acidosis and renal failure
- **Biot respirations** (**Fig. 15-6**)—Irregular, with varying depth and irregular, abrupt periods of apnea; caused by central nervous system disorders; however this pattern may be found in some healthy patients.

Ataxic breathing occurs when the pneumotaxic center takes over control of ventilation. The pattern is irregular, deep, shallow breathing with random periods of apnea of varying lengths (**Fig. 15-7**).

Inspect the patient's color for signs of cyanosis. Peripheral cyanosis has little clinical value and often is the result of peripheral vasoconstriction. When you assess oxygenation from the physical examination, look at the mucosa of the oral cavity and mouth for signs of **central cyanosis**.

Clubbing of the digits indicates chronic oxygen deficit. The distal phalanges of the fingers become widened. This is most often seen in patients with cystic fibrosis, pulmonary hypertension, and end-stage COPD.

Palpation

Palpation of the chest wall can help further assess findings suggested by inspection. It is used to assess thoracic

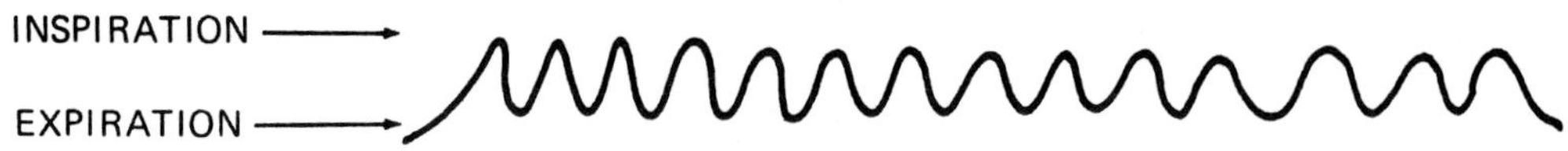

Figure 15-1. Spirometry pattern of normal ventilation.

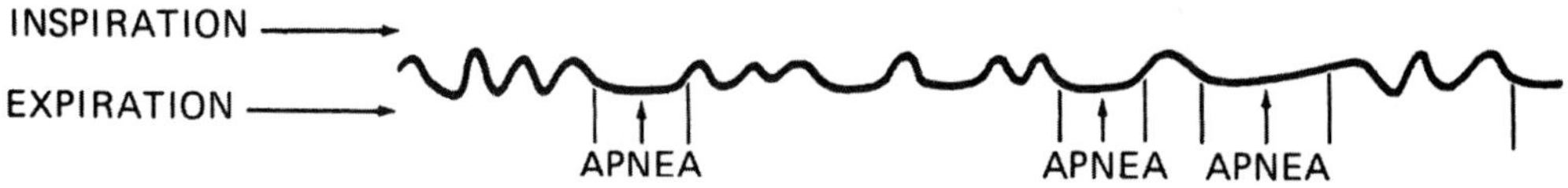

Figure 15-2. Spirometry pattern of apneustic breathing.

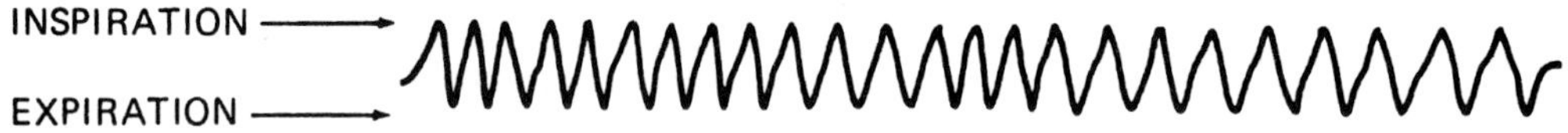

Figure 15-3. Spirometry pattern of central neurogenic hyperventilation.

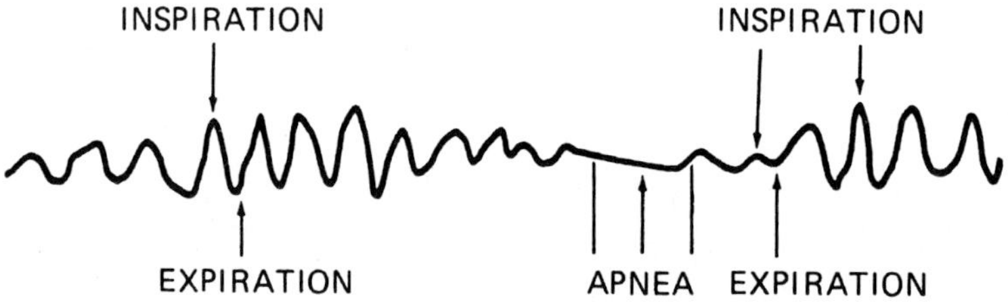

Figure 15-4. Spirometry pattern of Cheyne–Stokes breathing.

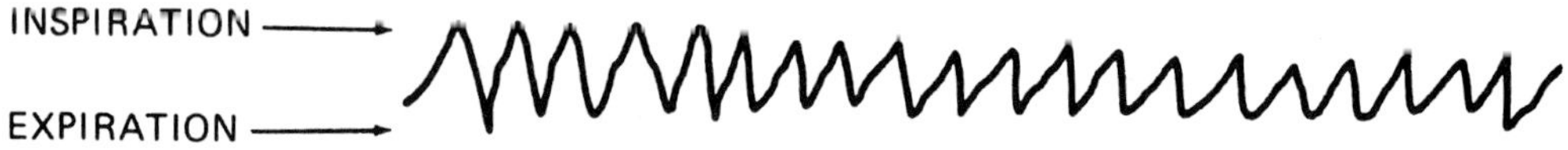

Figure 15-5. Spirometry pattern of Kussmaul breathing.

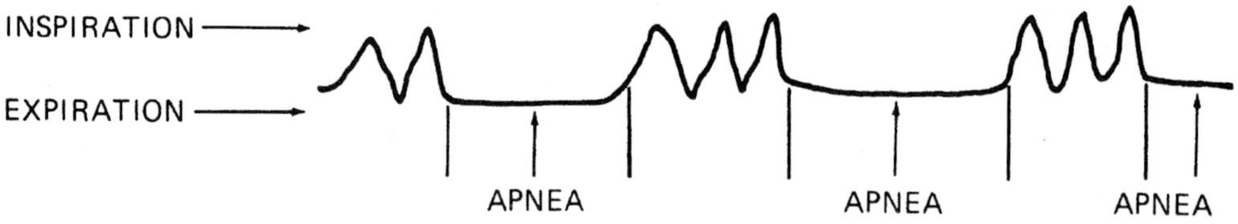

Figure 15-6. Spirometry pattern of Biot (cluster) breathing.

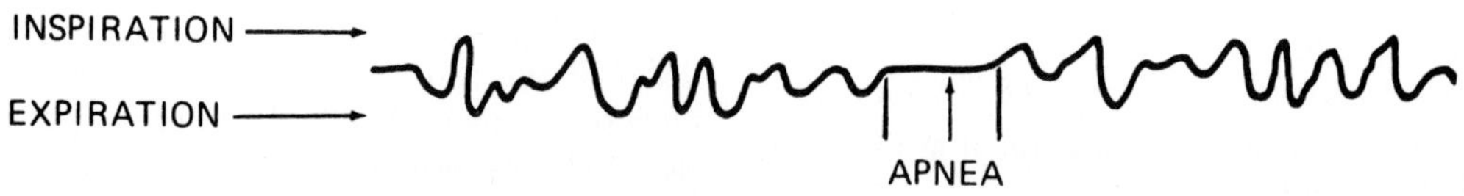

Figure 15-7. Spirometry pattern of pneumotaxic (ataxic) breathing.

expansion, tactile and vocal fremitus, and *crepitus (subcutaneous emphysema).*

Subcutaneous emphysema is assessed by the familiar crunching or popping that occurs on palpation. It is seen when a communication exists between the pleural space and subcutaneous tissue or the presence of a gas-producing bacteria. The presence of air in the skin may not be harmful, but it requires investigation as to its origin.

Percussion

Percussion is the assessment of the lung by striking or tapping on the thorax. It can help to identify areas of consolidation, hyperresonance, and diaphragmatic excursion. A flat or dull sound over the lung indicates that an air-filled space has been replaced with fluid or tissue.

Auscultation

Lung sounds are frequently described in general terms describing the quality of sound heard over each anatomic region. Tracheal and bronchial sounds reflect the airflow in the major airways. Bronchovesicular and vesicular sounds reflect the progression of airflow in more distal airways. The presence of bronchial sounds in the periphery or any place other than the bronchial area may reflect an abnormality. Any abnormal sound is referred to as an adventitious sound.

"Crackles" is the term used to describe the sounds heard during the reopening of airways secondary to changes in forces surrounding the airways. The airways collapse primarily on expiration and their sounds can be heard throughout the lungs. Crackles can have pulmonary or cardiac origins. Differentiation of pulmonary crackles from those of cardiovascular origin is based on the fact that **cardiac crackles are position dependent.**

Wheezes are due to either partial or complete airway obstruction. They can be high- or low-pitched. The presence of a wheeze is assessed by identifying the location of the loudest wheeze and listening to the airflow distal to this point. The presence of airflow distal to the location of the loudest wheeze indicates airflow past the obstruction. **If a wheeze disappears, the obstruction is either lessening or worsening.** If airflow is more easily heard as the wheeze diminishes, the lung is improving. **If airflow diminishes, the patient is worsening.**

KEY CLINICAL CONCEPT

When a wheeze disappears and airflow is diminishing, this is considered a potentially ominous sign on the exam, such as in a worsening asthma patient. In this case, immediate action would be required, possibly including intubation.

Lung sounds can be diminished by the presence of fluid or air between the lung and the stethoscope. For example, a pneumothorax or pleural effusion will diminish the intensity of lung sounds. On the other hand, consolidation of fluid in the lung itself will accentuate sound transmission. A pneumonia, for example, may accentuate the sound heard in the location of the pneumonia. A bronchial sound would be heard instead of the expected vesicular sound. Loss of airflow, as with bronchoconstriction or obstruction, differs from consolidation in that reduction in airflow generally diminishes breath sounds. For example, atelectasis or airway obstruction will reduce the intensity of breath sounds. It is up to the clinician to identify whether the source of the loss of breath sound is intrapulmonary (atelectasis, mucus plugs) or extrapulmonary (pneumothorax).

TABLE 15-1. NORMAL ARTERIAL BLOOD GAS VALUES AT SEA LEVEL

	Range	*Midpoint*	*Venous*
pH	7.35–7.45	7.40	7.36–7.41
Po_2	80–100 mm Hg	93	35–40 mm Hg
Pco_2	35–45 mm Hg	40	41–51 mm Hg
Hco_3^-	22–26 mEq/L	24	22–26 mEq/L
Sao_2	95%–100%	97%	70%–75%
Base excess	+2	0	+2

Interpreting Arterial Blood Gas Values

Basic acid–base disturbances can be identified by following a step-by-step procedure of analyzing ABG values. The important values used to interpret ABGs are shown in **Table 15-1**.

When the pH and the arterial carbon dioxide pressure ($PaCO_2$) move in *opposite* directions, the primary cause of acid–base disturbance is *respiratory*. If the pH and the $PaCO_2$ move in the *same* direction, the primary cause is *metabolic*.

Step 1: Look at the PaO_2 to assess for hypoxia.

- Normal range is 80 to 100 mm Hg for people 60 years or younger.
- For people 60 years old or older, to calculate their normal: from 80 mm Hg subtract 1 mm Hg for every year above 60.
- When PaO_2 is lower than the expected normal, it is called hypoxia.
- Any PaO_2 below 40 mm Hg is a life-threatening emergency.

Step 2: Look at the pH to identify the presence of acidosis or alkalosis.

- If it is 7.35 to 7.45, the pH is normal.
- If the pH is less than 7.35, an acidosis exists.
- If the pH is greater than 7.45, an alkalosis exists.

Step 3: Look at the $PaCO_2$ to determine the primary disturbance.

- If the $PaCO_2$ is between 35 and 45, a normal level exists.
- If the value is below 35, a respiratory alkalosis exists.
- If the value is above 45, a respiratory acidosis exists.
- If the $PaCO_2$ moves in the same direction as the pH, the primary cause is metabolic.

Example 1:

$$pH = 7.25$$
$$PaCO_2 = 26$$

Since the $PaCO_2$ and pH moved in the same direction, the primary problem is a metabolic one. The pH is acidotic, therefore a metabolic acidosis exists. A respiratory alkalosis exists as well, as evidenced by the low $PaCO_2$. The respiratory alkalosis is an attempt to compensate for the metabolic acidosis but is unable to correct the acidosis.

Example 2:

$$pH = 7.24$$
$$PaCO_2 = 59$$

Since the $PaCO_2$ and pH moved in opposite directions, the primary problem is respiratory. As the $PaCO_2$ is elevated and the pH is depressed, a pure respiratory acidosis exists.

Step 4: Look at the bicarbonate ion (HCO_3^-) value.

- If it is 22 to 26, consider it normal.
- If it is less than 22, a metabolic acidosis exists.
- If it is greater than 26, a metabolic alkalosis exists.

Example 3:

$$pH = 7.25$$
$$PaCO_2 = 26$$
$$HCO_3^- = 17$$

A metabolic acidosis exists because the pH and $PaCO_2$ moved in the same direction. The low HCO_3^- level confirms a metabolic acidosis.

	Example 1	*Example 2*	*Example 3*
pH	7.19	7.35	7.52
$PaCO_2$	30	62	25
HCO_3^-	14	40	25

Practice ABG Interpretation.

Example 1 Answer and Rationale: Since the $PaCO_2$ and pH moved in the same direction, the primary problem is metabolic. The pH and HCO_3^- confirm a metabolic acidosis. The low $PaCO_2$, a respiratory alkalosis, is an attempt to correct for the metabolic acidosis. Since the pH is very low, this situation requires intervention to correct the metabolic acidosis.

Example 2 Answer and Rationale: The $PaCO_2$ is elevated, indicating a respiratory acidosis, but the pH is normal. The only way this could occur would be if a compensation had occurred to offset the acidosis. The high HCO_3^- confirms that a metabolic alkalosis exists. The interpretation is respiratory acidosis compensated by a metabolic alkalosis. Since the pH is normal, no acute danger exists in this patient.

Example 3 Answer and Rationale: Since the $PaCO_2$ and pH moved in opposite directions, the primary problem is respiratory. Because of the low $PaCO_2$ and high pH, a respiratory alkalosis exists. No compensation has occurred, as evidenced by the normal HCO_3^- level. In this case, a pure respiratory alkalosis exists.

The body's ability to compensate will not take the pH beyond midpoint. The direction the pH takes from midpoint can provide the clinician with a clue as to the primary problem. Intervention from clinicians can result in overcompensation.

The combination of an acidosis and an alkalosis is tolerated better by the body than two acidoses or alkaloses, as they tend to block compensation for each other, resulting in a severe acid–base and electrolyte disturbance.

QUICK TIP! Using intravenous sodium bicarb drips to correct acidotic states is controversial unless the pH is extremely low. The best way to correct an acidotic state is to find and fix the cause of the acidosis. For example, diabetic ketoacidosis—administer insulin to decrease ketone production, or with lactic acidosis—reestablish oxygenation or perfusion to restore aerobic cell metabolism.

Pulmonary Function Tests

Pulmonary function tests are used to evaluate the volumes and flow rate of the respiratory system with spirometry (**Fig. 15-8**).

Measurement of the flow of exhaled gas and the exhalation time helps distinguish between restrictive and obstructive lung diseases (**Table 15-2**). **Forced vital capacity (FVC)** measures the volume of air that the patient can forcibly exhale (ie, his or her vital capacity) and suggests the maximum volume of air available for airway clearance.

FEV_1 is the forced expiratory volume in 1 second. The patient inhales as much as possible, holds his or her breath briefly, and then exhales as forcibly and quickly as possible. A decrease in the FEV_1 indicates obstruction to airflow.

Chest Radiography

The chest radiograph is used to evaluate the structures of the chest, the relationships between structures, and the presence of air and fluid. A systematic approach is essential to ensure the radiograph is fully assessed. One approach could be:

Step 1. Ensure you have the correct patient's film.

Step 2. Observe technique and quality of the film. Observe exposure, centering of patient image, and symmetry of clavicles.

Step 3. Assess bones, mediastinum, diaphragm, pleural space, and lung tissue.

Observations to make include: Determine that the major organs of the thorax are present and check their relationship to each other. The trachea is at the midline and tubular. Examine the cardiac silhouette for size and placement in the chest. The cardiac silhouette appears anteriorly as a white solid structure in the left mediastinum. The width of the normal heart is less than half that of the thorax. The lungs are examined for expansion and any increased densities, such as those caused by fluid or masses. Review of the chest film begins with the bony structures. Look for the presence of the ribs and observe any notching or calcifications. Recall the thoracic cage is made up of 12 ribs, seven attached (which are inserted in the sternum at a 45-degree angle) and five "floating" (not attached to the sternum). Review the position of the hemidiaphragm. It is a rounded silhouette at the base of the thorax. The right side is slightly higher than the left. Flattening of the diaphragm is seen with chronic air trapping, COPD, and asthma.

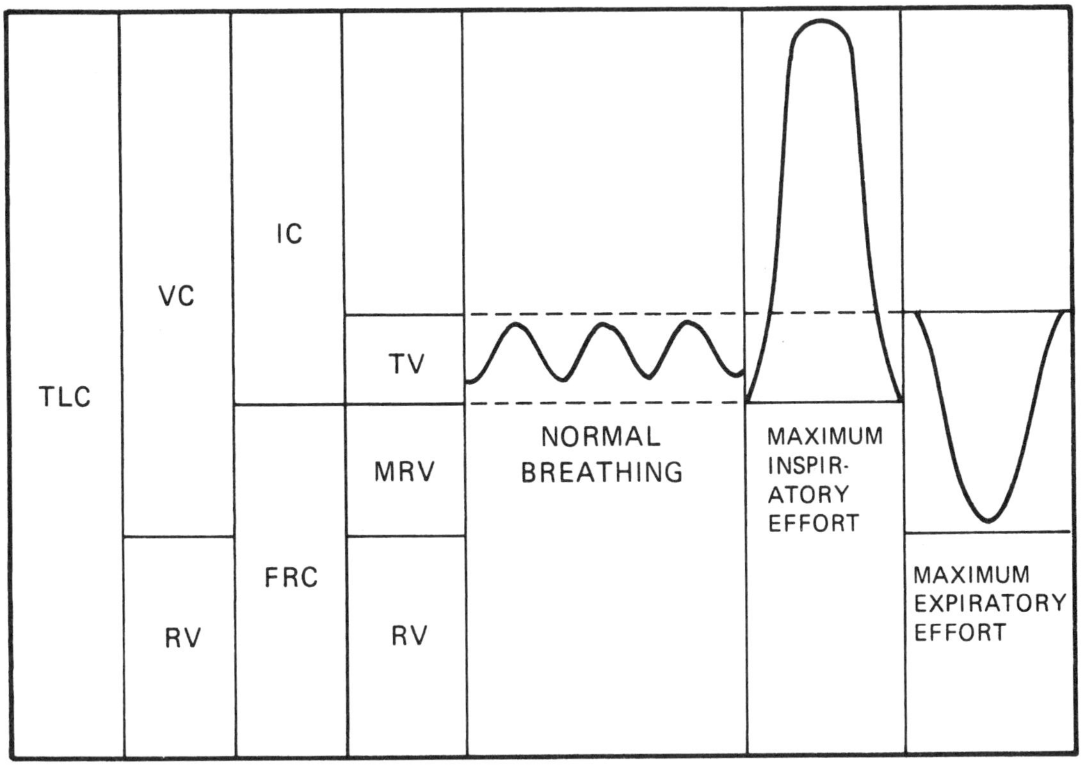

Figure 15-8. Lung volumes and capacities.

15.2 PULMONARY PHARMACOLOGY

Medications used in managing pulmonary disease include sympathomimetic bronchodilators, anticholinergic bronchodilators, corticosteroids, leukotriene inhibitors, mast cell stabilizers, and mucolytic agents.

Bronchodilators

Bronchodilators are divided into classes: adrenergic, anticholinergic, and methylxanthines.

The application of methylxanthine therapy remains controversial and somewhat unclear. Expert panels have not recommended it for acute use in the emergent patient, but admit to the potential benefits of chronic use in the brittle asthmatic. **Theophylline** (anhydrous), an example of a methylxanthine is usually given orally and metabolized in the liver. Its primary effect is bronchodilatation of the airways but is limited by its extensive list of toxicity-related side effects. The therapeutic range is 10 to 15 μg/mL although maintenance levels between 8 and 10 have shown to be adequate for chronic therapy in the nocturnally sensitive environment. Intravenous use is rare and reserved for the most extreme cases that are not responding to traditional therapy.

TABLE 15-2. DIFFERENTIATING OBSTRUCTIVE FROM RESTRICTIVE DISEASE

Parameter	*Obstructive*	*Restrictive*
Vital capacity	normal or ↓	↓
Functional residual capacity	↑	↓
Total lung capacity	↑	↓
Residual volume	↑	↓
FEV_1	↓	normal or ↓

Side effects of **theophylline** include tachycardia, tremor, nervousness, palpitations, dizziness, sweating, dysrhythmias, increased blood pressure, irritability, vomiting, nausea, headache, and restlessness. Toxicity can be minimized by keeping the dose low. Clinicians need to be familiar with drug interactions and other factors that inhibit metabolism and/or decrease elimination of theophylline.

Overdose of theophylline is critical, as there is no antidote. Early indicators of theophylline overdose include central nervous system changes, headache, confusion, gastrointestinal upset, palpitations, tachycardia, and tachypnea.

Adrenergic Sympathomimetic Bronchodilators. Sympathomimetic bronchodilators belong to the class of adrenergic receptor agonists that primarily stimulate $beta_2$ receptors in the lungs, relaxing smooth muscle constriction around the small airways of the lungs. As bronchospasm is reversed, a subsequent decrease in mucus production occurs along with increased mucociliary clearance, and stabilization of the mast cell.

Current therapy for bronchodilation is the use of selective short-acting $beta_2$ agonists such as **albuterol**, pirbuterol, metaproterenol, and levalbuterol. Short-acting sympathomimetics are preferentially administered via metered-dose inhalers (MDIs), or nebulized inhalation. Long-acting sympathomimetic agents are often given in metered dose, dry powder, or nebulized modalities. Parenteral and oral administration should generally be avoided.

Long-acting adrenergic bronchodilator agents such as Serevent, Brovana, and Foradil are classified as maintenance medications and are only given twice daily.

Side effects of short-acting beta$_2$ agonists are dose-dependent, are higher for oral preparations than inhaled ones, and include stimulation of heart rate, contractility, and automaticity. They should be used with caution in patients with a history of tachycardia, dysrhythmias, ischemic heart disease, or uncontrolled hyperthyroidism. Tachycardia can be precipitated by vasodilation and a fall in blood pressure. Patients with diabetes may have increased hyperglycemia. Pregnant women in the third trimester may have delayed or prolonged labor with the use of beta$_2$ agonists. Central nervous system side effects include anxiety, irritability, insomnia, and fine tremor.

Overdose of sympathomimetics can result in excessive cardiac stimulation. Carefully administered **beta blockers** *can be used to counteract the overdose;* however, be prepared for the resulting beta blockade in the lung.

Epinephrine, isoproterenol, and isoetharine are all catecholamine agents which lack beta$_2$ receptor specificity. **Epinephrine is the drug of choice for anaphylaxis** because of its vasoconstrictive and cardiovascular effects. *Subcutaneous epinephrine may be used to treat acute bronchospasm* but should be reserved for patients who are refractory to inhaled sympathomimetic and steroid therapy.

Anticholinergics

Anticholinergic drugs block the stimulation of cholinergic receptors by acetylcholine. Acetylcholine is a powerful bronchoconstrictor, stimulator of mucus production, and mast cell activator. Short-term anticholinergic bronchodilators like **Ipratropium (Atrovent)** are utilized as a first-line therapy in the treatment of COPD. Long acting anticholinergics like *Spiriva* are considered a maintenance medication only. Spiriva is a dry powder inhaled medication that is given once daily. Combination therapy, beta agonist, and anticholinergic are considered *synergistic medications*, and show positive outcomes in patients with COPD.

Corticosteroids

Corticosteroids are used to reduce inflammation in the airway. Steroids can be given orally, parenterally, inhaled, or nasally. Parenteral steroids, such as **hydrocortisone**, are used as "burst" therapy to treat severe exacerbations of asthma and COPD. However, if prolonged therapy is needed for persistent airway inflammation, oral steroids such as **prednisone** may be indicated. Both parenteral and oral steroids have a systemic effect and can cause many *side effects*. These include edema, weight gain, adrenal suppression, hypernatremia, hypokalemia, hypertension, redistribution of body fat, osteoporosis, muscle weakness, and increased risk of peptic ulcer disease.

Dosage for **hydrocortisone** is 20 to 240 mg/day, depending on the severity of the presenting symptoms. **Prednisone** dosage is 5 to 60 mg/day. The *tapering* of prolonged systemic steroids is done gradually to avoid withdrawal symptoms from *adrenal insufficiency*. Even 2 weeks of full-dose therapy can suppress the synthesis and release of cortisol into the bloodstream.

Inhaled steroids provide the same reduction of inflammation in the lung without the major systemic effects. They are supplied in a MDI, dry-powder inhaler (DPI), or nebulizer format. The most common inhaled steroids include **fluticasone (Flovent)**, mometasone furoate (Asmanex), budesonide (Pulmicort) beclomethasone dipropionate (QVAR), and triamcinolone acetonide (Azmacort). Inhaled steroids are used in conjunction with bronchodilator therapy. The effect of inhaled steroids may take days to weeks to achieve; therefore they are not used to treat acute exacerbations of airway inflammation. Inhaled steroids may reduce the need for oral maintenance of corticosteroids except in the most severe cases.

The major side effect of inhaled steroids is oropharyngeal fungal infections via *Candida albicans*. Instructing the patient to rinse his or her mouth with water and expectorate after using the inhaler will prevent fungal development.

Combination Medications

The maintenance and stabilization of most patients with asthma and COPD relies on the continual and compliant use of inhaled combination medications. Long-acting adrenergic agents combined with inhaled steroids have shown to be effective at reducing exacerbations. The most common inhaled combination medications are budesonide/formoterol (Symbicort), and fluticasone/salmeterol (Advair). New inhaler options continue to be developed such as the dry powder inhaler Ellipta. Ellipta inhalers can contain three medications, providing maintenance therapy for asthma and COPD patients in an easier-to-use form.

Mucolytic Agents

There are currently only two inhaled medications that directly have an effect on airway secretions. **Acetylcysteine (Mucomyst)** decreases secretion viscosity by breaking hydrogen bonds within the secretion, thereby thinning and improving mucociliary clearing. Mucomyst comes in two different percentage strengths (10%–20%); and is inhaled via a nebulizer modality. The clinician should be aware of the potential side effects of mucomyst. Of significance is the potential for bronchospasm, therefore it may be given with a beta$_2$ agonist. Dornase alfa (Pulmozyme) works by breaking down the DNA material of the neutrophils found in purulent airway secretions. This is a highly effective medication in reducing the viscosity of airway secretions. Pulmozyme is also given via nebulizer.

Leukotriene Inhibitors

Leukotrienes are taken orally to inhibit bronchospasm in the asthmatic reactive airway patient. They are antagonists of leukotriene receptors which cause bronchoconstriction and mucus secretion. The main role is to prevent exacerbations, which correlates to a maintenance category classification and not to be utilized for acute exacerbations. Zafirlukast (Accolate), montelukast (Singulair), and zileuton (Zyflo) are the most current medications available.

TABLE 15-3. NORMAL VALUES FOR PULSE OXIMETRY, VENOUS OXIMETRY, AND CAPNOGRAPHY

Parameter	*Value*	*Significance*
Pulse oximetry (SpO_2)	> 93% < 93%	Normal Hypoxemia
Venous oximetry (SvO_2)	60%–80% > 80% < 60%	Normal Decreased oxygen consumption Malposition of catheter Increased oxygen consumption or decreased oxygen delivery
($ScvO_2$)	70%–85%	Normal
Capnography ($PetCO_2$)	1–5 mm Hg < $PaCO_2$ > 5 mm Hg	Normal Widened gradient (Va/Q mismatch or increased dead space ventilation) can be due to pulmonary emboli, lung disease, or loss of cardiac output

Mast Cell Stabilizers

Cromolyn (Intal) and nedocromil sodium (Tilade) are inhaled medications used to stabilize the mast cells and reduce mast cell degranulation. They have no direct bronchodilator effect and are not used in acute situations. The drugs prevent the mast cells from releasing histamine and other mediators that lead to bronchoconstriction, edema, and inflammation of the airways. The dosage for cromolyn is 20 mg qid via nebulizer. Tilade is given in doses of 4 mg qid.

15.3 ADJUNCTIVE RESPIRATORY MONITORING

Adjunctive respiratory monitoring includes pulse oximetry, venous oximetry, and capnography (**Table 15-3**).

Oximetry

Pulse Oximetry. Pulse oximetry (Spo_2 is oxygen saturation as measured by pulse oximetry) is a commonly used and excellent indicator of arterial oxygen saturation (Sao_2) values. It can decrease the need to obtain ABGs; however, it is recommended that an ABG be obtained initially to verify the accuracy of the pulse oximeter and to determine $PaCO_2$ levels. Pulse oximetry is most useful in trending saturation levels during weaning from oxygen therapy or positive end-expiratory pressure (PEEP)/continuous positive airway pressure levels. Spot checks or one-time pulse oximetry readings have little value and are not recommended.

Pulse oximetry does not monitor ventilation (CO_2 levels). Monitoring for hypoventilation is only truly accurate if the patient is not wearing oxygen due to a masking effect that supplemental oxygen may have on patients with decreased respiratory effort.

Oximetry measures functional, not fractional Sao_2. Therefore the pulse oximetry reading is expected to be slightly higher than the Sao_2 measured by an ABG sample in the laboratory. Pulse oximetry must be used with caution when elevated values of abnormal hemoglobins are present. **For example, the Spo_2 functional measurement will mistake carboxyhemoglobin for oxyhemoglobin and will display a value that reflects the total of the two versus just the oxyhemoglobin.**

QUICK TIP! An exam question may include a patient with carbon monoxide poisoning with a seemingly normal SaO_2 of > 95%. However, these patients are still clinically hypoxic and benefit from 100% O_2. Symptoms also include headache, dizziness, confusion, and weakness.

Complications associated with the use of pulse oximetry are skin breakdown at the probe site and inaccurate readings due to venous stasis, low blood pressure (below 90 mm Hg systolic), and low perfusion states. Forehead or nasal alar oximetry can be used in low perfusion states when traditional pulse oximetry is not able to pick up a reliable signal. Other potential sources of error with pulse oximetry may be excessive movement, dark (blue or black) nail polish, artificial nails, and ambient light effect on a loose-fitting probe.

Venous Oximetry. Mixed venous oximetry utilizes blood from the pulmonary artery to estimate overall oxygenation. The balance between oxygen transport and consumption is estimated by levels of mixed venous oxygen saturation (SvO_2). As long as blood flow to the capillaries is relatively normal, SvO_2 levels provide relatively accurate reflections of cellular oxygenation. **Normal SvO_2 values, between 0.60 and 0.80,** indicate an adequate balance between oxygen delivery and consumption. **If the SvO_2 falls less than 0.60, either oxygen transport has *decreased* or oxygen consumption has *increased* indicating a risk for lack of oxygen at the tissue level (and the root cause should be investigated).** While limitations exist with SvO_2 use, it remains one of the more valuable tools in the assessment of global tissue oxygenation. The continuous SvO_2 levels will be higher, about 2%, than laboratory-measured values, because it measures only oxyhemoglobin and reduced hemoglobin.

Complications associated with continuous SvO_2 monitoring include inadequate calibration of the monitor, infection from long-term pulmonary artery catheter insertion, damage to the fiberoptics in the catheter, and possible malposition of the catheter.

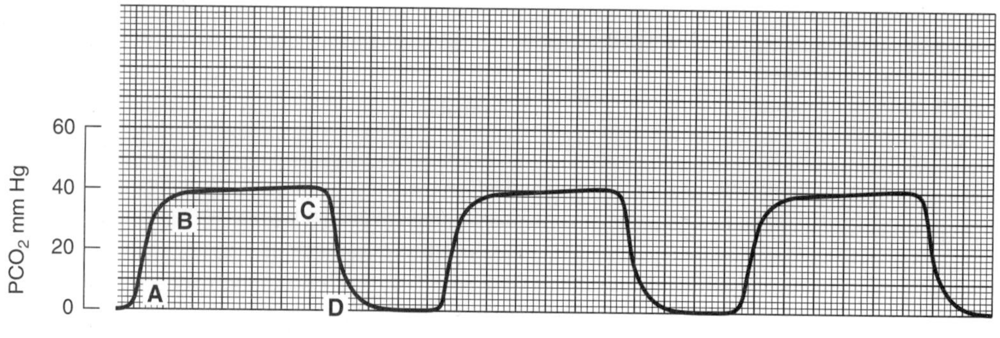

Figure 15-9. The normal capnogram. (A) Carbon dioxide concentration is zero, consists of gas from anatomic dead space. (B) Alveolar plateau, minimal rise in carbon dioxide near the end of exhalation. (C) End-tidal carbon dioxide level ($PetCO_2$). (D) Inspiration, rapid fall in carbon dioxide.

True SvO_2 values can be obtained only from the pulmonary artery. Venous saturations obtained from large vessels near the right heart, central venous oxygen saturation ($ScvO_2$), can provide a similar assessment of global tissue oxygenation. A normal $ScvO_2$ is 0.70 to 0.85. Intermittent lab samples may be drawn from the distal lumen of a central venous catheter placed in or near the right atrium. Some catheters have continuous $ScvO_2$ capability.

Capnography. Arterial carbon dioxide levels are the key to determining the adequacy of alveolar ventilation. Capnography is a noninvasive method of assessing exhaled carbon dioxide. The peak exhaled carbon dioxide value, end-tidal carbon dioxide level ($PetCO_2$), is a close approximation of arterial carbon dioxide values ($PaCO_2$). It is usually slightly lower than arterial values ($PaCO_2$) by 1 to 5 mm Hg and can be used to approximate $PaCO_2$.

When an increase in physiologic dead space exists, the $PetCO_2$ may not equal the $PaCO_2$. The clinician can monitor the $PaCO_2$–$PetCO_2$ gradient as an indicator of the severity of the pulmonary dead space; the greater the gradient, the greater the dead space. Trends in the gradient are useful to the clinician in following changes in dead space. *Some of the common clinical conditions that increase dead space are pulmonary embolism, low cardiac output states, overdistended alveoli from high PEEP or tidal volume and COPD.* In patients with COPD, the gradient may rise to 10 to 20 mm Hg or higher as a result of the ventilation/perfusion mismatch.

A capnogram is a display of the $PetCO_2$ values or a recorded waveform of carbon dioxide concentration. Fast-speed capnograms are used for breath-to-breath analysis, while slow-speed capnograms are used for trending over time (**Fig. 15-9**).

Capnography has many valuable uses. It is excellent at detecting tracheal intubations since it will reflect a CO_2 waveform. Capnography is a standard for intubation and ongoing monitoring of an artificial airway with mechanical ventilation. If an artificial airway becomes dislodged from the airway, the capnogram will reflect a loss of CO_2 waveform. Often the capnography alarm will alert the clinician before the ventilator alarm sounds. Capnography is also useful in assessing the effectiveness of cardiopulmonary resuscitation. Circulation is required to bring CO_2 from the cells to the lungs to be exhaled. When an arrest situation occurs, circulation will cease and the capnography waveform will reflect zero or a very low value. **As circulation is reestablished, the capnogram and $PetCO_2$ values will increase, reflecting the return of circulation.** During an arrest, lack of rise in capnography is indicative of a poor outcome, since effective circulation has not been restored. Capnography—mainstream or real-time measurement—**can be used to help** *identify end-exhalation on hemodynamic waveforms* **as well as indicate a decrease in cardiac output.** Capnography is useful for monitoring patients for hypoventilation during and after *procedural sedation, anesthesia, and opioid administration.*

KEY CONTENT CHECKLIST

- ❐ When a wheeze disappears and airflow is diminishing, this is considered a potentially ominous sign, such as in a worsening asthma patient. In this case, immediate action would be required, possibly including intubation.
- ❐ When interpreting ABGs, when the pH and the arterial carbon dioxide pressure ($Paco_2$) move in *opposite* directions, the primary cause of acid–base disturbance is *respiratory*. If the pH and the $Paco_2$ move in the *same* direction, the primary cause is *metabolic*.
- ❐ Pulse oximetry does not monitor ventilation (CO_2 levels). Monitoring for hypoventilation is only accurate if the patient is not wearing oxygen or with the use of capnography with or without oxygen administration.
- ❐ An exam question may include a patient with carbon monoxide poisoning with a seemingly normal SaO_2 of > 95%. However, these patients are still clinically hypoxic and benefit from 100% O_2. Symptoms also include headache, dizziness, confusion, and weakness.
- ❐ Using intravenous sodium bicarb drips to correct acidotic states is controversial unless the pH is extremely low. The best way to correct an acidotic state is to find and fix the cause of the acidosis. For example, diabetic ketoacidosis—administer insulin to decrease ketone production, or with lactic acidosis—reestablish oxygenation or perfusion to restore aerobic cell metabolism.

Review Questions:

Questions 1 and 2 refer to the following scenario:

After consulting with the physician, you have decided to begin weaning a 71-year-old woman from mechanical ventilation. She is placed on pressure-support ventilation (PSV) of 5 cm H_2O with a PEEP of +3 cm H_2O. After the weaning trial has been in progress for an hour, you obtain ABGs. The ABGs and vital signs are listed below:

Blood pressure 140/78 mm Hg
Pulse 94 (sinus rhythm)
Respiratory rate 22
Temperature 37.3
Spo_2 0.98
pH 7.23
$PaCO_2$ 59
Pao_2 91
HCO_3^- 24

1. Based on the above information, what is your interpretation of the ABGs?

a. Respiratory acidosis with a compensating metabolic alkalosis
b. Metabolic acidosis with a compensating respiratory alkalosis
c. Uncompensated respiratory acidosis
d. Uncompensated metabolic alkalosis

Answer: C. Rationale: The pH is acidotic at 7.23. The CO_2 is elevated at 59 indicating the respiratory acidosis as the source of the acid. Since the pH is not normal, it is not yet compensated.

2. Based on the above information, what action should you take?

a. Extubate at this time because she is doing well enough
b. Return to the ventilator since the ABGs indicate that she is failing the spontaneous breathing attempt
c. Continue the trial for another hour and then repeat the ABGs

Answer: B. Rationale: The increase in CO_2 indicates the patient is unable to maintain adequate ventilation and still requires the assistance of the ventilator to achieve adequate gas exchange.

16

Alternative Methods of Ventilatory Support

CHAPTER OVERVIEW AND OBJECTIVES

The CCRN exam will include questions related to ventilatory and oxygenation failure. This chapter reviews the treatment of these conditions. It is important to understand the concepts of mechanical ventilation, positive end-expiratory pressure (PEEP)/continuous positive airway pressure (CPAP), and oxygen therapy.

After studying this chapter, you should understand the following:

- The goal of oxygen therapy is to deliver a concentration of inspired oxygen to diffuse into the blood to provide adequate oxygen to body tissues. Recall that an adequate cardiac output and red blood cell concentration are also important for oxygen delivery to the tissues.
- Low-flow oxygen devices provide supplemental oxygen to be inhaled with patient inspirations.
- High-flow oxygen devices provide oxygen at greater concentrations accompanied by positive pressure airflow assisting with inspiratory efforts and volumes.
- Artificial airways and invasive mechanical ventilation provide a variety of settings to control respirations to assist with gas exchange according to the disease process in an individual patient.

16.1 OXYGEN THERAPY

Oxygen therapy is used to support oxygen transport while the underlying cause of oxygenation failure is being treated. There are two methods of delivering oxygen therapy: low- and high-flow systems (**Table 16-1**).

Low-Flow Oxygen Systems

Low-flow systems do not meet all inspiratory volume needs, requiring patients to entrain room air. The advantage of a low-flow oxygen system is its ease of use. In a low-flow oxygen system, the fraction of inspired oxygen level (FIO_2) fluctuates with varying depths of inspiration. A shallow breath has a higher FIO_2 than a deep one, even though the liter flow is the same, because less room air is entrained during inspiration. Low-flow systems provide FIO_2 levels between 24% and 44% with a nasal cannula or between 40% and 60% with a simple face mask (**Table 16-2**). Rebreathing masks can provide higher levels of inspired oxygen; however, they are not as reliable as high-flow systems.

Low-flow oxygen systems are useful in the less acutely ill or mouth-breathing patient. The oral inspiration of air draws nasal gases simultaneously into the lungs, allowing for effective oxygen therapy.

High-Flow Oxygen Systems

High-flow oxygen systems meet all inspiratory volume and flow requirements independent of inspiratory changes. High-flow oxygen systems can also now be delivered via nasal cannula and can provide stable FIO_2 levels, with oxygen concentrations 24% to 100% (**Table 16-3**). Critically ill patients with **oxygenation disturbances** will almost always require high-flow oxygen systems. *Oxygen therapy should not be removed until a stable SpO_2 or PaO_2/FIO_2 greater than 286 (60/0.21) is present.*

Complications

If oxygen therapy generates an arterial oxygen pressure (PaO_2) level more than 60 mm Hg or an arterial oxygen saturation (SaO_2) level more than 0.90, no further increases in oxygen therapy should be instituted. Oxygen therapy is not without risk.

TABLE 16-1. LOW- AND HIGH-FLOW OXYGEN THERAPY

Low-Flow
Nasal cannula
Simple face masks
Rebreather masks
Nonrebreather masks
High-Flow
High-flow nasal cannula
Oxymizer
Venturi masks
Nebulizer-regulated FIO_2 systems
Ventilator circuits

TABLE 16-3. OXYGEN DELIVERY WITH THE VENTURI MASK SYSTEM

FIO_2 Desired	*O_2 Liter Flow Required (L/min)*	*Air Entrainment Ratio*	*Total Gas Flow Delivered (L/min)*
0.24	4	1:25	104
0.28	4	1:20	44
0.31	6	1:7	48
0.35	8	1:5	48
0.40	8	1:3	32
0.50	12	1:1.7	32

An oxygen concentration in excess of 50% for more than 24 to 48 hours increases the potential for the development of oxygen toxicity and lung damage. Alveolar type II cells, *responsible for producing surfactant, are impaired by high oxygen levels.*

One of the factors promoting alveolar expansion is the presence of nitrogen, the most plentiful gas, making up approximately 79% of the barometric pressure. When 100% oxygen therapy is employed, nitrogen is completely displaced or washed out by the oxygen, resulting in a PaO_2 of 400 to 600 mm Hg. If perfusion exceeds ventilation, all oxygen can be absorbed from the alveoli, resulting in atelectasis.

High-Flow Nasal Cannula

High-flow nasal cannula (HFNC) provides oxygen in conjunction with compressed air and humidification delivered to the patient via a large bore nasal canula device at rates of air flow higher than can be delivered in traditional O_2 therapy. HFNC is more comfortable and generally well tolerated allowing the patient to eat, drink, and talk. Airflow and oxygen delivery can be independently titrated to provide up to 60 L/min of airflow and 100% FIO_2.

Continuous Positive Airway Pressure

CPAP is above atmospheric levels applied throughout the respiratory cycle for spontaneous breaths. CPAP stabilizes the airways during the expiratory phase. PaO_2 values can be increased if the functional residual capacity (FRC) can be increased and the time for gas exchange to occur is increased. CPAP increases FRC, improves distribution of ventilation, helps hold alveoli open, and opens smaller airways, improving oxygenation and potentially decreases **preload**. CPAP may help prevent microatelectasis and promote alveolar stability. For patients who have obstructive sleep apnea, CPAP is a common home treatment to hold the airway open and prevent collapse of the upper airway. Airway collapse and the negative changes in intrathoracic pressure are contributing factors to cardiac dysrhythmias, pulmonary hypertension, systemic hypertension, increasing risk of stroke, and other medical conditions.

TABLE 16-2. APPROXIMATE FIO_2 WITH NASAL CANNULA AND FACE MASK

	Liter Flow (L/min)	*Approximate FIO_2 (%)*
Nasal cannula	1	24
	2	28
	3	32
	4	36
	5	40
	6	44
Face mask	5–6	40
	6–7	50
	7–8	60

Bilevel Positive Airway Pressure

BiPAP, a form of noninvasive positive pressure ventilation (NPPV), is much like CPAP and may be seen more often in hospital settings but can also be a home treatment. In the hospital, patients in acute respiratory failure may need higher inspiratory pressures than CPAP can provide. BiPAP settings may include a minimum or backup respiratory rate and two pressure settings: a higher inspiratory pressure to increase tidal volume resulting in increased alveolar ventilation and a lower expiratory pressure that then provides a positive end-expiratory pressure (PEEP) to increase FRC resulting in an increased PaO_2 level. BiPAP reduces the work of breathing, is more like natural respirations, can deliver oxygen therapy, and is more effective at reducing CO_2 retention in hypercapnic respiratory failure. Additional information on NPPV is found later in this chapter.

Positive End-Expiratory Pressure

PEEP is the application of a positive airway pressure at end-exhalation while the patient is on mechanical ventilation. It improves oxygenation by the same mechanisms as CPAP and BiPAP. PEEP is effective at raising PaO_2 and SaO_2 levels by maintaining alveolar airflow during expiration. Airways tend to collapse during expiration because of increasing pressures outside the airway (**Fig. 16-1**).

Some clinicians believe in physiologic PEEP, a concept assuming that some PEEP is present in all people because of resistance of the airways. Low levels of PEEP, such as 3 to 5 cm H_2O, may be ordered even in patients without oxygenation problems to simulate physiologic PEEP.

PEEP is indicated to help reduce FIO_2 levels or to elevate PaO_2/SaO_2 values when high FIO_2 levels are unsuccessful, to drive lung water back into the vascular system, or to reduce mediastinal bleeding postoperatively.

Optimal PEEP levels are achieved by the lowest level of PEEP needed to raise the PaO_2/SaO_2 levels and do not result in

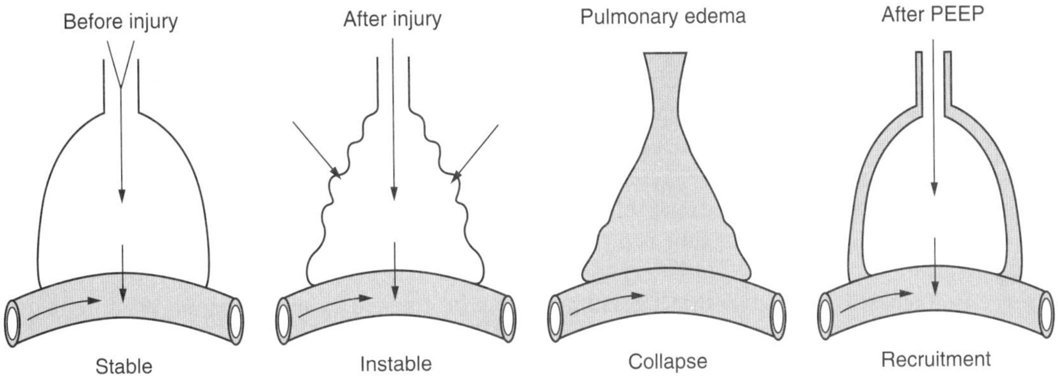

Figure 16-1. Effects of PEEP on airway stabilization, demonstrating recruitment of the alveoli.

cardiovascular compromise, such as decreased cardiac output, impeded right-heart filling, or tachycardia. The optimal PEEP level varies from patient to patient, although levels of PEEP higher than 20 cm H_2O are uncommon. Values between 5 and 15 cm H_2O are common in support of the patient with hypoxemia.

Auto-PEEP

Auto-PEEP, also known as intrinsic PEEP, is the trapping of air in the alveoli, producing PEEP as the result of early airway closure or insufficient exhalation time. Patients at risk for the development of auto-PEEP include those with chronic obstructive pulmonary disease (COPD) or asthma or patients with increased minute ventilation (VE) of 20 L/min or more; auto-PEEP may also develop with tachypnea, including overly aggressive Ambu-bagging. It can be measured by obstructing the exhalation port of a ventilator immediately prior to an inspiratory effort. Some mechanical ventilators will provide this assessment without manual occlusion of the exhalation port (**Fig. 16-2**).

Complications of auto-PEEP include increased work of breathing; barotrauma; hemodynamic compromise, such as decreased cardiac output and decreased venous return to the right heart; misinterpretation of filling pressure (PAOP/LA or CVP/RA) readings; increased intracranial pressure (ICP); decreased renal function; passive hepatic congestion; and increased intrapulmonary shunt.

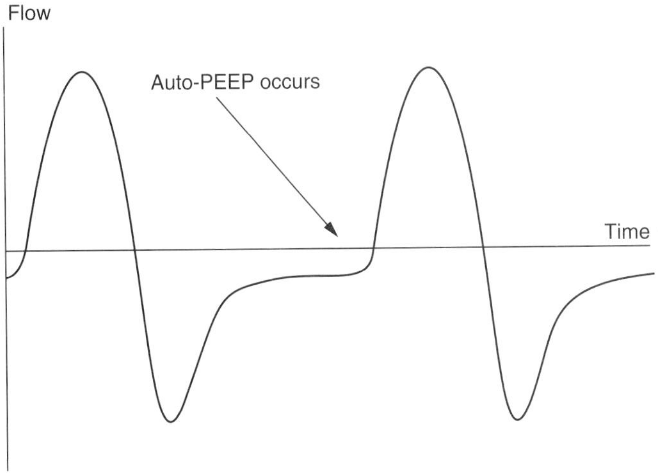

Figure 16-2. Airway flow showing incomplete exhalation and the presence of auto-PEEP.

Complications of PEEP, CPAP, and BiPAP

PEEP, CPAP, and BiPAP have potential side effects related to the increased airway pressures. When PEEP, CPAP, or BiPAP is applied, the cardiac output must be carefully monitored. **Cardiac output and stroke volume can fall because of the increased intrathoracic pressure, which impedes venous blood return to the right heart, producing a pseudohypovolemia.** If cardiac outputs are not available, the heart rate and systolic blood pressure are monitored. Increases in the heart rate and falls in systolic blood pressure may signal a reduction in cardiac output and stroke volume. In heart failure (HF), this reduction in venous blood return can actually be beneficial to reduce the fluid overload on the heart improving the heart's function until diuretics can reduce vascular fluid volume.

Barotrauma and pneumothorax are also complications of PEEP, CPAP, and BiPAP. Lung sounds should be monitored, and the thorax should be percussed for potential development of **pneumothorax and pneumomediastinum**. Sustained peak airway pressures (PAPs) greater than 40 cm H_2O increase the risk of barotrauma.

> **QUICK TIP!** The complications of PEEP, including the risk of pneumothorax frequently appear on the exam. This often involves a scenario of a ventilated patient with a drop in cardiac output or an abrupt onset of unilateral absence of lung sounds.

16.2 ARTIFICIAL AIRWAYS

To use an invasive ventilator, the patient must have an artificial airway, such as an endotracheal or a tracheostomy tube.

Endotracheal Tubes

Endotracheal tubes (ETTs) are used to establish and maintain an airway. They may be inserted nasally or orally by trained and experienced clinicians. Immediately after intubation, *placement of the ETT in the airway can be confirmed by the presence of CO_2 using **capnography***. All chest fields are auscultated to make sure that there are bilateral breath sounds. Physical examination should never substitute for CO_2 detection. Chest x-ray (CXR) is important to ensure whether the tip of the ETT is about 1 in. (2–3 cm) above the carina. Frequency of CXR is indicated postintubation and with worsening in condition. Reassessment of the ETT placement is mandatory. ETT position can change with coughing, patient movement, and suctioning. Continuous monitoring with *end-tidal CO_2 can detect a loss of airway early.* Nasotracheal intubation is contraindicated in patients with increased ICP, head trauma, or chronic sinusitis. Disadvantages include the possibility of tissue necrosis, nosebleed, rupture of nasal polyps, and submucosal dissection. Increased mucus production because of the irritant properties of the tube increases the patient's susceptibility to infection and the occurrence of ventilator-acquired pneumonia. Stabilization of the tube is difficult in the diaphoretic patient.

The advantages of orotracheal intubation are direct visualization and rapid intubation. Oral ETTs are repositioned every 2 to 4 hours to prevent necrosis of the lips or tongue. Disadvantages of oral intubation include increased dryness of oral mucosa, production of mucus, gagging, and susceptibility to infection.

Complications associated with intubation include laryngeal and tracheal trauma, ETT tube obstruction and displacement, **intubation of the right mainstem bronchus**, and infection.

Tracheostomy

Tracheostomy, the formation of an opening into the trachea, may be performed if long-term ventilatory support is expected. Tracheostomies bypass upper airway obstruction, decrease dead space, may help prevent aspiration and may decrease the possibilities of necrosis and/or tracheoesophageal (TE) fistula formation. Once a tracheostomy is in place, a sterile tracheostomy tube of the same size used in the patient must be at the patient's bedside for emergency replacement. An ETT of the same or smaller size is also acceptable for maintaining the airway in an emergency. Care must be taken when replacing a displaced tracheostomy tube since tubes can be placed into false tracks and may not actually be in the airway. Tube placement should be confirmed with capnography and CXR.

Suctioning

Maintaining patency of the airway can be facilitated through suctioning. Suctioning is a sterile procedure and can be accomplished with a closed-system multiple-use catheter or the traditional single-use catheter. **Suctioning should not be routinely performed. It should occur in situations such as secretions are blocking the airway, peak pressures are increased, oxygenation is decreased, or with respiratory distress.** Hyperoxygenation of the patient prior to suctioning reduces hypoxemia associated with suctioning. Patients who benefit from hyperoxygenation include those receiving an FIO_2 of 0.40 or higher, those who have demonstrated decreased SaO_2 with suctioning and those with cardiovascular compromise such as bradycardia or premature ventricular contractions (PVCs).

Suction pressures of less than 200 are generally adequate to remove secretions. The removal of viscous, thick secretions is difficult even with adequate suction. **The lack of benefit of instillation of saline in the endotracheal or tracheostomy tube has been well documented and such a maneuver increases the risk of ventilator-associated pneumonia (VAP).** Thinning of pulmonary secretions is accomplished by adequate fluid intake and the use of mucolytics. The stimulation of cough is a very effective aid to the clearance of secretions.

Cuff Management

Most ETTs and tracheostomy tubes for initiation of mechanical ventilation have inflatable cuffs. The cuff provides a closed system with a seal and reduces aspiration of fluids into the lungs. Soft, low-pressure cuffs are preferred because they minimize tracheal necrosis and fistula development. Pressure is distributed over a large area, and only sufficient pressure to provide a seal is necessary.

Policies vary from hospital to hospital regarding the measurement of cuff pressures. Generally, a minimal occlusive pressure is maintained at 25 cm H_2O or less, or 20 mm Hg, to prevent tracheal damage. If more pressure is required, the patient may need to have a larger tube inserted. Cuff pressure can be checked by using a blood pressure manometer, syringe and stopcock, or pressure manometer specifically designed for measuring cuff pressures. This may be a shared responsibility with the respiratory care practitioner.

Deflation of the cuff is not recommended while mechanical ventilation is in place. During the weaning process in a patient with a tracheostomy, the patient may have periods of time off ventilation when the tracheostomy tube cuff can be deflated. Before deflating the cuff, the patient should be suctioned carefully, especially orotracheally, to remove any secretions that may have accumulated on the top of the cuff. The patient must be monitored carefully for potential aspiration.

Complications

The major complication of a cuffed tube is obstruction from dried secretions (airway plugging). The increased production of mucus stimulated by the foreign body puts the patient at increased risk for airway plugging. The maintenance of adequate hydration and suctioning will help reduce the risk of plugging. Biofilm development on the artificial airway can lead to narrowing of the tube lumen. Additional potential complications include laryngeal edema, mucosal erosion, development of granulomas, vocal cord paralysis, and tracheal stenosis.

ETTs can become displaced easily, leading to loss of airway, carinal rupture, unilateral lung ventilation, tension pneumothorax, and atelectasis. *Signs of tube misplacement include loss of the end-tidal CO_2 waveform, diminished or absent lung sounds, loss of tidal volume, low-pressure alarm on the ventilator, little if any chest excursion on the contralateral side, expiratory wheezing, and sometimes uncontrollable coughing.* **Tension pneumothorax** *may occur in the lung that has become intubated; this is one of the most serious complications of ventilatory support. The only treatment is insertion of a chest tube to relieve the pressure and remove air. Without adequate treatment,* **tension pneumothorax** *can be rapidly fatal.*

If a tracheostomy tube's position fluctuates with the patient's pulse, it is possible that the tube is rubbing against the innominate artery; in such a case the physician is notified immediately. Erosion of the artery usually results in exsanguination and death. A tracheostomy tube may become misplaced, causing subcutaneous and/or mediastinal emphysema or pneumothorax. Progressively deteriorating blood gases, loss of capnography waveform, poor air movement, and/or difficulty in suctioning should alert the clinician to a possible shift in the tracheostomy tube.

Tracheal dilatation, ischemia, and necrosis may occur because tracheostomy tubes and ETTs are round whereas the trachea is oval. If ischemia and necrosis progress, a tracheal-esophageal (TE) fistula may occur. If suspected, this can be easily tested by instilling methylene blue into the mouth. If it is suctioned from the ETT or tracheostomy, a TE fistula may have developed. Confirmation of a TE fistula may be needed with either further imaging or endoscopic examination. This may be minimized using low-pressure cuffs.

The longer an ETT or tracheostomy tube is in place, the greater the danger of infection. *Frequent oral hygiene, including manual plaque removal with teeth brushing, use of chlorhexidine oral rinse,* and tube care, will make the patient more comfortable and help to reduce the risk of infection. **Keeping the head of bed elevated higher than 30 degrees can help prevent aspiration and decrease the risk of VAP.**

16.3 MECHANICAL VENTILATION

Respiratory failure occurs when the patient is unable to adequately oxygenate tissue—*Hypoxemic respiratory failure* or to remove CO_2 from tissues—*Hypercapnic respiratory failure* or a combination of both. Mechanical ventilation is indicated for one of three reasons: to improve or support alveolar ventilation, to reduce the work of breathing, or to aid in supporting oxygenation each of which cause respiratory failure. Improvement of alveolar ventilation (VA) is most obviously needed when $Paco_2$ levels are increasing along with a falling pH. Reducing the work of breathing may be necessary when respiratory rates are more than 30 breaths/min (**Table 16-4**). All modes of mechanical ventilation are designed to support one of these three functions. Mechanical ventilation should be considered early in the disease process to prevent the emergent need.

Mechanical ventilation is delivered by either negative or positive pressure. Negative-pressure ventilators include the iron lung or thoracic cuirass, which are no longer utilized in acute respiratory failure. Positive-pressure ventilators force air into the lungs, reversing normal breathing pressures and applying alveolar ventilation support.

The reversal of the normal negative inspiratory pressure to a positive pressure has a direct effect on the cardiovascular system. The increased intrathoracic pressure impedes venous return to the right heart, thus reducing stroke volume and cardiac output. The initial response may be a reflex increase in the heart rate to maintain cardiac output.

A complication of positive-pressure ventilation is pulmonary *barotrauma/volutrauma.* The PAP on the ventilator should be monitored to assess excessive airway pressures. The PAP reflects the pressure required to deliver the tidal volume (VT). It considers the resistance of the ventilator circuit, airway resistance, and compliance of the lungs. High PAPs can be monitored through dynamic compliance by dividing the PAP into the VT. Normal dynamic compliance is 40 to 55 cm/mL. Values lower than 30 cm/mL place the patient at increased risk for barotrauma/volutrauma. Plateau pressures are more reflective of alveolar pressure. Plateau pressures are measured at the end of inspiration and require a brief inspiratory hold or pause to be assessed. *Plateau pressures higher than 30 mm Hg place the patient at risk of barotrauma/volutrauma* (**Fig. 16-3**).

TABLE 16-4. SIGNS OF FAILURE OF SPONTANEOUS BREATHING

Respiratory rate	> 35 breaths per min
Tidal volume (VT)	< 2 mL/kg
Minute ventilation (VE)	< 5 or > 12 L/min
$PaCO_2$	Increasing by > 10 mm Hg from baseline
End-tidal CO_2	Rising trend
pH	< 7.30 with a rising $Paco_2$
Blood pressure	Increase in systolic of 20 mm Hg
Heart rate	Increase of > 20 bpm over resting heart rate

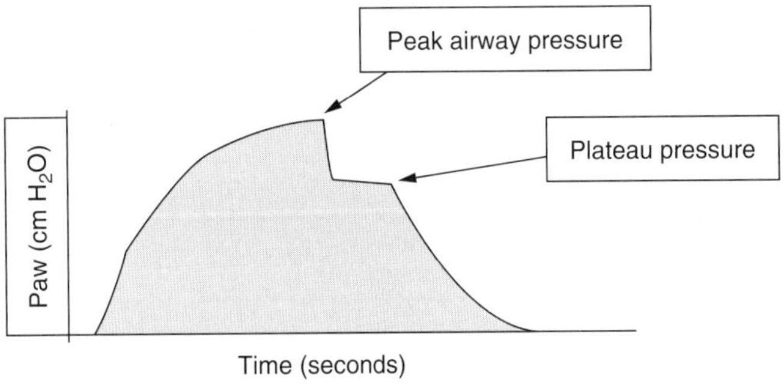

Figure 16-3. Peak and plateau airway pressure curves.

Modes of Mechanical Ventilation

Ventilator breaths can be delivered by several modes and are subdivided into categories that determine the method by which the breath is terminated: volume, pressure, or time. Some of the newer modes will blend these functions. Respiratory rate and VT are manipulated to achieve specific endpoints such as levels of oxygenation or minute ventilation.

Volume-Controlled Modes. The most common modes of mechanical ventilation are volume-controlled modes. The ventilator breath will be delivered until the preset volume (VT) is reached. The pressure required to deliver that breath will be variable. For safety, an upper pressure limit is set to prevent excessive pressures in the thoracic cavity. If the upper pressure limit is reached, the ventilator will cease delivering the breath. Continuous mandatory ventilation (CMV), assisted mandatory ventilation (AMV or assist/control), and synchronized intermittent mandatory ventilation (SIMV) are examples of volume modes (**Fig. 16-4**). *VT on all modes is initially set at 6 to 8 mL/kg of ideal body weight based on patient's height (not actual body weight)* with a respiratory rate between 8 and 20 breaths/min.

Continuous Mandatory Ventilation. CMV is used to support patients with little or no ventilatory drive or to gain control over excessive ventilatory drive. The ventilator delivers the preset VT at the preset rate without sensitivity to patient inspiratory effort. The patient is unable to initiate breaths or to change the breathing pattern in any way. CMV is rarely used.

Assisted Mandatory Ventilation. AMV (assist/-control) delivers constant preset VT and a minimum number of breaths determined by the preset respiratory rate. The patient can initiate a breath or more breaths than the minimum setting; however, they will be delivered at the preset VT. The patient can alter the respiratory rate and pattern, not the VT. The advantage of AMV is a reduction in the work of breathing. AMV can be used in weaning from mechanical ventilation by incorporating a spontaneous breathing trial (SBT) with T-piece or CPAP trials.

Synchronized Intermittent Mandatory Ventilation. SIMV delivers a preset respiratory rate and VT but allows the patient to breathe spontaneously between the preset VT and rate. The volume of the

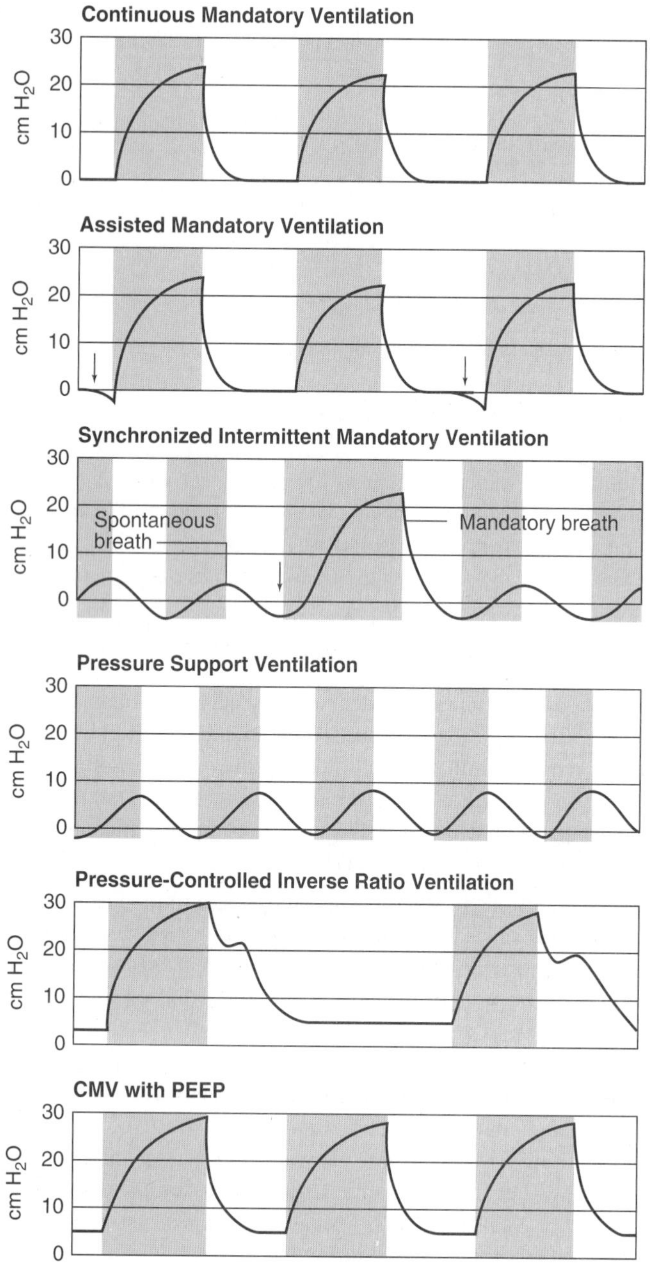

Figure 16-4. Pressure waveforms of differing modes of mechanical ventilation.

spontaneous breaths will vary depending on the patient's respiratory efforts. The patients work of breathing increases to strengthen their respiratory muscles in preparation for extubation. The ventilator is synchronized with the patient's ventilatory effort to reduce competition between the ventilator and the patient.

There are many controversies about SIMV. It may increase the work of breathing at a low respiratory rate of 6 breaths/min or less because the patient performs most of the work of breathing through the high-resistance ventilator circuit. High SIMV rates approximate AMV, as there is no time for the patient to initiate a spontaneous breath at his or her own VT. Many clinicians use a combination of SIMV and pressure-support ventilation (PSV). PSV will augment the spontaneous breaths over the set ventilator rate and decrease the work of breathing. Weaning can be accomplished by a gradual decrease in the set rate, allowing the patient to assume more of the work of breathing. SIMV does not offer an advantage in weaning over SBT and may lead to respiratory muscle fatigue.

Pressure-Limited Modes. Pressure-limited modes of mechanical ventilation will deliver a breath until a preset pressure is reached. Pressure becomes constant but the VT achieved is variable. The VT obtained is dependent on the compliance of the lungs. The more compliant the lung, the larger the VT obtained, and the less compliant the lower the VT obtained. PSV and pressure-control (PC) ventilation are the most common examples of this mode.

Pressure-Support Ventilation. In PSV, the ventilator delivers a preset positive pressure as the patient determines the inspiratory time, rate, and inspiratory flow rate. The patient is assisted during the inspiratory phase and must initiate a breath to receive the support. When inspiration ceases, the pressure support drops to ambient or PEEP. For safety, a backup apnea mode can be set on the ventilator; then, in case the patient fails to initiate a breath, the ventilator will revert to the backup mode after a predetermined time. The level of pressure support is set to achieve a VT of 6 to 8 mL/kg. Low levels of PSV, 3 to 6 cm H_2O, are valuable as an adjunct to overcoming ETT and ventilator circuit resistance. PSV can be used in weaning from mechanical ventilation by gradually decreasing its level. The combination of low levels of CPAP and PSV can be used for trials of spontaneous breathing. PSV can be added to spontaneous breaths in the SIMV mode.

Pressure-Control Ventilation. PC ventilation can be used to limit excessive airway pressures. If excessive airway pressures are being obtained during volume-limited modes of mechanical ventilation, switching to PC may be an option. Pressures will be capped or controlled and not allowed to go higher than the combination of the preset drive pressure plus the set PEEP. The drive pressure is the pressure that delivers the breath. VT and minute ventilation will be variable and must be closely monitored by the clinician. Lung compliance will affect the VT achieved. A respiratory rate can be set on PC to make the patient more comfortable while they are experiencing breathlessness or air hunger. However, PCV is more often used in critically ill patients when high peak pressures or low compliance is observed in volume cycled ventilation.

Inverse-Ratio Ventilation

In severe refractory hypoxemia, a more aggressive form of oxygenation support may be required. One of the most aggressive forms of support is inverse-ratio ventilation (IRV). In IRV, the inspiratory time from the ventilator is prolonged until it equals or exceeds expiratory time (the opposite of normal). *The primary advantage of IRV is an elevation of mean airway pressure. The elevation of mean airway pressure causes an opening of airways and a subsequent elevation of the Pao_2 and Sao_2.* Prolonging inspiratory time will increase the time oxygen must diffuse across the alveoli and attach to the hemoglobin. The increased inspiratory time may also help to open collapsed alveoli thus improving oxygenation. IRV can be delivered through either a volume- or pressure-limited mode.

In using IRV, several nursing considerations are essential. *This is an uncomfortable mode of mechanical ventilation.* First, the patient is usually **heavily sedated** and **may require paralytics** to decrease resistance to the ventilation and reduce oxygen consumption. Care must be taken to explain to the patient and family the nature of sedation and paralysis therapy that may be required. Second, the patient may not fully exhale, resulting in high levels of auto-PEEP and increasing the risk of barotraumas/volutrauma. Both a reduction in cardiac output and increased risk of lung injury **(including pneumothorax)** are present and should be monitored. The use of pressure control (PC-IRV) may decrease the risk of barotraumas/volutrauma. *Complications associated with IRV include the development of auto-PEEP, increased mean airway pressure, decreased right-heart filling, decreased cardiac output, and an increased respiratory rate.* Monitoring includes preload assessment (CVP, PAOP), cardiac output, blood pressure, exhaled V_T (PC-IRV), minute ventilation, auto-PEEP levels, compliance, Pa_{O_2}, Pa_{CO_2}, and continuous Sp_{O_2} and end-tidal CO_2 monitoring.

Blended Modes of Ventilation. Blended modes or dual modes of mechanical ventilation use elements from both volume- and pressure-limited modes. The desire is to achieve the guaranteed V_T and minimize the plateau pressure. *Currently, there is no clinical evidence to suggest that one mode of mechanical ventilation is superior to another.* As a note, different brands of ventilators will use different naming conventions, however, the method of ventilator support is the same.

Volume Control Plus. Breaths are pressure controlled with a guaranteed minimum volume, based on feedback with patient ventilation to ventilator logic. This can occur within a breath or breath-to-breath adjustment. The ventilator delivers test breaths, then adjusts pressure and flow to deliver a minimum tidal volume. Patients may experience less dyssynchrony with this mode since the flow of gas is adjusted to meet their demand. This mode is named differently by various ventilator manufacturers such as pressure-regulated volume control (PRVC), volume targeted pressure controlled, or autoflow.

Airway Pressure Release Ventilation. Airway pressure release ventilation (APRV) cycles between a high CPAP (P high) and a low CPAP (P low). A high CPAP (P high) is delivered for a long duration (T high) and then falls to a lower pressure (P low) for a shorter duration (T low). The transition from P high to P low deflates the lungs and eliminates carbon dioxide. Conversely, the transition from P low to P high inflates the lungs. Alveolar recruitment is maximized by the high CPAP. The difference between P high and P low is the driving pressure which, along with the lung compliance, will determine the V_T achieved. The time spent in T high and T low determines the rate or frequency of inflation and deflation. Spontaneous breathing can occur during the entire cycle of APRV. Further research is needed; however, APRV may decrease the PAP, improve alveolar recruitment, increase ventilation of the dependent lung zones, and improve oxygenation.

Noninvasive Ventilation. Noninvasive positive-pressure ventilation (NPPV), can be used to support a patient in hypercarbic or hypoxic respiratory failure. If successful, NPPV will allow the patient to avoid intubation and be supported until the acute event has been reversed. The earlier NPPV is applied, the greater its success. NPPV can also offer a transition for patients who require support following weaning, allowing for earlier weaning from mechanical ventilation and avoiding reintubation. NPPV is provided through a tight-fitting face mask or nasal mask. *Patients who are not candidates for NPPV are those that have an immediate need for intubation, are hypotensive, are unable to clear secretions, actively vomiting, increased ICP, or are unable to cooperate or tolerate the mask.* NPPV is given with portable ventilators that provide pressure support. Standard mechanical ventilators can also be used to provide NPPV; however, the circuits and alarms make their use more difficult. The inspiratory (IPAP) and expiratory (EPAP) pressures are set to provide the necessary level of support for each patient's need. The respiratory rate and inspiratory time can also be adjusted as per the patient's need. Patients requiring support for hypercarbic respiratory failure will require a higher IPAP to ensure adequate V_T and minute ventilation. Patients requiring support for hypoxemia will require higher EPAP levels. Initiation and titration of NPPV can be labor-intensive, as a properly fitting mask is essential as if patient cooperation . Complications of NPPV include mask discomfort; skin breakdown; facial, oropharyngeal, and eye dryness; sinus congestion; gastric insufflation; and aspiration. Hemodynamic compromise observed in positive-pressure ventilation may also be seen with NPPV.

Complications of Ventilator Support

Hypotension may occur secondary to decreased cardiac output when a patient is put on a ventilator or when ventilator adjustments are increased. *All positive-pressure ventilators exert a continuous positive pressure, which decreases venous return to the heart, thus decreasing cardiac output.* This may result in a decreased urine output and cardiac dysrhythmias. Cardiac monitoring is essential. Hypotension may be caused by hypovolemia; and intravenous fluids may correct this problem. Vasopressors are indicated if preload is increased and the cardiac output is decreased.

Infection is among the most common complications of mechanical ventilation. The warm, moist environment of the ventilator equipment makes it an ideal place for organism growth. Strict adherence to sterile technique with good hand hygiene, changing ventilator circuits only when grossly soiled, **keeping the head of bed elevated 30 degrees, aggressive oral hygiene, and weaning the patient as soon as possible are all important factors to decrease the risk of infection.** As soon as a culture identifies an infecting organism and not colonization, specific antibiotic therapy is started. Aggressive pulmonary hygiene procedures are vital nursing interventions in preventing infection.

Atelectasis often occurs with mechanical ventilation. Bronchial hygiene is extremely important to prevent further complications once atelectasis has developed. Accidental disconnection from the ventilator may occur. Immediately reconnect it or use a manual resuscitator. Continuous monitoring of **capnography** will alert the clinician early when disconnection occurs.

Pneumothorax is not unusual when PEEP is used with mechanical ventilation. Treatment is insertion of a chest tube, usually when a pneumothorax is 30% or greater or is causing tension. Without adequate treatment, pneumothorax can be rapidly fatal.

Overventilation may occur, decreasing Pa_{CO_2} more than desired. Reducing respiratory rate or V_T may be necessary to correct this problem.

16.4 WEANING FROM MECHANICAL VENTILATION

Weaning is the progressive removal of mechanical ventilatory support to spontaneous breathing. The first step in the weaning process is to determine whether the patient is ready for weaning. Assessment includes progress toward correction of the underlying reason for mechanical ventilation and respiratory mechanics; respiratory muscle endurance; and efficiency and work of breathing.

Lung-function tests used to assess readiness for weaning may include VT, vital capacity, minute ventilation, respiratory rate, and negative inspiratory force (NIF) or peak inspiratory effort (PIP), and the rapid-shallow-breathing index (respiratory frequency/VT). The routine use of these indexes is limited as they will not have a positive prediction as to which patients will be successfully weaned. Low indices can indicate a negative prediction and identify which patients may not be ready to wean. The most useful of the indices is the **rapid-shallow-breathing index**. Minute ventilation is the amount of air exchanged in 1 minute. *Normal minute ventilation is 5 to 10 L/min.* NIF or PIP is the maximal inspiratory effort the patient can generate as measured by an inspiratory manometer. Normal PIP or NIF is −70 to −90 cm H_2O (**Table 16-5**). *A NIF or at least −20 cm H_2O is the minimum for successful removal ventilatory support.* These assessments are limited by the effort the patient and therapist put into the assessment. It is important to correct as many of the patient's medical problems as possible before beginning the weaning process (**Table 16-6**).

QUICK TIP! Expect one or two questions regarding determining the appropriateness for weaning or extubation after being given a set of weaning parameters from a patient scenario.

There are several weaning techniques, including reduction of SIMV rates, reducing levels of PSV, alternating AMV with SBTs via T-piece trials, or CPAP/PSV. Weaning through the SIMV circuit may increase the work of breathing, promote respiratory muscle fatigue, and increase oxygen consumption. This method is the least successful method of weaning. *SBTs are the most effective method of liberating patients from the mechanical ventilator.* SBT should be brief, lasting from 30 to 120 min. Monitoring throughout the weaning process includes assessment of mental status, vital signs, respiratory muscle fatigue (RR, VT use of accessory muscles, rapid-shallow-breathing index), oxygenation (Spo_2), $Paco_2$ ($PetCO_2$), and electrocardiographic changes (**Table 16-7**). Care should be taken not to fatigue a patient through a prolonged SBT before extubation. Patients who fail SBTs after having the underlying process reversed may require a longer, slower wean along with physical reconditioning. **Daily readiness-to-wean assessment**, having clinician-driven weaning protocols, and using weaning teams have all been shown to decrease time spent on the ventilator.

TABLE 16-5. WEANING PARAMETERS

Muscle Efficiency	
Tidal volume (VT)	2–5 mL/kg
Minute ventilation (VE)	5–10 L/min
Vital capacity	> 10 mL/kg
Respiratory rate	< 30 breaths/min
NIF/PIP	> −20 cm H_2O
Rapid-shallow-breathing index	> 105 breaths/min/L
Oxygenation	
Pao_2	> 60 mm Hg on Fio_2 < 0.40
Hemoglobin	> 7 g/dL and not actively bleeding
Cardiac index	> 2.5 L/min
Pao_2/Fio_2 ratio	> 200
Carbon Dioxide Elimination	
$Paco_2$	35–45 mm Hg or at the patient's baseline level to maintain pH between 7.35 and 7.45
Dead space/tidal volume (VD/VT)	< 60%

TABLE 16-6. CONSIDERATIONS PRIOR TO INITIATING WEANING

Acid–base abnormalities
Airway secretion management
Cardiac abnormalities
- Arrhythmias
- Decreased cardiac output
- Anemia

Hyperglycemia
Infection
- Fever

Level of consciousness
Pain
Renal failure
- Electrolyte abnormalities
- Fluid imbalance
- Protein loss

Shock
Sleep deprivation

TABLE 16-7. CRITERIA FOR TERMINATION OF WEANING

Change in level of consciousness
Change in vital signs
- Diastolic blood pressure > 100 mm Hg
- Fall in systolic blood pressure
- Heart rate > 110 bpm or > 20 bpm increase over baseline
- Respiratory rate >30 breaths/min or > 10 breaths/min increase over baseline

Falling pulse oximetry saturation
Tidal volume < 250 mL
Rising end-tidal CO_2 values
Minute ventilation > 12 L/min (use caution and clinical judgement)
Electrocardiographic changes
- Premature ventricular contractions (PVCs) > 6/min
- Salvos of PVCs
- ST-segment elevation
- Ventricular conduction changes

Extubation

Once the patient has been successfully weaned from mechanical ventilation, the decision to extubate must be addressed. A contraindication to extubation is lack of a gag reflex and inability to protect the airway. Extubation should be done when clinical support is available to replace the ETT if necessary. Baseline vital signs, pulse oximetry, and PetCO_2 are obtained. The head of the bed is elevated 45 to 90 degrees. The airway is carefully suctioned to remove any secretions that may have accumulated on top of the cuff. After the cuff is deflated, the ETT is removed at the end of inspiration so that the patient will be able to cough and exhale forcefully to prevent the aspiration of secretions during tube removal.

The caregiver must be prepared for reintubation if upper airway obstruction, such as glottic edema, occurs. **Inspiratory stridor is treated with inhaled racemic epinephrine** 0.5 mL in 1 to 3 mL of normal saline to reduce edema. The dose is repeated at 20- to 30-minute intervals one or two times. *If this does not relieve the stridor, immediate intubation is recommended.*

The respiratory pattern will change following extubation for approximately 60 minutes. Minute ventilation increases by as much as 2 L/min, there is a slight increase in the Vt, an increase in the respiratory drive and rate, and a decrease in paradoxical abdominal movement. After about an hour, the respiratory pattern will return to preextubation patterns.

KEY CONTENT CHECKLIST

- ❒ When using BiPAP or mechanical ventilation, the reversal of the normal negative inspiratory pressure to a positive pressure has a direct effect on the cardiovascular system. The increased intrathoracic pressure impedes venous return to the right heart, and may reduce **stroke volume** and **cardiac output**. The initial response may be a reflex increase in the heart rate to maintain output.
- ❒ Suctioning an artificial airway is a sterile procedure performed only when the patient needs it such as secretions in the airway or increased PAPs.
- ❒ Patients receiving mechanical ventilation require additional monitoring for ventilator-patient interactions, as well as ventilator-related complications such as skin breakdown due to ETT or immobility, adequate nutrition, comfort, safety, patient and family interactions and support, delirium prevention, and weaning from the device.
- ❒ The complications of PEEP, including the risk of pneumothorax frequently appear on the exam. This often involves a scenario of a ventilated patient with a drop in cardiac output or an abrupt-onset of unilateral absence of lung sounds, And tracheal deviation away from the affected side.
- ❒ Expect one or two questions regarding determining the appropriateness for weaning or extubation after being given a set of weaning parameters from a patient scenario.

Review Questions:

1. Which of the following is the most common indication for PEEP therapy?

a. To improve carbon dioxide elimination
b. To treat a metabolic acidosis
c. To reduce postoperative bleeding
d. To allow reduction in F_{IO_2} levels

Answer: D. Rationale: PEEP is indicated to help reduce F_{IO_2} levels or to elevate Pa_{O_2}/Sa_{O_2} values when high F_{IO_2} levels are unsuccessful, to drive lung water back into the vascular system, or to reduce mediastinal bleeding postoperatively.

2. Which system gives more stable F_{IO_2} therapy?

a. Simple face mask
b. Nasal cannula
c. Rebreathing mask
d. Venturi mask

Answer: D. Rationale: High-flow oxygen systems meet all inspiratory volume and flow requirements independent of inspiratory changes. High-flow oxygen systems provide stable F_{IO_2} levels, with oxygen concentrations 24% to 100% (see Table 16-3). Critically ill patients with oxygenation disturbances will almost always require high-flow oxygen systems.

3. Which of the following is a complication of mechanical ventilation and PEEP therapy?

a. Atelectasis
b. Oxygen toxicity
c. Reduced cardiac output
d. ARDS

Answer: C. Rationale: The reversal of the normal negative inspiratory pressure to a positive pressure has a direct effect on the cardiovascular system. The increased intrathoracic pressure impedes venous return to the right heart, thus reducing stroke volume and cardiac output. The initial response may be a reflex increase in the heart rate to maintain output.

17

Acute Respiratory Dysfunction

CHAPTER OVERVIEW AND OBJECTIVES

Several questions on the CCRN exam can be expected to address the concepts of acute respiratory failure (ARF) and acute respiratory distress syndrome (ARDS). It is important to understand key physiologic events that produce the clinical symptoms of these conditions as well as the likely therapeutic events that might improve pulmonary function. This chapter provides a concise review of the major areas that the CCRN exam is likely to cover with respect to these topics.

After studying this chapter, you should understand the following:

- ARF occurs when the pulmonary system is unable to maintain adequate gas exchange.
- ARF occurs in many disease states and can be the primary problem or a complication of other disorders.
- It is necessary to identify the causative condition to provide appropriate treatment.

Recall that:

- Intrapulmonary shunting as areas of the lung alveoli that are inadequately ventilated but lung perfusion is adequate.
- Dead space as areas of the lung alveoli that are adequately ventilated but there is reduced pulmonary perfusion.

17.1 ACUTE RESPIRATORY FAILURE

Acute respiratory failure (ARF) is the result of abnormalities in ventilation, perfusion, or compliance or a combination of various pathologies, leading to hypercapnia and/or hypoxemia. Respiratory failure is a medical emergency that can result from long-standing, progressively worsening lung disease, or from severe lung disease that develops suddenly. The lungs are unable to maintain adequate oxygenation and carbon dioxide elimination to support metabolism, leading to respiratory acidosis. ARF develops rapidly over minutes to hours while chronic respiratory failure develops more slowly. It is necessary to identify the underlying condition in order to initiate appropriate treatment.

Pathophysiology

ARF presents as an **oxygenation or ventilation disturbance** that may be life-threatening. An alteration in **oxygenation** is the most common form of respiratory failure. Perfusion (Q) exceeds ventilation (V) (a low V/Q ratio or increased intrapulmonary **shunt**), causing decreased oxygenation of venous blood and a mixing of less oxygenated blood with arterial blood. The effect is a reduced arterial oxygen pressure ($Pa{O_2}$) value or hypoxic respiratory failure.

In ARF due to high V/Q ratios or increased **dead space** (V_D), there is a marked increase in the work of breathing. The patient increases minute ventilation (V_E) to compensate for an increased **dead space** in an effort to maintain adequate alveolar ventilation. Inadequate alveolar **ventilation** and failure to eliminate carbon dioxide cause acute increases in arterial carbon dioxide ($Pa{CO_2}$) levels, resulting in respiratory acidosis and subsequent hypercapnic respiratory failure.

Etiology and Risk Factors

Respiratory failure can arise from an abnormality in any of the components of the respiratory system, including the airways, alveoli, central nervous system (CNS), peripheral nervous system, respiratory muscles, and chest wall. Patients at risk for developing ARF include those with chronic obstructive pulmonary disease (COPD), restrictive lung disease, respiratory center depression, pulmonary edema, and pulmonary emboli, among many other conditions (**Table 17-1**).

TABLE 17-1. CAUSES OF ACUTE RESPIRATORY FAILURE
Oxygenation disturbances
Acute respiratory distress syndrome (ARDS)
Pulmonary edema
Pneumonitis
Pneumonia
Alveolar ventilation disturbances
Central nervous system depression
Medication or anesthetic effect
Head or cervical cord trauma
Cerebrovascular accident
Chronic obstructive pulmonary disease (COPD)
Interstitial pulmonary fibrosis
Pneumothorax
Ventilation/perfusion disturbances
Pulmonary emboli
Bronchiolitis
COPD
Lung trauma
Left-to-right shunt
Atelectasis
Oxygen toxicity
Pulmonary edema or emboli
Pneumonia

Chronic lung disease (COPD) complicated by a pneumonia, left ventricular (LV) failure resulting in pulmonary edema (cardiac), inhalation injuries, and ARDS are examples of ARF with alterations in oxygenation. ARF caused by a depressed CNS or a high V/Q ratio causes an increase in $Paco_2$.

Signs and Symptoms

Ventilation failure due to CNS depression presents with a slowed rate of breathing. Few other obvious physical symptoms may exist. If the ventilation failure is due to increased **dead space**, the respiratory rate (RR) and depth increase; the RR may exceed 30 breaths/min. The patient may also complain of shortness of breath and appear anxious.

Assessment findings include tachycardia, atrial cardiac dysrhythmias, pedal edema, tachypnea, dyspnea on exertion or at rest, labored breathing pattern, use of accessory muscles of respiration, crackles, wheezes, and a hyper resonant chest on percussion in patients with advanced COPD (**Table 17-2**).

Invasive and Noninvasive Diagnostic Studies

Arterial blood gas (ABG) values can deteriorate suddenly, indicating acute pulmonary insufficiency. Findings include a **Pao_2 less than 60 mm Hg**, requiring an increase in the fractional inspiratory oxygen pressure (Fio_2) and a **$Paco_2$ more than 45 mm Hg**. Other measures of oxygenation include a decreased a/A ratio (< 0.25), a widened A–a gradient, and a *decreased Pao_2/Fio_2 ratio (< 300)*. The patient may present with an elevated hematocrit (> 52%) and an elevated hemoglobin (> 18 g/dL) if this is a chronic problem and there is an underlying component of COPD. As the heart rate increases, cardiac output may fall.

TABLE 17-2. SYMPTOMS OF OXYGENATION-INDUCED RESPIRATORY FAILURE
Shortness of breath
Orthopnea
Pao_2 < 60 mm Hg
Sao_2 < 0.90
Spo_2 < 0.93
Anxiety
Increased respiratory rate (> 30 breaths/min)
Possible labored breathing
Increased intrapulmonary shunt
Pao_2/Fio_2 ratio < 300
Qs/Qt > 20%
a/A ratio < 25%
A–a gradient > 350 on 100% oxygen

The pulmonary artery diastolic pressure may be greater than 15 mm Hg if there is underlying lung disease.

Management of Patient Care

Management priorities include maintain adequate airway to optimize O_2 delivery and CO_2 removal, correction of hypoxia and acidosis, respiratory muscle rest, minimizing O_2 demand, control of shock, decreasing the risk of infection, and nutritional repletion.

Establishment or assurance of an adequate airway is needed to provide supportive treatment. Correction of hypoxia may require the use of oxygen therapy, continuous positive airway pressure (CPAP), noninvasive positive-pressure ventilation (NPPV) or endotracheal intubation with mechanical ventilation, and positive end-expiratory pressure (PEEP).

When medication is the cause of respiratory failure, discontinuation of the medication may reverse the respiratory depression and is the treatment of choice. When respiratory failure is due to trauma or increased intracranial pressure (ICP), treatment is focused on relieving the increased ICP.

When the problem is a **high V/Q ratio (increased dead-space ventilation)**, *reestablishing perfusion is the key.* If a *pulmonary embolism* exists, thrombolytic therapy may be indicated. If low perfusion is due to a low cardiac output, the cardiac output must be improved.

Supportive treatment includes oxygen therapy, PEEP, and mechanical ventilation. Treatment of LV failure producing pulmonary edema focuses on resolving the cardiac dysfunction. If a pulmonary infection is the underlying cause, antibiotic therapy is indicated.

Complications

Complications associated with ARF include severe respiratory and metabolic acidosis, infection, sequelae from use of artificial ventilation, immobility, medication administration, failure to wean from mechanical ventilation, infection, and lack of adequate nutritional support.

17.2 ACUTE RESPIRATORY DISTRESS SYNDROME

ARDS is an extreme form of respiratory failure and the most severe form of acute lung injury. It is a life-threatening condition *manifest by severe hypoxemia and decreased lung compliance.*

Pathophysiology

ARDS is the result of an acute inflammatory process where the lung becomes the target of the mediators released. There have been many mechanisms and mediators identified for the pathogenesis of ARDS. They include neutrophil activation, platelet activation, alveolar macrophage stimulation, complement activation, and the release of humoral vasoactive substances (**Fig. 17-1**).

ARDS can result from an inflammatory process that begins as a direct or indirect injury to the lung. Normally, the pulmonary capillaries allow only small amounts of fluid to leak into the interstitial compartment, which is readily drained by the pulmonary lymphatic system. Although ARDS is a *diffuse bilateral process*, it does not affect all alveoli equally. Some alveoli will remain undamaged even though they are surrounded by damaged alveoli.

Exudative Phase—Days 1 to 3. The pulmonary capillary membrane is damaged and *capillary leakage* results in a tremendous loss of fluid from the vascular space, primarily due to the loss of vascular proteins. As proteins leave the capillaries, they *pull large amounts of fluid into the pulmonary interstitial space*, overwhelming the capacity of the pulmonary lymphatic drainage and causing *alveolar flooding* and impaired oxygen transfer. Type I cells become swollen and injured. Protein, fibrin, and fluid create a membrane which contributes to collapse of the alveoli. The result is **severe intrapulmonary shunt** and hypoxemia.

Injury to the type II cells *results in* ***decreased surfactant*** *that further leads to the collapse of the alveoli,* and it becomes more difficult to open the alveoli that have collapsed. Atelectasis can result. This instability of the alveoli further increases the intrapulmonary shunt and hypoxemia.

Fibroproliferative Phase—Days 3 to 7. As healing occurs, remodeling and fibrosis occurs which can result in *stiff lungs* that can be permanent and disabling.

Resolution Phase—occurs over several weeks. Damaged lung capillaries and alveoli recover, fluid moves out of the alveoli and interstitial space. It is not understood why some patients have full recovery while others are left with a permanent respiratory disability.

Etiology and Risk Factors

The origin of ARDS is unclear, although it is felt to be the result of a severe inflammatory process. ARDS is due to direct or indirect injury to the lung. A *direct* injury process begins in the lung, *such as a pulmonary contusion or pneumonia* (**Table 17-3**). An *indirect* injury results from a process that began outside the lung, such as *pancreatitis*. ARDS will usually develop within 24 hours of the event. A few patients may develop ARDS up to 72 hours after the initial event. In those patients, for unclear reasons, it takes longer to upregulate the mediators from the inflammatory process.

Signs and Symptoms

ARDS presents with symptoms similar to those of acute hypoxic respiratory failure. Rapid deterioration of pulmonary function is a hallmark of ARDS. Clinical symptoms usually precede the change in the chest x-ray. The chest x-ray can change within an hour from relatively normal to showing **diffuse bilateral alveolar infiltrates (a whiteout picture)**, reflecting a large accumulation of lung water in a short period of time. **Hemodynamic parameters are used to differentiate ARDS from pulmonary edema due to LV failure. Generally, preload indicators will be normal or low in ARDS and high in LV failure. The pulmonary artery occlusive pressure (PAOP) is generally less than 18 mm Hg in ARDS, while LV failure presents with a high PAOP.**

QUICK TIP! A hallmark of ARDS is "noncardiogenic pulmonary edema." Diffuse, bilateral pulmonary edema is seen on the CXR; however, the PAOP is generally < 18 mm Hg.

Invasive and Noninvasive Diagnostic Studies

Early chest x-rays may appear normal. As the lung injury progresses, the chest film will initially show fine infiltrates that progress to diffuse bilateral alveolar and interstitial infiltrates, producing a "ground-glass" appearance.

ABGs will show a progressive deterioration with a falling Pao_2 that is not responsive to increases in Fio_2. As oxygenation worsens, the $Paco_2$ will begin to rise as compensatory mechanisms, such as an increased RR, fail. Other measures of oxygenation will reveal an increased V/Q mismatch (**$Pao_2/Fio_2 < 300$**), decreased oxygen delivery, and decreased oxygen consumption (VO_2).

Placement of a pulmonary artery catheter will reveal a normal, increased, or decreased cardiac output and cardiac index; normal central venous pressure (CVP); increased pulmonary vascular resistance (PVR); and normal, increased, or decreased systemic vascular resistance (SVR). **The PAOP will be normal or low, with a normal or increased pulmonary artery systolic (PAS) and diastolic (PAD) pressure.**

Management of Patient Care

Treatment of ARDS is supportive, primarily centering on supporting oxygenation through the use of mechanical ventilation, thus allowing the lung to heal while the underlying cause of the inflammatory process is treated. *Research has shown that an ARDS lung can be harmed further by improper management of the mechanical ventilator.* **Protective lung ventilation** strategies have been developed to support the patient and prevent further pulmonary damage.

Protective Ventilator Strategies

Patients with acute lung injury require changes in the management of mechanical ventilation. Since unaffected alveoli are intermingled with affected alveoli, the tidal breath will be delivered to them primarily. The amount of unaffected alveoli is small in relation to the affected alveoli. Some have compared this to the equivalent of having "baby lungs." *Care must be taken to avoid overdistention of the unaffected alveoli with each breath.* The upper inflection point on the pressure–volume curve reflects the point at which overinflation can occur (**Fig. 17-2**). To achieve this goal, *a lower tidal volume is used,* which will be below the upper inflection point. *A tidal volume of 4 to 6 mL/kg of ideal body weight* will prevent the overdistention of the alveoli that can result in further alveolar damage. *A lower pH and higher $Paco_2$ ("permissive hypercapnia")* may result from the lower minute ventilation due to use of the lower tidal volume. Patients can tolerate a moderate level of acidosis (pH 7.2 or higher) before intervention is necessary.

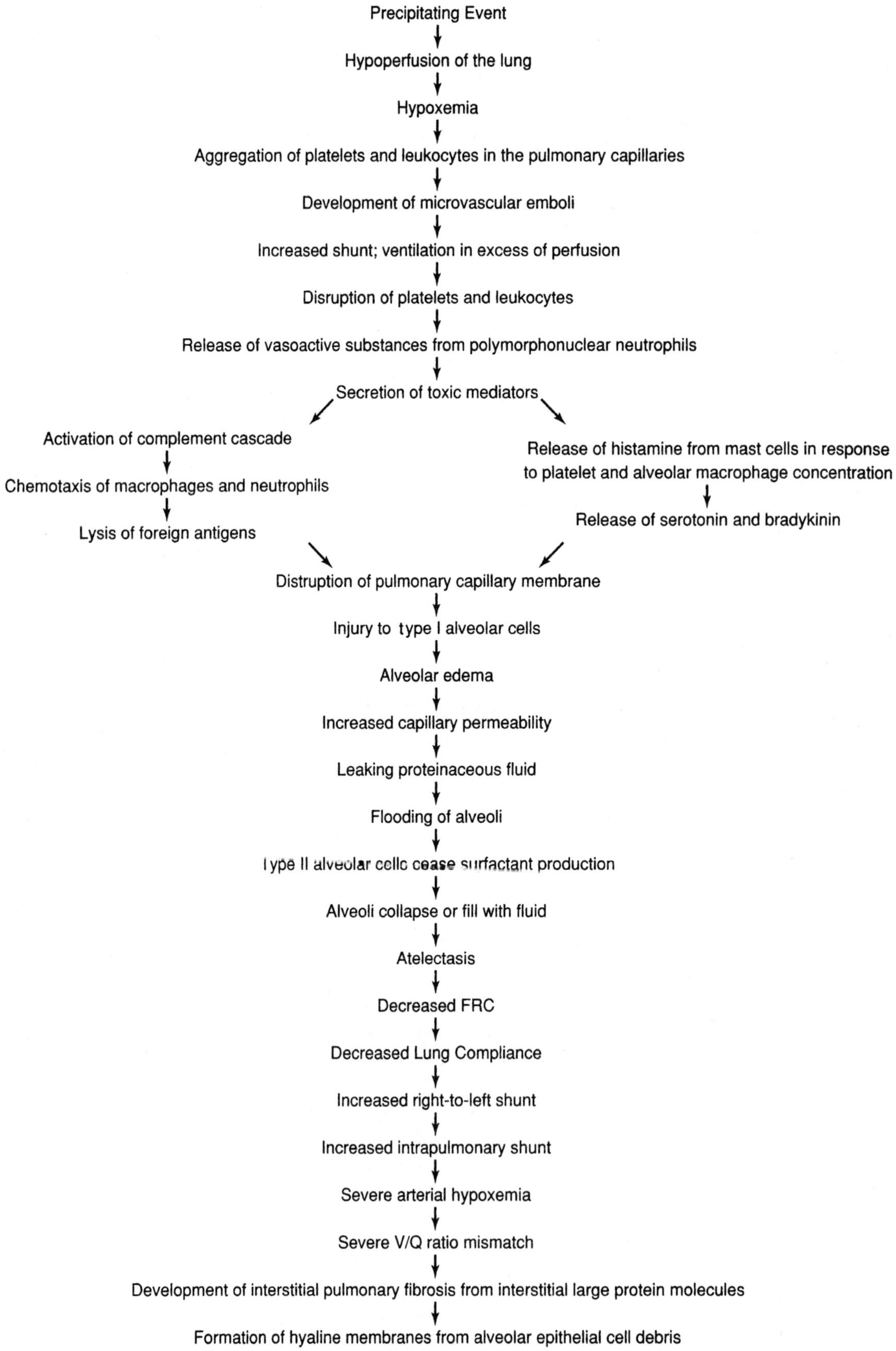

Figure 17-1. Pathogenesis of respiratory distress syndrome.

TABLE 17-3. CONDITIONS ASSOCIATED WITH THE DEVELOPMENT OF ACUTE RESPIRATORY DISTRESS SYNDROME (ARDS)	
Direct Injury	***Indirect Injury***
Pneumonia	Multiple blood transfusion
Pulmonary contusion	Shock
Aspiration	Multiple extremity trauma
Inhalation injury	Pancreatitis Sepsis

Careful monitoring of the plateau pressure is critical to assess the effect of the tidal volume. **A plateau pressure less than 30 is the desired goal.** *If the plateau pressure cannot be kept less than 30 cm H_2O with a tidal volume of 4 mL/kg or ideal body weight, switching to pressure control (PC) may be required.* PC will cap the thoracic pressures and prevent any further volutrauma or barotrauma.

Because of the *loss of surfactant*, the alveoli are stiff and harder to open. If the alveoli are allowed to open and close with each breath, further damage will result. The point at which the alveoli are open and remain open is called the lower inflection point on a pressure–volume curve (see Fig. 17-2). **PEEP** is used to stabilize the alveoli and keep them open throughout the entire respiratory cycle. PEEP levels of 10 to 15 cm H_2O will usually be required to reach this goal. **The goal for PEEP is to have enough to support oxygenation while enabling the down-titration of oxygen to FIO_2 less than 60% to decrease likelihood of oxygen toxicity.** The FIO_2 will initially be set high and titrated down to keep the SaO_2 more than 90 ($SpO_2 \geq 92\%$). Early recognition of acute lung injury and prompt institution of the lung-protective strategies can improve mortality by about 22% and prevent the development of pulmonary fibrosis.

Management of oxygenation is directed at preserving oxygen consumption and tissue perfusion. Since hypoxemia in ARDS can be severe, after ensuring lung-protective ventilation is in place, more aggressive treatment may be required to achieve minimum levels. Interventions include reduction of fever and prevention of hyperthermia and alkalosis. The use of sedatives and neuromuscular blockade (NMB) may be instituted to reduce muscle activity and improve ventilatory synchrony to further prevent excessive oxygen consumption. NMB may be used to decrease patient–ventilator dyssynchrony; however, it is avoided if at all possible so as not to risk the development of profound muscle weakness, which can lead to a prolonged recovery. *Analgesia and sedation should be optimized before initiation of NMB* **(PATIENT SHOULD BE DEEPLY SEDATED IF PARALYZED)**. If NMB is required, it should be kept to the lowest possible dose for the shortest length of time. *Daily interruption of NMB will allow for assessment of the sedation/analgesia level as well as the ongoing need for continued use of the NMB.* **Supplemental oxygen support at an FIO_2 of 0.50 or less with a PaO_2 of 60 to 70 mm Hg is preferred to limit the risk of oxygen toxicity while maintaining adequate oxygenation.**

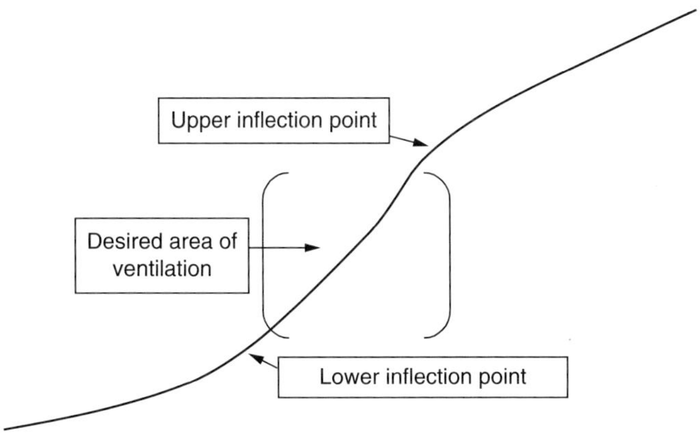

Figure 17-2. The point at which alveoli are open and remain open is called the lower inflection point on a pressure–volume curve.

Alternative ARDS Therapies

If severe hypoxemia remains despite the use of lung-protective strategies, other therapy may be necessary. Examples of these therapies are prone positioning, continuous lateral rotation bed therapy, PC combined with inverse-ratio ventilation (IRV), inhaled prostacyclins or nitric oxide, or extracorporeal membrane oxygenation (ECMO).

Prone positioning *has improved oxygenation and may improve survival in ARDS patients.* Placing a critically ill patient prone can be a difficult task. The prone position allows some of the collapsed alveoli to open, thus improving oxygenation, since more alveoli are available for gas exchange. If treatment is effective, it will be possible to decrease the FIO_2 while the SaO_2 remains more than 0.90. The effect can be temporary and may be lost when the patient is repositioned to supine. Care must be taken to protect the patient's eyes from abrasion and pooled secretions. Intravenous lines and the artificial airway must be well secured. While proned, patients may be able to be turned slightly side to side, have arms and head repositioned every 2 hours to relieve and assess skin pressure points. Pressure relief devices should be used to maintain skin integrity if the patient is proned for prolonged periods of time. Proning is contraindicated in patients with an unstable spine, open abdomen, or those with a large abdomen.

Continuous lateral rotation bed therapy may also provide an improvement in oxygenation. The exact degree of rotation that provides benefit is yet to be determined. Continuous rotation must generally go on for most of the day in order to provide benefit.

Inhalation medications that provide pulmonary artery vasodilatation can improve oxygenation. Long-term mortality benefit has not been shown, so their use is limited to rescue therapy. The inhalation medications (epoprostenol and nitric oxide) will be delivered via continuous nebulization or blended gas through the ventilator to open alveoli. These medications cross to the bloodstream and dilate blood vessels next to open alveoli. Improving blood flow to functioning alveoli will improve SaO_2.

Some centers have advocated the use of ECMO as a therapy for ARDS; however, it is not yet widely employed for this purpose.

High-frequency oscillatory ventilation (HFOV) is a method of mechanical ventilation that raises mean airway pressure and has the potential of reaching all of the lung protection ventilation goals. HFOV provides a bias flow of gas that allows for the dispersal of oxygen throughout the lung while preventing overdistention or collapse of alveoli. The RR is set very high, in hertz (1 Hz equaling 60 cycles), with a very small tidal volume (30–50 mL). Patients will require heavy sedation and possibly NMB to tolerate this method of ventilation. HFOV use may be considered controversial and recent research has shown it may even worsen mortality in the treatment of ARDS.

PC-IRV may provide another way to treat refractory hypoxemia of ARDS. The primary advantage of IRV is an elevation of mean airway pressure. This allows for the recruitment of alveoli and a subsequent elevation of the Pao_2 and Sao_2. (See Chapter 16 for more details on PC-IRV.)

Fluid administration should be monitored by effect on ***stroke volume*** *after initial fluid resuscitation, allowing for an adequate* ***preload*** *but avoiding further increases in lung water while maintaining an adequate* ***cardiac output***. Hemodynamic monitoring will be needed to adequately assess **preload and cardiac output**. Both crystalloids and colloids are used in fluid management.

Corticosteroid Therapy

Patients who do not show improvement in oxygenation after 5 to 7 days may be candidates for corticosteroid therapy. Patients with unresolving ARDS have been shown to have high levels of polymorphonuclear leukocytes (PMNs) in their bronchoalveolar lavage (BAL) fluid. This may represent an ongoing process of inflammation, which treatment with steroids may resolve. Care should be taken to assess for ongoing pulmonary or other infection prior to beginning steroids. The BAL is assessed in order to check for the presence of an ongoing untreated infectious process in the lung. Steroid treatment consists of methylprednisolone, 2 mg/kg loading dose, then 2 mg/kg per day from days 1 to 14, followed by a gradual decrease in the dose over 30 days. *The use of* **corticosteroid** *in ARDS is associated with a reduced mortality risk and an improvement in all morbidity outcomes.* Treatment is not accompanied by an increase in adverse events, such as infection, neuromyopathy, or other major complications. However, steroid administration does not prevent development of ARDS and late administration of steroids does not show benefit.

Complications

Complications associated with ARDS include metabolic and respiratory acidosis, cardiac arrest, barotrauma, and oxygen toxicity. Mortality associated with ARDS is decreasing because of improvements in care. Pulmonary function in many of these patients returns to normal. Other outcomes besides lung function should be considered. Owing to the severity of ARDS, profound muscle wasting and weakness can occur, which may require aggressive, long rehabilitation. This can be compounded by contractures or alterations in skin integrity that occur as the result of prolonged bed rest. Anxiety, cognitive impairment, and posttraumatic stress syndrome can occur. We are beginning to recognize that quality of life is as important as lung function. Often, patients do not return to the same quality of life they experienced prior to ARDS. Clinicians need to be meticulous in patient positioning, the prevention of nosocomial infection, and other complications of prolonged mechanical ventilation, illness, and bed rest. Long-term pulmonary complications can include a permanent reduction in pulmonary function (eg, decreased vital capacity and obstruction to airflow) due to fibrosis. Some patients may develop bronchopulmonary dysplasia—an obliteration of the bronchioles and formation of large cystic airspaces and thick fibrotic walls. Death is usually the result of the precipitating event of ARDS, not ARDS alone.

17.3 ACUTE RESPIRATORY INFECTIONS

Acute respiratory infection can lead to pneumonia, an acute inflammatory response of the lungs caused by a bacterial, fungal, or viral organism. The organisms can enter the lung directly by inhalation, by aspiration (micro or macro), or via the blood. Pneumonia can be community-acquired, healthcare-associated (dialysis centers, nursing homes), or hospital-acquired (nosocomial). Pneumonia is a common and potentially serious illness.

Community-Acquired Pneumonia

Common clinical features of community-acquired pneumonia (CAP) include cough, fever, pleuritic chest pain, dyspnea, and sputum production. A leukocytosis is often present. The presence of an infiltrate on plain chest radiograph is considered the "gold standard" for diagnosing pneumonia when clinical and microbiologic features are supportive. The causative agent of CAP remains unidentified in 30% to 50% of cases. *Streptococcus pneumoniae* is the most commonly identified pathogen in CAP, although many other organisms have been identified (**Table 17-4**). Community-associated methicillin-resistant *Staphylococcus aureus* (MRSA) typically produces a necrotizing pneumonia with high morbidity and mortality. Viral pneumonias, transmitted by airborne droplets, are usually community-acquired, although they can be nosocomial. Patients with a viral upper respiratory infection (URI) are at risk for the development of a secondary bacterial infection. Patients with comorbidities are at the highest risk of severe infection.

TABLE 17-4. ACUTE RESPIRATORY INFECTIONS: CAUSATIVE ORGANISMS
Community-acquired
Streptococcus pneumoniae
Moraxella catarrhalis
Haemophilus influenzae
Staphylococcus aureus **(MRSA or MSSA)**
Legionella species
Mycoplasma pneumoniae
Chlamydia pneumoniae
Viruses
Pneumocystis carinii
Hospital-acquired (Nosocomial)
Staphylococcus aureus **(MRSA or MSSA)**
Pseudomonas aeruginosa
Streptococcus pneumoniae
Klebsiella
Haemophilus influenzae
Escherichia coli
Serratia
Acinetobacter
Enterobacter
Stenotrophomonas maltophilia

Hospital-Acquired (Nosocomial) Pneumonia

Hospital-acquired pneumonia (HAP) can occur with or without mechanical ventilation and is defined as a pneumonia that occurs after a patient has been hospitalized for 2 or more days. Much attention has been given to the risk of *ventilator-associated pneumonia (VAP)*. VAP rates have decreased with the use of patient care bundles. The presence of an artificial airway predisposes a patient to aspiration and colonization of the airway with organisms. Development of HAP/VAP increases length of stay, hospital cost, and mortality. Risk factors for VAP include reintubation, self-extubation, prolonged mechanical ventilation, extremes of age (<6 years and >65 years), lying flat in bed, gastric distention, nasogastric tubes, inadequate endotracheal cuff pressure, routine changing of ventilator circuits, and H_2 blocker or antacid therapy (stress ulcer prophylaxis). Care must be taken to determine whether a positive sputum culture represents colonization or an actual infection before beginning antimicrobial treatment. Colonization is the presence of an organism in the sputum without the signs and symptoms of an infection. VAP can be prevented by clinician-driven protocols and *weaning as soon as possible, aggressive hand hygiene, maintaining the head of the bed at greater than 30 degrees of elevation or higher, draining ventilator circuits away from the patient, checking for gastric distention and preventing gastric residuals, careful oral suctioning to prevent pooling of secretions on top of the endotracheal tube cuff, and performing oral care.* Nonvented patients are also at risk of HAP (NVHAP). Aspiration is a major contributor to the development of NVHAP in the nonventilated patient as well. Prevention strategies similar to VAP prevention can be used to decrease the occurrence of NVHAP. Hospitals who have instituted oral care protocols for all patients have seen a decrease in NVHAP.

Pathophysiology

When an organism enters the lung, macrophages and the lymph system work to remove them and prevent infection. When the lungs' normal defense mechanisms fail, the organisms multiply, filling the alveoli with exudate. This results in areas of low ventilation and normal perfusion and increased **intrapulmonary shunt**. Hypoxic vasoconstriction reduces blood flow to the affected area. The organisms cause edema of the airway and stimulate goblet cells to increase mucus production. The increase in secretions and airway edema increase airway resistance, leading to an increased work of breathing.

Etiology and Risk Factors

Patients at risk for the development of pneumonia include older adults; persons with dehydration, immobility, malnutrition, or underlying lung disease; those on mechanical ventilation; the immunosuppressed; and those taking drugs that impair airway clearance.

Signs and Symptoms

Signs and symptoms of bacterial pneumonia include fever, shaking chills, possible pleuritic chest pain that is worse on inspiration, increased sputum production or purulence, and cough. Sputum ranges from reddish to green.

Viral pneumonia presents with a sudden onset of fever, dry cough, headache, myalgia, retrosternal chest pain unaffected by respiration, dyspnea, and cough.

Invasive and Noninvasive Diagnostic Studies

Chest x-ray will reveal lobar infiltrates and may show pleural effusion. *ABGs may show a decreased* Pao_2. Elevated leukocyte counts with a left shift and *elevated bands* may be seen on a complete blood count. Sputum may be cultured to identify the organism; however, routine sputum cultures are not recommended for CAP unless the patient does not respond to therapy or is immunocompromised. A positive sputum culture on a mechanically ventilated patient should be evaluated for colonization versus infection. Treatment is reserved for positive cultures when the patient has the additional signs of infection outlined above. A bronchial alveolar lavage (BAL) specimen examined for cell count can be useful in determining the presence of infection. A BAL specimen with **high polymorphonuclear neutrophil (PMN) indicates infection**.

Management of Patient Care

Management includes administration of the appropriate antibiotic by intravenous, oral, or intramuscular routes. The current recommendation regarding antibiotic therapy is to begin with broad coverage and narrow coverage as soon as an organism is identified. The more specific the antibiotic therapy given for the shortest possible duration, the less likely the patient is to develop resistance. Hydration is important to keep secretions thin and prevent them from becoming thick and tenacious. Aggressive pulmonary hygiene—such as deep breathing, coughing, early ambulation, and aerosol treatments—is used to help remove secretions. Bronchodilators are used to increase airway size and relax airway muscles. Analgesics are recommended to treat muscle aches and fever.

Complications

Complications of pneumonia include hypotension, sepsis, ARDS, and death.

17.4 STATUS ASTHMATICUS

Status asthmaticus is a severe continuing attack of asthma that fails to respond to conventional drug therapy. It can last for days to weeks; even with optimal therapy, it may be fatal.

Pathophysiology

Status asthmaticus is characterized by airway hyperreactivity or hyperresponsiveness, airway obstruction, and airway inflammation. The increased airway responsiveness is manifest by narrowing of the airways secondary to bronchial constriction and excessive mucus obstruction, thus increasing the work of breathing, interfering with gas exchange, and producing hypoxemia (**Fig. 17-3**). Air trapping with resulting hyperinflation of the lungs is a common clinical feature.

When an inhaled substance elicits a hypersensitivity response, immunoglobulin E (IgE) antibodies stimulate mast cells in the lung to release histamine. Histamine causes inflammation, irritation, and edema in the smooth muscles by attaching to receptor sites in the bronchi. There is a release of inflammatory mediators from the epithelial cells as well as the epithelial mast cells and macrophages. Eosinophils and neutrophils alter the

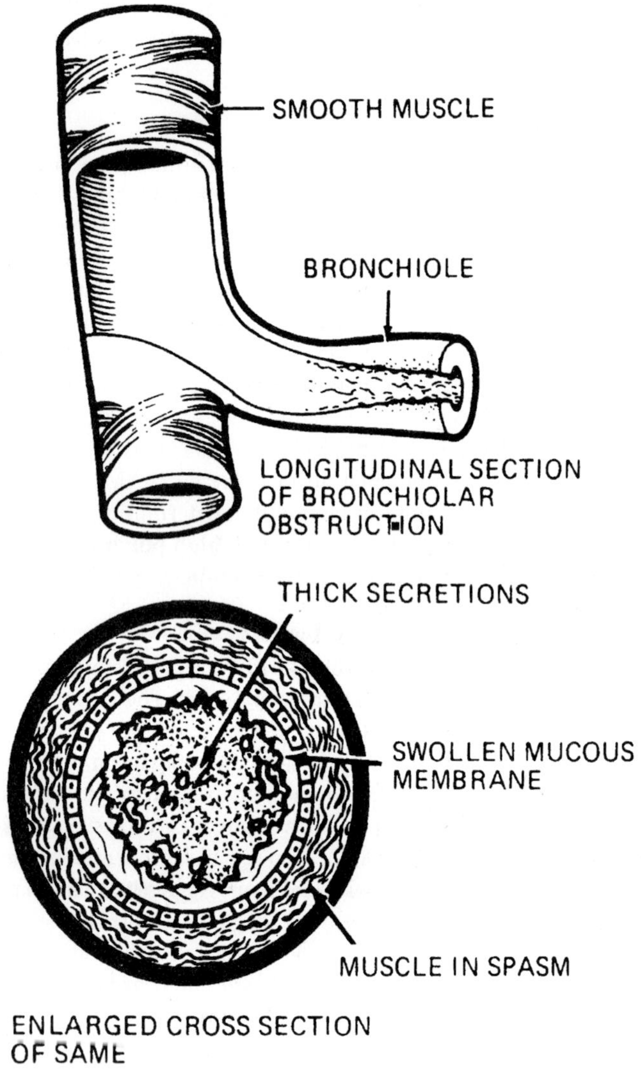

Figure 17-3. Appearance of respiratory bronchioles in asthma (bronchiolar obstruction on expiration by muscle spasm, swelling of mucosa, and thick secretions).

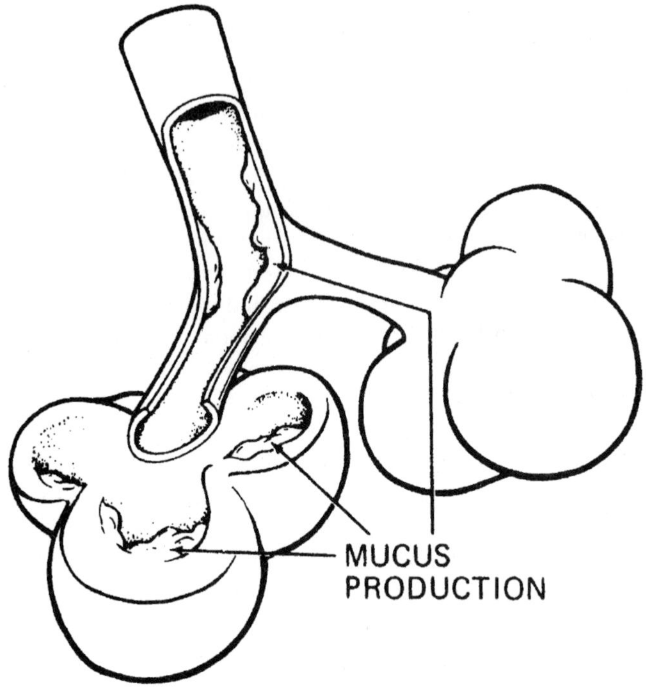

Figure 17-4. Airway lumen in bronchitis.

integrity of the epithelium, and changes occur in the autonomic neural control of the airway, mucociliary function, and airway responsiveness. Prostaglandin production is stimulated and further enhances the effects of histamine, stimulating goblet cells to secrete excessive tenacious mucus and leading to airway narrowing (**Fig. 17-4**).

As the attack continues unabated, the bronchial walls hypertrophy and the clearance of secretions is diminished, causing bronchiolar obstruction, reducing alveolar ventilation, and causing hyperinflation of the lung.

Early airway closure causes increased intrathoracic pressure on exhalation, thus inhibiting alveolar ventilation. As alveoli fill with the excessive mucus, blood is shunted by nonfunctioning alveoli and **intrapulmonary shunt** increases. Diminished ventilation results in a respiratory acidosis.

Etiology and Risk Factors

Status asthmaticus is a complication of asthma. The three most common causes of status asthmaticus are (1) exposure to allergens; (2) noncompliance with the medication regimen; and (3) respiratory infections. It can result from a reaction to an allergen or nonallergen such as exercise and can be precipitated by irritants such as cold air, odors, chemicals, or changes in the weather. Environments that become unusually hot, cold, or dusty often trigger status asthmaticus because of the effect of inspired air on the lungs. Other triggers include psychological and emotional stimuli, aspirin, nonsteroidal anti-inflammatory drugs, beta-adrenergic agents, overuse of bronchodilators, and autonomic nervous system imbalance.

Signs and Symptoms

Patients in status asthmaticus are extremely dyspneic, with a hyperpneic respiratory pattern and a sensation of chest tightness. Inspiratory and expiratory wheezing is usually audible, with a *prolonged expiratory phase* as the patient tries to exhale the trapped air through narrow airways. Physical examination reveals tachypnea; tachycardia; a rapid, thready pulse; use of accessory respiratory muscles; distant heart sounds; hyperresonance on percussion; flaring nares; pallor, cyanosis; increased work of breathing; and fatigue. **The disappearance of wheezing may be an ominous sign, as the airway may have become completely obstructed.** The patient may have **pulsus paradoxus**, a drop in the systolic blood pressure of 12 mm Hg or more during inspiration.

Invasive and Noninvasive Diagnostic Studies

ABGs initially show a low $Paco_2$ with a respiratory alkalosis. **When the $Paco_2$ normalizes or begins to rise that is an ominous sign since the patient is now tiring and generally requires intubation and mechanical support.** ABGs may reveal a normal or falling Pao_2. Chest x-ray will probably not be helpful, showing a hyperinflated lung that is normal or translucent. Pulmonary function tests are not useful during the acute phase, as the patient is unable to move enough air to complete the test.

Management of Patient Care

Management includes support of ventilation and respirations. Hypoxemia is the most common cause of death in asthma. Oxygen is the primary therapeutic modality. Supplemental oxygen must be provided for any patient who presents with status asthmaticus. Oxygen helps to correct V/Q mismatch. Beta-agonist agents, typically **albuterol** or salbutamol and terbutaline, are the mainstays of acute therapy in asthma. The nebulized inhaled route of administration is generally the most effective one, although some patients with severe refractory status asthmaticus may benefit from intravenous administration. Inhaled beta agonists can be administered intermittently or as continuous nebulized aerosol in a monitored setting. **Corticosteroids**, such as **methylprednisolone or prednisone**, are critical in the therapy of status asthmaticus and are used to decrease the intense airway inflammation and swelling in asthma as well as reduce mucous production and potentiate beta-agonists activity. Other treatments include anticholinergics, subcutaneous epinephrine, and magnesium. Helium and inhaled anesthetics may be used in severe cases. Helium is an inert gas that is less dense than nitrogen. *The administration of a helium–oxygen mixture (Heliox) reduces turbulent airflow across narrowed airways*, which can help to reduce and thus relieve the work of breathing and improve delivery of inhaled medication. Improved gas exchange with decreased respiratory acidosis will be seen. Heliox can be delivered via face mask or through a mechanical ventilator. Inhaled anesthetic agents, although potentially effective, are difficult to administer outside the operating room. Mechanical ventilation may be necessary to support respiration while the above therapies take effect. There are no widely agreed upon guidelines for when asthmatic patients require intubation. Intubation and mechanical ventilation are difficult and dangerous for the asthmatic and hence are avoided if at all possible. Intubation should be approached cautiously in patients with status asthmaticus because manipulation of the airway can cause increased airflow obstruction due to exaggerated bronchial responsiveness. The narrowed airways, positive-pressure ventilation, and delayed emptying can lead to dynamic hyperinflation (DHI), placing the patient at risk for barotrauma and cardiac compromise. Interstitial emphysema, pneumothorax, pneumomediastinum, subcutaneous emphysema, and/or pneumoperitoneum can result from barotrauma. To minimize the development of DHI, *a controlled hypoventilation should occur with settings that allow for a low minute ventilation, low RR, long exhalation time, and low tidal volume (6 mL/kg/ideal body weight). Care must be taken to assess for auto-PEEP, peak airway, and plateau pressures. Keeping plateau pressures less than 30 and auto-PEEP less than 10 cm H_2O is the goal.* Sedation is usually required, with NMB being necessary in extreme cases. Additional therapies include hydration, monitoring of oxygenation with ABGs or pulse oximetry, and antibiotics only if signs of infection are present.

Be aware of a decreasing level of consciousness, diminished wheezing, or a rising $Paco_2$. These may signal a worsening of the asthma episode.

Complications

Complications include pneumothorax, hypoxemia, respiratory acidosis, and hypoxia. Status asthmaticus can cause respiratory failure and death.

17.5 PULMONARY HYPERTENSION

Pulmonary hypertension (PH) is a condition in which pressure in the pulmonary arteries is abnormally high often leading to *right heart failure. PH is defined as a mean pulmonary artery pressure greater than 20 mm Hg as measured by right heart catheterization.*

Pathophysiology

PH can be idiopathic, familial, or associated with many other disease processes. The primary cause of significant PH is almost always increased PVR. Increased flow alone does not usually cause significant PH because the pulmonary vascular bed vasodilates and recruits vessels in response to increased flow, so that little, if any, increased pressure results. Similarly, increased pulmonary venous pressure alone does not usually cause PH. However, both increased flow and increased pulmonary venous pressure can increase PVR. The right ventricle hypertrophies in response to the pressure. If severe enough, the right ventricle dilates and cardiac output falls. A classification system based on the underlying cause of PH was developed to assist with treatment and management.

Classifications of Pulmonary Hypertension

Group 1. Pulmonary arterial hypertension (PAH)
Group 2. PH due to left heart disease
Group 3. PH due to lung disease or hypoxia or both
Group 4. Chronic thromboembolic PH or other artery obstructions
Group 5. PH with unclear multifactorial mechanisms

Etiology and Risk Factors

PAH is a rare disease with an incidence of about 15 to 50 per million per year. Adult women are almost three times as likely to present with PAH as adult men. The incidence of PH from other underlying causes is higher.

Clinical Manifestations

Patients with PH may initially complain of dyspnea on exertion, lethargy, and fatigue. As the disease progresses and right ventricular failure develops, exertional angina, exertional syncope, and peripheral edema may develop. The initial physical finding of PH is usually increased intensity of the pulmonic component of the second heart sound, which may even become palpable. Evidence of right ventricular hypertrophy or failure may also exist. *Patients may have signs of jugular venous distention, elevated CVP, right upper quadrant pain, and anorexia for gastrointestinal (GI) congestion. Prognosis relates to how well the right ventricle functions under this increased workload.* The prognosis is generally poor but varies according to the severity of the underlying cause, the functional abnormalities, and the hemodynamic abnormalities.

Invasive and Noninvasive Studies

Patients with PH undergo a variety of tests with the goal of confirming the diagnosis and to attempt to identify an underlying cause. Chest x-ray will show enlargement of central pulmonary arteries and, depending on the stage, may show enlarged right heart. The electrocardiogram may demonstrate signs of *right ventricular hypertrophy* or strain. Echocardiography is performed to estimate the pulmonary artery systolic (PAS) pressure and to assess right ventricular size, thickness, and function as well as valvular function. The echocardiogram is not the most precise way to determine pulmonary artery pressures. Echocardiography can be performed during exercise to identify patients with exercise-induced PH. Pulmonary function tests can identify possible underlying lung conditions (obstructive pattern is suggestive of COPD, while restrictive disease suggests interstitial lung disease, neuromuscular weakness, or chest wall disease) that are contributing to PH. Overnight oximetry can determine underlying causes such as obstructive sleep apnea that cause hypoxemia and pulmonary vasoconstriction. Thrombolytic components may be assessed by V/Q scan or CT scan/CTPA **(CT pulmonary angiography)**. *Right heart catheterization is necessary to confirm the diagnosis of PH and accurately determine the severity of the hemodynamic derangements as well as the presence of any congenital abnormalities.*

Management of Patient Care

There is no cure for PAH. Treatment, however, has improved dramatically during the past decade, offering both relief from symptoms and prolonged survival. Lung transplantation was the ultimate treatment option however with the improvement of vasodilator therapy, the need for transplantation has decreased. Treatment should be aimed at the causative underlying disease whenever possible. The mainstays of current medical therapy fall into several classes, including vasodilators, oxygen therapy, anticoagulants, antiplatelet agents, anti-inflammatory therapies, and vascular-remodeling therapies depending on the classification of PH. Continuous intravenous administration of the prostanoids carries with it a risk of thromboembolism or line infection. The endothelin receptor antagonists require frequent monitoring of liver enzymes given their association with hepatic damage. Also, medication interactions are a predominant concern with this class of drugs. As such, provision of care with many of these agents in these advanced-stage patients takes highly specialized care.

Lung transplantation remains a treatment option for patients who do not respond to the other therapies. The earlier PH is diagnosed the more responsive it will be to therapy. Patients should be referred to specialized treatment centers where clinicians have expertise in treating PH. Patients with PH should undergo an invasive hemodynamic assessment and an acute vasoreactivity test prior to the initiation of advanced therapy. Agents commonly used for vasoreactivity testing include **epoprostenol ("Flolan")**, adenosine, and inhaled nitric oxide. Patients with a positive vasoreactivity test are candidates for a trial of calcium channel blocker therapy. In contrast, patients with a negative vasoreactivity test should be treated with an alternative agent because calcium channel blockers have not been shown to be beneficial in these patients and may be harmful. Creation of a right-to-left shunt by atrial septostomy has been performed in some patients with syncope or severe right heart failure in an attempt to increase systemic blood flow by bypassing the pulmonary vascular obstruction.

Complications

Severe right heart failure (cor pulmonale) with resultant low cardiac output is the ultimate progression of PH. Chronic hepatic congestion from the *severe right heart failure* leads to hyperbilirubinemia and *cirrhosis*. Patients on intravenous medications are at risk for line infections. Patients with untreated PH have a median survival of 2 to 3 years from time of diagnosis.

KEY CONTENT CHECKLIST

- ❒ In ARDS, because of the loss of surfactant, the alveoli are stiff and harder to open.
  - Care must be taken to avoid overdistention of the unaffected alveoli with each breath by using smaller tidal volumes of 4 to 6 mL/kg of ideal body weight.
  - A lower pH and higher $Paco_2$ ("permissive hypercapnia") are often allowed.
  - Higher PEEP is usually needed to keep the stiff alveoli open to promote oxygenation.
- ❒ In Asthma, monitor for a decreasing level of consciousness, diminished wheezing, or a rising $Paco_2$ as these may signal a worsening of the asthma episode.
- ❒ A hallmark of ARDS is "noncardiogenic pulmonary edema." Diffuse, bilateral pulmonary edema is seen on the CXR; however, the PAOP is generally < 18 mm Hg.

Review Questions:

Questions 1 and 2 refer to the following scenario:

A 74-year-old 70-kg man is admitted to your unit with a diagnosis of respiratory failure secondary to pneumonia. He is currently intubated and on assisted mandatory ventilation (AMV), with a VT of 700 mL, ventilator respiratory rate of 10, total rate of 29. His blood gas values are as follows:

pH 7.48
$Paco_2$ 30
Pao_2 64
Fio_2 80%

1. Based on the preceding information, which type of respiratory failure exists?
a. Oxygenation failure
b. Ventilation failure
c. Combined oxygenation and ventilation failure
d. Neither oxygenation nor ventilation failure

Answer: A. Rationale: Normal range for Pao_2 is 80 to 100 mm Hg for people 60 years or younger. For people 60 years old or older, to calculate their normal: from 80 mm Hg subtract 1 mm Hg for every year above 60. For this patient, a normal Pao_2 would be 80 mm Hg – 14 to be the equivalent of 66, and his current Pao_2 value is 64. When Pao_2 is lower than the expected normal, it is called hypoxia.

2. Which treatment would be indicated based on the blood gas values given?

a. Increase the ventilator VT
b. Decrease the ventilator rate
c. Add PEEP therapy to reduce the F_{IO_2}
d. Reduce the F_{IO_2} while increasing the ventilator peak flow rate

Answer: C. Rationale: PEEP is effective at raising Pa_{O_2} and Sa_{O_2} levels by maintaining alveolar airflow during expiration. PEEP improves distribution of ventilation, helps hold alveoli open, and opens smaller airways, improving oxygenation by increasing the time for gas exchange to occur. PEEP is indicated to help reduce F_{IO_2} levels or to elevate Pa_{O_2}/Sa_{O_2} values when high F_{IO_2} levels are unsuccessful, to drive lung water back into the vascular system, or to reduce mediastinal bleeding postoperatively.

18

Acute Pulmonary Embolism and Aspiration

CHAPTER OVERVIEW AND OBJECTIVES

Pulmonary embolism is a likely content area for questions on the CCRN exam. Pulmonary emboli (PE) are best understood when applied to concepts in pulmonary physiology relative to disturbances of ventilation and perfusion (see Chapter 14). However, it is important to remember the physical presentation and treatment discussed in this chapter for purposes of the test.

After studying this chapter, you should understand the following:

- PE create disruption in blood flow to alveoli, eliminating exchange of carbon dioxide and oxygen, creating increased dead space.
- Obstruction of the pulmonary vasculature elicits neurohumoral stimuli, increasing pulmonary artery pressure and pulmonary vascular resistance. This can result in constriction of the distal airways, leading to alveolar collapse and atelectasis.
- Patients with PE will present with a variety of symptoms depending on the degree of hemodynamic compromise. They most often present with sudden dyspnea on the exam.

18.1 ACUTE PULMONARY EMBOLISM

An acute PE is a thrombus that occurs in the body, travels through the venous circulation typically from the lower extremities to the pulmonary circulation, and partially or completely occludes a pulmonary artery. A massive PE is one that occludes more than 50% of the pulmonary artery bed creating hemodynamic compromise.

Pathophysiology

The lung is capable of filtering small clots and other substances through fibrolytic mechanisms in the lung. The lung cannot dissolve large clots or multiple small clots. *Most PEs occur when a lower extremity, deep venous thrombus (DVT) breaks loose* from its attachment and flows through the venous circulation, entering the right ventricle and then lodging in small pulmonary arteries (**Fig. 18-1**). The embolus will most often lodge in the right lower lobe because of increased regional blood flow. Once in the lung, the embolus may be dissolved, grow, or fragment into many smaller pieces. An embolus can be composed of platelets, thrombin, erythrocytes, leukocytes, air, fat, fluid, tumors, or amniotic fluid (**Table 18-1**). Nonthrombotic emboli (NTPE) as seen with fat, amniotic fluid, tumor, sepsis, and particulate matter have a greater potential for entering the left heart because they can change shape easily and pass through the pulmonary capillary bed into the systemic circulation (although this is a rare complication). Respiratory and hemodynamic compromise will occur more readily if there is underlying chronic obstructive pulmonary disease (COPD), heart failure (HF), or other chronic conditions.

Obstruction of the pulmonary vasculature elicits neurohumoral stimuli, increasing pulmonary artery pressure and pulmonary vascular resistance. Because there is a disruption in the blood flow to alveoli, they become nonfunctioning units, not participating in the exchange of carbon dioxide and oxygen; there is therefore **increased dead space**. To maintain adequate gas exchange, ventilation is preferentially shifted to the uninvolved areas of the lung. This results in constriction of the distal airways, leading to alveolar collapse and atelectasis.

Etiology and Risk Factors

Patients at risk for the development of thrombus formation include those with three factors referred to as *Virchow's triad:* (1) damaged vascular endothelium; (2) venous stasis; and (3) hypercoagulability of the blood. Natural processes of clot dissolution may cause release of fragments; or external mechanisms such as direct trauma, muscle contraction, or changes in perfusion may contribute to the release of the thrombus.

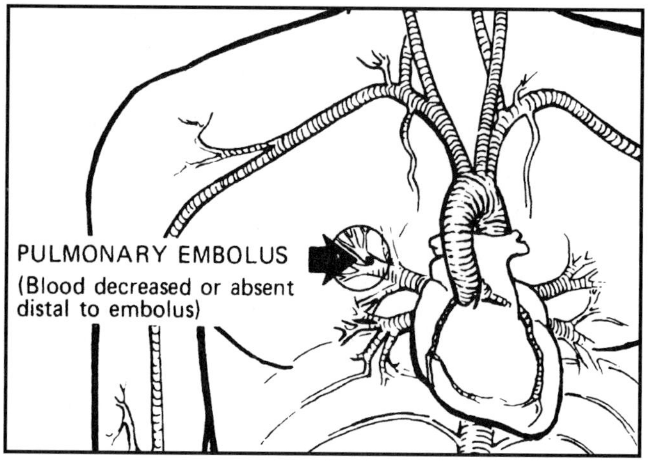

Figure 18-1. Pulmonary embolism.

PEs may develop in patients with no predisposing factors. Some acquired predisposing factors include stasis of venous blood resulting from immobilization, obesity, pregnancy, estrogen use, aging, major trauma or surgery within 4 weeks, malignancy, previous DVT, indwelling catheters or electrodes in the great veins or right heart, HF, and acquired thrombotic disorders (heparin-induced thrombocytopenia, postsplenectomy, antiphospholipid antibodies). Hereditary factors that can cause thromboembolic disease include deficiency of antithrombin, protein C or S, resistance to activated protein C (factor V Leiden), prothrombin gene mutation, raised plasminogen-activator inhibitor, plasminogen disorders, and high plasma concentration of factor VIII. Rare occasions of thrombus formation include thrombus formation in the heart secondary to acute myocardial infarction, atrial fibrillation, subacute bacterial endocarditis, and cardioversion.

Signs and Symptoms

Increased respiratory rate, dyspnea, and tachycardia are the most common signs of PE. These may present with or without pleuritic chest pain and hemoptysis. The signs and symptoms of PE must be divided into the clinical pictures of a massive embolism and a submassive embolism. **Massive embolism** (> 50% of pulmonary circulation obstructed) **occurs suddenly** and is associated with **hemodynamic compromise due to acute right HF (elevated pulmonary artery systolic pressure and pulmonary vascular resistance).** Cardiac output falls because of the right heart's inability to fill the left heart. The patient may have crushing substernal chest pain and appear to be in shock, with hypotension, elevated right heart pressures, dyspnea, cyanosis, apprehension, or coma. Respirations are rapid, shallow, and gasping. Arterial pulse is rapid and the volume is diminished. If awake, the patient may express feelings of impending doom.

If capnography is available to the patient, *the end-tidal CO_2 ($PETCO_2$) will suddenly decrease with a PE. The arterial CO_2 ($Paco_2$) may decrease as well due to hyperventilation.* However, the $PETCO_2$ decreases more due to a loss of blood flow in the lungs. This loss of blood flow causes an **increased dead space,** lowering the $PETCO_2$. Pao_2 levels may not change substantially. The difference between the $Paco_2$ and the $PETCO_2$ will widen. However, in large PEs, hypoxemia is common.

TABLE 18-1. ETIOLOGY OF PULMONARY EMBOLI
Deep venous thrombosis
Air embolus
Septic embolus
Fat embolus
Tumor embolus
Amniotic fluid embolus

KEY CLINICAL CONCEPTS

- The keyword "sudden" will often appear on the exam as a clue for considering PE. Also consider low Pao_2 and $Paco_2$ on the ABG and the type of hemodynamic compromise (right HF) that may be present.
- "Fat embolus" (usually after a long bone fracture) also presents very similar to PE.

Submassive PE may present only fleeting minimal symptoms or may be asymptomatic. If the submassive PE has occluded a medium-sized artery, tachypnea, dyspnea, tachycardia, generalized chest discomfort, and pleuritic-type chest pain may develop within a few hours. Fever, cough, and hemoptysis may occur over several hours or days. A pleural friction rub and a pleural effusion may develop. **Usually, no hemodynamic compromise is seen in minor or submassive PE since no right HF occurs.**

A subacute massive PE can develop because of multiple small emboli that accumulate over several weeks. Since the obstruction occurs gradually, the right heart has time to adapt and the degree of right HF is less than that which occurs with the sudden massive PE. Symptoms include dyspnea on exertion, exercise fatigue, elevated central venous pressure (CVP), and an S_3 gallop. Cardiac output is usually preserved unless the buildup of clot becomes unusually large; then the signs and symptoms will be like those of a sudden massive PE.

Invasive and Noninvasive Diagnostic Studies

No single noninvasive test is sufficient to diagnose PE in all patients. Diagnostic tests should be used, along with the degree of clinical suspicion given the patient's presentation and risk factors. Identifying a proximal lower extremity DVT can be helpful, since 70% of patients with PE are positive for DVT. If no DVT is identified, the patient is unlikely to have a PE (although a percentage of clots in the deep pelvis may not be seen on ultrasound). Routine chest films may be normal, but about 20% of such cases may show some area of consolidation. The chest film may be inconclusive within the first few hours after embolism. Things to look for on the chest film include pulmonary disease, atelectasis, pleural effusion, elevated diaphragm, and a *prominent pulmonary artery.*

D-Dimers are proteins released into circulation when a clot undergoes natural fibrinolysis. A positive D-Dimer result can occur in a number of medical conditions. A negative D-Dimer is often used to rule out PE. Age, clot-associated conditions, recent trauma, and procedures can increase D-Dimer, levels so results should be interpreted accordingly.

Electrocardiogram (ECG) may be normal but most often shows sinus tachycardia or *right ventricular (RV) strain.* In an extensive PE, the ECG may show *right axis deviation*, transient right bundle branch block, ST-segment depression, T-wave inversion in leads V_1 and V_4, and tall peaked P waves in leads II, III, and aVF. An "S1Q3T3" in the 12-Lead EKG may also be seen, however, the most common ECG finding is sinus tachycardia. If the embolus is massive, the ECG may show pulseless electrical activity (PEA).

Arterial blood gases (ABGs) are unreliable indicators of PE. If the arterial oxygen pressure (Pao_2) is less than 80 mm Hg on room air, a PE is less likely, although one may exist and not occlude major arteries. The ABGs may show a decrease in Pao_2 and $Paco_2$. Patients on a mechanical ventilator with continuous *end-tidal CO_2 monitoring will show a sudden decrease in the PETCO$_2$ value* and a widened PETCO$_2$ gradient due to **increase in dead-space** ventilation.

An elevated brain natriuretic peptide (BNP) or N-terminal pro-brain natriuretic peptide (NT-proBNP) predicts RV dysfunction and strain. An elevated troponin I or troponin T level is associated with an increased risk of short-term mortality.

Echocardiography can be useful in identifying *right HF* or strain that is associated with a massive PE. On rare occasions, a transesophageal echocardiography can see massive PE in the central pulmonary artery. Usually only the indirect signs of massive PE are noted; however, the echo can be useful in ruling out other causes of hemodynamic compromise (cardiac tamponade, aortic dissection, septal rupture) in an unstable patient.

Spiral/helical CT or computed tomography pulmonary angiogram (CTPA) with injection of contrast can provide valuable and reliable results for determining a PE and is the gold standard for detecting PE. It is faster, less complex, and less operator-dependent than pulmonary angiography. The Spiral/CTPA also provides the clinician with other valuable information about the lungs, such as pneumonia, detection of masses, and pleural effusions. RV dilation may be detected on spiral/CTPA, helping to identify the massive PE that is potentially fatal. Spiral/CTPA uses contrast limiting its use in patients with renal impairments, iodine/contrast allergies, or pregnancy; a V/Q scan is usually the preferred test for these patients.

A ventilation/perfusion (V/Q) lung scintigraphic scan that is normal or low probability usually rules out a PE. If a lung scan shows perfusion defects on segments that appear normal on chest imaging, PE is likely. A VQ scan may be abnormal simply because of COPD but will be a ventilation not a perfusion mismatch. The V/Q scan is reported in terms of probability of the scan being positive for PE. A V/Q scan with a high probability means that the patient has multiple perfusion defects with normal ventilation. This patient has an 85% chance of having a PE. Patients with low or intermediate probability on a V/Q scan must be viewed in light of clinical suspicion. A normal or low-probability V/Q scan in a patient with low clinical suspicion may not receive treatment for PE, while a patient with high clinical suspicion may still receive treatment and/or undergo other diagnostic evaluation.

Pulmonary angiography should be considered when other tests are inconclusive; however, this is rarely needed with new advances in CTPA technology. A positive angiogram will reveal filling deficits or sharp cutoffs in blood flow. A magnetic resonance imaging scan can also be used to detect changes in pulmonary blood flow or pinpoint an embolus although this is rarely utilized.

QUICK TIP! Select spiral/helical chest CT when asked to identify the gold standard diagnostic test for PE. However, select pulmonary angiography if the contrast chest CT option is not available.

Management of Patient Care

Treatment plans for PE are based on the amount of hemodynamic compromise. Patients with hemodynamic stability should receive anticoagulant therapy. Patients with hemodynamic instability should receive thrombolytic therapy followed by anticoagulant therapy.

Parenteral anticoagulants are administered to prevent clot progression. **Unfractionated heparin** (IV or subcutaneous), **low-molecular-weight heparin** (LMWH), and subcutaneous fondaparinux (a factor Xa inhibitor) impedes clotting by preventing fibrin formation. These medications are usually continued for several days until oral anticoagulation can be given.

Treatment with **unfractionated heparin** is based on body weight; the dosage is titrated based on the partial thromboplastin time (PTT) or anti-Xa levels. Each institution sets a range for therapeutic anticoagulation based on PTT results based on their available testing methods. A continuous infusion maintains a steady therapeutic blood level, in contrast to the heparin bolus every 4 to 6 hours. The bolus causes peak levels for short times and subtherapeutic levels for the remaining time before another bolus is due. **Heparin** is usually continued for several days or until oral anticoagulation can be administered. Adverse reactions associated with heparin therapy include bleeding and heparin induced thrombocytopenia.

Compared with unfractionated heparin, **LMWH** offers distinct advantages: it has a longer biological half-life, it can be administered subcutaneously once or twice daily, dosing is fixed, and laboratory monitoring is not required although anti Xa levels may be indicated in a subset of patients. One disadvantage of LMWHs is that their renal elimination precludes their use in individuals with severe renal dysfunction. Aside from bleeding risks that are equivalent to heparin, LMWH may offer fewer side effects for some patients.

Oral anticoagulants can be started when parenteral anticoagulation is started. Heparin or LMWH can be stopped after combined therapy with Xa inhibitors or with warfarin if the international normalized ratio (INR) of prothrombin clotting time exceeds 2.0. Oral anticoagulants are usually given for 3 to 6 months if the patient is asymptomatic. For multiple reasons, they may be given indefinitely or for the remainder of the patient's life. Oral anticoagulants that are factor Xa inhibitors **(rivaroxaban)** and direct thrombin inhibitors **(dabigatran)** can be used in place of **warfarin.** These medications provide anticoagulation within a few hours but have no antidote in the case of active bleeding.

Streptokinase, urokinase, and **tissue plasminogen activator (tPA)** are thrombolytic enzymes used to dissolve or lyse the emboli. These agents are administered only by intravenous infusion. Therapeutic action begins immediately and ceases with the interruption of the intravenous administration. *However, residual effects may last for as long as 12 to 24 hours. Thrombolytics are used in the treatment of patients with massive acute PE who are in acute right HF.*

Surgical embolectomy is reserved for those patients who are in fulminant shock, do not respond to anticoagulants, who have rebound effects to heparin, or who have recurrent emboli with chronic pulmonary hypertension. Procedures may include filter placement in the vena cava or embolectomy. Embolectomy is a serious operation and is usually reserved for massive emboli or for the decompensating patient who cannot be stabilized. The *vena cava filter* (inserted in the inferior vena cava) may filter emboli. The inferior vena cava filter (IVCF) will prevent further large emboli from reaching the lung, thus preventing further pulmonary and hemodynamic compromise, but may not filter very small emboli. The utilization of IVCFs has historically been the treatment of choice for DVT in those individuals with contraindications to standard anticoagulation or those with ongoing embolism despite appropriate anticoagulation therapy.

Prevention

Prevention of thrombus formation is critical. Patients should ambulate as much as their clinical condition allows. Elevating the legs, use of pneumatic devices, antiembolic hose, and active/passive range of motion will help prevent stasis of venous blood in nonambulating patients. Most hospitals have a venous thromboembolism (VTE) prevention program that assess risk factors for DVT development and bleeding risks. Based on the risk factors, the patient may also receive prophylactic low-dose **Heparin or LMWH**. It is important to educate the patient and family about risk factors of embolism development and preventive measures.

Complications

A complication of PE is pulmonary hypertension from pulmonary arterial obstruction. If the obstruction is partial or develops slowly, the patient may survive to be treated. However, if the obstruction is rapid and total, the patient may suffer *sudden death.* Chronic pulmonary hypertension does not usually occur with a single embolus. It usually results from multiple emboli of middle-sized vessels.

Complications of PE may include pulmonary infarction due to the extension of emboli. Any embolus that is large enough to alter hemodynamics can cause complications. These include stroke, myocardial infarction, cardiac dysrhythmias that are not amenable to therapy, liver failure and necrosis secondary to congestion, pneumonia, pulmonary abscesses, acute respiratory distress syndrome (ARDS), shock, and death.

18.2 PULMONARY ASPIRATION

Pulmonary aspiration is the inhalation of foreign fluid or particulate matter into the lower airways.

Pathophysiology

Aspiration occurs more often than realized and is not limited to the critically ill patients. Aspiration of foreign substances including oral secretions into the lung results in a chemical pneumonitis. When an acidic fluid is aspirated, it immediately causes alveolar–capillary breakdown, resulting in interstitial edema, intra-alveolar hemorrhage, atelectasis, increased airway resistance, and, commonly, hypoxia. These changes usually start within minutes of the initiating event and may worsen over a period of hours. Nonacidic fluid aspiration destroys surfactant and thus causes alveolar collapse, atelectasis, and hypoxia. Aspiration of particulate food matter causes both physical obstruction of the airway and a later inflammatory response caused by the presence of a foreign body. It can progress to a necrotizing process, resulting in lung abscess and empyema.

Etiology and Risk Factors

Pulmonary aspiration can be the result of inhalation of gastric contents, fluids (as in a near drowning), or saliva. Patients at risk for aspiration include the elderly and patients with neurologic compromise (eg, a cerebral vascular accident, seizures, or dementia). Head trauma, drug and alcohol overdose, vomiting, intestinal obstruction, hiatal hernia, and gastroesophageal reflux are all risk factors for aspiration.

Signs and Symptoms

Signs and symptoms include fever, breathlessness, tachycardia, tachypnea, wheezing, cough, increased work of breathing, and pleuritic pain.

Invasive and Noninvasive Diagnostic Studies

Chest imaging may reveal patchy infiltrates or large areas of fluid in the lung. **The right middle and/or lower lobes are the most common sites of infiltration.** ABGs may be normal or show a falling Pao_2, depending on the amount of the lung involved. Gram's stain and sputum cultures may be helpful to identify bacterial organisms.

Management of Patient Care

Treatment of aspiration pneumonitis is mainly supportive, consisting of oxygen and ventilatory support with positive end-expiratory pressure (PEEP). Patients with particulate aspirate may need bronchoscopy to remove large obstructing pieces. Management includes bronchodilators, intravenous fluids, and aggressive pulmonary hygiene. Empiric use of antibiotics is no longer recommended unless the patient is in the intensive care unit or has a prolonger hospitalization. Steroids are not recommended because they have not been shown to be effective.

Complications

The consequences of pulmonary aspiration depend on the type of material aspirated and its volume and pH. Complications include pneumonia, necrotizing pneumonitis, lung abscess, ARDS, and empyema.

KEY CONTENT CHECKLIST

- ❒ The key word "sudden" will often appear on the exam as a clue for considering PE. Also consider low Pao_2 and $Paco_2$ on the ABG and the type of hemodynamic compromise (right HF) that may be present.
- ❒ "Fat embolus" (usually after a long bone fracture) also presents very similar to PE.
- ❒ Due to the anatomy of the bronchial tree, the right middle and/or lower lobes are the most common sites of aspiration/infiltration but can occur in a variety of distribution patterns depending on the patient's position at the time of aspiration.
- ❒ Select spiral/helical chest CT when asked to identify the gold standard diagnostic test for PE. However, select pulmonary angiography if the contrast chest CT option is not available.

Review Questions:

1. Which of the following tests is most diagnostic for PE?

a. Blood gas analysis
b. V/Q scans
c. Pulmonary angiography
d. Pulmonary function tests

Answer: C. Rationale: There are several tests that can reveal how likely a PE is, but they are often not definitive. The angiogram will be most decisive although may be more difficult to perform. Pulmonary angiography should be considered when other tests are inconclusive. A positive angiogram will reveal filling deficits or sharp cutoffs in blood flow.

2. Effects from recurrent emboli due to DVT can be avoided by which one of the following therapies?

a. Use of a Greenfield (inferior vena cava) filter
b. Heparin
c. Warfarin
d. Use of lower extremity alternating compression devices

Answer: A. Rationale: When DVT(s) are present, the inferior vena caval filter (IVCF) will prevent further emboli from reaching the lung, thus preventing further pulmonary and hemodynamic compromise. The utilization of IVCFs has historically been the treatment of choice for DVT in those individuals with contraindications to standard anticoagulation or those with ongoing embolism despite appropriate anticoagulation therapy.

19

Thoracic Trauma and Air-Leak Syndromes

CHAPTER OVERVIEW AND OBJECTIVES

This chapter reviews chest trauma in order to give you the information you need about the assessment and treatment of chest injuries. Chest trauma, particularly from an assessment point of view, is also better understood if it is considered along with concepts in pulmonary physiology. The goal of this chapter is to provide enough information to help you understand how to assess and treat key pulmonary injuries but not overwhelm you with unnecessary information.

After studying this chapter, you should understand the following:

- Blunt lung injury develops over the course of 24 hours, leading to poor gas exchange, increased pulmonary vascular resistance, and decreased lung compliance.
- Pneumothorax symptoms depend on size of lung collapse.
- Tension pneumothorax produces symptoms that include dyspnea and restlessness, tachycardia, hypotension and potentially obstructive shock, diminished or absent breath sounds on the affected side, decreased chest wall movement, chest pain, and tracheal shift toward the unaffected side.
- Treatment of tension pneumothorax may require emergent insertion of a large bore needle into the second intercostal space, midclavicular line of the affected side.

19.1 THORACIC TRAUMA

Thoracic injuries are common in trauma. The more systems involved in trauma, the more critical each injury becomes. Thoracic injuries are especially serious in the elderly, the obese, and patients with cardiac or pulmonary disease. The older the patient, the more to have underlying health problems and diminished physiologic reserve. Thoracic trauma accounts for 25% of all trauma-related deaths. The injury can be the result of blunt or penetrating injury. Blunt trauma can result from direct injury to the chest or from deceleration injury. Airbag deployment may also cause thoracic trauma as well as aortic injury. Thoracic trauma occurs in 6 out of 10 motor vehicle accidents.

Pulmonary Contusion

The most common internal injuries are pulmonary contusion and result from direct compression of the chest. Pulmonary contusion can be self-limiting to causing critical illness due to complications such as pneumonia and atelectasis with resultant hypoxia.

Pathophysiology

Pulmonary contusion is damage to the lung parenchyma, resulting in localized edema and hemorrhage. The thorax hits an object, such as the steering wheel, compressing the thoracic cage, diminishing its size, and compressing the lungs because of the increased intrathoracic pressure. As the thorax rebounds from the steering wheel or other blunt trauma force, the thoracic cage increases in size, decreasing the intrathoracic pressure and the pressure on the lung parenchyma. The lung parenchyma, under pressure, expands, rupturing capillaries and results in hemorrhage (**Fig. 19-1**). Such **blunt lung injury develops over the course of 24 hours**, leading to poor gas exchange, increased pulmonary vascular resistance, and decreased lung compliance.

If the force of the injury is sufficient to lacerate the lungs, there is commonly bleeding, which is potentially dangerous. *Laceration may occur from tearing due to rib fractures or direct puncture.*

Etiology and Risk Factors. Contusions may result from blunt thoracic trauma or penetrating lung trauma. Motor vehicle crashes are the most common cause of lung contusion.

Signs and Symptoms. Depending on the severity of trauma, symptoms may include tachypnea, tachycardia, hypoxemia, and

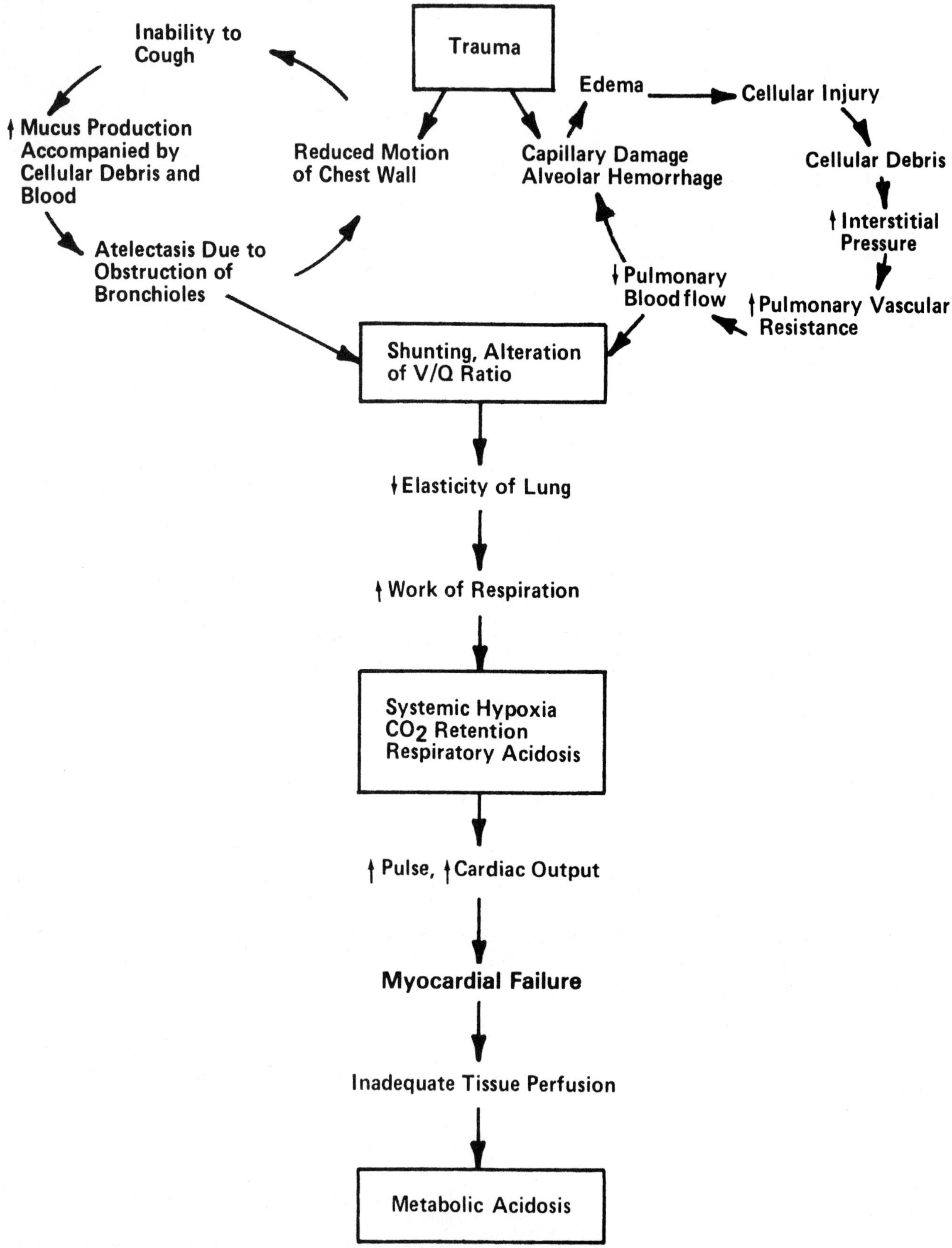

Figure 19-1. Mechanism of pulmonary contusion.

blood-tinged secretions. Crackles may be heard throughout all lung fields as a result of retained secretions. Obvious signs of chest wall damage may be present (bruising, abrasions, broken ribs, flail chest); however, these are often absent.

Invasive and Noninvasive Diagnostic Studies. The diagnosis of pulmonary contusion due to blunt trauma is difficult, since symptoms may not occur from 24 to 72 hours following trauma. Pulmonary contusion is rarely diagnosed by physical examination alone. The mechanism of injury should alert the clinician to the possibility of damage. Chest imaging may be normal or may reveal localized opacification in the injured area. The affected area may be larger than revealed by the chest film, with the film lagging behind the development of clinical symptoms. Computed tomography (CT) is very sensitive for identification of pulmonary contusion and may allow differentiation from areas of atelectasis or aspiration. The CT scan will accurately reflect the area of damage; however, most contusions that are visible only on a CT scan are not clinically relevant in that they are not large enough to impair gas exchange and do not worsen outcome. Arterial blood gases (ABGs) may show decreased carbon dioxide ($Paco_2$) and oxygen pressures (Pao_2) and **worsening of the Pao_2/Fio_2 ratio, indicating increasing intrapulmonary shunt (Qs/Qt).**

Management of Patient Care. Management of a pulmonary contusion is supportive, allowing for the injury to heal. If the contusion is mild, monitoring and supplemental oxygen by mask may be sufficient. *Severe pulmonary contusions are treated like acute respiratory distress syndrome (ARDS)* because of the large amount of lung tissue damage, refractory hypoxemia, and decreased lung compliance. An estimated 40% of patients with pulmonary contusion will require mechanical ventilation.

Agitation and anxiety may indicate the presence of hypoxia and may be a first sign of impending deterioration. Pain from chest wall injury will affect the ability to ventilate and clear secretions. Management of a blunt chest injury therefore includes adequate analgesia.

Since moderate to severe pulmonary contusions are often accompanied by multisystem injuries, fluid administration must be balanced against hemodynamic and pulmonary function. Fluid overload is associated with poor outcomes. Intake and output, **central venous pressure (CVP), and pulmonary artery pressure (PAP)** may be monitored. Steroids have been used to reduce lung edema; however, they are no longer recommended because they have been found to be ineffective.

Nasotracheal suctioning and humidification may help with removal of secretions.

Complications. Complications include pulmonary laceration, hemothorax, respiratory failure, atelectasis, pneumonia, and ARDS. A pulmonary contusion will usually resolve in 3 to 7 days provided that no secondary injury occurs. *A pulmonary laceration occurs when the force of the injury is sufficient to lacerate the lung from a rib fracture or direct puncture, causing bleeding and hemothorax.* Tracheal lacerations can occur, which may be life-threatening and require immediate expert consultation and possible surgery.

Rib Fractures

Rib fractures are common injuries, which occur most often following blunt thoracic trauma but can also result from severe coughing, athletic activities (eg, rowing, swinging golf club), or penetrating injury from gunshot wounds. Complications range from mild discomfort to life-threatening conditions such as **pneumothorax**, splenic laceration, and pneumonia.

Pathophysiology. It is not common to have a fracture of the first rib. Such a fracture is life-threatening and indicates severe force and possible underlying thoracic and/or abdominal injuries. Fractures in ribs 1, 2, or 3 may be associated with mediastinal injury. When a very strong force is applied to the upper thoracic cage, the result is a "starburst" fracture—that is, pieces of bone going in all directions. Sternal fracture is suspected when there is paradoxical movement of the anterior chest wall.

Middle ribs (ribs 4–8) are the most commonly fractured. If a single rib is fractured, pain relief is usually the only treatment necessary. The intact rib on each side of the fractured rib stabilizes the fracture and keeps it in alignment for healing. *Fractures of ribs 9 to 12 suggest possible laceration and/or rupture of the spleen (left) and/or liver (right) as well as diaphragmatic tears can occur.*

Etiology and Risk Factors. Rib fractures result from a blunt force that does not penetrate the chest wall. Motor vehicle collisions, falls, and violent assaults are the common causes of closed thoracic injury.

In an adult patient with blunt trauma, a **hemothorax**, **pneumothorax**, or pulmonary contusion seen on chest imaging will almost always be associated with a rib fracture, whether or not identified clinically or on imaging.

Signs and Symptoms. Symptoms include pain, dyspnea, ecchymosis, and splinting on movement. Often point tenderness is noted over the site of fracture. *Bony crepitus* may be present. The patient should be examined for neck injuries, brachial plexus injury, pneumothorax, aortic rupture or tear, and thoracic outlet syndrome.

Invasive and Noninvasive Diagnostic Studies. Rib fractures can be diagnosed by chest radiograph. It may be difficult to see hairline fractures initially. Simple rib fractures are more easily seen as they begin to repair and lay down additional calcium at the injury site. Compound rib fractures and fractures with overlying bone are more easily detected by chest imaging.

Patient Management. Management of chest wall injury is directed toward protecting the underlying lung and *allowing adequate oxygenation, ventilation, and pulmonary toilet.* Management includes *relief of pain* so that *pulmonary hygiene* can be achieved. A continual epidural is one of the most efficient forms of analgesia and may be placed in the thoracic or high-lumbar position. Epidurals will provide excellent *pain relief* with local anesthetic and/or opioid agents and *does not interfere with coughing, sighing, and deep breathing.* Patient-controlled analgesia (PCA) and intercostal nerve block can also be used in relieving pain.

Bronchial hygiene and physical therapy are used to prevent the development of atelectasis and pneumonia. Binders are not recommended because they decrease excursion over a wide area of the thorax, predisposing the patient to hypoxemia and atelectasis. Sternal fractures may be stabilized internally with endotracheal intubation, mechanical ventilation, and positive end-expiratory pressure (PEEP).

Complications. Complications of rib fractures include atelectasis, fever, pneumonia, retained pulmonary secretions, and ARDS.

Flail Chest

"Flail chest" refers to two or more adjacent ribs with two or more fractures, anteriorly or laterally. The flail thorax may be an especially severe injury if it is associated with a transverse fracture of the sternum. Sternal fracture is suspected when there is paradoxical movement of the anterior thoracic wall.

Pathophysiology. A section of the chest wall becomes detached from the thoracic cage. The involved portion of the thoracic wall may be so unstable that it will move paradoxically or opposite to the rest of the thoracic wall when the patient breathes (**Fig. 19-2**). During inspiration, negative intrathoracic pressure increases and the chest wall moves outward. With a **flail chest**, the injured segment moves inward. On expiration, intrathoracic pressure decreases, the chest wall moves inward, and the flail section moves outward. This results in atelectasis and alveolar collapse because the alveoli cannot fill with air.

> **QUICK TIP!** A flail chest pneumothorax scenario often appears on the exam in a patient after an MVA or blunt force trauma from playing sports. In this situation, prepare to identify the signs and symptoms of pneumothorax and treatments to anticipate.
>
> - Pneumothorax signs, symptoms, identification, and treatment often appear in many different questions and scenarios on the test.

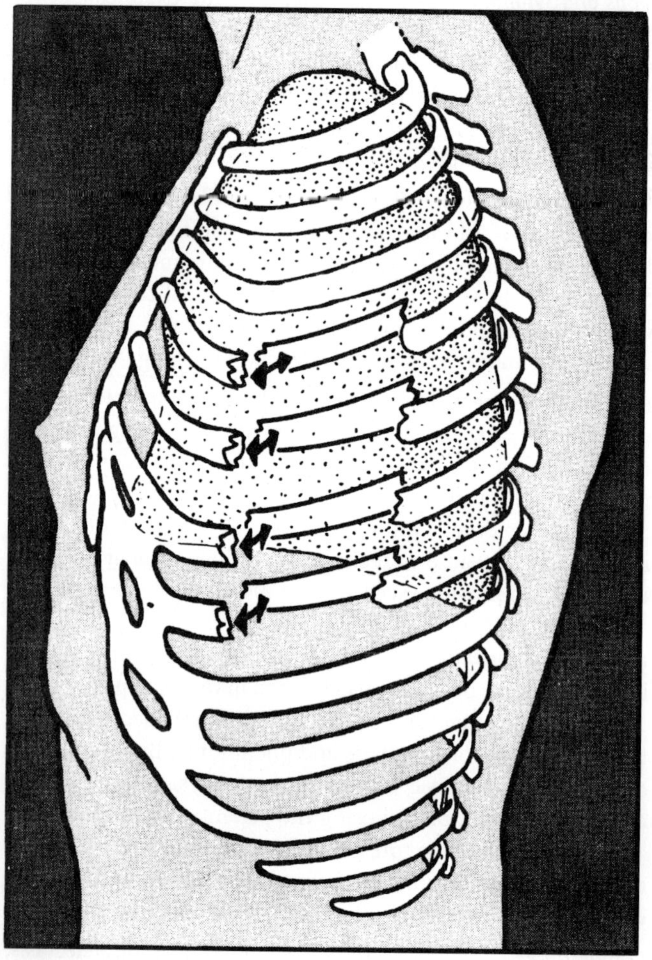

Figure 19-2. Flail chest segment.

Etiology and Risk Factors. Causes include fights, motor vehicle collisions, blast injuries, and athletic injuries.

Signs and Symptoms. Symptoms of flail injuries to the thorax include rapid, shallow respirations, cyanosis, severe thoracic wall pain, shock, *bony crepitation at the site of fracture,* and paradoxical thoracic movement. There may be signs of pulmonary contusion, bruised thorax, and tender chest on palpation. Hypotension, tachycardia, hypoxemia, and hemoptysis may also be present.

Invasive and Noninvasive Diagnostic Studies. Chest x-ray confirms the diagnosis of flail chest. ABGs may show a falling Pao_2, increasing $Paco_2$, and a pH below 7.35, indicating respiratory acidosis.

Patient Management. Specific treatment is stabilization of the flail segment and restoration of normal breathing. In an emergency, anything can be used to stabilize the thoracic wall and help *immobilize the segment* (eg, sandbags or hands). In the critical care unit, intubation, positive-pressure ventilation, and PEEP may be used to stabilize the flailing segment. *Neuromuscular blockade* may be used to paralyze the patient and allow ventilatory synchrony in order to help stabilize the chest wall. Adequate sedation and analgesia must be provided when neuromuscular blockade is used.

Pain control is a top priority. Patients are medicated to achieve adequate pain control and *reduce the work of breathing.* The strategies for controlling pain with rib fractures can also be utilized with a **flail chest**.

Complications. Complications include pulmonary contusion, pneumothorax, hypoxia, pulmonary laceration, and cardiac contusion.

Hemothorax

Hemothorax is an accumulation of blood in the thorax. It is often accompanied by a pneumothorax.

Pathophysiology. The three major effects of a hemothorax are the accumulation of blood in the lungs, collapsing alveoli, and systemic hypovolemia. Shock can occur quickly with the development of a hemothorax. Trauma to the thorax may cause bleeding from the intercostal, pleural, lung parenchymal, or mediastinal vessels or from the internal mammary artery. As blood fills the pleural space, the underlying lung tissue is compressed, causing alveolar collapse. A hemothorax may be self-limiting, especially if its origin is venous. As the blood accumulates in the chest, the increasing pressure may reduce or stop the source of bleeding. Arterial injury, which is less common, will not be self-limiting.

Etiology. Hemothorax is caused by blunt or penetrating thoracic trauma, iatrogenic causes, lacerated liver, or perforated diaphragm. It may also result from thoracic surgery, anticoagulant therapy, or a dissecting thoracic aneurysm.

Signs and Symptoms. The symptoms of a hemothorax depend on the size of the blood accumulation. *Small amounts* of blood *(ie, ≤ 400 mL)* will cause minimal symptoms. ***Larger amounts of blood (ie, ≥ 400 mL)*** usually present with signs of shock: tachycardia, tachypnea, hypotension, and anxiety. *Breath sounds may be diminished or absent, and the chest is dull on percussion.*

Invasive and Noninvasive Diagnostic Studies. The chest film may show pleural fluid or a *mediastinal shift. ABGs will show a*

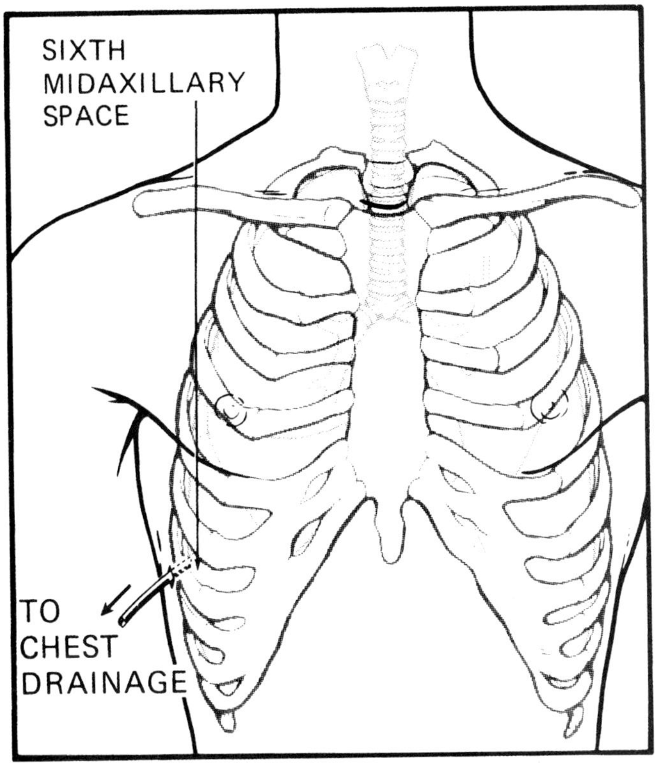

Figure 19-3. Chest tube insertion for hemothorax.

normal or decreased Pa_{O_2}, *an increased* Pa_{CO_2}, *and a falling pH.* If there has been a large amount of bleeding, the hematocrit and hemoglobin levels may be decreased. CVP or PAP may be low if fluid-volume depletion is evident. Ultrasound examination can detect smaller hemothoraces, although in the presence of a *pneumothorax or subcutaneous air,* ultrasound may be difficult or inaccurate. A CT scan will detect a hemothorax and is especially useful in identifying one in the presence of other multiple trauma.

Thoracentesis is used for both diagnosis and treatment. A soft catheter is inserted into the chest over a stylet and aspirated for blood or serosanguineous fluid.

Patient Management. Small hemothoraces may resolve spontaneously because of low pulmonary system pressure and the presence of thromboplastin in the lungs. Large hemothoraces are treated with the insertion of one or more chest tubes in the fifth or sixth intercostal space in the midaxillary line (**Fig. 19-3**). The chest tube is sutured in place and covered with a sterile dressing after being connected to a water-seal drainage system with suction. Autotransfusion may be used for patients with a blood loss of 1 L or more. Severe or uncontrollable hemothorax may require thoracotomy to remove the blood and fluid from the lung and correct the source of bleeding. Adequate venous access is critical so that fluid resuscitation and blood product administration can occur.

It is important to monitor the patient's ability to expel secretions and to suction when necessary so as to prevent hypoxia and atelectasis. Analgesics are recommended for relief of pain.

Complications. Complications of a hemothorax include atelectasis, lung collapse, hypoxemia, and mediastinal shift. Failure to adequately drain a hemothorax initially results in residual clotted hemothorax, which will not drain via a chest tube. If left untreated, these retained hemothoraces may become infected and lead to empyema formation.

Diaphragmatic Rupture

Pathophysiology. Diaphragm rupture is rare and often accompanied by other significant injuries of the thoracic or abdominal cavities. The integrity of the diaphragm is compromised allowing abdominal contents or air to enter the thoracic cavity, causing increasing intrathoracic pressure. In the majority of cases, the left hemidiaphragm is injured, perhaps because of the protection by the liver on the right side.

Etiology and Risk Factors. Rupture of the diaphragm is associated with both blunt and penetrating trauma, especially gunshot wounds of the lower abdomen and chest. The incidence of diaphragmatic rupture is doubled in patients with a fractured pelvis. It is almost always accompanied by intraperitoneal and multisystem injuries.

Signs and Symptoms. Symptoms are related to the amount of herniated viscera in the thorax. Primary symptoms of a ruptured or herniated diaphragm include auscultation of bowel sounds in the chest, increasing shortness of breath, unequal diaphragmatic movement on palpation, elevated diaphragm and hyperresonance to percussion, marked or increasing respiratory distress, severe shoulder pain (also called **Kehr's sign** due to referred pain carried by the phrenic nerve) on the same side as the tear, and shock.

Invasive and Noninvasive Diagnostic Studies. The initial chest imaging may be normal in 50% of cases or may reveal an elevated, arched shadow of a high left hemidiaphragm, a mediastinal shift to the right, shadows above the diaphragm, and abnormal air–fluid levels. The chest radiograph may also reveal a nasogastric tube in the left thorax or air bubbles in the left chest, indicating visceral herniation. Ultrasound and CT can also be useful in making the diagnosis. The *CT scan is the best available test to confirm the diagnosis.*

Management of Patient Care. Immediate treatment is to establish adequate respiratory function. This is most frequently accomplished by endotracheal intubation and mechanical ventilation. It may or may not be possible to stabilize a patient in shock prior to surgery, depending on the severity of the rupture. Definitive therapy consists of surgical repair of the torn diaphragm and replacement of the abdominal organs in the abdominal cavity.

The patient's respiratory status should be monitored to ensure adequate oxygenation. Increased intrathoracic pressure and abdominal contents in the thoracic cavity may cause marked hemodynamic compromise.

Complications. Complications include strangulation of the bowel or bowel obstruction, cardiovascular collapse, and death.

19.2 AIR-LEAK SYNDROMES

A **pneumothorax** *is accumulation of air in the pleural space.* It may be the result of blunt or penetrating trauma or rupture of a bleb or emphysematous bulla, or it may have an iatrogenic cause, such as **mechanical ventilation or high levels of PEEP** (**Table 19-1**). There are three types of pneumothorax: closed, open, and tension.

TABLE 19-1. SIGNS AND SYMPTOMS OF PNEUMOTHORAX
Inspection
Asymmetrical chest wall movement
Hyperexpansion
Chest wall rigidity on the affected side
Palpation
Subcutaneous emphysema
Decreased vocal fremitus
Mediastinal shift
Tracheal deviation
Tympany on the affected side
Percussion
Hyperresonance on the affected side
Auscultation
Decreased or absent breath sounds on the affected side

The closed or spontaneous pneumothorax occurs when air enters the pleural space through the airways. Spontaneous pneumothorax can be *primary*—occurring in healthy people *or secondary*—occurring due to underlying lung disease. If air cannot escape the chest, intrapleural pressure increases, pressure on the other lung and the heart will continue, and a *tension pneumothorax is possible.*

An open or traumatic pneumothorax is caused by a *penetrating injury* that allows air to enter and exit the pleural space (**Fig. 19-4**). The open pneumothorax is less dangerous than a closed pneumothorax because of the *reduced likelihood of developing a tension pneumothorax.*

Tension pneumothorax is potentially life-threatening. *Air accumulates in the pleural space but cannot escape.* During inhalation, air is sucked into the pleura through a tear; on exhalation, the torn pleura closes against the parenchyma, *creating a one-way valve that prevents air from being exhaled* (**Fig. 19-5**). The **tension pneumothorax** *quickly produces hemodynamic and cardiopulmonary compromise. The accumulation of air in the thorax causes increasing intrathoracic pressure that leads to severe hemodynamic imbalances.*

Pathophysiology. The lungs are contained in the visceral pleura. The parietal pleura line the thorax. The potential area between the two pleura, the pleural space, is lined by a thin layer of lubrication. If air or fluid enters the space, the surfaces are separated. The pressure of the intrapleural space is −5 cm H_2O. When air or fluid enters the pleural space, the pressure becomes positive. This positive pressure leads to lung collapse, decreased lung compliance, decreased total lung capacity, and decreased vital capacity. Hypoxia is the result of the increasing V/Q mismatch. If the pressure cannot escape, as in tension pneumothorax, the intrathoracic pressure continues to build, leading to hemodynamic compromise and cardiovascular collapse.

Signs and Symptoms. A simple pneumothorax may present with only mild respiratory distress, asymmetrical chest wall expansion, vague complaints of difficulty in catching the breath, and chest pain (see Table 19-1).

Tension pneumothorax produces symptoms that include dyspnea and restlessness, progressive cyanosis, tachycardia, hypotension, *diminished or absent breath sounds on the affected side,* decreased chest wall movement, signs of increasing respiratory distress, *chest pain and tracheal shift toward the* **unaffected** *side,* asymmetrical chest wall movement, and rigidity on the affected side. The *mediastinum, trachea, and point of maximum intensity (PMI) all shift away from the affected side.* If the patient is on volume-limited mechanical **ventilation the peak airway pressure will increase** and if the resistance is great enough the **high pressure alarm** *will activate and the patient will not receive the full set tidal volume.* Patients that are on pressure-limited mechanical ventilation will demonstrate a decreased tidal volume but since the pressure is limited it will remain unchanged. A tension pneumothorax is a medical emergency requiring immediate treatment.

Invasive and Noninvasive Diagnostic Studies. The chest radiograph will show an accumulation of air in the pleural space. *A mediastinal shift may be evident. ABGs will show a decreased*

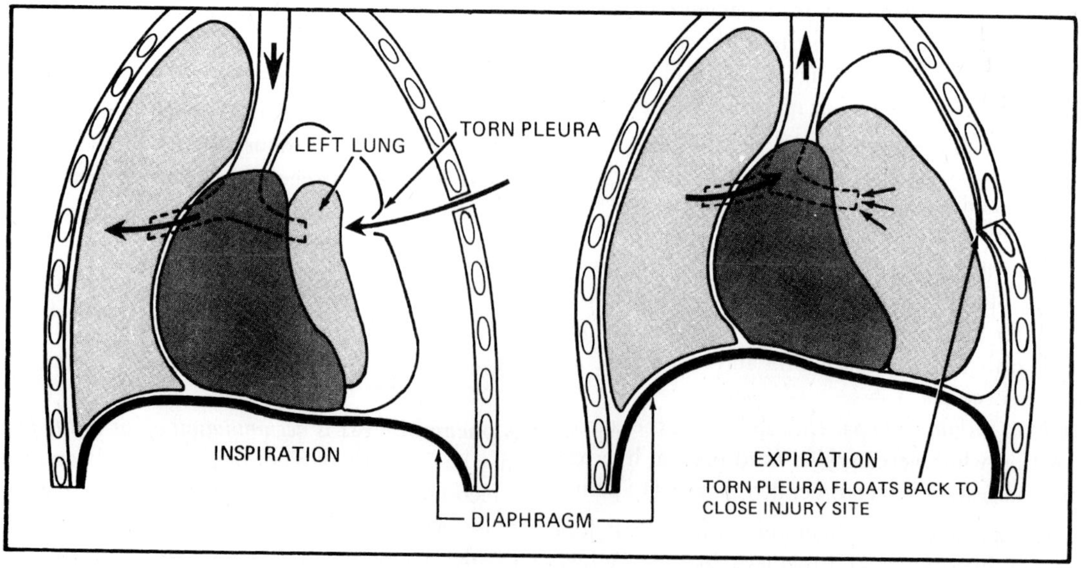

Figure 19-4. Open pneumothorax.

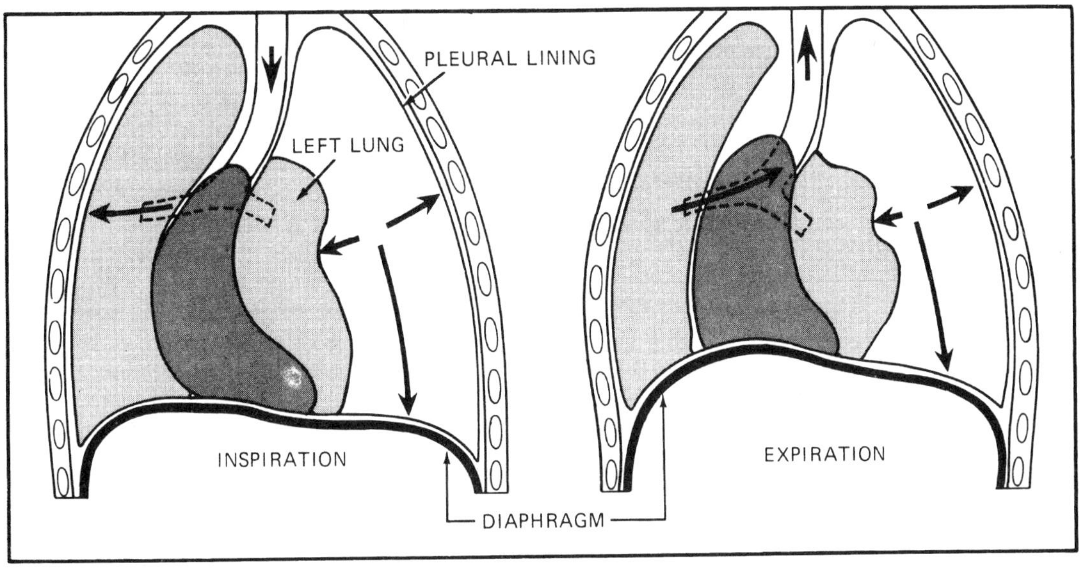

Figure 19-5. Tension pneumothorax.

Pao_2, and an increased pH (-respiratory alkalosis) due to the tachypnea. If respiratory compromise occurs, a rising $Paco_2$ and a falling pH will be seen.

Patient Management. A small pneumothorax may not require treatment. If no serious breathing problems occur, air will be reabsorbed in a few days. Drainage of air and fluid from the pleural space requires an evacuation system that allows air and fluids to exit but not to reenter. If the pneumothorax is small enough, needle aspiration or thoracentesis may be sufficient treatment to reexpand the lung. Small bore chest tubes (12–20 Fr) have been found to be as effective as large bore (24–Fr) to evacuate air, fluid, or blood from the thorax, resulting in less traumatic punctures and increased patient comfort. When hemothorax is present the larger bore chest tube may be more reliable in evacuating blood/clots.

If a **tension pneumothorax** is suspected and the patient is experiencing *hemodynamic compromise, decompression with a needle is necessary before placement of a chest tube.* **Tension pneumothorax** is a life-threatening condition that demands urgent management. If this diagnosis is suspected, do not delay treatment in the interest of confirming the diagnosis. Although a needle thoracostomy is not the definitive treatment for tension pneumothorax, **emergent needle decompression** may abate its progression and serve to restore cardiopulmonary function. *Insert a large-bore (ie, 14- or 16-gauge) needle with a catheter into the second intercostal space, just superior to the third rib at the midclavicular line, 1 to 2 cm from the sternal edge. Listen for the hissing sound of air escaping and remove the needle while leaving the catheter in place.*

If a chest tube is used, it is inserted in the second or third intercostal space at the midclavicular line to remove air (**Fig. 19-6**). Chest tubes are sutured in place and connected to a water-seal or suction drainage system. The insertion site of the tube is covered with a sterile dressing and connected to a water-seal drainage system.

The most common water-seal drainage systems are single units composed of three chambers to provide fluid collection, water seal, and suction control.

Air leaving the pleural space is readily seen by the bubbling in the water-seal chamber. When air has ceased leaking from the pleural space, this bubbling ceases. The water seal allows air to escape, but not return into, the pleural space. Evacuation of fluid is noted by measuring the amount of drainage in the fluid collection chamber.

For the evacuation of air, chest tubes are placed superiorly and anteriorly in a patient lying flat, near the second intercostal space in the midclavicular line. Chest tubes are placed in gravity-dependent positions, near the fifth intercostal space in the

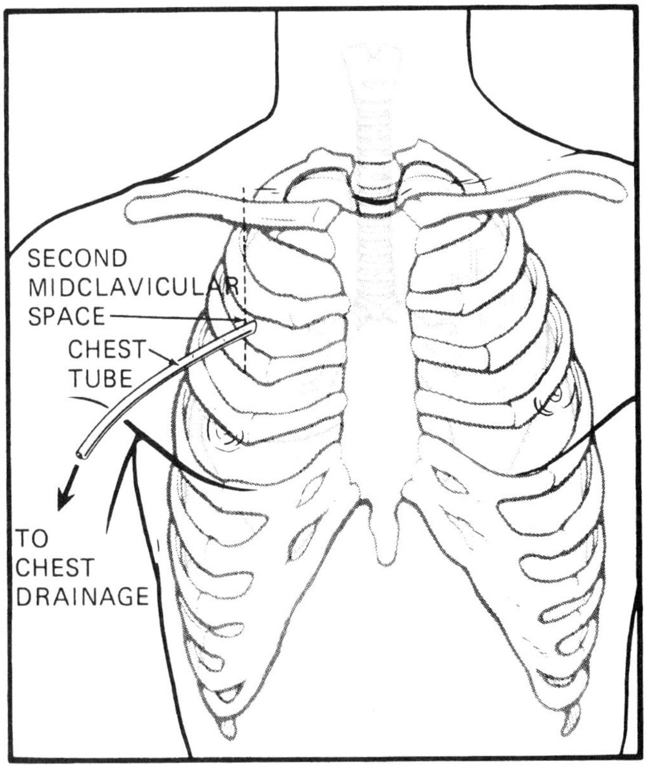

Figure 19-6. Chest tube insertion for removal of air.

midaxillary line, to facilitate fluid evacuation such as for pleural effusion or hemothorax. Placement lower than the fifth intercostal space increases the risk of puncturing abdominal viscera. Ultrasound may be utilized to identify fluid and the underlying structures prior to placement of a chest tube.

*Chest tubes should **NOT** be clamped if bubbling is present the water-seal chamber. There is the potential for a tension pneumothorax* in a situation where a tube is clamped while air is still exiting the pleural space. *If no air is leaking from the pleural space, the clamping of a chest tube is generally not a problem provided that there is no major accumulation of blood.* In the event the pleural drainage system is accidentally broken or severely cracked, emergently allowing atmospheric pressure into the system, apply a one-way valve (or stopcock) to the end of the tube or insert the uncontaminated end of the connective tubing into a bottle of sterile water or saline to a depth of 2 cm until a new unit can be set up. However, if the safety of the situation allows (ie, no tension pneumothorax), simply exchange the drainage system by clamping the existing system while setting up a new system.

Milking and stripping of chest tubes is generally not recommended, as it has been shown to create suction pressures of up to −400 cm H_2O. This can cause damage to lung tissue and disruption of suture lines.

Chest radiographs are used to verify the position of the chest tubes and monitor the reexpansion of the lung.

Complications. Complications of pneumothorax depend on the patient's size, rate of development, and underlying cardiopulmonary status. Cardiac and pulmonary failure can result from the sudden development of a large pneumothorax or a tension pneumothorax.

KEY CONTENT CHECKLIST

- ❒ Blunt lung injury develops over the course of 24 hours, leading to poor gas exchange, increased pulmonary vascular resistance, and decreased lung compliance.
- ❒ Tension pneumothorax quickly produces hemodynamic and cardiopulmonary compromise.
- ❒ The accumulation of air in the thorax causes increasing intrathoracic pressure that may lead to severe hemodynamic imbalances.
- ❒ A flail chest pneumothorax scenario often appears on the exam in a patient after an MVA or blunt force trauma from playing sports. In this situation, prepare to identify the signs and symptoms of pneumothorax and treatments to anticipate.
- ❒ Pneumothorax signs, symptoms, identification, and treatment often appear in many different questions and scenarios on the test.
- ❒ **Kehr's sign** is due to referred pain carried by the phrenic nerve to the left shoulder or above the clavicle as a result of diaphragmatic irritation or injury.
- ❒ Treatment of tension pneumothorax may require emergent insertion of a large bore needle into the second intercostal space, midclavicular line of the affected side.

Review Questions:

1. Which of the following findings would be an indication of a ruptured diaphragm?
a. Diminished bowel sounds
b. Tracheal shift toward the affected diaphragm
c. Irregular breathing
d. Bowel sounds in the chest

Answer: D. Rationale: Primary symptoms of a ruptured or herniated diaphragm include auscultation of bowel sounds in the chest, increasing shortness of breath, unequal diaphragmatic movement on palpation, elevated diaphragm and hyperresonance to percussion, marked or increasing respiratory distress, severe shoulder pain on the same side as the tear, and shock.

2. Which of the following would best support the diagnosis of pulmonary contusion?
a. Deteriorating Pao_2 value
b. 12-lead ECG
c. Distant heart tones and hyperventilation

Answer: A. Rationale: ABGs will show decreased carbon dioxide ($Paco_2$) and oxygen pressures (Pac_2) and worsening of the Pao_2/Fio_2 ratio, indicating increasing intrapulmonary shunt (Qs/Qt).

3. A 38-year-old man is admitted to your unit following a fall from a bicycle. He has sustained possible fractures of the sixth through ninth ribs on the right. Which of the following would NOT be a physical sign of fractured ribs without a pneumothorax?
a. Decreased breath sounds over the area
b. Shallow breathing
c. Splinting of the affected side
d. Crepitus palpated over the right chest and neck

Answer: D. Rationale: A pneumothorax is accumulation of air in the pleural space. An open or traumatic pneumothorax is caused by a penetrating injury that allows air to enter and exit the pleural space (see Fig. 19-4). The open pneumothorax is less dangerous than a closed pneumothorax because of the reduced likelihood of developing a tension pneumothorax. Since option D. is most closely associated with a pneumothorax, choose D.

REFERENCES

Alistair JE, Wachsmann J, Chamarthy MR, Panjikaran L, Tanabe Y, Rajiah P. Imaging of acute pulmonary embolism: an update. *Cardiovasc Diagn Ther.* 2018;8(3):225-243.

Devlin JW, Skrobik Y, Gélinas C, et al. Clinical Practice Guidelines for the Prevention and Management of Pain, Agitation/Sedation, Delirium, Immobility, and Sleep Disruption in Adult Patients in the ICU. *Crit Care Med.* 2018;46(9):e825-e873.

Frat JP, Coudroy R, Marjanovic N, Thille AW. High-flow nasal oxygen therapy and noninvasive ventilation in the management of acute hypoxemic respiratory failure. *Ann Transl Med.* 2017;5(14):297. doi: 10.21037/atm.2017.06.52.

Fernando SM, Ferreyro BL, Urner M, Munshi L, Fan E. Diagnosis and management of acute respiratory distress syndrome. *CMAJ.* 2021;193(21):E761-E768. doi: 10.1503/cmaj.202661.

Giri J, Akhilesh KS, Weinberg I, et al. Interventional Therapies for Acute Pulmonary Embolism: Current Status and Principles for the Development of Novel Evidence: a scientific statement from the American Heart Association. *Circulation.* 2019;140:e774-e801.

Humbert M, Kovacs G, Hoeper M, et al. 2022 ESC/ERS guidelines for the diagnosis and treatment of pulmonary hypertension. *Eur Respir J.* 2022. doi: 10.1183/13993003.00879-2022.

McNally E, Krisciunas GP, Langmore SE, et al. Oral Care Clinical Trial to Reduce Non-Intensive Care Unit, Hospital-Acquired Pneumonia: Lessons for Future Research. *J Healthc* Qual. 2019;41(1):1-9.

Metlay JP, Waterer GW, Long AC, et al. Diagnosis and treatment of adults with community-acquired pneumonia: an official clinical practice guideline of the American Thoracic Society and Infectious Diseases Society of America. *Am J Respir Crit Care Med.* 2019;200:e45-e67.

Saguil A, Fargo MV. Acute respiratory distress syndrome: diagnosis and management. *Am Fam Physician.* 2020;101(12):730-738.

PART II
Pulmonary Practice Exam

Questions 1 and 2 refer to the following scenario:
A 56-year-old woman is admitted to your unit with acute shortness of breath. She has a history of chronic obstructive pulmonary disease (COPD), congestive heart failure (CHF), and sleep apnea. Her current weight is 125 kg and she is 157 cm (5 ft. 2 in.) tall. On arrival in the emergency department, she is very short of breath and requires intubation. Her arterial blood gases (ABGs) and vital signs reveal:

pH	7.29
$PaCO_2$	74
PaO_2	59
HCO_3^-	35
Blood pressure	134/86 mm Hg
Pulse	122
Respiratory rate	33

She is placed on mechanical ventilation at the following settings:

Mode	assisted mandatory ventilation (AMV)
V_T	600
Respiratory rate	12
F_{IO_2}	0.40
PAP	42 cm H_2O
PEEP	+3 cm H_2O

She is given the following medications:

Albuterol	4 mg q 2 h
Dobutamine	3 μg/kg/min
IV fluids	50 mL/h
Propofol	20 mcg/kg/min

She is drowsy but responds to hearing her name called. After therapy, her vital signs are:

Blood pressure	98/56 mm Hg
Pulse	112 (atrial fibrillation)
Respiratory rate	12 (not breathing above the ventilator)
Temperature	37.80
Pulse oximetry (SpO_2)	0.95

Her ABGs reveal:

pH	7.55
$PaCO_2$	38
PaO_2	78
HCO_3^-	36

Her electrolytes are:

Sodium	136
Potassium	3.7
Chlorine	85

1. **Based on the above information, what is your interpretation of her current ABGs compared to her initial ABGs?**
   (A) respiratory alkalosis with a compensating metabolic acidosis and the presence of an increased anion gap
   (B) primary uncompensated metabolic alkalosis
   (C) respiratory acidosis corrected with mechanical ventilation; the compensating metabolic alkalosis remains
   (D) uncompensated respiratory acidosis
2. **What would be your response to the above ABGs?**
   (A) reduce the ventilator rate
   (B) increase the PEEP
   (C) change the albuterol from 4 to 5 mg
   (D) add pressure-support ventilation (PSV)

Questions 3 and 4 refer to the following scenario:
A 51-year-old man is in the intensive care unit with the diagnosis of acute respiratory failure (ARF), possibly secondary to sepsis. His last vital signs and laboratory data were as follows:

Blood pressure	108/60 mm Hg
Pulse	70 (normal sinus rhythm)
Respiratory rate	12
Temperature	38.8
Pulse oximetry (SpO_2)	0.99
pH	7.52
$PaCO_2$	29
PaO_2	109
HCO_3^-	29

He is currently on mechanical ventilation with the following settings:

Mode	Assisted mandatory ventilation
V_T	800
Respiratory rate	10
PAP	38 cm H_2O
PEEP	+5 cm H_2O
F_{IO_2}	100%

He also has an end-tidal carbon dioxide ($PetCO_2$) analyzer in place. It reads 27 mm Hg.

Based on the above information, the physician changes the V_T from 800 to 650. He requests ABGs in 30 min. Thirty minutes after the ventilator change, the $PetCO_2$ is 35.

3. **Are ABGs still necessary?**
   (A) Yes. Based on the widened CO_2 gradient, the $PetCO_2$ may not reflect change in $PaCO_2$ and pH.
   (B) No. The $PetCO_2$ will probably accurately trend the $PaCO_2$.
   (C) Yes, since the $PetCO_2$ does not reveal changes in blood gases.
   (D) No, since the $PetCO_2$ will accurately reflect changes in the PaO_2 and SpO_2 values.
4. **Based on the above ABGs, what is your interpretation of this patient's condition?**
   (A) uncompensated respiratory alkalosis
   (B) respiratory acidosis with a compensating metabolic alkalosis
   (C) compensated metabolic alkalosis
   (D) uncompensated respiratory acidosis
5. **The upper airway serves three of the key functions listed below. Select the one function that is NOT served by the upper airway.**
   (A) humidification of air
   (B) removal of particles
   (C) warming of inspired air
   (D) participation in gas exchange
6. **Which part of the trachea is relatively avascular, allowing for emergency placement of artificial airways in this area?**
   (A) thyroid cartilage
   (B) cricothyroid cartilage
   (C) laryngopharynx
   (D) glottis
7. **The left and right mainstem bronchi divide from the trachea at which of the following locations?**
   (A) carina
   (B) sternoclavicular junction
   (C) lingula
   (D) larynx
8. **Right mainstem bronchus intubations are more likely to be performed than left bronchus intubations for which of the following reasons?**
   (A) The right mainstem bronchus has more ciliary clearance of mucus, facilitating passage of the endotracheal tube.
   (B) The left mainstem bronchus is located several inches lower than the right.
   (C) The left mainstem bronchus, although wider than the right, sits posterior to the right mainstem bronchus.
   (D) The right mainstem bronchus is wider and has less angulation than the left.

Questions 9 through 11 refer to the following scenario:
A 69-year-old woman is admitted at 0700 with persistent right-sided chest pain that is not affected by respiration or position. She had a V/Q scan at 0900 that showed intermediate probability for a pulmonary embolism. The pain fluctuates and is now not very severe. She has crackles in her right middle lobe. Her ECG shows no signs of ischemia. She is not intubated but is on a 35% high-humidity face mask. She has the following vital signs and ABGs:

Blood pressure	94/56 mm Hg
Pulse	108 (sinus tachycardia)
Respiratory rate	26
Temperature	36.7
SpO_2	0.98
pH	7.26
$PaCO_2$	30
PaO_2	98
HCO_3^-	18
Lactate	4.8

Her physician has told you that he would call at about 1600 (4 PM). The current time is 1100.

9. **Based on the above information, interpret the ABGs.**
   (A) respiratory alkalosis with a compensating metabolic acidosis
   (B) metabolic acidosis with a partially (but not completely) compensating respiratory alkalosis
   (C) uncompensated respiratory alkalosis
   (D) uncompensated metabolic acidosis
10. **Based on the above information, what is your interpretation of the patient's oxygenation status?**
    (A) She shows signs of poor tissue oxygenation based on the elevated lactate, low HCO_3^-, and pH.
    (B) Her oxygenation is adequate at present based on the normal SpO_2 and PaO_2.
    (C) Her oxygenation is inadequate based on the FIO_2 of 0.35, generating a PaO_2 of only 98.
    (D) Her oxygenation is adequate at present based on the FIO_2 of 0.35, generating a PaO_2 of only 98 and an SpO_2 of 0.98.
11. **What intervention should you make at this time?**
    (A) Do not notify the physician but increase the FIO_2 per standing orders.
    (B) Notify the physician of abnormal values.
    (C) Wait until the physician calls at 1600 to report results of ABG.
12. **What is the name of the lipoprotein secreted by alveolar type II cells, which promotes alveolar expansion by reducing the surface tension of the alveoli?**
    (A) surfactant
    (B) phagocytes
    (C) alveolar epithelium
    (D) pulmonary parenchyma
13. **From which structure does the hypoxemic drive to breathe originate?**
    (A) aortic and carotid arteries
    (B) pons
    (C) medulla
    (D) basal ganglia

14. **Cheyne–Stokes breathing is characterized by which of the following respiratory patterns?**
(A) rapid shallow breathing
(B) short periods of apnea followed by respirations of increasing depth that then slow again to apnea
(C) regular deep breathing patterns that alternate with shallow-breathing patterns over a period of several minutes
(D) slow deep breaths

Questions 15 and 16 refer to the following scenario:
After receiving orders from the provider, you have decided to begin weaning a 71-year-old woman from mechanical ventilation. She is placed on PSV of 5 cm H_2O with a PEEP of +3 cm H_2O. After the weaning trial has been in progress for an hour, you obtain ABGs. The ABGs and vital signs are as listed below:

Blood pressure	140/78 mm Hg
Pulse	94 (sinus rhythm)
Respiratory rate	22
Temperature	37.3
SpO_2	0.98
pH	7.23
$PaCO_2$	59
PaO_2	91
HCO_3^-	24

15. **Based on the above information, what is your interpretation of the ABGs?**
(A) respiratory acidosis with a compensating metabolic alkalosis
(B) metabolic acidosis with a compensating respiratory alkalosis
(C) uncompensated respiratory acidosis
(D) uncompensated metabolic alkalosis

16. **Based on the above information, what action should you take?**
(A) Extubate at this time because she is doing well enough.
(B) Return to the ventilator since the ABGs indicate that she is failing the spontaneous breathing attempt.
(C) Continue the trial for another hour and then repeat the ABGs.

17. **In order to avoid ischemia of the trachea during endotracheal intubation, endotracheal cuff pressures should remain below venous drainage pressures. Normal pressures in the cuff should be kept in which range?**
(A) 0 to 5 mm Hg
(B) 5 to 10 mm Hg
(C) 10 to 15 mm Hg
(D) 15 to 20 mm Hg

18. **Normal arterial Po_2 levels (at sea level) fall within which of the following ranges?**
(A) 20 to 35 mm Hg
(B) 35 to 45 mm Hg
(C) 60 to 80 mm Hg
(D) 80 to 100 mm Hg

19. **Normal venous Po_2 levels (at sea level) fall within which of the following ranges?**
(A) 20 to 35 mm Hg
(B) 35 to 40 mm Hg
(C) 60 to 80 mm Hg
(D) 80 to 100 mm Hg

20. **Normal arterial hemoglobin saturation (Sao_2) falls within which of the following ranges?**
(A) 0.40 to 0.60
(B) 0.60 to 0.80
(C) 0.80 to 0.90
(D) more than 0.95

21. **Normal mixed venous hemoglobin saturation (SvO_2) falls within which of the following ranges?**
(A) 0.40 to 0.60
(B) 0.65 to 0.75
(C) 0.80 to 0.90
(D) more than 0.95

22. **In comparison of finger oximetry values (SpO_2) with Sao_2 levels, which of the following statements is most accurate?**
(A) SpO_2 values underestimate Sao_2 values.
(B) SpO_2 values overestimate Sao_2 values.
(C) SpO_2 values should equal Sao_2 values.
(D) SpO_2 values do not correlate with Sao_2 values.

Questions 23 and 24 refer to the following scenario:
A 75-year-old man is admitted to the unit with the diagnosis of pneumonia. He is short of breath and has circumoral cyanosis. He has crackles throughout both lungs. His initial ABGs and vital signs are:

Blood pressure	122/62	pH	7.25
Pulse	114	$PaCO_2$	53
Respiratory rate	30	PaO_2	34
Temperature	37.4	HCO_3^-	25
SpO_2	0.77		

The physician requests the following:

I. Place him on 40% oxygen via a face mask.
II. Start gentamicin 80 mg IV tid.
III. Do not give sedatives.

The physician asks that you inform her of any changes indicating that the patient's condition is worsening. After you start the oxygen, the circumoral cyanosis goes away. The patient states he feels about the same. His repeat ABGs and vital signs reveal:

Blood pressure	116/58	pH	7.21
Pulse	115	$PaCO_2$	59
Respiratory rate	30	PaO_2	61
Temperature	37.5	HCO_3^-	25
SpO_2	0.91		

23. **Based on the above information, what do you think of the patient's condition?**
(A) He is getting better based on his improved SpO_2 and PaO_2.
(B) He is about the same based on his blood pressure, pulse, respiratory rate, and HCO_3^-.
(C) He is getting worse based on his pH and $PaCO_2$.

24. What action is necessary, if any, for the above situation?
(A) No action is necessary, since he is improved.
(B) Call the physician based on the abnormal data.
(C) Repeat ABGs in 1 h but do not call the physician since the patient's condition has not markedly changed.

25. Which of the following does NOT worsen dynamic compliance?
(A) obesity
(B) airway secretions
(C) third-trimester pregnancy
(D) loss of airway rigidity

26. Which of the following best describes vital capacity?
(A) maximal inspiration followed by maximal expiration
(B) normal inspiratory volumes
(C) the amount of air vital to the person in 1 min
(D) the amount of air in the lungs at rest

27. The amount of air that does NOT participate in gas exchange is referred to by which of the following terms?
(A) minute ventilation
(B) alveolar ventilation
(C) dead-space ventilation
(D) bronchial ventilation

28. Alveolar ventilation is described by which of the following formulas?
(A) dead-space ventilation plus tidal volume
(B) minute volume minus dead-space ventilation
(C) tidal volume plus minute ventilation
(D) respiratory rate times tidal volume

29. Which level of dead space is considered normal?
(A) 25% to 35%
(B) 40% to 50%
(C) 55% to 65%
(D) 70% to 80%

Questions 30 and 31 refer to the following scenario:
A 28-year-old woman is admitted with acute shortness of breath. Her respiratory rate is 29, V_T 500, pulse 126, blood pressure 140/88. She has a history of asthma and is compliant with her medication regimen. Her ABGs reveal the following information:

pH	7.50
$PaCO_2$	27
PaO_2	71
HCO_3^-	24

30. Based on the preceding information, would the above laboratory values be reasonable to expect?
(A) No, the respiratory rate is increased in an attempt to increase the low $PaCO_2$.
(B) No, CO_2 is eliminated with each exhaled breath and with an increased respiratory rate, the $PaCO_2$ will be low.
(C) No, when the $PaCO_2$ is low due to the increased respirations eliminating the acidic CO_2, a respiratory alkalosis develops.
(D) All of the above are true.

31. What is her minute ventilation?
(A) elevated
(B) low
(C) normal
(D) cannot be estimated

32. Which of the following is the most common cause of hypoxemia?
(A) diffusion barriers
(B) hypoventilation
(C) changes in barometric pressure
(D) intrapulmonary shunts

33. Which of the following is an estimate of intrapulmonary shunting?
(A) PaO_2/FIO_2 ratio
(B) diffusion capacity
(C) mixed venous oxygen tensions
(D) FEV_1 (forced expiratory volume in 1 s)

34. Which of the following is the best description of FIO_2 (fraction of inspired oxygen)?
(A) the molecular weight of oxygen
(B) the percent of oxygen during inspiration
(C) the amount of oxygen (in milliliters) during inspiration
(D) the fraction of oxygen versus carbon dioxide during inspiration

35. Which of the following would be a normal oxygen tension (PaO_2) on exposure to 100% oxygen?
(A) 60 to 100 mm Hg
(B) 100 to 250 mm Hg
(C) 250 to 400 mm Hg
(D) 400 to 600 mm Hg

Questions 36 and 37 refer to the following scenario:
A 48-year-old man is admitted with the diagnosis of noncardiogenic pulmonary edema. Analysis of his ABGs reveals the following:

pH	7.37
$PaCO_2$	36
PaO_2	86
FIO_2	50%

36. Estimate the intrapulmonary shunt from the preceding data.
(A) normal
(B) low
(C) elevated
(D) cannot be estimated if the patient is on oxygen

37. Assume that the patient is on a regular diet. He is wondering if the HFNC will get in his way of eating and asks if he can take the HFNC off. Based on the preceding data, would it be safe to remove his oxygen in order to allow him to eat?
(A) no
(B) yes
(C) only if his nutritional status were depleted
(D) yes, providing he rests during the meal

38. Normal intrapulmonary shunts fall within which of the following ranges?
(A) 0% to 5%
(B) 6% to 15%
(C) 16% to 21%
(D) more than 21%

39. Which of the following is the most important determinant of oxygen transport?
(A) PaO_2
(B) Sao_2
(C) hemoglobin level
(D) cardiac output

40. Which of the following is an indicator of the balance between oxygen transport and consumption?
(A) PaO_2
(B) Sao_2
(C) SvO_2
(D) oxygen delivery

Questions 41 and 42 refer to the following scenario:
A 62-year-old woman is admitted to the unit with respiratory failure following hip replacement surgery. She complains of shortness of breath and orthopnea. She has the following laboratory data available:

PaO_2	61
Sao_2	0.91
SvO_2	0.65
$PaCO_2$	39
pH	7.35
FIO_2	60%

41. Based on the preceding information, which condition is likely to be developing?
(A) severe intrapulmonary shunt
(B) severe imbalance between oxygen transport and cellular oxygen demand
(C) increased oxygen extraction rates
(D) hypercarbic respiratory failure

42. Based on her oxygenation status, does the FIO_2 need to be increased?
(A) No, the SvO_2 indicates adequate oxygenation.
(B) Yes, the PaO_2 is low and warrants further oxygen therapy.
(C) Yes, the SvO_2 is low and warrants further oxygen therapy.
(D) No, since her intrapulmonary shunt is near normal.

43. If the SvO_2 level decreases, all of the following parameters but one should be investigated by the nurse. Which parameter does NOT warrant investigation?
(A) oxygen content (Cao_2)
(B) basic metabolic profile (electrolytes)
(C) cardiac output
(D) oxygen consumption

44. Which of the following corresponds most closely to the normal oxygen transport level?
(A) 250 to 550 mL/min
(B) 600 to 1000 mL/min
(C) 1200 to 1600 mL/min
(D) 1600 to 2000 mL/min

45. Which of the following exerts the primary chemical control over breathing?
(A) oxygen tension
(B) carbonic acid level
(C) carbon dioxide level
(D) bicarbonate level

46. Which of the following corresponds most closely to the normal minute ventilation (VE)?
(A) 1 to 4 L/min
(B) 5 to 10 L/min
(C) 11 to 15 L/min
(D) more than 15 L/min

47. The oxyhemoglobin dissociation curve is best described as illustrating which of the following?
(A) the ability of oxygen to dissociate into different ions
(B) the amount of oxygen carried in the blood per minute
(C) the amount of oxygen carried in the dissolved state
(D) the ability of hemoglobin to bind with oxygen

48. An acid is best described as which of the following?
(A) a substance that gives up a hydrogen ion
(B) a substance that accepts a hydrogen ion
(C) an entity preventing oxygen from taking the electron split from hydrogen
(D) a substance that depletes free-floating hydrogen from the blood

49. The pulmonary response to a change in hydrogen ion concentration occurs in which time frame?
(A) within 24 h
(B) within 48 h
(C) within 1 week
(D) within 5 min

50. The renal response to a change in hydrogen ion concentration occurs in which time frame?
(A) within 24 h
(B) within 48 h
(C) within 1 week
(D) within 5 min

51. Which of the following is the basis for the primary renal buffering mechanism for a change in hydrogen ion level?
(A) bicarbonate
(B) phosphate
(C) protein
(D) sulfate

Questions 52 through 57 require you to interpret a set of blood gas values.

52. What would be the correct interpretation of the following blood gas values?

pH	7.35
$PaCO_2$	72
HCO_3^-	41

(A) respiratory acidosis alone
(B) respiratory acidosis with compensating metabolic alkalosis
(C) metabolic alkalosis alone
(D) metabolic acidosis with compensating respiratory alkalosis

53. What would be the correct interpretation of the following blood gas values?

pH	7.22
$PaCO_2$	64
HCO_3^-	24

(A) respiratory acidosis alone
(B) respiratory acidosis with compensating metabolic alkalosis
(C) metabolic acidosis alone
(D) metabolic acidosis with compensating respiratory alkalosis

54. What would be the correct interpretation of the following blood gas values?

pH	7.53
$PaCO_2$	36
HCO_3^-	35

(A) respiratory acidosis alone
(B) respiratory alkalosis with compensating metabolic alkalosis
(C) metabolic alkalosis alone
(D) metabolic acidosis with compensating respiratory alkalosis

55. What would be the correct interpretation of the following blood gas values?

pH	7.55
$PaCO_2$	21
HCO_3^-	26

(A) respiratory alkalosis alone
(B) respiratory alkalosis with compensating metabolic acidosis
(C) metabolic alkalosis alone
(D) metabolic acidosis with compensating respiratory alkalosis

56. What would be the correct interpretation of the following blood gas values?

pH	7.36
$PaCO_2$	24
HCO_3^-	14

(A) respiratory acidosis alone
(B) respiratory acidosis with compensating metabolic alkalosis
(C) metabolic alkalosis alone
(D) metabolic acidosis with compensating respiratory alkalosis

57. What would be the correct interpretation of the following blood gas values?

pH	7.15
$PaCO_2$	37
HCO_3^-	11

(A) respiratory alkalosis alone
(B) respiratory acidosis with compensating metabolic alkalosis
(C) metabolic acidosis alone
(D) metabolic acidosis with compensating respiratory alkalosis

Questions 58 and 59 refer to the following scenario:
A 58-year-old man admitted with the diagnosis of COPD presents with shortness of breath, circumoral cyanosis, and orthopnea. He is alert and oriented, stating that his symptoms started a few days earlier. He presents with the following blood gas values:

pH	7.36
$PaCO_2$	66
PaO_2	50
HCO_3^-	37
FIO_2	room air

58. Based on the preceding information, which condition is likely to be developing?
(A) acute oxygenation failure
(B) acute ventilation failure
(C) metabolic acidosis
(D) pure respiratory acidosis

59. Which treatment would be indicated for this patient?
(A) intubation and mechanical ventilation
(B) PEEP therapy
(C) inverse-ratio ventilation
(D) high-flow low-FIO_2 oxygen therapy

60. A patient with the diagnosis of asthma is admitted to your unit. He has received initial bronchodilator therapy in the emergency room. His blood gas values at that time were as follows:

pH	7.39
$PaCO_2$	25
PaO_2	62
HCO_3^-	25
FIO_2	0.30

Which of the following sets of blood gas values would indicate a worsening of the asthmatic episode due to diminished alveolar air flow?
(A) pH 7.30, $PaCO_2$ 48, PaO_2 70, FIO_2 0.40
(B) pH 7.35, $PaCO_2$ 29, PaO_2 69, FIO_2 0.40
(C) pH 7.48, $PaCO_2$ 18, PaO_2 60, FIO_2 0.40
(D) pH 7.39, $PaCO_2$ 24, PaO_2 58, FIO_2 0.40

61. Which of the following parameters is used as an estimate of alveolar ventilation (VA)?
(A) PaO_2
(B) $PaCO_2$
(C) pH
(D) alveolar–arterial oxygen gradient

62. Considering the treatment strategy of "permissive hypercapnia," at which pH is a respiratory acidosis generally treated?
(A) less than 7.25
(B) 7.25 to 7.35
(C) 7.35 to 7.45
(D) any pH more than 7.45

63. Which of the following is NOT a cause of acute respiratory failure?
(A) CNS injury
(B) RV failure
(C) excessive use of narcotics
(D) LV failure

64. You are helping another nurse to move a patient up in bed when the low-pressure alarm on the ventilator goes off. It also indicates a low tidal volume. The patient is becoming short of breath and his SpO_2 has dropped from 0.95 to 0.84. The $PetCO_2$ waveform is absent. The endotracheal tube appears to be in place and there is no obvious disconnection from the ventilator. The other nurse goes to call respiratory therapy. What should you do?
(A) Increase the tidal volume on the ventilator while instructing the patient to remain calm.
(B) Increase the FIO_2 on the ventilator while instructing the patient to remain calm.
(C) Remove the ventilator and begin manual respiration (Ambu bag).
(D) Increase the ventilator respiratory rate and peak flow.

65. A 36-year-old female was admitted to the unit after a fall down a flight of stairs. She has fractures of the right fourth rib and the left fourth and fifth ribs. She calls to complain of feeling anxious and short of breath. Her respiratory rate has increased from 16 to 36. Her trachea is noted to deviate to the left, and diminished breath sounds are heard throughout the right lung fields. Subcutaneous emphysema over the site of the right chest is discovered. What condition is probably developing?
(A) tension pneumothorax
(B) cardiac tamponade
(C) hemothorax
(D) flail chest

66. How is the pulmonary artery occlusive pressure (PAOP) used in differentiating acute respiratory distress syndrome (ARDS) from cardiogenic-induced pulmonary edema?
(A) A low PAOP with large intrapulmonary shunts suggests ARDS.
(B) The PAOP rises in both ARDS and pulmonary edema but the PAOP in ARDS is usually more than 30 mm Hg.
(C) The PAOP is low in ARDS but the CVP is elevated.
(D) The PAOP equals the CVP in ARDS but not in pulmonary edema.

Questions 67 and 68 refer to the following scenario:
A 64-year-old woman is admitted to your unit 2 days after coronary artery bypass graft (CABG) surgery. Symptoms include severe shortness of breath, which has developed over the past 2 h; its cause is unknown. A chest roentgenogram shows marked amounts of fluid in both lungs. Blood gas and pulmonary artery catheter information is as follows:

Pulmonary Artery Catheter

Blood pressure	98/64 mm Hg
Pulse	114
PAP	44/23
PAOP	12
CVP	3
Cardiac output	5.4
Cardiac index	2.9

Blood Gases

pH	7.48
$PaCO_2$	25
PaO_2	73
FIO_2	70%

67. Based on the preceding data, which condition is likely to be developing?
(A) CHF-induced pulmonary edema
(B) sepsis from pulmonary infection
(C) hypovolemia-induced left heart failure
(D) ARDS

68. Which treatment is most likely indicated to support the preceding condition?
(A) oxygen and PEEP therapy and fluid administration
(B) oxygen and PEEP therapy
(C) mechanical ventilation and dobutamine
(D) intubation, bicarbonate administration, and dopamine

69. Mortality with ARDS can be high, as much as 50%. What is the usual cause of death?
(A) hypoxemia from the ARDS-induced intrapulmonary shunt
(B) LV failure induced by ARDS
(C) hypotension induced by the pulmonary capillary leak syndrome
(D) the precipitating event that initiated the ARDS

Questions 70 and 71 refer to the following scenario:
A 74-year-old 70-kg man is admitted to your unit with a diagnosis of respiratory failure secondary to pneumonia. He is currently intubated and on AMV, with a VT of 550 mL, ventilator respiratory rate of 10, total rate of 29. His blood gas values are as follows:

pH	7.48
$PaCO_2$	30
PaO_2	64
FIO_2	80%

70. Based on the preceding information, which type of respiratory failure exists?
(A) oxygenation failure
(B) ventilation failure
(C) combined oxygenation and ventilation failure
(D) neither oxygenation nor ventilation failure

71. Which treatment would be indicated based on the blood gas values given?
(A) increase the ventilator VT
(B) decrease the ventilator rate
(C) add PEEP therapy to reduce the FIO_2
(D) reduce the FIO_2 while increasing the ventilator peak flow rate

72. Which system gives more stable FIO_2 therapy?
(A) simple face mask
(B) nasal cannula
(C) rebreathing mask
(D) Venturi mask

73. At which level of FIO_2 support is oxygen toxicity thought to develop?
(A) 30% to 40% for longer than 48 h
(B) 40% to 50% for longer than 2 h
(C) more than 50% for longer than 24 h
(D) FIO_2 does not cause oxygen toxicity; high PaO_2 values are the cause of toxicity

74. Which of the following is the most common indication for PEEP therapy?
(A) to improve carbon dioxide elimination
(B) to treat a metabolic acidosis
(C) to reduce postoperative bleeding
(D) to allow reduction in FIO_2 levels

75. When PEEP or CPAP is used, which of the following values is monitored by the nurse to assess the effectiveness of therapy?
(A) mean arterial pressure
(B) right atrial pressure
(C) $PaCO_2$ levels
(D) SaO_2/SpO_2 values

76. During a code, the physician is attempting to intubate the patient but is concerned that the endotracheal tube may not be in the lungs. Breath sounds are present but difficult to hear. What should you do to help the physician?
(A) Call for a stat chest film and keep bagging the patient.
(B) Attach a carbon dioxide monitor to confirm tube placement.
(C) Call for someone in anesthesia to come intubate.
(D) Suggest that the physician pull the tube and start over.

Questions 77 and 78 refer to the following scenario:
A 38-year-old woman is admitted with respiratory failure secondary to viral pneumonitis. She is currently on assisted AMV with a ventilator rate of 12, total rate of 26, VT of 500, FIO_2 of 80%, and peak airway pressure of 38. Finger oximetry (SpO_2) values are about 0.93. She suddenly becomes restless and indicates that she is short of breath. Her SpO_2 decreases to 0.83. Breath sounds are diminished on the right with peak airway pressures of 52 cm H_2O.

77. Based on the preceding information, which condition is likely to be developing?
(A) ARDS
(B) pneumonia
(C) pneumothorax
(D) pericardial tamponade

78. Treatment would most likely include which of the following measures?
(A) administration of morphine and furosemide (Lasix)
(B) addition of 5 cm of PEEP
(C) administration of dobutamine
(D) insertion of a chest tube

79. Pressure-support ventilation (PSV) differs from synchronized intermittent mandatory ventilation (SIMV) and AMV in which of the following ways?
(A) PSV includes a level of PEEP with each breath.
(B) PSV is negative pressure regulated.
(C) SIMV and AMV are volume-limited, PSV is pressure-limited.
(D) SIMV and AMV do not reduce the work of breathing, whereas PSV reduces the work of breathing and is therefore a better weaning tool.

80. Which of the following is an indication of a patient's potential ability to breathe spontaneously when removed from the ventilator?
(A) vital capacity of 5 mL/kg
(B) tidal volume of 1 to 2 mL/kg
(C) peak inspiratory pressures less than 20 cm H_2O
(D) minute ventilation of 5 to 10 L/min

Questions 81 and 82 refer to the following scenario:
A 58-year-old 80-kg man is recovering from acute respiratory failure. He has been on mechanical ventilation for 24 hours and was previously in good health. He currently has no shortness of breath and is on AMV of 12, with a total respiratory rate of 18. His FIO_2 is 0.40 with a PaO_2 of 98, a $PaCO_2$ of 36, pH of 7.42. He has the following weaning parameters:

VT	410 mL
VC	950 mL
PIP/NIF	−29 cm H_2O
VE	9 L/min
Respiratory rate	22

81. Based on the preceding information, which form of weaning is most likely to be implemented?
(A) SIMV
(B) IRV
(C) T-piece trial
(D) PSV

Before answering question 82, read the following additional information:

After 1 h on a CPAP trial, the following additional information about this patient is available:

VT	450 mL
VC	950 mL
PIP	−38 cm H_2O
VE	8.3 L/min
Respiratory rate	18
SaO_2	96%
PaO_2	85
$PaCO_2$	39
pH	7.39

82. Based on the additional information, what should be the next step in weaning this patient?
(A) Place him back on the ventilator and repeat the attempt later.
(B) Change to PSV weaning.
(C) Extubation is indicated.
(D) Rest one more day, then extubate.

Questions 83 through 85 refer to the following scenario:
A 63-year-old man is admitted with acute respiratory distress. Symptoms include marked shortness of breath and circumoral cyanosis. He is awake but is beginning to be less responsive. He has a history of COPD. Blood gases reveal the following information:

pH	7.22
$PaCO_2$	62
PaO_2	54
Sao_2	0.81
HCO_3^-	25
FIO_2	30%

83. Based on the preceding information, which condition is likely to be developing?
(A) CHF
(B) ARDS
(C) ARF
(D) pulmonary emboli

84. What would be the first treatment indicated at this time?
(A) increase the FIO_2
(B) intubate and place on mechanical ventilation
(C) postural drainage treatment
(D) aminophylline aerosol treatment

85. A 42-year-old man is in the unit with hepatic failure secondary to ETOH (alcohol) abuse. He is currently intubated for airway protection and requires sedation to keep him from fighting the ventilator. He has the following ventilator settings and vital signs:

Mode	AMV
Blood pressure	124/76 mm Hg
Rate	12
Pulse	92
V_T	550
Respiratory rate	18
FIO_2	0.30
SpO_2	0.97

He is combative (or restless) at times and requires restraints. When you go into the room to check on him, he is in the process of extubating himself. He yells "Thank God that is out." His vital signs are:

Blood pressure	148/88 mm Hg
Pulse	112
Respiratory rate	22
SpO_2	0.98

You tell the secretary to call the physician. It will take 10 min for the physician to get there. What should you do in the meantime?
(A) Attempt to reintubate with a new endotracheal tube.
(B) Manually bag him with 100% oxygen.
(C) Place a 40% face mask on him and observe his response.
(D) Give a midazolam (Versed) bolus to sedate him in preparation for reintubation.

86. Which of the following is a complication of mechanical ventilation and PEEP therapy?
(A) atelectasis
(B) oxygen toxicity
(C) reduced cardiac output
(D) ARDS

87. What is the highest FIO_2 that can generally be achieved with a nasal cannula?
(A) 30%
(B) 40%
(C) 60%
(D) 100%

Questions 88 and 89 refer to the following scenario:
A 70-year-old man is in your unit with a diagnosis of exacerbation of COPD, probably a pneumonia-induced event. He has very thick secretions, which have been difficult to remove during endotracheal suctioning.

88. Which of the following is the best method to aid in removal of thick secretions?
(A) instillation of saline
(B) increasing the suction pressure
(C) stimulating his cough reflex
(D) increasing the humidity of his oxygen

89. Failure to remove the secretions will produce which effect on blood gases?
(A) decrease in $PaCO_2$
(B) decrease in PaO_2
(C) increase in pH
(D) increase in HCO_3^- levels

90. What is the optimal level of PEEP therapy?
(A) the highest level of PEEP that increases cardiac output
(B) the highest level of PEEP that stabilizes $PaCO_2$ and PaO_2
(C) the lowest level of PEEP that improves cardiac output and Sao_2
(D) the lowest level of PEEP that increases the PaO_2 without depressing the cardiac output

91. Which of the following is an example of the bronchodilator category of methylxanthines?
(A) terbutaline
(B) albuterol
(C) metaproterenol
(D) theophylline

92. Low PaO_2 levels produce at least three physiologic reactions. Which of the following is NOT a consequence of low PaO_2 levels?
(A) pulmonary hypertension
(B) increased drive to breathe
(C) low Sao_2 levels
(D) left shift of the oxyhemoglobin dissociation curve

93. If the finger oximeter is reading 0.97 and the PaO_2 is 63, what may we infer about the oxyhemoglobin dissociation curve?

(A) A left shift in the oxyhemoglobin dissociation curve exists.
(B) A right shift in the oxyhemoglobin dissociation curve exists.
(C) The oxyhemoglobin dissociation curve is in a normal position.
(D) The oxyhemoglobin dissociation curve cannot be correlated with SaO_2 and PaO_2 values.

94. If the oxyhemoglobin dissociation curve shifts to the right, what is the clinical implication?

(A) Oxygen is more readily dissociated from hemoglobin.
(B) Hemoglobin binds oxygen more tightly.
(C) Erythropoietin stimulation will increase hemoglobin levels.
(D) Phosphate levels will be depleted.

95. What will shift the oxyhemoglobin dissociation curve to the right?

(A) hypothermia
(B) fever
(C) alkalosis
(D) multiple transfusion

96. Which of the following treatments would most improve oxygen transport status in an COPD/emphysema patient?

(A) oxygen therapy
(B) blood transfusion
(C) CPAP therapy
(D) intermittent positive-pressure breathing (IPPB) treatment

97. Which combination of treatments would be most effective in treating status asthmaticus?

(A) corticosteroids and bronchodilators
(B) methylxanthines and antibiotics
(C) postural drainage and bronchodilators
(D) incentive spirometry and bronchodilators

Questions 98 through 100 refer to the following scenario:
A 24-year-old woman is admitted to your unit in acute respiratory distress with the diagnosis of asthma. Lung auscultation reveals generalized wheezing. She is compliant with medications at home. She has received epinephrine, oxygen, and albuterol in the emergency department with no improvement in her symptoms. Her blood gases reveal the following:

pH	7.48
$PaCO_2$	27
PaO_2	59
FIO_2	4 L/min via nasal cannula
HCO_3^-	23

98. Based on the preceding information, which condition is likely to be developing?

(A) pneumonia
(B) status asthmaticus
(C) pulmonary emboli
(D) ARDS

99. Assume that the FIO_2 is increased to 6 L/min. Which of the following blood gas values would be an indication of a worsening status?

	(A)	(B)	(C)	(D)
pH	7.36	7.52	7.44	7.44
$PaCO_2$	40	24	27	29
PaO_2	70	64	72	59

100. Physical assessment by the nurse is one of the keys to the evaluation of therapy. During auscultation of the patient's lungs, what should the nurse be aware of if a reduction in the degree of wheezing were to occur?

(A) The patient's condition may be worsening or improving.
(B) Reduction in wheezing always indicates improvement.
(C) RV failure is developing.
(D) Pulmonary hypertension is being alleviated.

101. What is the definition of status asthmaticus?

(A) the first episode of a newly diagnosed asthmatic
(B) the preterminal asthmatic episode
(C) an asthma episode that has failed to improve with conventional treatment
(D) an asthma episode that is complicated by CHF

102. Pulmonary emboli produce all of the following physiologic changes but one. Which of the following is NOT likely to occur with pulmonary emboli?

(A) pulmonary hypertension
(B) arterial hypoxemia
(C) hypocarbia (low $PaCO_2$)
(D) LV heart failure

103. Which of the following tests is most diagnostic for pulmonary emboli?

(A) blood gas analysis
(B) V/Q scans
(C) pulmonary angiography
(D) pulmonary function tests

104. Effects from recurrent emboli due to deep venous thrombosis can be avoided by which one of the following therapies?

(A) use of a Greenfield (inferior vena cava) filter
(B) heparin
(C) warfarin
(D) use of lower extremity alternating compression devices

Questions 105 and 106 refer to the following scenario:
A 34-year-old woman is admitted to your unit 3 weeks after a cesarean delivery with acute shortness of breath and right chest pain. She has no prior cardiopulmonary medical history. Her vital signs are blood pressure 90/55 mm Hg, heart rate 140, respiratory rate 36. A stat transthoracic echocardiogram shows acute right heart failure and pulmonary hypertension. She has the following blood gas values:

pH	7.46
$PaCO_2$	30
PaO_2	62
FIO_2	3 L/min

105. Based on the preceding information, which condition is likely to be developing?
(A) ARDS
(B) dissecting thoracic aneurysm
(C) pleuritis
(D) pulmonary emboli

106. Which treatment would most likely improve her immediate symptoms?
(A) heparin
(B) oxygen therapy
(C) tissue plasminogen activator (tPA) or streptokinase
(D) aminophylline

107. Which of the following features of pleural drainage systems indicates an active pleural leak?
(A) bubbling in the water-seal chamber
(B) bubbling in the suction control chamber
(C) fluctuation of water level in the water-seal chamber with respiration
(D) no fluctuation of water level in the water-seal chamber with respiration

108. Which type of condition can lead to a tension pneumothorax?
(A) closed pneumothorax
(B) open pneumothorax
(C) subcutaneous emphysema
(D) pneumomediastinum

109. Which type of rib fracture has the highest complication rate?
(A) first rib
(B) third rib
(C) fifth rib
(D) seventh rib

110. Which of the following findings would be an indication of a ruptured diaphragm?
(A) diminished bowel sounds
(B) tracheal shift toward the affected diaphragm
(C) irregular breathing
(D) bowel sounds in the chest

111. A 56-year-old male has a right lower lobe pneumonia and has been receiving 40% oxygen via a face mask. The patient is complaining of dyspnea and has developed an increased respiratory rate with a decreased SpO_2. An arterial blood gas (ABG) is obtained. ABG results show: pH 7.29, $PaCO_2$ 51, PaO_2 57, Sao_2 87%, and HCO_3^- 27. The patient remains alert and denies any additional discomfort. What intervention would benefit the patient?
(A) intubate the patient and initiate mechanical ventilation
(B) increased the FIO_2 per face mask
(C) initiate non-invasive ventilation (NIV)
(D) re-evaluate antibiotic therapy

112. A 66-year-old female is receiving NIV for acute respiratory failure secondary to pneumonia. The patient has increased secretions, is getting restless and removing the face mask resulting in Sao_2 less than 88%. What intervention would you anticipate for this patient?
(A) administer anxiolytic
(B) increase the FIO_2
(C) apply restraints
(D) intubation and mechanical ventilation

Questions 113 through 115 refer to the following scenario:
A 41-year-old woman is admitted to your unit having landed on her left chest after a fall from the roof of her single-story house. She complains of left chest pain, which increases in intensity with deep inspiration. An admission chest roentgenogram is unremarkable. She is coughing up small amounts of blood-tinged sputum. Her trachea is midline. Her ECG and heart tones are normal. Blood pressure is 140/80 mm Hg, pulse 120, respiratory rate 28. Sao_2 is 92% on room air.

113. Based on the preceding information, which condition would need to be ruled out?
(A) cardiac rupture
(B) cardiac tamponade
(C) pulmonary contusion
(D) pneumomediastinum

Four hours after admission, the patient appears agitated and complains of increasing shortness of breath. Her pulse rate is now 140 and her respiratory rate is 38. The pulse oximeter displays a reading of 85% on room air.

114. What further treatment would be indicated based on this scenario?
(A) repeat chest film and supplemental oxygen
(B) insertion of a left chest tube
(C) pericardiocentesis
(D) emergent intubation

115. Which of the following would best support the diagnosis of pulmonary contusion?
(A) a deteriorating PaO_2 value
(B) 12-lead ECG
(C) distant heart tones and hyperventilation

Questions 116 and 117 refer to the following scenario:
A 23-year-old woman is admitted to your unit from the emergency department following a motor vehicle collision. She has no apparent injuries, although a chest film indicated a fourth-rib fracture on the left and a fifth-rib fracture on the right. Shortly after arrival in the unit, she develops marked shortness of breath and manifests a rightward deviation of the trachea and diminished breath sounds on the left. Her blood pressure is 94/62 mm Hg, pulse 120, respiratory rate 32.

116. Based on the preceding information, what condition is likely to be developing?
(A) open pneumothorax
(B) tension pneumothorax
(C) cardiac tamponade
(D) flail chest

117. What would be the best treatment for this condition?
(A) insertion of pleural chest tubes
(B) insertion of mediastinal chest tubes
(C) open thoracotomy
(D) pericardiocentesis

PART II
Pulmonary Practice Exam

Practice Fill-Ins

1. ______
2. ______
3. ______
4. ______
5. ______
6. ______
7. ______
8. ______
9. ______
10. ______
11. ______
12. ______
13. ______
14. ______
15. ______
16. ______
17. ______
18. ______
19. ______
20. ______
21. ______
22. ______
23. ______
24. ______
25. ______
26. ______
27. ______
28. ______
29. ______
30. ______
31. ______
32. ______
33. ______
34. ______
35. ______
36. ______
37. ______
38. ______
39. ______
40. ______
41. ______
42. ______
43. ______
44. ______
45. ______
46. ______
47. ______
48. ______
49. ______
50. ______
51. ______
52. ______
53. ______
54. ______
55. ______
56. ______
57. ______
58. ______
59. ______
60. ______
61. ______
62. ______
63. ______
64. ______
65. ______
66. ______
67. ______
68. ______
69. ______
70. ______
71. ______
72. ______
73. ______
74. ______
75. ______
76. ______
77. ______
78. ______
79. ______
80. ______
81. ______
82. ______
83. ______

84. ______________________
85. ______________________
86. ______________________
87. ______________________
88. ______________________
89. ______________________
90. ______________________
91. ______________________
92. ______________________
93. ______________________
94. ______________________
95. ______________________
96. ______________________
97. ______________________
98. ______________________
99. ______________________
100. ______________________
101. ______________________
102. ______________________
103. ______________________
104. ______________________
105. ______________________
106. ______________________
107. ______________________
108. ______________________
109. ______________________
110. ______________________
111. ______________________
112. ______________________
113. ______________________
114. ______________________
115. ______________________
116. ______________________
117. ______________________

PART II
Answers

1. **C** Chapter 15 Rationale: The first ABG showed pH is acidotic at 7.29. The $PaCO_2$ is elevated at 74 indicating respiratory acidosis. The HCO_3 is 35 indicating a metabolic alkalosis is also present. The ventilator was set to increase her breathing to eliminate CO_2 and her follow-up ABG shows pH 7.55, which is alkalotic and $PaCO_2$ of 38, which is now within normal range. The HCO_3 remains elevated at 36.
2. **A** Chapter 16 Rationale: Reduce the ventilator rate to decrease respirations thereby decreasing the elimination of CO_2, encouraging the pH to return to normal.
3. **B** Chapter 15 Rationale: With validation that the $PetCO_2$ is very similar to the ABG CO_2, you can now trend the CO_2 by observing the $PetCO_2$ for changes.
4. **A** Chapter 15 Rationale: The pH is alkalotic at 7.52, the $PaCO_2$ is low at 29 indicating the alkalosis is due to respiratory. When the pH and the $PaCO_2$ move in opposite directions, the primary problem is often respiratory.
5. **D** Chapter 14 Rationale: Gas exchange takes place in the lower airways in the alveoli.
6. **B** Chapter 14 Rationale: The cricoid cartilage is a complete ring located just below the thyroid cartilage, where the vocal cords are located. The cricothyroid membrane is an avascular structure that connects the thyroid and cricoid cartilages. It is through this membrane that an airway may be established in an emergency. In this way, the posterior wall of the larynx and vocal cords are not injured.
7. **A** Chapter 14 Rationale: The trachea divides into the right and left mainstem bronchi at the carina, located at the angle of Louis at the sternomanubrial junction, at about the second intercostal space.
8. **D** Chapter 14 Rationale: The right mainstem bronchus comes off the trachea in almost a straight line, while the left mainstem bronchus comes off the trachea at an angle of approximately 40 degrees. The right mainstem bronchus is wider in diameter than the left.
9. **B** Chapter 15 Rationale: The pH is acidotic at 7.26 and the HCO_3 is low at 18 indicating a metabolic acidosis. The lungs try to compensate by increasing respirations to rid the body of acid, CO_2, resulting in a $PaCO_2$ that is low at 30, thus creating a partially compensating degree of respiratory alkalosis.
10. **A** Chapter 14 Rationale: The body's cells require oxygen for energy production. When perfusion/oxygenation is inadequate, the cells begin anaerobic metabolism, which produces lactate. Lactate is one of the most common causes of metabolic acidosis and is an acid causing the HCO_3, and subsequently the pH, to decrease.
11. **B** Chapter 14 Rationale: An elevated lactate level of more than 4 mmol/L is a critical finding. It indicates poor perfusion or a shock state. It is important to find and correct the source of the acid/lactate as quickly as possible to prevent deterioration of the patient's condition.
12. **A** Chapter 14 Rationale: Surfactant is the lipoprotein that decreases surface tension and facilitates alveolar expansion. Phagocytes simply engulf and absorb other particles. The alveolar epithelium has a role in actually secreting the surfactant. Pulmonary parenchyma is a general term for pulmonary tissue.
13. **A** Chapter 14 Rationale: Chemoreceptors are located at the bifurcation of the internal and external carotid arteries, carotid bodies, and aortic bodies at the aortic arch. These highly vascular neural bodies are stimulated by any decrease in oxygen supply, such as decreased blood flow, decreased hemoglobin, increased pH, or increased $PaCO_2$. Stimulation of the carotid and/or aortic bodies will increase cerebral cortical activity, resulting in tachycardia, hypertension, and increased respiratory rate, tidal volume, pulmonary resistance, bronchial smooth muscle tone, and adrenal gland secretions.
14. **B** Chapter 15 Rationale: Classic Cheyne–Stokes breathing is characterized by a crescendo–decrescendo pattern that is associated with intermittent apneic periods. This description allows quick elimination of options A and D. The key distinguishing factor between B and C is that option C does not mention apnea. Choose B.
15. **C** Chapter 15 Rationale: The pH is acidotic at 7.23. The CO_2 is elevated at 59 indicating the respiratory system as the source of the acid. Since the pH is not normal, it is not yet compensated.
16. **B** Chapter 16 Rationale: The increase in CO_2 indicates the patient is unable to maintain adequate ventilation and still requires the assistance of the ventilator to achieve adequate gas exchange.
17. **D** Chapters 14 and 16 Rationale: Estimates of venous drainage pressures are approximately 40 mm Hg. Inflation of the endotracheal tube cuff to 15 to 20 mm Hg should be enough to prevent an air leak, but low enough to avoid occluding the circulation. An easy way to remember this would be, "Inflate up to twenty and that is plenty."

18. **D** Chapter 15 Rationale: Normal arterial PO_2 levels are 80 to 100 mm Hg, somewhat similar to SaO_2 levels (see "oxyhemoglobin dissociation curve" for examples regarding how PO_2 levels correlate exactly with SaO_2 values). Any PO_2 value less than 80 mm Hg may be associated with hypoxia.

19. **B** Chapter 15 Rationale: If in doubt with a question such as this, a helpful approach may be to eliminate the extremes such as A and D. 20 to 35 mm Hg may be too low to be associated with any O_2 level and 80 to 100 mm Hg is more closely associated with a PaO_2 level. 60 to 80 mm Hg is more closely associated with an SvO_2 level. The correct answer is 35 to 40 mm Hg. Choose B.

20. **D** Chapter 15 Rationale: In healthy patients, a normal SaO_2 is more than 95%. Remember that moving a decimal point two places to the right will change a fraction to a percentage. Choose D.

21. **B** Chapter 15 Rationale: The SvO_2 is the oxygen saturation of "mixed venous" blood that is aspirated from the tip of the pulmonary artery catheter. Remember that a normal SaO_2 (fully oxygenated blood) is more than 95% and in normal circumstances the body's tissues extract approximately 25% of this via one circuit through the body by the time the blood reaches the pulmonary artery. Thus, 0.25 subtracted from 0.95 = 0.75. Choose B.

22. **B** Chapter 15 Rationale: Oximetry measures functional, not fractional SaO_2. Therefore the pulse oximetry reading is expected to be 2% to 4% higher than SaO_2 measured by an ABG sample in the laboratory.

23. **C** Chapter 15 Rationale: $PaCO_2$ levels are increasing resulting in increased acidosis as shown by a decrease in pH. The patient is experiencing inadequate and worsening ventilation.

24. **B** Chapters 15 and 17 Rationale: The patient's condition and degree of ventilation are deteriorating; the physician needs to be notified of the change in condition.

25. **D** Chapter 14 Rationale: Dynamic compliance is the measurement of the lungs when in motion, at the end of inspiration and expiration. Obesity, airway secretions, and pregnancy can limit the volume of air taken into the lungs. Loss of rigidity in the airways may actually improve compliance measurements. Choose D.

26. **A** Chapter 14 Rationale: Vital capacity (VC) is the amount of gas that can be forcefully exhaled after a maximum inspiration (VC = VT + IRV + ERV). Normal is about 4000 to 5000 mL.

27. **C** Chapter 14 Rationale: Gas exchange occurs only in the terminal bronchioles and alveoli. A portion of the inhaled air remains in the trachea and larger airways (referred to as dead space), unable to participate in gas exchange.

28. **B** Chapter 14 Rationale: The amount of inhaled air that reaches the alveoli and takes part in gas exchange is alveolar ventilation. Minute ventilation (VE) is obtained by multiplying the RR by the tidal volume. However, since dead-space gas does not participate in gas exchange, it must be subtracted from the MV, with the result being the alveolar ventilation. Choose B.

29. **A** Chapter 14 Rationale: Anatomic dead space is estimated to be 150 mL or 1 mL/lb of ideal body weight (25% to 35% of VT).

30. **D** Chapter 14 Rationale: Dead space consists of any length of the airway that does not participate in gas exchange. This patient's dead space is expected to be increased, therefore all of the parameters in A, B, and C would be reasonable to expect. Choose D.

31. **A** Chapter 14 Rationale: Minute ventilation (VE) is normally 5 to 10 L/min and is measured by multiplying VT × respiratory rate. In this case, 29 × 0.5 L = 14.5 L, indicating the VE to be elevated.

32. **D** Chapter 14 Rationale: Intrapulmonary, or physiologic, shunt occurs when there is adequate pulmonary capillary blood flow but a portion of the alveoli are not being ventilated, making them unable to participate in gas exchange. Accumulated secretions, atelectasis, pulmonary edema, pneumonia, ARDS, neoplasms, and foreign objects are only a few of many common causes of obstruction.

33. **A** Chapter 14 Rationale: Intrapulmonary shunt is measured by shunt equations or estimated from oxygen tension indices, such as the PaO_2/FIO_2 ratio or a/A ratio. Normal PaO_2/FIO_2 ratio is more than 286. The lower it becomes, the worse the intrapulmonary shunt. Clinically significant shunt typically does not respond to increasing levels of FIO_2.

34. **B** Chapter 16 Rationale: The FIO_2 of room air is approximately 21%. As a general rule, approximately 4% of FIO_2 can be added for every one liter (1 L) of supplemental O_2 delivered, contributing to the total percent of oxygen during inspiration (ie, FIO_2).

35. **D** Chapters 14 and 16 Rationale: When 100% oxygen therapy is employed, nitrogen is completely displaced or washed out by the oxygen, resulting in a PaO_2 of 400 to 600 mm Hg.

36. **C** Chapter 14 Rationale: Intrapulmonary shunt is measured by shunt equations or estimated from oxygen tension indices, such as the PaO_2/FIO_2 ratio or a/A ratio. Normal PaO_2/FIO_2 ratio is more than 286. The lower it becomes, the worse the intrapulmonary shunt. The hypoxemia of patients with intrapulmonary shunt will not respond dramatically to oxygen therapy, since the shunted blood will not come in contact with the increased alveolar PO_2. In this case, the PaO_2/FIO_2 ratio is 86/0.5 = 172, suggesting the degree of shunt is increased.

37. **A** Chapter 16 Rationale: Generally, if the PaO_2/FIO_2 ratio is below 200 the patient will not be able to maintain adequate oxygen levels in their blood without some form of supplemental oxygen therapy. Since this patients PaO_2/FIO_2 ratio is 172, it is not safe to remove supplemental oxygen during meals.

38. **A** Chapter 14 Rationale: Normal pulmonary anatomy accounts for the 2% to 5% of the blood flowing through the lung that does not come in contact with inspired air for gas exchange.

39. D Chapter 14 Rationale: Once oxygen has penetrated the erythrocyte membrane, it is carried through the systemic circulatory system to all body tissues. The transport of oxygen to body tissues is influenced most by cardiac output, hemoglobin concentration, and oxygen–hemoglobin binding and releasing factors. As the cardiac output varies, the quantity of blood oxygenated in the lungs also varies. A markedly decreased cardiac output will alter oxygen content, although the available blood will be maximally oxygenated. If hemoglobin is low, cardiac output will increase to help compensate and maintain an adequate oxygen content. The amount of oxygen transported per minute is determined by the cardiac output, even though there are other contributing factors.

40. C Chapter 15 Rationale: Mixed venous oximetry utilizes blood from the pulmonary artery to estimate overall oxygenation. The balance between oxygen transport and consumption is estimated by levels of mixed venous oxygen saturation (SvO_2). As long as blood flow to the capillaries is relatively normal, SvO_2 levels provide relatively accurate reflections of tissue oxygenation. Normal SvO_2 values, between 0.60 and 0.80, indicate an adequate supply–demand balance, between oxygen delivery and consumption. If the SvO_2 falls less than 0.60, either oxygen transport has decreased or oxygen consumption has increased indicating a risk for lack of oxygen at the tissue level.

41. A Chapters 14 and 15 Rationale: The PaO_2/FIO_2 ratio indicates a significant pulmonary shunt. This patient's increased FIO_2 coupled with decreased PaO_2 and SaO_2 also suggests shunt.

42. A Chapter 16 Rationale: The best metric of oxygen supply–demand balance and overall indicator of tissue oxygenation is the SvO_2 level. This patient's SvO_2 is within normal limits, indicating that oxygenation is adequate and that the rate of FIO_2 delivery can remain the same at this time.

43. B Chapters 14 and 15 Rationale: SvO_2 depends on the oxygen content in the blood, oxygen consumption by the body's cells, and cardiac output/delivery of the blood to the lungs and body's cells. If any one of these three are abnormal, it will contribute to the SvO_2 being abnormal. The basic metabolic profile has the least significant impact on oxygenation given the options available.

44. B Chapter 14 Rationale: Oxygen transport/oxygen delivery (D^{O}_2) is the amount of oxygen delivered to the cells expressed as milliliters of oxygen per minute. Oxygen transport (D^{O}_2) = CaO_2 × cardiac output × 10, expressed in milliliters per minute. Normal oxygen transport is between 600 and 1000 mL/min or 10 to 12 mL/kg.

45. C Chapter 14 Rationale: $PaCO_2$ provides the normal neurochemical control of the respiratory cycle because of its effect on the CSF pH. A rise in CSF hydrogen ion concentration will first increase respiratory depth and then the respiratory rate. Oxygen tension would be an example of a secondary chemical control over breathing (eg, advanced COPD) if the primary level of control fails. Choose C.

46. B Chapter 14 Rationale: VE is normally 5 to 10 L/min and is measured by multiplying VT × respiratory rate. VE of 10 to 12 L/min is often considered criteria for extubation, making option C (11–15 L/min) too high, eliminating option C. Choose B.

47. D Chapter 14 Rationale: Factors affecting oxygen–hemoglobin binding and releasing include temperature, pH, PCO_2, acidosis or alkalosis, and 2,3-diphosphoglycerate (2,3-DPG). The oxyhemoglobin curve is an S-shaped curve representing the nonlinear relationship of the PaO_2 and the SaO_2.

48. A Chapter 14 Rationale: An acid is a chemical substance that dissociates into positive or negative electrically charged ions and gives up a hydrogen (H^+) proton to the solution.

49. D Chapter 14 Rationale: If the buffering system has not rectified an acid–base disturbance within minutes, the respiratory system will become active. Because of this, the respiratory system can act as a much quicker acid–base buffer than the kidneys (which may take days).

50. B Chapter 14 Rationale: The kidneys provide the strongest defense against acid–base disturbances by increasing hydrogen ion elimination and increasing bicarbonate ion reabsorption. Unfortunately, it takes from several hours to several days for the kidneys to rebalance the hydrogen ion concentration.

51. A Chapter 14 Rationale: The bicarbonate buffer system is the most important system because the end products of the chemical buffer are regulated by both the kidneys and the lungs. The chemical reaction in this system is reversible and occurs extremely rapidly: $H^+HCO_3^- \leftrightarrow H_2\,CO_3\,3 \leftrightarrow CO_2 + H^+$ If the buffering moves toward the left, the bicarbonate ion is the end product, regulated by the kidneys.

52. B Chapter 15 Rationale: The pH is low indicating acidosis and the $PaCO_2$ is elevated indicating that respiratory is the source. The HCO_3 is also elevated indicating the kidneys are attempting to compensate metabolically.

53. A Chapter 15 Rationale: The pH is low indicating acidosis and the $PaCO_2$ is elevated indicating that respiratory is the source. The HCO_3 is normal indicating that the kidneys have not yet begun to compensate for the acidosis.

54. C Chapter 15 Rationale: The pH is high indicating alkalosis and the $PaCO_2$ is normal indicating it is not contributing to the alkalosis. The HCO_3 is elevated indicating metabolic as the source of the alkalosis.

55. A Chapter 15 Rationale: The pH is high indicating alkalosis and the $PaCO_2$ is low indicating a respiratory alkalosis is present. The HCO_3 is normal indicating that no metabolic compensation has occurred.

56. **D** Chapter 15 Rationale: The pH is normal or compensated. The $PaCO_2$ is low indicating a compensating respiratory alkalosis. The HCO_3 is low indicating a metabolic acidosis is present. The pH is within normal because the respirations increased to rid the body of CO_2 to compensate for the metabolic acidosis. Remember, the body will not overcompensate; this likely began as an acidosis. The pH of 7.36 being so close to the acidosis threshold is also a clue. Choose D.

57. **C** Chapter 15 Rationale: The pH is low indicating acidosis and the $PaCO_2$ is normal indicating it is not contributing to the acidosis. The HCO_3 is low indicating a metabolic acidosis. The $PaCO_2$ is low normal, indicating the respiratory system has likely increased respirations to rid the body of CO_2 to compensation for the metabolic acidosis.

58. **A** Chapter 17 Rationale: Acute respiratory failure (ARF) is the result of abnormalities in ventilation, perfusion, or compliance, leading to hypercapnia and/or hypoxemia. Respiratory failure is a medical emergency that can result from long-standing, progressively worsening lung disease or from severe lung disease that develops suddenly. The lungs are unable to maintain adequate oxygenation and carbon dioxide elimination to support metabolism, leading to respiratory acidosis. It is necessary to identify the underlying condition in order to initiate appropriate treatment. Re-establishing adequate oxygenation is a priority. This patient's hypercapnia is likely chronic (given his elevated HCO_3^-).

59. **D** Chapter 16 Rationale: The patient is awake, alert, and oriented, which indicates stability in this unhealthy state. Beginning with noninvasive oxygen therapy is the treatment of choice. The oxygen therapy can be escalated to a more invasive form if needed.

60. **A** Chapters 15 and 17 Rationale: ABGs initially show a low $PaCO_2$ with a respiratory alkalosis. When the $PaCO_2$ normalizes or begins to rise, that is an ominous sign since the patient is now tiring and generally requires intubation and mechanical support. ABGs may reveal a normal or falling PaO_2.

61. **B** Chapter 14 Rationale: The only option available that indicates ventilation is $PaCO_2$, option B. The PaO_2 measures oxygenation and the pH is an indicator of acid–base balance. The alveolar–arterial gradient measures intrapulmonary shunt. Choose B.

62. **A** Chapters 14 and 15 Rationale: A *respiratory* acidosis requires active treatment only if the increase in $PaCO_2$ results in a pH of about 7.25. Treatment with an alkali should be reserved for severe *metabolic* acidosis, pH less than 7.20. Either source of acidosis can be corrected with correction of the underlying cause.

63. **B** Chapter 17 Rationale: Patients at risk for developing ARF include those with COPD, restrictive lung disease, respiratory center depression, pulmonary edema, and pulmonary emboli, among many other conditions (Table 17-1). Chronic lung disease (COPD) complicated by a pneumonia, left ventricular (LV) failure resulting in pulmonary edema (cardiac), inhalation injuries, and ARDS are examples of ARF with alterations in oxygenation. ARF caused by a depressed central nervous system (CNS) or a high V/Q ratio causes an increase in $PaCO_2$.

64. **C** Chapters 14 and 16 Rationale: When a patient's ventilator is alarming or does not seem to be working properly, remove the ventilator tubing from the ET tube and begin providing manual respirations with the Ambu bag. This will provide you with additional assessment of the airway such as how easy it is to instill air into the ET tube.

65. **A** Chapter 19 Rationale: Tension pneumothorax produces symptoms including dyspnea and restlessness, progressive cyanosis, diminished or absent breath sounds on the *affected side* decreased chest wall movement, signs of increasing respiratory distress, chest wall pain, and tracheal shift *toward the unaffected side.* A hemothorax is often accompanied by a pneumothorax but a hemothorax alone or a cardiac tamponade would not produce crepitus. Flail chest involves two or more adjacent ribs with two or more fractures, creating a section of rib that is not attached to the rib cage.

66. **A** Chapter 17 Rationale: Hemodynamic parameters are used to differentiate ARDS from pulmonary edema due to LV failure. Generally, preload indicators will be normal or low in ARDS and high in LV failure. The PAOP is generally less than 18 mm Hg in ARDS, while LV failure presents with a high PAOP.

67. **D** Chapter 17 Rationale: Hemodynamic parameters are used to differentiate ARDS from pulmonary edema due to LV failure. Generally, preload indicators will be normal or low in ARDS and high in LV failure. The PAOP is generally less than 18 mm Hg in ARDS, while LV failure presents with a high PAOP.

68. **B** Chapter 17 Rationale: Treatment of ARDS is supportive, primarily centering on supporting oxygenation through the use of mechanical ventilation, thus allowing the lung to heal while the underlying cause of the inflammatory process is treated. PEEP is used to stabilize the alveoli and keep them open throughout the entire respiratory cycle. PEEP levels of 10 to 15 cm H_2O will usually be required to reach this goal. The FIO_2 will initially be set at high and titrated down to keep the SaO_2 more than 90 ($SpO_2 > 93$). Management of oxygenation is directed at preserving oxygen consumption and tissue perfusion. Neuromuscular blockade (NMB) is avoided if at all possible so as not to risk the development of profound muscle weakness, which can lead to a prolonged recovery. Fluid administration is kept to a minimum, allowing for an adequate preload but avoiding further increases in lung water while maintaining an adequate cardiac output.

69. **D** Chapter 17 Rationale: Complications associated with ARDS include metabolic and respiratory acidosis, cardiac arrest, barotrauma, and oxygen toxicity; however, death is usually the result of the precipitating event of ARDS, not ARDS alone.

70. **A** Chapter 15 Rationale: Normal range for PaO_2 is 80 to 100 mm Hg for people 60 years or younger. For people 60 years old or older, to calculate their normal: from 80 mm Hg subtract 1 mm Hg for every year above 60. For this patient, a normal PaO_2 would be 80 mm Hg minus 14, to be the equivalent of 66, and his current PaO_2 value is 64. When PaO_2 is lower than the expected normal, it is called hypoxia.

71. **C** Chapter 16 Rationale: PEEP is effective in raising PaO_2 and Sao_2 levels by maintaining alveolar airflow during expiration. PEEP improves distribution of ventilation, helps hold alveoli open, and opens smaller airways, improving oxygenation by increasing the time for gas exchange to occur. PEEP is indicated to help reduce FIO_2 levels or to elevate PaO_2/Sao_2 values when high FIO_2 levels are unsuccessful, to drive lung water back into the vascular system, or to reduce mediastinal bleeding postoperatively.

72. **D** Chapter 16 Rationale: High-flow oxygen systems meet all inspiratory volume and flow requirements independent of inspiratory changes. High-flow oxygen systems provide stable FIO_2 levels, with oxygen concentrations 24% to 100% (Table 16-3). Critically ill patients with oxygenation disturbances will almost always require high-flow oxygen systems.

73. **C** Chapter 16 Rationale: An oxygen concentration in excess of 50% for more than 24 h increases the potential for the development of oxygen toxicity and lung damage. Alveolar type II cells, responsible for producing surfactant, are impaired by high oxygen levels.

74. **D** Chapter 16 Rationale: PEEP is indicated to help reduce FIO_2 levels or to elevate PaO_2/Sao_2 values when high FIO_2 levels are unsuccessful, to drive lung water back into the vascular system, or to reduce mediastinal bleeding postoperatively.

75. **D** Chapter 16 Rationale: Optimal PEEP levels are achieved by the lowest level of PEEP needed to raise the PaO_2/Sao_2 levels, and do not result in cardiovascular compromise such as decreased cardiac output, impeded right-heart filling, or tachycardia.

76. **B** Chapter 16 Rationale: Immediately after intubation, placement of the endotracheal tube in the airway can be confirmed by the presence of CO_2 through the use of a capnography. All chest fields are auscultated to make sure that there are bilateral breath sounds. Physical examination should never substitute for CO_2 detection.

77. **C** Chapters 16 and 19 Rationale: Pneumothorax can be due to trauma or rupture of bleb or emphysematous bulla, or it may have an iatrogenic cause, such as mechanical ventilation or high levels of PEEP. Hypoxia is the result of the increasing V/Q mismatch due to the collapsing lung. Hypoxia causes restlessness and shortness of breath. The breath sounds will be diminished over the lung that is collapsed and the peak airway pressure will increase because of the decreased compliance.

78. **D** Chapters 16 and 19 Rationale: Drainage of air and fluid from the pleural space requires an evacuation system that allows air and fluids to exit but not to reenter.

79. **C** Chapter 16 Rationale: Continuous mandatory ventilation (CMV), assisted mandatory ventilation (AMV or assist/control), and synchronized intermittent mandatory ventilation (SIMV) are examples of volume-limited modes (Fig. 16-4). Pressure-limited modes of mechanical ventilation will deliver a breath until a preset pressure is reached. Pressure-support ventilation and pressure control ventilation are the most common examples of this mode.

80. **D** Chapter 16 Rationale: The most useful of the indices is the rapid–shallow-breathing index. Minute ventilation is the amount of air exchanged in 1 min. Normal minute ventilation is 5 to 10 L/min. Negative inspiratory force or peak inspiratory effort is the maximal inspiratory effort the patient can generate as measured by an inspiratory manometer. Normal PIP or NIF is −70 to −90 cm H_2O (Table 16-5). A NIF or at least −20 cm H_2O is the minimum for successful removal ventilatory support.

81. **C** Chapter 16 Rationale: This patient's weaning trial parameters indicate he is likely to be able to maintain respirations without the help of the ventilator. Placing him on a T-piece will give him the chance to breathe on his own for a period of time before removing the endotracheal tube.

82. **C** Chapter 16 Rationale: After breathing "on his own" through the endotracheal tube, the patient's weaning trial parameters continue to indicate he is likely to maintain his respirations without the ET tube in place or the use of the ventilator.

83. **C** Chapters 15 and 17 Rationale: Arterial blood gas (ABG) values can deteriorate suddenly, indicating acute pulmonary insufficiency. Findings include a PaO_2 less than 60 mm Hg, requiring an increase in the fractional inspiratory oxygen pressure (FIO_2) and a $PaCO_2$ more than 45 mm Hg. Other measures of oxygenation include a decreased a/A ratio (<0.25), a widened A–a gradient, and a decreased PaO_2/FIO_2 ratio (<200). The patient may present with an elevated hematocrit (above 52%) and an elevated hemoglobin (>18 g/dL).

84. **B** Chapters 15 and 16 Rationale: This patient's condition is deteriorating; aggressive treatment is needed. Intubating the patient to control and improve his respiratory status is important.

85. **C** Chapter 16 Rationale: The patient is tolerating the removal of his ET tube. Support his respirations with oxygen and observe for the need to reintubate. Consider discontinuing his sedation taking into account his EtOH withdrawal and lack of an airway protectant device.

86. **C** Chapter 16 Rationale: The reversal of the normal negative inspiratory pressure to a positive pressure has a direct effect on the cardiovascular system. The increased intrathoracic pressure impedes venous return to the right heart, thus reducing stroke volume and cardiac output. The initial response may be a reflex increase in the heart rate to maintain output.

87. **B** Chapter 16 Rationale: Low-flow systems provide FIO_2 levels between 24% and 44% with a nasal cannula or between 40% and 60% with a simple face mask (Table 16-2). Rebreathing masks can provide higher levels of inspired oxygen; however, they are not as reliable as high-flow systems.

88. **C** Chapter 16 Rationale: Suction pressures of less than 200 are generally adequate to remove secretions. The removal of viscous, thick secretions are difficult even with adequate suction. The lack of benefit of instillation of saline in the endotracheal or tracheostomy tube has been well documented, and such a maneuver increases the risk of ventilator-associated pneumonia (VAP). Thinning of pulmonary secretions is accomplished by adequate fluid intake. The stimulation of cough is a very effective aid to the clearance of secretions.

89. **B** Chapters 14 and 15 Rationale: Blockage of airways with secretions will not allow inhaled air to reach the alveoli, thereby decreasing the PaO_2. Additionally, the inability to achieve gas exchange will also increase the $PaCO_2$.

90. **D** Chapter 16 Rationale: Optimal PEEP levels are achieved by the lowest level of PEEP needed to raise the PaO_2/SaO_2 levels and do not result in cardiovascular compromise, such as decreased cardiac output, impeded right-heart filling, or tachycardia.

91. **D** Chapter 15 Rationale: Bronchodilators are divided into classes: adrenergic, anticholinergic, and methylxanthines. Theophylline (anhydrous) is a methylxanthine. The following are short-acting beta2 agonists: albuterol, pirbuterol, metaproterenol, and levalbuterol. Short-acting sympathomimetics are preferentially administered via metered-dose inhalers (MDIs), or nebulized inhalation.

92. **D** Chapter 14 Rationale: A low PaO_2 (<60 mm Hg) can produce pulmonary hypertension, increased breathing, and low SaO_2 levels. Low PaO_2 does not directly alter the oxyhemoglobin curve.

93. **A** Chapter 14 Rationale: PaO_2 is the amount of oxygen dissolved in plasma. SaO_2 is the percentage of hemoglobin binding sites that are bound with oxygen. In a shift to the left, hemoglobin binds oxygen much more tightly and releases less oxygen to the tissues, thus the PaO_2 will be lower than the SaO_2.

94. **A** Chapter 14 Rationale: A shift to the right means that there is less oxygen in the blood. It also means that oxygen is more readily given up to the tissues by the hemoglobin, preventing hypoxia. If shift persists, eventually the decreased oxygen content will not prevent tissue hypoxia.

95. **B** Chapter 14 Rationale: All the other conditions listed will shift the curve to the left.

96. **A** Chapters 14 and 15 Rationale: In emphysema, the alveolar septa collapse, destroying the alveolar structure and decreasing the surface area available for diffusion. Decreased alveolar ventilation (VA) results in rising $PaCO_2$, causing the displacement of oxygen and lowering of PaO_2. Hypoventilation-induced hypoxemia is easily treated with oxygen therapy; however, the decreased VA must be improved or respiratory failure will occur.

97. **A** Chapter 17 Rationale: Corticosteroids, such as methylprednisolone or prednisone, are critical in the therapy of status asthmaticus and are used to decrease the intense airway inflammation and swelling in asthma. Beta-agonist agents, typically albuterol or salbutamol and terbutaline, are the mainstays of acute therapy in asthma. The nebulized inhaled route of administration is generally the most effective one, although some patients with severe refractory status asthmaticus may benefit from intravenous administration.

98. **B** Chapter 17 Rationale: Status asthmaticus is a severe continuing attack of asthma that fails to respond to conventional drug therapy. It can last for days to weeks; even with optimal therapy, it may be fatal. Status asthmaticus is characterized by airway hyperreactivity or hyperresponsiveness, airway obstruction, and airway inflammation. The increased airway responsiveness is manifest by narrowing of the airways secondary to bronchial constriction and excessive mucus obstruction, thus increasing the work of breathing, interfering with gas exchange, and producing hypoxemia.

99. **A** Chapter 17 Rationale: ABGs initially show a low $PaCO_2$ with a respiratory alkalosis. When the $PaCO_2$ normalizes or begins to rise, that is an ominous sign since the patient is now tiring and generally requires intubation and mechanical support.

100. **A** Chapter 17 Rationale: Inspiratory and expiratory wheezing is usually audible, with a prolonged expiratory phase as the patient tries to exhale the trapped air through narrow airways. The disappearance of wheezing may be an ominous sign, as the airway may have become completely obstructed.

101. **C** Chapter 17 Rationale: Status asthmaticus is a severe continuing attack of asthma that fails to respond to conventional drug therapy. It can last for days to weeks; even with optimal therapy, it may be fatal.

102. **D** Chapter 18 Rationale: Massive embolism (>40% of pulmonary circulation obstructed) occurs suddenly and is associated with acute right heart failure (elevated pulmonary artery systolic pressure and pulmonary vascular resistance). Cardiac output falls as a result of the right heart's inability to fill the left heart. The end-tidal CO_2 ($PetCO_2$) will suddenly decrease with a PE. The arterial CO_2 ($PaCO_2$) may decrease as well due to hyperventilation. However, the $PetCO_2$ decreases more due to a loss of blood flow in the lungs. This loss of blood flow causes an increased dead space, lowering the $PetCO_2$. PaO_2 levels may not change substantially; however, in large PEs, hypoxemia is common. Obstruction of the pulmonary vasculature elicits neurohumoral stimuli, increasing pulmonary artery pressure and pulmonary vascular resistance.

103. **C** Chapter 18 Rationale: There are several tests that can reveal how likely a PE is, but they are often not definitive. The angiogram will be most decisive although may be more difficult to perform. Pulmonary angiography should be considered when other tests are inconclusive. A positive angiogram will reveal filling deficits or sharp cutoffs in blood flow.

104. **A** Chapter 18 Rationale: When DVT(s) are present, the inferior vena caval filter (IVCF) will prevent further emboli from reaching the lung, thus preventing further pulmonary and hemodynamic compromise. The utilization of IVCFs has historically been the treatment of choice for DVT in those individuals with contraindications to standard anticoagulation or those with ongoing embolism despite appropriate anticoagulation therapy.

105. **D** Chapter 18 Rationale: Increased respiratory rate, dyspnea, and tachycardia are the most common signs of PE. Cardiac output falls as a result of the right heart's inability to fill the left heart. The patient may have crushing substernal chest pain and appear to be in shock, with hypotension, elevated right heart pressures, dyspnea, cyanosis, apprehension, or coma. Respirations are rapid, shallow, and gasping. Arterial pulse is rapid and the volume is diminished.

106. **C** Chapter 18 Rationale: Thrombolytics are used in the treatment of patients with massive acute PE who are in acute right heart failure. Streptokinase, urokinase, and tissue plasminogen activator (tPA) are thrombolytic enzymes used to dissolve or lyse the emboli. Therapeutic action begins immediately and ceases with the interruption of the intravenous administration.

107. **A** Chapter 19 Rationale: Air leaving the pleural space is readily seen by the bubbling in the water-seal chamber. When air has ceased leaking from the pleural space, this bubbling ceases. Evacuation of fluid is noted by measuring the amount of fluid in the collection chamber.

108. **A** Chapter 19 Rationale: The closed or spontaneous pneumothorax occurs when air enters the pleural space through the airways. Spontaneous pneumothorax can be primary—occurring in healthy people, or secondary—occurring due to underlying lung disease. If the air cannot escape the chest, intrapleural pressure increases, pressure on the other lung and the heart will continue, and a tension pneumothorax is possible.

109. **A** Chapter 19 Rationale: Although it is not common to have a fracture of the first rib, such a fracture is life threatening and indicates severe force and possible underlying thoracic and/or abdominal injuries. Fractures in ribs 1, 2, or 3 may be associated with mediastinal injury. When a very strong force is applied to the upper thoracic cage, the result is a "starburst" fracture—that is, pieces of bone going in all directions. Sternal fracture is suspected when there is paradoxical movement of the anterior chest wall.

110. **D** Chapter 19 Rationale: Primary symptoms of a ruptured or herniated diaphragm include auscultation of bowel sounds in the chest, increasing shortness of breath, unequal diaphragmatic movement on palpation, elevated diaphragm and hyperresonance to percussion, marked or increasing respiratory distress, severe shoulder pain on the same side as the tear, and shock.

111. **C** Chapter 16 Rationale: The ABG shows oxygenation and ventilation abnormalities. NIV can address both issues without the associated complications of invasive mechanical ventilation in a patient that is alert, cooperative, and can protect his/her own airway. An increase in the FIO_2 alone will not address the hypoventilation. The described scenario does not indicate the need to re-evaluate antibiotics.

112. **D** Chapter 16 Rationale: Securement of an airway and adequate oxygenation are a priority. A NIV mask is not appropriate for patients with large amounts of secretions or who are not cooperative in wearing the NIV mask. The ETT also allows suctioning of secretions that can assist with increasing oxygenation. While sedation, increased FIO_2, and restraints are helpful they are not adequate to increase oxygenation without the presence of an ETT.

113. **C** Chapter 19 Rationale: Pulmonary contusion is damage to the lung parenchyma, resulting in localized edema and hemorrhage. The thorax hits an object, such as the steering wheel, compressing the thoracic cage, diminishing its size, and compressing the lungs as a result of the increased intrathoracic pressure.

114. **A** Chapter 19 Rationale: Agitation and anxiety may indicate the presence of hypoxia and may be a first sign of impending deterioration. Pain from chest wall injury will affect the ability to ventilate and clear secretions. Management of a blunt chest injury therefore includes adequate analgesia. If the contusion is mild, monitoring and supplemental oxygen by mask may be sufficient.

115. **A** Chapter 19 Rationale: Arterial blood gases (ABGs) will show decreased carbon dioxide ($PaCO_2$) and oxygen pressures (PaC_2) and worsening of the PaO_2/FIO_2 ratio, indicating increasing intrapulmonary shunt (Qs/Qt).

116. **B** Chapter 19 Rationale: If the air cannot escape the chest, intrapleural pressure increases, pressure on the other lung and the heart will continue, and a tension pneumothorax is possible.

117. **A** Chapter 19 Rationale: If a tension pneumothorax is suspected and the patient is experiencing hemodynamic compromise, decompression with a needle is necessary before placement of a chest tube. Tension pneumothorax is a life-threatening condition that demands urgent management. If a chest tube is used, it is inserted in the second or third intercostal space at the midclavicular line to remove the air.

PART III

ENDOCRINE

Jennifer MacDermott

20

Introduction to the Endocrine System

CHAPTER OVERVIEW AND OBJECTIVES

Endocrine concepts make up about 4% (6–8 questions) of the CCRN exam. According to the CCRN guideline, the key areas of endocrine dysfunction covered in the exam primarily include the following:

1. Diabetes insipidus
2. Inappropriate secretion of antidiuretic hormone (SIADH)
3. Hyperosmolar Hyperglycemia Syndrome (HHS), formerly referred to as Hyperglycemic hyperosmolar nonketotic coma (HHNK)
4. Diabetic ketoacidosis (DKA)
5. Acute hypoglycemia

Considering that these five areas will be covered in only six to eight questions on the CCRN exam, it is unlikely that detailed attention will be given to any one (or different) content area.

After studying this chapter, you should be able to:

- Describe the primary function of general hormones whose dysfunctional secretion may result in admission to a critical care unit.
- Discuss how a negative feedback system provides precise control of hormones when functioning properly.

20.1 HORMONAL PURPOSE AND FUNCTION OF THE ENDOCRINE SYSTEM

The primary function of the endocrine system is to regulate the metabolic functioning of the body. The term "endocrine" refers to the internal secretion of biologically active substances, such as hormones, that help to regulate the functions of cells and organs. The endocrine system controls metabolic functions of the body to include cellular metabolism, transport of substances through cell membranes, and rates of cellular chemical reactions.

There is a close interrelationship between the nervous system (responsible for integrating body processes) and the endocrine system (responsible for appropriate metabolic activity). Neuronal stimulation is required for some specific hormones to be secreted and/or to be secreted in adequate amounts.

The endocrine system is composed of specific glands (**Fig. 20-1**) that secrete chemical substances directly into the bloodstream. The major single endocrine glands are the pituitary (also called the hypophysis) (**Fig. 20-2**) and the thyroid. The parathyroids consist of four glands, not two sets of paired glands. The adrenals form one pair of endocrine glands. Other glands containing endocrine components and function in both the endocrine system and another system are the ovaries and testes (collectively termed the gonads) and the pancreas. The thymus gland has a major role in immunology but is sometimes included in discussions of the endocrine system.

All endocrine glands are very vascular. They function by extracting substances from the blood to synthesize into complex hormones. Hormones are released from the specific endocrine glands into the veins that drain the glands themselves. The circulatory system transports endocrine substances to target glands and tissues throughout the body.

KEY CLINICAL CONCEPTS

As you review the following chapters on the endocrine system, focus on key concepts rather than minor details. Endocrine dysfunction is a difficult area for many nurses taking the CCRN exam.

20.2 CLASSIFICATION OF HORMONES

The substances secreted by endocrine glands are chemicals called hormones. Hormones exert physiologic control over body cells. They bind specifically to hormone receptors expressed on

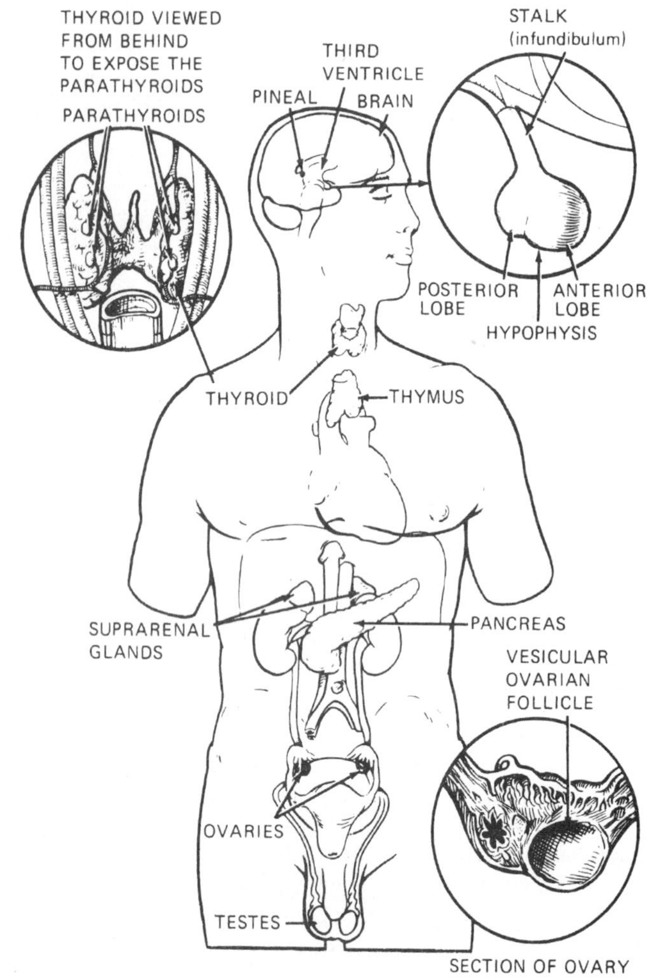

Figure 20-1. Overview of the endocrine system.

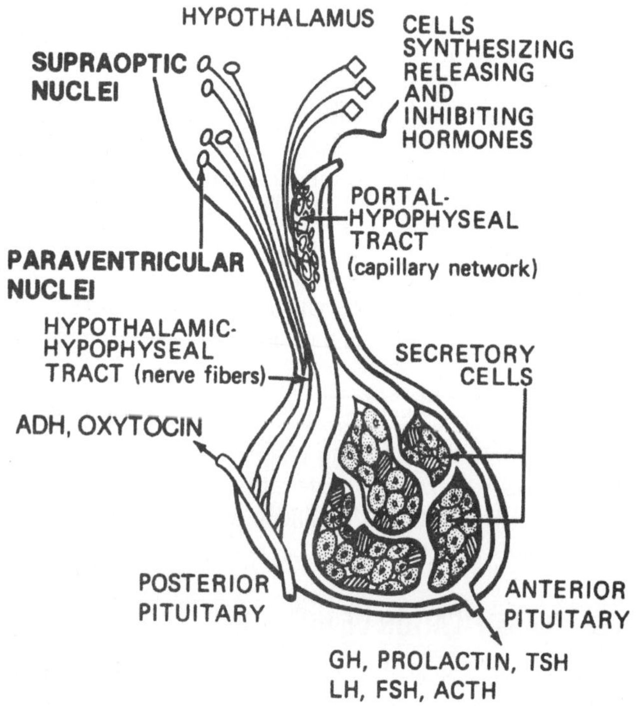

Figure 20-2. Paraventricular and supraoptic nuclei of the hypothalamus.

TABLE 20-1. ENDOCRINE GLANDS AND HORMONES OF SIGNIFICANT IMPORTANCE

Glands	Hormones
Adenohypophysis (anterior pituitary)	Adrenocorticotropin, somatotropin or growth hormone, thyroid-stimulating hormone
Neurohypophysis (posterior pituitary)	Antidiuretic hormone, oxytocin
Thyroid	Thyroxine, triiodothyronine, calcitonin
Parathyroid	Parathyroid hormone (parathormone)
Adrenal medulla	Epinephrine, norepinephrine
Adrenal cortex	Glucocorticoids (cortisol), mineralocorticoids (aldosterone)
Pancreas	Insulin, glucagons

the cell surface or within the cell. Local hormones are those released in specific areas (or tissues) and they exert a limited, local effect. Acetylcholine is an example of a local hormone having physiologic control at some synapses in the nervous system. General hormones are secreted by a specific endocrine gland and transported by the vascular system to a specific, predetermined site.

Important General Hormones

All of the general hormones play important roles in regulating various functions of the body. However, dysfunctional secretion of certain hormones would rarely, if ever, be a reason for admission to a critical care unit. General hormones include oxytocin, follicle-stimulating hormone (FSH), luteinizing hormone (LH), prolactin, melanocyte-stimulating hormone (MSH), corticosterone, deoxycorticosterone, and androgens (including estrogens, progesterone, and testosterone). These hormones are not discussed in detail in this text.

Those general hormones whose dysfunctional secretion may precipitate admission to a critical care area are listed in **Table 20-1** and are covered in Chapters 21, 22, 23, and 24.

20.3 TYPES OF HORMONES

Hormones are classified based on their class of action on a receptor (eg, glucocorticoid, mineralocorticoid) and ligand or action type (eg, agonist, partial agonist, antagonist). Hormones may be amines, peptides, proteins (or protein derivatives), or steroids.

Prostaglandins are often considered tissue hormones. The first three types of hormones, amine, protein, and peptide, are water-soluble and do not require a carrier molecule for transportation throughout the body. Steroids and thyroxine are not water-soluble and must rely on a carrier substance to transport them to their site of action, the target cell.

Prostaglandins are unsaturated fatty acids, of which three types have been identified based on their chemical structure. They are synthesized in the seminal vesicles, brain, liver, iris, kidneys, lungs, and other areas. Prostaglandins have a potent effect but are considered local hormones, not general hormones.

20.4 ACTIONS OF HORMONES

Amine, Protein, and Peptide Hormones

Amine, protein, and peptide hormones include growth hormone (GH), adrenocorticotropin hormone (ACTH), thyroid-stimulating hormone (TSH), parathyroid hormone (PTH), calcitonin, insulin, the catecholamines, glucagon, antidiuretic hormone (ADH), FSH, LH, and prolactin. Since these hormones are water-soluble and do not require a carrier substance, their concentrations may fluctuate rapidly and widely. These hormones are thought to react with specific surface receptors on the target-cell membrane. This alters the membrane's enzymes and leads to a change in the intracellular concentration of an enzyme. The hormone is called the first messenger and the intracellular enzyme is called the second messenger. The second messengers are cyclic 3′, 5′ adenosine monophosphate (cAMP), cyclic guanosine monophosphate (cGMP), calcium–calmodulin complex, and prostaglandins. Cyclic AMP (within the cell) activates enzymes, causes protein synthesis, alters cell permeability, causes muscle relaxation/contraction, and causes secretion. It is by the action of cAMP that many hormones exert control over the cells.

Steroids and Thyroxine

Steroids (sex hormones, aldosterone, and cortisol) and thyroxine are non-water soluble hormones. These hormones are able to cross the cell membrane easily and then bind with an intracellular receptor. The hormone–receptor complex reacts with chromatin in the cell nucleus to synthesize specific proteins. Because these hormones are lipid chemicals, the reactions take longer to occur but are no less potent than the amine, protein, and peptide hormone reactions.

20.5 THE NEGATIVE-FEEDBACK SYSTEM

Some hormones are needed in very minute amounts in the body for variable amounts of time; some have prolonged action periods and some affect and interact with other hormones, producing a very complex, intricate system. A control system must exist to maintain this complex system.

Most control systems, including the endocrine system, act by a negative-feedback mechanism. When there is an increased hormone concentration, physiologic control is increased. The stimulus for hormone production received in the hypothalamus is decreased. This results in an inhibition of hormone-releasing factors that is negative in relation to the stimulus. In the same manner, when hormone concentrations are deficient or absent, a stimulus is received in the hypothalamus that results in an increased release of hormone-stimulating factors. This again is a negative (or opposite) response to the stimulus sent to the hypothalamus. The greater the need for the hormone, the greater the intensity of the stimulus; similarly, the greater the concentration of the hormone, the lower the intensity of the stimulus.

When a hormone concentration is deficient, the physiologic control of the body cells increases as more hormone is produced and/or secreted. With an increase in physiologic control, the feedback stimulus relayed to the endocrine gland decreases in intensity, and release of the hormone decreases as homeostasis is achieved. The reverse process applies when the hormone concentration is excessive.

TABLE 20-2. RELEASING AND INHIBITING FACTORS PRODUCED BY THE HYPOTHALAMUS

Releasing Hormones	Inhibiting Hormones	Peripheral Hormones
Growth hormone–releasing hormone	Growth hormone–inhibiting hormone	Growth hormone
Prolactin-releasing hormone	Prolactin-inhibiting hormone	Prolactin
Corticotropin-releasing hormone	—	Adrenal steroids
Follicle-stimulating hormone–releasing hormone	—	Gonadal steroids
Luteinizing hormone–releasing hormone	—	Gonadal hormones
Thyrotropin-releasing hormone	—	Thyroid hormones

It is known that the hypothalamus produces releasing and inhibiting hormones (or factors) whose single target is the adenohypophysis, the so-called master gland. It is believed that all hormones have releasing and inhibiting factors produced by the hypothalamus, but only eight are known at this time (**Table 20-2**).

The principles of achieving regulatory control are similar for all the hormones listed in Table 20-1 except for the hormones of the adrenal medulla.

The **hormones of the adrenal medulla, epinephrine and norepinephrine**, are under control of the autonomic nervous system. The hormones of the neurohypophysis (the posterior pituitary) are controlled by the concentration of the substance released from the target-cell "feeding back" on the hypothalamus. The release of the hormone leads to a change in a plasma constituent that regulates hypothalamic activity rather than a change in the gland itself. Tropic hormones, secreted only by the adenohypophysis (the anterior pituitary), cause an increase in size and secretion rates of other endocrine glands and are controlled by the negative-feedback system as well as other factors.

QUICK TIP! If a patient presents with HTN, headache, palpitations, and elevated circulating catecholamines (such as epinephrine and norepinephrine), you may be asked what test may be anticipated. The answer is often an abdominal CT to check for **pheochromocytoma** that may manifest as a mass on the adrenal glands.

All adenohypophyseal hormone-releasing and inhibiting factors (except the adrenal medulla) are carried by the hypothalamic–hypophyseal tract from the hypothalamus into the median eminence (**Fig. 20-3**) and then into the hypophyseal stalk.

In the stalk, the hypophyseal portal system carries the releasing and inhibiting factors into the adenohypophysis for storage until needed.

The two neurohypophyseal hormone-releasing and inhibiting factors are formed in the paraventricular and supraoptic nuclei in the hypothalamus (see Fig. 20-3). They are then carried by nerve fibers into the neurohypophysis for storage.

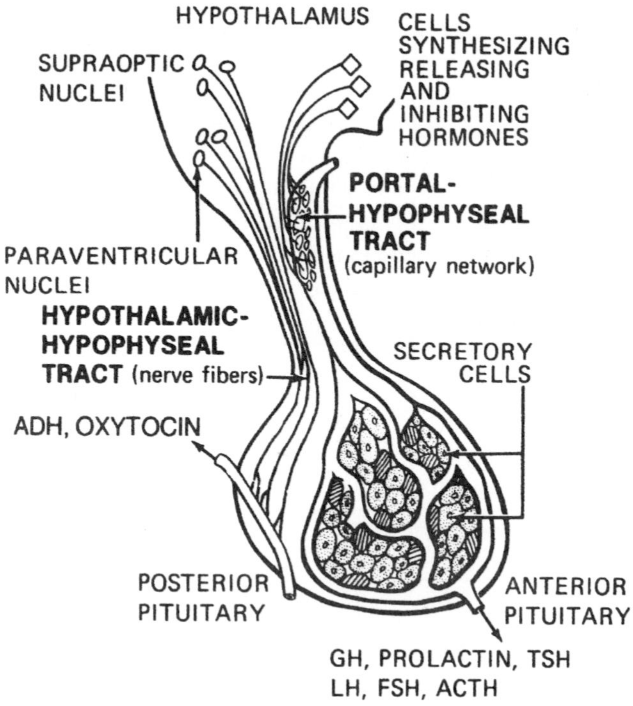

Figure 20-3. Portal–hypophyseal and hypothalamic–hypophyseal tracts of the hypothalamus.

KEY CONTENT CHECKLIST

- ❒ Remember, concepts of basic anatomy, such as the structure of the pituitary stalk, are usually not addressed on the CCRN exam. It may, in general, be helpful to understand such concepts, but do not spend too much time trying to memorize this type of detail.
- ❒ Instead, most, if not all of your endocrine questions will focus on:
  - DKA versus HHNK
  - Signs and symptoms of acute hypoglycemia
  - SIADH
  - Diabetes insipidus
- ❒ If a patient presents with HTN, headache, palpitations, and elevated circulating catecholamines (such as epinephrine and norepinephrine), you may be asked what test may be anticipated. The answer is often an abdominal CT to check for **pheochromocytoma** that may manifest as a mass on the adrenal glands.

Review Questions:

1. **All of the adenohypophyseal (anterior pituitary) hormones have an effect on a target gland EXCEPT:**
   a. Adrenocorticotropin
   b. Growth hormone
   c. Thyroid-stimulating hormone
   d. Luteinizing hormone

Answer: B. Rationale: Growth hormone (somatotropin) has a general effect on bones, organs, and soft tissues. It is essentially considered a peripheral hormone that influences growth of body tissues. Thyroid-stimulating hormone acts on the thyroid, adrenocorticotropin stimulates the adrenals to produce cortisol, and luteinizing hormone acts on the ovaries and testes.

2. **Which hormone(s) does the thyroid gland NOT secrete?**
   a. Thyroxine
   b. Triiodothyronine
   c. Calcitonin
   d. ADH

Answer: D. Rationale: In this negatively stated question, all the options are secreted from the thyroid EXCEPT one. Thyroxine and triiodothyronine are secreted by the thyroid. Calcitonin, also known as "thyrocalcitonin," is secreted by the thyroid. ADH is secreted by the posterior pituitary.

3. **Calcitonin is released by which organ?**
   a. Pituitary gland
   b. Adrenal gland
   c. Parathyroid gland
   d. Thyroid gland

Answer: D. Rationale: The thyroid gland is the only option available that releases calcitonin. Remember that a rare complication in patients post-thyroidectomy is tetany which is influenced by the alteration in calcitonin levels after the procedure.

REFERENCE

White BA, Harrison JR, Mehlmann LM, eds. *Endocrine and Reproductive Physiology.* 5th ed. St. Louis, MO: Elsevier Inc; 2019.

21

Anatomy, Physiology, and Dysfunction of the Pituitary Gland

CHAPTER OVERVIEW AND OBJECTIVES

As you review the functions of the pituitary gland, do not attempt to memorize basic anatomic features. Rarely would questions on anatomy, such as the type of tissue from which the pituitary arises, be on the CCRN exam.

After studying this chapter, you should understand the following:

- Describe the signs and symptoms associated with diabetes insipidus along with the hallmarks of management.
- Discuss the etiology of the syndrome of inappropriate section of antidiuretic hormone (SIADH) and how to safely correct the associated hyponatremia.

21.1 ANATOMY OF THE HYPOPHYSIS

The pituitary gland, or hypophysis, is a small gland about 1 cm in diameter and weighing about 0.5 g. It is located in the sella turcica, a depression in the sphenoid bone of the skull (**Fig. 21-1**), and is attached to the hypothalamus by the hypophyseal stalk. The hypophysis is often referred to as the body's master gland because the hormones it secretes regulate many other endocrine glands.

Structure of the Adenohypophysis

The adenohypophysis is composed of epithelial-type cells (embryologic extensions of pharyngeal tissue). Many different types of epithelial cells have been identified for each hormone formed.

The hypothalamic–hypophyseal portal vessels in the adenohypophysis are made up of microscopic blood vessels (**Fig. 21-2**). These vessels connect the hypothalamus and the adenohypophysis (by passage through the pituitary stalk) and terminate in the anterior pituitary sinuses.

Substances carried in the hypothalamic–hypophyseal vessels are actually hormone factors and not hormones per se. These factors are releasing and inhibiting factors (see Table 20-2). For each adenohypophyseal hormone, there is an associated releasing factor. For some adenohypophyseal hormones, there are inhibitory factors.

Structure of the Neurohypophysis

Many cells of the neurohypophysis are called pituicytes, which are like the glial cells of the nervous system. The pituicytes provide supporting tissue for nerve tracts arising from the supraoptic and paraventricular nuclei of the hypothalamus. These nuclei form the neurohypophyseal hormones, which are carried by the nerve tracts through the hypophyseal stalk, a structure terminating in bulbous knobs in the neurohypophysis. The hormone is thus secreted from the bulbous knobs onto the capillaries and is absorbed into the vascular system. The adenohypophysis has a vascular relationship to the hypothalamus, whereas the neurohypophysis has a neural relationship.

21.2 PHYSIOLOGY

The various hormones control the activity of the target glands and target tissues. They exert an effect on target tissues by altering the rates at which cellular processes occur. There are two basic mechanisms of hormone action: cyclic 3′,5′-adenosine monophosphate (cAMP) and genetic activation. cAMP initiates actions characteristic of the target cell. For example, parathyroid hormone cells activated by cAMP form and secrete parathyroid hormone (parathormone); specific cells in the pancreas activated by cAMP form and secrete glucagon. Known hormones

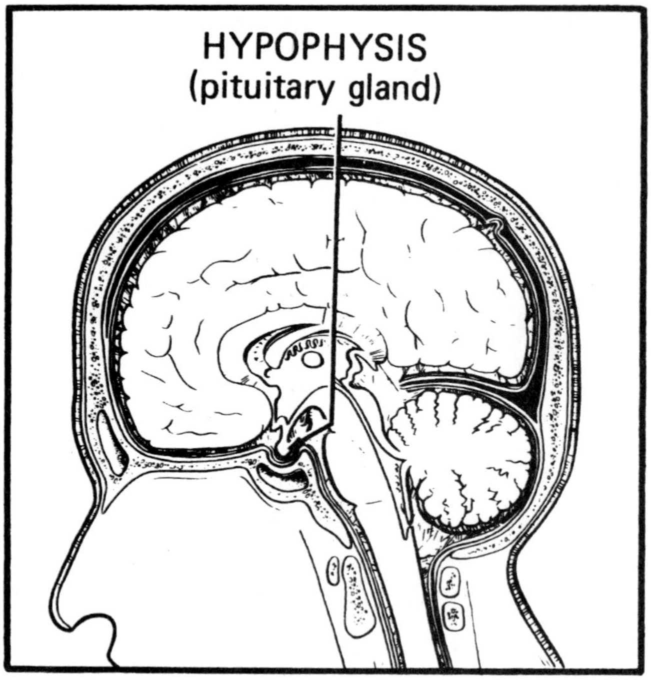

Figure 21-1. Location of the hypophysis (pituitary gland).

affected by cAMP include secretin, glucagon, parathormone, vasopressin, catecholamines, adrenocorticotropin, follicle-stimulating hormone (FSH), thyroid-stimulating hormone (TSH), and hypothalamic-releasing factors.

Hormones of the Adenohypophysis

Hormone factors, all formed in the hypothalamus, are secreted by the adenohypophysis.

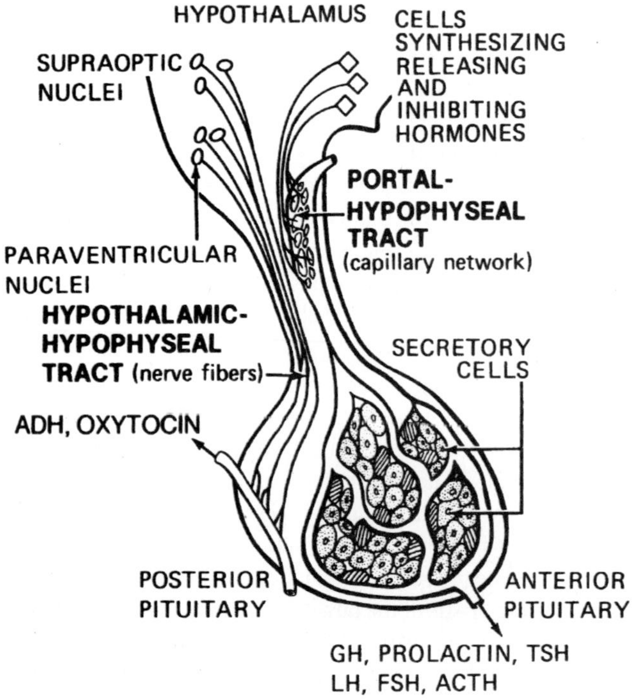

Figure 21-2. The hypothalamic–hypophyseal portal vessel.

1. Thyrotropin-releasing hormone (TRH) causes the release of TSH.
2. Growth hormone–releasing hormone (GRH) causes release of growth hormone (GH) or somatotropin (STH). Growth hormone–inhibiting factor (GIF), or somatostatin, inhibits the release of GH.
3. Corticotropin-releasing hormone (CRH) causes release of adrenocorticotropin (ACTH).
4. Gonadotropin-releasing hormone (GnRH) causes release of luteinizing hormone (LH) and FSH.
5. Prolactin-inhibiting hormone (PIH) causes inhibition of prolactin secretion.
6. Human chorionic gonadotropin (HCG).
7. Human placental lactogen (HPL).

All of the major adenohypophyseal hormones have an effect upon a target gland except GH.

Growth Hormone and Metabolism. GH is also called somatotropin. Somatotropin has a general effect on bones, organs, and soft tissues; it is therefore considered a peripheral hormone. It influences the growth of body tissues.

GH has an important role in all aspects of metabolism. GH increases the rate of intracellular protein synthesis throughout the body. It is a factor in the mobilization of fatty acids from adipose tissue and in the conversion of these fats into energy. GH conserves carbohydrates by decreasing glucose utilization in the body.

Growth Hormone Factors. There are specific factors that stimulate or inhibit the release of GH.

- Inhibit release: hyperglycemia, sustained corticosteroid therapy at high levels, release of GIF from the hypothalamus.
- Promote release: pituitary tumors, hypoglycemia, exercise, decreased amino acid levels, release of GRH from the hypothalamus

GH secretion follows a diurnal pattern, with most release occurring in the first 2 hours of deep sleep. This follows the pattern of the nonrapid eye movement (non-REM) stage of sleep.

Hormones of the Neurohypophysis

Two hormones are released by the neurohypophysis: antidiuretic hormone (ADH), also called vasopressin, and oxytocin. Oxytocin is not discussed in this text.

> QUICK TIP! Injury to the neurohypophysis and subsequent effect on ADH is a reason why patients with neurosurgical transsphenoidal hypophysectomy patients and traumatic brain injury are subject to diabetes insipidus (DI).

ADH is formed mainly in the supraoptic nuclei of the hypothalamus. ADH is transported from the supraoptic nuclei by neurophysins. Neurophysins are protein carriers that bind very loosely with ADH and oxytocin to transport these hormones to the neurohypophysis for storage until needed.

Action of Antidiuretic Hormone. ADH works on the distal convoluted tubules and the collecting ducts of the kidney, altering the permeability of these tubules and ducts. Without ADH, the tubules and ducts are impermeable to water. In the presence of ADH, they become permeable to water, thus allowing large quantities of water to leave the tubules and collecting ducts and to reenter the hypertonic medullary interstitial fluid. This helps conserve and balance the fluid content of the body.

Control of Antidiuretic Hormone. **Serum sodium levels and extracellular fluid osmolality exert a major influence on ADH.** Osmoreceptors shrink when hypertonicity of the extracellular fluid exists. The osmoreceptors emit impulses to the hypothalamus, and ADH is released from the neurohypophysis to reabsorb water from the kidneys and to reestablish homeostasis. **When body fluids become diluted, stimulated osmoreceptors result in the inhibition of ADH,** and water is not reabsorbed from the kidneys. Many factors control ADH in addition to the serum sodium and extracellular osmolality.

- **Inhibit release (decrease ADH):** decreased plasma osmolality, **increased intravascular volume**, alcohol ingestion, pituitary surgery
- **Promote release (increase ADH):** inadequate blood volume including **hemorrhagic states**, trauma, stress, anxiety, exercise, pain, exposure to heat, nausea, hypoxia, nicotine, diphenylhydantoin (Dilantin)

KEY CLINICAL CONCEPT

One or two questions may be expected on the influence of ADH on clinical conditions.

21.3 NEUROHYPOPHYSEAL DYSFUNCTION

There are two main neurohypophyseal disorders: diabetes insipidus (DI) and the syndrome of inappropriate ADH (SIADH).

Diabetes Insipidus (DI)

DI is a disease of impaired renal conservation of water, resulting from either **inadequate secretion of vasopressin** from the neurohypophysis (central DI) or to an insufficient renal response to vasopressin (nephrogenic DI). When there are decreased levels of ADH, diuresis and dehydration occur. Decreased levels of ADH are found when there is damage to or destruction of the ADH neurons in the supraoptic and paraventricular neurons of the hypothalamus. DI then results.

Symptoms. The symptoms of DI include:

- Polyuria, nocturia
- Polydipsia, unless the thirst center has been damaged
- Dilute urine (specific gravity between 1.001 and 1.005 and urine osmolality < 300 mOsm/kg)
- Urinary output between 2 and 15 L/day regardless of fluid intake
- Increased serum osmolality (> 295 mosmol/kg)

Polyuria may not occur until 1 to 3 days postinjury due to the utilization of stored ADH in the neurohypophysis. *Urine output greater than 200 mL/h for 2 hours should be reported to a physician.*

Etiology: Central DI. The two leading causes of central DI are resection of hypothalamic or pituitary tumors and closed head injuries with damage to the supraoptic nuclei and/or hypothalamus. Postoperative DI is usually transient. Other causes include infectious, inflammatory, and degenerative systemic conditions, but these are not common. Nephrogenic DI is often caused by hypercalcemia, hypokalemia, renal disease, and certain medications and certain medications, such as lithium. Central DI can be distinguished from nephrogenic DI by the administration of **desmopressin (DDAVP),** which will increase urine osmolality in patients with central DI but have little or no effect in patients with nephrogenic DI.

Treatment. In central DI, the objective of therapy is first to prevent dehydration and electrolyte imbalances while determining and treating the underlying cause.

- In patients who have intravascular volume depletion, volume status should first be restored with 0.9% sodium chloride.
- Fluid support with hypotonic dextrose in water (D_5W) IV or oral or nasogastric water administration is essential to match daily fluid losses and fix the estimated fluid deficit, with a goal to return the urine volume milliliter for milliliter plus any insensible loss.
- Exogenous **vasopressin (Pitressin)** is the treatment of choice for polyuria. It is a short-acting ADH therapy with vasopressor activity. **Desmopressin** is a synthetic ADH that can be used as an intravenous (central line only), subcutaneous, or nasal spray therapy. The advantage of DDAVP is a longer duration of action and negligible vasoactive properties. Following head trauma or neurosurgery, an aqueous **vasopressin** infusion of 5 to 10 units subcutaneously may be used to decrease the risk of dehydration and hypotension.
- **Desmopressin** therapy should be continued as long as DI persists. The duration of DI is dependent on its cause. If DI is related to pituitary manipulation during surgery or other neurosurgeries, DI may resolve in only a few days. If it is idiopathic, it may be permanent.
- Serum sodium must be monitored closely, every 4 hours during fluid resuscitation to monitor for the development of hyponatremia. The frequency of monitoring can extend to every 12 hours once the patient stabilizes. The correction of hypernatremia must be controlled, limited to no more than 10 mmol/L in 24 hours.

Etiology: Nephrogenic DI. In nephrogenic DI, the kidneys are partially or completely resistant to ADH. Nephrogenic DI in children is caused by hereditary gene mutations. In adults, nephrogenic DI is most commonly caused by chronic **lithium** ingestion or hypercalcemia. Hypokalemia, kidney disease, pregnancy, other drugs, or other rare inherited disorders may also cause nephrogenic DI.

Treatment. In nephrogenic DI, the goal of treatment is to correct the underlying cause or discontinue the offending medication. In addition, a low salt diet, diuretics, and nonsteroidal anti-inflammatory medications (NSAIDs) may be used.

Nursing Interventions

- Monitor intake and output accurately
- Daily weights
- Monitor electrolytes (especially potassium and sodium), urine-specific gravity, osmolality, blood urea nitrogen
- Monitor for signs of dehydration and hypovolemic shock, which will allow for early intervention in patients who are at risk for deterioration.

QUICK TIP! Remember SIADH is the **over**-secretion of ADH, whereas DI is the **under**-secretion of ADH. In DI, the urine does not look yellow anymore, it tends to just be clear like water.

The Syndrome of Inappropriate Secretion of Antidiuretic Hormone

SIADH is a condition of impaired water excretion caused by the inappropriate secretion of ADH resulting in hypotonic hyponatremia. In SIADH there is either increased secretion or increased production of ADH. This increase is unrelated to osmolality and causes a slight increase in total body water. Sodium and osmolar concentration in extracellular fluid and serum are severely decreased resulting in hypo-osmolar hyponatremia. SIADH is a diagnosis of exclusion, it occurs in absence of thyroid, adrenal, or kidney dysfunction.

Etiology

- **Malignancy:** small cell carcinoma of the lung, central nervous system, head/neck, gastrointestinal and urologic
- **Central nervous system disorders:** head trauma, infections (encephalitis, meningitis), vascular insult (stroke, subarachnoid or subdural hemorrhage), inflammation (lupus, Guillain-Barre syndrome)
- **Pulmonary disorders:** infections (pneumonia, tuberculosis, empyema, abscess), acute respiratory failure, positive pressure ventilation, asthma, cystic fibrosis, chronic obstructive pulmonary disease (COPD)
- **Other:** pain, severe nausea, prolonged exercise, postoperative state, human immunodeficiency syndrome (HIV) infections, drugs, or idiopathically

Symptoms and Complications. Symptoms produced by SIADH reflect the interaction between the underlying condition and excessive water retention. Symptoms are mainly neurologic and nonspecific. The most common symptoms of SIADH are weakness, headache, decreased mentation, lethargy, nausea, vomiting, diarrhea, anorexia, and gait disturbances. Complications of SIADH include cerebral edema, seizures, coma, brain herniation, respiratory arrest, permanent brain damage, and death.

Laboratory Recognition. SIADH occurs, by definition, in a euvolemic state. SIADH is present when the following criteria are met in the absence of thyroid, adrenal, or kidney dysfunction:

- Serum sodium < 135 mmol/L and osmolality < 275 mOsm/kg
- Urine sodium > 30 mEq/L and osmolality > 100 mOsm/kg H_2O

Acute hyponatremia requires confirmation of hyponatremia present < 48 hours, whereas chronic hyponatremia is when duration is either unknown or > 48 hours. Central nervous system symptoms are more evident as the serum sodium drops below 125 mmol/L. **Seizures and coma are more likely to be present in the patient with a serum sodium less than 115 mmol/L.**

QUICK TIP! A serum osmolality level is approximately the serum sodium level multiplied by two. For example, sodium of 140 × 2 = 280 serum osmolality.

Treatment. The first step in treating SIADH is to treat the underlying cause should there be a treatable cause. Conditions that can be treated include SIADH due to infections, drugs, adrenal insufficiency, or hypothyroidism. First-line treatment of SIADH in most patients is fluid restriction to prevent water intoxication. Fluid limitation may be set by utilizing the Furst equation. A ratio < 1 indicates the need for mild fluid restriction of < 1.5 L/day versus a ratio > 1 a severe fluid restriction < 1 L/day. In patients with low urine output and highly concentrate urine, sodium levels are less likely to respond to fluid restriction. Severity of symptoms and chronicity of hyponatremia will determine the rate of correction of the hyponatremia. In severe cases (serum sodium < 125 mEq/L), 3% hypertonic saline will be administered if associated symptoms are moderate to severe. If the hyponatremia is confirmed to be acute in nature, there is no restriction in the rate of sodium correction. If the chronicity is unknown or > 48 hours, **rapid correction of sodium should be avoided to prevent osmotic demyelination.** In chronic hyponatremia with moderate to severe symptoms, the initial rate of correction is 1 mEq/L/h in the first 3 to 4 hours but no more than 8 mEq/L in 24 hours. Patients who have mild symptoms or are asymptomatic may receive 3% hypertonic saline or alternative therapy. **Maximum rate of correction should be 8 mEq/L.** If the patient is at high risk for ODS, a correction rate of 6 to 8 mEq/L/24 h is recommended. Notable risk factors for ODS include present serum sodium < 105 mEq/L, alcoholism, advanced liver disease, and malnutrition. In all patients, supplemental potassium is usually necessary, with follow-up frequent monitoring of serum potassium and sodium levels every 2 to 4 hours until the patient is stable. Additional therapies that may be utilized include salt tablets, urea tablets, and loop diuretics. Daily weights are important measures of fluid gain. Vasopressin receptor antagonist may be given intravenously (conivaptan) or orally (tolvaptan) when other measures have proven to be ineffective. They produce a selective water diuresis without affecting sodium and potassium excretion.

Nursing Interventions

- **Maintain strict fluid restrictions as ordered.**
- Administer 3% hypertonic saline IV infusions as ordered.
- If a nasogastric tube is inserted, it should be irrigated with normal saline instead of water and enemas should be avoided.
- Monitor vital signs, intake and output, daily weights, and laboratory monitoring of urine-specific gravity and electrolyte levels.
- Cardiac monitoring will allow for early identification of arrhythmias or electrocardiographic (ECG) changes associated with hyperkalemia or hypokalemia.
- Monitor neurologic status for subtle signs of decreasing level of consciousness.
- Seizure precautions.
- For a comatose patient, turning, suctioning as needed, and standard nursing care procedures are required.
- Provide frequent oral care, mouth-rinsing without swallowing.
- Provide hard candy and chilled beverages in patients without altered mental status or dysphagia as it will be helpful in coping with fluid restriction.
- Avoid mouthwashes with an alcohol base and lemon and glycerin swabs because of their drying effects.
- Provide emotional support to the alert patient, offering reassurance that his or her condition can be treated successfully.

KEY CONTENT CHECKLIST

- ❐ Injury to the neurohypophysis and subsequent effect on ADH is a reason why patients with neurosurgical transsphenoidal hypophysectomy patients and traumatic brain injury are subject to DI.
- ❐ Remember SIADH is the **over**-secretion of ADH, whereas DI is the **under**-secretion of ADH. In DI, the urine does not look yellow anymore; it tends to just be clear like water.
- ❐ A serum osmolality level is approximately the serum sodium level multiplied by two. For example, sodium of $140 \times 2 = 280$ serum osmolality.
- ❐ **Inhibit release (decrease ADH):** decreased plasma osmolality, **increased intravascular volume,** alcohol ingestion, pituitary surgery
- ❐ **Promote release (increase ADH):** inadequate blood volume including **hemorrhagic states,** trauma, stress, anxiety, exercise, pain, exposure to heat, nausea, hypoxia, nicotine, diphenylhydantoin (Dilantin)

Review Questions:

1. **Common clinical findings of SIADH may include which symptom?**
   a. Mental status changes
   b. Tachycardia
   c. Polyuria
   d. Polydipsia

Answer: A. Rationale: Symptoms produced by SIADH reflect the interaction between the underlying condition and excessive water retention. Symptoms are mainly neurologic and nonspecific. The most common symptoms of SIADH are personality changes, headache, decreased mentation, lethargy, nausea, vomiting, diarrhea, anorexia, decreased tendon reflexes, seizures, and coma. Complications of SIADH include seizures, coma, and death. Options B, C, and D are all associated with dehydration and can be ruled out as potential answers. Choose A.

2. **What is the dominant effect of ADH on the kidneys?**
   a. It causes them to excrete water and sodium.
   b. It causes them to reabsorb water and concentrate urine.
   c. It causes them to reabsorb sodium and excrete potassium.
   d. It causes them to reabsorb potassium and excrete sodium.

Answer: B. Rationale: ADH ("antidiuretic hormone") works on the distal convoluted tubules and the collecting ducts of the kidney, altering the permeability of these tubules and ducts. Without ADH, the tubules and ducts are impermeable to water. In the presence of ADH, they become permeable to water, thus allowing large quantities of water to leave the tubules and collecting ducts and to reenter the hypertonic medullary interstitial fluid. This helps conserve and balance the fluid content of the body and results in reabsorption of water and subsequent concentration of urine. Choose B.

3. **ADH release is inhibited by which of the following?**
   a. Increased serum osmolality
   b. Decreased serum osmolality
   c. Increased serum sodium
   d. Increased potassium level

Answer: B. Rationale: When a patient is hydrated, serum osmolality (ie, blood concentration) will decrease, followed by a decrease in ADH due to the body's decreased need to retain sodium and water. Options A and C can be ruled out because they are associated with dehydration, which would stimulate release of ADH. Potassium level does not directly impact ADH. Choose B.

REFERENCES

Adrogué HJ, Tucker BM, Madias NE. Diagnosis and management of hyponatremia: a review. *JAMA*. 2022 Jul 19;328(3):280–291. doi: 10.1001/jama.2022.11176.

Baldeweg SE, Ball S, Brooke A, et al; Society for Endocrinology Clinical Committee. Society for Endocrinology Clinical Guidance: inpatient management of cranial diabetes insipidus. *Endocr Connect*. 2018 Jul;7(7):G8–G11. doi: 10.1530/EC-18-0154.

Christ-Crain M, Winzeler B, Refardt J. Diagnosis and management of diabetes insipidus for the internist: an update. *J Intern Med*. 2021 Jul;290(1):73–87. doi: 10.1111/joim.13261. Epub 2021 Mar 13.

Levy M, Prentice M, Wass J. Diabetes insipidus. *BMJ*. 2019 Feb 28;364:l321. doi: 10.1136/bmj.l321.

Martin-Grace J, Tomkins M, O'Reilly MW, Thompson CJ, Sherlock M. Approach to the patient: hyponatremia and the syndrome of inappropriate antidiuresis (SIAD). *J Clin Endocrinol Metab*. 2022 Jul 14;107(8):2362–2376. doi: 10.1210/clinem/dgac245.

Seay NW, Lehrich RW, Greenberg A. Diagnosis and management of disorders of body tonicity-hyponatremia and hypernatremia: *Core Curriculum*. 2020. Am J Kidney Dis. 2020 Feb;75(2):272–286. doi: 10.1053/j.ajkd.2019.07.014. Epub 2019 Oct 10.

White BA, Harrison JR, Mehlmann LM, eds. *Endocrine and Reproductive Physiology*. 5th ed. St. Louis, MO: Elsevier; 2019.

22

Anatomy, Physiology, and Dysfunction of the Thyroid and Parathyroid Glands

CHAPTER OVERVIEW AND OBJECTIVES

The most recent CCRN guidelines do not discuss the care of patients with thyroid and parathyroid disturbances as part of the CCRN exam. However, understanding of thyroid and parathyroid function is useful for understanding other clinical conditions, particularly electrolyte and cardiovascular responses.

After studying this chapter, you should understand the following:

- Discuss the signs and symptoms associated with myxedema coma versus thyroid storm.
- Describe the hallmarks of the treatment of myxedema coma and thyroid storm.
- List the diagnostic criteria for hypoparathyroidism along and complications of the condition if left untreated.

22.1 ANATOMY OF THE THYROID GLAND

Location and Shape

The thyroid gland is in the anterior portion of the neck at the lower part of the larynx and the upper part of the trachea (**Fig. 22-1**). The thyroid has two lobes, which resemble a butterfly's wings. The lobes lie on either side of the trachea and are connected by a narrow band of tissue called the isthmus, which lies anteriorly across the second and third tracheal rings.

Internal Structure

Each lobe of the thyroid is divided into lobules by dense connective tissue. Each lobule (**Fig. 22-2**) is composed of sac-like structures called *follicles*. The follicles are lined with cuboidal epithelium.

The follicular sacs are filled with a thick, viscous material called colloid. Colloid is thyroglobulin, which is converted to thyroxine (T_4) as needed. Storage, synthesis, and release of thyroxine are controlled by the hypothalamic-releasing hormone (factor) and the thyroid-stimulating hormone (TSH) of the adenohypophysis.

22.2 PHYSIOLOGY OF THE THYROID GLAND

The thyroid gland secretes three important hormones: T_4, triiodothyronine (T_3), and thyrocalcitonin. Approximately 90% of the hormone is T_4 and 10% is T_3. In peripheral tissues, T_4 is converted to T_3. The functions of these two hormones are essentially the same. Thyroid hormones stimulate metabolism of all body cells and produce effective function of multiple body systems. The intensity, speed of action, and formation of these hormones differ.

Iodide Trapping (the Iodide Pump)

To form thyroid hormones, iodides must be removed from blood and extracellular fluids and transported into the thyroid gland follicles. The iodide then diffuses throughout the thyroid cells and follicular sacs in a process known as iodide trapping.

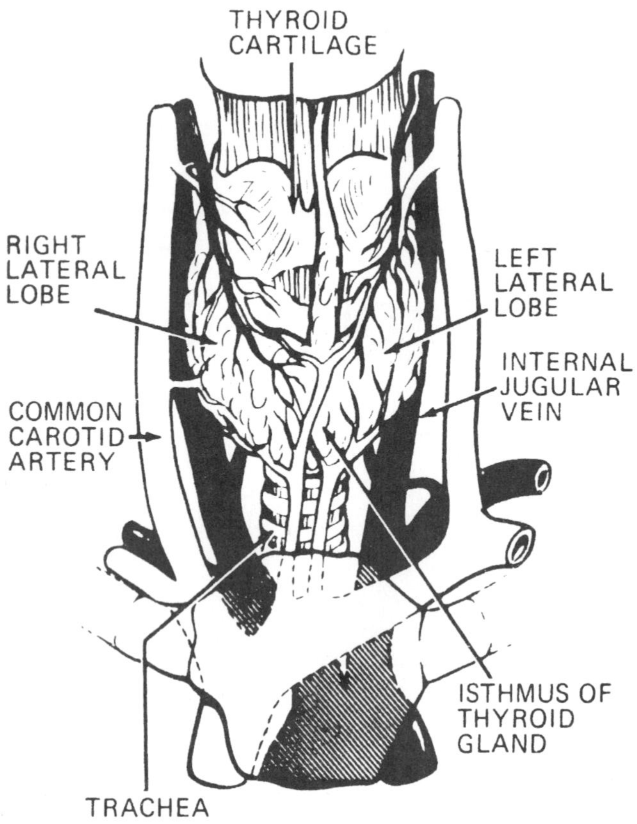

Figure 22-1. Location and shape of the thyroid gland.

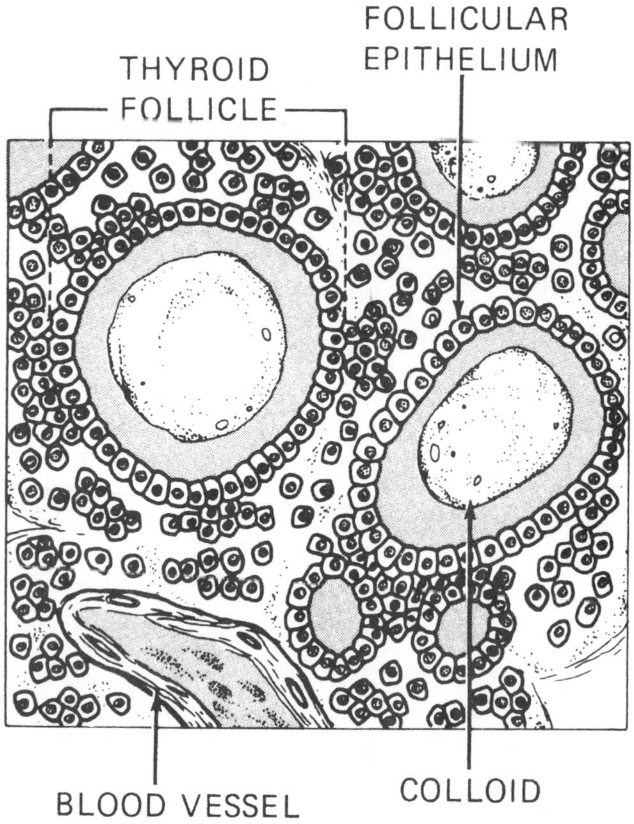

Figure 22-2. Internal structure of the thyroid follicles.

Organification of Thyroglobulin

Thyroglobulin is the major component reacting with iodide to form T_4. Thyroid cells synthesize the glycoprotein thyroglobulin, which is the colloid filling the follicular sacs. Iodide is stored until thyroglobulin is needed. It then becomes ionized by enzymes, converting the iodide into iodine at the point where thyroglobulin is released intracellularly. The binding of iodide with the glycoprotein is termed the organification of thyroglobulin. The iodide is then oxidized iodine. The oxidized iodine bonds with tyrosine (an amino acid) and chemical reactions progress to yield T_4 and T_3. The thyroid hormones are stored in an amount that is equal to the normal body requirements for 1 to 3 months.

Release of Thyroxine and Triiodothyronine

These two thyroid hormones separate from the thyroglobulin molecule. Separation is a multistep process involving several intermediate chemicals. The result is that T_4 and T_3 are lysed from the glycoprotein. Once freed, these thyroid hormones enter the venous circulatory system of the thyroid gland itself and are carried into the systemic circulation. The strongest stimulation to release these hormones is cold temperature. Thyrotropin-releasing hormone (TRH) factors will stimulate release of TSH, and T_4 and T_3 will be released from the thyroid gland (but not as rapidly as in response to cold).

The release of these hormones is inhibited by heat, insufficient hypothalamic-releasing factors (resulting in insufficient TSHs), and/or increases in plasma glucocorticoids.

Action of Thyroxine and Triiodothyronine

An interesting "rule of four" exists. Once these two hormones are in the peripheral tissues, T_3 is four times as strong in initiating metabolic activities as T_4. Thyroxine's effect on the tissues will last four times as long as triiodothyronine's effect. So, these two hormones balance each other very well.

Thyroxine Function

Approximately 1 mg of iodine per week is needed for normal T_4 formation. Iodides are absorbed from the gastrointestinal tract. Two-thirds of ingested iodides are excreted in the urine, and the remaining one-third is used by the thyroid gland to form the glycoprotein thyroglobulin.

The major effect of the thyroid hormones is to increase all metabolic activities of the body excluding those of the brain, spleen, lungs, retina, and testes. In children, the thyroid hormones also promote growth.

Production, Release, and Action of Calcitonin

Calcitonin is manufactured in special thyroid cells called parafollicular cells, or C cells. These cells are found in the interstitial tissue between the follicles of the thyroid gland.

An increase in the plasma concentration of calcium stimulates the release of calcitonin, as will the ingestion or administration of magnesium and/or glucagon.

Calcitonin's major effect is on bones. Calcitonin reduces plasma calcium levels by immediate decrease in osteoclastic activity, a transient increase in osteoblastic activity, and a prolonged prevention of new osteoclast formation.

22.3 ANATOMY OF THE PARATHYROID GLANDS

Size and Location

The parathyroid glands are four small, flat, roundish glands located on the posterior surface of the lateral lobes of the thyroid (**Fig. 22-3**). Usually, one parathyroid gland is located at the superior end of each thyroid lobe and another gland at the inferior end of each lateral lobe of the thyroid. This location may vary considerably. It is normal to have four glands; however, there may be fewer or more than four glands.

Internal Structure

Two types of cells have been identified in the adult parathyroid gland. Chief cells (**Fig. 22-4**) are the main cells in the adult. Oxyphil cells (Fig. 22-4) are present in adults but are frequently absent in children. The function of oxyphil cells is unknown. There is a possibility that oxyphil cells are modified chief cells.

22.4 PHYSIOLOGY OF THE PARATHYROID GLANDS

Hormone Secretion

The parathyroid glands secrete a hormone termed *parathyroid hormone* (PTH). Chief cells in the parathyroid gland are responsible for the secretion of PTH. If two of the glands are inadvertently removed during a subtotal thyroidectomy, the remaining glands will produce sufficient PTH for the body's needs. Some parathyroid tissue should be preserved. This tissue will hypertrophy and continue to secrete PTH.

When hypothalamic-releasing factors are stimulated by a decreased serum calcium level or an increased serum magnesium/phosphate concentration, a series of reactions occur, resulting in the secretion of PTH. PTH release is inhibited by hypothalamic factors when serum calcium is increased or when there is an excessive concentration of vitamin D.

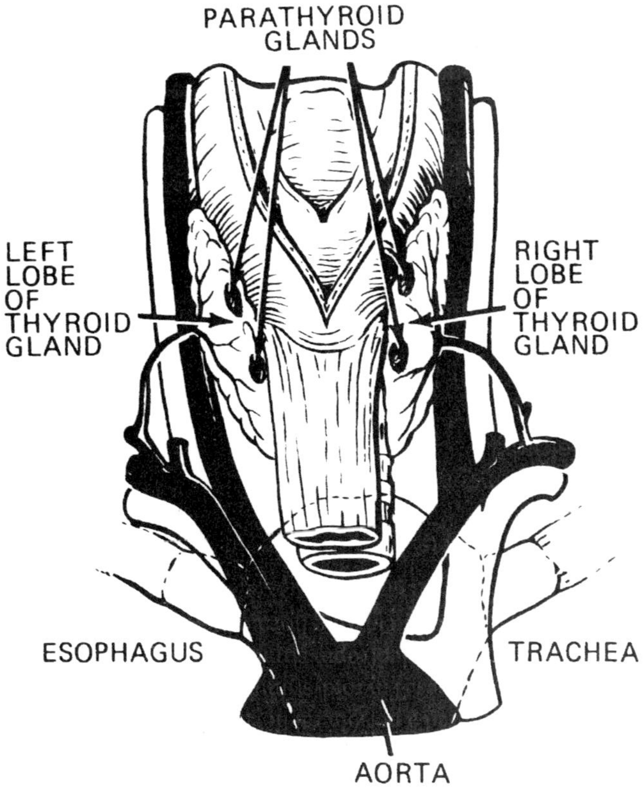

Figure 22-3. Location of the parathyroid glands (posterior view).

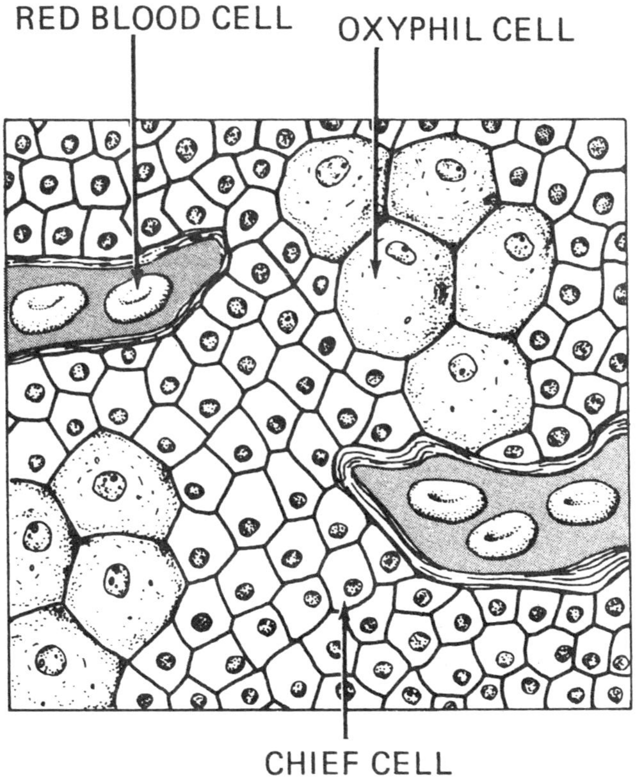

Figure 22-4. Chief cells and oxyphil cells of a parathyroid gland.

QUICK TIP! Calcium and phosphate levels change in opposite of each other. When calcium is increased, phosphate decreases. When phosphate levels increase, calcium decreases.

Action of Parathyroid Hormone

The main action of PTH and calcitonin is conservation of normal blood calcium levels. PTH decreases renal tubular reabsorption of phosphates, sodium, potassium, and amino acids. It increases reabsorption of calcium, magnesium, and hydrogen ions. Calcitonin's major effect is on bones. Calcitonin reduces plasma calcium levels by immediate decrease in osteoclastic activity, a transient increase in osteoblastic activity, and a prolonged prevention of new osteoclast formation.

Activated vitamin D is essential for PTH to function appropriately. The release of PTH is controlled by a negative-feedback mechanism between the blood calcium levels, the hypothalamus, and the parathyroid glands.

Target cells of the parathyroid glands include those of all bones (in a reciprocal relationship with calcium), the kidneys, and the gastrointestinal tract if there is sufficient ingestion of vitamin D.

22.5 THYROID DYSFUNCTION

Common disorders of the thyroid gland result primarily from autoimmune processes that either stimulate the overproduction of thyroid hormones (thyrotoxicosis) or cause glandular destruction and hormone deficiency (hypothyroidism). *Hypothyroidism*, also called **myxedema**, results from a lack of thyroid hormones. **Myxedema coma** is the result of severe deficiency or total absence of thyroid hormones. *Hyperthyroidism* may be due to **Graves disease**. The fulminant form of hyperthyroidism is called **thyroid storm** or **thyrotoxic crisis.**

Hypothyroidism (Myxedema)

Hypothyroidism is present when there is insufficient secretion of thyroid hormone. In hypothyroidism, the thyroid gland is usually small and consists of large amounts of fibrous tissue.

Hypothyroidism is a chronic disease that is eight to nine times more common in women than in men and occurs in all age groups but peak incidence between age 30 and 50 years.

Etiology. Hypothyroidism affects up to 5% of the general population The most common cause of hypothyroidism worldwide is iodine deficiency. Autoimmune disease (*Hashimoto thyroiditis*) and iatrogenic causes (excess treatment of hyperthyroidism) can also result in hypothyroidism. Hypothyroidism occurs after a thyroidectomy. Certain medications such as **amiodarone,** interleukin-2 inhibitors, and lithium have also been implicated.

Signs and Symptoms

- Edema of the face and a puffiness of the eyelids (**Fig. 22-5**)
- Weakness, fatigue weight gain, depression, menstrual irregularities, constipation, paresthesia of the fingers
- Lack of concentration, failing memory, and alteration in mentation occur
- Dry, scaly skin and friable, dry hair that falls out

Complications. **The most serious complication of hypothyroidism is its progression to myxedema coma and death if untreated.** Hypothyroidism is associated with an increased incidence of early severe arteriosclerosis. Angina and myocardial infarction are especially common after starting replacement thyroid therapy. The therapy improves and increases myocardial action, but the arteriosclerosis prevents increased delivery of oxygen to the myocardium that can result in ischemia and infarction. Anemia and increased sensitivity to hypnotic and sedative drugs may become serious problems. Resistance to infection is suppressed and response to treatment of infection is poor.

Treatment. The optimal treatment for hypothyroidism is early intervention with the goal of restoring a euthyroid state. The only possibility for the prevention of complications is the early recognition of hypothyroidism and close monitoring of medical therapy for the remainder of the patient's life. This, of course, necessitates the patient's compliance with the medical regimen.

The treatment of choice is synthetic T_4. The advantage of T_4 is it allows a patient's own physiologic mechanisms to control the production of active hormone. T_4 is a prohormone with very little activity. It is deiodinated in the peripheral tissues to make the active form of thyroid hormone T_3. Most of the drug is absorbed and has a long plasma half-life, so only once-daily treatment is necessary. **Levothyroxine (T_4)** preparations exist under several brand names. Hormone levels checked as a follow-up to assess if dose adjustments are required. It should always be taken on an empty stomach either 60 minutes before breakfast or at bedtime, at least 3 hours after an evening meal. It should also be taken separately from other potentially interfering medication, including calcium carbonate, proton pump inhibitors, bile acid sequestrants, phosphate binders, ferrous sulfate, aluminum-containing antacids, and sucralfate. The usual dose starting dose is 1.6 µg/kg/day. The elderly may need to start low and

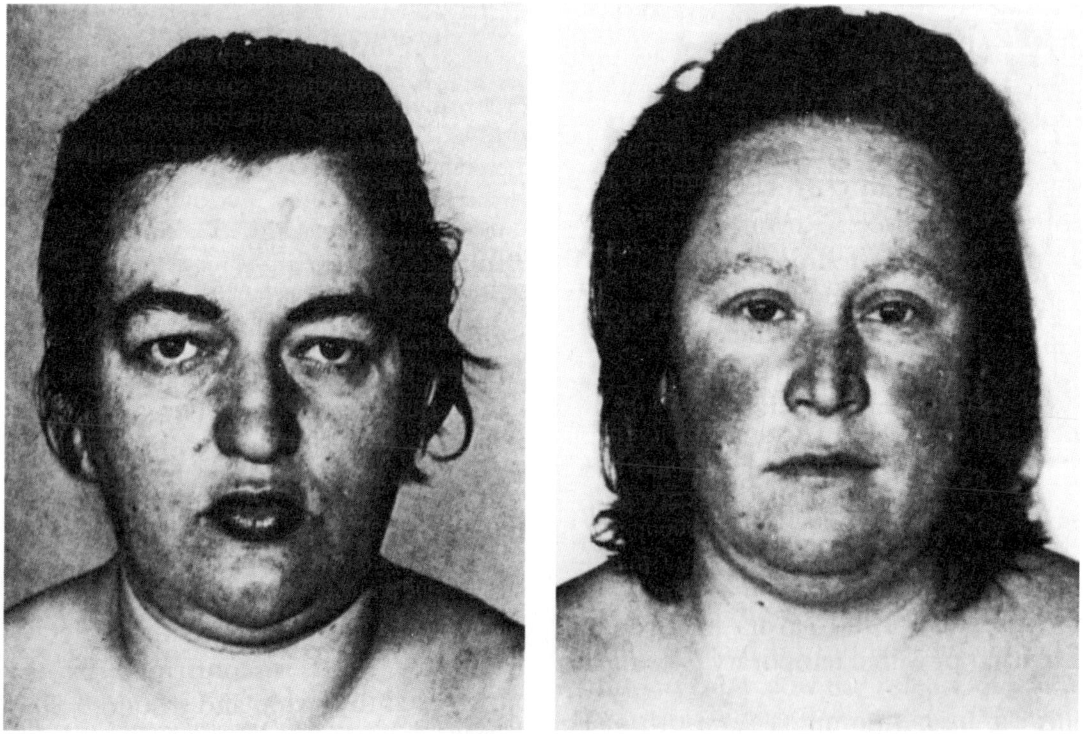

Figure 22-5. Facial appearance of two patients with myxedema.

titrate up to the desired level. Other thyroid hormone therapies include T_3 (Cytomel), desiccated thyroid, and/or mixtures of T_4 and T_3. In general, these should be avoided because they can vary in their bioavailability, thus causing wide fluctuations in serum T_3 levels.

KEY CLINICAL CONCEPT

Do not attempt to remember all these dosages. For the CCRN exam, keep in mind basic concepts such as that hypothyroidism (if it is addressed at all) simply requires thyroid hormone replacement.

Myxedema Coma

Myxedema coma is a life-threatening emergency that is fatal without treatment. Myxedema coma results from untreated or inadequately treated hypothyroidism and can be precipitated by severely cold weather or hypothermia, hypoglycemia, hyponatremia, hypercalcemia, acidosis, infections, cerebrovascular accident, trauma, burns, gastrointestinal bleeding, hypoxemia, hypercapnia, or administration of an anesthetic, sedative, narcotic, or potent diuretic drug. In addition, **myxedema coma** is most frequently associated with discontinuation of thyroid hormone therapy by the patient.

Clinical Presentation. **Myxedema coma** presents with a myriad of symptoms across multiple body systems.

- Hypothermia, hyporeflexia, coma, seizure
- Bradycardia, heart block, hypotension, pericardial effusion
- Hypoventilation, hypoxemia, hypercapnia, pleural effusion
- Anorexia, ascites, reduced motility, constipation, paralytic ileus, megacolon
- Slow speech, hoarse voice, macroglossia, perilaryngeal edema
- Dry and scaly skin; nonpitting edema of face, hands, and feet; thinning or sparce body hair

There are no laboratory tests that indicate presence of **myxedema coma**. The free T_4 level may be low and can be undetectable while TSH levels may vary widely. Often, hypoglycemia, hypochloridemia, hypercalcemia, and mildly elevated creatinine and blood urea nitrogen (BUN) levels can be seen.

Treatment. A multiple-systems approach must be used in treating this emergency.

- Mechanical ventilation is used to control hypoventilation, carbon dioxide narcosis, and respiratory arrest
- Thyroid replacement with **levothyroxine sodium** (L-thyroxine sodium) an intravenous dose of 200 to 400 μg is given initially based on clinical suspicion alone and should not be delayed awaiting test results. Subsequent daily oral replacement dose of L-thyroxine 1.6 μg/kg body weight (reduced to 75% dose if being administered intravenously). Utilization of liothyronine in conjunction with L-thyroxine is a controversial topic as **myxedema coma** is rare and there are no clinical trials.
- Intravenous 3% hypertonic saline and glucose will correct the dilutional hyponatremia and hypoglycemia
- Warming techniques should be used to increase temperature gradually. Recommendations for use of ordinary warm blankets rather than electric heating blankets.

KEY CLINICAL CONCEPT

Caution to avoid warming to raise the body temperature too quickly. Warming faster than 0.25°C to 0.5°C/h could result in vasodilation, drop in blood pressure, and neurologic injury.

- **Empiric stress dose hydrocortisone (100–300 mg daily) should be used to treat a possible adrenocortical insufficiency**
- *Empiric broad-spectrum antibiotics to treat a possible infection if sepsis is suspected. Remember due to the clinical presentation of myxedema coma, typical signs of infection like fever and tachycardia are not likely to be seen.*
- Vasoactive drugs may be used to support blood pressure
- Bradycardia may require treatment with drugs or with a temporary pacemaker

Hyperthyroidism

Toxic goiter and thyrotoxicosis are synonyms for hyperthyroidism. Hyperthyroidism due to **Graves disease** is the most common cause of thyrotoxicosis and is thought to be an autoimmune process, although the terms are used interchangeably. Graves disease results in the formation of autoantibodies that bind to the TSH receptor in thyroid cell membranes and stimulate the gland to hyperfunction.

Etiology. In hyperthyroidism, the thyroid gland enlarges, usually to two or more times the normal size. This releases excess thyroid hormones into the body, increasing the systemic adrenergic activity. Hyperthyroidism is thought to be caused by a failure of the negative-feedback system. Some cases are due to toxic adenomas, toxic-multinodular goiter, thyroiditis, or familial traits.

Clinical Presentation. Thyrotoxicosis of any cause produces many different clinical signs and symptoms.

- Nervousness, restlessness, emotional lability, irritability, heat intolerance, increased sweating
- Fatigue, insomnia, weakness, muscle cramps, weight change
- Tachycardia, palpitations
- *Exophthalmos* (protruding eyeballs) (**Fig. 22-6**).

Diagnosis and Treatment. The diagnosis is confirmed with increased T_4 and T_3 levels and a subnormal TSH. Treatment may be medical or surgical.

- Beta blockers ameliorate the symptoms of hyperthyroidism that result from increased beta-adrenergic tone (palpitations, tachycardia, tremulousness, anxiety, and heat intolerance) and should be started as soon as the diagnosis has been made unless there is a contraindication for their use.
- Thionamides (propylthiouracil [PTU] or methimazole) are the primary drugs to treat **Graves' hyperthyroidism** with the goal of achieving a euthyroid state in 3 to 8 weeks.
- ^{131}I, Ablative therapy with radioiodine or a subtotal thyroidectomy may be used as definitive therapy. After surgery, the patient usually requires daily thyroid medication for life.

Complications. Complications of hyperthyroidism include Heart failure, malnutrition, and ventilatory failure (due to exhaustion) are common. A more life-threatening complication is **thyroid storm**.

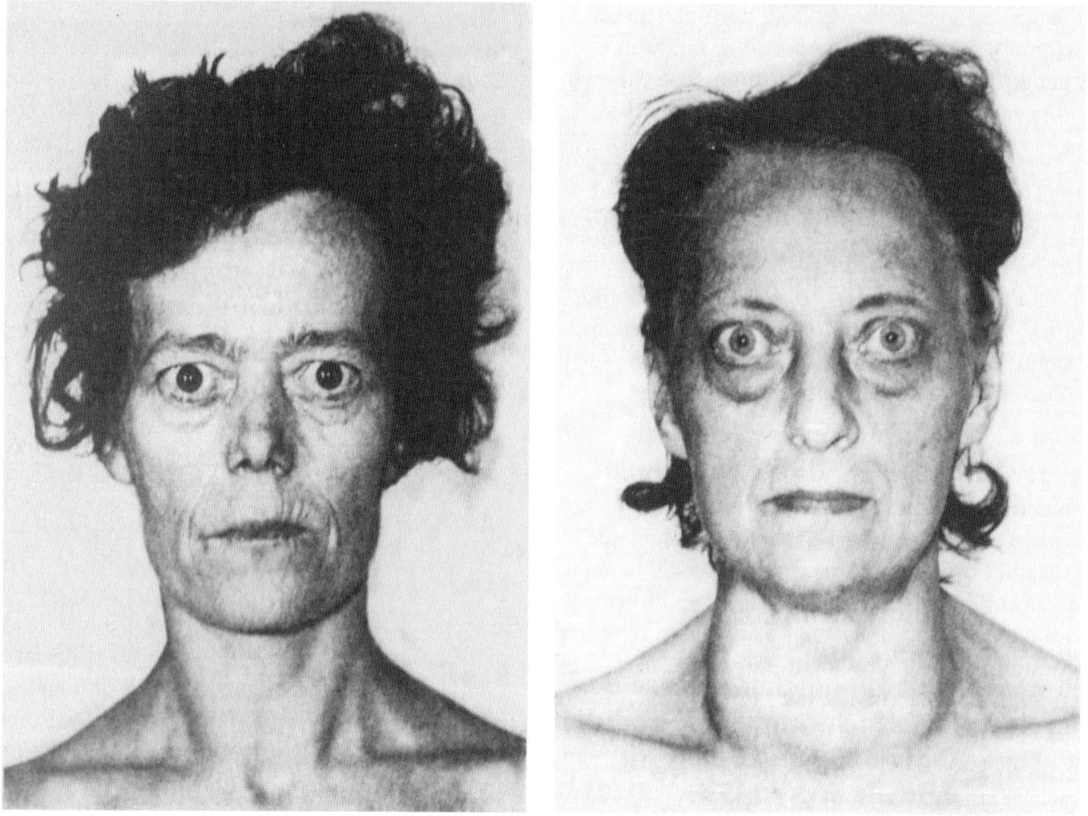

Figure 22-6. Facial appearance of two patients with hyperthyroidism.

Thyrotoxic Crisis (Thyroid Storm)

Thyrotoxic crisis, or thyroid storm, is a life-threatening hypermetabolic state due to hyperthyroidism. Thyrotoxic crisis is a metabolic emergency and has a more than 20% mortality rate.

Pathophysiology. This is the same as for hyperthyroidism.

Etiology. Any factor that increases the synthesis and secretion of thyroid hormones may cause a storm. Classically, thyroid storm occurs because of either previously unrecognized or poorly treated hyperthyroidism. Etiologic factors include subtotal thyroidectomy (due to release of thyroid hormones during the surgery), ketoacidotic states, abruptly stopping antithyroid drugs, or overdosing on thyroid medications (intentional or otherwise). Trauma, stress, infection, or an acute iodine load may precipitate a crisis.

Clinical Presentation. The **thyroid storm** syndrome characteristically includes:

- **Hyperthermia (up to 106°F)** diaphoresis, dehydration, fatigue
- Hypertension with widened pulse pressure, tachydysrhythmias (atrial fibrillation and paroxysmal atrial tachycardia), an S_3 gallop may appear with pulmonary edema
- Nausea, vomiting, diarrhea, jaundice, weight loss, increased appetite
- Altered neurologic status, including agitation, tremors, hyperkinesia, delirium, stupor/coma; seizure
- Proximal muscle weakness, atrophy, and amenorrhea

Due to volume depletion, laboratory results may reveal hemoconcentration, hypercalcemia, hyperglycemia, elevated creatinine and BUN, and elevated aspartate aminotransferase (AST) and alanine aminotransferase (ALT).

> QUICK TIP! Whenever the S_3 heart sound is observed on the exam, consider it associated with, or an early sign of pulmonary edema and HF.

Treatment. Initial treatment of thyroid storm includes stabilization, airway protection, oxygenation, intravenous fluids, and monitoring. Treatment of thyroid storm is of an emergency nature. Treatment is started without waiting for laboratory confirmation of the diagnosis.

- Therapy directed against systemic disturbances includes treatment of fever with **acetaminophen** and external cooling measures. (The core temperature should be monitored.)
- Correction of hypovolemia with intravenous fluids and electrolyte replacement should be administered.
- A reduction in the peripheral effects of excessive thyroid hormone is achieved by intravenous beta blockers **(propranolol, esmolol)** to decrease the hypermetabolic activity, glucocorticoids **(hydrocortisone)** that decrease conversion of T_4 to T_3 and serve as prophylaxis against relative adrenal insufficiency, and in severe cases cholestyramine, plasmapheresis, hemodialysis, or hemoperfusion to remove T_4 and T_3 from the serum.
- A reduction in thyroid hormone production and secretion is accomplished with the use of thionamides (methimazole, PTU) which block new hormone synthesis within 1 to 2 hours after administration. However, they will not block release of hormone from the thyroid gland. Iodine solutions may slow

the release of thyroid hormones. They should be administered about 1 hour after a thionamide has been given. The two most commonly used are Lugol's solution and potassium iodide.

- Treatment of any precipitating or underlying illness is paramount.

Nursing Interventions. General symptomatic supportive care is appropriate. A quiet environment with limited visitors helps decrease external stress. Physiologic stress is often treated daily with **hydrocortisone**.

Cooling therapy is useful in hyperpyrexia. Cooling can be achieved with a variety of cooling blankets or intravascular catheters. Cooling to the extent of shivering and piloerection (hair on arms standing up, ie, goose bumps) may have a rebound effect of raising the temperature even higher and increasing metabolic activity. Adjustment of room temperature is necessary; a cool room is desirable.

Fluids, electrolytes, and glucose are given to prevent dehydration and imbalances and to provide energy to meet metabolic needs.

Complications. **If untreated, thyroid storm results in heart failure, hepatic necrosis, coma, and death**. Mortality rate ranges from 8% to 25%. The presence of stress, infection, nonthyroid surgery, diabetic ketoacidosis, and trauma may result in thyroid storm so intense that it is not amenable to reversal.

22.6 PARATHYROID DYSFUNCTION

Hypoparathyroidism

A major parathyroid dysfunction is hypoparathyroidism. This state is a metabolic crisis when it results in severe hypocalcemia.

Pathophysiology. A deficiency of the PTH causes a hypocalcemia state, resulting in abnormal neuromuscular activity (calcium level < 8.5 mg/dL). It is thought that this deficiency occurs secondary to a dysfunction in the calcium and phosphate concentration feedback loops' control systems.

Etiology. Hypoparathyroidism generally occurs following neck surgery, usually secondary to ischemia or damage of the parathyroid gland. Hypomagnesemia caused by malnutrition and malabsorption, increased renal secretion, and chemotherapeutic agents may also cause hypoparathyroidism. Several genetic conditions, hemochromatosis, Wilson disease, and certain metastases have been implicated. Hypoparathyroidism may also be idiopathic.

Clinical Presentation

- Nausea, vomiting, abdominal cramps
- Dyspnea, laryngeal stridor, cyanosis
- Dry, scaly skin, brittle nails, coarse and thin hair
- Confusion, emotional lability, paresthesias of fingers and toes, and muscular twitching, tetany, hyperreflexia, seizures

KEY CLINICAL CONCEPT

Hypocalcemia is associated with **over-excitation**, for example tetany, cramps, convulsions, and seizure. Hypercalcemia is associated with **over-relaxation,** for example hyporeflexia, coma, bradycardia, fatigue, etc. Similarly, these same excitation versus relaxation tendencies also exist with serum potassium and magnesium.

Diagnosis

- Hypocalcemia, serum calcium corrected for albumin or ionized calcium
- Urine hypophosphaturia and perhaps hypocalciuria
- Low or undetectable PTH level
- Low 1,25-dihydroxyvitamin D level

Two signs are a positive **Trousseau's and Chvostek's signs**, although these signs are not always present. **Trousseau's sign** is elicited by occluding circulation to the arm. This is done by inflating a blood pressure cuff to just above the systolic pressure level. If positive, the patient's hand will develop a carpopedal spasm within 3 minutes. A carpopedal spasm results in a hollow palm position and fingers rigid and flexed at the metacarpophalangeal joints. **Chvostek's sign** is elicited by lightly tapping the facial nerve in front of the ear. If positive, there is a unilateral contraction of the facial muscles.

QUICK TIP! Be familiar with Trousseau's and Chvostek's signs for the exam.

Treatment. The objective of treatment is to raise serum calcium levels to normal. Infusion of **10% calcium gluconate** (93 mg of elemental calcium per 10 mL of solution) infused over 10 to 15 minutes followed by continuous infusion of 0.5 to 1.5 mg/kg/h over 8 to 10 hours while initiating oral calcium replacement.

Chronic hypoparathyroidism management includes **calcium and vitamin D supplementation** along with recombinant human PTH 1-84.

- *Cardiac status must be monitored, especially if the patient is on digitalis.* Digitalis and calcium have a synergistic action, and *hypocalcemia can decrease the effects of digitalis.*

Complications. Complications include seizures, tetany, laryngeal spasm, shock, and death. Long-term complications include chronic kidney disease due to calcification and reduced bone turnover with unclear significance,

Nursing Interventions. Preventive nursing care in hypoparathyroidism may avoid the complications of seizures and tetany. The environment should be modified to be as quiet as possible, including the limiting of visitors until the patient is well stabilized.

- *Administration of calcium as ordered, with special attention to possible infiltration and precipitation if being given intravenously. Avoiding milk products* if being given orally will help ensure maximum benefit with minimal side effects of the drugs. Monitor for hypoventilation or deteriorating respiratory status. Emotional and physical stress often causes hyperventilation. In turn, hyperventilation causes alkalosis, which may precipitate tetany.
- Monitor closely with continuous cardiac monitoring since calcium therapy may alter cardiac conduction times, with resultant dysrhythmias.
- Monitor intake/output, response to medication therapy, neurologic status, and such is applicable to these patients, as the medication therapy will cause a change in their electrolytes and fluid balance.

KEY CONTENT CHECKLIST

- ❒ Be familiar with Trousseau's and Chvostek's signs for the exam.
- ❒ Calcium and phosphate levels change in opposite of each other. When calcium is increased, phosphate decreases. When phosphate levels increase, calcium decreases.
- ❒ Caution to avoid warming to raise the temperature too quickly. Warming faster than 0.25°C to 0.5°C/h could result in vasodilation, drop in blood pressure, and neurologic injury.
- ❒ Hypocalcemia is associated with **over-excitation**, for example tetany, cramps, convulsions, and seizure. Hypercalcemia is associated with **over-relaxation**, for example hyporeflexia, coma, bradycardia, fatigue, etc. Similarly, these same excitation versus relaxation tendencies also exist with serum potassium and magnesium.
- ❒ Whenever the S_3 heart sound is observed on the exam, consider it associated with, or an early sign of pulmonary edema and HF.

Review Questions:

1. Which of the following is a symptom of hypothyroidism?
   a. Paresthesia of the fingers
   b. Sensitivity to cold
   c. Dry scaly skin
   d. All of the above

Answer: D. Rationale: Sensitivity to cold, paresthesia, and dry scaly skin are symptoms of hypothyroidism. This question is a good example of the need to read through all available options, because all may be correct. Since metabolism is downregulated, additional symptoms of hypothyroidism may include weight gain, fatigue, cramps, inattention or memory problems, constipation, thinning hair, brittle nails, and depression. Choose D.

2. Which of the following is NOT associated with hypoparathyroidism?
   a. Trousseau's sign
   b. Thyroidectomy
   c. Hypocalcemia
   d. Gastric ulcers

Answer: D. Rationale: Since parathormone increases calcium levels, hypoparathyroidism is associated with hypocalcemia. This helps eliminate option C. Trousseau's sign is a tetany-like spasm of the muscles of the hand and forearm that occurs with blood pressure cuff inflation in the presence of hypocalcemia, also eliminating option A. Risks of thyroidectomy include manipulation of the parathyroid due to proximity of the glands, which may precipitate hypoparathyroidism and thus, hypocalcemia, eliminating option B as well. Choose D.

3. The goals of treatment for hyperthyroidism include which of the following?
   a. A reduction in the peripheral effects of excessive circulating thyroid hormone
   b. A reduction in the production and secretion of thyroid hormone
   c. Treatment of a precipitating or underlying illness
   d. All of the above

Answer: D. Rationale: Graves disease often results in the weight loss, tachycardia, hyperthermia, warm skin, muscle wasting, exophthalmos, etc. associated with hyperthyroidism. A and B essentially say the same thing. Treatment of the underlying cause is also a key guiding principle for all exam questions. Choose D.

REFERENCES

Bilezikian JP. Hypoparathyroidism. *J Clin Endocrinol Metab.* 2020 Jun 1; 105(6):1722–1736. doi: 10.1210/clinem/dgaa113..

Chiovato L, Magri F, Carlé A. Hypothyroidism in context: where we've been and where we're going. *Adv Ther.* 2019 Sep;36(suppl 2):47–58. doi: 10.1007/s12325-019-01080-8. Epub 2019 Sep 4.

Gafni RI, Collins MT. Hypoparathyroidism. *N Engl J Med.* 2019 May 2; 380(18):1738–1747. doi: 10.1056/NEJMcp1800213.

Jonklaas J, Bianco AC, Bauer AJ, et al. Guidelines for the treatment of hypothyroidism: prepared by the American thyroid association task force on thyroid hormone replacement. *Thyroid.* 2014;24:1670–1751.

Ross DS, Burch HB, Cooper D, et al. 2016 American thyroid association guidelines for diagnosis and management of hyperthyroidism and other causes of thyrotoxicosis. *Thyroid.* 2016;26:1343–1421.

White BA, Harrison JR, Mehlmann LM, eds. *Endocrine and Reproductive Physiology.* 5th ed. St. Louis, MO: Elsevier; 2019.

Ylli D, Klubo-Gwiezdzinska J, Wartofsky L. Thyroid emergencies. *Pol Arch Intern Med.* 2019 Aug 29;129(7-8):526–534. doi: 10.20452/pamw.14876. Epub 2019 Jun 25.

23

Anatomy, Physiology, and Dysfunction of the Pancreas

CHAPTER OVERVIEW AND OBJECTIVES

Focus your attention on disturbances in blood glucose and the clinical conditions associated with abnormal blood glucose levels. Bear in mind, however, that only a few (ie, two to four) questions are likely in the content area covered by this chapter.

After studying this chapter, you should understand the following:

- Compare the diagnostic criteria for diabetic ketoacidosis (DKA) and hyperosmolar hyperglycemic state (HHS).
- Discuss the hallmarks in the treatment of DKA and HHS.
- Describe the common etiologies for hyperglycemia and hypoglycemia in critical care and the associated complications of each.

23.1 ANATOMY

The pancreas has a dual classification. It is considered an accessory digestive gland because it produces many enzymes essential to digestion. These enzymes are released through exocrine glands (glands that release substances through ducts). The pancreas (**Fig. 23-1**) is also classified as an endocrine gland because it releases two hormones, insulin and glucagon, directly into the bloodstream.

Two major types of tissues are found in the pancreas: the acini and the islets of Langerhans. The acini secrete digestive enzymes into the duodenum via exocrine glands. The islets of Langerhans are scattered throughout the pancreas; they may be called pancreatic islets in some texts. Several structurally and functionally different cells make up the islets of Langerhans. The majority of the cells include alpha (20%), beta (68%), and delta cells (10%) (**Fig. 23-2**).

- Alpha cells are located within the clusters of islet cells. They secrete the hormone **glucagon,** which is often called the *hyperglycemic factor*. Alpha cells secrete directly into the venous system of the pancreas.
- Beta cells are located within the clusters of islet cells and are slightly smaller than alpha cells. They secrete **insulin.** The insulin molecules are very complex amino acid structures.
- Delta cells are located within the clusters of the islet cells. They secrete a hormone called somatostatin. Somatostatin has an effect upon the secretion of glucagon and insulin.

23.2 PHYSIOLOGY

Glucagon

The alpha cells of the islets of Langerhans secrete the hormone glucagon, which affects many body cells, especially those of the liver. **Glucagon is secreted when blood amino acid levels rise and in the presence of a decreased blood glucose level.**

Glucagon acts primarily as an antagonist to insulin; its primary site of function is the liver. The most important aspect of this action is to increase blood glucose levels. Glucose metabolism is altered by two important actions of glucagon:

1. Glycogenolysis (the breakdown of liver glycogen stores) and the release of glucose.
2. Gluconeogenesis (the formation of glucose from other substances) provides new glucose.

There is also an increase in fatty acid oxidation and in urea formation as a natural response to glucagon.

Insulin

Insulin is a small protein of two amino acid chains. If the chains become separated, insulin loses its effectiveness. Once secreted into the circulatory system, insulin is removed by the liver and

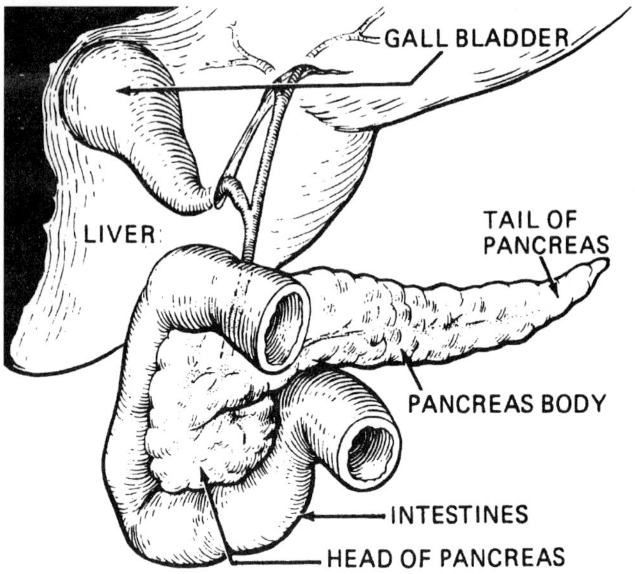

Figure 23-1. The pancreas.

degraded. Most insulin circulates for only about 10 minutes before the degradation process occurs. This allows control and rapid initiation or cessation of insulin's action when it is being administered intravenously.

Insulin's action includes transporting glucose across cell membranes, increasing fatty acid storage, enhancing protein synthesis, facilitating the transport of potassium, and decreasing the breakdown of triglycerides in cells. Factors that facilitate the secretion of insulin are an increase in blood glucose levels and growth hormone levels. Decreased insulin levels result in hyperglycemia, ketosis, and acidosis.

23.3 DYSFUNCTION OF GLUCOSE METABOLISM

The American Diabetes Association (ADA) recommends all hospitalized patients with diabetes or a hyperglycemia (> 140 mg/dL) should undergo $HgbA_{1C}$ testing if not performed in the prior 3 months. States of dysfunctional glucose metabolism that are treated in critical care areas include **diabetic ketoacidosis (DKA), hyperglycemic hyperosmolar state (HHS), hyperglycemia of critical illness, and hypoglycemia.**

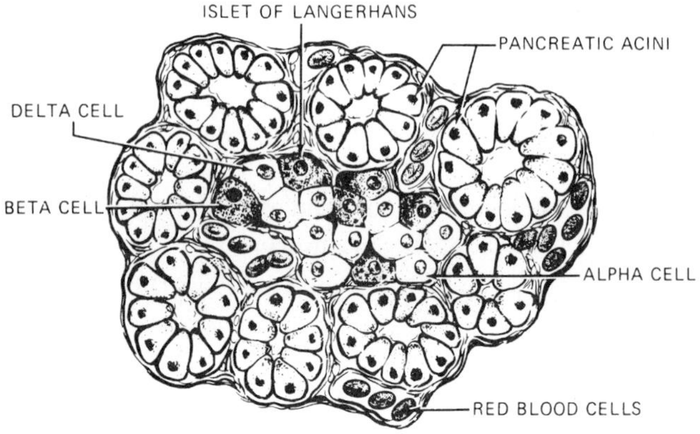

Figure 23-2. Cells of the pancreas.

Diabetic Ketoacidosis

DKA is an acute, life-threatening complication of diabetes, occurring most commonly in patients with type 1 (insulin-dependent) diabetes mellitus but can occur in patients with type 2 diabetes mellitus. DKA represents a state of relative insulin deficiency which is most commonly caused by omission of insulin or infection. The digestion of carbohydrates raises the blood glucose level, which stimulates the pancreas to secrete insulin. If insulin cannot be secreted or secreted in sufficient amounts, hyperglycemia develops. In addition, increased release of cortisol, glucagon, growth hormone, and catecholamines leads to dehydration, ketosis, and electrolyte imbalance.

Pathophysiology. A lack of insulin prevents peripheral cells from utilizing available blood glucose. The liver inhibits the production of glycogen, and such glycogen that is available is rapidly degraded. This releases free glucose into the blood, further raising the blood sugar level.

Since the cells cannot utilize the free glucose, protein stores release amino acids and adipose tissue releases fatty acids. The amino acids and free fatty acids are synthesized by the liver, which is producing excessive amounts of acetyl-CoA. The acetyl-CoA is rapidly degraded into keto, acetoacetic, and beta hydroxybutyric acids. These acids are produced faster than the kidneys and lungs can dispose of them, **causing a metabolic acidosis. Ketones** (keto acids or ketoanions) are excreted by the kidneys, producing a positive urine acetone test. Acetoacetic acid and beta hydroxybutyric acid are oxidized into acetone. **The acetone is exhaled and is responsible for the sweet, fruity smell of the breath in these patients.** Both hyperglycemia and circulating ketones result in an osmotic diuresis, leading to hypovolemia along with electrolyte loss.

Etiology

- Inadequate insulin.
- Increased stress due to illness, infection, trauma, surgery, cardiac conditions, pancreatitis and occasionally psychogenic trauma.
- Pregnancy.
- Certain medications such as glucocorticoids, diuretics, sympathomimetic agents, and atypical antipsychotics may predispose patients to severe hyperglycemia and DKA.
- **Previously undiagnosed type 1 diabetes mellitus can also present with DKA.**

Clinical Presentation

- Rapid presentation, typically over 24 hours.
- Polydipsia, polyuria, polyphagia (usually with weight loss).
- Dyspnea **respirations are Kussmaul in character and may have an acetone smell.**
- Nausea, vomiting, anorexia, and abdominal pain.
- Generalized malaise, dehydration.
- Tachycardia, orthostatic hypotension, and weakness are usually present.
- Neurological symptoms progressing from lethargy to coma, visual disturbances.

Diagnosis. Criteria that help distinguish DKA from HHS are illustrated in **Table 23-1**.

TABLE 23-1 CRITERIA THAT DISTINGUISH DKA FROM HHS

	Diabetic Ketoacidosis (DKA)	*Hyperosmolar Hyperglycemia Syndrome (HHS)*
Plasma glucose level	250–600 mg/dL	> 600 mg/dL
Ketones	present	absent
pH	< 7.3	> 7.30
Bicarbonate	< 18 mEq/L	> 18 mEq/L
Anion gap	> 16	variable
Osmolality	variable	>320 mOsm/kg
Underlying diabetes, commonly	Type 1	Type 2
Symptom onset	acute	days to weeks
Typical age at presentation	Child, teenager, or young adult	Usually middle-aged or older adult

Ketones should be measured via direct measurement. Serum β-hydroxybutyric acid (BHB) is recommended *with elevated levels defined as > 3, but urine ketones may be tested if serum BHB is unavailable. Metabolic acidosis can also result in potentially life-threatening electrolyte imbalances including hyper- or hypokalemia.* A mild leukocytosis and lipase and serum creatinine elevation may be present as a result of ketosis, catecholamine activity, and hypovolemia. DKA should be ruled out in any patient who is comatose, dehydrated, and having deep, labored respirations.

Euglycemic ketoacidosis can occur in certain circumstances resulting in normal plasma glucose levels in the presence of the other features of DKA including ketosis and an anion gap metabolic acidosis. Patients taking sodium-glucose co-transporter 2 (SGLT2) inhibitors, patients with poor PO intake, and pregnant women may present with euglycemic DKA.

Treatment. Treatment goals include correcting and treating the underlying cause, addressing the metabolic abnormalities, monitoring for and treating complications, and addressing patient disposition.

Management of metabolic abnormalities include the following:

- Intravenous fluids
  - Rapid administration of isotonic IV fluid bolus 1000 mL/kg followed by 250 to 500 mL/h. **Dextrose should be added to IVF once serum glucose < 250 mg/dL.**
  - Controversy exists over recommended fluid type (NS vs LR), the most recent recommendations from the ADA Standards of Care do not recommend a specific IVF.
  - **The goal is to correct the extracellular volume depletion without inducing cerebral edema due to too rapid reduction is serum osmolality.**
- Insulin
  - Intravenous insulin should be initiated at 0.1 mL/kg/h. An insulin bolus may or may not be administered prior to infusion initiation.
  - Administration of basal insulin within 12 hours of the insulin infusion may be considered at the patient's usual home dose or a starting weight-based dose on 0.25 units/kg. Alternatively, if basal insulin is initiated at the time of transition from insulin infusion to subcutaneous administration, basal insulin should be administered 2 to 4 hours prior to intravenous insulin discontinuation.
  - Rapid-acting subcutaneous insulin can be used to successfully treat mild-to-moderate DKA if the patient is not in a state of shock.
  - **The goal is 50 to 75 mg/dL reduction in serum glucose each hour. A slow decrease is desired to prevent cerebral edema.**
- Potassium replacement
  - Insulin replacement will result in the shifting of potassium from the serum into the cell, so it is recommended that insulin administration be held until after the potassium level is at least 3 mmol/L.
  - Potassium may be added to intravenous fluids or administered separately.
  - *The serum potassium should be maintained between 4 and 5 mEq/L.*

KEY CLINICAL CONCEPT

The same physiologic concept can also be utilized in different clinical situations. For example, insulin and glucose (D_{50}) can be administered IVP in the event of suspected life-threatening hyperkalemia to shift potassium back into the cells. Calcium chloride IVP may also be given in combination with this to stabilize the cardiac cell membranes.

- **Bicarbonate** use has not been found to make a difference in resolution of acidosis or improvement in hospital outcomes, so it is generally not recommended. Controversy exists over the use of bicarbonate to correct the acidosis present in DKA. Typically, fluid and insulin administration will resolve any acidosis, making bicarbonate administration unnecessary. Bicarbonate given intravenously causes a shift in the bicarbonate/carbonic acid ratio, releasing carbon dioxide. Carbon dioxide crosses the blood–brain barrier, dissolving in the spinal fluid. This increases cerebral acidosis, which may prolong diabetic coma, and also results in need for increased minute ventilation to blow off additional carbon dioxide. Bicarbonate may be considered if pH is less than 7 and if the patient shows signs of cardiac dysfunction or signs of life-threatening hyperkalemia. Venous or arterial pH may be used to monitor effect and to adjust dosing.

Complications. The most common complication of treatment of DKA is hypoglycemia and can be significantly reduced with low-dose insulin and careful monitoring of blood glucose. Acidosis, electrolyte imbalances, acute renal failure, rhabdomyolysis, pulmonary edema, cerebral edema, seizures, shock, coma, and death are the major complications of DKA.

Nursing Interventions

- Blood glucose monitoring hourly to guide the administration of regular insulin infusion.
- Administration and titration of insulin to correct hyperglycemia as indicated by the blood glucose level. Continuous insulin infusion is used with caution to prevent hypoglycemia. The ADA guidelines recommend a patient can be *switched from IV to SQ insulin when the serum glucose is less than 200 mg/dL, serum anion gap is normal, serum bicarbonate is more than 18 mEq/L, and venous pH is more than 7.30.*
- Monitor respiratory status to identify potential impending hypoxia.
- Frequent auscultation of lung sounds to identify pulmonary edema, especially in the presence of underlying cardiac diseases.
- Cardiac monitoring for potential arrhythmias due to electrolyte imbalances. **With hypokalemia, U waves are normally present. In hyperkalemia, peaked or tented T waves are present.** There may be tachycardia, which converts to bradycardia if the hyperkalemia increases.
- Monitor urine output.
- Monitor potassium levels closely due to potassium shifts into and out of the cell. **Initially potassium moves from the cells into blood, and much is excreted in the urine. When insulin is given, potassium shifts back into the cells.**
- Assess neurologic status frequently. Hyperglycemia does not have a deleterious effect on brain cells, but other electrolyte imbalances and cerebral edema will do so. Symptoms of cerebral edema usually appear 12 to 24 hours after the initiation of treatment for DKA. Headache is the earliest symptom, followed by behavior changes and lethargy. Deterioration can be rapid with seizures, pupillary changes, bradycardia, incontinence, and respiratory arrest. *Mortality can be high in patients that develop cerebral edema.*

Hyperglycemic Hyperosmolar State

HHS (formerly known as hyperosmolar, hyperglycemic, nonketotic coma [HHNK]) is classified as **hyperglycemia with profound dehydration without ketosis**. *In HHS, enough insulin is being released to prevent ketosis, but there is not enough to prevent hyperglycemia.*

Pathophysiology. Hyperglycemia increases the solutes in the extracellular fluid, causing a hyperosmolality. As a result, cellular dehydration occurs, which is also the cause of diuresis. Without treatment, an osmotic gradient develops between the brain and the plasma, resulting in dehydration and central nervous system dysfunction. The end result of dehydration is a decreased glomerular filtration rate and the development of azotemia.

Typically, the HHS patient is older, becomes ill, and experiences general malaise. Because of this, the patient is anorexic and eats and drinks poorly, which leads to dehydration. Since the patient is not eating, the body uses protein and fat for energy to maintain body processes. Almost the same pathophysiologic pattern of DKA appears in HHS. The difference is that in HHS, a sufficient amount of insulin is released to prevent the development of ketosis. The patient may be stuporous or comatose before being seen by a physician.

Etiology. The most common causes of HHS are inadequate insulin therapy or undiagnosed diabetes. Frequently, a mild diabetic state exists without any problems until the diabetic is under stress from an infection or other acute condition such as a stroke, myocardial infarction, or trauma. The risk is greater in patients with inadequate fluid intake due to altered thirst mechanism. Similar to DKA, medications such as glucocorticoids may also contribute.

Clinical Presentation. Patients may present with the following:

- Lethargy, coma, seizures
- Polyuria, polydipsia, nausea, vomiting, and weight loss
- Low urine output as fluid depletion becomes more severe, glucosuria
- Signs of dehydration such as dry skin and mucous membranes
- Tachypnea, tachycardia, hypotension
- **Urine and plasma are both negative for ketones.**

Complications of HHS are similar to those of DKA. Death can result with HHS coma if treatment is not quickly initiated.

Treatment

The goal of HHS treatment is to correct of volume deficit and electrolyte abnormalities and to lower blood glucose.

- Intravenous fluids
  - Administration of isotonic IV fluid bolus 1000 mL followed by 250 to 500 mL/h. Dextrose should be added to IVF once serum glucose < 250 mg/dL.
  - Controversy exists over recommended fluid type (NS vs LR), the most recent recommendations from the ADA Standards of Care do not recommend a specific IVF.
  - **The goal is to correct the extracellular volume depletion without inducing cerebral edema due to too rapid reduction is serum osmolality.**
- Insulin
  - Intravenous insulin should be initiated at 0.1 mL/kg/h. An insulin bolus may or may not be administered prior to infusion initiation.
  - Administration of basal insulin within 12 hours of the insulin infusion may be considered at the patient's usual home dose or a starting weight-based dose on 0.25 units/kg. Basal insulin should be administered 2 to 4 hours prior to intravenous insulin discontinuation.
  - Rapid-acting subcutaneous insulin can be used to successfully treat mild-to-moderate HHS if the patient is not in a state of shock.
  - **The goal is 50 to 75 mg/dL reduction in serum glucose each hour. A slow decrease is desired to prevent cerebral edema.**
- Potassium replacement
  - Insulin replacement will result in the shifting of potassium from the serum into the cell, so it is recommended that insulin administration be held until after the potassium level is at least 3 mmol/L.

- Potassium may be added to intravenous fluids or administered separately.
- *The serum potassium should be maintained between 4 and 5 mEq/L.*

- Bicarbonate
  - If metabolic acidosis is present, it is usually corrected by the administration of intravenous fluids.
  - The use of sodium bicarbonate is controversial for the same reasons as it is in DKA.

Nursing Interventions

- Administer intravenous fluids to correct dehydration and hyperosmolality while avoiding complications such as pulmonary edema.
- Hourly blood glucose monitoring.
- Administration and titration of IV insulin to correct hyperglycemia as indicated by blood glucose level. Continuous insulin infusion is used with caution to prevent hypoglycemia.
- Monitor respiratory status frequently to assess for pulmonary edema.
- Continuous cardiac monitoring to identify dysrhythmias due to electrolyte imbalances, especially hypo-/hyperkalemia.
- Assess neurologic status frequently.

Hyperglycemia of Critical Illness. *Stress-induced hyperglycemia in critically ill nondiabetic patients is a common occurrence.* The release of stress hormones—including glucagon, catecholamines, cortisol, and growth hormone, as well as their catabolic effects—causes increased gluconeogenesis and glycogenolysis and resultant hyperglycemia. In addition, these catabolic hormones induce tissue resistance to insulin. A number of additional factors including cytokines, epinephrine, and reactive oxygen species are also involved in initiating hepatic insulin resistance. The reported effects of hyperglycemia in critical illness include impaired immune function, increased inflammation, impaired wound healing, and endothelial cell dysfunction. Hyperglycemia in critically ill patients has been associated with increased intensive care unit (ICU) and hospital length of stay, increased incidence of infections, and increased mortality.

Research on the benefits of moderate glycemic control has led to closer control of hyperglycemia in critically ill patients. **Intravenous insulin protocols to maintain moderate glycemic control, with serum glucose levels 140 to 180 mg/dL, have been shown to significantly reduce mortality rates and improve outcomes for critically ill medical-surgical patients.** As a result, the management of hyperglycemia with the use of insulin protocols has become a standard in critical care. Nursing implications include oversight of intravenous administration of insulin, often with the use of protocols, and close monitoring of serum glucose levels. The risk of hypoglycemia from tight glucose control carries a significant mortality and should be avoided *(except for special populations such as cardiac surgery, which benefit from tight glycemic control).*

More recently glycemic variability (GV) has become an important concept in critical care. GV refers to the oscillations in glucose levels that happen throughout the day. Clinical studies demonstrate glucose fluctuations are associated with oxidative stress, endothelial dysfunction, and inflammation. High GV has been shown to be associated with increased incidence of hypoglycemia, microvascular and macrovascular complications, and increased mortality.

Hypoglycemia

Pathophysiology. A decreased blood level of glucose (< 70 mg/dL) is the criterion for the diagnosis of a hypoglycemia or insulin shock. The decrease may be due to a defect in the process of forming glucose, either gluconeogenesis or glycogenolysis or by the removal of glucose by the use of adipose, muscle, or liver tissues.

Etiology. A broad range of substances such as alcohol, insulin, and sulfonylurea drugs may cause hypoglycemia. A sudden reduction in corticosteroid dose, emesis, reduced oral intake, unexpected interruption of enteral or parenteral feeding, reduced rate of IV dextrose, inappropriate timing of mealtime insulin administration, endocrine dysfunction, liver disease, severe congestive heart failure, and pregnancy may also cause hypoglycemia. Postgastrectomy patients may experience hypoglycemia as well.

Clinical Presentation. The clinical presentation of hypoglycemia can vary among patients. The early signs and symptoms are restlessness, diaphoresis, tachycardia, and hunger. **Beta blockers** may hide these signs and symptoms. *If the hypoglycemia progresses to less than 40 mg/dL, which is referred to as severe hypoglycemia, the central nervous system will be affected and the patient may exhibit bizarre behavior that can progress to a comatose state.* **Headache, dizziness, irritability, fatigue, poor judgment, confusion, visual changes, hunger, weakness, tremors, seizures, nausea, and personality changes are common signs and symptoms.**

> QUICK TIP! Although signs and symptoms of hypoglycemia may sound very basic, a question regarding signs and symptoms of hypoglycemia often shows up on the exam.

Diagnosis and Treatment. A glucose level less than 70 mg/dL warrants intervention. If the hypoglycemia is mild and the patient is able to take oral nutrition, oral glucose may be administered. If the glucose is less than 45 mg/dL administration of 50 mg of 50% dextrose intravenously is preferred. The patient will usually respond within 1 to 2 minutes. A sample of blood may be drawn prior to giving the glucose so that the diagnosis can be confirmed by laboratory tests but should not delay treatment. If hypoglycemia is present in a patient who is *not* diabetic, additional tests must be performed to determine etiology. If hypoglycemia is present in a known diabetic, the underlying cause must be identified and corrected. If the patient is on an insulin regimen, it should be reviewed and adjustments made as appropriate.

Complications. The brain obtains almost all of its energy from glucose metabolism. *If the glucose level is maintained below 50 mg/dL, cerebral ischemia, edema, and neuronal hyperexcitability occur.* If it is not promptly reversed, the low blood glucose levels may cause clonic convulsions and coma, irreversible brain damage, myocardial ischemia or infarction, stroke, and death. Additionally, patients experiencing hypoglycemia are at increased risk of in-hospital falls and longer hospital stay.

The Somogyi Effect

When too much insulin is administered, hypoglycemia occurs. This alerts the body's defense systems, which overreact. With hypoglycemia, certain anti-insulin hormones are secreted. These include epinephrine, glucagon, glucocorticoids, and growth hormones. The secretion of these hormones causes hyperglycemia. A cyclical pattern may develop as a result of hypoglycemia. One day may be followed by 1 or more days of hyperglycemia. In some patients, the cycle is so short that periods alternate within the same day. Symptoms of hypoglycemia in a hyperglycemic patient may indicate a Somogyi effect. Blood sugar levels may reach dangerously high levels because of this rebound effect.

The Dawn Phenomenon

Early-morning increases in blood glucose concentration can occur with no corresponding hypoglycemia during the night. This phenomenon is thought to be secondary to the nocturnal elevations of growth hormone.

KEY CONTENT CHECKLIST

- ❒ Although signs and symptoms of hypoglycemia may sound very basic, a question regarding signs and symptoms of hypoglycemia often shows up on the exam.
- ❒ The combination of insulin and glucose moves potassium from the extracellular to the intracellular space. For example, insulin and glucose (D_{50}) can be administered IVP in the event of suspected life-threatening hyperkalemia to shift potassium back into the cells. Calcium chloride IVP may also be given in combination with this to stabilize the cardiac cell membranes.
- ❒ Know the difference between DKA versus HHS. This always shows up on the exam.
- ❒ Intravenous insulin protocols to maintain moderate glycemic control, with serum glucose levels 140 to 180 mg/dL, have been shown to significantly reduce mortality rates and improve outcomes for critically ill medical-surgical patients.

Review Questions:

1. Which term best describes gluconeogenesis?
   a. Utilization of oxygen stores due to deficits of serum glucose
   b. Breakdown of protein
   c. Formation of glucose from noncarbohydrate precursors
   d. Breakdown of glycogen stores in the liver

Answer: C. Rationale: Gluconeogenesis is the formation of glucose from other substances and provides new glucose. Choose C.

2. Initial insulin therapy for DKA is usually administered by which route?
   a. Intravenous bolus
   b. Intravenous bolus followed by a continuous infusion
   c. Subcutaneously
   d. Intramuscularly

Answer: B. Rationale: Normally, an intravenous bolus of insulin is administered, followed by a slow continuous intravenous infusion. Insulin may be administered by subcutaneous or intramuscular injections; however, this is not advocated in the crisis stage of DKA because of poor peripheral absorption. Rapid-acting subcutaneous insulin can be used to successfully treat mild to moderate DKA if the patient is not in a state of shock. Choose B.

3. HHS coma is differentiated from DKA by which of the following?
   a. Hyperglycemia
   b. Absence of ketosis
   c. Serum osmolality
   d. Serum potassium levels

Answer: B. Rationale: HHS coma follows almost the same pathophysiologic pattern of DKA. The difference is that in HHS coma, a sufficient amount of insulin is released to prevent the development of ketosis; however, there is not enough insulin produced to prevent hyperglycemia. Choose B.

REFERENCES

American Diabetes Association. 16. Diabetes Care in the Hospital: Standards of Medical Care in Diabetes-2023. *Diabetes Care.* 2023;46(suppl 1):S267–S278.

Cruz P. Inpatient hypoglycemia: the challenge remains. *J Diabetes Sci Technol.* 2020 May;14(3):560–566. doi: 10.1177/1932296820918540.

Karslioglu French E, Donihi AC, Korytkowski MT. Diabetic ketoacidosis and hyperosmolar hyperglycemic syndrome: review of acute decompensated diabetes in adult patients. *BMJ.* 2019 May 29;365:l1114. doi: 10.1136/bmj.l1114.

Kreider KE, Gabrielski AA, Hammonds FB. Hyperglycemia syndromes. *Nurs Clin North Am.* 2018 Sep;53(3):303–317. doi: 10.1016/j.cnur.2018.04.001.

Long B, Willis GC, Lentz S, Koyfman A, Gottlieb M. Evaluation and management of the critically ill adult with diabetic ketoacidosis. *J Emerg Med.* 2020 Sep;59(3):371–383. doi: 10.1016/j.jemermed.2020.06.059.

Martinez M, Santamarina J, Pavesi A, Musso C, Umpierrez GE. Glycemic variability and cardiovascular disease in patients with type 2 diabetes. *BMJ Open Diabetes Res Care.* 2021 Mar;9(1):e002032. doi: 10.1136/bmjdrc-2020-002032.

White BA, Harrison JR, Mehlmann LM, eds. *Endocrine and Reproductive Physiology.* 5th ed. St. Louis, MO: Elsevier; 2019.

24

Anatomy, Physiology, and Dysfunction of the Adrenal Glands

CHAPTER OVERVIEW AND OBJECTIVES

Like thyroid disturbances, adrenal dysfunction is less likely to be specifically addressed on the CCRN exam; questions pertaining to adrenal dysfunction will usually appear in the context of another system. Consequently, read this chapter to introduce yourself to key concepts and to familiarize yourself with major functions of the adrenal glands.

24.1 ANATOMY

The adrenal glands are a pair of glands located on the top of each kidney (**Fig. 24-1**). Each of the two glands is identical to the other.

The adrenal gland is composed of two separate parts (**Fig. 24-2**): the adrenal cortex, the outer two-thirds of the gland, and the adrenal medulla, the inner one-third of the gland. A mnemonic for remembering where each part lies is the letter "M," standing for "medulla" and "middle."

The Adrenal Cortex

The adrenal cortex is composed of three distinct regions or zones (**Fig. 24-3**). The outermost zone is the zona glomerulosa. The middle zone is the zona fasciculata. The innermost zone is the zona reticularis. The zona glomerulosa functions by itself. The zona fasciculata and zona reticularis function together as a unit.

The zona glomerulosa is a thin zone located on the outer part of the cortex, directly under the capsular covering. The cells in this zone are arranged in clumps. The regulation of the hormone (aldosterone) secreted in the zona glomerulosa is completely independent of the regulatory controls over the zona fasciculata and the zona reticularis. The regulatory control of the zona glomerulosa is the release of adrenocorticotropic hormone (ACTH), releasing factors from the hypothalamus and ACTH-stimulating factors from the adenohypophysis.

The zona fasciculata is the largest of the three zones. Its cells are arranged in straight rows. The zona reticularis is composed of an anastomosing network of cells. These two zones function together to regulate cortisol and androgen hormones and are controlled by the same regulatory mechanisms of the adenohypophysis.

The Adrenal Medulla

Cells of the adrenal medulla (Fig. 24-2) develop from the same embryologic source as the sympathetic neurons. These cells are also called chromaffin cells because of their histologic staining characteristics. Because of their origin, *the cells of the adrenal medulla are related functionally to the sympathetic nervous system.*

24.2 PHYSIOLOGY

Functionally, the adrenal cortex and the adrenal medulla are totally different. Without adrenocortical hormones or replacement therapy, death occurs in 3 to 14 days.

Adrenocortical Hormones

The hormones secreted by the adrenal cortex are classified as corticosteroids, since they are synthesized from the steroid cholesterol. As a group, more than 30 corticosteroids may be referred to as corticoids.

The adrenal cortex secretes three classes of hormones: the glucocorticoids, the mineralocorticoids, and the androgenic hormones.

The Glucocorticoids. Glucocorticoids play a major role in utilization of carbohydrates, proteins, and fats.

Cortisol. This glucocorticoid is responsible for 95% of the adrenocortical secretory actions. Cortisol is the most important

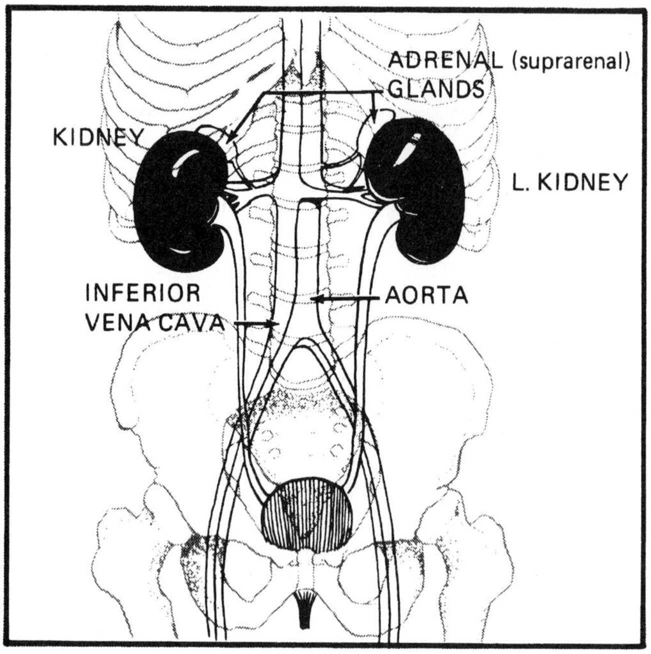

Figure 24-1. Location of the adrenal glands.

hormone of this class of steroid hormones, affecting all body cells (especially the liver). *It is secreted by the zona fasciculata and the zona reticularis in response to stress (both physical and psychogenic), trauma, and infection.*

> **QUICK TIP!** Cortisol secretion during stress is associated with the same physiologic rationale for why stress-dose hydrocortisone is given during vasopressor-refractory septic shock.

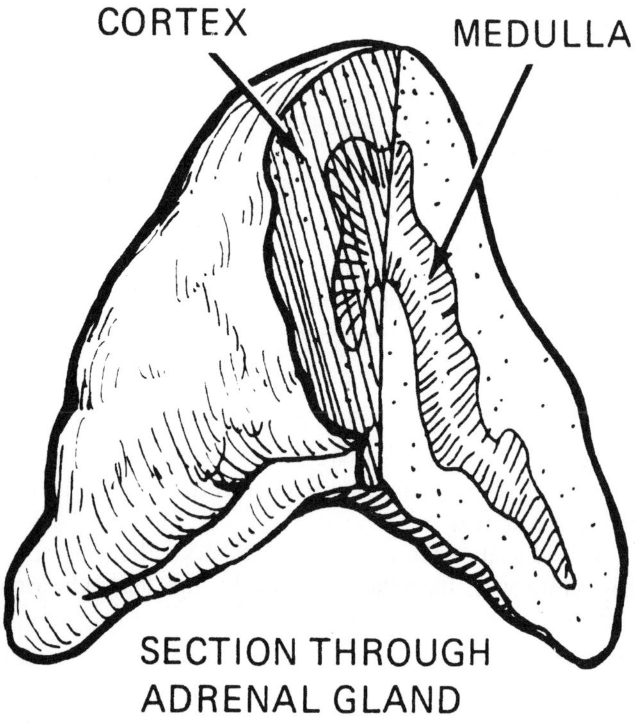

Figure 24-2. Section showing cortex and medulla of the adrenal gland.

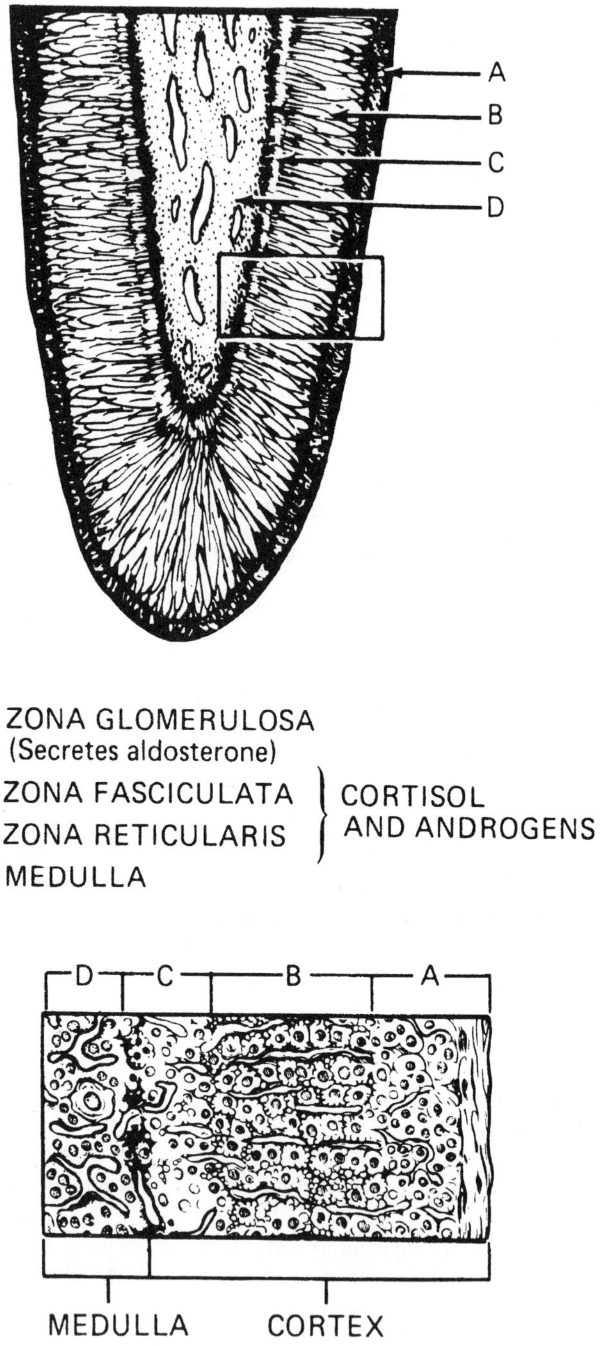

Figure 24-3. Zones and medulla of the adrenal gland.

Cortisol is active in all metabolic processes.

- Stimulates gluconeogenesis by the liver at up to 10 times its normal rate and decreases the rate of glucose utilization by the cells, *causing blood glucose concentration to rise during stress states.*
- Decreases protein storage in all body cells except the liver, resulting in muscle weakness and decreased functions of immunity in the lymphoid tissues. The proteins stored in tissues are shifted to the liver, which results in decreased protein synthesis.
- Promotes fatty acid mobilization weakly, but that mobilization is sufficient to provide some fat for body energy.
- Possesses a strong anti-inflammatory effect and, in sufficient amounts, may block and/or reverse the inflammatory process.

Secretion of the glucocorticoids is controlled almost entirely by ACTH secreted by the anterior pituitary gland. The hypothalamus provides the negative feedback mechanism responsible for cortisol-releasing factors (CRFs) and cortisol-inhibitory factors (such as exogenous intake of corticosteroids).

The Mineralocorticoids. Mineralocorticoids are named as such since their action is chiefly with the extracellular fluid electrolytes (minerals) sodium and potassium. The most important mineralocorticoid is **aldosterone,** which is secreted in the zona glomerulosa.

Aldosterone. This mineralocorticoid's most important function is regulating the movement of sodium and potassium through the renal tubular walls. It also plays a minor role in hydrogen ion transport.

Aldosterone exerts its action on the distal convoluted tubules and the collecting ducts. There is a slight effect on sweat glands (to conserve salt in hot conditions). *The primary action of aldosterone is to cause an increase in sodium reabsorption and potassium and hydrogen ion excretion by the kidney.* Since water follows sodium, **aldosterone** secretion tends to change the extracellular fluid volume in proportion to its secretion.

Aldosterone excess may rapidly cause severe hypokalemia and alkalosis, including muscle weakness, and muscle paralysis if the potassium level is reduced to half of its normal value. Hypertension may occur as a result of the increase in extracellular fluid volume.

The release of **aldosterone** is stimulated by an increased serum potassium level, the renin–angiotensin cascade, decreased serum sodium levels, and ACTH.

QUICK TIP! Increased aldosterone may cause hypokalemia and sodium retention. Decreased aldosterone levels may cause hyperkalemia and hyponatremia.

Decreased levels of **aldosterone** allow the extracellular level of potassium to rise to double the normal potassium level, resulting in severe hyperkalemia and cardiac toxicity, as evidenced by weakness of contractions. A concurrent decrease in serum sodium and increase in water loss occurs. A potassium level only slightly higher will cause a cardiac death.

The Androgens. Several androgens are secreted by the adrenal cortex, but their alterations are not usually a primary cause for treatment in a critical care area and are not covered in this text except to mention that they are secreted by the zona fasciculata and the zona reticularis.

Adrenal Medullary Hormones

The hormones secreted by the adrenal medulla are classified as catecholamines and have very far-reaching effects. Catecholamines are synthesized in the adrenal medulla as well as by the endings of sympathetic adrenergic nerve fibers, the brain, and some peripheral tissues. *Both of the catecholamines secreted by the adrenal medulla have an effect on the adrenergic (sympathetic) receptor sites. There are three sites: termed alpha, beta$_1$ (b$_1$), and beta$_2$ (b$_2$).* **Table 24-1** lists the adrenergic receptors and their functions.

TABLE 24-1. ADRENERGIC RECEPTORS AND THEIR FUNCTIONS

Alpha Receptor	*Beta Receptor*
Vasoconstriction (α_1, α_2)	Vasodilatation (β_2)
Iris dilatation (α_1)	Cardioacceleration (β_1)
Intestinal relaxation (α_1, α_2)	Increased myocardial strength (β_1)
Intestinal sphincter contraction (α_2)	Intestinal relaxation (β_2)
Pilomotor contraction (α_1)	Uterine relaxation (β_2)
Bladder sphincter contraction (α_1)	Bronchodilatation (β_2)
Ureter (α_1)	Colorigenesis (β_2)
Vas deferans (α_1)	Glycogenolysis (β_2)
Uterus (α_1)	Lipolysis (β_1)
Urethral (α_1)	Bladder relaxation (β_2)
Bronchioles (α_1)	
Inhibit insulin release (α_2)	
Glucagon release from pancreas (α_2)	
Platelet aggregation (α_2)	

Ordinarily, the norepinephrine secreted directly in a tissue by adrenergic nerve endings remains active for only a few seconds, illustrating that its reuptake and diffusion away from the tissue are rapid. However, the norepinephrine and epinephrine secreted into the blood by the adrenal medulla remain active until they diffuse into some tissue, where they are destroyed by enzymes. This occurs mainly in the liver. Therefore, the effects last about 10 times as long as compared to direct sympathetic stimulation.

Epinephrine (Adrenaline). Epinephrine (adrenaline) accounts for 80% of the total catecholamine secreted by the adrenal medulla; *it excites both alpha- and beta-adrenergic receptor.*

A major action of epinephrine is the "fight or flight" body response to stress. These actions would include positive effects on the cardiac muscle, shifting of blood to certain muscles, decreasing gastrointestinal function, bronchiolar dilatation accompanied by hyperpnea and tachypnea, and an increase in serum glucose level.

Epinephrine is released by sympathetic nervous system stimulation and other hormones, such as insulin and histamine.

Norepinephrine. Norepinephrine accounts for 20% of catecholamines secreted by the adrenal medulla. **Norepinephrine excites alpha receptors** and to a slight degree beta receptors. The action of norepinephrine is similar to that of epinephrine with two notable exceptions. The effect of norepinephrine on cardiac and metabolic functions is not as intense as that of epinephrine. Also, norepinephrine has a more intense action than epinephrine on skeletal muscle vasculature. *This increases peripheral vascular resistance as a result of the increased vasoconstriction.*

The sites of action for norepinephrine are body cells and vascular beds, and releasing factors for norepinephrine are the same as for epinephrine.

24.3 DYSFUNCTION OF THE ADRENAL CORTEX

Adrenal insufficiency is a major life-threatening dysfunction of the adrenal cortex. It is also known as hypoadrenalism and/or hypocorticism.

Addison Disease

Addison disease is a chronic dysfunction of the adrenal glands, resulting in an inadequate adrenal secretion of cortisol and aldosterone *(adrenal insufficiency)*. Addison disease results from progressive destruction of the adrenals, with up to 90% or more of the glands being affected before adrenal insufficiency appears. Mineralocorticoid decrease results in an aldosterone deficiency, leading to increased excretion of sodium, chloride and water in the urine and subsequent dehydration. A decrease in glucocorticoids results in a cortisol deficiency. This results in stimulation of the hypophysis to secrete ADH unrestrained. Resistance to both physical and psychogenic stress is decreased. Acquired forms of primary adrenal insufficiency are relatively rare, may occur at any age, and affect both sexes.

Symptoms. Adrenal cortex dysfunction results in a deficiency of mineralocorticoids and glucocorticoids. Symptoms are nonspecific and include weakness, fatigue, musculoskeletal pain, weight loss, abdominal pain, postural dizziness, depression, and anxiety. On examination, the patient may have hyperpigmentation especially in sun-exposed areas, skin creases, dry mucus membranes, and scars. Melanin pigmentation (**Fig. 24-4**) is increased in most cases of Addison disease. This pigmentation is unevenly distributed and is probably due to increased secretion of melanocyte-stimulating hormone (MSH) and ACTH from the adenohypophysis. Low blood pressure with orthostatic hypotension is also often found. *Laboratory abnormalities include hyponatremia and hyperkalemia.*

Etiology. The most common cause of Addison disease is autoimmune destruction of the adrenals. Adrenal infiltration or injury secondary to adrenal hemorrhage, metastasis, infection (tuberculosis, human immunodeficiency virus [HIV], cytomegalovirus [CMV], candidiasis, histoplasmosis, syphilis), hemochromatosis, amyloidosis, or bilateral adrenalectomy can also cause Addison disease. Autoimmune Addison disease can be associated with thyroid disease, diabetes mellitus, celiac disease, premature ovarian failure, autoimmune gastritis, and pernicious anemia.

Treatment. If untreated, the patient dies within a few days to a few weeks from circulatory shock. Replacement therapy with glucocorticoids, generally **hydrocortisone** three times daily, and a mineralocorticoid, **fludrocortisone** are necessary. Medication dosages are titrated based on clinical assessment.

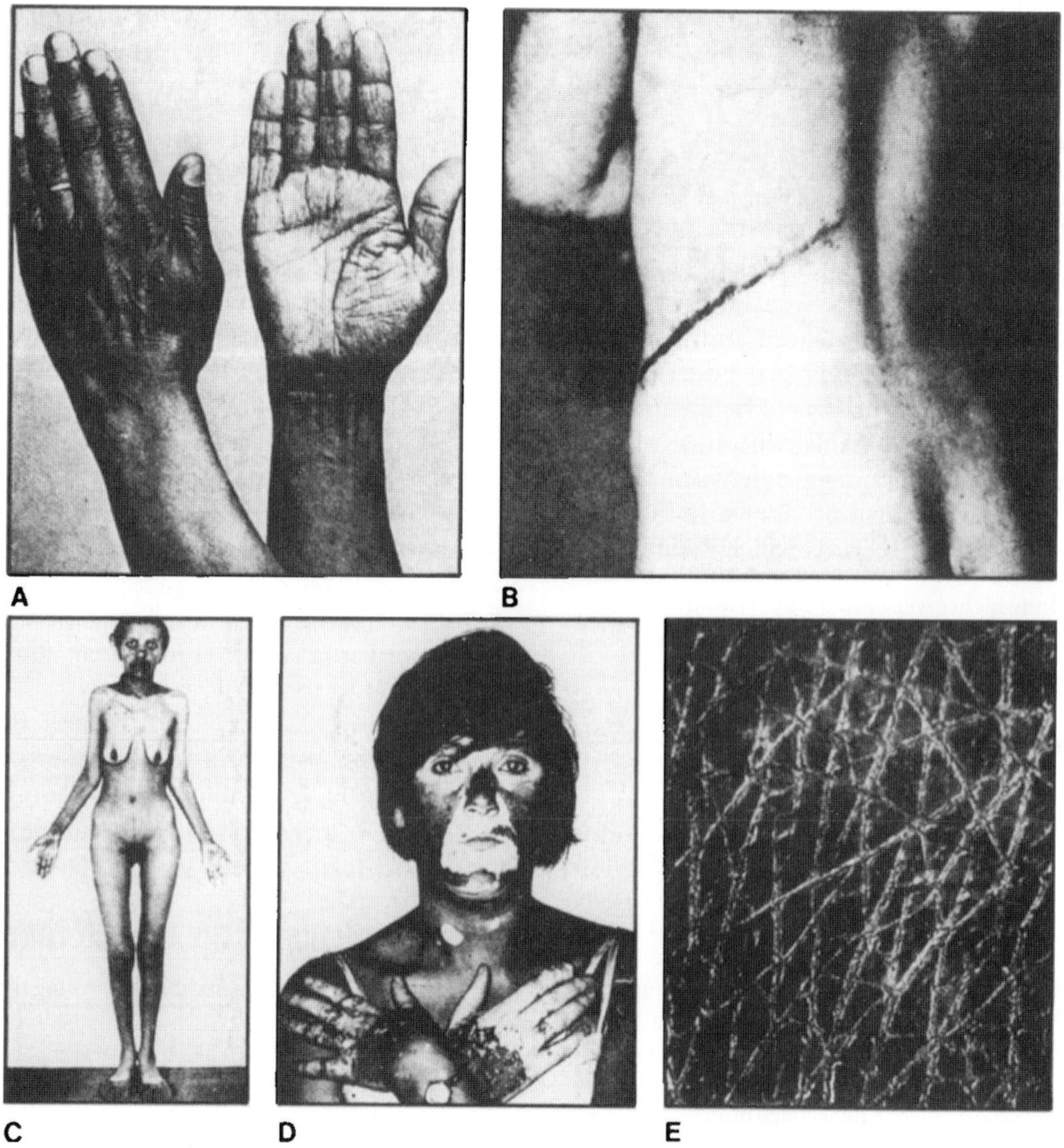

Figure 24-4. Melanin oversecretion in Addison disease.

Strict adherence to a diet low in potassium and high in sodium may help prevent complications. If a tumor is the etiologic factor, surgery is performed.

Complications. Without appropriate identification and treatment, Addison disease can lead to an *acute adrenal insufficiency (crisis),* which may be fatal. Such a crisis may occur any time if there is an increase in stress, since the adrenal cortex cannot increase its production of cortisol. Steroids should be increased in patients with Addison disease who are under stress from infection, trauma, surgery, or other types of stress. Even a slight cold necessitates increased steroid hormone levels.

Acute Adrenal Insufficiency

Acute adrenal insufficiency is an emergency medical condition caused by insufficient cortisol. It is often referred to as an adrenal crisis.

Etiology. Patients typically have the diagnosis of Addison disease before presenting with adrenal crisis precipitated by stress from infection, trauma, surgery, or another physical or psychological stressor. However, Addison disease is notoriously difficult to diagnose due to nonspecific presenting signs and symptoms, so patients may present in adrenal crisis with the undiagnosed underlying disease. Less commonly, the initiation of thyroxine (T_4) replacement may induce crisis due to increased cortisol metabolism or carbamazepine, mitotane, or St. John's wort which increase cortisol clearance.

Clinical Presentation

- Severe weakness, back pain, confusion , reduced consciousness, delirium, syncope, coma
- Nausea, vomiting, and abdominal pain which may mimic an acute abdomen
- Hypotension, shock

Diagnosis. Patient history, physical examination, presenting symptoms, and laboratory abnormalities are usually sufficient to provide a tentative diagnosis and indicate the need for immediate treatment. Hyponatremia, hyperkalemia, hypoglycemia, and hypercalcemia are generally present. Definitive laboratory studies for the diagnosis of Addison disease are generally not completed when a patient is in crisis but a baseline cortisol and ACTH level can be obtained prior to treatment; however, treatment should not be held while awaiting test results.

Complications. Death is the common complication, although it is usually preceded by dysrhythmias, hypovolemia, shock, and coma.

Treatment

- Rapid administration of 1 L isotonic saline or 5% glucose in isotonic saline followed by continuous isotonic saline based on patient need
- **Hydrocortisone** 100 mg IV immediately followed by 200 mg/day as continuous infusion for 24 hours, reduced to 100 mg/day the following day

Nursing Interventions

- Monitor respiratory status. If serial arterial blood gases show deteriorating respiratory status, the patient may be intubated and placed on a ventilator. Standard nursing procedures for all artificially ventilated patients should be followed.
- Continuous cardiac and hemodynamic monitoring for dysrhythmias, hypotension, and shock.
- Monitor intake and output.
- Monitor laboratory values for renal function and electrolyte abnormalities.
- Providing emotional support of the patient and family is of utmost importance in an attempt to decrease exogenous stress as much as possible.

Adrenal Insufficiency in Critical Illness

Adrenal insufficiency in critical illness is also referred to as critical illness-related corticosteroid insufficiency (CIRCI). As a part of the normal stress response, the hypothalamic–pituitary–adrenal (HPA) axis is activated, causing the release of cortisol. *During critical illness states, adrenal insufficiency can develop* due to dysfunction at the hypothalamic, pituitary, and/or adrenal level (HPA axis). The integrity of the HPA axis can be assessed with a random cortisol level. Dysfunction at the HPA axis will result in low circulating cortisol levels. *A random cortisol level of less than 10 μg/dL in a moderately stressed (vasopressor-independent) critically ill patient is suggestive of HPA dysfunction.* A corticotropin stimulation test can also be used to diagnose adrenal insufficiency in critically ill patients. A delta serum cortisol level of less than 9 μg/dL 60 min after a high-dose corticotropin (250 μg) test is suggestive of adrenal insufficiency.

Current evidence recommends administration of steroids in patients with septic shock that is not responsive to fluid and moderate to high-dose vasopressor therapy may reduce the risk of death. No specific steroid is recommended over another, but **hydrocortisone** 200 mg/day divided as 50 mg IV q6h is the most commonly used regimen.

Hypercortisolism (Cushing Syndrome)

Hypercortisolism is a marked increase in the production of mineralocorticoids, glucocorticoids, and androgen steroids, resulting in the condition known as Cushing syndrome **(not to be confused with Cushing triad, which is associated with brain herniation)**.

Etiology. Cushing syndrome is usually due to an adrenocorticotropin (ATH)-secreting pituitary tumor. It occurs more frequent in women than men. A pituitary tumor causes increased release of ACTH, which results in hyperplasia of the adrenal cortex. An ectopic ACTH-secreting adenoma of the lungs (most common), pancreas, thyroid, or thymus and carcinoma of the gallbladder, cervix, or prostate may also cause hypercortisolism.

Clinical Presentation

- Increased gluconeogenesis, resulting in hyperglycemia
- Increased protein catabolism resulting in severe weakness, suppressed immune system, osteoporosis, and thin, fragile skin.
- Increased fatty tissue deposits, resulting in the typical "moon face," and increased trunk fat or "buffalo hump" (**Fig. 24-5**).
- Increased mineralocorticoids (aldosterone) result in increased potassium excretion, causing dysrhythmias, renal disorders, and muscle weakness.
- Increased cortisol may cause mood swings ranging from euphoria to depression. It can also cause insomnia, short-term memory deficits, decreased attention span, or severe psychotic paranoia.

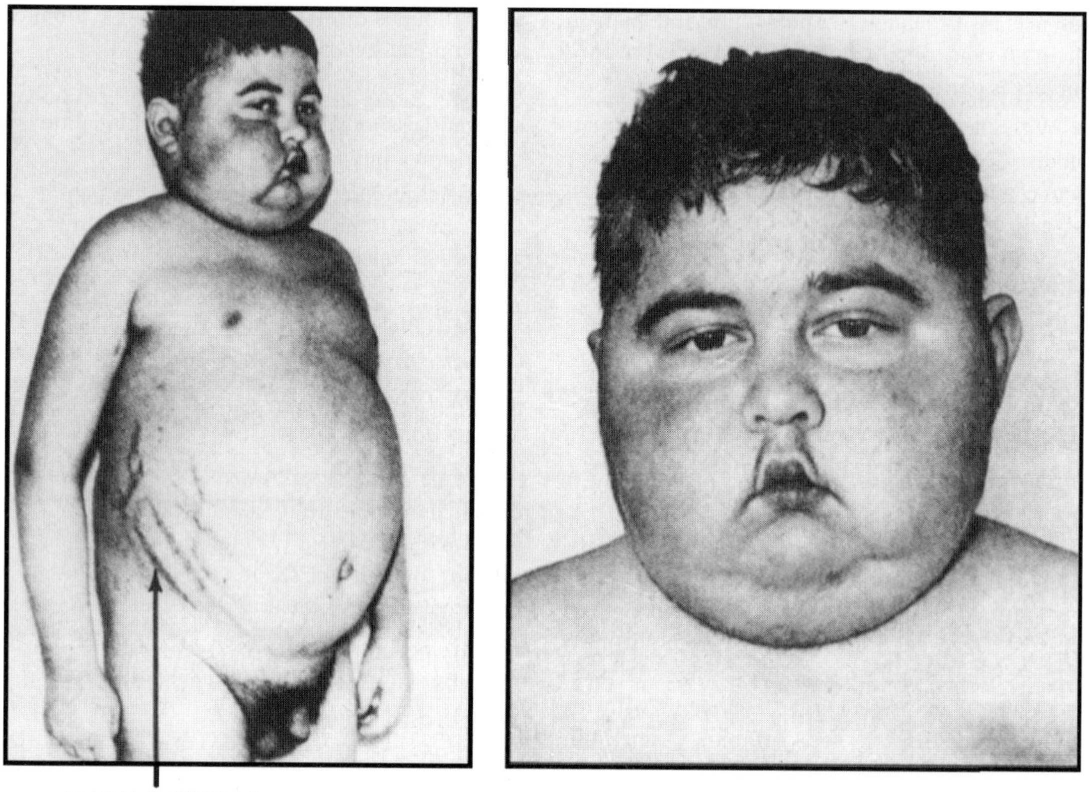

Figure 24-5. Cushing syndrome, showing "moon face," trunk fat, and purple striae.

- Increased **aldosterone** causes a decrease in sodium secretion, resulting in an *increase in fluid retention, resulting in edema and usually an increase in blood pressure and weight.*
- Increased sex hormones (androgens) cause increased facial hair and acne.
- Pink and purplish striae of the abdomen, underarms, and buttocks may be seen. There is easy bruising and hematoma formation.

Diagnosis. Patient history, physical examination, and presenting symptoms are usually sufficient to provide a tentative diagnosis. Definitive laboratory studies are those evaluating endocrine function and identifying resultant system dysfunction or imbalance. Magnetic resonance imaging (MRI) is most sensitive for evaluating for presence of a pituitary tumor. Hyperglycemia, acidosis, and increased cortisol levels are present.

Treatment. Treatment consists of removing the tumor if possible, which will necessitate steroid replacement. A diet low in sodium and high in potassium is required.

> QUICK TIP! Diet questions are rare on the exam. Perhaps only one diet question will be asked, if any. Do not focus exam preparation on diet modifications if this is not an area of strength.

Nursing Interventions

- Routine postsurgical nursing care is required
- Monitor for endocrine imbalance, indicating a need for replacement therapy.
- Monitor for signs of infection.
- Providing education relating to diet therapy and medication regimens is essential to prevent recurrent endocrine crises.

Note: The increase in mineralocorticoids may also cause Conn syndrome (increased sodium and blood pressure and decreased potassium levels due to a benign aldosterone-secreting tumor).

Hypofunction of the Adrenal Medulla

Hypofunction of the adrenal medulla does not cause systemic problems because the sympathetic nervous system will compensate for decreases in epinephrine and norepinephrine.

Hyperfunction of the Adrenal Medulla

Hyperfunction of the adrenal medulla can be life-threatening primarily because of the severe persistent or paroxysmal hypertension that leads to cerebrovascular accident and congestive heart failure. In hyperfunction, epinephrine increases blood pressure, cardiac output, pulse, and metabolism. Norepinephrine increases the blood pressure more than epinephrine does. Hyperfunction may be precipitated by stress and/or exertion, ingestion of tyrosine-containing foods, increased caffeine intake, external pressure on the tumor, and anesthesia.

Pheochromocytoma

Pheochromocytomas produce, store, and secrete catecholamines. Hyperfunction of the adrenal medulla is the most common cause of pheochromocytoma. Pheochromocytoma is an encapsulated, vascular tumor of chromaffin tissue of the adrenal medulla.

Diagnosis. Signs and symptoms are the major diagnostic clues. However, hyperfunction of the adrenal medulla often resembles other disorders that must be ruled out. These include diabetes mellitus, essential hypertension, and psychoneurosis. Although pheochromocytoma occurs in less than 0.6% of hypertensive individuals, it is an important correctable cause of hypertension.

The initial testing is recommended to be measurements of urinary and plasma fractionated metanephrine. **Diagnosis may be confirmed via CT scan.**

Clinical Presentation. The outstanding symptom is episodes of extremely high blood pressure secondary to the excessive medullary hormones. Other signs and symptoms include increased sympathetic nervous activity, sweating, headache, palpitations and dysrhythmias, postural hypotension, apprehension, nausea/vomiting, tremor, pallor or flushing of the face, abdominal and/or chest pain, and hyperglycemia.

Treatment

- Surgical removal of the pheochromocytoma, performed either laparoscopically or via an open laparotomy for very large, invasive tumor.
- Preoperative **alpha-adrenergic blocking agents** to control hypertension. **Calcium channel blockers** can be added to alpha blockers if needed. A **beta blocker** may be added to help control tachycardia
- Prognosis is dependent on the timing of diagnosis and the presence of malignancy, which cannot be determined by histologic examination, but a tumor is considered malignant if metastases are present. Lifetime surveillance is usually required, as metastases may occur years afterward.

Nursing Interventions

- Promote rest and reassure the patient
- Monitor blood pressure closely.
- Routine postoperative procedures are instituted
- Monitor for shock, hypotension (due to decreased levels of **epinephrine** and **norepinephrine**), hypoglycemia, and hemorrhage (the adrenal glands being very vascular).

KEY CONTENT CHECKLIST

- ❒ Diet questions are rare on the exam. Perhaps only one diet question will be asked, if any. Do not focus exam preparation on diet modifications if this is not an area of strength.
- ❒ *Pheochromocytomas produce, store, and secrete catecholamines.* Hyperfunction of the adrenal medulla is the most common cause of pheochromocytoma. Pheochromocytoma symptomatic hypertension (HTN), urgent, or emergent HTN. Diagnosis is made via computed tomography (CT) scan.
- ❒ Increased aldosterone levels may cause hypokalemia and hypernatremia. May be found in Cushing disease.
- ❒ Decreased aldosterone levels may cause hyperkalemia and hyponatremia. May be found in Addison disease.
- ❒ Cortisol secretion during stress is associated with the same physiologic rationale for why stress-dose hydrocortisone is given during vasopressor-refractory septic shock.

Review Questions:

1. Hyperfunction of the adrenal medulla is associated with which of the following?

a. Pheochromocytoma
b. Addison disease
c. Graves disease
d. Cushing syndrome

Answer: A. Rationale: Hyperfunction of the adrenal medulla is the most common cause of pheochromocytoma. Pheochromocytoma is an encapsulated, vascular tumor of chromaffin tissue of the adrenal medulla. Choose A.

2. The clinical situation of large fluctuations in blood glucose, such as hypoglycemia symptoms in a patient with hyperglycemia, is described by which term?

a. Somogyi effect
b. Addison response
c. Adams syndrome
d. Pancreatic flash

Answer: A. Rationale: A cyclical pattern may develop. Hypoglycemia 1 day may be followed by 1 or more days of hyperglycemia. In some patients, the cycle is so short that periods alternate within the same day. Symptoms of hypoglycemia in a hyperglycemic patient may indicate a Somogyi effect. Choose A.

REFERENCES

Annane D, Pastores SM, Rochwerg B, et al. Guidelines for the diagnosis and management of critical illness-related corticosteroid insufficiency (CIRCI) in critically ill patients (part I): Society of Critical Care Medicine (SCCM) and European Society of Intensive Care Medicine (ESICM) 2017. *Intensive Care Med.* 2017 Dec;43(12):1751–1763. doi: 10.1007/s00134-017-4919-5. Epub 2017 Sep 21.

Bornstein SR, Allolio B, Arlt W, et al. Diagnosis and treatment of primary adrenal insufficiency: an endocrine society clinical practice guideline. *J Clin Endocrinol Metab.* 2016 Feb;101(2):364–89. doi: 10.1210/jc.2015-1710. Epub 2016 Jan 13.

Fleseriu M, Auchus R, Bancos I, et al. Consensus on diagnosis and management of Cushing's disease: a guideline update. *Lancet Diabetes Endocrinol.* 2021 Dec;9(12):847–875. doi: 10.1016/S2213-8587(21)00235-7. Epub 2021 Oct 20.

Lenders JWM, Kerstens MN, Amar L, et al. Genetics, diagnosis, management and future directions of research of phaeochromocytoma and paraganglioma: a position statement and consensus of the Working Group on Endocrine Hypertension of the European Society of Hypertension. *J Hypertens.* 2020 Aug;38(8):1443–1456. doi: 10.1097/HJH.0000000000002438.

White BA, Harrison JR, Mehlmann LM, eds. *Endocrine and Reproductive Physiology.* 5th ed. St. Louis, MO: Elsevier; 2019.

PART III
Endocrine Practice Exam

1. **An increase in hormone concentration will cause which of the following?**
   (A) an inhibition of hormone-releasing factors
   (B) an increase of hormone-releasing factors
   (C) increased production by the pituitary
   (D) increased production by the hypothalamus

2. **The hormones of the adrenal medulla are under the control of which of the following?**
   (A) hypothalamus
   (B) posterior pituitary (neurohypophysis)
   (C) anterior pituitary (adenohypophysis)
   (D) autonomic nervous system

3. **All of the adenohypophyseal (anterior pituitary) hormones have an effect on a target gland EXCEPT:**
   (A) adrenocorticotropin
   (B) growth hormone
   (C) thyroid-stimulating hormone
   (D) luteinizing hormone

4. **The anterior pituitary receives stimulation from the hypothalamus through which of the following?**
   (A) vascular system
   (B) sympathetic nervous system
   (C) parasympathetic nervous system
   (D) central nervous system

5. **Which of the following is NOT secreted by the anterior pituitary gland?**
   (A) ACTH (adrenocorticotropic hormone)
   (B) thyroid-stimulating hormone
   (C) growth hormone
   (D) ADH (antidiuretic hormone)

6. **Which of the following is a factor inhibiting the release of growth hormone?**
   (A) hypoglycemia
   (B) exercise
   (C) hyperglycemia
   (D) decreased amino acid levels

7. **ADH release is inhibited by which of the following?**
   (A) increased serum osmolality
   (B) decreased serum osmolality
   (C) increased serum sodium
   (D) increased potassium level

Questions 8 and 9 refer to the following scenario:

A 25-year-old man is admitted to the intensive care unit with a diagnosis of brainstem contusion. Two days after admission, the patient is consistently thirsty. You note that the urine output is nearly 2000 mL in 8 h with an intake of 950 mL. Blood pressure is 140/74 mm Hg, pulse 84, and respiratory rate 22. The following laboratory data are available:

Serum		Urine	
Na^+	155	Na^+	14
K^+	3.7	Osmolality	312
Cl^-	114	Specific gravity	1.005
HCO_3^-	23		

8. **Based on the preceding information, which condition is likely to be developing?**
   (A) syndrome of inappropriate antidiuretic hormone secretion (SIADH)
   (B) adult-onset diabetes mellitus
   (C) anterior pituitary stimulation
   (D) diabetes insipidus

9. **Which treatment could you expect to be given to this patient?**
   (A) Desmopressin acetate (DDAVP, 1-desamino-8-D-arginine vasopressin)
   (B) D_5W in a 200-mL/h fluid bolus
   (C) diuretics
   (D) fluid restriction

10. **A patient is admitted to the intensive care unit with a diagnosis of SIADH. Which laboratory data would be expected if this diagnosis is correct?**
    (A) hyponatremia
    (B) hypernatremia
    (C) increased serum osmolality
    (D) hyperkalemia

11. **Common clinical findings of SIADH may include which symptom?**
    (A) mental status changes
    (B) tachycardia
    (C) polyuria
    (D) polydipsia

12. **Which of the following treatment modalities would NOT be an appropriate treatment modality for SIADH?**
    (A) fluid restriction
    (B) diuretic administration
    (C) administration of 3% hypertonic saline
    (D) sodium polystyrene sulfonate (Kayexalate) enemas

13. **The critical care nurse should recognize that the major complications of diabetes insipidus could include:**
    (A) dehydration
    (B) hyponatremia
    (C) hyperkalemia
    (D) bradycardia and hypertension

14. What is the dominant effect of ADH on the kidneys?
(A) It causes them to excrete water and sodium.
(B) It causes them to reabsorb water and concentrate urine.
(C) It causes them to reabsorb sodium and excrete potassium.
(D) It causes them to reabsorb potassium and excrete sodium.

15. Which hormone(s) does the thyroid gland NOT secrete?
(A) thyroxine
(B) triiodothyronine
(C) calcitonin
(D) ADH

16. The release of thyroxine is inhibited by which situation?
(A) hyperthermia
(B) hypothermia
(C) hypokalemia
(D) hypernatremia

17. Calcitonin is released by which organ?
(A) pituitary gland
(B) adrenal gland
(C) parathyroid gland
(D) thyroid gland

18. The goals of treatment for hyperthyroidism include which of the following?
(A) a reduction in the peripheral effects of excessive circulating thyroid hormone
(B) a reduction in the production and secretion of thyroid hormone
(C) treatment of a precipitating or underlying illness
(D) all of the above

Questions 19 and 20 refer to the following scenario:
A 48-year-old woman is admitted to your unit with a possible syncopal episode. She is currently awake although she is nervous and anxious. Vital signs are as follows:

Blood pressure	178/108
Pulse	129
Respiratory rate	28
Temperature	39°C

During your initial examination, you note that she has exophthalmos and that her skin is warm and wet.

19. Given the preceding information, which condition could be present?
(A) myxedema coma
(B) parathyroid crisis
(C) thyroid storm
(D) aldosterone crisis

20. Which of the following would be administered in this situation?
(A) calcitonin
(B) propranolol (Inderal)
(C) normal saline
(D) parathyroid hormone

21. On which organ does calcitonin exert its major effect?
(A) kidney
(B) bone
(C) parathyroid
(D) liver

22. Parathormone release is inhibited by which serum situation?
(A) increased calcium
(B) decreased magnesium
(C) increased phosphate
(D) increased magnesium

23. Parathormone secretion is stimulated by which humoral event?
(A) decreased calcium
(B) increased sodium
(C) increased phosphate
(D) Both A and C

24. Which of the following is a symptom of hypothyroidism?
(A) paresthesia of the fingers
(B) sensitivity to cold
(C) dry scaly skin
(D) all of the above

25. Which of the following is NOT a symptom of myxedema coma?
(A) hypothermia
(B) hypoventilation
(C) hyponatremia
(D) hyperthermia

Questions 26 and 27 refer to the following scenario:
A 51-year-old woman is admitted to your unit with hypotension, bradycardia, and a decreased level of consciousness. Her core temperature is 35.5°C. The temperature in her apartment was 25°C (77°F). No history is available regarding prior medical problems. She appears to be overweight, with dry scaly skin and puffy face and lips. Blood gas analysis reveals the following information:

pH	7.25
$PaCO_2$	56
PaO_2	63

Shortly after admission, she has a grand mal seizure. She is intubated and placed on mechanical ventilation.

26. Based on the preceding information, which condition is likely to be developing?
(A) acute congestive heart failure (CHF)
(B) acute respiratory distress syndrome (ARDS)
(C) thyroid crisis
(D) myxedema coma

27. Which treatment would be required to correct the condition?
(A) dobutamine (50 mg/kg/min)
(B) cooling blanket
(C) levothyroxine (0.2 mg)
(D) calcitonin (2 mg/kg/h)

28. Which of the following is NOT a common precipitating factor of myxedema coma?
(A) stress
(B) exposure to heat
(C) infection
(D) exposure to cold

29. Which of the following is NOT a common symptom of hyperthyroidism?
(A) marked fatigue
(B) cold intolerance
(C) tachycardia
(D) weight loss

30. Which of the following is NOT associated as a precipitating factor with thyrotoxic crisis?
(A) diabetic ketoacidosis
(B) trauma
(C) increased intracranial pressure
(D) infection

31. A deficiency of parathormone causes which clinical sign?
(A) hypocalcemia
(B) hypercalcemia
(C) hyponatremia
(D) hyperkalemia

32. Appropriate response to treatment of myxedema coma would be illustrated by which of the following changes in physiologic parameters?
(A) increase in $PaCO_2$
(B) reduction in heart rate
(C) increase in body temperature
(D) decrease in pH

33. Which of the following is NOT associated with hypoparathyroidism?
(A) Trousseau sign
(B) thyroidectomy
(C) hypocalcemia
(D) gastric ulcers

34. Which part of the endocrine system secretes aldosterone?
(A) zona glomerulus of the adrenal cortex
(B) zona fasciculata of the adrenal cortex
(C) adrenal medulla
(D) zona reticularis of the adrenal cortex

35. Which category of hormone is NOT secreted by the adrenal cortex?
(A) glucocorticoids
(B) mineralocorticoids
(C) androgenic hormones
(D) adrenergic hormones

36. Primary adrenal insufficiency is characterized by which of the following?
(A) hyperpigmentation
(B) hypertension
(C) bradycardia
(D) skeletal tremors

Questions 37 and 38 refer to the following scenario:
A 35-year-old man is admitted to your unit with hypotension and probable dehydration. He is confused and it is difficult to obtain a history regarding past medical problems. He has multiple hyperpigmented areas on his body. He complains of nausea, abdominal pain, and marked fatigue. Laboratory data reveal the following:

Na^+	154
K^+	5.9
Cl^-	109
HCO_3^-	20
Glucose	46

37. Based on the preceding information, which condition is likely to be developing?
(A) myxedema coma
(B) adrenal insufficiency
(C) hyperparathyroid storm
(D) Cushing syndrome

38. What treatment would most likely be initiated to reverse all of the above symptoms?
(A) parathormone administration
(B) thyronine administration
(C) glucocorticoid administration
(D) pituitary extract administration

39. Which of the following is another term for adrenal insufficiency?
(A) Graves' disease
(B) myxedema crisis
(C) Addison disease
(D) Cushing syndrome

40. Aldosterone exerts its action on the distal convoluted tubule to cause which effect?
(A) potassium reabsorption
(B) sodium excretion
(C) sodium reabsorption
(D) chloride excretion

41. Aldosterone release is stimulated by all of the following EXCEPT:
(A) decreased potassium level
(B) renin–angiotensin cascade
(C) increased potassium level
(D) decreased sodium level

42. Which term best describes gluconeogenesis?
(A) utilization of oxygen stores due to deficits of serum glucose
(B) breakdown of protein
(C) formation of glucose from noncarbohydrate precursors
(D) breakdown of glycogen stores in the liver

Questions 43 and 44 refer to the following scenario:
A 67-year-old man is admitted to your unit with a decreased level of consciousness. He was brought to the hospital by the police after being found in a shopping mall "acting strange." He complains of fatigue but is generally disoriented as to time and place. His respiratory rate is deep and rapid. Vital signs and laboratory data are as follows:

Blood pressure	96/58
Pulse	114
Respiratory rate	34
Glucose	760
Osmolality	307
pH	7.28
$PaCO_2$	20
PaO_2	91
Na^+	156
K^+	5.0
HCO_3^-	14

The blood pressure also decreases when the patient changes from a lying to a sitting position.

43. Based on the preceding information, which condition is likely developing?
(A) adrenal crisis
(B) thyroid storm
(C) hyperosmolar, hyperglycemic, nonketotic (HHNK) coma
(D) diabetic ketoacidosis (DKA)

44. Which of the following would most likely be administered to this patient?
(A) glucocorticoids
(B) thyroxine
(C) sodium bicarbonate
(D) insulin and normal saline

45. Which blood gas change is usually present in DKA?
(A) respiratory acidosis alone
(B) metabolic acidosis alone
(C) respiratory alkalosis alone
(D) respiratory acidosis and metabolic alkalosis

46. Initial insulin therapy for DKA is usually administered by which route?
(A) intravenous bolus
(B) intravenous bolus followed by a continuous infusion
(C) subcutaneously
(D) intramuscularly

47. Presenting signs and symptoms of DKA could include which of the following?
(A) shallow slow respirations
(B) decreased urine output
(C) tachycardia and orthostatic hypotension
(D) peripheral edema and dependent pulmonary crackles

48. Insulin therapy brings about which electrolyte change?
(A) increased serum potassium
(B) decreased serum sodium
(C) increased intracellular potassium
(D) decreased intracellular calcium

49. HHS (hyperosmolar hyperglycemic syndrome) coma is differentiated from DKA by which of the following?
(A) hyperglycemia
(B) absence of ketosis
(C) serum osmolality
(D) serum potassium levels

Questions 50 and 51 refer to the following scenario:
A 57-year-old woman is admitted to the unit following a seizure at home. She has no history of seizures. The family describes the patient as not feeling well for several days and as having not eaten or taken fluids normally during this time. Her vital signs and laboratory data are as follows:

Blood pressure	92/54
Pulse	108
Respiratory rate	31
Glucose	1089
Osmolality	389
pH	7.37
$PaCO_2$	30
PaO_2	79
Na^+	149
K^+	3.0
HCO_3^-	20

50. Based on the preceding information, which condition is likely to be developing?
(A) adrenal crisis
(B) thyroid storm
(C) HHS coma
(D) DKA

51. Which treatment would most likely be initially administered to this patient?
(A) glucocorticoids
(B) continuous insulin drip and isotonic crystalloids
(C) sodium bicarbonate
(D) D50 bolus and intermittent IM insulin

52. Hyperfunction of the adrenal medulla is referred to as which of the following?
(A) pheochromocytoma
(B) Addison disease
(C) Graves' disease
(D) Cushing syndrome

53. Dehydration in HHS coma is primarily due to which event?
(A) lack of ADH
(B) inability of the kidney to concentrate urine
(C) nausea and vomiting
(D) osmotic diuresis from the high glucose level

54. HHS coma is partially differentiated from DKA by which laboratory result?
(A) hyperglycemia
(B) absence of ketosis
(C) hyperkalemia
(D) serum osmolality

Questions 55 and 56 refer to the following scenario:

A 69-year-old overweight man is in your unit following resection of a perforated bowel. He has a history of adult-onset diabetes and mild hypertension. The patient is alert and oriented with stable vital signs at the beginning of your shift. During your shift he becomes disoriented. His skin is cool and clammy; he has muscle tremors and complains of nausea. Serum electrolytes are drawn. The laboratory results are as follows:

Na^+	133
K^+	3.7
Cl^-	100
HCO_3^-	25
Glucose	43
Osmolality	282

55. Based on the preceding information, which condition is likely to be developing?
(A) hyperosmolar hyperglycemic nonketotic acidosis
(B) hypoglycemia
(C) diabetic ketoacidosis
(D) diabetes insipidus

56. Which treatment would most likely be given to this patient?
(A) insulin bolus followed by infusion
(B) glucose (dextrose) bolus (D50)
(C) normal saline bolus with potassium
(D) glucocorticoids

57. The clinical situation of large fluctuations in blood glucose, such as hypoglycemia symptoms in a patient with hyperglycemia, is described by which term?
(A) Somogyi effect
(B) Addison response
(C) Adams syndrome
(D) pancreatic flash

58. Which of the following physical signs are seen in hypoglycemia and hyperglycemia?
(A) cool skin
(B) rapid breathing
(C) drowsiness
(D) tachycardia

59. At which blood glucose level does change in mentation begin?
(A) 10 to 20 mg/dL
(B) 20 to 30 mg/dL
(C) 30 to 40 mg/dL
(D) any level below 50 mg/dL

60. High serum glucose levels can directly cause which physical symptom?
(A) increased urine output
(B) decreased urine output
(C) hypotension
(D) decreased respiratory rate

61. Which of the following are symptoms of a pheochromocytoma?
(A) hypertension, tachycardia, and hyperglycemia
(B) hypertension, hypoglycemia, and bradycardia
(C) hyperglycemia, hypotension, and tachycardia
(D) hypotension, headache, and hyperglycemia

Questions 62 and 63 refer to the following scenario.

A 70-year-old woman was admitted to the surgical ICU 3 days ago for intestinal obstruction, which has since resolved. She has a history of hyperthyroidism with sub-partial thyroidectomy and hypertension. She is alert and oriented with stable vital signs. Today's morning labs reveal a serum glucose of 210 mg/dL; a repeat level at 10 am was 203 mg/dL.

62. Based on the preceding information, which condition is likely to be developing?
(A) hyperthyroidism
(B) hyperosmolar hyperglycemic nonketotic acidosis
(C) critical illness hyperglycemia
(D) thyroid storm

63. Which treatment would most likely be indicated?
(A) Lugol's solution
(B) high-dose hydrocortisone
(C) insulin infusion
(D) desiccated thyroid extract

PART III
Endocrine Practice Exam

Practice Fill-Ins

1. ______
2. ______
3. ______
4. ______
5. ______
6. ______
7. ______
8. ______
9. ______
10. ______
11. ______
12. ______
13. ______
14. ______
15. ______
16. ______
17. ______
18. ______
19. ______
20. ______
21. ______
22. ______
23. ______
24. ______
25. ______
26. ______
27. ______
28. ______
29. ______
30. ______
31. ______
32. ______
33. ______
34. ______
35. ______
36. ______
37. ______
38. ______
39. ______
40. ______
41. ______
42. ______
43. ______
44. ______
45. ______
46. ______
47. ______
48. ______
49. ______
50. ______
51. ______
52. ______
53. ______
54. ______
55. ______
56. ______
57. ______
58. ______
59. ______
60. ______
61. ______
62. ______
63. ______

PART III
Answers

1. **A** Chapter 20 Rationale: Most control systems, including the endocrine system, act by a negative-feedback mechanism. When there is an increased hormone concentration, physiologic control is increased. The stimulus for hormone production received in the hypothalamus is decreased. This results in an inhibition of hormone-releasing factors that is negative in relation to the stimulus. As a test-taking strategy, also note that options B, C, and D all emphasize increased production. Choose A.
2. **D** Chapter 20 Rationale: The hormones of the adrenal medulla are epinephrine and norepinephrine, also known as the "fight or flight" catecholamines. These hormones are stimulated in states of fear or danger, as well as during critical illness, by the autonomic nervous system. Choose D.
3. **B** Chapter 21 Rationale: Growth hormone (somatotropin) has a general effect on bones, organs, and soft tissues. It is essentially considered a peripheral hormone that influences growth of body tissues. Thyroid-stimulating hormone acts on the thyroid, adrenocorticotropin stimulates the adrenals to produce cortisol, and luteinizing hormone acts on the ovaries and testes. Choose B.
4. **A** Chapter 21 Rationale: Hypothalamic-releasing factors are secreted and carried to the anterior pituitary by the bloodstream. As a test-taking strategy, note that options B, C, and D all relate to the nervous system, helping to eliminate them. An example of nervous system stimulation would be the autonomic nervous system influence on the adrenal medulla, stimulating the release of epinephrine and norepinephrine. Choose A.
5. **D** Chapter 21 Rationale: In this negatively stated question, we note that A, B, and C are all influenced by the anterior pituitary. Option D, ADH, is influenced by the posterior pituitary. Choose D.
6. **C** Chapter 21 Rationale: This initially appears as a straight knowledge question. However, if in doubt, consider the physiologic factors influencing rebound, restoration, or repair of tissue. A, B, and D are all associated with increased growth. Hyperglycemia, such as in diabetes, is usually associated with muscle wasting. Choose C.
7. **B** Chapter 21 Rationale: When a patient is hydrated, serum osmolality (ie, blood concentration) will decrease, followed by a decrease in ADH due to the body's decreased need to retain sodium and water. Options A and C can be ruled out because they are associated with dehydration, which would stimulate release of ADH. Potassium level does not directly impact ADH. Choose B.
8. **D** Chapter 21 Rationale: The symptoms of diabetes insipidus include dilute urine (until severe dehydration occurs) with a specific gravity between 1.001 and 1.005. Urinary output varies from 2 to 15 L/day regardless of fluid intake. Polyuria is often of sudden onset. Polyuria may not occur until 1 to 3 days postinjury due to the utilization of stored ADH in the neurohypophysis. In this case, head injury is a precipitating factor. Choose D.
9. **A** Chapter 21 Rationale: Diabetes insipidus is a condition characterized by rapid volume loss through the urine potentially leading to hypovolemic shock if not detected and treated appropriately. In this case, diuretics would exacerbate the hypovolemic situation, so eliminate C. Fluid challenges and fluid restriction may be included in the supportive care, however, would not help correct the underlying problem. Option A is the only option that helps treat the underlying problem. Choose A.
10. **A** Chapter 21 Rationale: SIADH is a condition of impaired water excretion with accompanying hyponatremia and hypoosmolality caused by the inappropriate secretion of ADH and associated volume overload. Options B, C, and D are all associated with dehydration. Choose A.
11. **A** Chapter 21 Rationale: Symptoms produced by SIADH reflect the interaction between the underlying condition and excessive water retention. Symptoms are mainly neurologic and nonspecific. The most common symptoms of SIADH are personality changes, headache, decreased mentation, lethargy, nausea, vomiting, diarrhea, anorexia, decreased tendon reflexes, seizures, and coma. Complications of SIADH include seizures, coma, and death. Options B, C, and D are all associated with dehydration and can be ruled out as potential answers. Choose A.
12. **D** Chapter 21 Rationale: The first step in treating SIADH is to restrict fluid intake to prevent water intoxication. The objective of therapy is to correct electrolyte imbalances. Severity of symptoms will determine the rate of correction of the hyponatremia. In severe cases (severe hyponatremia with serum sodium levels <105 mEq/L), 3% hypertonic saline and intravenous furosemide (Lasix) are used. Enemas would not be indicated. Choose D.
13. **A** Chapter 21 Rationale: Monitoring body weight, electrolytes (especially potassium and sodium), urine specific gravity, osmolality, blood urea nitrogen, and being alert for signs of dehydration and hypovolemic shock will allow for early intervention in patients who are at risk for deterioration. Choose A.
14. **B** Chapter 21 Rationale: ADH ("antidiuretic hormone") works on the distal convoluted tubules and the collecting ducts of the kidney, altering the permeability of these tubules and ducts. Without ADH, the tubules and ducts

are impermeable to water. In the presence of ADH, they become permeable to water, thus allowing large quantities of water to leave the tubules and collecting ducts and to reenter the hypertonic medullary interstitial fluid. This helps to conserve and balance the fluid content of the body and results in reabsorption of water and subsequent concentration of urine. Choose B.

15. **D** Chapter 22 Rationale: In this negatively stated question, all the options are secreted from the thyroid EXCEPT one. Thyroxine and triiodothyronine are secreted by the thyroid. Calcitonin is also known as "thyrocalcitonin," and is secreted by the thyroid. ADH is secreted by the posterior pituitary. Choose D.
16. **A** Chapter 22 Rationale: For this question, just remember that thyroid hormone is associated with metabolism and that upregulation and downregulation operate on a negative feedback loop. Hyperthermia would suggest a hypermetabolic state, which would stimulate a downregulation thyroxine (thyroid) hormone. Hypothermia would cause an increase in thyroxine, so eliminate B. Potassium and sodium levels have little influence on thyroxine production. Choose A.
17. **D** Chapter 22 Rationale: The thyroid gland is the only option available that releases calcitonin. Remember that a rare complication of patients who are post-thyroidectomy is tetany, which is influenced by the alteration in calcitonin levels after the procedure. Choose D.
18. **D** Chapter 22 Rationale: Goals of treatment not only include managing the physiologic effects of hyperthyroidism, but also the underlying cause (which may also include regulating the level of circulating thyroid hormone). Remember to always consider the underlying cause as a general rule. All are reasonable goals of treatment. Choose D.
19. **C** Chapter 22 Rationale: The thyroid storm syndrome characteristically includes hyperthermia (up to 106°F), hypertension with widened pulse pressure, and tachydysrhythmias (atrial fibrillation and paroxysmal atrial tachycardia). Choose C.
20. **B** Chapter 22 Rationale: A reversal of the peripheral effects of excessive thyroid hormone is achieved through administration of intravenous beta blockers (propranolol, esmolol) to decrease the hypermetabolic activity. Beta blockers block the increased sympathetic nervous system ("fight or flight") activity associated with hyperthyroidism. Choose B.
21. **B** Chapter 22 Rationale: Calcitonin exerts its primary effect on the bones, while generally lowering serum calcium. Calcitonin exerts a lesser effect on the renal cell reabsorption of calcium; however, this is not as much as the effect on the bones, eliminating A. Parathyroid hormone increases serum calcium, opposing the effect of calcitonin, which helps eliminate C. The liver is not affected at all. Choose B.
22. **A** Chapter 22 Rationale: Calcitonin (secreted from the thyroid) and parathyroid hormone (from the parathyroid) counterbalance one another to regulate serum calcium. Parathyroid hormone increases serum calcium. Therefore, when the calcium level is increased, parathormone is inhibited. The calcium level and the serum phosphorus level also have a "see-saw" relationship. When the level of one is increased, the level of the other is decreased, and vice versa—this helps eliminate option C. Magnesium does not influence parathormone, ruling out B and D. Choose A.
23. **D** Chapter 22 Rationale: Decreased calcium levels stimulate parathormone to increase serum calcium, largely through its effect on bone tissue. Also remember the "see-saw" relationship that exists between calcium and serum phosphate. When calcium is decreased, phosphate will be increased. Choose D.
24. **D** Chapter 22 Rationale: Sensitivity to cold, paresthesia, and dry scaly skin are symptoms of hypothyroidism. This question is a good example of the need to read through all available options, because all may be correct. Since metabolism is downregulated, additional symptoms of hypothyroidism may include weight gain, fatigue, cramps, inattention or memory problems, constipation, thinning hair, brittle nails, and depression. Choose D.
25. **D** Chapter 22 Rationale: Myxedema coma is a state of extreme hypothyroidism. This downregulated metabolic state precipitates hypothermia and hypoventilation. Increased ADH levels and decreased free water clearance result also in hyponatremia. Hyperthermia is more closely associated with hyperthyroidism. Choose D.
26. **D** Chapter 22 Rationale: Myxedema coma is characterized by hypothermia, hypoventilation, hyponatremia, hyporeflexia, hypotension, and bradycardia. This patient's weight gain, dry scaly skin, and decreased level of consciousness also help confirm myxedema coma. Choose D.
27. **C** Chapter 22 Rationale: Many examination questions will expect ability to demonstrate identification and treatment of the underlying condition. Since this patient is in myxedema coma, the best treatment for the underlying cause is thyroid hormone supplementation, levothyroxine, option C. Dobutamine may temporarily improve the hypotension and bradycardia, however the underlying cause is not cardiogenic and the dobutamine dose is extremely high, eliminating A. A cooling blanket would exacerbate the symptoms. Calcitonin is secreted by the thyroid; however, it is not primary thyroid hormone supplementation, eliminating D. Choose C.
28. **B** Chapter 22 Rationale: If the answer to this question does not seem clear, consider options that may tax or place increased demand on metabolism, which would exacerbate myxedema coma. A stressor, infection, or exposure to cold may all do this. Choose B.
29. **B** Chapter 22 Rationale: This is a negatively stated question, saying that all of the following are symptoms of hyperthyroidism EXCEPT one option. Hyperthyroidism is a state of upregulated metabolism, making A, C, and D all likely associated symptoms. Option B, cold intolerance, is a classic sign of HYPOthyroidism. Choose B.

30. **C** Chapter 22 Rationale: In this negatively stated question, it is saying that all of the following options are potential precipitating factors for thyrotoxic crisis EXCEPT one. Trauma, DKA, and infection can all be etiologic factors for a crisis (or "storm"). Increased intracranial pressure (particularly associated with head trauma) may precipitate diabetes insipidus, but not thyrotoxic crisis. Choose C.
31. **A** Chapter 22 Rationale: Parathormone increases serum calcium levels. Therefore, parathormone deficiency often results in hypocalcemia, option A. This also eliminates option B. Parathormone has a negligible influence on sodium and potassium levels. Choose A.
32. **C** Chapter 22 Rationale: Myxedema coma is a severely downregulated, hypo-metabolic state. Symptoms may include hypothermia, hypoventilation with an associated respiratory acidosis, and bradycardia. Therefore, treatment of the underlying cause would increase heart rate, body temperature, and ventilation which would result in decreased $Paco_2$ with associated increased pH. Choose C.
33. **D** Chapter 22 Rationale: Since parathormone increases calcium levels, hypoparathyroidism is associated with hypocalcemia. This helps eliminate option C. Trousseau sign is a tetany-like spasm of the muscles of the hand and forearm that occurs with blood pressure cuff inflation in the presence of hypocalcemia, also eliminating option A. Risks of thyroidectomy include manipulation of the parathyroid due to proximity of the glands, which may precipitate hypoparathyroidism and thus hypocalcemia, eliminating option B as well. Choose D.
34. **A** Chapter 24 Rationale: Mineralocorticoids are named as such since their action is chiefly with the extracellular fluid electrolytes (minerals) sodium and potassium. The most important mineralocorticoid is aldosterone, which is secreted in the zona glomerulosa. The adrenal cortex is composed of three distinct regions or zones (Fig. 24-3). The outermost zone is the zona glomerulosa. The middle zone is the zona fasciculata. The innermost zone is the zona reticularis. Choose A.
35. **D** Chapter 24 Rationale: The hormones secreted by the adrenal cortex are classified as corticosteroids, since they are synthesized from the steroid cholesterol. As a group, more than 30 corticosteroids may be referred to as corticoids. The adrenal cortex secretes three classes of hormones: the glucocorticoids, the mineralocorticoids, and the androgenic hormones. The hormones secreted by the adrenal medulla are classified as catecholamines or adrenergic hormones. Choose D.
36. **A** Chapter 24 Rationale: Melanin pigmentation is increased in most cases of Addison disease. This pigmentation is unevenly distributed and is probably due to increased secretion of melanocyte-stimulating hormone (MSH) and ACTH from the adenohypophysis.
37. **B** Chapter 24 Rationale: A mineralocorticoid decrease results in an aldosterone deficiency. Without aldosterone, there is an increased excretion of sodium, chloride, and water in the urine. The depletion of sodium leads to dehydration and hypotension. At the same time, there is a retention of potassium. Choose B.
38. **C** Chapter 24 Rationale: Replacement therapy of small amounts of mineralocorticoids and glucocorticoids may prolong life for years. Choose C.
39. **C** Chapter 24 Rationale: Addison disease is a chronic dysfunction of the adrenal glands, resulting in an inadequate adrenal secretion of cortisol and aldosterone (adrenal insufficiency). Hypercortisolism is a marked increase in the production of mineralocorticoids, glucocorticoids, and androgen steroids, resulting in the condition known as Cushing syndrome. Choose C.
40. **C** Chapter 24 Rationale: Aldosterone exerts its action on the distal convoluted tubules and the collecting ducts. The primary action of aldosterone is to cause an increase in sodium reabsorption and potassium and hydrogen ion excretion by the kidney. The release of aldosterone is stimulated by an increased serum potassium level, the renin–angiotensin cascade, decreased serum sodium levels, and ACTH. Choose C.
41. **A** Chapter 24 Rationale: The release of aldosterone is stimulated by an increased serum potassium level, the renin–angiotensin cascade, decreased serum sodium levels, and ACTH. Choose A.
42. **C** Chapter 23 Rationale: Gluconeogenesis is the formation of glucose from other substances and provides new glucose. Choose C.
43. **D** Chapter 23 Rationale: Three distinct clinical features are seen in DKA: hyperglycemia, ketonuria/ketonemia, and metabolic acidosis. Serum glucose levels are above 300 mg/dL. Serum ketones are present, identified through the anion gap. Arterial pH less than 7.30 and serum bicarbonate less than 15 mEq/L are also seen. Metabolic acidosis can also result in potentially life-threatening electrolyte imbalances including hyperkalemia or hypokalemia. Additionally, rapid and deep breathing, or Kussmaul respirations, are a feature of DKA. Choose D.
44. **D** Chapter 23 Rationale: The objectives of treatment in DKA are to correct acidemia, hyperglycemia, hypovolemia, hyperosmolality, potassium deficit, and ketonemia. Underlying conditions responsible for DKA, such as infections, must be identified and treated concurrently. Glucocorticoids are administered for adrenal crisis. Thyroxine is administered during myxedema coma. Sodium bicarbonate should only be administered when hyperglycemia and hypovolemia are corrected and the patient continues to experience a metabolic acidosis, not as a part of initial DKA treatment. Choose D.
45. **B** Chapter 23 Rationale: Three distinct clinical features are seen in DKA: hyperglycemia, ketonuria/ketonemia, and metabolic acidosis. Choose B.
46. **B** Chapter 23 Rationale: Normally, an intravenous bolus of insulin is administered followed by a slow continuous intravenous infusion. Insulin may be administered by subcutaneous or intramuscular injections; however, this is not advocated in the crisis stage of DKA because of poor peripheral absorption. Rapid-acting subcutaneous insulin can be used to successfully treat mild to moderate DKA if the patient is not in a state of shock. Choose B.

47. **C** Chapter 23 Rationale: The most common symptoms of DKA are polydipsia, polyuria, polyphagia (usually with weight loss), dyspnea, and a generalized malaise. Nausea, vomiting, anorexia, and abdominal pain may be present. Signs of dehydration, tachycardia, orthostatic hypotension, and weakness are usually present. Respirations are Kussmaul (rapid and deep) in character and may have an acetone smell. Mentation ranges from lethargy to coma. Choose C.
48. **C** Chapter 23 Rationale: When insulin is administered, potassium shifts into the cells. In addition to laboratory results, cardiac monitoring may show whether the patient's serum potassium is low, normal, or high. Choose C.
49. **B** Chapter 23 Rationale: HHS coma follows almost the same pathophysiologic pattern of DKA. The difference is that in HHS coma, a sufficient amount of insulin is released to prevent the development of ketosis; however, there is not enough insulin produced to prevent hyperglycemia. Choose B.
50. **C** Chapter 23 Rationale: Usually the patient with HHS, who is typically older than 50 years, is lethargic or comatose. Symptoms include polyuria, polydipsia, nausea, vomiting, and weight loss. Eventually, the urinary output begins to fall as fluid depletion becomes more severe. Dehydration is apparent, with dry skin and mucous membranes. Tachypnea as well as tachycardia, hypotension, and glycosuria are present. Choose C.
51. **B** Chapter 23 Rationale: Correction of the fluid balance is one of the first objectives of treatment. It is essential that fluids be administered to correct hyperosmolality and hypovolemia. If the patient has a cardiac history, slow administration of fluid (300 mL/h) may be performed. Hypoinsulinemia may be corrected through the administration of intravenous of insulin. Hyperglycemia is not known to have deleterious effects on the brain, but hyperosmolar dehydration may cause seizures. Choose B.
52. **A** Chapter 24 Rationale: Hyperfunction of the adrenal medulla is the most common cause of pheochromocytoma. Pheochromocytoma is an encapsulated, vascular tumor of chromaffin tissue of the adrenal medulla. Choose A.
53. **D** Chapter 23 Rationale: Hyperglycemia increases the solutes in the extracellular fluid, causing a hyperosmolality and cellular dehydration. This is also the cause of diuresis. Without treatment, an osmotic gradient develops between the brain and the plasma, resulting in dehydration and central nervous system dysfunction. The three most outstanding signs are an elevated blood sugar level (commonly >1000 mg), plasma hyperosmolarity (>350 mOsm/kg), and an extremely elevated hematocrit. Choose D.
54. **B** Chapter 23 Rationale: In HHS, urine and plasma are both negative for acetone or ketones compared to DKA. The blood urea nitrogen is usually elevated and there is marked leukocytosis. The remaining lab results are similar in both conditions. Choose B.
55. **B** Chapter 23 Rationale: If the hypoglycemia progresses to less than 50 mg/dL, the central nervous system will be affected and the patient may exhibit bizarre behavior that can progress to a comatose state. Headache, dizziness, irritability, fatigue, poor judgment, confusion, visual changes, hunger, weakness, tremors, seizures, nausea, and personality changes are common signs and symptoms. HHS and DKA are associated with high glucose values. Diabetes insipidus is associated with hypernatremia. Choose B.
56. **B** Chapter 23 Rationale: A glucose level less than 45 mg/dL with blood glucose monitoring is sufficient to require infusion of 50 mg of 50% dextrose intravenously. Insulin administration would exacerbate hypoglycemia. Hypoglycemia is not usually associated with dehydration so normal saline administration is not indicated. Glucocorticoids provide no therapeutic effect for hypoglycemia reversal. Choose B.
57. **A** Chapter 23 Rationale: A cyclical pattern may develop: hypoglycemia one day may be followed by one or more days of hyperglycemia. In some patients, the cycle is so short that periods alternate within the same day. Symptoms of hypoglycemia in a hyperglycemic patient may indicate a Somogyi effect. Choose A.
58. **D** Chapter 23 Rationale: The early signs and symptoms of hypoglycemia are restlessness, diaphoresis, tachycardia, and hunger. Symptoms of hyperglycemia include polyuria, polydipsia, nausea, vomiting, and weight loss. Hyperglycemia progresses to increasing dehydration with dry skin and mucous membranes. Tachypnea as well as tachycardia, hypotension, and glycosuria are present. Choose D.
59. **D** Chapter 23 Rationale: When the glucose level is below 50 mg/dL, cerebral ischemia, edema, and neuronal hyperexcitability occur. If the blood glucose level drops to 20 to 40 mg/dL, clonic convulsions may occur. If the blood glucose level drops below 20 mg/dL, coma develops. If it is not promptly reversed, the low blood glucose levels may cause irreversible brain damage, myocardial ischemia, infarction, and death. Choose D.
60. **A** Chapter 23 Rationale: Hyperglycemia increases the solutes in the extracellular fluid, causing a hyperosmolality. As a result, cellular dehydration occurs, which is also the cause of diuresis. Subsequently, there is an increase in urine output. Choose A.
61. **A** Chapter 24 Rationale: The outstanding symptom is the extremely high blood pressure. Other signs and symptoms include increased sympathetic nervous activity such as sweating, headache, palpitations, dysrhythmias, postural hypotension, apprehension, nausea/vomiting, tremor, pallor or flushing of the face, abdominal and/or chest pain, and hyperglycemia. Choose A.
62. **C** Chapter 23 Rationale: Stress-induced hyperglycemia in critically ill nondiabetic patients is a common occurrence. The release of stress hormones—including glucagon, catecholamines, cortisol, and growth hormone, as well as their catabolic effects—causes increased gluconeogenesis

and glycogenolysis and resultant hyperglycemia. In addition, these catabolic hormones induce tissue resistance to insulin. A number of additional factors including cytokines, epinephrine, and reactive oxygen species are also involved in initiating hepatic insulin resistance. Choose C.

63. C Chapter 23 Rationale: Intravenous insulin protocols to maintain moderate glycemic control, with serum glucose levels 140 to 180 mg/dL, have been shown to significantly reduce mortality rates and improve outcomes for critically ill patients. Choose C.

PART IV

IMMUNOLOGY AND HEMATOLOGY

Ashley N. Thompson

Section Overview

Immunologic and hematologic concepts account for 3% (approximately four to five questions) of the CCRN exam. The major content areas covered under immunology and hematology include immunosuppression, life-threatening coagulopathies such as disseminated intravascular coagulation (DIC), sickle cell crisis, and organ transplantation. To answer the questions on anaphylactic shock and immunosuppression correctly, one must have a working knowledge of immune response principles. To answer questions on DIC, normal coagulation concepts must be known. This chapter presents key information normally encountered on the CCRN exam regarding both the four major concepts and the principles necessary to achieve the understanding required for the CCRN exam.

25

Physiology of the Immunologic and Hematologic Systems

CHAPTER OVERVIEW AND OBJECTIVES

As with most other chapters, concentrate on key principles rather than on details or points of pure anatomy and physiology. Nurses often find immunology and hematology to be a difficult area of the CCRN exam because of their lack of clinical familiarity with the concepts. Study this chapter and then try to apply the information during your work. The more you can integrate the information after reading it, the more likely you will be to retain the information for the test.

After studying this chapter, you should be able to:

- Describe the pathophysiology related to the immunologic and hematologic systems.
- Define and explain immunologic responses to changes in clinical condition.
- Define and explain alterations in hematologic system related to interventions.
- Describe the elements related to normal coagulation.
- Discuss the significance of anticoagulation as it relates to homeostasis.

25.1 IMMUNE SYSTEM

Alterations in hemostasis and coagulation are common problems during critical illness. Therefore, understanding the immune system and hematologic and immunologic disorders is important for the early detection and treatment.

The mature immune system can perform following three general types of functions:

- Defense: Resistance to infection is facilitated by both nonspecific innate mechanisms and acquired immune responses that bring about the destruction of foreign antigens (anything recognized by the body as nonself, eg, microorganisms, proteins, and cells of transplanted organs). Although the function of the immune system is inherently protective, there are conditions in which natural immune responses may become destructive to the host. Examples of conditions that are destructive to the host are the numerous autoimmune diseases, as well as allergic and anaphylactic reactions.
- Homeostasis: The maintenance of immunologic homeostasis involves keeping a balance between immune protective and destructive responses, as well as the removal of aging immune cells from the body.
- Surveillance: Involves the recognition of microorganisms or cells bearing foreign antigens on their membranes. Some of the immune cells, lymphocytes, are highly mobile and travel throughout the vascular and lymphatic systems in search of potentially harmful antigens. Some types of cancer cells are sought out and destroyed by immune cells in this way.

Innate Immune System

The innate immune system consists of natural mechanisms for the protection of an individual against foreign antigens. The body's first line of defense consists of anatomic, chemical, and cellular defenses against microbial invasion. Anatomic defenses include the skin, mucous membranes, and ciliated epithelia. Chemical defenses include gastric acid, lysozymes, natural immunoglobulins, and the interferons. Cellular defenses include leukocytes.

Anatomic and Chemical Defenses. The skin provides the initial physical barrier to external environmental antigens. The outermost skin layer, the stratum corneum, is the main barrier to microbial invasion. Certain conditions (pH, humidity, and temperature) influence the growth of potentially pathogenic organisms on the skin. When the acid–base balance of the skin is altered in favor of a higher pH, this protective mechanism is lost. When water loss from epidermal cells exceeds intake, the stratum corneum can dry and crack, predisposing the host

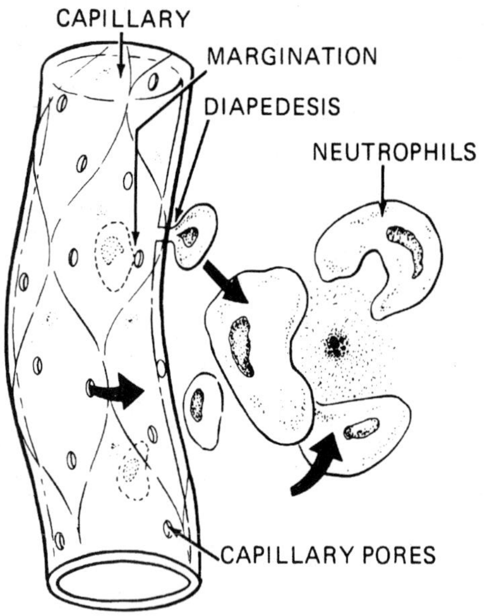

Figure 25-1. Phagocytosis of WBCs.

to microbial invasion. On the other hand, excessive moisture decreases barrier efficiency.

Skin cells are constantly exfoliating, and in this process organisms are sloughed along with dead skin cells. In addition, the skin is colonized with normal flora (mainly aerobic cocci and diphtheroids), which prevents the colonization of potentially pathogenic organisms. The resident flora maintains the skin's pH in the acidic range and competes effectively for nutrients and binding sites on epidermal cells, making it difficult for nonresident flora to survive. When the normal flora is altered, as occurs with long-term or broad-spectrum antibiotic therapy and with the use of disinfectants or occlusive dressings, opportunistic organisms take advantage of the lack of competition for nutrients and epidermal binding sites and multiply to cause infection.

Leukocytes. All leukocytes (white blood cells [WBCs]) develop as stem cells in the bone marrow. Leukocytes develop along two major lineages: the myeloid lineage and the lymphoid lineage.

- The myeloid lineage includes all leukocytes except the lymphocytes.
- The lymphoid lineage consists of T and B lymphocytes.

Myeloid cells make up the backbone of the natural or innate defense system. Myeloid leukocytes can be further classified into two major groups: granulocytes and monocytes. These cells are also phagocytes. Phagocytes are a type of cell within the body capable of engulfing and absorbing bacteria and other small cells and particles (**Fig. 25-1**). Phagocytosis is the process by which excess antigen and dead cells are removed from the body. Phagocytosis is also essential in the initiation of cellular and humoral immune responses by T and B lymphocytes.

Granulocytes. Granulocytes, commonly referred to as polymorphonuclear granulocytes (PMNs) or polymorphs, are produced in the bone marrow at the rate of approximately 80 million per day, and their average life span is about 2 to 3 days. Some 60% to 70% of all leukocytes are PMNs. These cells are sometimes called polymorphs because their nuclei are multilobed; they are called granulocytes because they contain intracellular granules. These intracellular granules contain hydrolytic enzymes that are cytotoxic to foreign organisms. Furthermore, granulocytes are classified into three more distinct types according to the histologic staining reactions of the granules: neutrophils, eosinophils, and basophils. Granulocytes may leave the circulation to become tissue phagocytes (**Fig. 25-2**).

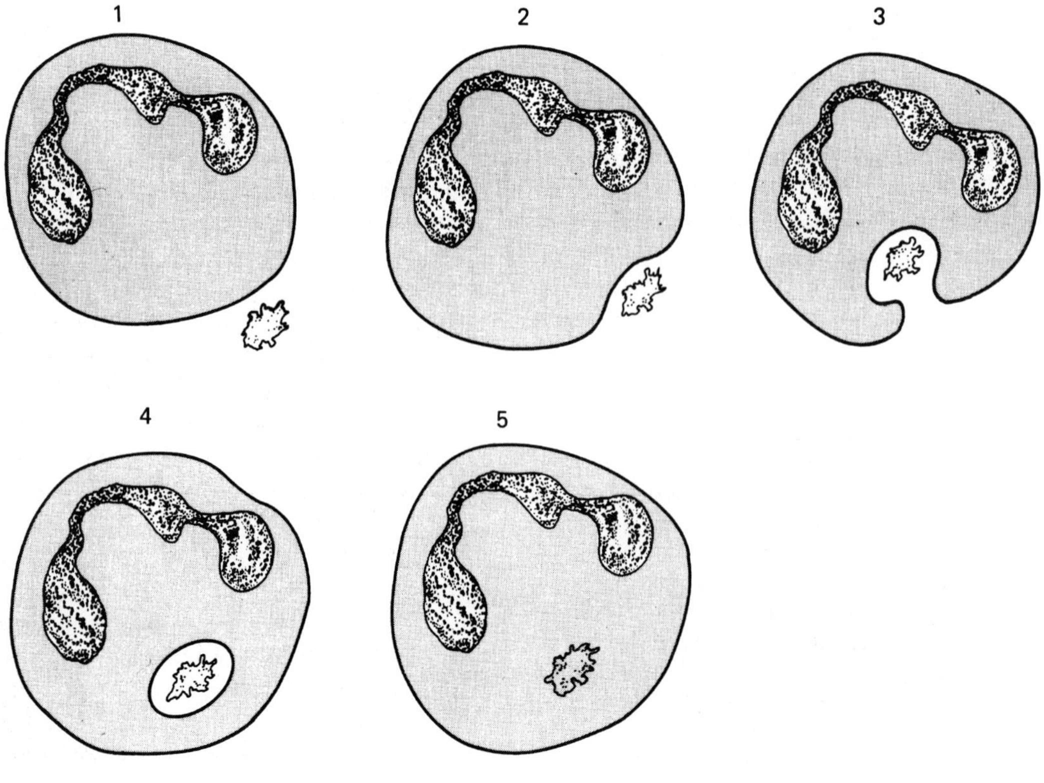

Figure 25-2. Diapedesis of WBCs.

Neutrophils are the most abundant cells in the bone marrow and blood, comprising about 90% of all granulocytes. Three forms of neutrophils can be identified in the peripheral blood: segmented neutrophils, bands, and metamyelocytes. Segmented neutrophils are fully mature, **bands are slightly immature**, and metamyelocytes are completely immature neutrophils. Neutrophils are strongly phagocytic: that is, they ingest microorganisms or other cells and foreign particles, and they digest the ingested material within their phagocytic vacuoles.

QUICK TIP! Bandemia (> 10%) may be suggestive of infection and can be used as a surrogate for WBC when considering sepsis systemic inflammatory response syndrome (SIRS) criteria.

In conditions such as infection, there is an increased demand for neutrophils. The bone marrow responds by releasing more neutrophils into the circulation, and in this process, immature cells, or band cells, are released along with the mature cells. Thus, the percentage of bands in the peripheral blood is increased. This condition is referred to as a *"shift to the left"* and indicates acute inflammation or infection. In more serious conditions, metamyelocytes will also appear in increased numbers in the peripheral blood. The normal neutrophil count in the adult is between 1000 and 6000/mm^3 blood, or approximately 60% of the differential WBC count. Bands normally number about 600/mm^3 blood, or approximately 0% to 5% of the differential WBC count. Metamyelocytes should not be present in the peripheral blood.

Eosinophils are weakly phagocytic cells that are seen in increased numbers in the circulation specifically during parasitic infections and allergic reactions. Eosinophils degranulate (release their cytotoxic granules) on antigenic stimulation and kill organisms extracellularly. The normal eosinophil count is about 200/mm^3 blood, or between 2% and 5% of the differential WBC count.

Basophils are responsible for anaphylactoid reactions to allergens. Like eosinophils, basophils can release their cytotoxic granules when stimulated by certain antigens to effect extracellular killing. Basophils are morphologically identical to mast cells but can be differentiated from mast cells in that basophils are blood-borne and mast cells reside in tissues outside of the circulation. In other words, when a basophil migrates out of the circulation to reside in tissue, it becomes a mast cell. The normal basophil count is about 100/mm^3 blood, or about 0.2% of the differential WBC count.

Monocytes. PMNs can be differentiated from monocytes by their multilobed nuclei and many intracellular granules. Monocytes are mononuclear cells and do not contain cytotoxic intracellular granules. They do, however, release the prostaglandin PGE2, which is a mediator of the inflammatory response. The normal monocyte count is about 200 to 1000/mm^3 blood, or about 5% of the differential WBC count.

A specific type of monocyte is the antigen-presenting cell (APC). APCs are formed in the epidermis, where they are called Langerhans cells, and in the lymphoid system. APCs play an important role in linking the innate immune system with the acquired immune system. APCs carry foreign antigens that enter the host via the respiratory or gastrointestinal tract, or the skin, through the lymphatic system and present them to lymphocytes in the lymph nodes and spleen, thereby triggering cellular and humoral immune responses.

Response to Injury. Tissue injury provides the initial stimulus for activation of inflammatory mechanisms and results in the cellular release of vasoactive substances such as histamine, bradykinin, and serotonin. The circulatory effects are:

- Vasodilatation and increased bloodflow to the affected site
- Increased vascular permeability, facilitating diapedesis of immune cells from the circulation to the tissues
- Pain

The clotting system is activated to "plug up" the injury. Increased bloodflow and capillary permeability lead to local interstitial edema and swelling. Leukocyte migration occurs as phagocytes are attached to the affected site (chemotaxis), and dying leukocytes release pyrogens, which stimulate the hypothalamus to produce a state of fever. Pyrogens also stimulate the bone marrow to release more leukocytes, thus perpetuating the process.

Finally, the complement system is activated. The complement system consists of a complex set of approximately 20 interacting proteolytic enzymes and regulatory proteins found in the plasma and body fluids that attack antigens. The complement system is conceptually similar to the coagulation system in that complement proteins react sequentially in a series of enzymatic reactions in a cascading manner. Several factors are responsible for the activation of the complement system: the formation of antigen–antibody complexes, aggregated immunoglobulin, platelet aggregation, release of endotoxins by gram-negative bacteria, the presence of viruses or bacteria in the circulation, and the release of plasmin and proteases from injured tissues. Complement proteins can mediate the lytic destruction of cells, including erythrocytes (red blood cells [RBCs]) and WBCs, platelets, bacteria, and viruses.

The inflammatory response can be altered or suppressed in many situations: the administration of **corticosteroids** or other *immunosuppressive drugs, malnutrition, advanced age, chronic illness, and prolonged stress.* Conversely, the inflammatory response can become exaggerated in conditions such as **anaphylaxis** and **septic shock**.

The innate immune mechanisms just discussed will be called on as the first line of defense in ridding the host of foreign antigens. However, if these mechanisms are not entirely successful, a second set of defenses, the acquired immune system, is activated to work in concert with the innate immune system. The acquired immune system is composed of lymphocytes and other lymphoid structures necessary for specific immune responses.

Acquired Immune System

The lymphoid system matures during the fetal and neonatal periods when lymphoid stem cells differentiate into T and B lymphocytes. Now, the mechanisms for conferring genetic specificity to lymphocytes develop. This property of specificity is what differentiates the lymphoid cell from the myeloid cell, which can react with any antigen. The process of lymphopoiesis (lymphocyte origination and differentiation into functional effector cells) begins in the yolk sac and then continues later in life in the thymus gland, the liver, the spleen, and finally the bone marrow, which is the primary site of lymphopoiesis in the full-term neonate.

Primary Lymphoid Tissue. Primary lymphoid tissue consists of central organs that serve as major sites of lymphopoiesis. Lymphoid stem cells originate in the bone marrow. These cells give rise to the various components of the acquired immune system.

Secondary Lymphoid Tissue. Secondary lymphoid tissue is peripheral tissue that provides an environment for lymphocytes to encounter antigens and proliferate if necessary. Secondary lymphoid tissue consists of the bone marrow, spleen, lymph nodes, thymus, liver, and mucosa-associated lymphoid tissue in the tonsils, respiratory tract, gut, and urogenital tract. Localization of secondary lymphoid tissue is not coincidental, as these structures provide major portals for the entry of foreign microorganisms into the body. Once in secondary lymphoid tissue, lymphocytes may migrate from one lymphoid structure to another by vascular and lymphatic channels.

Lymphatics. The lymphatic system consists of:

- A capillary network, which collects lymph (a clear, watery fluid in the interstitial spaces)
- Collecting vessels, which carry lymph from the lymphatic vessels back to the vascular system
- Lymph nodes
- Lymphatic organs, such as the tonsils

Lymphatic channels provide a major transit system for lymphocytes while they carry out immunologic surveillance. Both superficial and deep lymphatics empty into the large thoracic duct, which drains into the left subclavian vein (**Fig. 25-3**).

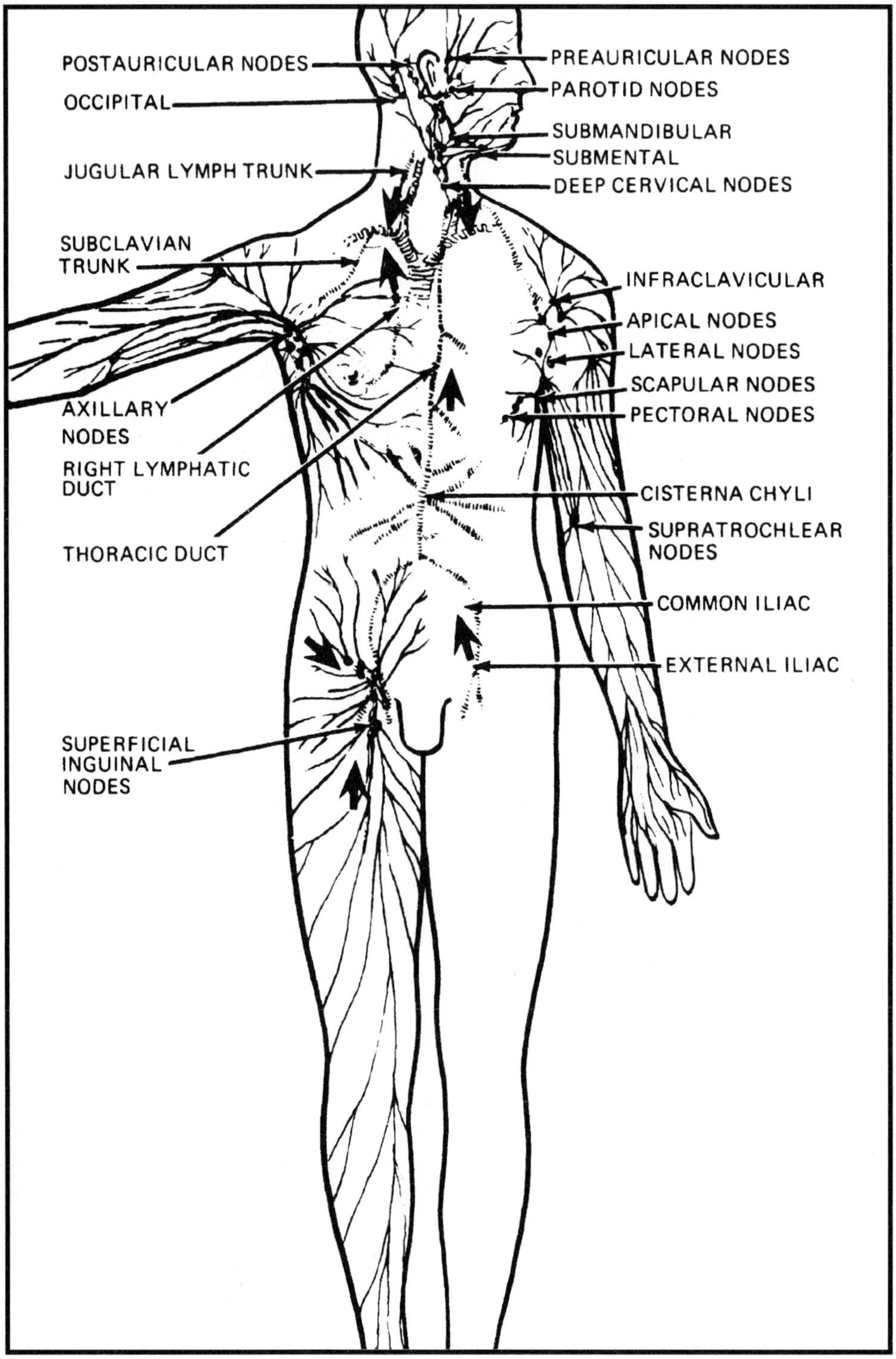

Figure 25-3. Location of lymph nodes in the body.

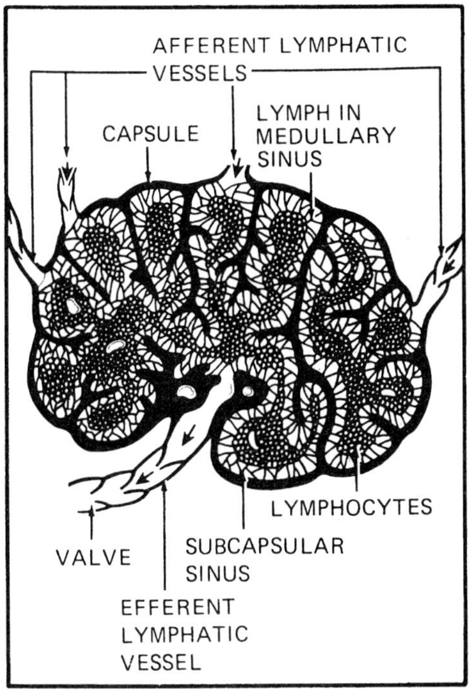

Figure 25-4. Typical lymph node.

Lymph Nodes. Lymph nodes are small oval bodies of lymphatic tissue encapsulated by fibrous tissue that are situated along the path of lymphatic vessels. The interior of the lymph nodes resembles a matrix of connective tissue that forms compartments densely populated with lymphocytes. Afferent lymphatics carry lymph to the lymph nodes, and efferent lymphatics serve as exit routes for lymphocytes from lymph nodes (**Fig. 25-4**). Lymph nodes are located at the junctions of lymphatic vessels and form a complete network for the draining and filtering of extravasated lymph from interstitial fluid spaces.

Spleen. The spleen is a soft, purplish, highly vascular, coffee bean-shaped organ in the left upper quadrant. It lies between the fundus of the stomach and the diaphragm. It is covered by a fibroelastic membrane that causes the organ at the hilum to form fibrous bands (trabeculae) that constitute the internal framework of the spleen and contain the splenic pulp.

KEY CLINICAL CONCEPT

- The spleen serves as a blood reservoir and stores approximately 8 ounces of blood that can be released in trauma or bleeding.
- **Kehr's sign:** Left shoulder pain that may occur due to splenic injury during abdominal trauma. Diaphragmatic irritation and shoulder pain manifests as referred pain via the phrenic nerve.

During fetal and neonatal life, the spleen gives rise to RBCs. The physiologic function of the spleen in adult life is not completely understood. However, a major function of the spleen seems to be the removal of particulate matter from the circulation. The spleen produces monocytes, lymphocytes, opsonins, and IgM antibody-producing plasma cells.

Bloodflow within the spleen is sluggish, which allows phagocytosis to occur. The spleen clears the blood of encapsulated organisms (*Neisseria meningitidis*, *Haemophilus influenzae*, *Streptococcus pneumoniae*), and antigens in the rest of the body are phagocytosed and carried to the spleen to be eradicated by antibodies.

Postsplenectomy sepsis syndrome is seen predominantly in young immunosuppressed individuals who have been splenectomized, but this syndrome can occur in the healthy adult after splenectomy. The etiology of this often-fatal syndrome is the loss of particulate filtering, coupled with the loss of IgM and opsonin production by the spleen. Patients that undergo surgical splenectomy are vaccinated against these encapsulated organisms to help prevent future infections.

Normally about 30% of the total platelet population is sequestered in the spleen, but this can increase to 80% with splenomegaly. In addition, increased numbers of RBCs and WBCs are sequestered in splenomegaly, therefore pancytopenia (anemia, leukopenia, and thrombocytopenia) occurs during splenomegaly.

Thymus. The thymus is a prominent organ in the infant, occupying the ventral superior mediastinum. In the older adult, it may be scarcely visible because of atrophy. The thymus is composed mostly of lymphocytes. Its only known function is the production of lymphocytes.

Lymphocytes. Lymphocytes are the primary defenders of the acquired immune system. Lymphocytes have surface receptors that are specific for surface molecules (antigens) located on the surfaces of foreign proteins. Lymphoctyes are the only cells that have the intrinsic ability to recognize specific antigens.

There are two major types of lymphocytes: T lymphocytes (T cells) and B lymphocytes (B cells). *T cells are involved in immunologic regulation and mediate what is called the cellular immune response. B cells produce antibodies and mediate what is called the humoral immune response.*

T Lymphocytes (T Cells). Under the influence of thymic hormones, immature T cells develop. As mediators of the cellular immune response, T cells defend against viruses, fungi, some neoplastic conditions, and they destroy transplanted organs by mediating accelerated and acute rejection responses. T-cell function is inhibited by viral and parasitic infections, malnutrition, prolonged general anesthesia, radiation therapy, uremia, Hodgkin disease, and advanced age.

T cells are divided into four functionally distinct but interactive cell populations or subsets: cytotoxic, helper (T4), suppressor (T8), and memory T cells.

Cytotoxic and memory T cells are referred to as *effector cells* because they have a specific cytotoxic effect on antigen-bearing cells. Cytotoxic T cells bind to target cells and facilitate their destruction via substances known as lymphokines, which stimulate inflammatory cells, and via the production of cytolytic proteins.

Lymphokines are one of the two soluble products of lymphocytes, the other being antibodies. Lymphokines are inflammatory and regulatory hormones of the immune system that serve a variety of functions, such as the recruitment of macrophages to antigen sites (chemotaxis), augmentation of T-cell function in general, and inhibition of viral replication.

- Lymphokines carry molecular signals between immunocompetent cells to amplify the immune response. Their role in amplification of the T-cell response is crucial to cellular immunity.

- IL-1 stimulates T-cell proliferation, induces fever, stimulates the liver to produce acute-phase proteins, and stimulates the release of prostaglandin.
- IL-2 (T-cell growth factor) also stimulates T-cell proliferation. The reaction of T cells with IL-1 is necessary to produce IL-2.

Memory T cells are T cells that have been sensitized to a specific antigen and then cloned to remember the antigen. Memory cells remain present in the body for many years and are therefore available for defense on repeated exposure to an antigen. Repeated exposure to an antigen that the host has been previously sensitized to will result in a more rapid and accelerated immune response than on the first exposure.

Helper and suppressor T cells are *regulatory* in nature. Helper T cells are active in lymphokine-mediated events. They produce multiple lymphokines that promote the proliferation and activation of other lymphocytes and macrophages. Although the B cell can produce antibody by direct interaction with surface antigen on a macrophage, the assistance of helper T cells is required for most antibody production. They recruit cytotoxic T cells to antigen sites and interact with macrophages in the spleen and lymph nodes to facilitate antibody production by B cells.

B Lymphocytes (B Cells). B cells are effector cells that mediate the humoral immune response through the production of antibodies, which is their major function. B cells are important in defense against pyrogenic bacterial infections and can destroy transplanted organs by mediating hyperacute graft rejection. When a B cell is stimulated by a particular antigen, it differentiates into a lymphoblast. The lymphoblast differentiates into a plasmablast, which further differentiates into a plasma cell. Plasma cells, which can produce and release antibodies, do so until the antigen is destroyed. Memory of the offending antigen is retained for at least several months.

Antibodies are also referred to as immunoglobulins (**Table 25-1**). Immunoglobulins are specifically modified proteins present in serum and tissue fluids that are capable of selectively reacting with inciting antigens. The body produces millions of antibodies, each is specific and can usually recognize only one antigen. When viruses or bacteria, for instance, enter the body, their structural surface features are recognized by the body as foreign. Antibodies are then formed and attracted to these foreign structures, for which they have identical matching receptors. In this way, antibodies can bind with antigens in a process called antigen–antibody complex formation. Mechanisms of antigen interaction by antibody include agglutination, precipitation, neutralization, and lysis.

TABLE 25-1. TYPES AND FUNCTIONS OF IMMUNOGLOBULINS

Type	*Function*
IgM	First antibody in fetal life First antibody after exposure to a new antigen
IgG	Major antibody of adult life Produced after repeated exposure to the same antigen
IgA	Found in secretions: tears, saliva, mucous secretions in gastrointestinal and respiratory tracts Meets antigen at port of entry
IgE	Mediates allergic reactions
IgD	Function unclear; may be regulatory in nature

Antibodies can be divided into five major classifications: **IgM, IgG, IgA, IgD, and IgE. IgM** is the principal mediator of the primary immune response.

- **IgM** is a natural antibody; that is, there is no known contact with the antigen that stimulated its production. About 10% of all antibodies are of the **IgM** type.
- **IgG** is the principal mediator of the secondary immune response, which requires repeated exposure to the same antigen. **IgG** is the major antibody against bacteria and viruses. *About 75% of all antibodies are of the **IgG** type.*
- **IgA** is the secretory immunoglobulin present in bodily secretions and offers natural protection against nonspecific foreign antigens. About *15% of all antibodies* are of the **IgA** type.
- The function of **IgD** is not known, but about 1% of antibodies are of this type.
- Only about 0.002% of antibodies are of the immunoglobulin E **(IgE)** type, **IgE** antibodies present on basophils and mast cells play a significant role in inflammatory and immune reactions.

Lymphocyte Responses. All cells express foreign antigens. Foreign cells, of course, express antigens that are genetically different from those of the host. It is through specific receptors on the surfaces of lymphocytes that B and T cells can be differentiated, and it is also through these receptors that B and T cells can recognize foreign antigens. During lymphocyte maturation, each B and T cell acquires specific cell membrane surface receptors that allow the cell to "match up" with certain foreign antigens. This matching between host lymphocytes and foreign antigens is the recognition phase of the acquired immune response. When this occurs, lymphocytes are activated to differentiate, proliferate, and then quickly mount an effective immune response against the offending antigen.

Cellular Immune Response. The cellular immune response is the immune response mediated by T cells. T cells recognize foreign antigens only after they are displayed on the surfaces of macrophages or APCs. The cellular immune response can be summarized as follows:

- The presence of a foreign antigen is necessary to initiate the response.
- Initially, macrophages encounter the antigen and begin to phagocytize it. Antigenic fragments are released and then carried to T cells in the lymph nodes by APCs.
- Resting virgin or memory T cells are activated when the antigen–APC complex binds with the T-cell surface receptor.
- APCs are stimulated to produce IL-1, which summons helper T cells.
- Helper T cells are then responsible for a few actions, including the release of IL-2, which causes the differentiation and proliferation of T cells. The helper T cells also stimulate antibody production by B cells.

- Clonal expansion greatly increases the sensitized T-cell population.
- Ultimately, the antigen-bearing cells are destroyed by the direct cytotoxic effect of effector T cells. Some sensitized T cells are returned to the lymphoid system with the memory of the antigen for future challenge.

Examples of cellular immune responses include tumor cell surveillance, defense against viral and fungal infections, acute organ rejection, graft-versus-host disease, and autoimmune diseases.

Humoral Immune Response. The humoral immune response is mediated by B cells. Antigens trigger B cells by stimulating immunoglobulins on their surfaces. The humoral immune response can be summarized as follows:

- As with the cellular immune response, the presence of a foreign antigen is necessary to initiate the process. Unlike T cells, B cells can recognize an antigen in its native configuration.
- Macrophages encounter the antigen and begin to phagocytize it. Antigenic fragments are released and then carried to B cells in the lymph nodes and spleen by APCs. Resting virgin or memory B cells are activated when antigen binds to surface immunoglobulin.
- IL-1 is released by APCs, and helper T cells stimulate the sensitization and clonal proliferation of effector B cells. B cells are activated to differentiate and produce antibody when antigen binds to their receptors.
- Antigen–antibody complexes form, and ultimately the antigen-bearing cells are destroyed.
- As in the cellular immune response, some of the plasma cells with specific memory of the antigen are cloned and returned to the lymphoid system.

In addition, B cells can process and present antigen to T cells. Examples of humoral immune responses include resistance to encapsulated pyrogenic bacteria such as pneumococci, streptococci, meningococci, and *H. influenzae*, hemolytic transfusion reactions, and hyperacute organ rejection.

The first exposure of an antigen to an activated lymphocyte evokes a primary immune response. Repeated exposure of the identical antigen to activated lymphocytes evokes an accelerated secondary response. In the secondary immune response, the latent period is shorter and the amount of antigen required to initiate the response is less.

The differences between cell and humoral responses are listed in **Table 25-2**.

Hypersensitivity Reactions

When an adaptive immune response occurs in an exaggerated or inappropriate form, causing tissue damage, a hypersensitivity reaction is said to occur. Hypersensitivity reactions occur on second exposure to the causative antigen. Four types of hypersensitivity reactions are described.

Type I. *Type I hypersensitivity reactions (allergic or anaphylactic) are immediate in nature. This antibody (IgE)-mediated response results in the release of histamine by mast cells, which produces an*

TABLE 25-2. COMPARISON OF B- AND T-CELL IMMUNITY

Characteristic	*B Lymphocyte*	*T Lymphocyte*
Type of immunity	Humoral	Cell-mediated
Immune functions	Antibody formation Immediate hypersensitivity	Direct cytotoxicity Delayed hypersensitivity Immune surveillance (destruction of cancer cells) Graft rejection Immune regulation
Organisms protective against	Pyogenic bacteria *Staphylococcus* *Haemophilus* *Neisseria* Viruses Hepatitis B virus Adenovirus Enterovirus Echovirus	Intracellular bacteria *Pseudomonas* *Listeria* *Mycobacteria* Viruses Herpes simplex virus Herpes zoster and varicella zoster viruses Cytomegalovirus Epstein–Barr virus Retrovirus (excluding HIV) Fungi *Candida* *Cryptococcus* *Aspergillus* Protozoa *Pneumocystis carinii* *Toxoplasma gondii*

acute inflammatory reaction. The distinguishing clinical feature of a type I hypersensitivity reaction is an immediate wheal-and-flare reaction.

Type II. Type II hypersensitivity reactions are caused by the presence of preformed circulating cytotoxic antibodies. These antibodies destroy the target cells on contact.

Examples of type II hypersensitivity reactions are transfusion reactions, autoimmune hemolytic anemia, and hemolytic disease of the newborn (HDNB). In a transfusion reaction, antibodies (IgM) to ABO antigens cause agglutination, complement fixation, and intravascular hemolysis. A direct Coombs test will confirm the presence of antibody on the RBCs. An indirect Coombs test measures the degree of hemolytic activity. In autoimmune hemolytic anemia, antibodies against the body's own RBCs are produced. This reaction is provoked by allergic reactions to drugs, when a drug and antibody to the drug form a complex that attacks the RBCs. HDNB occurs during the pregnancy of a mother who has been sensitized to blood group antigens on a previous infant's RBCs and makes IgE antibodies to them. The antibodies cross the placenta and react with the fetal RBCs, causing destruction. Rhesus D (Rh factor) is the most commonly involved antigen.

Type III. Type III hypersensitivity reactions are immune complex-mediated reactions. In this condition, large quantities of antigen–antibody complexes are deposited in the tissues and cannot be cleared from the body by the reticuloendothelial system. This leads to a condition known as serum sickness. Causes are persistent infection, autoimmune disease, and environmental antigens.

Type IV. In type IV (delayed-type) hypersensitivity reactions, when the host meets a foreign antigen, antigen-sensitized T cells release lymphokines that destroy the antigen. Allergic contact dermatitis, acute allograft rejection, and delayed hypersensitivity skin testing are examples of type IV hypersensitivity reactions.

Anaphylaxis

Anaphylaxis is an acute, generalized, and violent antigen–antibody reaction that may be rapidly fatal even with prompt emergency treatment.

Pathophysiology. *Anaphylaxis results from a reaction to an allergen that causes the release of IgE. On first exposure to an antigen, IgE* antibodies are formed and attached to *mast cells* in tissues and *basophils* in the vascular system. Once antibodies have been formed, a second exposure to the antigen results in an immune reaction (*releasing histamine*) that may vary from mild to fatal. In its severe form, the reaction is called anaphylactic shock.

The reaction of anaphylactic shock is primarily a histamine reaction, setting off a chain of multiple chemical reactions that cause further reactions. The more reactions that occur, the more severe the anaphylaxis and the greater the mortality.

The release of histamine results in vasodilatation of the capillaries (causing hypotension) and a markedly increased cellular permeability. The increase in intracellular fluid alters the cell shape, leaving spaces between the previously compact cells. This promotes movement from the vascular system, thus increasing the colloid osmotic pressure. As more **colloids** move into interstitial spaces, edema and a decreased circulating volume of blood occur. This has the effect of decreasing **cardiac output**.

TABLE 25-3. COMMON ANAPHYLAXIS ALLERGENS

Foods	*Food Additives*	*Medications*	*Others*
Eggs Peanut butter Fish Shellfish Milk Cheese Tomatoes Chocolate Nuts and seeds	Monosodium glutamate Autolyzed yeast Natural flavorings Yeast extract Food coloring	Antibiotics Aspirin Contrast dye Blood products Vaccines Narcotics Local anesthetics	Latex Exercise Insect venom Animal hair/dander Dust Pollen

Histamine occurs in two forms: H_1 and H_2. H_1 causes vasoconstriction of the bronchi and intestines. H_2 increases gastric acid secretion and minor cardiac stimulation. Both H_1 and H_2 are responsible for vasodilatation.

The release and action of histamines result in the release of other amines into the bloodstream. Bradykinin, serotonin, slow-reacting substances, a chemotactic factor attracting eosinophils, prostaglandins, and acetylcholine all play a role in the physiologic development of anaphylaxis. These chemicals may also activate the complement system. These amines increase arteriolar and venous dilatation, capillary permeability, and abnormal shift of fluid from the vascular tree into the interstitial compartment. This shift decreases circulating blood volume but does not decrease total blood in the body. With blood remaining in the microcirculation, decreased systolic and diastolic pressure occurs. These substances and H_1 and H_2 cause an intense bronchiolar constriction that leads to a general hypoxemia.

Etiology. Many substances known as allergens can cause anaphylaxis. *Allergens can range from foods and food additives to drugs and insect-sting venom, including bee, wasp, and hornet* (**Table 25-3**). Routes of entry for an allergen can include injection, ingestion, inhalation, and skin absorption. *Drugs, especially antibiotics, are the major allergens in anaphylaxis.* Other drugs, iodine-based contrast dye, and blood transfusions are also involved in anaphylaxis. More recently, food preservatives and additives have been attributed to an increasing number of cases of anaphylaxis.

Clinical Presentation. **Clinical signs of anaphylaxis include generalized pruritus, respiratory distress, syncope, and apprehension, and can appear within several minutes of exposure to the antigen (Table 25-4).** The severity of the reaction is directly related to the onset of symptoms, with early signs appearing with a severe reaction. Occasionally, biphasic reactions occur in which symptoms recur several hours after the initial reaction.

Angioedema *is edema in membranous tissues and is most easily seen in the eyes and mouth.* It also occurs in the tongue, hands, feet, and genitalia. There is a diffuse erythema occurring more in the upper body parts than in the lower. Occasionally, abdominal cramps, vomiting, and/or diarrhea may occur. Unconsciousness occurs early in severe anaphylaxis.

As fluid shifts from the capillaries into the interstitial tissue, edema of the uvula and larynx occurs. This edema may produce

TABLE 25-4. CLINICAL SIGNS AND SYMPTOMS OF ANAPHYLAXIS

Less Severe or Initial	Severe and Emergent
Pruritus (generalized itching)/Hives/Rash	Confusion or decreased LOC
Flushing	Shortness of breath
Chest tightness	Stridor
Wheezing/Coughing	Bronchospasm
Angioedema (edema of the lips/tongue)	Laryngeal edema
Generalized or localized swelling	Hypotension/Shock
Restlessness/Feeling of impending doom	Weak, thready pulse/Tachycardia
Nausea/vomiting/diarrhea	
Difficulty swallowing (dysphagia)	
Abdominal pain or cramps	

Source: *clevelandclinic.org, Anaphylaxis—"What are the symptoms of anaphylaxis?" (6/5/23)*

an acute respiratory obstruction. *Laryngeal edema is accompanied by impaired phonation and a barking or high-pitched cough.* If the patient is alert, he or she will show *signs of increased anxiety and complain of air hunger.*

Cardiovascular effects of anaphylaxis are the same as those associated with other types of shock—mainly hypotension, tachycardia, and changes in the electrocardiogram similar to those that occur in myocardial injury. Temporary changes in the ST segment and the T wave suggest coronary ischemia. However, the serum enzymes are normal.

Life-threatening signs and symptoms include respiratory distress, stridor, bronchospasm, and laryngeal edema. The changes in ventilation (causing hypoxia) and decreased circulating blood may result in convulsions and unconsciousness. Circulatory failure and respiratory distress are the usual causes of death in anaphylaxis.

Complications. Myocardial infarction (MI) secondary to venous dilatation and a decreased blood pressure may occur. With decreased blood pressure, increased tissue hypoxia occurs. This results in increased tissue anoxia and destruction. Hypoventilation occurs because of the *decreased venous return of blood to the heart and increased tissue hypoxia.*

Pulmonary status, already compromised by bronchiolar constriction, may be further damaged because of over administration of the intravenous fluids used to compensate for the decreased vascular volume. Chemical reactions causing further imbalances may lead to central nervous system convulsions and coma. If the pulmonary, cardiac, or vascular system is refractory to treatment, anaphylaxis results in a shock state and can lead to cardiac, renal, pulmonary, and multisystem organ failure. Death in anaphylaxis can result from cardiovascular or respiratory distress.

QUICK TIP! Questions related to how you would prioritize the "ABCs" are not uncommon on the exam.

Treatment. The treatment goals for anaphylactic shock include the "ABCs" of emergency care (airway, breathing, and circulation) along with volume expansion. Hypotension can be managed with intravenous fluids to promote intravascular volume expansion. Vasoconstrictor agents may be required to reverse the effects of severe vasodilation and depressed myocardial function. **Epinephrine is a first-line drug given to patients with anaphylaxis because it promotes bronchodilation and vasoconstriction and inhibits further mediator release.** *The primary objective of treatment is to dilate the bronchioles, which is accomplished by the administration of epinephrine* either subcutaneously or intramuscularly. *Antihistamines* are used simultaneously to help control local edema and itching, but they cannot alter the circulatory failure and bronchoconstriction to a significant degree. After administration of **epinephrine**, the respiratory system may need to be supported by mask, intubation, or tracheostomy with the use of a ventilator.

The second goal of therapy is to improve the patient's circulatory status. Promoting the movement of fluid from the interstitial compartment back into the vascular compartment is usually achieved using intravenous fluids. Vasopressors may be used to cause constriction of the blood vessels. However, this can make tissue anoxia more severe, and use of vasopressors is controversial. The third-space loss of fluid is believed to be caused by leakage through the injured capillary walls. **Glucocorticoids** help to decrease cellular damage, reduce the severity of anaphylaxis, and prevent inflammation of the damaged tissues. **Hydrocortisone** given intravenously is typically administered. Steroids stabilize the membrane of the basophils, reducing the chemical reactions in anaphylaxis.

Nursing Intervention. Assessment of the signs and symptoms of anaphylaxis, especially respiratory distress and life-threatening hemodynamic instability, is extremely important. *Research has shown that laryngeal edema and hypotension are major factors causing death.*

Anaphylaxis may occur in susceptible patients immediately or as much as an hour after injection of an antigen (eg, drug, blood). Respiratory assessment includes:

- Identifying stridor
- Observing accessory muscle use
- Identifying the presence of cyanosis
- Auscultating lung fields for crackles, rhonchi, or wheezes
- Pulse oximetry monitoring and/or measuring arterial blood gases

Mechanical ventilation should be on standby if not already in use. Normal nursing interventions for patients on ventilators are applicable for these patients.

The patient's cardiac and circulatory status should be monitored closely, as hypotension can precede the onset of anaphylactic shock. Death can occur within minutes if there is circulatory failure or pulmonary edema. Vital signs—including heart rate, blood pressure, respiratory rate, and pulse oximetry—should be observed continuously until the patient is stable and then at very frequent intervals (at least every 15 minutes for four times, then every 30 minutes for four times, and then every 1–2 hour).

If **epinephrine** is used intravenously, it is essential to monitor for hypertension and cardiac dysrhythmias.

Renal status is monitored by Foley catheter to prevent fluid overload as the extracellular fluid moves back into the vascular system with appropriate drugs. In severe anaphylaxis, the patient may be unconscious, as the patient's condition stabilizes and his or her level of consciousness returns to normal, emotional support is essential. Explaining to the patient what has happened, what all the monitoring equipment is being used for, and that these monitors will be removed as his or her condition improves will help to alleviate the patient's fear. In addition, prevention of anaphylactic shock through identification of patients at risk and careful monitoring of patient response to potential allergens including drugs, blood products, and blood are important components of nursing care.

25.2 HEMATOLOGIC SYSTEM

Red Blood Cell Formation and Anemias

Hematopoiesis. Blood cells mature in the bone marrow. In the adult, bone marrow is primarily located in the long, flat bones (skull, ribs, sternum, pelvis, shoulder girdles, vertebrae, innominates). The mature erythrocyte, leukocyte, and thrombocyte all begin as primitive cells called stem cells. In response to specific stimuli, called colony-stimulating factors, a stem cell becomes "committed" to a particular cell line and matures to perform the functions of either an RBC, WBC, or platelet. Once the stem cell is committed, it is no longer capable of mitosis. It matures within the bone marrow and is released into the peripheral blood. Stem cells increase in number during times of increased demand (hypoxia, infection) to increase production of the needed blood cell type.

RBC production is stimulated by the hormone erythropoietin. *Erythropoietin is released by the kidney in response to tissue hypoxia.* This hormone results in increased erythrocyte production by:

- Increasing the number of stem cells placed into the maturational process
- Decreasing maturation time
- Increasing hemoglobin synthesis
- Causing a premature release of reticulocytes from the bone marrow

Reticulocytes may appear in the peripheral blood within 2 days of increased demand, but an increase in mature erythrocytes is not apparent until 6 to 8 days. An increase in the peripheral reticulocyte count is an indication of increased RBC production.

The primary function of the RBC is the transportation of oxygen and carbon dioxide. This transport occurs via the hemoglobin molecule. Normal hemoglobin production depends on a sufficient iron supply, protoporphyrin, and globin. The life span of the mature RBC in the circulation is approximately 120 days. As the cell becomes older, it is no longer able to traverse the microvasculature, and then it is phagocytized by the reticuloendothelial tissue.

Platelet Production. Platelet production is thought to be regulated by the hormone thrombopoietin. Platelets mature in the bone marrow and migrate to the spleen. Platelets contribute to hemostasis by forming a plug over an area of damaged endothelium. Plug formation requires an adequate number of functioning platelets as well as vascular integrity. Platelets are a source of phospholipids, which are necessary in the coagulation process.

Normal Coagulation and Pathologic Hematologic Conditions

Several actions occur to halt and prevent bleeding. Vasoconstriction and platelet aggregation are the first two events in hemostasis. Primary hemostasis is the process of platelet plug formation at the site of injury. This occurs within seconds of injury. Secondary hemostasis involves the reactions of the plasma coagulation system resulting in fibrin formation. This occurs within several minutes of injury.

Normal Coagulation. Blood clotting is a complex process that controls bleeding when tissues are injured. Normal coagulation depends on the presence of all clotting factors and the appropriate functioning of other separate but interrelated components. These components are the extrinsic cascade, the intrinsic cascade, and the common final pathway.

Within the circulating blood, there is a plethora of clotting factors to continue a cascade once initiated. It is interesting to note that there is at least one specific spot in each of the three cascades (extrinsic, intrinsic, and final common pathway) that requires calcium ions (Ca^{2+}, factor IV) to continue activation of these cascades. These sites are identified in **Fig. 25-5**, which shows the normal coagulation process.

Extrinsic Cascade. The extrinsic cascade (**Fig. 25-6**) is activated by injury to vessels and tissue. The result of this cascade is the release of thromboplastin into the circulatory system.

A second mechanism for activating clotting factors is the release of phospholipids from platelets and damaged tissue. This is thought to increase the rate of blood coagulation through both the extrinsic and intrinsic cascades.

Intrinsic Cascade. The intrinsic cascade (**Fig. 25-7**) is initiated when factor XII (the Hageman factor, or the surface substance) encounters collagen or the basement membrane of the blood vessel's damaged endothelium.

Common Final Pathway Cascade. Both the extrinsic and intrinsic cascades react to completion and, in the presence of calcium ions, join to form the common final pathway cascade shown in **Fig. 25-8**.

Syneresis is the final step in coagulation and the first step in clot stability. Syneresis is the process of particle suspension in a gel that begins to aggregate and form a compact mass—the clot. Clot retraction occurs soon after syneresis is complete. Platelets contain an enzyme called thromboplastin that causes the fibrin strands and cells in the clot to be drawn together, expressing a clear, serous fluid. Clot retraction is responsible for drawing the edges of damaged vessels together, which fosters healing.

Anticoagulation. When the vascular damage has been repaired, dissolution of the clot begins. This is termed fibrinolysis. Up to this point, the various cascades have clotted the injured vessels but have not caused massive intravascular clotting. Massive clotting is avoided because excess thrombin is carried away from the clot site by the circulating blood and antithrombin III is released from mast cells.

There are two mechanisms to prevent excessive clotting: the antithrombin system and the fibrinolytic system.

Antithrombin System. This system protects our bodies from excessive intravascular clotting by neutralizing the clotting capability of thrombin. Antithrombin III is the neutralizing

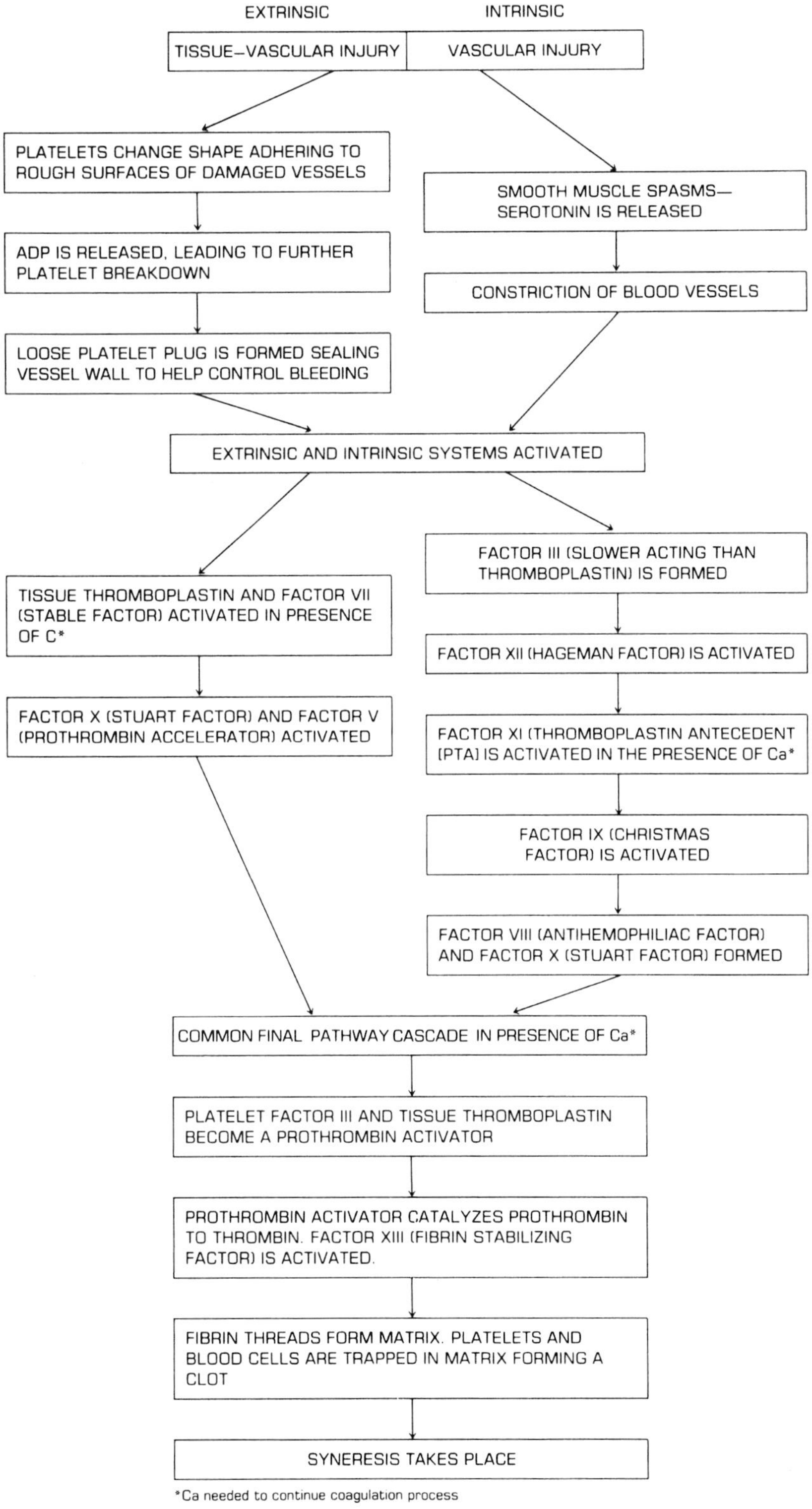

Figure 25-5. Normal coagulation process.

agent. Heparin functions as an antithrombin III and inhibits all serine proteases in all cascades. These include Xa, Ha, Vt12, and thrombin. Heparin interrupts the action of thrombin on fibrinogen.

When clot retraction is complete, profibrinolysis is activated by factor XII. This activation results in fibrinolysin (plasmin), which phagocytizes the clot and other clotting factors present more than the normal amount. In this way, both intravascular clotting and bleeding are controlled.

Fibrinolytic System. Fibrinolysis, or clot lysis, begins immediately after the formation of a hemostasis plug. Three potential activators of the fibrinolytic system are Hageman factor (factor XII) or plasma protein fragments, *urinary plasminogen activator or urokinase, and tissue plasminogen activator.*

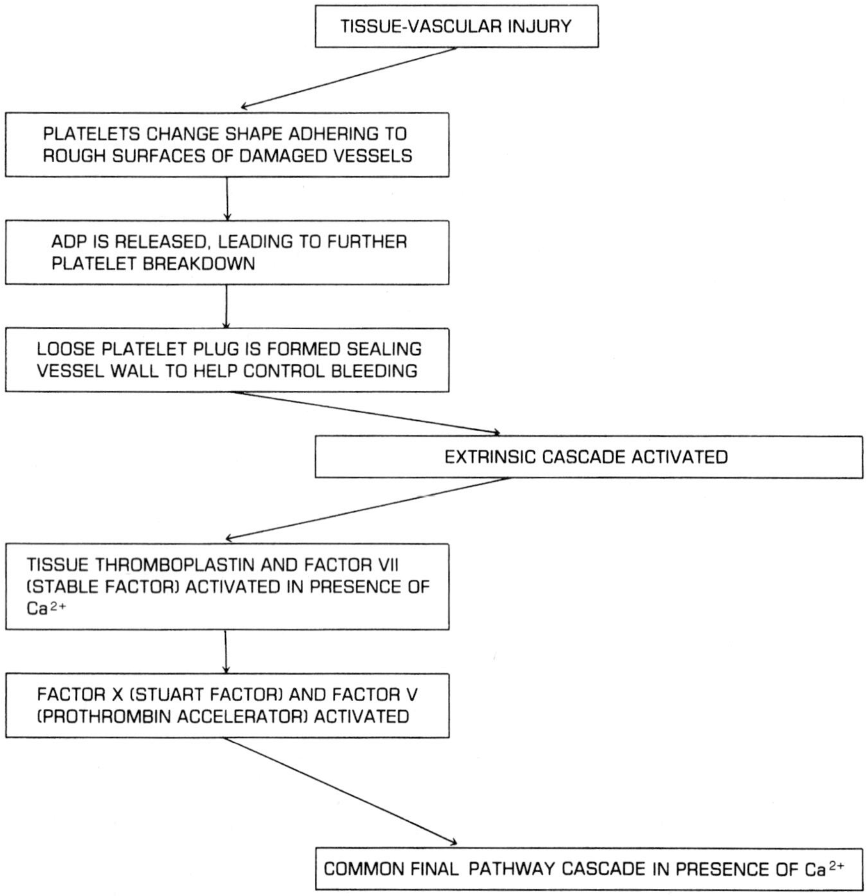

Figure 25-6. Extrinsic cascade segment of the overall normal coagulation process.

These activators convert plasminogen, adsorbed to the fibrin clot, to plasmin, which lyses the clot. Clot lysis (fibrinolysis) is accomplished by two mechanisms: clearance of activated clotting factors by the reticuloendothelial system and the actual lysis of the fibrin structure in the clot. Lysis of the clot is initiated by either the internal or external pathway. In the internal pathway, factor XII is activated to XIIa on contact with an abnormal or irregular vascular lining. At the same time, XIIa catalyzes prekallikrein to kallikrein (a blood plasminogen activator). The extrinsic system provides tissue plasminogen activators from damaged vascular areas. Both types of plasminogen activators convert plasminogen to plasmin. Plasmin breaks the fibrin structure, causing the mesh holding blood components, such as platelets, to weaken and dissociate as a stable unit. The breakdown of the fibrin structure causes an increase in fibrin degradation products (or fibrin split products). **An increase in fibrin degradation products may signal the onset of a coagulopathy such as DIC.**

KEY CLINICAL CONCEPT

There is often more than one question related to DIC. Remember lab findings associated with DIC: ↑PT increased, ↑INR increased, ↑Ptt increased, ↓Platelets decreased, ↓Fibrinogen decreased, ↑Fibrin split products (FSPs) increased. Increased FSPs indicate that the fibrinolytic system has been initiated, which is specific to DIC. Remember that FSP is the most important laboratory test for DIC.

Antiplatelet, Anticoagulant, and Fibrinolytic Therapy. Antithrombotic agents—including antiplatelet drugs, anticoagulants, and fibrinolytic agents—are used to prevent thrombotic events, prevent or minimize complications of thrombotic events, and restore vascular patency. **Table 25-5** outlines anticoagulant agents commonly used in critical care. Fibrinolytic therapy in the treatment of acute MI and pulmonary emboli employs the principles of normal clot lysis. Normally, the fibrinolytic system converts plasminogen to plasmin, which degrades fibrin into soluble fragments. In the presence of large thrombi, this system cannot dissolve the fibrin mass. However, the introduction of exogenous plasminogen activators produces more plasmin, which depletes circulating fibrinogen and promotes lysis. Exogenous plasminogen activator also destroys coagulation factors V and VIII, causing a systemic lytic state that increases the potential risk of bleeding.

The fibrinolytic agents used most frequently include **reteplase (rPA), alteplase (tPA),** and **streptokinase (SK).** SK is derived from beta-hemolytic streptococci and activates the fibrinolytic process by forming an activator complex with plasminogen. SK depletes fibrinogen and other coagulant factors, predisposing the patient to systemic bleeding. Allergic anaphylactic reactions can be induced on a second exposure to the drug due to its nature as a bacterial protein. **Alteplase (tPA, Activase)** was the first recombinant tissue-type plasminogen activator and is identical to a native tissue plasminogen activator. It is the fibrinolytic agent most often used for the treatment of coronary artery thrombosis, pulmonary embolism, and acute stroke. **Reteplase (rPA, Retavase)** is a

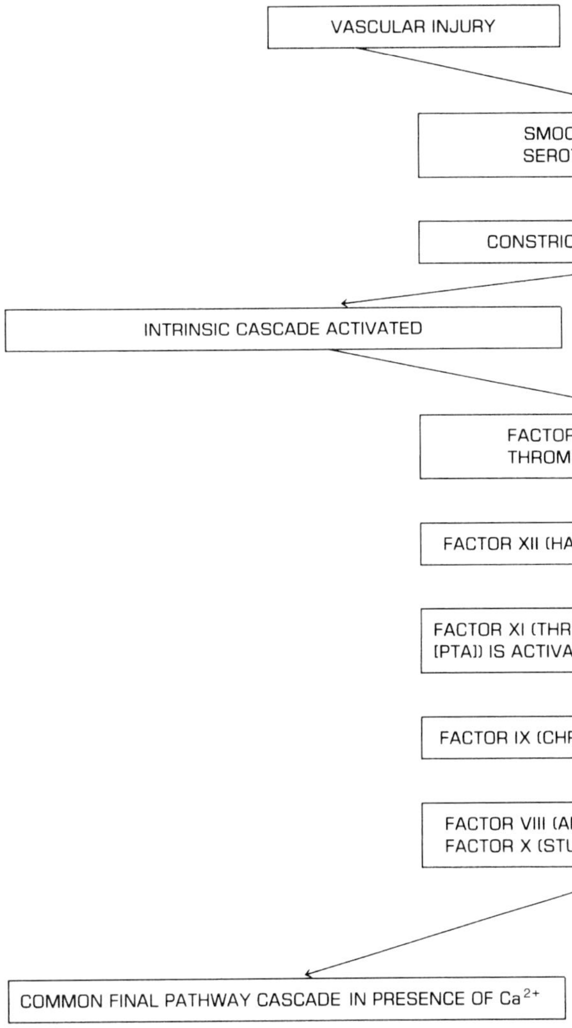

Figure 25-7. Intrinsic cascade segment of the overall normal coagulation process.

synthetic second-generation recombinant tissue-type plasminogen activator that works more quickly and has a lower bleeding risk than the first-generation agent alteplase.

Fibrinolysis is indicated for acute MI (if the patient presents within 12 hours of symptom onset), coronary artery thrombosis, pulmonary embolism, acute stroke, and acute peripheral arterial occlusions. Bleeding complications can occur with fibrinolysis. *For serious bleeding complications, the fibrinolytic agent should be stopped and supportive therapy instituted.* Volume and/or transfusion may be indicated if blood or

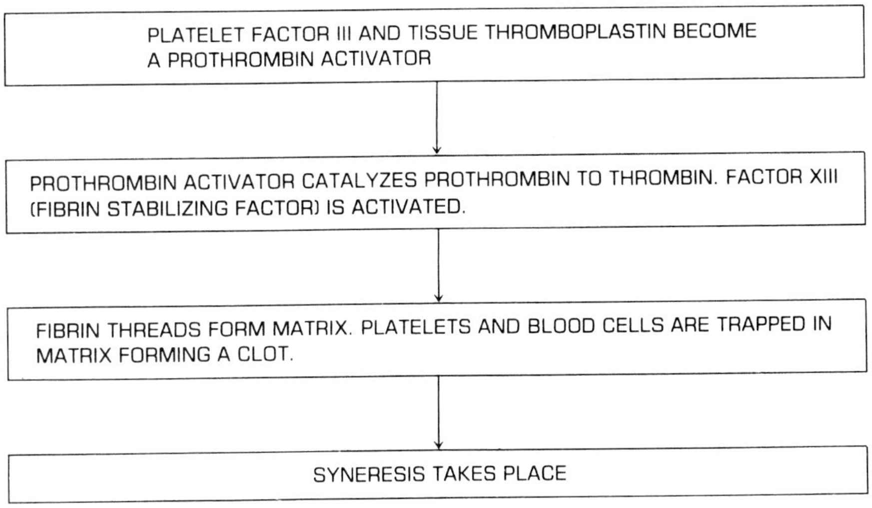

Figure 25-8. Common final pathway (cascade) segment of the normal coagulation process.

TABLE 25-5. ANTICOAGULANT AGENTS COMMONLY USED IN CRITICAL CARE

Antiplatelet agents	Aspirin Clopidogrel bisulfate (Plavix) Ticagrelor (Brilinta) Prasugrel (Effient) Dipyridamole (Persantine) Ticlopidine (Ticlid)
Glycoprotein IIb/IIIA inhibitors	Abciximab (Reopro) Eptifibatide (Integrilin) Tirofiban hydrochloride (Aggrastat)
Unfractionated heparin	Heparin sodium
Low-molecular-weight heparins	Enoxaparin sodium (Lovenox) Dalteparin sodium (Fragmin)
Fibrinolytic agents	Recombinant plasminogen activator (rPA, reteplase) Alteplase (tPA, Activase) Tenecteplase (TNKase) Streptokinase (Streptase) (less frequent)

Source: *Adapted with permission from Chulay M, Burns S. Hematology and Immunology Systems.* AACN Essentials of Critical Care Nursing. *New York: McGraw-Hill; 2006.*

blood factors such as fresh frozen plasma and/or cryoprecipitate are needed to replenish fibrin and clotting factors. *If the patient has also been receiving heparin,* **protamine sulfate** *may be used to reverse the heparin effect.* **Aminocaproic acid (Amicar)**, *a specific antidote to fibrinolytic agents, may also be indicated.*

KEY CONTENT CHECKLIST

- ❒ Bandemia (> 10%) may be suggestive of infection and can be used as a surrogate for WBC when considering sepsis SIRS criteria.
- ❒ Questions related to how you would prioritize the "ABCs" are not uncommon on the exam.
- ❒ The spleen serves as a blood reservoir and stores approximately 8 ounces of blood that can be released in trauma or bleeding.
- ❒ **Kehr's sign:** Left shoulder pain that may occur due to splenic injury during abdominal trauma. Diaphragmatic irritation and shoulder pain manifests as referred pain via the phrenic nerve.
- ❒ There is often more than one question related to DIC. Remember lab findings associated with DIC: ↑PT increased, ↑INR increased, ↑Ptt increased, ↓Platelets decreased, ↓Fibrinogen decreased, ↑Fibrin split products increased. Increased FSPs indicate that the fibrinolytic system has been initiated, which is specific to DIC. Remember that FSP is the most important laboratory test for DIC.

Review Questions:

1. Which of the following components of the immune system is referred to as "cell-mediated" in its immune response?

a. Segmented neutrophils
b. Band neutrophil
c. T lymphocytes
d. B lymphocytes

Answer: C. Rationale: There are two major types of lymphocytes: T lymphocytes (T cells) and B lymphocytes (B cells). T cells are involved in immunologic regulation and mediate what is called the cellular immune response. B cells produce antibodies and mediate what is called the humoral immune response. Neutrophils are phagocytic, early responders to a pathogen. Choose C.

2. Which term is used to describe a substance regarded as foreign in terms of the immune response?

a. Antibody
b. Antigen
c. Complement
d. Cytotoxic

Answer: B. Rationale: By definition, an antigen is a substance that is regarded as foreign in terms of the immune response. Antibodies are released to fight antigens, eliminating A. Complement is released to aid antibodies, eliminating C as well. Cytotoxic is a nonspecific term used to describe a toxin-induced threat to cellular viability. Choose B.

3. Which of the following types of cells produce antibodies?

a. Segmented neutrophils
b. Monocytes
c. B lymphocytes through plasma cells
d. Reticuloendothelial cells

Answer C. Rationale: B cells are effector cells that mediate the humoral immune response through the production of antibodies, which is their major function. B cells are important in defense against pyrogenic bacterial infections and can destroy transplanted organs by mediating hyperacute graft rejection.

26

Diagnosis and Treatment of Immunologic and Hematologic Problems

CHAPTER OVERVIEW AND OBJECTIVES

This chapter is supplemental to other chapters in Part IV. It provides additional information on diagnostic tests, pharmacology, and treatments for immunologic and hematologic problems. No specific questions will be derived from this chapter, although questions may be derived indirectly from the content of this chapter. Read this chapter to improve your general understanding of diagnostic tests and treatments related to hematology, immunology, and human immunodeficiency virus (HIV) testing.

After studying this chapter, you should understand the following:

- Describe the elements of the complete blood count panel and hemostatic screening tests.
- Define the disease influences that impact the blood cell count.
- Describe the elements and rationale for product selection during blood and component therapy.
- Describe the nursing interventions related to a transfusion reaction and related clinical implications.
- Identify key treatment of immunologic and hematologic problems.

26.1 COMPLETE BLOOD COUNT

The red blood cell (RBC) count consists of the total number of circulating RBCs, the part of the blood that transports oxygen. **Table 26-1** lists normal values. The hemoglobin (Hb) measures the oxygen-carrying capacity of the RBC, while the hematocrit (Hct) compares the RBC volume to the plasma volume. Other RBC indices include mean corpuscular volume (MCV), which is the average size of the RBC, and the mean corpuscular hemoglobin (MCH), which measures the average weight of the Hb per RBC. Finally, the mean corpuscular hemoglobin concentration (MCHC) measures the average percentage of Hb in an RBC. A peripheral smear allows the practitioner to examine the RBC and get data on composition, size, and shape.

Another useful test in evaluating the hematologic system is the reticulocyte count. This test identifies the bone marrow's ability to produce young erythrocytes. Reticulocytes are matured into RBCs in just under 24 hours. The life span of an RBC is approximately 120 days, after which it dies and releases Hb into the circulation; this is transported to the liver and spleen and ultimately broken down. Iron is then stored in the liver and spleen for future use and the remaining heme molecule is converted into bilirubin and excreted in the urine or stool.

The white blood cell (WBC) count measures the total number of white cells or leukocytes. Further breakdown of the WBC

TABLE 26-1. NORMAL LABORATORY VALUES FOR THE COMPLETE[a] BLOOD COUNT	
Red cell count (RBC)	
Women	3.8–5.2 × 10/mL
Men	4.4–5.9 × 10/mL
Hemoglobin (Hb)	
Women	11.7–15.7 g/dL
Men	13.3–17.7 g/dL
Hematocrit (Hct)	
Women	34.9%–46.9%
Men	39.8%–52.2%
Platelets (Plt)	150,000–400,000
White cell count (WBC)	3500–11,000/mL
Neutrophils	39%–79%
Lymphocytes	10%–40%
Monocytes	3%–8%
Basophils	0%–2%
Eosinophils	0%–5%
Reticulocyte count	0.5%–1.5%
Erythrocyte sedimentation rate (ESR)	
Women	1–20 mm/h
Men	1–13 mm/h
Prothrombin time (PT)	11–16 s
Activated partial thromboplastin time (aPTT)	20–35 s
Bleeding time	< 4 min
INR	1.0–2.0
Fibrinogen	200–400 mg/dL
Fibrin split products (FSP)	2–10 μg/mL
D-dimer	< 200 mg/mL

[a]*Normal values may vary between laboratories. Refer to local laboratory standard values in interpreting test results.*

count is called the *differential*. Components of the differential include neutrophils, monocytes, lymphocytes, basophils, and eosinophils. Absolute counts in the differential are more important because they are in direct relation to the WBC count. Abnormal components and causative agents of the differential are listed in **Table 26-2**.

The erythrocyte sedimentation rate (ESR) is often used in evaluating infectious diseases. It is a nonspecific test that examines the volume of RBCs that settle in 1 hour. Elevation is usually seen with inflammation, infection, or malignancy.

26.2 HEMOSTATIC SCREENING TESTS

Normal clotting has three stages: (1) vascular injury activates thromboplastin activity in both the extrinsic and intrinsic pathways, (2) thromboplastin converts prothrombin to thrombin, and (3) thrombin converts fibrinogen in the plasma at the site of injury to form a fibrin plug.

Specific tests can be performed to evaluate blood-clotting activity, identify abnormalities, and ascertain patient response to therapy.

Prothrombin Time

The prothrombin time (PT) measures the activity level and patency of the extrinsic clotting cascade and the common final pathway. The PT measures factors I, II, V, VII, and X. Normal values are the same as control values (should be 11–16 s). *The effectiveness of warfarin (Coumadin) is assessed with the PT.*

Activated Partial Thromboplastin Time

The activated partial thromboplastin time (aPTT) measures the activity level and patency of the intrinsic clotting cascade and common final pathway. Normal values of 20 to 35 seconds are used to assess all clotting factors except VII and XIII. *The effectiveness of heparin is assessed with the aPTT.*

Bleeding Time

Platelet plug formation time is measured with the bleeding time. Normal values are less than 4 minutes (Ivy), 1 to 4 minutes (Duke), and 1 to 9 minutes (Mielke). *Bleeding times predominantly reflect platelet function*, and conditions causing poor platelet function produce abnormal results.

Platelet Count

This is a specific count of platelets seen in a blood smear. Normal values are 150,000 to 450,000 platelets per microliter (mcL). Values below 100,000 are pathognomonic for thrombocytopenia, the cause of which must be determined. *A platelet count less than 50,000 results in excessive bleeding*, since there is an insufficient number of platelets to clot. *Prior to performing an invasive procedure (eg, CVL insertion) a platelet count of at least 50,000 should be present.* **Counts less than 20,000 are associated with spontaneous bleeding.** *A higher than normal platelet count, more than 450,000, can result in an increased risk of forming blood clots.*

26.3 HUMAN IMMUNODEFICIENCY VIRUS SCREENING TESTS

New recommendations related to the HIV are consistently being reviewed. The current recommendations include an initial fourth-generation antigen/antibody combination immunoassay. If this initial result is negative, then there is no need for further testing. However, if this initial test is reactive, then an HIV-1/HIV-2 differentiation immunoassay should be performed. The only differentiation assay laboratory test approved by the Food and Drug Administration (FDA) is the Multispot HIV1/2 Rapid test. If there is a reactive test on the initial fourth-generation combination immunoassay and a nonreactive result on the differentiation assay, an HIV-1 nucleic acid test (NAT) should be performed to confirm the diagnosis. Previously, the Western Blot was considered the confirmatory test for a diagnosis of HIV; however, this test is no longer part of the recommended screening algorithm for HIV testing. Other diagnostic studies that have proven useful in tracking the progression of HIV and response to therapy are CD4 counts and HIV viral load. The CD4 cell is the primary target and binding site of HIV. As the virus progresses, the CD4 count drops, although with the new antiretroviral therapy available today, it is not uncommon to see the CD4 count rise significantly. A diagnostic marker called HIV viral load is available and measures the free virus in the plasma. This test can also show response to new therapy or indicate the need for a treatment change.

TABLE 26-2. INFLUENCE OF DISEASE ON BLOOD CELL COUNT

Cell Type	*How Affected*
Neutrophils	Increased by: • Infections: osteomyelitis, otitis media, salpingitis, septicemia, gonorrhea, endocarditis, smallpox, chickenpox, herpes, Rocky Mountain spotted fever • Ischemic necrosis due to myocardial infarction, burns, carcinoma • Metabolic disorders: diabetic acidosis, eclampsia, uremia, thyrotoxicosis • Stress response due to acute hemorrhage, surgery, excessive exercise, emotional distress, third trimester of pregnancy, childbirth • Inflammatory disease: rheumatic fever, rheumatoid arthritis, acute gout, vasculitis, and myositis Decreased by: • Bone marrow depression due to radiation or cytotoxic drugs • Infections: typhoid, tularemia, brucellosis, hepatitis, influenza, measles, mumps, rubella, infectious mononucleosis • Hypersplenism: hepatic disease and storage diseases • Collagen vascular disease, such as systemic lupus erythematosus • Deficiency of folic acid or vitamin B_{12}
Eosinophils	Increased by: • Allergic disorders: asthma, hay fever, food or drug sensitivity, serum sickness, angioneurotic edema • Parasitic infections: trichinosis, hookworm, roundworm, amebiasis • Skin diseases: eczema, pemphigus, psoriasis, dermatitis, herpes • Neoplastic diseases: chronic myelocytic leukemia, Hodgkin disease, metastases, and necrosis of solid tumors • Miscellaneous: collagen vascular disease, adrenocortical hypofunction, ulcerative colitis, polyarteritis nodosa, postsplenectomy, pernicious anemia, scarlet fever, excessive exercise Decreased by: • Stress response due to trauma, shock, burns, surgery, mental distress • Cushing syndrome
Basophils	Increased by: • Chronic myelocytic leukemia, polycythemia vera, some chronic hemolytic anemias, Hodgkin disease, systemic mastocytosis, myxedema, ulcerative colitis, chronic hypersensitivity states, nephrosis Decreased by: • Hyperthyroidism, ovulation, pregnancy, stress
Lymphocytes	Increased by: • Infections: pertussis, brucellosis, syphilis, tuberculosis, hepatitis, infectious mononucleosis, mumps, German measles, cytomegalovirus • Other: thyrotoxicosis, hypoadrenalism, ulcerative colitis, immune diseases, lymphocytic leukemia Decreased by: • Severe debilitating illness, such as congestive heart failure, renal failure, advanced tuberculosis • Defective lymphatic circulation, high levels of adrenal corticosteroids, immunodeficiency due to immunosuppressives
Monocytes	Increased by: • Infections: subacute bacterial endocarditis, tuberculosis, hepatitis, malaria, Rocky Mountain spotted fever • Collagen vascular disease: systemic lupus erythematosus, rheumatoid arthritis, polyarteritis nodosa • Carcinomas, monocytic leukemia, lymphomas

26.4 TESTS FOR OTHER INFECTIOUS DISEASES

Diagnostic tests often ordered for patients with a suspected infectious disease include cultures, susceptibility, and Gram's stain. Samples for these procedures will be collected by the nurse or physician and sent to the microbiology lab. Sources include blood, sputum, urine, and drainage from wounds. In addition, the nurse should review subjective and objective assessments and be aware of the various signs of hematologic and immunologic disease (**Table 26-3**).

26.5 BLOOD AND COMPONENT THERAPY

The primary reason for transfusing blood is to increase the amount if circulating oxygen in order to prevent tissue hypoxia. **Blood is administered primarily when the Hb/Hct levels are**

TABLE 26-3. SIGNS AND SYMPTOMS OF HEMATOLOGIC AND IMMUNOLOGIC DISEASES

Subjective
Fatigue
Dyspnea
Inability to perform activities of daily living
Objective
Altered mental status
Fever
Tachycardia
Hypotension
Tachypnea
Cough
Dysrhythmia
Abnormal lab values
Positive cultures
Skin lesions
Poor urine output
Lymphadenopathy

low (generally when Hb levels are < 7 g/dL), when intravascular volume is low, and to replace deficient or utilized substances such as protein, platelets, and clotting factors.

QUICK TIP! Common RBC transfusion criteria are Hb <7 g/dL or < 8 to 10 g/dL in the setting of acute coronary syndrome (ACS), or actively bleeding.

Whole Blood

One unit of whole blood is approximately 500 mL of blood cells, plasma, platelets, proteins, and other intravascular nutrients and substances. Whole blood is the best substance to transfuse in hemorrhage, since it replaces both volume and elements. Due to supply shortages, the transfusion of whole blood is rare. Whole blood can be divided into **packed RBCs (PRBCs), fresh frozen plasma (FFP), and cryoprecipitate,** making it possible for more than one patient to benefit from the donation of 1 unit of whole blood. Whole blood can be stored for 5 weeks; however, factors V and VIII are labile and are significantly decreased after 7 days.

Normally, during the administration of a blood transfusion, the cold donor blood (due to storage) is rapidly warmed as it mixes with circulating blood at normal infusion rates. Rapid replacement with cold blood predisposes the patient to cardiac arrest, hypothermia, and coagulopathies. When massive, rapid transfusions are necessary, the blood can be passed through a warmer to reach body temperature, thus reducing these dangers.

QUICK TIP! Hypothermia associated with PRBC transfusion would also shift the oxyhemoglobin dissociation curve to the left.

Packed Red Blood Cells

PRBCs provide the advantage of less blood volume (200–300 mL) to infuse, thereby decreasing the chance of fluid overload. PRBCs are used in severe anemias without blood loss and hemorrhage. **One unit of PRBCs raises Hb concentration about 1 g/dL.** PRBCs are given cautiously in patients with congestive heart failure (HF), cardiac disease, or with renal failure related to the increased risk of fluid overload. **In the average adult, 1 unit of RBCs raises the Hct by 3% and the Hb by 1 g/dL.**

Fresh Frozen Plasma

FFP is the fluid portion of blood after centrifugation to remove the RBCs. When the plasma is frozen, all clotting factors (especially V and VII) except the platelets are preserved.

Administration of plasma is indicated when there is a coagulopathy or hypovolemia with little or no actual blood loss, for example in burns and crush injuries. In an emergency, FFP may be used as a volume expander in hypovolemic bleeds until fresh whole blood is available. One unit of FFP can raise coagulation factors by 5% to 8% and fibrinogen by 13 mg/dL in the average patient.

Cryoprecipitates

Cryoimmunoglobulins must be obtained and processed at temperatures more than 20°C and ideally before refrigeration, which may cause cryoproteins to be caught in the blood clots. Cryoprecipitates usually compose 20 to 30 mL/unit of blood and must be infused immediately after thawing. Cryoprecipitates contain factors VIII and XIII and fibrinogen. One unit (20–50 mL) raises fibrinogen by about 75 mg/dL. **Cryoprecipitate is useful to quickly raise the fibrinogen level in patients with disseminated intravascular coagulation (DIC).** The administration of cryoprecipitates is also indicated in hemophilia A and von Willebrand disease.

Platelets

Less than 50,000 platelets per cubic microliter (mcL) is considered inadequate for hemostasis. **Abnormalities in coagulation time are a better index of the need for platelet transfusion than an actual platelet count.** Bleeding time is a test that can be performed to determine how long a patient takes to form a clot. Thromboelastogram (TEG) may be utilized in certain settings to measure how long it takes for a clot to form and what is the strength of the clot that is formed. These measurements are used to determine whether platelets or other blood products should be provided. In patients with renal dysfunction, **DDAVP** may be provided to neutralize the effects of uremia and allow circulating platelets to function appropriately. *Uremia inhibits platelet aggregation.*

In thrombocytopenia, splenomegaly, and DIC, platelet transfusions are useful until more definitive therapy can be instituted. Alloimmunity may require cross-matching to have any value for platelet transfusion. One unit of single donor (pheresis) platelets is equivalent to 5 to 6 platelet concentrates. *One concentrate of platelet can raise the platelet count by 5000 to 7000/mcL.* Platelets can be safely kept at room temperatures for up to 3 days and *are inactivated if refrigerated.*

Blood Substitutes. Several synthetic blood products have been proposed for use in transfusion therapy to increase oxygen-carrying capacity. Hemopure is a bovine-based oxygen carrier fluid. It is compatible with all blood types and has been utilized with special patient populations that that do not accept blood products due to religious reasons (Jehovah's witnesses). This fluid serves a volume expander and transports and delivers oxygen. This therapy is not FDA approved. Human polymerized hemoglobin (PolyHeme) is an oxygen-carrying resuscitative fluid that has been tested in the treatment of acute blood loss. Currently, there are no blood substitutes that have been approved by the FDA.

Granulocytes

Centers performing leukapheresis can filter out granulocytes. Each unit is about 200 to 300 mL, and the recipient must be compatible with the donor. An infusion of granulocytes improves phagocytosis from the marginal cells without increasing the already circulating pool of WBCs. The marginal cells are those being released from the bone marrow. Patients that are neutropenic have demonstrated a strong response to granulocyte infusions in combination with antibiotics.

Patients may experience a mild to moderate reaction to the transfusion as evidenced by fever, chills (rigors), and oxygen desaturation during granulocyte infusion. **Acetaminophen** and **diphenhydramine** are administered prior to the transfusion to minimize these reactions.

Reactions to Blood and Component Therapy

Despite meticulous procedures for blood and component therapy, reactions do occur. There are four major reactions.

1. **Circulatory overload** occurs when too much fluid or too rapid an infusion is administered to patients with underlying cardiac, renal, liver, pulmonary, or hematologic disease. With proper monitoring and assessment, circulatory overload should not occur. If it does occur, prompt and appropriate intervention to remove sufficient fluid and support the ABCs until homeostasis is achieved.
2. **A bacterial reaction** to transfusion therapy is the most common reaction and is characterized by the development of a fever in a previously afebrile patient. If the patient is febrile, a rising temperature may indicate a reaction.
3. **Allergic reactions** may occur with almost any product transfused. A slight reaction may be manifested by a mild urticaria. A severe allergic reaction is indicated by anaphylaxis.
4. **A hemolytic reaction** usually occurs within the first 30 minutes of the transfusion. It results in actual hemolysis of the RBCs, and the transfusion must be stopped. A Coombs test will diagnose this problem.

Clinical Presentation. The signs and symptoms will differ with the type of reaction, length of transfusion, substance being infused, and intensity of the reaction. Common signs and symptoms may include chills, fever, hives, hypotension, cardiac palpitations, tachycardia, flushing of the skin, headache, loss of consciousness, nausea and vomiting, shortness of breath, back pain, and hemoglobinuria. In some instances, warmth along the vein carrying the infusion may be detected.

Nursing Intervention. **The nurse must immediately stop the infusion** (saving the substance being transfused) and keep the vein open with 0.9 normal saline. Accurate assessment of patient status must be completed quickly and efficiently for comparison with pretransfusion baseline data. The physician and the blood bank are notified of the reaction, and the physician's orders are carried out. If the reaction is anaphylactic, emergency resuscitative measures are instituted while personnel contact the physician and laboratory. The blood product being infused at the time of reaction must be saved for further testing.

Nursing support of the patient and family is best achieved by rapid but efficient and professional conduct in instituting all necessary interventions. Education as to the cause of the reaction may prevent a recurrence.

TABLE 26-4. CLOTTING FACTORS AND THEIR SYNONYMS

Factors	*Synonym*
I	Fibrinogen
Ia	Fibrin
II	Prothrombin
IIa	Thrombin
III	Thromboplastin
IV	Calcium
V	Ac-globulin (labile factor, proaccelerin)
VII	Proconvertin (autoprothrombin I)
VIIa	Convertin
VIII	Antihemophilic globulin
IX	Christmas factor (autoprothrombin II), plasma thromboplastin component
IXa	Activated plasma thromboplastin component
X	Stuart–Prower factor (autoprothrombin III)
XI	Plasma thromboplastin antecedent
XII	Hageman factor
XIIa	Activated Hageman factor
XIII	Fibrin-stabilizing factor

Clotting Factors. Confusion often occurs with the nomenclature assigned to the specific clotting factors. Consequently, an international committee agreed that all clotting factors would be designated by roman numerals for the inactive clotting factors. It was further agreed that once activated, the clotting factors would be identified by the roman numeral and a lower case "a." **Table 26-4** lists the clotting factors and their synonyms. There is no designated factor VI.

Most of the clotting factors are found in circulating blood, the blood elements, and tissues surrounding and within the microcirculatory system. Clotting factors I (fibrinogen), II (prothrombin), and V, VII, IX, and X are synthesized in the liver. Factors XII and XIII may also be synthesized in the liver. Site of production of factor VIII is not entirely understood but is thought to be from endothelial cells.

Four clotting factors—factors II, VII, IX, and X—are dependent on vitamin K for synthesis by the liver. It is known that at least 30 substances may relate to the clotting process; however, the 17 listed in Table 26-4 are the most significant.

26.6 TREATMENTS FOR HEMATOLOGIC AND IMMUNOLOGIC DISORDERS

Neutropenia

Treatment for neutropenia involves administering colony-stimulating factors such as **filgrastim (*Neupogen*).** This medication stimulates granulocyte precursors and must be given intravenously or subcutaneously. The dosage is 5 to 7.5 μg/kg three to seven times per week.

Anemia

Certain anemias can be treated with **epoetin alfa (*Epogen*)** injections. This is the erythropoietin hormone produced by recombinant DNA technology. The usual dosage is 100 units/kg three times a week. The route must be intravenous or subcutaneous because of poor bioavailability by the oral route.

Infection

At the first indication of infection, blood urine and /or respiratory cultures are obtained based upon the suspected source (ie concern for pneumonia, respiratory culture is obtained). Antibiotics are provided initially to cover a broad range of organisms. After culture data results, antibiotics are narrowed to agents that are specific to the culture results. Many antibiotics require specific monitoring to achieve therapeutic range and monitoring for toxicity. Peak and trough levels may be required as well as routine monitoring of renal and hepatic function.

Included in treatment should be appropriate infection control. Isolation should be used per disease specifications. The goal is to decrease nosocomial infections (**Table 26-5**).

Immunodeficiency

Finally, the treatment for HIV/AIDS is ever-changing. Combination antiretroviral therapy, or HAART, is the cornerstone of management of patients with HIV infection. Currently, agents used for the treatment of HIV infection fall into five categories: (1) reverse transcriptase inhibitors, or those that inhibit the viral reverse transcriptase enzyme; (2) protease inhibitors, those that inhibit the viral protease; (3) fusion inhibitors; (4) entry inhibitors; and (5) integrase inhibitors. The reverse transcriptase inhibitors were the first class of drugs licensed for the treatment of HIV infection and are indicated for this use as part of combination regimens. Reverse transcriptase inhibitors include the *nucleoside analogues* zidovudine, didanosine, zalcitabine, stavudine, lamivudine, abacavir, and emtricitabine; the *nucleotide analogue* tenofovir; and the *nonnucleoside reverse transcriptase inhibitors* nevirapine, delavirdine, efavirenz, and etravirine. Protease inhibitors (saquinavir, indinavir, ritonavir, nelfinavir, amprenavir, lopinavir/ritonavir, atazanavir, tipranavir, darunavir) are used as part of initial regimens in combination with reverse transcriptase inhibitors and are effective in suppressing HIV replication. Enfuvirtide, the only FDA-approved fusion inhibitor, is administered as a subcutaneous injection. It works by inhibiting fusion of the HIV envelope to the target cell membrane. Entry inhibitors (maraviroc) inhibit the binding of HIV to the chemokine receptor CCR5, which is the coreceptor used by monotropic strains of HIV. Its use is restricted to persons who are infected with monotropic, rather than T-cell tropic, strains of HIV. Integrase inhibitors (raltegravir) inhibit the viral integrase enzyme which mediates integration of the viral genome into the target cell DNA. Often, three-drug regimens are used in the treatment of HIV, and all require close monitoring because of their potential for causing numerous side effects, including bone marrow suppression, peripheral neuropathy, hepatomegaly, renal toxicity, and gastrointestinal upset.

TABLE 26-5. RISK FACTORS FOR IMMUNOCOMPROMISE

Age extremes: neonates and elderly
Malnutrition
Known diseases involving the immune system, such as HIV infection
Chronic disease, such as diabetes, renal, or hepatic failure
Immunosuppressive agents: steroids, cancer chemotherapeutic agents, and transplant immunosuppressive agents
Radiation therapy
Invasive catheters, such as intravascular catheters, indwelling urinary catheters, wound drains, ventricular shunts
Prosthetic devices such as synthetic vascular grafts
Cardiovascular devices such as pacemakers, implantable defibrillators
Orthopedic hardware such as pins, plates, screws, artificial joints
Loss of skin integrity because of wounds, burns, presence of decubitus ulcers
Loss of protective epithelial barriers because of oral or nasogastric intubation

Source: *Adapted with permission from Chulay M, Burns SM.* AACN Essentials of Critical Care Nursing. *New York, NY: McGraw Hill; 2005.*

QUICK TIP! Bactrim is a key drug of choice for pneumocystis carinii pneumonia (PCP) prophylaxis in the setting of HIV/AIDS

KEY CONTENT CHECKLIST

- ❒ The effectiveness of warfarin (Coumadin) is assessed with the PT.
- ❒ The effectiveness of heparin is assessed with the aPTT.
- ❒ In the average adult, 1 unit of RBCs raises Hct by 3% and Hb by 1 g/dL.
- ❒ Prior to performing an invasive procedure (eg, CVL insertion) a platelet count of at least 50,000 should be present. Counts less than 20,000 are associated with spontaneous bleeding. Less than 50,000 platelets per cubic microliter (mcL) is considered inadequate for hemostasis.
- ❒ Cryoprecipitate is useful to quickly raise the fibrinogen level in patients with DIC.
- ❒ Administration of plasma is indicated when there is a coagulopathy or hypovolemia with little or no actual blood loss
- ❒ In the setting of any type of transfusion reaction, the nurse must immediately stop the infusion (saving the substance being transfused)
- ❒ Hypothermia associated with PRBC transfusion would also shift the oxyhemoglobin dissociation curve to the left
- ❒ Common RBC transfusion criteria are Hb <7 g/dL or < 8 to 10 g/dL in the setting of acute coronary syndrome (ACS), or actively bleeding.

Review Questions:

1. **Which test is best employed to assess the effectiveness of heparin therapy?**
   a. Partial thromboplastin time (PTT)
   b. Prothrombin time (PT)
   c. Platelet levels
   d. Bleeding time

Answer: A. Rationale: The activated partial thromboplastin time (aPTT) measures the activity level and patency of the intrinsic clotting cascade and common final pathway. Normal values of 20 to 35 s are used to assess all clotting factors except VII and XIII. The effectiveness of heparin is assessed with the aPTT.

2. **Which antibody is naturally present in bodily secretions (eg, saliva)?**
   a. IgG
   b. IgQ
   c. IgA
   d. IgE

Answer: C. Rationale: IgA is the secretory immunoglobulin present in bodily secretions and offers natural protection against nonspecific foreign antigens. About 15% of all antibodies are of the IgA type. Reference Table 25-1 for further detail.

3. **What is the first stage in the coagulation process?**
   a. Conversion of plasminogen to plasmin
   b. Conversion of fibrinogen to fibrin
   c. Activation of thrombin
   d. Activation of thromboplastin

Answer: D. Rationale: Syneresis is the final step in coagulation and the first step in clot stability. Syneresis is the process of particle suspension in a gel that begins to aggregate and form a compact mass—the clot. Clot retraction occurs soon after syneresis is complete. Platelets contain an enzyme called thromboplastin that causes the fibrin strands and cells in the clot to be drawn together, expressing a clear, serous fluid. Clot retraction is responsible for drawing the edges of damaged vessels together, which fosters healing.

27

Hematologic and Immunologic Failure and Its Effects on Other Organ Systems

CHAPTER OVERVIEW AND OBJECTIVES

The CCRN exam may contain approximately two to five questions on disorders of the immune system. Although specifics of different types of diseases, such as cancers, are not likely to be addressed on the exam, it is important to understand the general concepts presented in this chapter. Immunologic concepts are sometimes difficult to apply clinically, but the major concepts are important to the assessment and therapeutic interventions associated with critical-care immunology.

After studying this chapter, you should understand the following:

- Define the disorders of the hematologic system and associated clinical and nursing implications for care.
- Describe the elements of the immunologic system.
- Define the disorders of the immunologic system and associated clinical and nursing implications for care.

27.1 DISORDERS OF THE HEMATOLOGIC SYSTEM

Anemia

Definition and Etiology. Anemia is the most common problem of the erythrocyte (red blood cell [RBC]). Anemia is a clinical condition where this is a reduction in the number of RBCs, quantity of hemoglobin (Hb) and/or reduction in the volume of RBCs. Anemia is measured with an RBC count, Hb concentration, and hematocrit (Hct) concentration.

Causes of anemia (**Table 27-1** outlines the classification of anemias) include the following:

- Heredity
- Nutritional deficiencies
- Blood loss
- Immunologic and idiopathic causes
- Exogenous (medications) causes
- Chronic diseases
- Infections
- Neoplasms

Clinical Presentation. The signs and symptoms of anemia are the result of tissue hypoxia or the compensatory mechanisms activated to prevent damage resulting from hypoxia. Persons are symptomatic at varying levels. Someone with mild anemia may be asymptomatic. Anemia may be the first indication of a serious underlying disease such as cancer or renal failure. If it occurs gradually, adaptation allows for minimal signs and symptoms. A person with a rapid onset of anemia may be very symptomatic. The signs and symptoms associated with anemia are as follows: increased pulse, respiration, and pulse pressure; decreased blood pressure; palpitations; chest pain; dyspnea on exertion; fatigue; weakness; vertigo; bone tenderness; and delayed wound healing.

TABLE 27-1. CLASSIFICATION OF ANEMIA

I. Blood loss
   A. Acute
   B. Chronic
II. Deficient RBC production
   A. Iron deficiency
   B. Vitamin B_{12} deficiency
   C. Folic acid deficiency
   D. Bone marrow failure or suppression
      1. Myelofibrosis
      2. Aplastic anemia
      3. Malignant infiltration of marrow by tumor
      4. Marrow toxin (drugs, radiation)
      5. Infectious agents
III. Excessive RBC destruction
   A. Hemolytic anemia
   B. Defective glycolysis (glucose-6-phosphate dehydrogenase [G6PD] deficiency)
   C. Membrane abnormalities
   D. Physical causes (prosthetic heart valves)
IV. Defective hemoglobin synthesis
   A. Thalassemias
   B. Sickle cell anemia
V. Anemias of chronic disease
   A. Renal disease
   B. Inflammatory disease
   C. Liver disease
   D. Endocrine disorders
   E. Cancers

KEY CLINICAL CONCEPT

Sometimes a general rule of thumb applies in critical care, "If it occurs slowly, you can correct it slowly. If it occurs quickly, you must correct it quickly." Examples of this include electrolyte balances and anemia.

Diagnosis. Anemia laboratory findings are as follows:

- Decreased Hb and Hct
- Decreased RBC indices
- Increased reticulocyte count (presence depends on cause of anemia)
- Decreased erythrocyte count.

Nursing Intervention. Nursing interventions for the patient with anemia minimize complications, conserve energy, and implement medical therapies. The key interventions include the following:

1. History
   a. Signs of blood loss
   b. Bleeding tendencies
   c. Exposure to marrow toxins (drugs, radiation, chemicals)
   d. Previous history of anemia
   e. Surgical history (eg, gastric resection)
   f. Comorbid conditions
   g. Changes in nutritional status
2. Physical assessment
   a. Oxygenation: vital signs, lung sounds, tolerance of activity
   b. Skin, mucous membranes: pallor, jaundice, purpura, petechiae, IV-line sites, wounds, indwelling catheters, stomatitis
   c. Gastrointestinal (GI): ascites, splenomegaly
   d. Mobility: paresthesias, impaired sensation, bone pain (sternum, ribs, vertebrae)
3. Administer therapy to correct anemia
   a. Packed RBC infusion
   b. Iron replacement
   c. Hematopoietic hormone (erythropoietin alfa, EPO [Epogen, Procrit], darbepoetin alfa [Aranesp]).
4. Minimize energy expenditure by
   a. Organizing activities per patient tolerance
   b. Planning rest periods
   c. Limiting external stimulation
   d. Preventing chills
5. Maintain skin integrity
6. Promote a diet adequate in protein, iron, vitamins, and minerals
7. Maintain physical safety (eg, assist with ambulation if the patient is dizzy)
8. Institute an appropriate oral hygiene program

Thrombocytopenia

Thrombocytopenia is defined as quantitative decrease in the number of circulating platelets. Causes include

- Decreased bone marrow production
- Increased sequestration of platelets in the spleen
- Accelerated destruction of platelets.

Drug-induced thrombocytopenia can result from many common drugs including antibiotics (sulfonamides, penicillins, cephalosporins), **heparins** (highest incidence is with unfractionated products), cardiovascular drugs (thiazide diuretics), and chemotherapeutic agents (carboplatin, alkylating agents, anthracyclines, antimetabolites). Normal platelet count is 150,000 to 300,000/mm^3. The risk of bleeding increases as the platelet count decreases.

KEY CLINICAL CONCEPT

Usually, persons are placed on bleeding precautions when the platelet count falls below 50,000/mm^3. **The risk of spontaneous bleeding increases at a platelet count of less than 20,000/mm^3.**

Table 27-2 outlines common causes of thrombocytopenia.

Clinical Presentation. Signs and symptoms associated with thrombocytopenia include petechiae, ecchymosis, hematemesis, hemoptysis, hematuria, vaginal bleeding, rectal bleeding, blood in stool, anemia, and active bleeding from mucous membranes, wounds, indwelling catheters, and sites of invasive procedures. Additionally, presentation may include complaints of frequent nose bleeds, unresolved hematomas, and fatigue.

TABLE 27-2. CAUSES OF THROMBOCYTOPENIA

Symptom	*Cause*
Decreased production	Leukemia Lymphoma Multiple myeloma Metastatic cancer Chemotherapy Radiation therapy Drugs (thiazides, estrogen) Alcohol
Increased destruction	Autoimmune disorders Idiopathic thrombocytopenic as in purpura Malignant disorders Disseminated intravascular coagulation Infectious agents
Abnormal platelet function	Aspirin (ibuprofen) qualitative dysfunction but not thrombocytopenia
Decreased availability	Sequestration in spleen

Treatment. Platelet transfusions are administered to thrombocytopenic patients who are actively bleeding, undergoing invasive procedures, or at increased risk of spontaneous bleeding. Platelet transfusions can be from a random donor pooling or a single-donor human including those from a leukocyte antigen (HLA)-matched product. Upon exposure to an increasing number of platelet transfusions, the patient may become refractory to the benefits of the transfusion because of antibody formation to platelets. A person with fever usually has increased destruction of platelets. A 1- to 2-hour posttransfusion platelet count is performed to document the effectiveness of the platelet transfusion. Reactions or complications of platelet transfusions are like those of whole-blood transfusions but also include a higher risk of reaction than transfusion of packed RBCs secondary to the coadministration of plasma.

If the patient is experiencing immune or idiopathic thrombocytopenia (generally related to immunosuppression from chemotherapy), an additional series of medications may be initiated. Treatment is initiated with corticosteroids, which can result in a short-term recovery of the platelet count. Additive therapies may include rituximab, immune globulin, and anti-Rh (D) immunoglobulin. A splenectomy may be performed if thrombocytopenia is not responsive to medications. *While removing, the spleen will stop the destruction of platelets, it will increase the risk of infection.*

Nursing Intervention. Nursing interventions are based on (1) protection of the patient from bleeding and associated complications and (2) early detection of bleeding. *Most institutions have policies (bleeding precautions, platelet precautions) that are instituted when the platelet count is less than 50,000/mm^3.* A sign is placed near the patient to alert all health team members that the patient is at risk for bleeding. Key interventions include

1. *Bleeding precautions for a platelet count of less than 50,000/mm^3*
2. Assessment of sites of potential bleeding
   a. Skin
   b. Mucous membranes
   c. Indwelling catheter sites
3. Assessment of bodily excrement for occult and frank bleeding
   a. Urine
   b. Stool
   c. Sputum
   d. Pad count in menstruating women
4. Routine neurologic assessment
5. Prevention of trauma
   a. Use soft toothbrushes or toothettes for oral hygiene
   b. Use electric razors
   c. Coordinate blood sampling to avoid multiple venipunctures
   d. Institute bowel routine to prevent constipation
   e. Avoid intramuscular injections
   f. Avoid prolonged use of tourniquets
   g. Avoid use of urinary catheters, rectal tubes
   h. Use soft restraints only when absolutely necessary
   i. Use padded side rails when the patient is in bed
   j. Assist the patient with ambulation if indicated
   k. Institute measures to minimize vomiting
6. Avoid use of aspirin, aspirin-containing compounds, and ibuprofen
7. Control of temperature elevations
8. Monitor pertinent laboratory data
   a. Hb
   b. Hct
   c. Platelet count
   d. Pre- and postplatelet transfusion counts

QUICK TIP! *It is unlikely that hemophilia and von Willebrand disease will be on the CCRN exam. This section is included simply to provide a more complete description of abnormal coagulation concepts.*

27.2 HEMOPHILIA AND VON WILLEBRAND DISEASE

Hemophilia can refer to three inherited bleeding disorders. The bleeding is due to a deficiency in a plasma clotting factor. von Willebrand disease is included in this section since it also involves a deficient clotting factor.

Etiology

Hemophilia A and B are sex-linked recessive disorders. They affect men mainly but do occur rarely in women. Women are often a "carrier" and genetically transmit these diseases to male offspring. Hemophilia C is an autosomal trait. von Willebrand disease has an autosomal dominant mode of inheritance, so it should occur equally among men and women. It is an actual lack of factor VIII. A complete absence of this factor may occur, or there may be a reduced amount of structurally normal factor.

A common clinical presentation includes spontaneous muscle hemorrhage that leads to hematoma formation. These collections of blood press against nerves, resulting in transient motor and/or sensory loss. Epistaxis and GI bleeding, without a history or presence of ulcers, are the next most common symptoms. Patients may also present with hemarthrosis (bleeding into their joints).

Hemorrhage into the central nervous system (CNS) is rare in hemophiliacs but often results in death when it does occur. Most often, the bleeding episode is due to trauma.

Diagnosis

The clinical condition can be verified by laboratory tests. The partial thromboplastin time (PTT) is prolonged. Factor assays reveal decreased factor VIII in hemophilia A and normal to decreased factor VII in von Willebrand disease. Factor IX is decreased in hemophilia B. Platelet aggregation is normal in hemophilia but decreased in von Willebrand disease. A familial tendency for excessive bleeding is usually known, even if they are unable to name the exact disorder. Testing is performed on individuals with family history or after presenting with the clinical symptoms discussed above.

Treatment

The goal of therapy is to prevent severe deformities and prolong life expectancy.

In hemophilia A, cryoprecipitated antihemolytic factor (AHF) is administered to raise the factor to 25% of normal to allow coagulation. Surgery requires increasing the AHF to 50% of normal. If the AHF is not available, fresh frozen plasma or plasma fraction, rich in AHF, may be administered. In hemophilia B, administration of fresh frozen plasma or of factor IX itself will increase the blood level of factor IX. In von Willebrand disease, the infusion of cryoprecipitates or blood fractions rich in factor VIII and von Willebrand factor (VWF) will shorten the bleeding time. Prior to surgery or in bleeding states, an intravenous infusion of cryoprecipitate or fresh frozen plasma is needed to raise the factor VIII level to 50% of normal. A patient with hemophilia or von Willebrand disease needs the care of a hematologist prior to surgical procedures and dental extraction.

Nursing Intervention

During hemophiliac bleeds, administration of the deficient clotting factor or plasma is ordered. AHF is effective for 48 to 72 hours. Repeat transfusions may be required to stop the bleed.

Apply cold compresses to the injured area, raise the injured area if possible, and cleanse any wounds. Thrombin-soaked fibrin or sponge may be utilized for wound care in some institutions. Restrict activity for 48 h after the bleeding is controlled to prevent recurrence. Control pain with analgesics such as acetaminophen (Tylenol), propoxyphene hydrochloride (Darvon), codeine, or meperidine hydrochloride (Demerol). *Avoid intramuscular injections to prevent a hematoma* at the injection site. *Aspirin and ibuprofen are contraindicated because they impair platelet aggregation.* If the patient bleeds into a joint, immediately elevate the joint and immobilize it in a slightly flexed position. Watch for signs of further bleeding such as increased pain and swelling, fever, or possible shock-like symptoms. *Monitor the patient's PTT.*

In von Willebrand disease, monitor the patient's bleeding time for 24 to 48 hours after surgery and observe for signs bleeding. *During a new bleed, elevate the injured part and apply cold compresses and gentle pressure to the bleeding site.* Education as to the causative factors and treatment of minor injuries is indicated, as well as discussion of conditions for which the patient should seek medical attention.

Educate the patient and parents (if the patient is a child) in how to control minor trauma and warn against using aspirin or aspirin-containing drugs. Refer the parents to a genetic counseling service.

The National Hemophilia Society, local hemophilia groups, genetic evaluation, or psychotherapy may be useful for fostering better acceptance of the disease and forming an association with other patients who are managing successfully.

27.3 SICKLE CELL DISEASE

Sickle cell disease is an autosomal recessive disorder in which an abnormal Hb leads to chronic hemolytic anemia. Sickle cell disease is also referred to as sickle cell anemia because of the pathophysiology.

Pathophysiology

Those with sickle cell disease have an abnormal Hb molecule, known as hemoglobin S. This Hb molecule causes the RBCs to become insoluble when hypoxic and with continued hypoxia these cells become crescent- or sickle-shaped. Sickling decreases the cells' flexibility and impairs their ability to easily travel through blood vessels as well as impairs their oxygen carrying capacity. The sickling occurs because of a mutation in the Hb gene.

Sickling has a hemolyzing effect, and altered cells collect in the capillaries and small vessels. This impairs normal circulation and results in pain, swelling, tissue infarctions, and anoxia. Blood viscosity is therefore increased, causing further impairment of circulating blood. Blockages extend in the capillaries and small vessels, leading to further sickling obstruction. A vicious cycle is thus begun.

Etiology

Congenital hemolytic anemia occurs most often in African Americans and is due to genetic inheritance. The causative factor is a defect in the hemoglobin S molecule.

There is a homozygous and a heterozygous inheritance. Homozygous inheritance involves the substitution of the amino acid valine for glutamic acid in the beta-hemoglobin chain, resulting in the disease itself. In heterozygous inheritance, the patient carries the sickle cell trait but may be asymptomatic.

Clinical Presentation

Common symptoms and physical findings observed include tachycardia, cardiomegaly, murmurs, pulmonary infarctions, chronic fatigue, dyspnea (with or without exertion), hepatomegaly, jaundice, pallor, aching bones, chest pain, ischemic leg ulcers, and increased susceptibility to infection. Infection, stress, dehydration, and hypoxic states (eg, strenuous exercise) may induce a crisis.

Sickle cell disease may lead to various acute and chronic complications, including vaso-occlusive crises that are caused by sickle-shaped RBCs that obstruct capillaries and restrict blood flow to an organ, resulting in ischemia, pain, and often organ damage.

The frequency, severity, and duration of these crises vary considerably. They do not usually develop for the first 5 years but then appear sporadically. They are due to the obstruction of blood vessels by rigid, tangled sickle cells. Tissue anoxia and possibly also necrosis occur, causing severe thoracic, abdominal, muscular, and bone pain. Jaundice may occur along with dark urine and a low-grade fever. After a crisis resolves, infection may occur within 4 days to several weeks secondary to occlusion and necrosis of the blood vessels.

Autosplenectomy occurs with long-standing disease. The spleen suffers infarction, scarring, and then shrinkage to the point that the organ is no longer palpable. At this stage the spleen ceases to perform its normal functions and places the individual at risk for infection.

Aplastic (megaloblastic) crisis is a result of bone marrow suppression and is often associated with a viral infection. Signs and symptoms include fever, markedly decreased bone marrow activity, pallor, lethargy, dyspnea, possible coma, and RBC hemolysis.

Acute sequestration develops in some children aged 8 months to 2 years. There is a sudden, massive entrapment of RBCs in the liver and spleen. Symptoms of this rare crisis are lethargy and pallor. If not treated, it progresses to hypovolemic shock and death. This is the leading cause of death in sickle cell children younger than 1 year. Following the first episode, splenectomy is usually performed. Sequestration is often associated with aplastic crisis and parvovirus B19 infection.

A hemolytic crisis is rare and is usually confined to those who have a G6PD deficiency. This crisis usually occurs as an infectious response to complications of sickle cell disease rather than to the disease itself.

Diagnosis

A family history and the clinical presentation typically point toward sickle cell disease. A blood smear shows sickle-celled RBCs rather than normal RBCs. Hb electrophoresis showing hemoglobin S is pathognomonic.

Treatment

There is no specific treatment for the primary disease; palliative measures are used to manage care. Painful crises are treated with hydration and analgesics. Pain management requires opioid administration at regular intervals until the crisis has been resolved. For milder crises, some patients can be managed on nonsteroidal anti-inflammatory drugs (NSAIDs). For more severe crises, most patients require inpatient management for intravenous opioids. Oral hydroxyurea (Hydrea), which increases hemoglobin F concentration, thus preventing the formation of hemoglobin S polymers, has been found to be an effective pharmacologic treatment to reduce pain events and the need for transfusions. Hydroxyurea decreases thrombotic events/crisis and is often used for patients with a history of severe vaso-occlusive events and acute chest syndrome. Treatment of aplastic crisis includes transfusion of packed RBCs, oxygen, and supportive therapies. In sequestration crisis, treatment includes whole-blood transfusion, oxygen, and large amounts of oral or intravenous fluids. Folic acid supplementation and transfusions may be used for aplastic or hemolytic crises. The use of pneumococcal vaccination can reduce the incidence of infections with pneumococcus.

Nursing Intervention

Supportive care during exacerbations will help avoid such crises and provide a more normal life. Pain management is a key area of focus. *During the crisis, apply warm compresses to painful areas and cover the child with a blanket. Avoid cold compresses, since their use may result in vasoconstriction and prolong the crisis.* Encourage bed rest and hydration, administer analgesics, antipyretics, and antibiotics as ordered.

> **KEY CLINICAL CONCEPT**
>
> Be aware of the impact of heat versus cold. Cold reduces inflammation as well as swelling and blood flow. Heat vasodilates and improves blood flow. Warming blankets may help raise the patient's temperature but may also cause vasodilation and induce hypotension.

Education of the patient and family will help avoid some crises. Such education would include avoidance of drinking large amounts of cold fluids, swimming in cold water, clothing that restricts circulation, and any activity that would produce hypoxia, such as flying in small (unpressurized) aircraft. A large fluid intake will prevent dehydration and decrease blood viscosity, reducing the chance of another crisis. Stress the importance of childhood immunizations and prompt treatment for infections.

27.4 THE IMMUNE SYSTEM

Cells of the Immune System

The ultimate effect of immunodeficiency is an impaired ability of the body to defend against foreign antigens. This leads to an increased susceptibility to infection and certain other diseases believed sometimes to be linked to an impaired immune status, such as cancer and autoimmune disorders. The incidence of infection, the most common complication of immunosuppression, increases with both the duration and the severity of the immunodeficiency. In fact, *the highest risk of infection occurs when the leukocyte (white blood cell [WBC]) count is less than 1000/mm^3 and the neutrophils number less than 500/mm^3*. The infections that develop are related to the underlying immune defect and the organisms to which the individual is now most susceptible. Most infections associated with immunosuppression are opportunistic or secondary to endogenous organisms that do not cause infection in the presence of a normally functioning immune system. However, many of the organisms colonizing a hospitalized patient are acquired during the hospitalization. Additionally,, the infections that develop in the immunosuppressed tend to be more severe. The lung is the most common site of serious infectious

TABLE 27-3. COMMON INFECTIONS IN THE IMMUNOCOMPROMISED HOST

Site of Infection	*Bacteria*	*Viruses*	*Fungi*	*Protozoa*
Skin	*Staphylococcus aureus*	Herpes simplex virus	*Candida*	
	Staphylococcus epidermidis	Herpes zoster and varicella zoster viruses		
Oropharynx		Herpes simplex virus	*Candida*	
Gastrointestinal tract	Gram-negative rods	Herpes simplex virus (esophagitis)	*Candida*	*Giardia lamblia*
	Mycobacterium avium-intracellulare	Cytomegalovirus		*Cryptosporidium* *Entamoeba histolytica*
Urinary tract	Gram-negative rods		*Candida*	
Lungs	Gram-negative rods	Cytomegalovirus	*Candida*	*Pneumocystis carinii*
	Mycobacterium tuberculosis		*Aspergillus, Mucor*	*Toxoplasma gondii*
	Mycobacterium avium-intracellulare		*Histoplasma capsulatum*	
CNS	*Listeria monocytogenes*	Herpes zoster and varicella zoster viruses	*Cryptococcus neoformans*	*Toxoplasma gondii*
	Streptococcus pneumoniae	Herpes simplex virus	*Aspergillus*	
	Pseudomonas aeruginosa			
	Haemophilus influenzae			
Blood	Gram-negative rods		*Candida*	

complications. **Table 27-3** reviews common infections in the immunocompromised host.

27.5 IMMUNOSUPPRESSION

The immune system serves many functions, such as surveillance, homeostasis, and defense. Immunosuppression is an alteration, a decrease, in normal immune protective responses. Immunosuppression can also occur because of injury, surgery, shock, infection, or sepsis. Alterations in cell-mediated immunity can result from underlying disease (eg, congenital defects in cell-mediated immunity, Hodgkin disease, acquired immunodeficiency syndrome [AIDS]), or they may occur because of malignancies (such as acute leukemias) or antineoplastic or immunosuppressive treatment (eg, treatment of lymphoma or transplant rejection).

Opportunistic Infection

Immunosuppressed individuals are vulnerable to opportunistic infections. These infections are caused by organisms that are ubiquitous in the environment (internal and external) but rarely cause disease in the immunocompetent host. Patients with alterations in cell-mediated immunity are especially susceptible to infections caused by intracellular pathogens such as *Listeria monocytogenes, Mycobacterium* spp., *Cryptococcus neoformans,* other fungi (such as *Aspergillus* and *Candida*), herpes viruses [herpes simplex virus (HSV), cytomegalovirus (CMV)], as well as ***Pneumocystis carinii.*** Patients with humoral immune dysfunction (eg, untreated multiple myeloma, patients who have undergone splenectomy) are susceptible to infections caused by encapsulated organisms, particularly *Streptococcus pneumoniae* and *Haemophilus influenzae.*

The three major determinants of nosocomial infection are the hospital environment, microorganisms, and host defense. Hospitalization and the critical care environment predispose an individual to an increased risk of infection. Hospitalization initiates the conversion of normal cutaneous flora to colonization of a new microbial population that is prevalent in the hospital. Colonization by itself is not harmful to the individual, however, when the first lines of defense are broken or bypassed, colonization opens the way to infection.

Some 50% of patients admitted to intensive care units (ICUs) become colonized with gram-negative bacteria within 72 hours. The major vector of these bacteria is the human hand. Nosocomial infections occur in 25% to 50% of patients admitted to ICUs. The most frequent types of nosocomial infection are urinary tract infections, wound infections, respiratory infections, and septicemia, in that order. Other factors that predispose critically ill patients to infection include surgery, trauma, endotracheal intubation, shock, malnutrition, renal failure, liver failure, splenectomy, broad-spectrum antibiotic or corticosteroid therapy, and obesity.

Immunosuppressed individuals are usually neutropenic (see Chapter 25 for a discussion of the anatomy and physiology of neutrophils; see Chapter 26 for treatment). The longer the patient is neutropenic, the greater the chance for mortality (**Table 27-4**). This is because some of the signs and symptoms of infection—redness, tenderness, swelling, and erythema—are often absent as a result of the lack of granulocytes. *Patients with circulating granulocyte counts below 500 are especially susceptible to infections caused by gram-negative bacilli*

TABLE 27-4. CAUSES OF DEATH IN NEUTROPENIC PATIENTS

Complication	*Percent of Patients*
Infection	35
Hemorrhage	27
Progression of disease	18
Other Renal insufficiency Myocardial infarction Pulmonary edema	20

(including *Pseudomonas aeruginosa*) *and staphylococci.* Immunosuppressed patients may not present display symptoms of illness in the same way an immunocompetent patient would; sometimes, the only sign is a low-grade fever. Patients treated with **corticosteroids** are at significantly increased risk for bacterial, fungal, and ***P. carinii*** infections.

Nursing Care. Nursing care of the patient who is immunosuppressed is based on the nursing diagnosis of potential for infection (**Table 27-5**). The patient requires frequent and thorough physical assessments because the signs and symptoms of infection are often subtle in the immunocompromised host. Important points regarding assessment and interventions are outlined here.

Assessment

1. History
   a. Age
   b. Past infections
   c. Medications, noting those that are immunosuppressive
   d. History of immunosuppressive treatments (eg, radiation therapy)
   e. Presenting signs and symptoms
   f. Coexisting systemic symptoms (weight loss, malaise, etc)
2. Physical examination
   a. Inspect skin carefully, particularly noting conditions of skin folds, pressure points, and perirectal area (frequent site of infection in the immunocompromised host). Observe for
      i. Localized redness or swelling (may not be present with neutropenia or lymphopenia)
      ii. Excoriation
      iii. Rash suggestive of HSV or herpes zoster
      iv. **Lesions, infections, or Kaposi sarcoma**
      v. Lymphadenopathy
   b. *Closely inspect the mouth and throat, a frequent site of infection in the immunocompromised host.* Note:
      i. Condition of teeth and gums (if infected, can cause sepsis)
      ii. **Lesions (candidiasis, herpes simplex, Kaposi sarcoma)**
   c. Monitor temperature and note pattern of elevation.
      i. *An elevated temperature is the best indication of infection in the immunosuppressed.*
      ii. A temperature over 38°C is probably indicative of infection.
      iii. Fever is also part of the disease process of some disorders associated with immuno-suppression (leukemia, lymphoma, human immunodeficiency syndrome [HIV] infection).
   d. Assess central line and peripheral intravenous lines for signs of infection.
   e. Assess breath sounds.
      i. Adventitious sounds are frequently absent or minimal at the onset of infection in the immunosuppressed patient.
      ii. Note respiratory rate, presence of cough, and character of sputum.
      iii. Be prepared with ventilator support, since rapid deterioration in respiratory status can occur.
   f. Note complaints of tenderness and localized pain, as they may be indicators of infection.
      i. Back pain
      ii. Burning on urination
      iii. Rectal discomfort with bowel movements
3. Laboratory data
   a. WBC (leukopenia or leukocytosis)
      i. WBC differential
      ii. *Absolute granulocyte (or absolute neutrophil count) count, especially if less than 500/mm^3*
      iii. Lymphocyte count
   b. T_4 count; T_4:T_8 ratio (indicators of immune status in patients with AIDS)

Interventions.

1. Meticulous personal hygiene
   a. Prevent skin breakdown by turning the patient and using pressure-relieving devices.
   b. Avoid injury (will provide a port of entry for microorganisms), keep nails trim, use electric razor.
   c. Provide meticulous perirectal care.
      i. *Avoid taking rectal temperatures* and using rectal suppositories and enemas because of fragile rectal mucosa and the possibility of causing a break in the mucosa.
      ii. Initiate a bowel regimen to avoid constipation and/or control diarrhea.
2. Good oral hygiene
   a. Brush oral cavity, using a soft toothbrush or toothettes.
   b. Moisturize lips and mucosa with water-soluble lubricant.
   c. If stomatitis is present, rinse mouth with normal saline every 2 to 4 h.
   d. Avoid commercial mouthwashes as the alcohol content can be harsh and irritate oral mucosa.
   e. Advise patient to avoid smoking and use of alcohol.
   f. Encourage a soft bland diet and cool foods or provide nutritional support.
   g. Control pain.
      i. Viscous lidocaine.
      ii. Peridex mouth rinse (chlorhexidine gluconate) (not used for pain control but to decrease colonization).
      iii. Mixture of sodium bicarbonate (5 mL), Maalox (5 mL), 2% viscous lidocaine (5 mL), and diphenhydramine (5 mg). Every 4 hours, swish in mouth for 3 minutes and then swallow.
   h. Obtain order for appropriate antimicrobials if secondary infection is present.

TABLE 27-5. ETIOLOGY OF ACQUIRED IMMUNODEFICIENCY

Etiologic Condition	*Immune Defect*
	Injury/Disease
Burns	Disruption of natural barrier Impaired phagocytosis Deficient/delayed hypersensitivity
Uremia	Abnormal neutrophil function Impaired cell-mediated immunity
Diabetes mellitus	Impaired neutrophil function
Cancer	
Solid tumors	Deficiency in cell-mediated immunity Impaired neutrophil function
Leukemias	Deficiency in humoral and cell-mediated immunity
Hodgkin disease	Impaired cellular immunity
Non-Hodgkin's lymphoma	Impaired humoral or cellular immunity (depends on type of lymphocyte involved)
Multiple myeloma	Impaired humoral immunity
AIDS	Impaired cell-mediated immunity with subsequent deficiency in humoral immunity
Certain infections (influenza, cytomegalovirus, Epstein–Barr virus, mononucleosis, tuberculosis, candidiasis)	Depression of lymphocyte and monocyte function
	Treatment/Medication
Surgery	Disruption of natural barriers Lymphopenia
Splenectomy	Impaired humoral immunity
Radiation therapy	Neutropenia Lymphopenia
Anesthetic agents	Inhibition of phagocytosis Impaired humoral and cell-mediated immunity
Cytotoxic drugs (cancer chemotherapy)	Disruption of natural barriers (mucositis) Neutropenia/lymphopenia Deficiencies in humoral and cell-mediated immunity
Steroids	Anti-inflammatory Suppressed functioning of neutrophils Deficiencies in humoral and cell-mediated immunity
Immunosuppressive agents (azathioprine, cyclosporine, *tacrolimus*, antilymphocyte globulin)	Impaired cell-mediated immunity
Certain antibiotics (pentamidine gentamicin, Septra)	Leukopenia Neutropenia
	Miscellaneous
Extremes of age	Deficiencies in humoral and cell-mediated immunity
Protein–calorie malnutrition	Impaired phagocytosis Deficiencies in humoral and cell-mediated immunity
Stress	Exact mechanism of immunodeficiency unknown

3. Aseptic technique
   a. Minimize invasive procedures.
   b. Use smallest-gauge lumens possible on all invasive devices.
   c. Provide meticulous care of vascular access.
   d. Coordinate blood studies.
   e. Keep all systems closed as much as possible.
   f. Avoid transparent, occlusive dressings over drainage wounds (the presence of WBCs collecting under the dressing is required to clean out the wound).

4. Manipulation of the environment to minimize exposure to organisms
   a. Eliminate sources of stagnant water (sources of gram-negative bacteria).
      i. Change disposable tubing on ventilators daily.
      ii. Avoid cold-mist humidifiers.
   b. Remove live plants and flowers from the room (sources of *Aspergillus*).
   c. Institute protective isolation when the WBC count is less than $1000/mm^3$ or the absolute granulocyte count is less than $500/mm^3$.
   d. Restrict exposure to persons with infection.
   e. Evaluate the appropriateness of a low bacterial diet.
      i. Eliminate raw, unpeeled fruits and vegetables and uncooked eggs and meat from the diet.
      ii. Effectiveness in decreasing the incidence of infection is controversial.
5. Adequate nutrition
   a. Nutritional intake may be compromised by anorexia, fatigue, stomatitis, dysphagia, nausea, vomiting, and taste changes caused by some medications, including chemotherapy.
   b. Encourage a high-calorie, high-protein diet.
   c. **Enteral feedings are preferable to parenteral nutrition because of decreased risk of infection, namely bacterial translocation from ischemic bowel.**
6. Alleviation of stress
   a. Allow rest periods.
   b. Maintain day/night schedule as much as possible.
   c. Minimize environmental noise.
   d. Maximize comfort.
   e. Attend psychosocial needs.

27.6 DISORDERS OF THE IMMUNE SYSTEM

Acquired Immunodeficiency Syndrome

AIDS is the endpoint of infection by HIV, a retrovirus found in the body fluids of infected individuals. HIV disease is a spectrum ranging from primary infection, with or without the acute syndrome, to the asymptomatic stage, to advanced disease. HIV is transmitted by sexual contact, exchange of bloods and body fluids, and perinatally. The profile of the high-risk groups affected by the disease to date include intravenous drug users, hemophiliacs, blood transfusion recipients prior to 1985, male homosexuals and bisexuals, and sexual partners of any of these individuals.

Since recognition of the disease in 1981, much has been learned about the spectrum of HIV infection. Individuals who are infected may range from being asymptomatic to having systemic symptoms such as generalized persistent lymphadenopathy, fever, night sweats, diarrhea, and weight loss. AIDS itself is diagnosed when specific "indicator" diseases (ie, diseases that indicate an underlying immunodeficiency) are present. Under most circumstances, the diagnosis also requires the person to be HIV-seropositive. The antibody develops an average of 6 to 12 weeks after exposure to the virus. The pattern of disease will vary from person to person. Some people experience rapid progression of the disease, while others are considered long-term survivors.

Clinical Presentation. The immunodeficiency of AIDS is multifaceted. HIV primarily infects the T_4 cell, and because of the role of the T cell as the main coordinator of the immune response, devastating deficiencies occur in both the cell-mediated and humoral immune responses. The viral effects on the immune system include a profound lymphopenia and a reverse T_4:T_8 ratio (< 1). Thus, the person with AIDS develops opportunistic infections. These infections tend to be severe and become disseminated, but they also tend to recur upon discontinuation of antimicrobial therapy. Most patients with AIDS die because of infection due to an organism normally protected against by T cells.

Some of the infections frequently seen with AIDS include CMV retinitis, cryptococcal meningitis, toxoplasmosis, mycobacterial infections and, **most commonly, *P. carinii* pneumonia (PCP)**. The onset of PCP is usually insidious, characterized by a gradually increasing shortness of breath, dry cough, fever, and—on chest roentgenography—pulmonary infiltrates. *The respiratory status of a patient with PCP can deteriorate rapidly*, necessitating admission to a critical-care unit. Hypoxemia and dyspnea may require ventilatory support. Drug therapy usually includes administration of a 21-day course of **intravenous pentamidine or trimethoprim/sulfamethoxazole (Bactrim)**. Occasionally high-dose steroids are given. In many patients, it may take 7 to 10 days for a clinical response to be seen. It is not unusual for a relapse of PCP to occur; when it does, it is often fulminant in nature and associated with a mortality rate of approximately 40%. For this reason, patients are commonly started on **prophylactic therapy, which may consist of maintenance doses of oral trimethoprim/sulfamethoxazole (Bactrim)** or aerosolized pentamidine.

Secondary cancers, namely, **Kaposi sarcoma and non-Hodgkin lymphoma (NHL)**, can also occur in association with AIDS. Kaposi sarcoma, which arises from the endothelium of either lymphatic or blood vessels, is characterized by *skin and mucosal lesions* ranging in color from dark red or purple to nearly black. The lesions typically develop in the oropharynx, lymph nodes, GI tract, lungs, and skin. NHL is typically high grade, of B-cell origin, and present in extranodal sites. In approximately 20% of those with NHL, the cancer presents as a primary lymphoma of the brain—a very rare occurrence in the general population. Generally, the AIDS-related malignancies are much more aggressive and respond more poorly to therapy than the same cancers in the general population.

Neuropsychiatric manifestations accompany AIDS in over 60% of patients and in some cases, are diagnostic of the disease. The most common disorder of this type is AIDS dementia complex, a subcortical dementia manifested by changes in cognition, behavior, and motor functioning. Symptoms initially include memory loss, difficulty in concentrating, and lethargy; these may progress to withdrawal, aphasia, ataxia, paresis, and seizures. The condition is thought to occur secondary to HIV infiltration of the brain. The virus is known to infect macrophages, which themselves are not destroyed by the virus but serve to transport HIV across the blood–brain barrier.

Also, identified as part of the clinical picture associated with AIDS is the HIV wasting syndrome. This is defined as loss of over 10% of the usual body weight, accompanied by diarrhea, weakness, or fever of a chronic nature. Multiple factors may contribute to development of the syndrome, including difficulty in maintaining adequate nutrition. However, like the cachexia seen with cancer, muscle wasting seems to exceed what would be expected.

Treatment. Upon initial diagnosis, the treatment of an HIV-positive diagnosis is a series of antiretroviral drugs. These drugs work to suppress the virus to low levels and may even suppress the virus to the point that it is no longer detectable. The person is not cured at this point, but via a more robust immune system, has increased their ability to lead a longer life. Currently, there are 31 antiretrovirals that have been approved by the Food and Drug Administration (FDA). The process of using a series of antiretrovirals for treatment and management is referred to as highly active antiretroviral treatment or HAART therapy. In addition to HAART therapy, additional medications may be prescribed to manage the disease including nucleoside reverse transcriptase inhibitors, protease inhibitors, and nonnucleoside reverse transcriptase inhibitors.

Additional treatment is generally aimed at the secondary diseases that develop with AIDS. Systemic NHL, usually widely disseminated at the time of diagnosis, necessitates treatment with an intensive chemotherapy regimen that is fairly toxic and usually poorly tolerated by the patient with AIDS. Primary lymphoma of the brain usually has a good initial response to cranial radiation, but relapse soon occurs, generally within the CNS. Therapy for **Kaposi sarcoma,** commonly initiated when the patient develops pain or lymphatic obstruction or when the lesions are cosmetically disturbing, is palliative and consists of chemotherapy and/or radiation. These cancer therapies, particularly chemotherapy, induce myelosuppression and compound the already existing immunodeficiencies of AIDS, making the patient even more susceptible to the development of infection (see Chapter 26 for specific medication treatment).

Nursing Intervention. In addition to requiring nursing care relevant to immunosuppression, patients with AIDS, especially those with PCP, require aggressive pulmonary care and close monitoring of arterial blood gases. Decisions regarding intubation and ventilation should be made prior to severe respiratory dysfunction. As cognitive impairment can occur secondary to hypoxemia, AIDS dementia, opportunistic infection, or CNS malignancy, a close assessment of mental status is required to detect any changes from baseline. If impaired concentration and memory are noted, it is necessary to give the patient simple explanations and directions and to maintain a safe environment. Nutritional support must also be addressed. If diarrhea is present—a common problem due to either HIV enteropathy or opportunistic infection—enteral feedings may not be possible. Continues assessment and intervention is required to support these patients during their critical illness.

Leukemias

Leukemias are a group of malignancies that occur when immature WBCs proliferate uncontrollably and accumulate in the bone marrow and peripheral blood. Leukemias are classified according to the type of cell that is predominant and whether the disease is acute or chronic. The four general categories of leukemia are acute lymphocytic or lymphoblastic (ALL), acute nonlymphocytic or myelogenous (ANLL or AML), chronic lymphocytic (CLL), and chronic myelogenous (CML).

TABLE 27-6. MANIFESTATIONS OF LEUKEMIA

Rationale	*Signs and Symptoms*
Bone marrow failure	Anemia Thrombocytopenia Leukocytosis (primarily blast cells) Granulocytopenia (if ALL, CLL) Lymphopenia (if ALL, CML)
Organ infiltration	Bone pain Lymphadenopathy Splenomegaly Hepatomegaly Testicular mass or swelling Headache, nausea, vomiting (CNS involvement)
Hyperleukocytosis	Stroke Adult respiratory distress syndrome Splenic infarction
Hypercatabolism and rapid cell turnover (tumor lysis syndrome)	Disseminated intravascular coagulation Hyperuricemia Hyperkalemia Hypocalcemia Weight loss

The accumulation of leukemic cells, which do not function normally, impedes the adequate production of normal RBCs, WBCs, and platelets. This, along with infiltration of other organs by the leukemic cells, underlies the clinical presentation of leukemia. **Table 27-6** presents a summary of the signs and symptoms.

Complications. The patient with leukemia requires a critical-care setting when complications arise. Both the disease itself and the intensive chemotherapy used to treat it are associated with severe and often prolonged myelosuppression. The total WBC count may be less than $100/mm^3$ for a period of a week or more after high-dose chemotherapy. Thus, infection is the major cause of morbidity and mortality in the patient with leukemia. Common pathogens causing infection in immunocompromised patients are Gram-negative bacteria (*Escherichia coli*, *Klebsiella*, *Pseudomonas*) and fungi (*Candida*, *Aspergillus*). Frequent presentations include cellulitis, pneumonia, and perirectal infections. Sepsis is common and must be treated immediately and aggressively.

Also, contributing to the likelihood of infection is the disruption that can occur in the natural barriers of the skin and mucous membranes, allowing easy entry to microorganisms. The chemotherapy, depending on the drugs and the doses, can cause severe stomatitis and mucositis. In patients who have received bone marrow from a donor, graft-versus-host disease (GVHD) can occur as the transplanted marrow recognizes the host tissue as foreign. One of the tissues that the engrafted T cells attempt to reject is the skin. In acute GVHD, this usually starts as a rash and may progress to desquamation. The treatment for GVHD includes immunosuppressive drugs, thus compounding the already existing immunodeficiencies. Target tissues for acute GVHD are skin, liver, GI tract, and immune system.

Another reason for admission of a leukemia patient to the critical-care unit is severe bleeding and hemorrhage. This can occur secondary to thrombocytopenia induced by the disease process and/or the chemotherapy. *It is not unusual for the platelet count to be less than 20,000/mm^3, which puts the patient at risk for spontaneous bleeding. Of particular concern is the possibility of a pulmonary or intracranial hemorrhage.* Because of the multiple platelet transfusions required, single-donor leukocyte-poor products are administered. Random donor versus single donor is controversial. Products should be irradiated due to immunosuppression.

Bleeding may also be seen in association with disseminated intravascular coagulation (DIC), a complication of leukemia, especially progranulocytic leukemia, a subtype of acute myeloid leukemia (AML). It is caused by the release of tissue thromboplastin from tumor cells. The clotting cascade is triggered, leading to accelerated coagulation and the formation of excessive thrombin. With the ongoing coagulation, the fibrinolytic system is activated. Thus, clotting and bleeding continue until the cycle is interrupted by treatment of the cause. *Besides hemorrhage, organ dysfunction can occur because of thromboemboli.* Chemotherapy should be initiated immediately; however, initiation of chemotherapy can potentially exacerbate DIC due to the destruction of promyelocytes. Heparin, although it's use is controversial with other etiologies of DIC, has been found to be an effective supportive therapy in acute progranulocytic leukemia. Newer therapies for acute promyelocytic leukemia (APL), a subtype of AML, include the use of all-transretinoic acid (ATRA). ATRA is a form of "differentiation therapy" as it activates a retinoid receptor and causes promyelocytes to differentiate (to mature), which deters them from proliferating. There is a differentiation syndrome associated with ATRA (and arsenic used for relapsed APL) which consists of leukocytosis fever, weight gain, edema, pulmonary infiltrates, pleural and pericardial effusions, hypotension, and renal dysfunction. Treatment should be initiated with dexamethasone 10 mg q12h.

Leukostasis can also be life-threatening. Leukostasis can occur with a WBC count of more than 100,000/mm^3, consisting mostly of blasts. Leukemia blasts plug capillaries, causing rupture, bleeding, and organ dysfunction. Intracerebral hemorrhage is the most common and most lethal complication. Management includes the administration of fluids and allopurinol to counteract the hyperuricemia associated with cell lysis. Appropriate chemotherapy must be initiated. As an emergency measure, leukapheresis may be necessary.

Treatment. A first step in treatment of the acute leukemias is to obtain complete remission. Remission is defined as normal peripheral blood with resolution of cytopenias, normal bone marrow with no excess blasts, and normal clinical status. The acute leukemias require immediate treatment with chemotherapy, and the type of initial chemotherapy depends on the subtype of leukemia. Treatment is approached in three phases. The initial phase, called induction therapy, consists of a combination of chemotherapy drugs given in high doses to achieve remission. Complete remission occurs when the number of leukemic cells is below detection, hematopoiesis is restored, and signs and symptoms of the disease are no longer present. However, because leukemic cells remain, even though they are microscopically undetectable, a consolidation phase of therapy is necessary to further decrease or eliminate these cells, which often involves multiple cycles (two to three). This cycle of chemotherapy, also very intensive, is usually administered 6 to 8 weeks after induction. The third phase, maintenance therapy, involves the administration of moderate doses of chemotherapy over a prolonged time. It is given with the intent of maintaining remission, but its effectiveness is controversial (not indicated with AML but is used with ALL).

By comparison, chronic leukemia is treated with oral chemotherapy agents, which are associated with much less toxicity. More aggressive therapy may be initiated as the disease progresses, particularly in patients with CML who undergo an end-stage blast crisis, which resembles an acute leukemia. Patients with CLL are often treated with intravenous chemotherapy, which can increase the risk of infection.

The rate of relapse—ie, the recurrence of detectable leukemic cells either in the bone marrow, peripheral blood, or extramedullary sites—varies with the type of leukemia. However, once relapse occurs, it is more difficult to induce a second remission. One treatment alternative that is available to patients with ALL, ANLL, and CML who meet specific criteria is bone marrow transplantation. This involves the administration of dosages of chemotherapy and radiation therapy that, although ablative to the bone marrow, are also more cytotoxic to cancer cells. Prior to the cytotoxic therapy, bone marrow cells are harvested from the patient or a matched donor. If the patient is to receive his or her own marrow, special techniques are used in an attempt to completely eliminate all leukemic cells before infusion. The bone marrow is reinfused at the time the blood counts reach their lowest point. Engraftment of the bone marrow and functional immune recovery takes approximately 4 weeks, but patients often remain immunosuppressed for a period of 1 year or more.

Nursing Intervention. In the patient with leukemia, nursing care centers on monitoring for potential infection and injury (bleeding), discussed elsewhere in this chapter. In addition to the assessments previously reviewed, assessment of neurologic status is important because of the possibility of CNS complications, including intracranial bleeding or stroke. Fluid and electrolyte balance must also be carefully monitored because of the large volume of fluids given and the possibility of tumor lysis syndrome or septic shock. Multisystem failure can occur secondary to leukemic infiltration, leukostasis, DIC, sepsis, or the toxicity of cancer chemotherapy. In addition to the continual assessments, the nurse will administer the extensive supportive therapy required, including multiple antibiotics, blood and blood product transfusions, and usually total parenteral nutrition. Nursing care of the patient with leukemia is a challenge, particularly in terms of protecting the patient from infection amid all the critical-care interventions.

Other Malignancies Associated with Immunodeficiency

Lymphomas. Lymphoma is a group of cancers that affect the cells that play a role in the immune system, and primarily represents cells involved in the lymphatic system of the body. Lymphomas, in which the malignant cell is either a lymphocytes B or T cell or their subtypes, are broadly classified in one of two major categories: Hodgkin lymphoma ([HL], previously called Hodgkin disease) and all other lymphomas (NHLs). These two types occur in the same places, may be associated with the same symptoms, and often have similar gross physical characteristics. However, they are readily discriminated via microscopic examination.

Hodgkin disease develops from a specific abnormal B-lymphocyte lineage. NHL may derive from either abnormal B or T cells and are distinguished by unique genetic markers.

Though similar in many respects, the distinguishing feature of HL is the presence of Reed–Sternberg cells, whose origin and nature are uncertain. The incidence of HL peaks during the second and third decades and again after 60 years of age. NHL occurs primarily in older individuals and is four times more common than HL.

Lymphoma is the most common type of blood cancer in the United States. It is the sixth most common cancer in adults and the third most common in children. NHL is far more common than HL. Lymphoma can occur at any age, including childhood. HL is most common in two age groups: young adults aged 16 to 34 years and in older adults aged 55 years and older. NHL is more likely to occur in older persons.

The disease usually presents as one or more enlarged lymph nodes, usually in the cervical region (cervical region predisposition is normally seen in HL). Occasionally, the initial site of disease is the GI tract. Approximately one-third of patients also exhibit systemic symptoms consisting of fever, night sweats, and loss over 10% of the usual body weight. Staging procedures are done to determine the extent of disease, as this has implications for treatment. HL tends to spread from one lymph node group to an adjacent group, whereas NHL tends to skip to noncontiguous groups. The workup must determine the involvement, if any, of lymph node groups, the bone marrow, liver, and spleen. Sometimes an exploratory laparotomy may be necessary, especially with HL.

The "staging" or evaluation of extent of disease, for both HL and NHL, are similar.

- Stage I (early disease)—Lymphoma located in a single lymph node region or in one area or organ outside the lymph node.
- Stage II (locally advanced disease)—Lymphoma located in two or more lymph node regions all located on the same side of the diaphragm or in one lymph node region and a nearby tissue or organ. (The diaphragm is a flat muscle that separates the chest from the abdomen.)
- Stage III (advanced disease)—Lymphoma affecting two or more lymph node regions, or one lymph node region and one organ, on opposite sides of the diaphragm.
- Stage IV (widespread or disseminated disease)—Lymphoma outside the lymph nodes and spleen that has spread to another area or organ such as the bone marrow, bone, or CNS.

Both HL and NHL are further classified with letters.

- An "A" or "B" designation indicates whether the person with lymphoma had symptoms such as fevers, night sweats, and/or weight loss at the time of diagnosis. "A" indicates no such symptoms, and "B" indicates symptoms.
- An "E" designation indicates that the tumor spread directly from a lymph node into an organ or that a single organ outside the lymphatic system is affected with no apparent lymphatic involvement.

Treatment for lymphoma depends on the type and stage. If the lymphoma is localized, radiation therapy is initiated and is usually given with or after chemotherapy to disease sites. In HL, this consists of total nodal irradiation and radiation to the spleen (if not removed at laparotomy). For early-stage disease, radiation is given with curative intent, although it is generally more effective in HL than in NHL. Chemotherapy is given for more widespread systemic disease, and sometimes, in the case of NHL, is recommended as the treatment of choice for localized disease. Both chemotherapy and radiation therapy, if given to areas of major bone marrow activity, are myelosuppressive. Another side effect that is sometimes associated with the chemotherapeutic treatment of NHL is tumor lysis syndrome.

Cure is expected in over 65% of patients with lymphoma. However, if the disease recurs, therapy is more poorly tolerated because of the depressed bone marrow reserve because of the initial therapy. Potential complications representing oncologic emergencies that can occur with progressive disease are superior vena cava syndrome, tumor lysis syndrome, and spinal cord compression. In superior vena cava syndrome, the vena cava is obstructed by tumor or enlarged nodes. The impaired venous drainage causes cough, dyspnea, neck vein distention, and facial, trunk, and arm edema. Immediate treatment with radiation is required to relieve pressure on the superior vena cava. The other complication treated on an emergency basis is spinal cord compression, usually due to lymph node extension into the epidural space. Paraplegia can result if treatment is not initiated with radiation therapy or, if the neurologic deterioration is rapid, a decompression laminectomy.

Multiple Myeloma. Multiple myeloma is a relatively uncommon malignancy of the plasma cell, the antibody-producing form of the B cell. A disease of older adults (median age at presentation is 65 years), multiple myeloma is a malignancy of plasma cells characterized by replacement of the bone marrow, bone destruction, and paraprotein formation. In this disease, excessive amounts of a single type of immunoglobulin are produced. **Table 27-7** lists the clinical manifestations of myeloma. The disease, commonly advanced at the time of diagnosis, is treated palliatively. Most commonly patients require treatment because of bone pain or other symptoms related to the disease. Renal dysfunction and failure are common. The treatment of myeloma is rapidly changing. Although combination chemotherapy has frequently been used, nonchemotherapy options with new and investigative agents are being tested. Autologous stem cell transplantation can be used for management after the initial disease has been controlled. Clinical trials employing combination therapy of new biologic agents are also under way. Although the disease is not curable, most patients survive for many years.

TABLE 27-7. CLINICAL MANIFESTATIONS OF MULTIPLE MYELOMA

Rationale	*Signs and Symptoms*
Bone marrow involvement by plasmacytomas (plasma Leukopenia cell tumors)	Anemia (common) Thrombocytopenia
Skeletal involvement by plasmacytomas and tumor activation of osteoclasts	Bone pain Osteolytic lesions
Pathologic fractures	Hypercalcemia
Production of light chains called Bence–Jones protein (part of immunoglobulin)	Proteinuria Renal insufficiency due to tubular damage
Hyperviscosity	Occlusion of small vessels Headache Mental status changes Visual disturbances Retinal hemorrhage Intermittent claudication
Hypervolemia	Congestive heart failure

KEY CONTENT CHECKLIST

- ❒ It is unlikely that hemophilia and von Willebrand or sickle cell disease will be on the CCRN exam. This section is included simply to provide a more complete description of abnormal coagulation concepts.
- ❒ Bleeding precautions are used when the platelet count falls below 50,000/mm^3. The risk of spontaneous bleeding increases at a platelet count of less than 20,000/mm^3.
- ❒ Impact of heat versus cold to muscles/skin. Cold reduces inflammation as well as swelling and blood flow. Heat vasodilates and improves blood flow. Warming blankets may help raise the patient's temperature but may also cause vasodilation and induce hypotension.
- ❒ Nursing interventions for immunosuppressed patients includes prevention and monitoring for infection. Remember that an immunocompromised patient may have fewer or less intense clinical symptoms because they are not able to mount an immune response.
- ❒ *The highest risk of infection occurs when the leukocyte (WBC) count is less than 1000/mm^3 and the neutrophils number less than 500/mm^3.*
- ❒ Enteral feedings are preferable to parenteral nutrition because of decreased risk of infection, namely bacterial translocation from ischemic bowel,
- ❒ HIV patients are at risk of developing a type of cancer called Kaposi sarcoma,
- ❒ PCP, an opportunistic infection, is often treated with Bactrim (TMP/SMX),

Review Questions:

1. HIV works through inhibition of which aspect of the immune system?

a. B-cell lymphocytes
b. T-cell lymphocytes
c. Neutrophils
d. Complement

Answer: B. Rationale: HIV primarily infects the T4 cell, and because of the rule of the T cell as the main coordinator of the immune response, devastating deficiencies occur in both the cell-mediated and humoral immune responses. The viral effects on the immune system include a profound lymphopenia and a reverse T_4:T_8 ratio (< 1).

2. Which of the following is/are common clinical presentation(s) of multiple myeloma?

a. Bone pain
b. Pathologic fractures and bone pain
c. Stomatitis and bone pain
d. Stomatitis and pathologic fractures

Answer: B. Rationale: A disease of older adults (median age at presentation is 65 years), multiple myeloma is a malignancy of plasma cells characterized by replacement of the bone marrow, bone destruction, and paraprotein formation. In this disease, excessive amounts of a single type of immunoglobulin are produced. Table 27-7 lists the clinical manifestations of myeloma. Stomatitis is inflammation of the mouth and lips that is a common complication of chemotherapy. Choose B.

3. An 18-year-old African American woman is admitted to your unit with complaints of shortness of breath and severe joint pain. She has a history of sickle cell anemia. Measures to reduce patient discomfort should include which of the following?

a. Analgesics
b. Oxygen therapy
c. Normal saline fluid challenge
d. All of the above

Answer: D. Rationale: Painful crises are treated with hydration and analgesics; pain management requires opioid administration at regular intervals until the crisis has been resolved. Oxygen should be administered as the carrying capacity on the RBC is diminished during crisis.

28

Life-Threatening Coagulopathies

CHAPTER OVERVIEW AND OBJECTIVES

Hematology and immunology comprise approximately 2% (two to four questions) of the CCRN exam. The exam is likely to focus on life-threatening coagulopathies, so expect one to three questions on this content.

After studying this chapter, you should understand the following:

- Discuss the pathophysiology associated with disseminated intravascular coagulation (DIC).
- Discuss the treatment and care of the patient experiencing DIC.
- Define thrombocytopenic conditions.

28.1 DISSEMINATED INTRAVASCULAR COAGULATION

DIC is a state of *hypercoagulability* that is triggered by activation of the clotting cascade with resultant generation of excess thrombin, deposition of fibrin in the microcirculation, and activation of the *fibrinolytic* system. DIC is not a specific disease but rather an acquired disorder that occurs in a wide variety of clinical disorders. Although many diseases can be complicated by DIC, it is most frequently associated with massive trauma, infection, sepsis, metastatic malignancy, and obstetric syndromes (abruptio placentae, amniotic fluid embolism, retained fetus, second-trimester abortion).

Pathophysiology

Regardless of the cause, specific pathophysiologic signs occur in DIC. The common denominator is the release of procoagulants into the circulatory system. Free hemoglobin, cancer tissue fragments, amniotic fluid, and bacterial toxins are some of the procoagulants that may activate the clotting cascade. Activation of the cascade results in diffuse intravascular fibrin formation. Fibrin is then deposited in the microcirculation.

With the *clotting of the capillaries*, blood is shunted to the arteriovenous anastomoses. This shunting causes the capillary tissue to use *anaerobic metabolism. With the production of lactic and pyruvic waste products and blood stagnation in the microcirculation, acidemia develops.*

Three procoagulant factors develop in capillary blood because of the DIC disease process. Acidosis acts as a strong procoagulant along with the "normal" procoagulants in the blood. The third factor is the concentration of procoagulants, which increases secondary to the stagnation of blood. These processes result in massive sequestration of clotted blood in the capillaries (**Fig. 28-1**).

DIC develops rapidly, so that coagulating factors are depleted in the microcirculation faster than the clotting factors can be replenished. Without circulating coagulant factors, hemostasis cannot be maintained (**Fig. 28-2**) and the patient begins to bleed.

Etiology

Many factors may precipitate DIC, including multiple trauma, crush injuries, hemorrhagic shock, malignant hypertension, incompatible blood transfusion, any and all cancers, burns, and coronary bypass surgery. DIC does not occur in isolation; it is always a sequela to some initiating event. All the major physiologic anticoagulants including antithrombin III, protein C, and tissue factor pathway inhibitor appear to be affected in DIC. The systemic formation of fibrin results from increased generation of thrombin and the simultaneous suppression of anticoagulation, and delayed removal of fibrin due to impaired fibrinolysis.

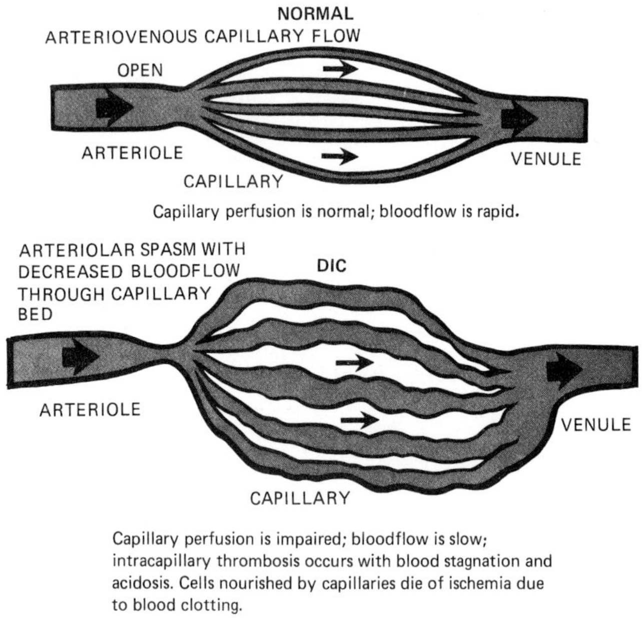

Figure 28-1. Sequestration of clotted blood in the capillaries.

Clinical Presentation

In most cases of DIC, arterial hypotension occurs secondary to the arteriovenous anastomoses. The anastomoses are caused by arterial vasoconstriction of the precapillary sphincter and vasodilatation of the capillaries.

Bleeding occurs after injections or venipunctures, from incisions, in the mucosa of the mouth, in the respiratory system, in the gastrointestinal system, and in the genitourinary system. It is common for several of these systems to be bleeding simultaneously; rarely is only one system involved.

Despite the complete depletion of circulating fibrinogen, some circulating thrombin still exists, since fibrinogen is not present to convert it to fibrin. Activation of the clotting process produces thrombin and thereby fibrin. Fibrin and thrombin convert plasminogen to plasmin. Antithrombins (especially antithrombin III) destroy thrombin function. In DIC, thrombin production exceeds antithrombin III production and thereby promotes uncontrolled coagulation.

The initiation of fibrinolysis results in the dissolution of clots and degrades fibrin into its fractions, which further adds to the bleeding. **Laboratory results suggestive of DIC include a decreased platelet count and fibrinogen level, a prolonged prothrombin time/international normalized ratio (PT/INR), partial thromboplastin time (PTT), activated partial thromboplastin time (APTT), and an increased fibrin degradation product (FDP) and D-dimer.**

QUICK TIP! At least one question will appear regarding laboratory tests (and which are increased vs decreased) to determine DIC.

Pulmonary compromise may require intubation. Following the trend of arterial blood gases (ABGs) and observing for signs and symptoms of hypoxemia will show when suctioning and/or mechanical ventilation is indicated.

Monitor fluid balance, especially if the patient receives multiple blood transfusions and other fluids or if the patient has another preexisting disease.

Skin care to preserve skin integrity is very important. Care must be taken to treat the patient very gently and to maintain good body alignment with adequate support. Sufficient but not excessive pressure is applied to sites of intramuscular injection or venipuncture by laboratory personnel to prevent hematoma formation.

Petechiae are pinpoint, flat lesions that appear as reddish-purple spots on the skin, buccal mucosa, and conjunctivae. Purpura is characterized by reddish brown spots usually evidencing presence of fluid. Ecchymoses are black-and-blue bruises.

Psychosocial support is extremely important to decrease the anxiety of the patient, who is aware and frightened by all the lost blood and the flurry of activity around him or her. Very brief explanations should be given; for example, "I'm giving you some medicine through the vein to help stop your bleeding." Providing an explanation of DIC in terms that the patient and family can understand will help to decrease anxiety and foster positive relationships among all parties.

Treatment

The primary treatment of DIC is to treat the underlying disease, which is easier said than done in the face of hemorrhaging. DIC can cause life-threatening hemorrhage and measures to control bleeding or thrombosis may require emergency measures. Treatment will vary with the clinical presentation. Patients with bleeding may require blood products and antithrombotic factors.

- Fresh-frozen plasma (FFP) or cryoprecipitate, to replace depleted clotting factors.
- Platelets may be transfused if counts are less than 5000 to 10,000/mm^3, especially with active bleeding.
- Infusion with antithrombin is controversial and has not demonstrated improvement in patient mortality.

It is necessary to replace the clotting factors and the effects of thrombin must be stopped. Correction of acidosis, hypotension, hypovolemia, and hypoxia must occur as these four conditions act as procoagulants and continue the utilization/-depletion of clotting factors. **Vitamin K** (-formation of prothrombin) and folic acid (thrombocytopenia) are administered to correct these deficiencies.

The use of heparin remains controversial because it is difficult to assess its effectiveness. Heparin neutralizes free circulating thrombin by combining with antithrombin III, which inactivates the thrombin. Heparin functions as an anticoagulant to prevent further thrombus formation in the microcirculatory system. (It does not alter the thrombi already formed.) Heparin prevents the activation of factor X. Heparin also inhibits platelet aggregation.

Caution: If used, heparin should be given intravenously, not subcutaneously. Factors affecting subcutaneous heparin include the absorption rate, which is dependent on the amount injected, the depth of injection, body temperature, and cardiovascular status. If a hematoma develops at the injection site, absorption is markedly altered. The amount of heparin needed may be too great for subcutaneous administration. The delay in reaching

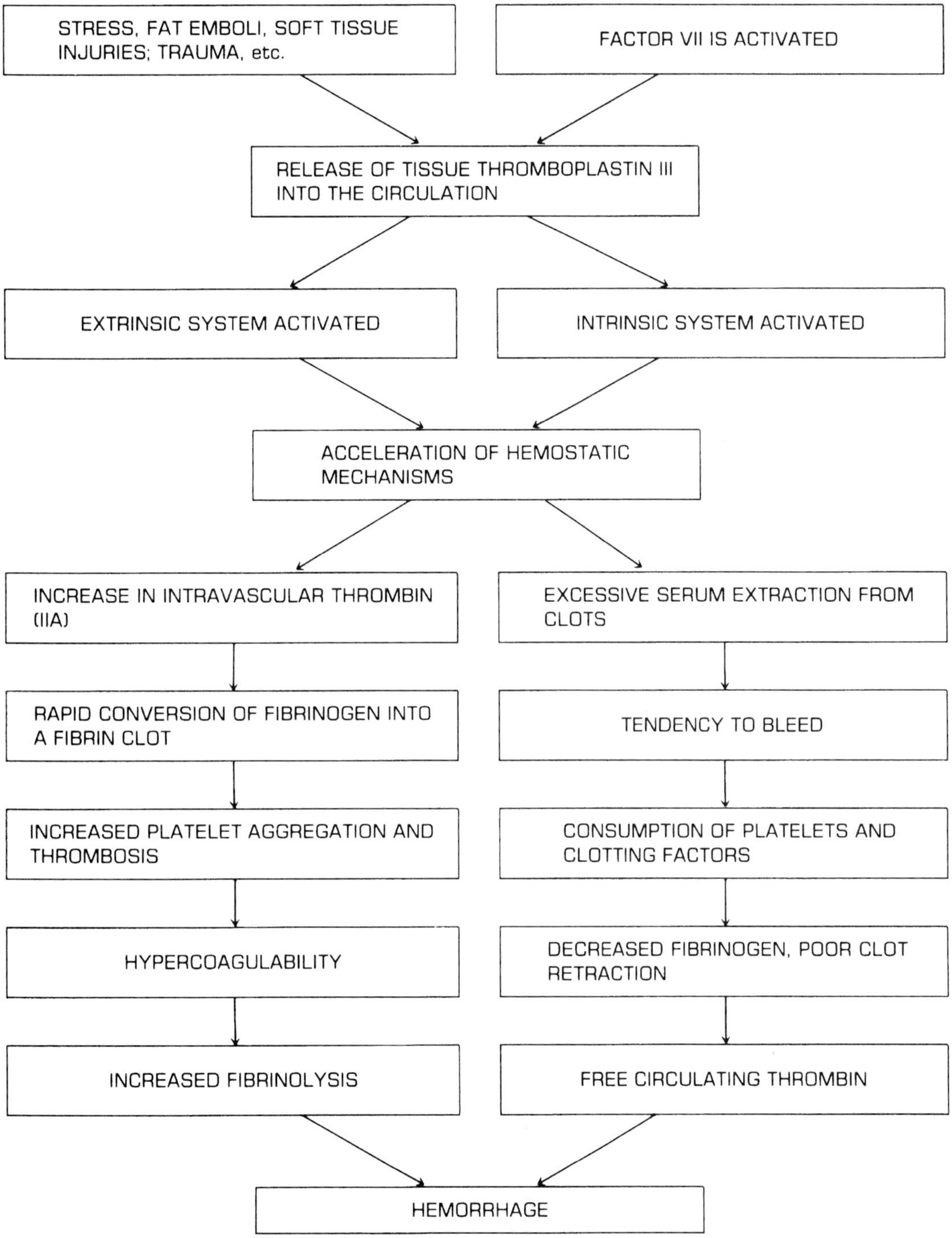

Figure 28-2. Alteration of the coagulation process in DIC.

a therapeutic blood level may be too long with subcutaneous administration.

Complications

Prognosis varies depending on the underlying disorder. DIC may become an exsanguinating hemorrhage. Death is not uncommon.

Nursing Interventions

Assessment of patients at high risk for DIC includes looking for the development of petechiae, purpura, and ecchymoses. Oozing of blood from injection sites, intravenous lines, and invasive monitoring lines may indicate the onset of DIC.

Cardiac status must be monitored for dysrhythmias secondary to acidosis, hypovolemia, hypervolemia, and electrolyte imbalances. Early recognition and treatment of dysrhythmias may prevent progression to more serious dysrhythmias. Renal problems develop as a consequence of impaired cardiac output, fluid depletion, and hypotension. The oliguric or anuric patient cannot eliminate heparin adequately, so the dose must be titrated to match the patient's utilization and excretion of the drug.

Monitor the amount of bleeding and identify the system involved. Observe for frank bleeding and notify the provider at the onset of bleeding.

Watch for signs of thrombus formation. If thrombi develop, the symptoms will vary according to the system involved. The kidneys are most often involved (oliguria or anuria).

Intracranial bleeding may be identified by changes in the neurologic exam. Signs and symptoms may include altered level of consciousness, disorientation to person, place, and/or time, changes in pupil reactions and changes in strength or extremity movement. Components of this exam must be checked frequently. Any change will indicate a possible bleed.

28.2 THROMBOTIC THROMBOCYTOPENIC PURPURA

Thrombotic thrombocytopenic purpura (TTP) can cause multisystem complications requiring critical care during the acute phase. It is characterized by thrombocytopenia, hemolytic anemia, fever, neurologic complications, and renal failure. The etiology is unknown, but TTP appears to involve a deficiency of a von Willebrand factor-cleaving protease, ADAMTS13. In some cases, it is due to an antibody directed against the protease. TTP is occasionally precipitated by estrogen use, pregnancy, drugs (quinine, ticlopidine), or infections. It can also occur as a complication of bone marrow transplantation or the use of cyclosporine or tacrolimus. The pathophysiology of TTP includes widespread deposition of platelet microthrombi that occlude the arteries and capillaries. This is especially evident in the brain, bone marrow, and kidneys. The result is bleeding and petechiae. Treatment is aimed at managing the manifestations of the syndrome, including severe thrombocytopenia and hemolytic anemia. The use of plasmapheresis, corticosteroids, and immunosuppression has been effective, and splenectomy may prevent subsequent relapses. The complexity and severity of this disease make it a challenge for the critical care nurse.

28.3 IDEOPATHIC THROMBOCYTOPENIA PURPURA

Idiopathic thrombocytopenia purpura (ITP) is defined as thrombocytopenia that occurs without any specific cause; however, many cases are due to an autoimmune response with antibodies against platelets developing. ITP is also known as immune thrombocytopenia purpura or immune-mediated thrombocytopenia purpura. ITP is usually chronic in adults and is more frequent in women. Symptoms of ITP include the development of bruising and petechiae, usually on the extremities, or bleeding from the nostrils or gums (especially when the platelet count is < 20,000/mm^3). Bleeding time is prolonged, but a normal bleeding time does not exclude the diagnosis. The diagnosis is often one of exclusion. *Treatment is generally indicated for a platelet count less than 20,000/mm^3, and a level less than 10,000/mm^3 is a potential medical emergency as the patient is at risk for spontaneous bleeding as well as subarachnoid or intracerebral hemorrhage if moderate head trauma were to occur.* Treatment may include intravenous steroids (methylprednisolone or prednisone), intravenous immunoglobulin, thrombopoietin receptor agonists to simulate platelet production, platelet infusion, and surgical removal of the spleen.

28.4 HEPARIN-INDUCED THROMBOCYTOPENIA

Heparin-induced thrombocytopenia (HIT) occurs due to an immune response because of heparin administration, either unfractionated or low-molecular weight. HIT has been designated as the most frequent drug-induced immune-mediated type of thrombocytopenia. In HIT, the platelet count falls below the normal range (< 150,000/mm^3) within 5 to 14 days after heparin administration. Patients at higher risk for developing HIT include those status postcardiovascular surgery, orthopedic surgery, and general surgery. In HIT, the immune system forms antibodies against heparin and results in platelet activation and blood clot formation resulting in a decreased platelet count and a predisposition to thrombosis. *Heparin therapy should be stopped*, and alternate non-heparin forms of anticoagulation should be used in patients with confirmed HIT or while awaiting confirmatory tests. The diagnosis of HIT is confirmed by measuring the platelet factor 4 (PF4) antibody levels. The PF4 antibody that causes HIT can disappear after approximately 3 months; however, the patient should avoid heparin products and notify their medical team that they have a heparin allergy. If an arterial or venous thrombus occurs as a result of HIT, the patient should be treated with a nonheparin anticoagulant for at least 3 months. *The serum platelet count should recover in approximately 7 days after cessation of heparin products.* Monitoring the patient for bleeding and minimizing bleeding risks are areas of focus for nursing care for both ITP and HIT.

KEY CONTENT CHECKLIST

- ❒ DIC develops rapidly, so that coagulating factors are depleted in the microcirculation faster than the clotting factors can be replenished. Without circulating coagulant factors, hemostasis cannot be maintained.
- ❒ Laboratory results suggestive of DIC include a decreased platelet count and fibrinogen level, a prolonged PT/INR, PTT, APTT, and an increased fibrin degradation product (FDP) and D-dimer.
- ❒ Patients with bleeding in DIC may require blood products (FFP, cryoprecipitate, and platelets) and antithrombotic factors.
- ❒ In addition to low platelet count, TTP is characterized by thrombocytopenia, hemolytic anemia, fever, neurologic complications, and renal failure.
- ❒ In HIT, the platelet count falls below the normal range (< 150,000/mm^3) within 5 to 14 days after heparin administration, monitor for signs of thrombus in addition to monitoring platelet count.

Review Questions:

1. **Causes of DIC do not include**
   a. Sepsis
   b. Crush injury
   c. Rhinovirus
   d. Cancer

Answer: C. Rationale: Sepsis, crush injury, and cancer are all known causes of DIC. The common cold that is caused by rhinovirus has not been associated with initiating DIC.

2. **Clinical manifestations of HIT**
   a. Occur as early as 3 days post heparin administration
   b. Begin with a single hemorrhage event
   c. Include new-onset thrombocytopenia
   d. Include cerebral hemorrhage

Answer: C. Rationale: HIT is seen with a fall of platelet count below 150,000 after 5 days and up to 14 days after exposure to heparin medication. Hemorrhage is not a common presentation of HIT and occurs in rare cases.

REFERENCES

Accessmedicine.com: Disseminated intravascular coagulation. In: *Schwartz Surgery Online*. New York, NY: McGraw-Hill; 2005. Accessed July 28, 2009.

Accessmedicine.com: Transplantation. In: *Schwartz Surgery Online*. New York, NY: McGraw-Hill; 2005:chap 10. Accessed July 30, 2009.

American Association of Allergy, Asthma, and Immunology. Media resources: Position statement 26. The use of epinephrine in the treatment of anaphylaxis. http://www.aaaai.org/media/resources/academy_statements/advocacy_statements/ps26.asp. Accessed August 10, 2009.

Baroletti SA, Goldhaber SZ. Heparin-induced thrombocytopenia. *Circulation*. 2006;114:e355–e356.

Branson BM, Owen SM, Wesolowski LG, et al. *Laboratory Testing for the Diagnosis of HIV Infection: Updated Recommendations*. Center for Disease Control National Center for HIV/AIDS, Viral Hepatitis, STD, and TB Prevention. 2014.

Cardenas AM, Baughan E, Hodinka RL. Evaluation of the Bio-Rad Multispot HIV-1/HIV-2 Rapid Test as an alternative to Western blot for confirmation of HIV infection. *J Clin Virol*. 2013;58(Suppl 1):e97–e103.

Cook J. Diagnosis and management of iron-deficiency anemia. *Clin Haematol*. 2005;18:319–332.

Creteur J, Sibbald W, Vincent, JL. Hemoglobin solutions—not just red blood cell substitutes. *Crit Care Med*. Aug 2000;28(8):3025–3034.

Cuker A, Crowther MA. 2013. Clinical Practice Guideline on the Evaluation and Management of Adults with Suspected Heparin-Induced Thrombocytopenia (HIT). American College of Hematology. http://www.hematology.org/practiceguidelines.

Cuker A, Arepally G, Chong B, et al. American Society of Hematology 2018 Guidelines for management of venous thromboembolism: heparin-induced thrombocytopenia. *Blood Adv* 2018;2(22): 3360–3392. doi: https://doi.org/10.1182/bloodadvances.2018024489.

Dellinger RP. Deep vein thrombosis. In: *Adult Multiprofessional Critical Care Review*. Chicago, IL: Society of Critical Care Medicine; 2007:243–252.

DeLoughery TG. Blood component therapy. In: *Adult Multiprofessional Critical Care Review*. Chicago, IL: Society of Critical Care Medicine; 2007: 379–392.

Dressler DK. *Hematology and immunology systems*. In: Chulay M, Burns SM, eds. *AACN Essentials of Critical Care Nursing*. New York, NY: McGraw Hill; 2006:305–315.

Dressler DK. Death by clot: Acute coronary syndromes, ischemic stroke, pulmonary embolism, and disseminated intravascular coagulation. *AACN Adv Crit Care* 2009;20(2):166–176.

Dudeck MA, Weiner LM, Allen-Bridson K. National Healthcare Safety Network (NHSN) Report, Data Summary for 2012, Device-Associated Module. *Am J Infect Control*. 2013;41:1148–1166.

Ellis AK, Day JH. Diagnosis and management of anaphylaxis. *Can Med Assoc J*. 2003;169:307–312.

Ellis K, Brener S. New fibrinolytic agents for MI: as effective as current agents but easier to administer. *Cleve Clin J Med*. 2004;71(1):20–37.

Fauci AS, Lane HC. Human immunodeficiency virus disease: AIDS and related disorders. *Harrison's Online*. New York, NY: McGraw-Hill; 2005. Accessed July 28, 2009.

Feied C, Handler JA. Thrombolytic therapy. 2004. E-Medicine. http://www.emedicine.com/emerg/topic831.htm. Accessed August 10, 2009.

Franchini M. Heparin-induced thrombocytopenia: an update. *Thromb J*. 2005;3:14.

Glass M, Spitrey J. Heparin-induced thrombocytopenia: your questions answered. *AACN Adv Crit Care*. 2009;20(1):5–11.

Greenberg AG, Kim HW. Hemoglobin-based oxygen carriers. *Crit Care*. 2004;8(Suppl 2):S61–S64.

Harrison's Online. Clinical immunology; hematology; disorders of hemostasis [online]. www.harrisonsonline.com. Accessed July 30, 2009.

Harrison's Online. Shock [online]. www.harrisonsonline.com. Accessed July 30, 2009.

Hirnschall G, Harries AD, Easterbrook PJ, et al. The next generation of the World Health Organization's global antiretroviral guidance. *J Int AIDS Soc*. 2013;16:18757.

Holcomb S. Recognizing and managing anemia. *Nurse Pract*. 2005;30:16–31.

Hübel K, Dale DC, Engert A, Liles WC. Current status of granulocyte (neutrophil) transfusion therapy for infectious diseases. *J Infect Dis*. 2001;183:321.

James SH. Hematology pharmacology: anticoagulant, antiplatelet, and procoagulant agents in practice. *AACN Adv Crit Care*. 2009;20(2):177–192.

Katz EA. Blood transfusion: friend or foe. *AACN Adv Crit Care*. 2009;20(2): 155–163.

Leichtman AB. Balancing efficacy and toxicity in kidney-transplant immunosuppression. *N Engl J Med*. 2007;357:2625.

Malm K, von Sydow M, Andersson S. Performance of three automated fourth-generation combined HIV antigen/antibody assays in large-scale screening of blood donors and clinical samples. *Transfus Med*. 2009;19(2):78–88.

Medline Plus Health Information. Anaphylaxis. National Institute of Health [online]. http://www.nlm.nih.gov/medlineplus/ency/article/000844.htm. Accessed August 10, 2009.

Merrill AA, Roth D, O'Nan P, et al. Nephrology nurses in a new role: diagnostic and interventional nephrology. *Nephrol Nurs J*. 2004;31(4):390:395–396.

Moyer VA, U. S. Preventive Services Task Force. Screening for HIV: U.S. Preventive Services Task Force Recommendation Statement. *Ann Intern Med*. 2013;159(1):51–60.

Munro N. Hematologic complications of critical illness: anemia, neutropenia, thrombocytopenia, and more. *AACN Adv Crit Care*. 2009;20:145–154.

Pandori MW, Westheimer E, Gay C, et al. The Multispot rapid HIV-1/HIV-2 differentiation assay is comparable with the Western blot and an immunofluorescence assay at confirming HIV infection in a prospective study in three regions of the United States. *J Clin Virol*. 2013;58(Suppl 1):e92–e96.

Patel P. Acute kidney failure. http://www.nlm.nih.gov/medlineplus/ency/article/000501.html. Accessed August 10, 2009.

Powderly WG, Mayer KH. Centers for Disease Control and Prevention revised guidelines for human immunodeficiency virus (HIV) counseling, testing and referral: Targeting HIV specialists. *Clin Infect Dis*. 2003;37(6):813–819.

Quillen K, Yau YY, Leitman SF. The determinants of granulocyte yield in 1198 granulocyte concentrates collected from unrelated volunteer donors mobilized with dexamethasone and granulocyte-colony-stimulating factor: a 13-year experience. *Transfusion*. 2009;49:421.

Raab MS, Podar K, Breitkreutz I, et al. Multiple myeloma. *Lancet*. 2009; 374:324–339.

Salinitri F, Berlie H, Desai N. Pharmacotherapeutic blood pressure management in a chronic kidney disease patient. *AACN Adv Crit Care*. 2009;20:205–213.

Silverman MA. Idiopathic thrombocytopenia purpura. EMedicine 2009. http://emedicine.medscape.com/article/779545. Accessed September 5, 2009.

Tefferi A, Hanson C, Inwards D. How to interpret and pursue an abnormal complete blood cell count in adults. *Mayo Clin Proc.* 2005;80:923–936.

Thompson MA, Aberg JA, Hoy JF, et al. Antiretroviral treatment of adult HIV infection: 2012 recommendations of the International Antiviral Society-USA panel. *JAMA.* 2012;308:387.

Umbreit J. Iron deficiency: a concise review. *Am J Hematol.* 2005;78:225–231.

Van Hemerlrijck, J, Levien LJ, Veeckman, L, et al. A safety and efficacy evaluation of hemoglobin-based oxygen carrier HBOC-201 in a randomized, multicenter red blood cell controlled trial in noncardiac surgery patients. *Anesth Analg.* Oct 2014;119(4):766–776.

Vernon S, Pfeifer GM. Blood management strategies for critical care patients. *Crit Care Nurse.* 2003;6:34–41.

Weinstein, R. Clinical practice guide on red blood cell transfusion. *Ann Intern Med.* 2012;157:49–58.

PART IV
Immunology and Hematology Practice Exam

1. **Which cell, known as the "helper cell," is vital in activating the immune response?**
   (A) segmented neutrophil
   (B) band neutrophil
   (C) T4 lymphocyte
   (D) T8 lymphocyte
2. **Which of the following components of the immune system is referred to as "cell-mediated" in its immune response?**
   (A) segmented neutrophils
   (B) band neutrophil
   (C) T lymphocytes
   (D) B lymphocytes
3. **Which of the following components of the white blood cell count makes up the largest percent of the differential?**
   (A) segmented neutrophils
   (B) band neutrophils
   (C) monocytes
   (D) lymphocytes
4. **Which term is used to describe a substance regarded as foreign in terms of the immune response?**
   (A) antibody
   (B) antigen
   (C) complement
   (D) cytotoxic
5. **Which of the following are NOT considered macrophages?**
   (A) segmented neutrophils
   (B) band neutrophils
   (C) monocytes
   (D) lymphocytes
6. **A 71-year-old man is admitted to your unit with recurrent pneumonia. Since the pneumonia was present before, which of the following type of cells would have the ability to remember the *Haemophilus* antigen from a prior infection?**
   (A) segmented neutrophils
   (B) band neutrophils
   (C) lymphocytes
   (D) eosinophils
7. **A 23-year-old woman is in your unit following a motor vehicle accident. During the admission, she develops a urinary tract infection. If this were her first exposure to the bacteria causing the infection, which component of the white blood cell count would be the first to respond to the antigen?**
   (A) segmented neutrophils
   (B) eosinophils
   (C) T4 lymphocytes
   (D) T8 lymphocytes
8. **Which of the following types of cells produce antibodies?**
   (A) segmented neutrophils
   (B) monocytes
   (C) B lymphocytes through plasma cells
   (D) reticuloendothelial cells
9. **Which of the following components of the immune system is referred to as "humorally mediated" in its immune response?**
   (A) segmented neutrophils
   (B) band neutrophils
   (C) T lymphocytes
   (D) B lymphocytes

Questions 10 and 11 refer to the following scenario:
A 21-year-old man is in your unit for respiratory distress caused by reaction to chemotherapy for Hodgkin disease. The following laboratory information is available:

White blood cells	1300/mm^3
Segmented neutrophils	25%
Banded neutrophils	10%
Lymphocytes	25%
Platelets	15,000/mm^3
Activated partial thromboplastin time	100 seconds

10. **Based on the preceding information, which complications should you be aware may occur in this situation?**
    (A) bleeding and infection
    (B) infection and hypercoagulation
    (C) hypercoagulation
    (D) infection
11. **Which of the following measures would potentially be most helpful in this scenario?**
    (A) placing the patient on respiratory isolation
    (B) placing the patient on bodily secretion isolation
    (C) drawing blood only from arteries
    (D) placing the patient on reverse isolation
12. **Which cell secretes lymphokines (biological response modifiers)?**
    (A) segmented neutrophil
    (B) band neutrophil
    (C) T lymphocyte
    (D) B lymphocyte
13. **Which of the following is NOT a lymphokine?**
    (A) interferon
    (B) interleukin
    (C) granulocyte-macrophage colony-stimulating factor (GM-CSF)
    (D) cyclosporine

14. Which antibody mediates allergic reactions?
(A) IgD
(B) IgM
(C) IgE
(D) IgG

15. Which is the most dominant antibody in adult life?
(A) IgA
(B) IgB
(C) IgC
(D) IgG

16. Which of the following would be given to provide passive immunity from accidental puncture with a needle contaminated with hepatitis?
(A) IgA
(B) IgB
(C) IgC
(D) IgG

17. The human immunodeficiency virus (HIV) works through inhibition of which aspect of the immune system?
(A) B-cell lymphocytes
(B) T-cell lymphocytes
(C) neutrophils
(D) complement

18. Which of the following agents is used to treat *Pneumocystis carinii* pneumonia?
(A) Septra (Bactrim)
(B) acyclovir
(C) amphotericin B
(D) vancomycin

19. Bone marrow failure occurring with leukemia can present with which of the following symptoms?
(A) bleeding, increased risk of infection, and anemia
(B) increased risk of infection and hypercoagulation
(C) anemia and hypercoagulation
(D) decreased risk of infection and anemia

20. In which organ system does much of the development of antibodies take place?
(A) hepatic
(B) respiratory
(C) gastrointestinal
(D) splenic

21. Which of the following is/are common clinical presentation(s) of multiple myeloma?
(A) bone pain
(B) pathologic fractures and bone pain
(C) stomatitis and bone pain
(D) stomatitis and pathologic fractures

Questions 22 and 23 refer to the following scenario:
A 37-year-old man is admitted to your unit for investigation of the cause of his hypotension. He has a history of weight loss, night sweats, and cervical lymph node enlargement. Laboratory data and vital signs reveal the following information:

Blood pressure	88/60 mm Hg
Pulse	118
Respiratory rate	31
Temperature	38.7°C
White blood cells	6000
Platelets	400,000

Reed–Sternberg cells are noted in the laboratory analysis.

22. Based on the preceding information, which condition is likely to be developing?
(A) sepsis
(B) multiple myeloma
(C) Hodgkin disease
(D) acute lymphocytic leukemia

23. Which treatment modality or modalities could be employed in this patient?
(A) splenectomy and chemotherapy
(B) radiation therapy and chemotherapy
(C) chemotherapy and splenectomy
(D) splenectomy, radiation therapy, and chemotherapy

24. Which phase of chronic myelocytic leukemia can resemble an acute leukemia?
(A) blast crisis
(B) recombinant phase
(C) hematopoiesis phase
(D) myelosuppressive phase

Questions 25 and 26 refer to the following scenario:
A 27-year-old man is admitted to your unit with shortness of breath, weight loss, and nonproductive cough. Current vital signs are:

Blood pressure	118/74 mm Hg
Pulse	114
Respiratory rate	34
Temperature	38.4°C

HIV serum testing is positive.

25. Based on the preceding information, which condition is likely to be present?
(A) Kaposi sarcoma
(B) non-Hodgkin's lymphoma
(C) *Klebsiella pneumoniae*
(D) *Pneumocystis carinii* pneumonia

26. What is the likely cause for the shortness of breath?
(A) noncardiogenic pulmonary edema
(B) lymphocytic infiltration into the bronchi
(C) V/Q disturbance from pneumonia
(D) high $PaCO_2$ levels

27. Which side effect of chemotherapy can affect nutritional status?
(A) loss of serum proteins
(B) stomatitis
(C) increased oxygen consumption
(D) loss of gastrointestinal function

28. Which condition occurs with the graft-versus-host response to transplanted bone marrow?
(A) The body rejects the transplanted marrow.
(B) The transplanted cells reject normal cells.
(C) The donor cells mutate into abnormal host cells.
(D) Both graft cells and normal cells reject each other.

29. At what point does spontaneous bleeding become a nursing concern in the patient receiving chemotherapy?
(A) white blood cell count less than $3000/mm^3$
(B) fibrin split product level less than 400
(C) platelet count less than $20,000/mm^3$
(D) platelet count more than $50,000/mm^3$

30. Which is the first response in coagulation following trauma to a blood vessel?
(A) vasoconstriction
(B) platelet aggregation
(C) fibrin formation
(D) thrombin formation

31. Which electrolyte is an integral part of the coagulation process?
(A) sodium
(B) potassium
(C) magnesium
(D) calcium

Questions 32 and 33 refer to the following scenario:
A 41-year-old woman is admitted to your unit with an exacerbation of chronic lymphocytic leukemia. She states that she has had small amounts of vaginal bleeding. Ecchymotic areas are noted on her arms and legs. Laboratory data reveal the following:

Platelets	$15,000/mm^3$
White blood cells	$4100/mm^3$
Granulocytes	50%

32. Which of the following nursing measures should be employed on this patient?
(A) place on bleeding precautions
(B) place on reverse isolation and bleeding precautions
(C) avoid fresh plants and vegetables in the room and place on reverse isolation
(D) place on reverse isolation

33. Which treatment would most likely be ordered for this patient?
(A) platelet transfusions
(B) initiation of aerosolized pentamidine
(C) low-dose heparin therapy
(D) amphotericin B

34. Which of the following characterizes disseminated intravascular coagulation?
(A) decreased prothrombin time
(B) increased levels of fibrinogen degradation products
(C) antithrombin formation
(D) platelet proliferation

35. A patient admitted with a diagnosis of pulmonary embolism is to receive a thrombolytic agent. Which of the following is NOT considered a thrombolytic medication?
(A) tissue plasminogen activator (tPA)
(B) urokinase
(C) streptokinase
(D) heparin

36. Which test is best employed to assess the effectiveness of heparin therapy?
(A) partial thromboplastin time (PTT)
(B) prothrombin time (PT)
(C) platelet levels
(D) bleeding time

37. The thrombolytic effect of plasmin is due to which action?
(A) prevention of platelet aggregation
(B) blocking of the intrinsic pathway
(C) breaking down of fibrin
(D) ionization of calcium

38. Which cell is characteristic of Hodgkin disease?
(A) Kaposi
(B) Reed–Sternberg
(C) promyelocyte
(D) Stevens

39. Which lymphoma tends to progress along adjacent groups of lymph nodes, as opposed to skipping to noncontinuous groups?
(A) lymphocytic leukemia
(B) multiple myeloma
(C) non-Hodgkin's lymphoma
(D) Hodgkin disease

Questions 40 and 41 refer to the following scenario:
A 35-year-old man is admitted to your unit with the diagnosis of Hodgkin disease. He is admitted because of dyspnea, upper trunk edema, jugular venous distention, and cough.

40. Based on the preceding information, which condition is likely to be developing?
(A) right ventricular failure
(B) lymphocytic infiltration into the myocardium
(C) superior vena cava syndrome
(D) venous congestion secondary to splenic enlargement

41. Which treatment would most likely improve the symptoms?
(A) diuretics
(B) radiation therapy
(C) administration of fluorouracil (5-FU)
(D) surgery to remove lymphatic obstructions.

42. An 18-year-old African American woman is admitted to your unit with complaints of shortness of breath and severe joint pain. She has a history of sickle cell anemia. Measures to reduce patient discomfort should include which of the following?
(A) analgesics
(B) oxygen therapy
(C) normal saline fluid challenge
(D) all of the above

43. **Which of the following tests is used to diagnose a hemolytic transfusion reaction?**
    (A) Coombs test
    (B) prothrombin time (PT)
    (C) activated partial thromboplastin time (aPTT)
    (D) fibrinogen level

44. **What is another name for factor I?**
    (A) fibrinogen
    (B) thrombin
    (C) prothrombin
    (D) thromboplastin

45. **The extrinsic pathway for coagulation is initiated by which mechanism?**
    (A) irregularity of the blood vessel wall
    (B) presence of atherosclerotic plaques, causing increased turbulent blood flow
    (C) exposure to interstitial tissue following trauma to the blood vessel
    (D) introduction of an extrinsic substance into the blood

46. **What is the cause of superior vena cava syndrome?**
    (A) obstruction of the superior vena cava by thrombi
    (B) compression of the vena cava by enlarged lymph nodes
    (C) failure of the left and right heart due to lymphocytic infiltration
    (D) bronchial obstruction due to tumor growth

47. **Advantages of having "normal flora" of bacteria on the skin include which of the following?**
    (A) They maintain the acidic pH of the skin.
    (B) They compete successfully for nutrients with pathologic organisms.
    (C) They maintain the skin's acidic pH and compete for nutrients with pathologic organisms.
    (D) They produce oxygen for use by superficial cell layers and they compete for nutrients with pathologic organisms.

48. **Which antibody is naturally present in bodily secretions (eg, saliva)?**
    (A) IgG
    (B) IgQ
    (C) IgA
    (D) IgE

49. **What is the primary purpose of the complement system?**
    (A) to aid in the coagulation process
    (B) to assist antibodies in destroying antigens
    (C) to prevent the development of tumor cells
    (D) to act as scavengers to clear antigenic debris

50. **What is the first stage in the coagulation process?**
    (A) conversion of plasminogen to plasmin
    (B) conversion of fibrinogen to fibrin
    (C) activation of thrombin
    (D) activation of thromboplastin

51. **Nursing care of the patient receiving thrombolytic therapy includes which of the following?**
    (A) avoiding intramuscular injections and using a soft toothbrush
    (B) avoiding intramuscular injections and using oximetry rather than blood gas studies for SaO_2 determination
    (C) using a soft toothbrush and using oximetry rather than blood gas studies for SaO_2 determination
    (D) all of the above

52. **Which component is primarily stored in the spleen?**
    (A) platelets
    (B) neutrophils
    (C) lymphocytes
    (D) factor VIII

53. **Which hormone is thought to regulate bone marrow production of platelets and red blood cells?**
    (A) growth hormone
    (B) erythropoietin
    (C) thyroid-stimulating hormone
    (D) adrenocorticotropic hormone (ACTH)

PART IV
Immunology and Hematology Practice Exam

Practice Fill-Ins

1. ______
2. ______
3. ______
4. ______
5. ______
6. ______
7. ______
8. ______
9. ______
10. ______
11. ______
12. ______
13. ______
14. ______
15. ______
16. ______
17. ______
18. ______
19. ______
20. ______
21. ______
22. ______
23. ______
24. ______
25. ______
26. ______
27. ______
28. ______
29. ______
30. ______
31. ______
32. ______
33. ______
34. ______
35. ______
36. ______
37. ______
38. ______
39. ______
40. ______
41. ______
42. ______
43. ______
44. ______
45. ______
46. ______
47. ______
48. ______
49. ______
50. ______
51. ______
52. ______
53. ______

PART IV
Answers

1. **C** Chapter 25 Rationale: T cells are divided into four functionally distinct but interactive cell populations or subsets: cytotoxic, helper (T4), suppressor (T8), and memory T cells. Neutrophils are phagocytic, early responders to a pathogen. Choose C.
2. **C** Chapter 25 Rationale: There are two major types of lymphocytes: T lymphocytes (T cells) and B lymphocytes (B cells). T cells are involved in immunologic regulation and mediate what is called the cellular immune response. B cells produce antibodies and mediate what is called the humoral immune response. Neutrophils are phagocytic, early responders to a pathogen. Choose C.
3. **A** Chapter 25 Rationale: Neutrophils are the most abundant cells in the bone marrow and blood, comprising about 90% of all granulocytes. Three forms of neutrophils can be identified in the peripheral blood: segmented neutrophils, bands, and metamyelocytes. Segmented neutrophils are fully mature, bands are slightly immature, and metamyelocytes are completely immature neutrophils. Neutrophils are strongly phagocytic: that is, they ingest microorganisms or other cells and foreign particles, and they digest the ingested material within their phagocytic vacuoles.
4. **B** Chapter 25 Rationale: By definition, an antigen is a substance that is regarded as foreign in terms of the immune response. Antibodies are released to fight antigens, eliminating A. Complement is released to aid antibodies, eliminating C as well. Cytotoxic is a nonspecific term used to describe a toxin-induced threat to cellular viability. Choose B.
5. **D** Chapter 25 Rationale: Macrophages are cells that participate in phagocytosis or recruit other cells to support this process such as lymphocytes. These cells are part of the innate immune system; lymphocytes are distinct in that they are part of the acquired immune system. Even if you were not sure of the answer, consider using the "cluster technique" and rule out option A & B since they are both neutrophils to narrow down your choices.
6. **C** Chapter 25 Rationale: Lymphocytes will be the cells that recognize the *Haemophilus* antigen. Memory T cells are T cells that have been sensitized to a specific antigen and then cloned to remember the antigen. Memory cells remain present in the body for many years and are therefore available for defense upon repeated exposure to an antigen. Repeated exposure to an antigen that the host has been previously sensitized to will result in a more rapid and accelerated immune response than on the first exposure.
7. **A** Chapter 25 Rationale: In conditions such as infection, there is an increased demand for neutrophils. The bone marrow responds by releasing more neutrophils into the circulation, and in this process immature cells, or band cells, are released as early responders to infection along with the mature cells.
8. **C** Chapter 25 Rationale: B cells are effector cells that mediate the humoral immune response through the production of antibodies, which is their major function. B cells are important in defense against pyrogenic bacterial infections and can destroy transplanted organs by mediating hyperacute graft rejection.
9. **D** Chapter 25 Rationale: In this question, if the answer is not readily known and lymphocytes is a suspected correct answer, a cluster technique may be used. Since option A and B are both associated with neutrophils, consider eliminating them. T cells are associated with cellular-mediated immunity, eliminating option C as well. B cells produce antibodies and mediate what is called the humoral immune response; choose D.
10. **A** Chapter 25 Rationale: The normal neutrophil count in the adult is between 1000 and 6000/mm^3 blood, or approximately 60% of the differential WBC count. Bands normally number about 600/mm^3 blood, or approximately 0% to 5% of the differential WBC count. Normal values are 150,000 to 450,000 platelets per microliter (mcL). Values below 100,000 are pathognomonic for thrombocytopenia, the cause of which must be determined. A platelet count less than 50,000 results in excessive bleeding, since there is an insufficient number of platelets to clot. Counts less than 20,000 are associated with spontaneous bleeding.
11. **D** Chapter 25 Rationale: Patient is at risk for infection. Placing the patient on reverse isolation will help protect the patient from potential exposure.
12. **C** Chapter 25 Rationale: Cytotoxic T cells bind to target cells and facilitate their destruction via substances known as lymphokines, which stimulate inflammatory cells, and via the production of cytolytic proteins.
13. **D** Chapter 25 Rationale: Cytotoxic T cells bind to target cells and facilitate their destruction via substances known as lymphokines, which stimulate inflammatory cells, and via the production of cytolytic proteins. Cyclosporine is an immunosuppressive drug often given to prevent posttransplant rejection; choose D.
14. **C** Chapter 25 Rationale: IgE mediates allergic reactions. Although only about 0.002% of antibodies are of the IgE type, IgE antibodies present on basophils and mast cells play a significant role in inflammatory and immune reactions.

15. **D** Chapter 25 Rationale: IgG is the principal mediator of the secondary immune response, which requires repeated exposure to the same antigen. IgG is the major antibody against bacteria and viruses. About 75% of all antibodies are of the IgG type.
16. **D** Chapter 25 Rationale: IgG is the principal mediator of the secondary immune response, which requires repeated exposure to the same antigen. IgG is the major antibody against bacteria and viruses.
17. **B** Chapter 25 Rationale: HIV primarily infects the T4 cell, and because of the rule of the T cell as the main coordinator of the immune response, devastating deficiencies occur in both the cell-mediated and humoral immune responses. The viral effects on the immune system include a profound lymphopenia and a reverse T4:T8 ratio (<1).
18. **A** Chapter 25 Rationale: Drug therapy for *Pneumocystis carinii* pneumonia (PCP) usually includes administration of a 21-day course of intravenous pentamidine or trimethoprim/sulfamethoxazole (Septra).
19. **A** Chapter 27 Rationale: Table 27-6. Clinical presentations associated with bone marrow failure include bleeding, increased risk of infection, and anemia.
20. **D** Chapter 27 Rationale: The spleen produces monocytes, lymphocytes, opsonins, and IgM antibody-producing plasma cells.
21. **B** Chapter 27 Rationale: A disease of older adults (median age at presentation is 65 years), multiple myeloma is a malignancy of plasma cells characterized by replacement of the bone marrow, bone destruction, and paraprotein formation. In this disease, excessive amounts of a single type of immunoglobulin are produced. Table 27-7 lists the clinical manifestations of myeloma. Stomatitis is inflammation of the mouth and lips that is a common complication of chemotherapy. Choose B.
22. **C** Chapter 26 Rationale: The disease usually presents as one or more enlarged lymph nodes, usually in the cervical region (cervical region predisposition is normally seen in HL [Hodgkin's Lymphoma]). Occasionally, the initial site of disease is the gastrointestinal (GI) tract. Approximately one-third of patients also exhibit systemic symptoms consisting of fever, night sweats, and loss of over 10% of the usual body weight.
23. **D** Chapter 26 Rationale: Treatment for lymphoma depends on the type and stage. If the lymphoma is localized, radiation therapy is initiated and is usually given with or after chemotherapy to disease sites. In HL, this consists of total nodal irradiation and radiation to the spleen (if not removed at laparotomy).
24. **A** Chapter 26 Rationale: During a blast crisis the patient may present with symptoms that closely resemble symptoms of acute leukemia. During this phase the cells are more sensitive to chemotherapy, and remission can be induced in about 50% of these patients. The patient may experience a fever, bone pain, and fatigue during this time.
25. **D** Chapter 26 Rationale: PCP onset is usually insidious, characterized by a gradually increasing shortness of breath, dry cough, fever, and—on chest roentgenography—pulmonary infiltrates. The establishment of a chronic, persistent infection is the hallmark of HIV disease. Some of the infections frequently seen with AIDS include cytomegalovirus retinitis, cryptococcal meningitis, toxoplasmosis, mycobacterial infections and, most commonly, *P. carinii* pneumonia.
26. **C** Chapter 26 Rationale: The V/Q disturbance occurs in these patients as a result of the disease attacking the interstitial tissue of the lungs, creating intrapulmonary shunt. This attack leads to a thickening of the tissue of the alveoli and alveolar septa. This complication results in significant hypoxia as gas exchange is compromised and carbon dioxide levels rise. The cysts that form in the lungs are aggressive and prolific—often found in aggregates of 2 to 8.
27. **B** Chapter 26 Rationale: Stomatitis often occurs in the mucous membranes of the mouth. During this time, patients will often experience extreme discomfort when trying to take in food or drink. Many times the discomfort will result in the patient refusing to eat or drink.
28. **B** Chapter 26 Rationale: In patients who have received bone marrow from a donor, graft-versus-host disease (GVHD) can occur as the transplanted marrow recognizes the host tissue as foreign and begins to reject normal cells. One of the tissues that the engrafted T cells attempt to reject is the skin.
29. **C** Chapter 26 Rationale: Another reason for admission of a leukemia patient to the critical care unit is severe bleeding and hemorrhage. This can occur secondary to thrombocytopenia induced by the disease process and/or the chemotherapy. It is not unusual for the platelet count to be less than 20,000/mm^3, which puts the patient at risk for spontaneous bleeding.
30. **A** Chapter 26 Rationale: Vasoconstriction is the first response to maintain hemostasis. The blood vessel experiences a spasm to constrict the vessel and prevents blood loss. B, C, and D all relate to subsequent clot formation. Choose A.
31. **D** Chapter 25 Rationale: Both the extrinsic and intrinsic cascades react to completion and, in the presence of calcium ions, join to form the common final pathway cascade shown in Fig. 25-7.
32. **A** Chapter 26 Rationale: It is not unusual for the platelet count to be less than 20,000/mm^3, which puts the patient at risk for spontaneous bleeding. Of particular concern is the possibility of a pulmonary or intracranial hemorrhage. Infection is not as significant concern since the granulocytes and WBC are within normal range. B, C, and D all include tactics to reduce infection risk. Choose A.
33. **A** Chapter 26 Rationale: Treatment would be focused on reversing the risk of spontaneous bleeding associated with the low platelet count. This will likely require multiple platelet transfusions. Special consideration should be made to administer single-donor leukocyte-poor products. Random donor vs single donor is controversial. Products should be irradiated due to immunosuppression.
34. **B** Chapter 29 Rationale: Disseminated intravascular coagulation (DIC) is a state of hypercoagulability, which is triggered by activation of the clotting cascade with

resultant generation of excess thrombin, deposition of fibrin in the microcirculation, and activation of the fibrinolytic system. Characteristic lab values include prolonged prothrombin time-international normalized ratio (PT-INR) and partial thromboplastin time (PTT), decreased platelet count and fibrinogen level, and increased fibrinogen degradation products (FDPs).

35. D Chapter 25 Rationale: Heparin is considered an anticoagulant that is used to prevent the formation of blood clots. Urokinase, streptokinase, and tPA are all thrombolytics. Choose D.

36. A Chapter 26 Rationale: The activated partial thromboplastin time (aPTT) measures the activity level and patency of the intrinsic clotting cascade and common final pathway. Normal values of 20 to 35 s are used to assess all clotting factors except VII and XIII. The effectiveness of heparin is assessed with the aPTT.

37. C Chapter 26 Rationale: Plasmin is an enzyme within the blood that degrades the fibrin clot through fibrinolysis.

38. B Chapter 27 Rationale: Though similar in many respects, the distinguishing feature of Hodgkin's lymphoma is the presence of Reed–Sternberg cells, whose origin and nature are uncertain. Kaposi's sarcoma is an oncology condition that can occur in end-stage AIDS, and Stevens-Johnson syndrome is a rare skin reaction. Choose B.

39. D Chapter 27 Rationale: Hodgkin's lymphoma is characterized by progressing along adjacent groups of lymph nodes accompanied by the development of systemic symptoms.

40. C Chapter 27 Rationale: Superior vena cava syndrome is characterized by enlarged veins in neck and head, shortness of breath, chest pain, difficulty swallowing, and cough. The origin of the disease is often linked to an obstruction due to cancer or lymphoma.

41. B Chapter 27 Rationale: Treatment to improve symptoms would include radiation to reduce the size of the tumor causing the obstructions.

42. D Chapter 27 Rationale: Painful crises are treated with hydration and analgesics; pain management requires opioid administration at regular intervals until the crisis has been resolved. Oxygen should be administered. as the carrying capacity on the red blood cell is diminished during crisis.

43. A Chapter 26 Rationale: A hemolytic reaction usually occurs within the first 30 min of the transfusion. It results in actual hemolysis of the RBCs, and the transfusion must be stopped. A Coombs test will diagnose this problem.

44. A Chapter 25 Rationale: Factor I is also known as fibrinogen. Prothrombin is coagulation factor II, which gives rise to thrombin, eliminating options B and C. Thromboplastin is often associated with factor III, eliminating D as well. Choose A.

45. C Chapter 25 Rationale: The extrinsic cascade (Fig. 25-6) is activated by injury to vessels and tissue. The end result of this cascade is the release of thromboplastin into the circulatory system.

46. B Chapter 27 Rationale: The cause of superior vena cava syndrome is the compression of the vena cava by enlarged lymph nodes in lymphoma or from lung or metastatic cancer.

47. C Chapter 25 Rationale: The resident flora maintains the skin's pH in the acidic range and competes effectively for nutrients and binding sites on epidermal cells, making it difficult for nonresident flora to survive.

48. C Chapter 25 Rationale: IgA is the secretory immunoglobulin present in bodily secretions and offers natural protection against nonspecific foreign antigens. About 15% of all antibodies are of the IgA type. Reference Table 25-1 for further detail.

49. B Chapter 25 Rationale: The complement system consists of a complex set of approximately 20 interacting proteolytic enzymes and regulatory proteins found in the plasma and body fluids that attack antigens.

50. D Chapter 25 Rationale: Syneresis is the final step in coagulation and the first step in clot stability. Syneresis is the process of particle suspension in a gel that begins to aggregate and form a compact mass—the clot. Clot retraction occurs soon after syneresis is complete. Platelets contain an enzyme called thromboplastin that causes the fibrin strands and cells in the clot to be drawn together, expressing a clear, serous fluid. Clot retraction is responsible for drawing the edges of damaged vessels together, which fosters healing.

51. D Chapter 25 Rationale: Nursing interventions are based upon (1) protection of the patient from bleeding and associated complications and (2) early detection of bleeding.

52. A Chapter 25 Rationale: Normally about 30% of the total platelet population is sequestered in the spleen, but this can increase to 80% with splenomegaly.

53. B Chapter 25 Rationale: RBC production is stimulated by the hormone erythropoietin. Erythropoietin is released by the kidney in response to tissue hypoxia. This hormone results in increased erythrocyte production by (1) increasing the number of stem cells placed into the maturational process, (2) decreasing maturational time, (3) increasing hemoglobin synthesis, and (4) causing a premature release of reticulocytes from the bone marrow.

PART V

NEUROLOGY

Anne C. Lindstrom

Section Overview

The following section outlines neurologic concepts often encountered in critical care.

- In its present format, about 14% of the CCRN exam is devoted to neurologic concepts.
- Neurology concepts are often difficult to apply due to the complexity. The following section will focus on neurologic disorders commonly seen in critical care nursing.
- The content will review key concepts and identify quick tips for supporting patients.
- The key content areas include
  - Acute spinal cord injury
  - Acute brain injuries: Ischemic stroke, hemorrhage, increased intracranial pressure, brain herniation, and brain death
  - CNS infections
  - Neuromuscular conditions
  - Seizures

29

Anatomy and Physiology of the Nervous System

CHAPTER OVERVIEW AND OBJECTIVES

The neurologic principles are often difficult concepts to apply in the CCRN exam due to the complexity of central and autonomic nervous system dysfunction. The neurologic aspect of the CCRN exam does not require that you be knowledgeable about every potential disturbance of the nervous system; rather, the primary focus is on problems commonly seen in general critical nursing practice.

After studying this chapter, you should understand the following:

- The basic anatomy and physiology of the central nervous system (CNS).
- Describe the function of the autonomic nervous system and the role of neurotransmitters.
- Understand the metabolic demands of the brain and its impact on body systems.

29.1 ANATOMY

It is customary to divide the nervous system into three segments to facilitate comprehension of the system and its dysfunctions. The three segments are the central nervous system ([CNS]—composed of the brain and spinal cord), the peripheral nervous system (composed of the cranial, spinal, and peripheral nerves), and the autonomic nervous system (composed of the sympathetic and parasympathetic systems).

Extracerebral Structures

Extracerebral structures include the scalp, skull, and meninges. These structures provide protection to the brain.

Scalp. The letters in SCALP form a mnemonic for remembering the cranial coverings (**Fig. 29-1**). "SCA" stands for the single layer of Skin and Cutaneous and Adipose tissue that contains blood vessels.

Skull. The bony calvarium (skull) comprises eight bones fused to form a solid, nondistensible unit. The cranium, which is the skull minus the mandible, is hollow and has a volume of 1400 to 1500 mL. It consists of an outer and an inner layer of regular bone and a middle layer, called the diploe (or diploic space), which is spongy and lightweight.

The bones comprising the cranium are the frontal (single), occipital (single), and pairs of parietal, temporal, sphenoid, and ethmoid bones (**Fig. 29-2**). The main function of the bony calvarium is to protect the brain from external forces. The fusion of these bones, at around 18 to 24 months of age, forms three suture landmarks:

- The coronal suture is the fusion of the frontal and parietal bones.
- The sagittal suture is the fusion of the two parietal bones.
- The lambdoid suture is the fusion of the parietal bones and the occipital bone.

The internal surface of the cranium has three distinct ridges on it that serve to divide the brain into anterior, middle, and posterior segments called *fossae* (plural; singular is fossa).

Meninges. The three membranes covering the entire brain surface, the spinal cord, and the spinal canal below the cord are the meninges (**Fig. 29-3**). The mnemonic "PAD" may help you to remember the meningeal coverings and their purpose: the *p*ia mater, *a*rachnoid, and *d*ura mater are the meningeal layers, and they absorb shocks from sudden movements or trauma; they literally "PAD" the brain.

Starting from the brain itself, the first meningeal layer is the pia mater. The pia mater touches the brain's surface and its convolutions.

The arachnoid layer of the meninges is a delicate, avascular membrane between the dura and pia mater. It looks much like a lacy spider web with projections onto the pia mater. The space between the arachnoid layer and pia mater, called the *subarachnoid space*, contains many cerebral arteries and veins. These arteries and veins are bathed in cerebrospinal fluid (CSF).

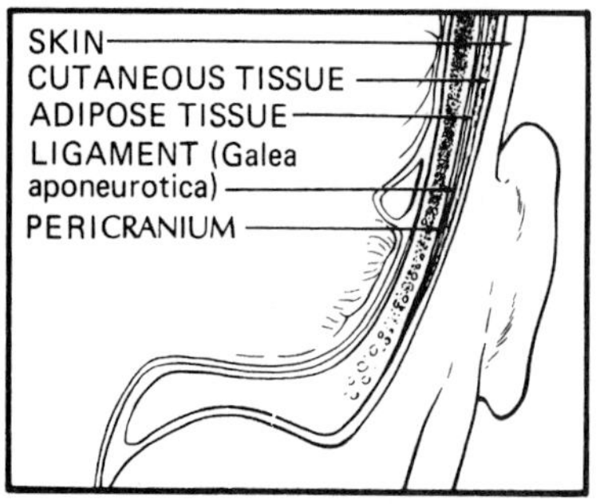

Figure 29-1. Layers of the scalp.

The arachnoid membrane also has projections into the venous sinuses called arachnoid villi, which allow for the reabsorption of CSF from the subarachnoid space to the venous system. The subarachnoid space enlarges at the base of the brain to form the subarachnoid cisterns.

The outermost layer of the meninges is the dura mater. The dura mater is composed of two layers of tough fibrous membrane that protect the underlying brain tissue. Between the two layers are clefts, which form the dural venous sinuses. The inner layer also gives rise to several folds, which divide the cranial cavity into compartments. There are four important compartments that are significant landmarks in the brain:

- The falx cerebri (separating the cerebral hemispheres)
- The falx cerebelli (separating the right and left cerebellar hemispheres)
- The tentorium cerebelli (separating the cerebral hemispheres from the cerebellum)
- The diaphragm sellae, which forms a tent-like covering or roof over the pituitary gland (which sits in a part of the bony skull called the sella turcica) (**Fig. 29-4**).

The extradural space, also called the *epidural space*, is a potential space between the inner table of the skull and the outermost meningeal layer, the dura mater. This potential

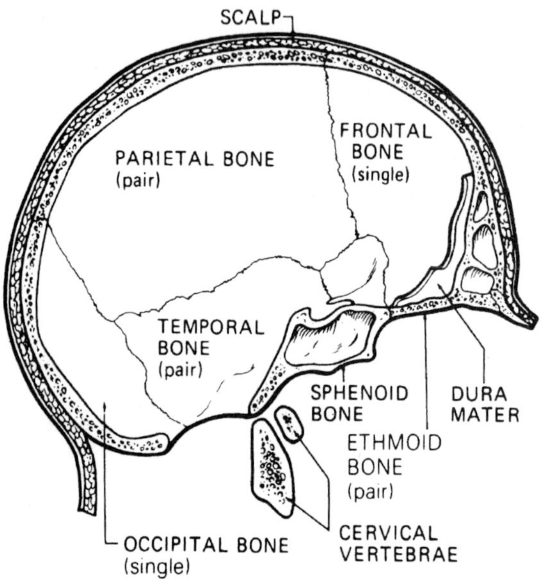

Figure 29-2. Cranium.

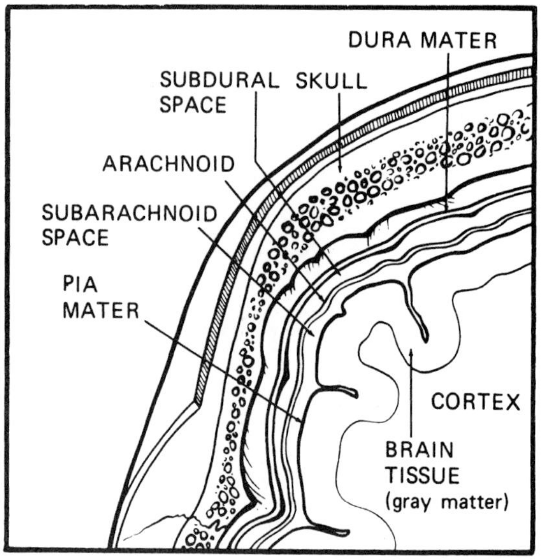

Figure 29-3. Meninges.

space may become real when an individual experiencing a blow to the head develops an epidural hematoma. **Epidural hematomas** *commonly result from a laceration of the middle meningeal artery in association with a skull fracture* at the parietotemporal junction.

Another potential space, the subdural space, lies between the dura mater and the arachnoid. This is the site of **subdural hematomas**. *This type of hematoma is most often venous in origin and results from tearing of the bridging dural veins.*

QUICK TIP! Epidural hematomas are usually associated with arterial bleeding and subdural hematomas are associated with venous bleeding. (See also Chapter 32 for additional key distinguishing factors.)

Central Nervous System

The brain is made up of nervous tissue that fills up the cranial vault. It weighs about 3 lb in the adult male. Although it is an integrated unit, the brain is divided into three major sections:

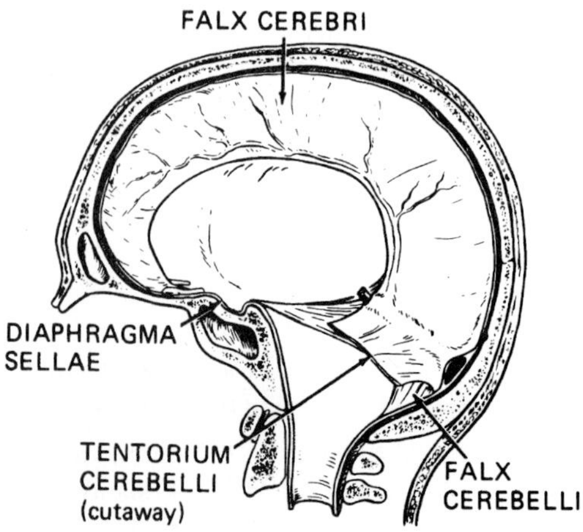

Figure 29-4. Sagittal section showing processes formed by the inner layer of the dura mater.

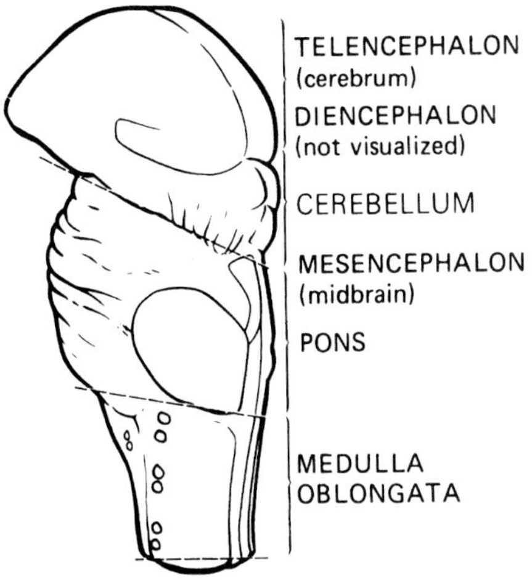

Figure 29-5. Gross anatomic sections of the brain.

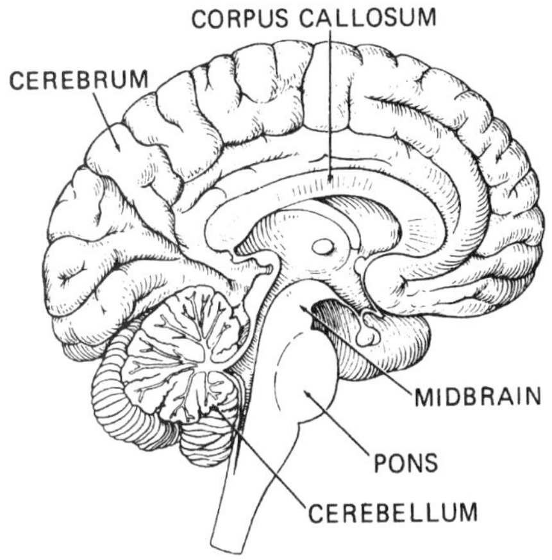

Figure 29-6. Midsagittal section showing the corpus callosum.

- The cerebrum
  - Cerebral hemispheres
  - White matter fibers
  - Limbic system
  - Basal ganglia
  - Diencephalon
- The brainstem
  - Midbrain
  - Pons
  - Medulla
- The cerebellum(**Fig. 29-5**).

Cerebrum

The cerebrum (also called the telecephalon) is contained in the anterior and middle fossae of the cranium. The left and right cerebral hemispheres are incompletely separated by a deep medial longitudinal fissure, called the *falx cerebri*, formed by the sagittal folds of the dura mater. The two cerebral hemispheres are joined by the corpus callosum (**Fig. 29-6**). It provides a path for fibers to cross from one hemisphere to the other.

The cerebral surface is covered with convolutions, which give rise to gyri (raised portions) and sulci or fissures (depressions in the surface). The cerebral surface is about six cells deep and called the cerebral cortex. It normally appears gray; thus, these six layers (**Fig. 29-7**) are called *gray matter*.

From a lateral view, two fissures divide each hemisphere (**Fig. 29-8**). The lateral fissure (also called the fissure of Sylvius) divides the temporal lobe from the parietal and frontal lobes and contains the primary auditory center The central sulcus, also known as the *fissure of Rolando*, divides the frontal lobe from the parietal lobe. Immediately in front of the central sulcus is the precentral gyrus, which is the primary motor area. Immediately posterior to the central sulcus is the postcentral gyrus, which is the primary sensory cortical area.

For descriptive purposes, the lateral surface of the hemisphere is divided into four lobes.

- The frontal lobe (approximately the anterior one-third of the hemisphere) is anterior to the central sulcus and above the lateral fissure. The frontal lobe is responsible for voluntary motor function and higher mental functions such as judgment and foresight, affect, personality,

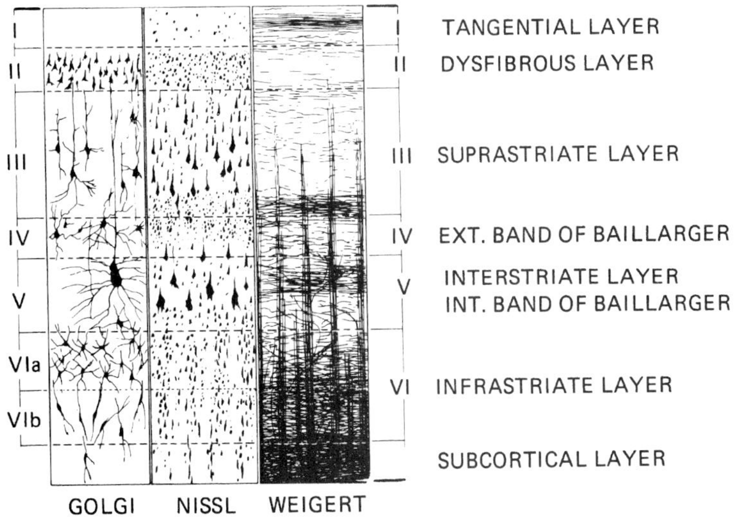

Figure 29-7. Six layers of the cerebral cortex.

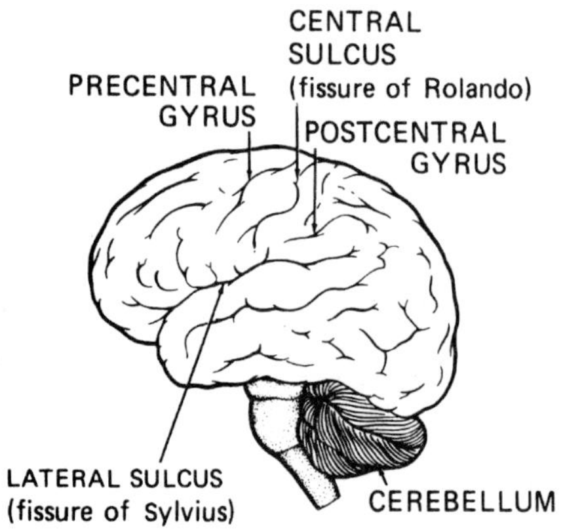

Figure 29-8. Fissures, sulci, and gyri dividing the cerebral hemisphere.

inhibition, abstract thinking, and motor speech (dominant hemisphere).

- The parietal lobe extends from the central sulcus to the parietooccipital fissure. This lobe is responsible for sensory function, sensory association, and higher-level processing of general sensory modalities.
- The occipital lobe is lying behind, or caudal to, an arbitrary line drawn from the parietooccipital fissure to the preoccipital notch. The function of the occipital lobe is visual reception and visual association.
- The temporal lobes are located under the lateral fissures of Sylvius. The temporal lobes are each divided into a primary auditory receptive area (in dominant hemisphere), a secondary auditory association area, and a tertiary visual association area.

The basal ganglia, or basal nuclei, are also part of the telencephalon and include the caudate nucleus, putamen, globus pallidus, claustrum, subthalamic nucleus, and substantia nigra (**Fig. 29-9**).

Specific functions of the brain segments are listed in **Table 29-1**.

Diencephalon. The diencephalon is composed of the thalamus, epithalamus, subthalamus, and hypothalamus (**Fig. 29-10**). It is a paired structure with a thin fluid space between the two sides. The thalamus is the largest structure in the diencephalon. It is the major relay area for all neuronal impulses and integrates all body sensations except smell. The hypothalamus connects with the limbic system, thalamus, mesencephalon, and pituitary gland. The hypothalamus is also responsible to produce antidiuretic hormone (ADH) and oxytocin as well as influence body temperature, water balance, and the intake of food.

Brainstem

Midbrain. The midbrain (also known as the *mesencephalon*) is located between the diencephalon and the pons. It contains the major motor nerves for eye movement, carries impulses down from the cerebrum, and controls the wakefulness of the brain through the reticular-activating system (RAS; **Fig. 29-11**). RAS fibers connect with the thalamus, cerebral cortex, cerebellum, and spinal cord. They contain nuclei of the third and fourth cranial nerves.

Pons. The pons is situated between the midbrain and the medulla oblongata. It forms a bridge (thus its name comes from the Latin word for bridge) between the cerebellar hemispheres and contains the neurons for sensory input and motor output for the face. It contains the nuclei of the fifth, sixth, seventh, and eighth cranial nerves. The pons in conjunction with the medulla controls the rate and length of respirations.

Medulla Oblongata. The medulla oblongata is located between the pons and spinal cord. It marks the change between the spinal cord and the brain itself. The corticospinal tracts, which mediate voluntary motor function, descend through the medulla and intersect in the lower medulla. They are responsible for specific symptoms of dysfunction occurring ipsilaterally (same side as the lesion or injury) or contralaterally (opposite side). Regulation of respiratory rhythm, rate, and strength of heartbeat and blood vessel diameter are controlled by the medulla. The nuclei for reflex activities such as coughing, sneezing, swallowing, and vomiting and the 9th to 12th cranial nerves are found here.

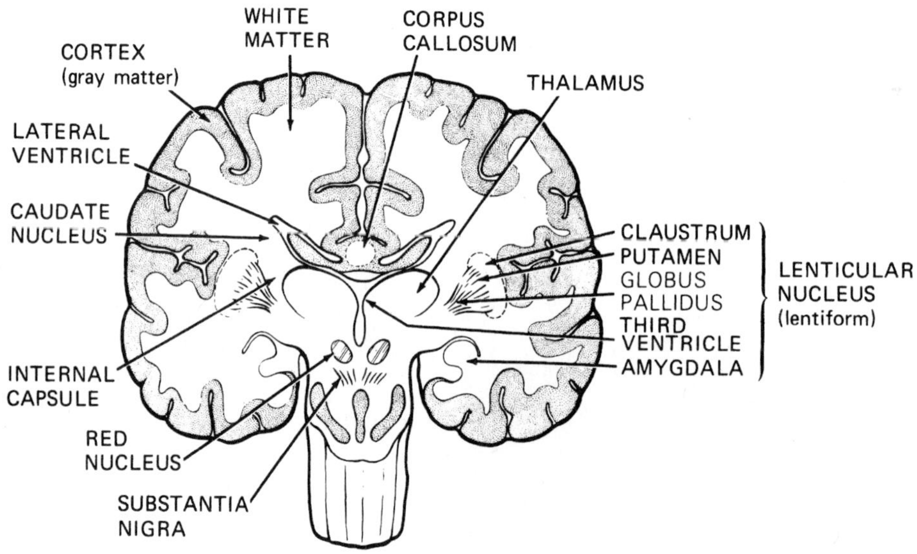

Figure 29-9. Coronal section of the brain showing internal parts of basal ganglia of the telencephalon.

TABLE 29-1. FUNCTIONS OF SPECIFIC BRAIN STRUCTURES

Structure	*Function*
Cerebrum (divided into cerebral hemispheres)	Governs all sensory and motor thought and learning; analyzes, associates, integrates, and stores information
Cerebral cortex (four lobes)	
Frontal lobe	Motor function; motor speech area; controls morals, values, emotions, and judgment
Parietal lobe	Integrates general sensation; governs discrimination; interprets pain, touch, temperature, and pressure
Temporal lobe	Auditory center; sensory speech center
Occipital lobe	Visual area
Basal ganglia	Central motor movement
Thalamus (diencephalon)	Screens and relays sensory impulses to cortex; lowest level of crude conscious awareness
Hypothalamus (diencephalon)	Regulates autonomic nervous system, stress response, sleep, appetite, body temperature, water balance, and emotions
Midbrain (mesencephalon)	Motor condition, conjugates eye movements
Pons	Contains projection tracts between spinal cord, medulla, and brain
Medulla oblongata	Contains all afferent and efferent tracts, most pyramidal tracts, and cardiac, respiratory, vasomotor, and vomiting centers
Cerebellum	Connected by cerebellar peduncles to other parts of CNS; coordinates muscle movement, posture, equilibrium, and muscle tone
Limbic system	Regulation of some visceral activities; some function in emotional personality

Cerebellum

The cerebellum is situated in the posterior fossa of the cranial cavity. It is separated from the cerebrum by dura mater folds forming the tentorium cerebelli. The cerebral hemispheres are above the tentorium cerebelli and are thus supratentorial structures. The two cerebellar hemispheres are connected to each other by a structure called the *vermis*. They are connected to the brainstem by cerebellar peduncles. There are three cerebellar peduncles (**Fig. 29-12**).

- The superior cerebellar peduncles send impulses from the cerebellum to the thalamus.
- The middle cerebellar peduncles receive cerebral cortex information from nuclei in the pons.
- The inferior cerebellar peduncles receive impulses that reveal body and extremity positions.

Gray and white matters compose the cerebellum. The cerebellum receives input from the brainstem and spinal cord nuclei, whose axons project to the cerebellar cortex. These tracts carry excitatory impulses to cerebellar cortex.

Equilibrium, posture, muscle tone, and, ultimately, muscle coordination are mediated by the cerebellum.

Circulation and Formation of Cerebrospinal Fluid

Four ventricles (cavities) are involved in the CSF system (**Fig. 29-13**). The two largest ventricles are the lateral ventricles, which are in the cerebral hemispheres. The lateral ventricles are connected to the third ventricle via the interventricular

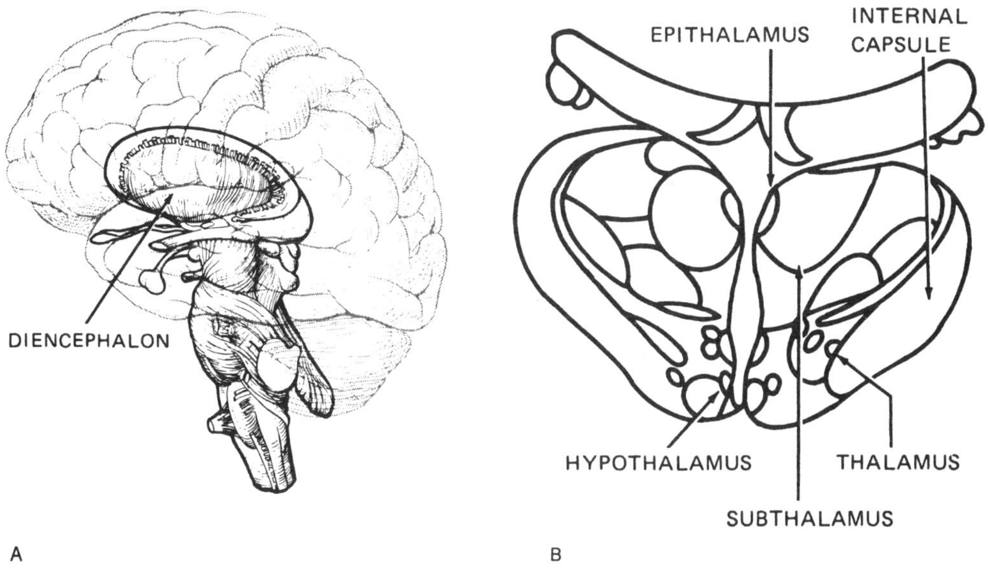

Figure 29-10. Position of the diencephalon (**A**) and the internal components of the diencephalon (**B**).

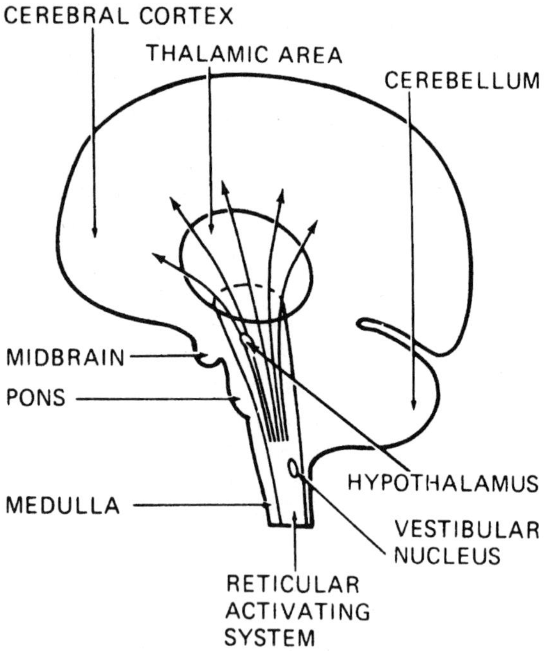

Figure 29-11. Reticular-activating system.

foramen, or the foramen of Monro. The cerebral aqueduct of Sylvius exits from the floor of the third ventricle. This channel passes down through the brainstem to the fourth ventricle, which is continuous with the central canal of the spinal cord. *CSF is synthesized at approximately 20 mL/h by the choroid plexus.* This is an area of modified epithelial cells covering tufts of capillaries found in all ventricles but predominating in the anterior segment of the lateral ventricles. *CSF is a clear, colorless liquid having a few cells, some protein, glucose,* and a large amount of sodium chloride.

The foramen of Monro allows the CSF to leave the lateral ventricles and flow into the third ventricle. *Obstruction at this point will produce hydrocephalus.* The most common site of obstructive hydrocephalus occurs in the aqueduct of Sylvius at or above the fourth ventricle, obstruction at the foramen of Monro, or at the outlets of the fourth ventricle. From the third ventricle, CSF flows through the aqueduct of Sylvius into the fourth ventricle. Foramina of Luschka and Magendie direct the CSF from the fourth ventricle into the cisterns and subarachnoid space.

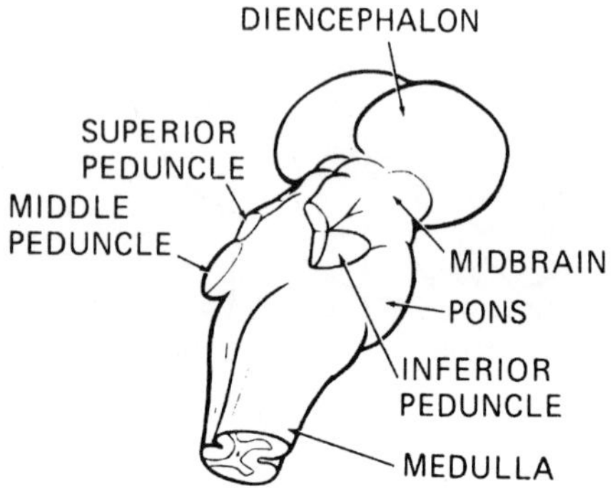

Figure 29-12. Cerebellar peduncles.

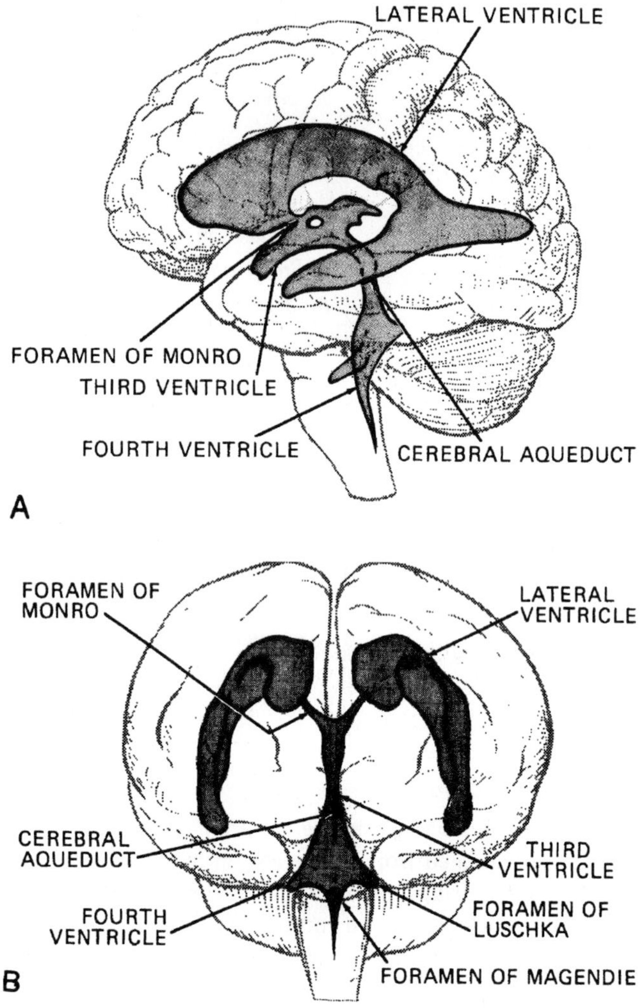

Figure 29-13. Lateral **(A)** and anterior **(B)** views of the ventricular system of the brain.

After circulating (in the subarachnoid space) over the entire brain and spinal cord, the CSF is reabsorbed by the arachnoid villi in dural sinuses and by pacchionian bodies found in the superior sagittal sinus.

The CSF "cushions" the brain and spinal cord to protect them from colliding with the cranium and vertebrae in response to moving forces. The CSF also reduces the gravitational weight of the brain. *To a limited extent, the CSF adjusts to changes in the intracranial vault's pressure and volume. If the pressure or volume in the vault increases, more CSF will be absorbed and/or pushed into the spinal canal to maintain normal pressure.* Normally, 125 to 150 mL of CSF is in the ventricles and the subarachnoid space. *An average of 500 mL of CSF is produced in a 24-hour period or approximately 22 mL/h.* The CSF also participates in the exchange of nutrients and waste material between blood and the cells of the CNS.

KEY CLINICAL CONCEPT

Obstruction of CSF will lead to hydrocephalus and can increase intracranial pressure. External ventricular drainage (or "ventriculostomy") is often required to drain excess CSF. (Chapter 31 has additional information.)

Cerebral Blood Supply. The brain is supplied with oxygenated blood from two arterial systems: the anterior circulation originating with the carotid arteries and the posterior circulation which originates with the vertebral arteries. The common carotid arteries bifurcate, forming the external and internal carotid arteries. As a reserve to these two systems, the circle of Willis helps to provide adequate circulation through its anastomoses. The circle of Willis anastomoses is between the two vertebral arteries and the two carotid arteries (**Fig. 29-14**). Only about 50% of people have a complete circle of Willis. The internal carotid carries about two-thirds of the blood that flows to the brain. The right and left vertebral arteries branch off the subclavian arteries. They pass through the foramen magnum as they enter the skull.

Arterial Blood Supply. External cerebral blood supply. The external carotid arteries feed the external face, head, and neck. The external carotid arteries bifurcate and form the occipital, temporal, and maxillary arteries.

- The occipital arteries supply the posterior fossa.
- The temporal arteries supply the temporal region.
- The maxillary arteries form the middle meningeal arteries, which supply the anterior, middle, and posterior portions of the meninges and the fossae.

Internal cerebral blood supply. On entering the skull, the internal carotid artery follows the carotid groove upward through the cavernous sinus and the sphenoid bone and into the circle of Willis at the base of the brain. Before this, smaller vessels originate, one of which is the ophthalmic artery. Temporary blockage of the ophthalmic artery by microemboli may cause amaurosis fugax (temporary blindness in one eye).

Each internal carotid artery bifurcates to form several major branches, including the posterior communicating artery, anterior cerebral artery, anterior choroidal artery, and middle cerebral artery.

- The anterior communicating artery connects the left and right anterior cerebral arteries, forming a bridge to join the right and left anterior circulation. This bridge creates the front portion of the circle of Willis.
- The posterior communicating artery connects the internal carotid artery to the posterior cerebral artery and joins the anterior to the posterior circulation of the brain. These communicating arteries do not supply any part of the brain directly, but some are collateral channels helping to form the back portion of the circle of Willis.
- The vertebral arteries enter the posterior fossa and join to form the basilar artery.
- The basilar artery gives off several major branches, including the superior cerebellar arteries and the anterior inferior cerebellar arteries, and bifurcates to form the posterior cerebral arteries.
  - The superior cerebellar arteries supply the pons, midbrain, and cerebellum.
  - The anterior inferior cerebellar arteries feed the cerebellum and the pons.
  - The posterior cerebral arteries supply the posterior one-third of the cerebrum as well as parts of the midbrain and choroid plexus of third and fourth ventricles.
- The circle of Willis contains the anterior cerebral artery, the anterior communicating artery, the posterior communicating arteries, and the posterior cerebral arteries. These arteries are involved in supplying blood to the anterior two-thirds of the cerebrum.

Veins run parallel with many of the arteries. The middle meningeal arteries are special in that the veins that accompany these arteries are positioned between the arteries and the bones of the cranium. This helps protect the middle meningeal artery, which is frequently torn in skull fractures of the temporal bones.

Venous Blood Supply. As there is an internal and external arterial blood supply, there is a corresponding internal and external venous return system. Many of the veins are important in aneurysms and as surgical landmarks. The veins that drain the dura mater and diploe of the skull (external) empty into the venous sinuses, which are located between the layers of the dura mater. Internal cerebral veins also empty into venous sinuses.

Venous sinuses are lined with epithelium; they have no valves and no muscle in their walls. The sinuses connect with emissary veins, which in turn connect with external cranial veins that empty into the internal jugular veins.

- The superior sagittal sinus receives venous blood from the superior cerebral veins.
- The inferior sagittal sinus receives venous blood from the veins of the medial cerebral hemisphere.
- The straight sinus receives venous blood from the internal cerebral veins.

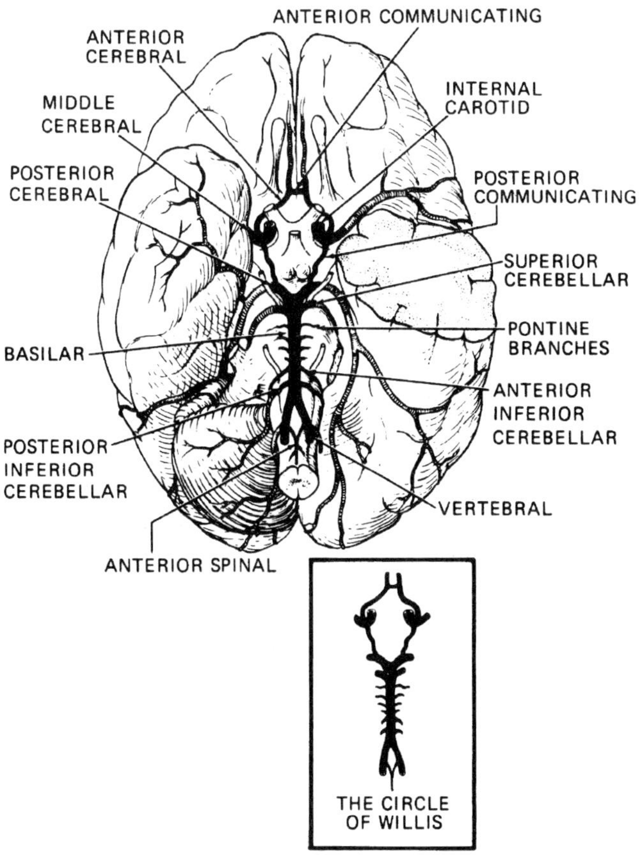

Figure 29-14. Circle of Willis.

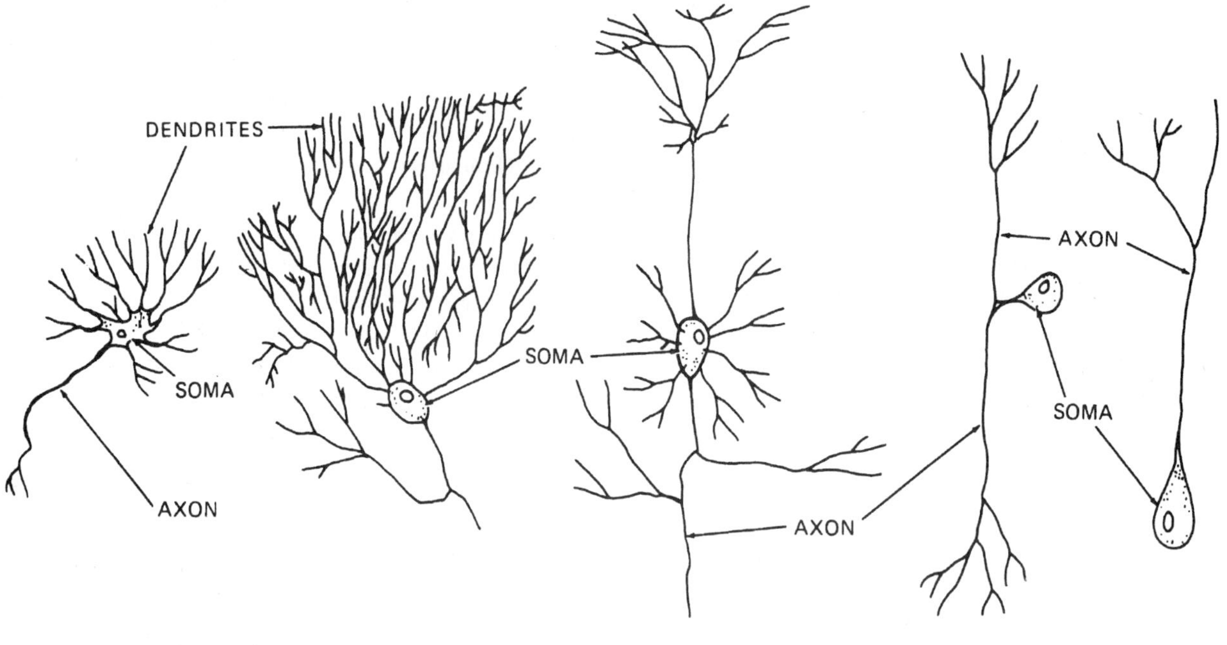

Figure 29-15. Various shapes of neurons and neuroglia.

There are many other sinuses that receive venous blood from other areas of the brain.

Components of Nervous Tissue. There are two main types of cells in the brain: neurons (**Fig. 29-15**) and neuroglia (glial cells). The neuron is the functioning unit of the nervous system; its job is to transmit impulses. There are more than 10 billion neurons in the CNS and three-fourths of them are in the cerebral cortex.

Neurons. Neurons are categorized in two ways: by the direction of impulse flow and/or by the number of processes emanating from the neuronal cell's body. Neurons that transmit impulses to the spinal cord or brain are afferent sensory neurons. Those transmitting impulses away from the brain or spinal cord are called efferent motor neurons. Interneurons transmit impulses from sensory neurons to motor neurons. The mnemonic *SAME* can help you to remember the direction and type of neuron: *SA* stands for sensory afferent and *ME* stands for motor efferent.

Neurons will be one of three types, per the number of processes that exist:

- Unipolar neurons have one process coming from the cell body. After a short distance, this one process will split to form one axon and one dendrite (typical of both cranial and spinal nerves).
- Bipolar neurons have one axon and one dendrite coming from the cell body (rod and cone cells of the optic system to the CNS).
- Multipolar neurons have one axon and multiple dendrites (typical of motor neurons).

Regardless of the category of neurons, they all have certain unique structures unique to neurons (**Fig. 29-16**), that is, axons, dendrites, neurofibrils, Nissl bodies, myelin, neurilemma, and nodes of Ranvier.

The cell body of a neuron is called a *soma* or *perikaryon*.

There is one axon per neuron responsible for transmitting impulses away from the soma. Myelin is a protein–lipid compound that covers some axons. In the CNS, myelin is produced by oligodendrocytes. In the peripheral nervous system, myelin is produced by Schwann cells. Myelin covers axons of nerve cells in between the nodes of Ranvier. The nodes of Ranvier are bare spots at regular intervals that speed the conduction of impulses.

Dendrites are short processes that transmit impulses to the soma. The branching of dendritic processes is termed *arborization* since the processes look like tree branches.

The neurilemma is an outer coating of the neurons outside of the CNS. The neurilemma encompasses all structures, even myelin. It is the neurilemma that provides for the regeneration of peripheral nerves. Since neurilemma is not found on neurons in the brain and spinal cord, these cells cannot regenerate.

Neuroglia. Neuroglias provide an extensive support system to help neurons maintain optimal function (**Fig. 29-17**).

Neuroglias are composed of glial cells, and they outnumber the neurons by 10 to 1.

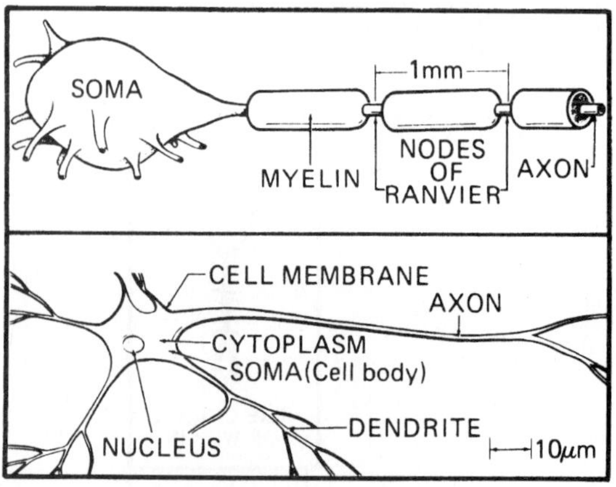

Figure 29-16. Schematic diagram of neuronal structures.

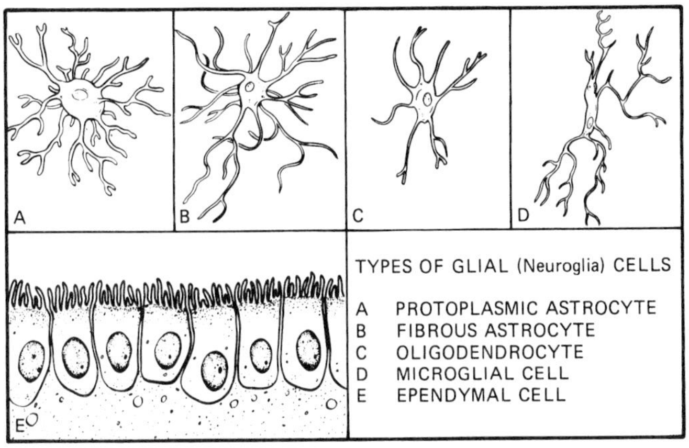

Figure 29-17. Types of glial cells (neuroglia).

Four types of cells compose the glial support system:

- Astrocytes are star-shaped cells that form the actual tissue support system. and constitute part of the blood–brain barrier by sending foot processes to the blood vessels.
- Microglia are tiny cells that lie dormant until nervous tissue is damaged. They wander in and out of the CNS in response to need. When damage occurs, the microglia mobilize and travel to the damaged tissue where they phagocytize the debris.
- Oligodendroglia primary function is the original formation of myelin in the CNS during fetal, neonatal, and early childhood years. Once the myelin has been formed, the oligodendroglia cannot form it again.
- Ependyma are special glial cells found lining the ventricles of the brain and the central canal of the spinal cord. They plan a critical role in CSF secretion, circulation, and homeostasis.

The spinal cord is the second part of the CNS. It is examined in Chapter 34.

Peripheral Nervous System. The peripheral nerves, the spinal nerves, and the cranial nerves form the peripheral nervous system. There are 31 pairs of spinal nerves and 12 pairs of cranial nerves.

Instead of being named, the 31 pairs of spinal nerves are numbered in relation to the vertebral level at which they emerge from the spinal cord. Spinal nerves do not attach directly to the spinal cord. Instead, they attach to a short anterior (ventral, motor) root and a short posterior (dorsal, sensory) root (**Fig. 29-18**). The posterior root has a bulge called the *spinal ganglion*, which consists of neuronal cell bodies. There are 8 cervical, 12 thoracic, 5 lumbar, 5 sacral, and 1 coccygeal pairs of spinal ganglia.

Peripheral nerves often encompass more than one spinal nerve root. The sciatic nerve is a good example. It includes all the spinal nerve roots in the sacrum.

Spinal Nerve Fibers. Four types of nerve fibers compose the spinal nerves:

- Motor fibers, which originate in the ventral (anterior) horn of the spinal cord, with efferent fibers relaying motor impulses from the CNS to peripheral skeletal muscles
- Sensory fibers, which originate in the dorsal (posterior) horn of the spinal cord, with afferent fibers relaying sensory impulses from organs and muscles to the CNS

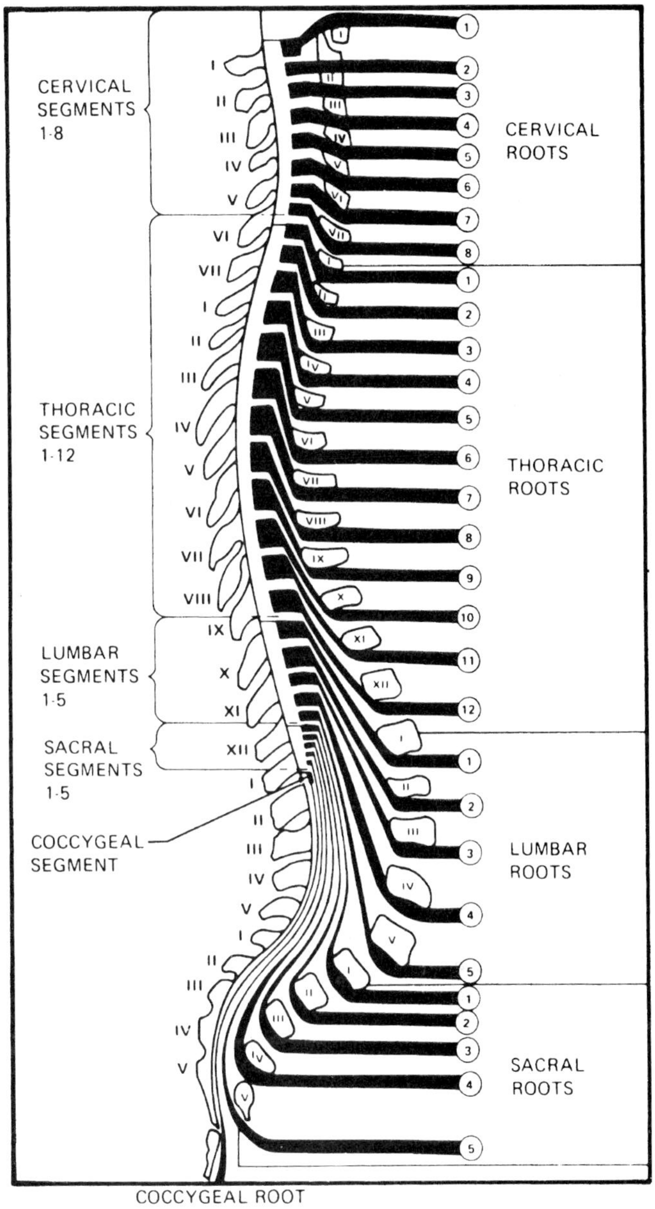

Figure 29-18. Spinal nerve roots and their attachment to the spinal cord.

- Meningeal fibers, which transmit sensory and vasomotor innervation to the spinal meninges
- Autonomic fibers, which are considered separately further on

Dermatomes. Each spinal nerve's dorsal root innervates a specific portion of skin. These skin regions are called *dermatomes* (**Fig. 29-19**). They are clinically important in identifying areas of spinal cord injury.

Plexuses. The spinal nerves interweave in three areas called the cervical, brachial, and lumbosacral plexuses (**Fig. 29-20**).

- The cervical plexus involves spinal nerves C1 to C4. It sends motor impulses to neck muscles and the diaphragm and receives sensory impulses from the neck and head.
- The brachial plexus is composed of spinal nerves C4 to C8 and T1. It innervates the arms.
- The lumbosacral plexus is formed by spinal nerves L1 to L5 and S1 to S3. It innervates the legs.

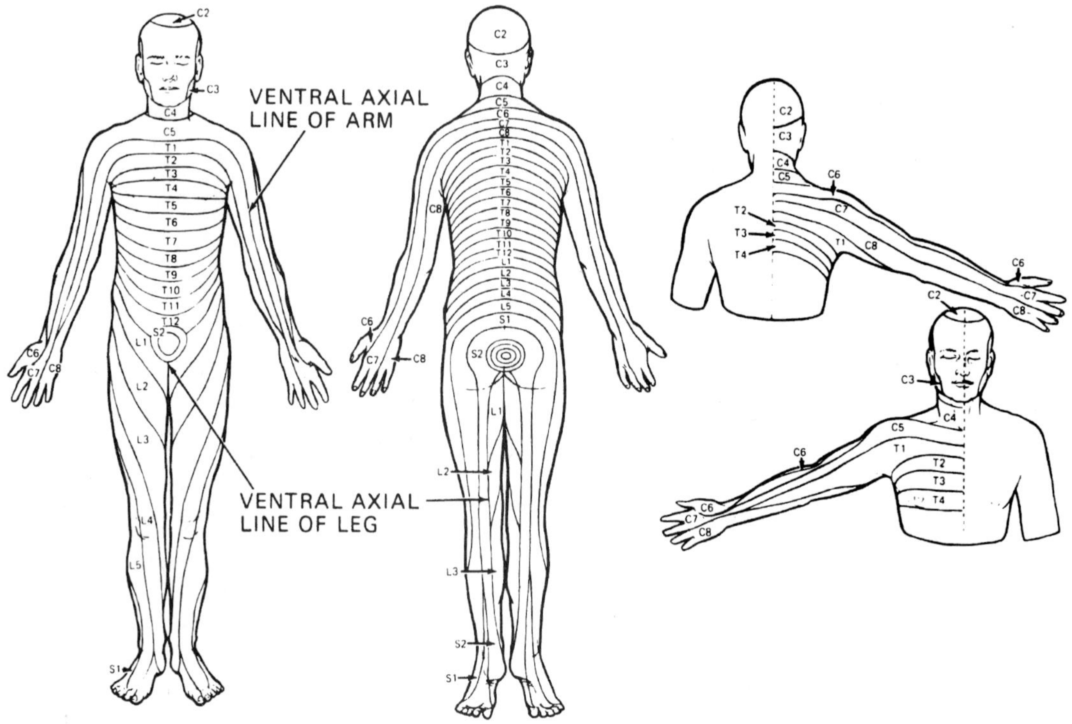

Figure 29-19. Dermatomes.

Cranial Nerves. Twelve pairs of cranial nerves complete the peripheral nervous system. Three pairs of cranial nerves are totally sensory, five pairs are totally motor, and four pairs are combined sensorimotor. The origins of the nerves are seen in **Fig. 29-21**. By convention, the cranial nerves are numbered by roman numerals as well as named.

The cranial nerves are summarized in **Table 29-2**. *The following mnemonic may help to keep them in order: On Old Olympus' Towering Tops, A Finn and German Viewed Some Hops.*

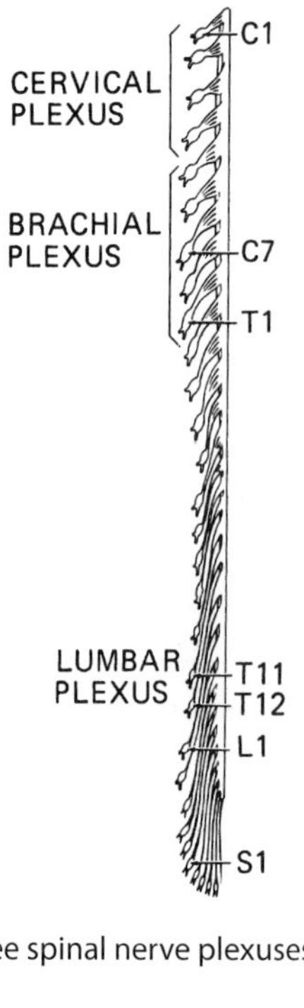

Figure 29-20. The three spinal nerve plexuses.

QUICK TIP! There will almost certainly be at least one question on the cranial nerves. If you have trouble remembering them, consider using the mnemonic and write them down on the scratch sheet of paper before your exam starts.

The Autonomic Nervous System

The sympathetic nervous system and the parasympathetic nervous system together form the autonomic nervous system.

Sympathetic Nervous System. The **sympathetic nervous system** releases norepinephrine, which stimulates and prepares the body for "fight, fright, or flight." *Norepinephrine* and *epinephrine* are categorized as adrenergic chemicals (hormones). Fibers originating in the thoracic and lumbar areas form the peripheral sympathetic nervous system division. The sympathetic nervous system has a chain of ganglia situated on both sides of the vertebrae (**Fig. 29-22**). Nerve fibers between the spinal cord and the ganglia are termed preganglionic fibers (or axons). The nerve fibers between the ganglia and visceral end organ are called postganglionic fibers (or axons). The norepinephrine that is released to maintain body functions is not easily or rapidly neutralized, so the effect is sustained for a period of time.

Parasympathetic Nervous System. The **parasympathetic nervous system** releases acetylcholine, which is categorized as a cholinergic chemical (hormone). The parasympathetic system is an antagonist to the sympathetic system and mediates or slows body responses when the "fight, fright, or flight" situation no longer exists. Fibers originating in the cranial and sacral areas form the peripheral parasympathetic nervous system division (**Fig. 29-23**). The parasympathetic nervous system does not have a chain of ganglia next to the vertebral column.

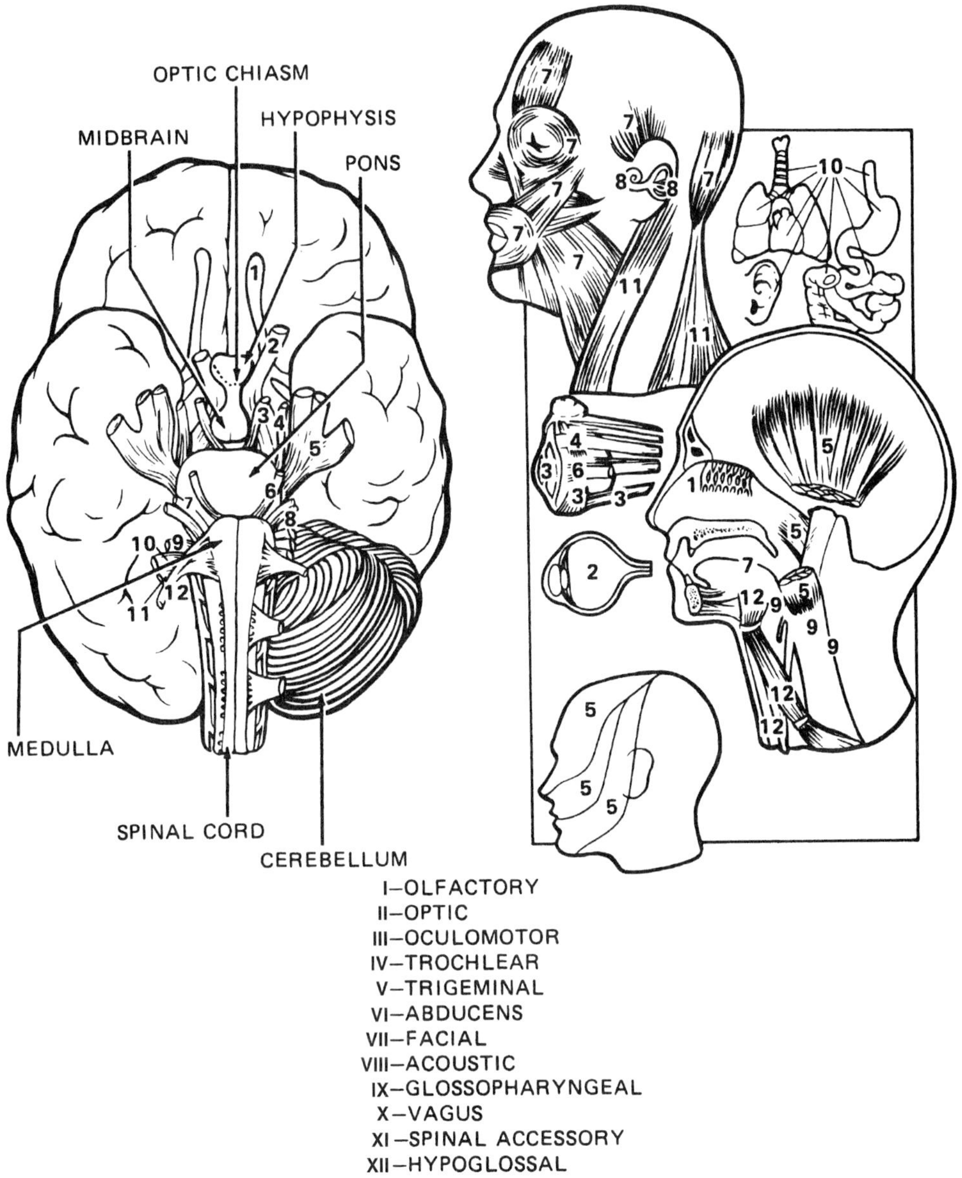

Figure 29-21. Origins of the cranial nerves.

TABLE 29-2. SUMMARY OF CRANIAL NERVES

Number	*Name*	*Major Functions*
I	Olfactory	Sense of smell
II	Optic	Central and peripheral vision
III	Oculomotor	Eye movement; elevation of upper eyelid; pupil constriction
IV	Trochlear	Downward and inward eye movement
V	Trigeminal	Touch, pain, temperature; jaw and eye muscle proprioception; mastication
VI	Abducens	Abduction of the eye
VII	Facial	Close eyelid, muscles of facial expression; secretion by glands of mouth and eyes; taste (anterior two-thirds of tongue)
VIII	Acoustic Vestibular branch Cochlear branch	Equilibrium Hearing
IX	Glossopharyngeal	Movement of pharyngeal muscles; secretion by parotid glands; pharyngeal and posterior tongue sensation
X	Vagus	Pharyngeal and laryngeal movement; visceral activities; pharyngeal and laryngeal sensation; taste
XI	Spinal accessory	Pharyngeal, sternocleidomastoid, and trapezius movement
XII	Hypoglossal	Tongue movement

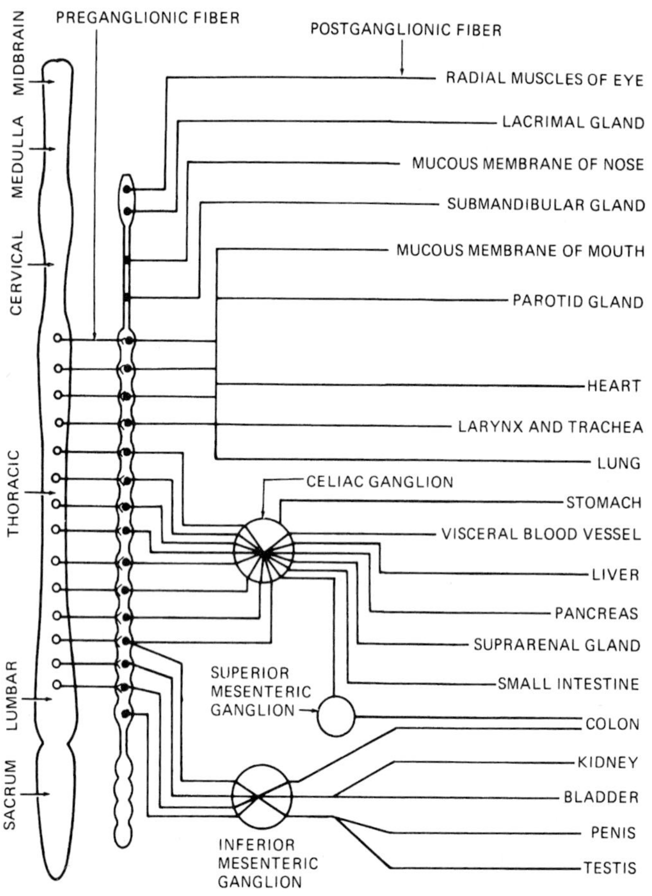

Figure 29-22. Ganglia of the sympathetic nervous system.

Postganglionic fibers (or axons) are therefore short. The chemical released by the parasympathetic system, acetylcholine, is rapidly neutralized by cholinesterase. Because of this, the parasympathetic effect is brief and must be renewed regularly to counter the sympathetic stimulation. **Atropine** is an example of a parasympathetic inhibitor, which is why it increases the heart rate. It allows for more sympathetic nervous system stimulation by parasympatholytic activity.

Neural Cell Depolarization and Repolarization

Depolarization and repolarization of the nerve cell follow the same principles as depolarization and repolarization of the cardiac cell.

Depolarization. The neuron in a resting state (resting membrane potential [RMP]) is positively charged outside the cell membrane and negatively charged on the inner surface of the cell membrane. When the cell is stimulated, sodium rapidly enters the cell and potassium leaves the cell. This produces a positive ionic charge at the entry site and decreases the RMP. This positive ionic charge is transmitted along the length of the neuron and is termed a wave of depolarization.

Repolarization. As soon as potassium reenters the cell and sodium leaves it, the resting state of the cell is reestablished. This is called **repolarization**. A specific mechanism exists to force the sodium ions that entered the cell's cytoplasm back into the extracellular fluid. This is termed the *sodium pump*. Without the sodium pump, ion homeostasis could not be preserved. At the same time, a potassium pump exists to maintain potassium ion homeostasis by forcing potassium ions back into the cell.

An **action potential** occurs when an ionic charge on one side of the membrane is different from an ionic charge on the other. **Depolarization** occurs when a stimulus is strong enough (threshold) to alter the cell membrane's permeability to sodium, allowing a change in the ionic charge. *(Sodium ions enter and potassium ions leave the cell's interior.)* Once an action potential exists and a stimulus of threshold-level magnitude occurs, the neuron totally depolarizes, following the **all-or-none principle.** It depolarizes in its entirety or else it does not depolarize at all. As with the cardiac cell, the neuron has a ***complete** refractory period* during which it is repolarizing and cannot be stimulated. Also like the cardiac cell, the neuron has a ***relative** refractory period.* During this period, it can be stimulated (or excited), but only when the stimulus is at a threshold level.

Two terms are important in relation to action potentials. "Summation" refers to repetitive, accumulated discharges that eventually reach threshold levels (much like placing building blocks one on top of the other until the top is reached). Action potential occurs in summation. "Facilitation" is an increase in every subsequent neuronal stimulus even though the stimulus remains below threshold levels. No action potential occurs in facilitation. The rapid velocity at which the impulse is conducted is due in part to the neuron's structure (**Fig. 29-24**) and the size of the nerve fiber.

Chemical Synapses

A *synapse* is a point of junction but not of contact between one neuron and another, a muscle cell, or a gland cell. Synapses differ in shape and size but function similarly in transmitting impulses.

The neuron's axon enlarges at its end, forming a synaptic knob. This knob may be called a terminal button or a presynaptic terminal (**Fig. 29-25**). The synaptic knob contains vesicles filled with specific neurotransmitter chemicals. When the axonal knob is stimulated, these chemicals are released. The presynaptic terminal is separated from the postsynaptic side by a minute space termed the synaptic cleft. The postsynaptic membrane is slightly thicker at the synaptic cleft than elsewhere and is termed the subsynaptic membrane. The extra thickness is thought to be due to an increased number of receptor sites for the neurotransmitter.

Neurotransmitters

Acetylcholine. Acetylcholine is a cholinergic neurotransmitter chemical found in the vesicles of neuromuscular junctions and in the parasympathetic system and is considered the primary neurotransmitter of the peripheral nervous system. It acts on the postsynaptic membrane briefly before it is neutralized by the enzyme acetylcholinesterase (ACH). ACH is found in abundance in skeletal muscles and blood, so it very rapidly breaks down acetylcholine into acetic acid and choline. This rapid degradation of acetylcholine ensures that only one action potential occurs at a time at the receptor sites on the postsynaptic membrane. The end products (acetic acid and choline) are resynthesized in the synaptic vesicles for use again.

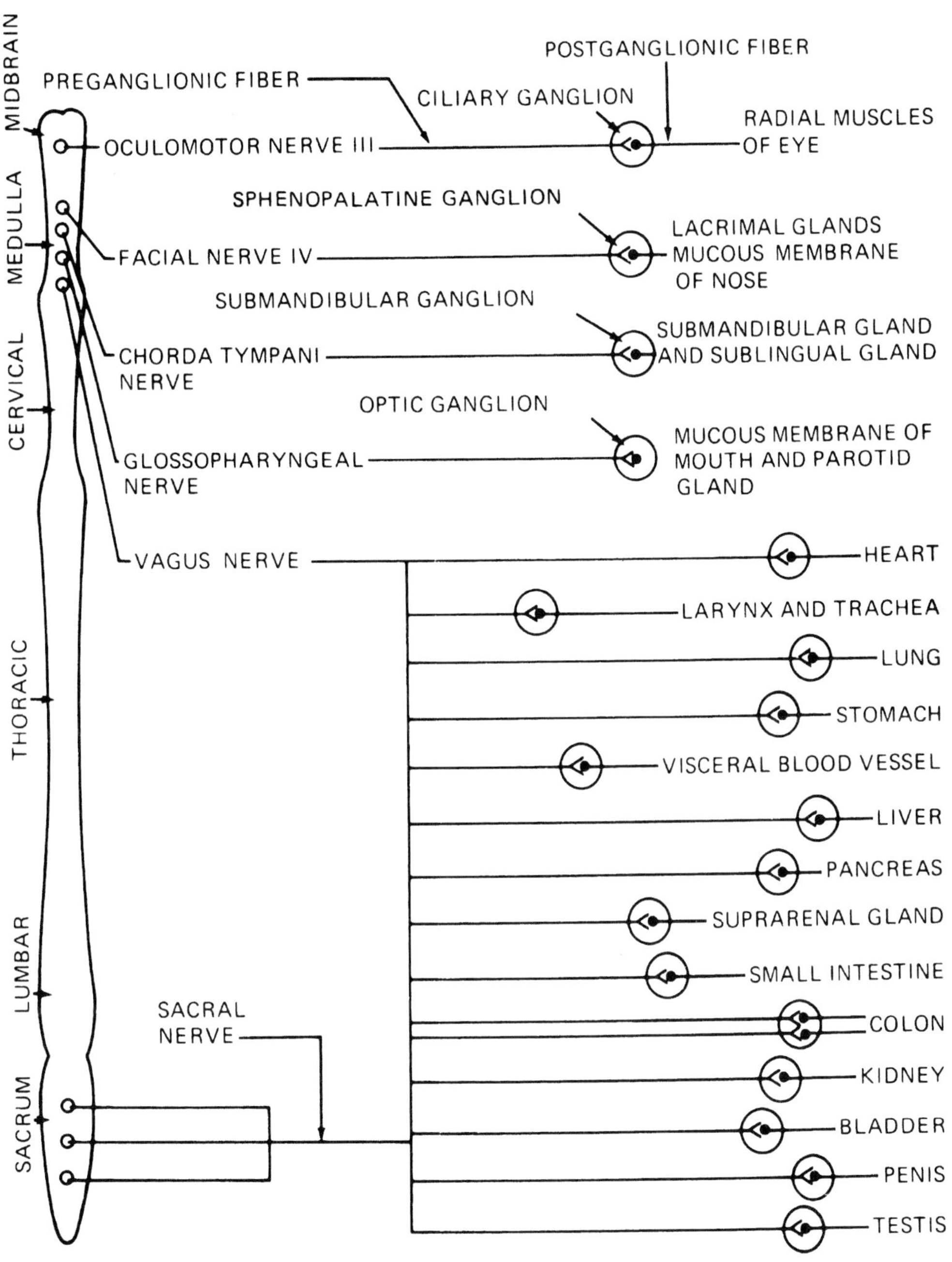

Figure 29-23. Ganglionic fibers of the parasympathetic nervous system.

The result of the release of acetylcholine at many peripheral synapses is muscular contraction. The amount of acetylcholine released is determined in part by the diffusion of calcium ions into the presynaptic terminal. Calcium ions are necessary for depolarization at other peripheral synapses, so it is assumed that calcium plays a similar role at all chemical synapses.

Monoamines. The monoamines that have been identified as neurotransmitters in the CNS include the catecholamines; dopamine, norepinephrine, and epinephrine and the indolamine serotonin. The activity of the monoamine neurotransmitters in the synaptic cleft is limited by their reuptake into the presynaptic ending, where they are recycled into vesicles for future release.

Dopamine. Dopamine is a precursor of epinephrine and norepinephrine. Dopamine acts as an inhibitory chemical transmitter and is among the most important chemicals involved in basal ganglionic functions. It may play a role in eating, drinking, and sexual behavior.

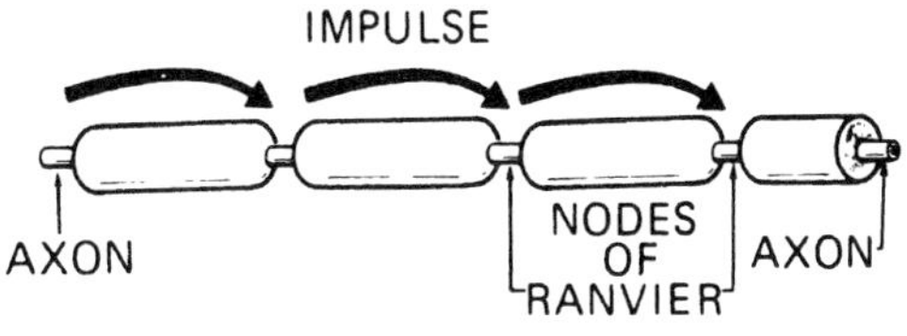

Figure 29-24. Nodes of Ranvier providing saltatory conduction.

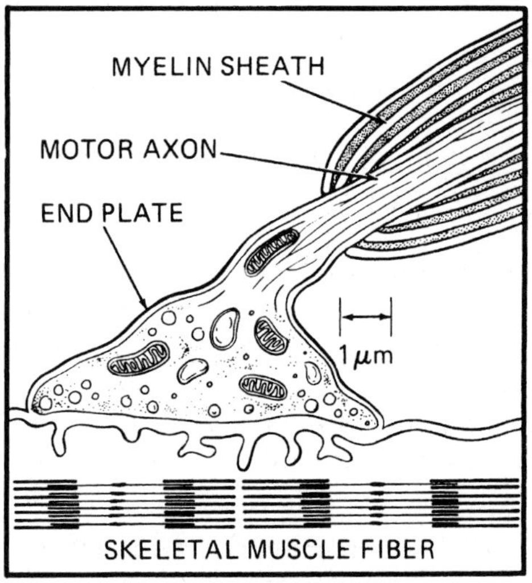

Figure 29-25. Chemical synapse.

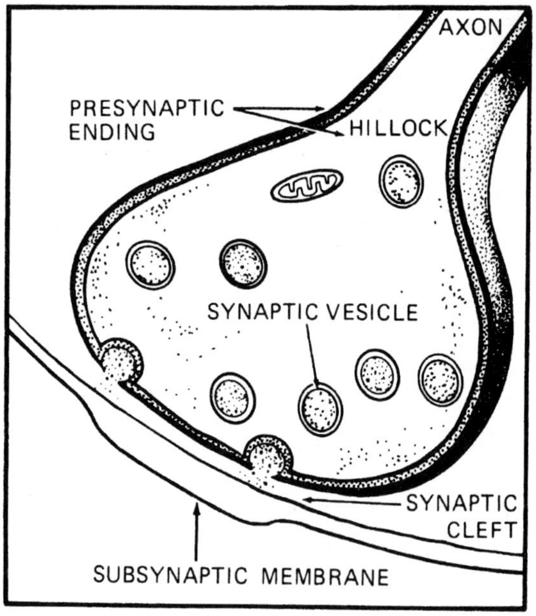

Figure 29-26. Neuromuscular junction or neuromuscular endplate.

KEY CLINICAL CONCEPT

Dopamine is decreased in the brains of patients with Parkinson's Disease. Treatment consists of medications to increase dopamine concentration. If this appears on the exam, it is unrelated to anything regarding a dopamine infusion.

Epinephrine and Norepinephrine. Epinephrine and norepinephrine are found in adrenergic fibers of the sympathetic nervous system.

Like dopamine, norepinephrine has been found to have inhibitory influences on postsynaptic neurons. Little is known of the action of epinephrine as a central neurotransmitter. Within the sympathetic nervous system, epinephrine and norepinephrine are found in adrenergic fibers. They are responsible for exerting a generalized "fight, flight, or fright" response.

Serotonin. Serotonin is also a monoamine chemical. It is an inhibitory transmitter and is linked to slow-wave sleep patterns. Although it has been suggested that serotonin plays a physiologic role in sleep, psychotic states, pain transmission, and response to hallucinogenic drugs, little is known about its specific functions.

Gamma-Aminobutyric Acid (GABA). GABA is a neutral amino acid that has an inhibitory effect on synaptic function. It functions to reduce neuronal excitability by inhibiting nerve transmission.

Reflexes

A reflex is a stereotypical reaction of the CNS to specific sensory stimuli. There are two types of reflexes: monosynaptic and polysynaptic.

Monosynaptic Reflex Arc

This constitutes the simplest reflex in the body and is depicted in **Fig. 29-27**. Inside every group of muscles is a structure called a muscle spindle, which is made up of small fibers bound together by afferent sensory fibers (**Fig. 29-28**). As a muscle spindle is stretched, an action potential develops and a sensory

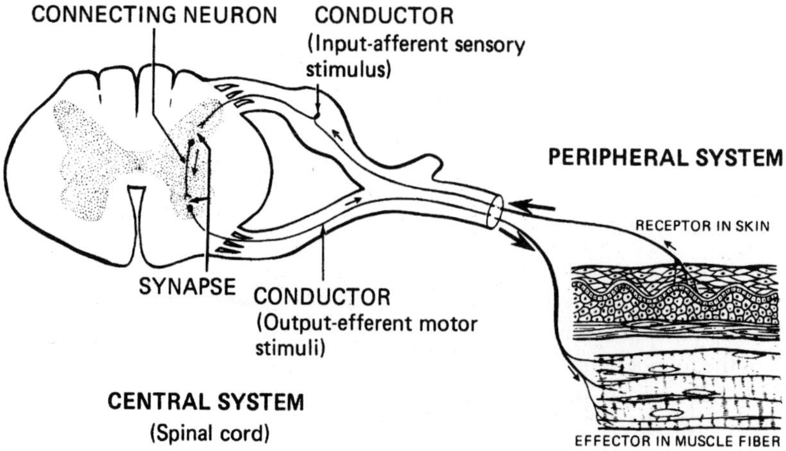

Figure 29-27. Monosynaptic reflex arc.

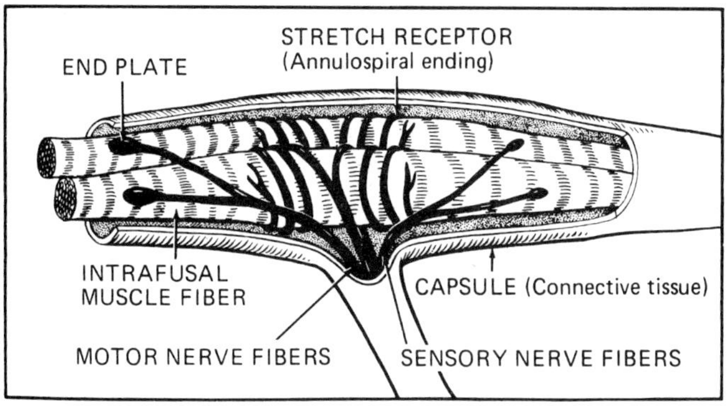

Figure 29-28. Muscle spindle.

impulse travels to the dorsal root ganglion. From the ganglion, the impulse enters the spinal cord. In the gray matter (unmyelinated) of the spinal cord, the impulse synapses with interneurons in the anterior portion of the cord. These interneurons have efferent (motor) fibers that leave the spinal cord through the anterior (ventral) root. The efferent fibers carry an impulse back to the original muscle. The muscle contracts upon receiving this impulse. The muscle stretch reflex (knee jerk) is the one most commonly tested.

Polysynaptic Reflex Arcs. The withdrawal reflex is a common example of the polysynaptic reflex (**Fig. 29-29**). Afferent nerve fibers in the peripheral muscles are excited producing an impulse. This impulse enters the spinal cord via a dorsal root ganglion. This excited neuron will synapse with appropriate interneurons within the gray matter of the spinal cord.

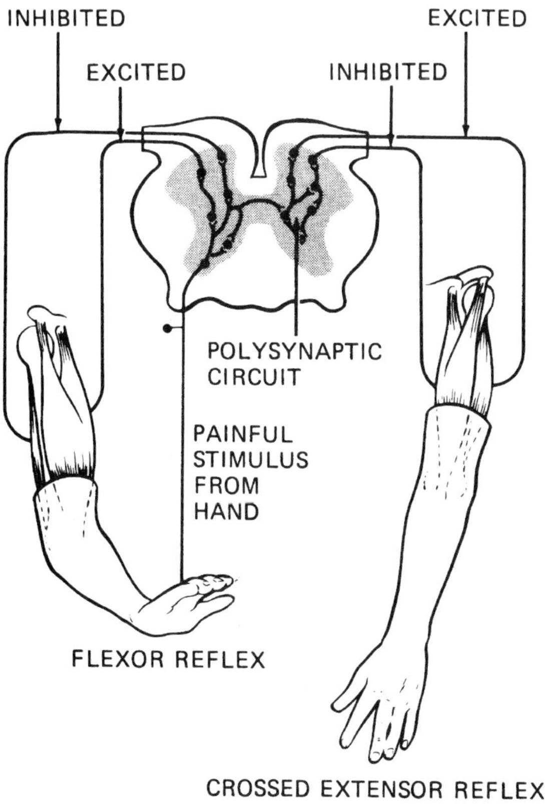

Figure 29-29. Polysynaptic reflex arc.

The interneurons in the anterior (ventral) horn emerge from the spinal cord through efferent (motor) fibers. These fibers transmit the motor impulse to the original muscle that produced the sensory impulse. The muscle then contracts.

Metabolism in the Brain

Both white matter (myelinated) and gray matter (unmyelinated) have the same metabolic needs.

The cerebral need for oxygen does not decrease in a resting state. Even though it weighs only about 3 lb (2% of the body weight), brain tissue requires about 20% of the body's oxygen supply. *The brain needs a constant supply of oxygen and is unable to store oxygen for future use.* The energy necessary for the brain's metabolic functions is obtained from the oxidation of glucose. All oxidative reactions require oxygen. Hypoxia may occur without irreversible anoxic injury to brain cells. *If the anoxic state lasts 4 minutes or more at normal body temperature, cerebral neurons are destroyed.* Once destroyed, cerebral neurons cannot regenerate. The area of the brain most sensitive to hypoxia is the telencephalon, particularly the hippocampus, which is most likely to be damaged by small amounts of decreased oxygen. However, the entire cerebral cortex is very sensitive to decreases in oxygen (Fig. 29-7).

The brainstem is the area most resistant to hypoxic damage. If hypoxia occurs in this area beyond the 4- to 5-minute limit, irreversible coma or a persistent vegetative state usually develops.

Nutritional Needs

The extensive, continuous activity of the brain results in very high metabolic energy needs. Glucose, a carbohydrate, is the main source of energy (adenosine triphosphate, or ATP) for cellular activity. Glucose and oxygen are essential for reestablishing electrochemical gradients for impulse transmission, for the synthesis of neurotransmitters, and for maintaining cellular integrity. *If the cerebral glucose level is less than 70 mg/100 mL, confusion results. With a glucose level of less than 20 mg/100 mL, coma develops, followed by death if there is no treatment.* Whereas hypoglycemia causes confusion, coma, and death, *hyperglycemia does not appear to have a direct influence on nervous system functions.* Certain vitamins are essential in adequate amounts to ensure normal CNS functions.

Vitamin B_1 (thiamine) is important in the Krebs cycle of energy production. Insufficient B_1, common in alcoholics, causes the Wernicke–Korsakoff syndrome, which in late stages causes cerebellar degeneration.

The function of vitamin B_{12} is not understood. However, insufficient B_{12} results in a gradual degeneration of the brain, optic nerves, spinal cord (especially posterior and lateral columns), and dorsal root entry zone of the peripheral nerves. Degeneration often starts with the spinal cord. Pernicious anemia is the dominant systemic disease of vitamin B_{12} deficiency however, it is also present in alcoholism and other malnutritional states.

Pyridoxine is a coenzyme that participates in many enzymatic reactions in the CNS. Pyridoxine deficiencies produce polyneuropathies, seborrheic dermatitis, glossitis, and conjunctivitis.

Nicotinic acid is needed for synthesis of coenzymes. Insufficient nicotinic acid results in altered mentation, leading to coma, extrapyramidal rigidity, and tremors of the extremities.

This form of encephalopathy seems to be becoming nonexistent in the United States.

Circulatory Needs

The brain needs a more continuous supply of oxygenated blood, even during sleep, than any other organ because the brain's needs are never decreased. The cerebral blood flow (CBF) is the **cerebral perfusion pressure (CPP)** divided by cerebrovascular resistance, the difference between mean arterial (systemic) pressure (MAP) and ICP **(CPP = MAP – ICP)**. The size of the cerebrovascular system, activity, disease, fever, injury, and other factors determine the actual amount of blood needed at any given time.

Autoregulation. Hypercapnia ($Paco_2$ > 45 mm Hg) and to a lesser extent hypoxia (Pao_2 < 60 mm Hg) will cause an arteriolar dilatation of the cerebral arteries, thus increasing the amount of blood flowing into the brain regardless of the actual amount needed. This may cause an increase in ICP that the healthy brain can accommodate but that an injured or diseased brain may not be able to accommodate. The brain has its own autoregulatory mechanism, which functions mainly by increasing (constricting arteries) resistance to blood flow or by decreasing (dilatation of arteries) resistance to blood flow, thus altering the diameter of the vessels. **Autoregulation** maintains constant blood flow over a range of perfusion pressures. *The limits of autoregulation are generally thought to be a MAP between 50 and 150 mm Hg.* This system works well until the ICP increases beyond a certain unknown point, when compensatory mechanisms fail. Hypocapnia ($Paco_2$ < 35 mm Hg) causes arteriolar constriction of the cerebral arteries and may be harmful to the brain due to a decrease in delivery of oxygenated blood. Balancing the $Paco_2$ is imperative in optimizing CBF.

Increases in ICP will result in a decrease in blood perfusion to the brain because of compression of the arteries, veins, and brain mass.

QUICK TIP! In the setting of emergently high ICP, bagging and hyperventilating the patient to induce hypocapnia, can cause arteriolar vasoconstriction and induce ICP reduction. This should only be used in the initial, acute period and not as a sustained treatment.

Blood–Brain Barrier

A barrier is known to exist between the blood and brain, which controls the diffusion of substances from the blood into the extracellular fluid or CSF of the brain. The location and structure of this barrier is thought to be related to the "tight junctions" of cerebral endothelial cells. The permeability of cerebral capillaries and the choroid plexus controls the movement of specific substances.

Water, oxygen, glucose, and carbon dioxide move quickly through the blood–brain barrier. Other substances either move slowly or not at all across the barrier. This control determines the level of metabolism, ionic composition, and homeostasis of cerebral tissue.

In addition to a blood–brain barrier, there is a blood–CSF barrier that functions like the blood–brain barrier in controlling the composition of the CSF. This is a vitally important function, because substances in the CSF are rapidly absorbed into the interstitial brain fluid.

KEY CONTENT CHECKLIST

- ❒ **Epidural** hematomas are usually associated with **arterial** bleeding and **subdural** hematomas are associated with **venous** bleeding.
- ❒ Obstruction of CSF will lead to hydrocephalus and can increase intracranial pressure. External ventricular drainage is often required to drain excess CSF.
- ❒ The following mnemonic may help to keep the cranial nerves in order: "On Old Olympus' Towering Tops, A Finn and German Viewed Some Hops." Consider writing these down prior to the exam.
- ❒ Dopamine is decreased in the brains of patients with Parkinson disease. Treatment consists of medications to increase dopamine concentration (unrelated to situations involving a dopamine infusion).
- ❒ The CBF is the **CPP** divided by cerebrovascular resistance, the difference between MAP and ICP (**CPP = MAP – ICP**).
- ❒ In the setting of emergently high ICP, bagging and hyperventilating the patient to induce hypocapnia, can cause arteriolar vasoconstriction and induce ICP reduction. This should only be used in the initial, acute period and not as a sustained treatment.
- ❒ The **sympathetic** nervous system releases norepinephrine, which stimulates and prepares the body for "fight, fright, or flight." The **parasympathetic** system is an antagonist to the sympathetic system and mediates or slows body responses when the "fight, fright, or flight" situation no longer exists. The parasympathetic system can also be called the "rest and digest" side of the nervous system.
- ❒ Repolarization happens as potassium reenters the call and sodium leaves it, reestablishing the resting state of the cell. An action potential occurs when an ionic charge on one side of the membrane is different from an ionic charge on the other. Depolarization occurs when a stimulus is strong enough (threshold) to alter the cell membrane's permeability to sodium, allowing a change in the ionic charge.

Review Questions:

1. Which cerebral component is responsible for reabsorbing cerebrospinal fluid (CSF)?

a. Lateral ventricle
b. Dura mater
c. Arachnoid villi
d. Subarachnoid cisterns

Answer: C. Rationale: After circulating (in the subarachnoid space) over the entire brain and spinal cord, the CSF is reabsorbed by the arachnoid villi in dural sinuses and by pacchionian bodies found in the superior sagittal sinus.

2. A patient in your unit has suffered frontal head injuries from a motor vehicle accident. Which type of impairment may result from injury to the frontal lobe?

a. Loss of sensation
b. Loss of vision
c. Alterations in hearing
d. Alterations in personality

Answer: D. Rationale: The frontal lobe is responsible for voluntary motor function and higher mental functions such as judgment and foresight, affect, personality, inhibition, abstract thinking, and motor speech (dominant hemisphere).

3. **Autoregulation of the cerebral circulatory system is most sensitive to changes in which of the following parameters?**
   a. Mean arterial pressure
   b. Pao_2
   c. pH
   d. Glucose level

Answer: A. Rationale: The brain has its own autoregulatory mechanism, which functions mainly by increasing (constricting arteries) resistance to blood flow or by decreasing (dilatation of arteries) resistance to blood flow, thus altering the diameter of the vessels. Autoregulation maintains constant blood flow over a range of perfusion pressures. The limits of autoregulation are generally thought to be a mean arterial pressure (MAP) between 50 and 150 mm Hg. This system works well until the ICP increases beyond a certain unknown point, when compensatory mechanisms fail.

REFERENCES

American Association of Critical-Care Nurses, AANN, and American Association of Critical-care Nurses. *AACN Protocols for Practice: Monitoring Neuroscience Patients.* Sudbury, MA: Jones and Bartlett; 2009.

American Association of Neuroscience Nursing. *Care of the Patient with Myasthenia Gravis.* Glenview, IL: AANN; 2013.

American Association of Neuroscience Nursing. *Care of the Patient Undergoing Intracranial Pressure Monitoring/External Ventricular Drain or Lumbar Drainage.* Glenview, IL: AANN; 2011.

American Association of Neuroscience Nursing. *Care of the Adult Patient with a Brain Tumor.* Glenview IL: AANN; 2014.

American Association of Neuroscience Nursing. *Nursing Management of Adults with Severe Traumatic Brain Injury.* Glenview, IL: AANN; 2020.

American Association of Neuroscience Nursing. *Care of the Patient with Aneurysmal Subarachnoid Hemorrhage.* Glenview, IL: AANN; 2018.

American Association of Neuroscience Nursing. *Guide to the Care of the Patient with Seizure.* 2nd ed. Glenview, IL: AANN; 2007.

American Association of Neuroscience Nursing. *Care of the Adult Patient with a Brain Tumor.* Glenview, IL: AANN; 2014.

American Association of Neuroscience Nursing. *Cervical Spine Surgery: A Guide to Preoperative and Postoperative Patient Care.* Glenview, IL: AANN; 2014.

American Association of Neuroscience Nursing. *Evidence-Based Strategies for Care of the Patient with Movement Disorders and Deep Brain Stimulation.* Glenview, IL: AANN; 2019.

American College of Surgeons. *Best Practice Guidelines: Spine Injury 2022.* [online] https://www.facs.org/media/k45gikqv/spine_injury_guidelines.pdf.

Arbour R. Intracranial hypertension: monitoring and nursing assessment. *Crit Care Nurse.* 2004;24:19–32.

Bader MK, Stutzman SE, Palmer S, et al. The Adam Williams Initiative: collaborating with community resources to improve care for traumatic brain injury. *Crit Care Nurse.* 2014;34(6):39–47.

Bader MK. Gizmos and gadgets for the neuroscience intensive care unit. *J Neurosci Nurs.* 2006;38:248–260.

Bader MK, Arbour R, Palmer S. Refractory increased intracranial pressure in severe traumatic brain injury: barbiturate coma and bispectral index monitoring. *AACN Clin Issues.* 2005;16:526–541.

Bader MK, Littlejohns LR., Olson, DM. *AANN Core Curriculum for Neuroscience Nursing.* 6th ed. Philadelphia, PA: Saunders; 2016.

Bader MK, Littlejohns LR, March K. Brain tissue oxygen monitoring in severe brain injury: II. Implications for critical care teams and case study. *Crit Care Nurse.* 2003;23(4):29–38, 40–42, 44.

Brophy GM, Bell R, Claassen J, et al; Neurocritical Care Society Status Epilepticus Guideline Writing Committee. Guidelines for the evaluation and management of status epilepticus. *Neurocrit Care.* 2012;17(1):3–23. doi: org/10.1007/s12028-012-9695-z.

Carney N, Totten AM, O'Reilly C, et al. Guidelines for the Management of Severe Traumatic Brain Injury, 4 ed. *Neurosurgery.* 2017;80(1):6–15.

Censullo JL, Sebastian S. Pentobarbital sodium coma for refractory intracranial hypertension. *J Neurosci Nurs.* 2003;35:252–262.

Connolly ES, Rabinstein AA, Carhuapoma JR et al. *Guidelines for the Management of Aneurysmal Subarachnoid Hemorrhage.* [online] https://www.ahajournals.org/doi/10.1161/str.0b013e3182587839. Accessed 27 May 27, 2022.

Cook AM, Morgan Jones G, Hawryluk G, et al. Guidelines for the acute treatment of cerebral edema in neurocritical care patients. *Neurocrit Care.* 2020;32(3):647–666. doi: org/10.1007/s12028-020-00959-7.

Fehlings MG, Tetreault LA, Wilson JR, et al. A clinical practice guideline for the management of acute spinal cord injury: introduction, rationale, and scope. *Global Spine J.* 2017;7(3 Suppl):84S–94S. doi: org/10.1177/2192568217703387.

Farahvar A, Gerber LM, Chiu YL, Carney N, Hartl R, Ghajar J. Increased mortality in patients with severe traumatic brain injury treated without intracranial pressure monitoring. *J Neurosurg.* 2012;117(4):729–734.

Fisher RS, Cross JH, French JA, et al. Operational classification of seizure types by the International League Against Epilepsy: position paper of the ILAE Commission for Classification and Terminology. *Epilepsia.* 2017 Apr;58(4):522–530. doi: 10.1111/epi.13670. Epub 2017 Mar 8.

Fisher RS. The new classification of seizures by the International League Against Epilepsy 2017. *Curr Neurol Neurosci Rep.* 2017 Jun;17(6):48. doi: 10.1007/s11910-017-0758-6.

Faul M, Coronado V. Epidemiology of traumatic brain injury. In: Grafman J, Salazar AS, eds. *Handbook of Clinical Neurology.* Vol 127. Waltham, MA: Elsevier BV; 2015:3–13.

Frizzell JP. Acute stroke: pathophysiology, diagnosis and treatment. *AACN Clin Issues.* 2005;16:421–440.

Glauser T, Shinnar S, Gloss D, et al. Evidence-based guideline: treatment of convulsive status epilepticus in children and adults: report of the Guideline Committee of the American Epilepsy Society. *Epilepsy Curr.* 2016;16(1):48–61. doi: org/10.5698/1535-7597-16.1.48.

Greenberg SM, Ziai WC, Codronnier C, et al. *2022 Guideline for the Management of Patients with Spontaneous Intracerebral Hemorrhage: A Guideline From the American Heart Association/American Stroke Association.* [online] https://www.ahajournals.org/doi/10.1161/STR.0000000000000407. Accessed May 27, 2022.

Hickey JV, Strayer AL. *The Clinical Practice of Neurological and Neurosurgical Nursing.* 8th ed. Philadelphia, PA: Lippincott Williams & Wilkins; 2019.

Kamel H, Navi BB, Nakagawa K, Hemphill JCIII, Ko NU. Hypertonic saline versus mannitol for the treatment of elevated intracranial pressure: a meta-analysis of randomized clinical trials. *Crit Care Med.* 2011;39(3):554–559.

Kirkness CJ. Cerebral blood flow monitoring in clinical practice. *AACN Clin Issues.* 2005;16:476–487.

Kleindorfer DO, Towfighi A, Chaturvedi S, et al. *2021 Guideline for the Prevention of Stroke in Patients with Stroke and Transient Ischemic Attack: A Guideline From the American Heart Association/American Stroke Association.* [online] https://www.ahajournals.org/doi/10.1161/STR.0000000000000375. Accessed May 27, 2022.

Krumholz A, Wiebe S, Gronseth GS, et al. The ILAE classification of seizures and evidence-based guideline: management of an unprovoked first seizure in adult. Report of the Guideline Development Subcommittee of the American Academy of Neurology and the American Epilepsy Society. *Neurology.* Apr 2015;84(16):1705–1713. doi:10.1212/WNL.0000000000001487.

Luke AM. Critical care management of the patient with elevated intracranial pressure. *Crit Care Alert.* 2009;9: 44–47.

March K. Intracranial pressure monitoring: why monitor? *AACN Clin Issues.* 2005;16(4):456–475. McGraw Hill's Access Medicine. *Critical Care Neurology.* http://www.accessmedicine.com/content.aspx?aID=86945&searchStr=neurology 86945. Accessed August 22, 2009.

Medline Plus. *ICP Monitoring*. http://www.nlm.nih.gov/medlineplus/ency/article/003411.htm. Accessed August 22, 2009.

Narayanaswami P, Sanders DB, Wolfe G, et al. International Consensus Guidance for Management of Myasthenia Gravis 2020 Update. *Neurology*. 2021 Jan;96(3):114–122. doi: 10.1212/WNL.0000000000011124.

Oertel M, Kelly D, Lee J, et al. Efficacy of hyperventilation, blood pressure elevation, and metabolic suppression therapy in controlling intracranial pressure after head injury. *J Neurosurg*. 2002;97:1045–1053.

Powers WJ, Alejandro AR, Ackerson T, et al. *Guidelines for the Early Management of Patients with Acute Ischemic Stroke: 2019 Update to the 2018 Guidelines for the Early Management of Acute Ischemic Stroke: A Guideline for Healthcare Professionals from the American Heart Association/American Stroke Association.* [online] https://www.ahajournals.org/doi/10.1161/STR.0000000000000211. Accessed May 27, 2022.

Prasad M, Krishnan PR, Sequeira R, Al-Roomi K. Anticonvulsant therapy for status epilepticus. *Cochrane Database Syst Rev*. 2014;9:CD003723. doi: 10.1002/14651858.CD003723.pub3.

Saherwala AA, Bader MK, Stutzman SE, et al. Increasing adherence to brain trauma foundation guidelines for hospital care of patients with traumatic brain injury. *Crit Care Nurse*. 1 Feb 2018;38(1): e11–e20. doi: org/10.4037/ccn2018691.

Spenser SS. Seizures and epilepsy. In: Goldman L, Ausiello D, eds. *Cecil Medicine*. 23rd ed. Philadelphia, PA: Saunders Elsevier; 2007:chap 426.

Stocchetti N, Maas AI, Chieregato A, et al. Hyperventilation in head injury. *Chest*. 2005;127:1812–1827.

Strayer A. Lumbar spine: common pathology and interventions. *J Neurosci Nurs*. 2005;37:181–193.

Summers D, Leonard A, Wentworth D, et al. Comprehensive overview of nursing and interdisciplinary care of the acute ischemic stroke patient: a scientific statement from the 87. *Stroke*. 2009;40:2911–2944.

Venkatasubramanian C, Lopez GA, O'Phelan KH, et al. Emergency Neurological Life Support: Fourth Edition: Updates in the approach to early management of a neurological emergency. *Neurocrit Care*. 2020;32:636–640. doi: org/10.1007/s12028-019-00810-8.

Vincent JL, Berre J. Primer on medical management of severe brain injury. *Crit Care Med*. 2005;33:1392–1399.

Wang Y, Lim L, Levi C, et al. Influence of admission body temperature on stroke mortality. *Stroke*. 2000;31: 404–409.

Wijdicks EF, Varelas PN, Gronseth GS, Greer DM, et al; American Academy of Neurology. Evidence-based guideline update: determining brain death in adults: report of the Quality Standards Subcommittee of the American Academy of Neurology. *Neurology*. 2010;74(23):1911–1918. doi: org/10.1212/WNL.0b013e3181e242a8.

Williams L, Rotich J, Fineber N, et al. Effects of admission hyperglycemia on mortality and costs in acute ischemic stroke. *Neurology*. 2002;59:67–71.

30

Intracranial Pressure

CHAPTER OVERVIEW AND OBJECTIVES

In this chapter, the concepts of intracranial pressure (ICP) are covered. Expect one to three questions on the CCRN exam to refer to the contents of this chapter.

After studying this chapter, you should understand the following:

- Describe the two compensatory mechanisms for increasing ICP.
- Define cerebral perfusion pressure (CPP).
- Differentiate between obstructive and nonobstructive hydrocephalus.
- Identify indications for ICP monitoring.
- Identify the three trend waveforms seen in ICP monitoring.

The concepts of ICP are fundamental to caring for any critical neurology patient. Whether patients have sustained a severe traumatic brain injury, experienced a stroke, brain tumors, hemorrhage, hydrocephalus, or undergone a craniotomy, the pathophysiologic changes may lead to cerebral edema and increased ICP.

30.1 PHYSIOLOGY OF INTRACRANIAL PRESSURE

The volume of the cranial vault is about 80% brain tissue, 10% cerebrospinal fluid (CSF), and 10% intravascular fluid (blood).

The adult cranial vault is nondistensible (it is bone), and the components of the vault are essentially noncompressible. Based on these tenets, a relationship between the vault and its contents is construed. The **Monro–Kellie doctrine** provides the framework for reviewing physiology and treatments for elevated ICP. The hypothesis states that brain tissue, blood volume, and CSF are balanced in a state of dynamic equilibrium. *If an increase occurs in the relative volume of one component, such as CSF, the volume of one or more of the other components must decrease or an elevation in ICP will result.* Within a very narrow range, the contents of the cranial vault can adjust to increases in ICP. When the limits of range and time are exceeded, the ICP rises precipitously.

Compensatory Mechanisms for Increasing Intracranial Pressure

Initial increases in the volume of the cranium are compensated for by two mechanisms: compression of the low-pressure venous system and the displacement of CSF.

1. A decrease in intravascular fluid (blood) occurs by compression of the low-pressure venous system. Intravascular volume is the most alterable of the three components of the cranium (brain tissue, CSF, and blood). There is a specific limit to the extent of compressibility. When this limit is exceeded, ICP rises.
2. Displacement of CSF is the compensatory mechanism for increasing ICP. As the ICP rises, CSF is displaced from the cranial vault into the spinal subarachnoid space. When maximal displacement of CSF has occurred, there is probably an increase in CSF absorption, which aids compensatory mechanisms.

These mechanisms function to keep the ICP constant. They function well when the ICP increases slowly. Even then, the mechanisms will lose their compensatory function at a certain point (variable with the individual). *If the ICP rises rapidly, the compensatory mechanisms cannot function.*

QUICK TIP! As a rule of thumb, when a problem develops slowly, it can be corrected slowly (eg, with ICP increases, electrolyte imbalances, etc). However, if the problem develops rapidly, it must be corrected rapidly.

Intracranial Compliance

The brain's ability to adjust to increases in its contents refers to *compliance*. This is the relationship of change in volume for a given change in pressure. When the brain is compliant (*compliance is high*), increases in the volume of the content do not produce increases in ICP. When a state of noncompliance occurs (*compliance is low*), small increases in the contents of the cranial vault result in a large increase in ICP.

ICP represents the ever-changing relationship between the brain, blood, and CSF inside the cranial vault. *In adults, the normal ICP range is 5 to 15 mm Hg. Increase in ICP greater than 20 mm Hg is considered elevated, and treatment measures are generally initiated. Intracranial hypertension is defined as an ICP greater than 20 mm Hg that persists for 5 minutes or longer.* The control of ICP elevations is an important aspect of the management of severe traumatic brain injury and other intracranial pathologies, since sustained increases in ICP can result in decreases in the delivery of oxygenated blood to the brain as well as herniation and compression of the brain and brainstem.

> **QUICK TIP!** On the exam, increased ICP will appear as obviously high or normal. You will generally not be asked to manage a situation in a question with a "borderline" ICP value.

Cerebral Blood Flow

The brain requires approximately 50 mL/100 g/min of arterial blood flow. Decreases below 18 mL/100 g/min cause ischemia. If such conditions are not corrected, intracellular chaos will ensue, leading to edema and destruction of cells. Cerebral blood flow (CBF) is calculated by measuring the CPP and dividing it by the cerebrovascular resistance. CPP is used as a primary means to approximate the delivery of blood flow. **CPP is the difference between the mean arterial pressure (MAP) and the mean ICP (CPP = MAP – ICP). Normal CPP is 80 mm Hg.** *In severe head injury, the minimal acceptable CPP is 50 to 70 mm Hg.* When CPP declines below this threshold, there is a risk that the cerebrovasculature will vasodilate, leading to worsening of ICP. Optimal or target CPP for patients should be individualized.

Many factors influence CBF besides the CPP. Autoregulation controls CBF through many mechanisms. Globally, **autoregulation** *maintains a constant CBF by vasodilating or vasoconstricting cerebral arteries normally during MAP of 50 to 150 mm Hg despite increases or decreases in blood pressure.* CBF is altered due to metabolic changes in arterial carbon dioxide (CO_2) and oxygen (O_2). When $PaCO_2$ is high, vasodilation occurs, while a low $PaCO_2$ causes vasoconstriction of the cerebral arteries. A PaO_2 below 50 mm Hg leads to vasodilation. In addition, the blood's pH influences CBF, with acidosis causing vasodilation and alkalosis causing vasoconstriction. All of these influences contribute to the delivery of blood to the cranium. By keeping the ICP low, an adequate CBF is promoted. With elevated ICP, the CBF is manipulated in an attempt to reduce blood volume and thus to decrease ICP.

30.2 CAUSES OF INCREASED ICP

A number of pathologies can potentially increase ICP. The volume of the brain can increase with tissue swelling from trauma, stroke, or surgical manipulation; mass lesions such as brain tumors; or bleeding into the parenchyma. Alteration in the amount of CSF inside the cranium is caused by obstruction of CSF pathways, inability to reabsorb CSF, or overproduction of CSF. Increase in the blood content in the cranium occurs as a result of tearing of arteries/veins, creating hematomas, impairment in venous drainage from the brain by compression of neck veins, positioning the head of bed flat, increased intrathoracic or intra-abdominal pressure, and in response to the injury where CBF dramatically rises, creating hyperemia. Other pathologies may lead to increased ICP, such as hypoxic brain injury, electrolyte abnormalities, infectious disease processes, and toxins. When any of these etiologies occur, it is prudent to measure the pressure inside the cranial vault.

Intracranial Mass Lesions

Intracranial mass lesions include intracranial space-occupying lesions such as tumors or abscesses that occur within the cranium or skull, vascular lesions (thrombosis, emboli, etc), and lesions due to trauma. The symptoms of intracranial mass lesions are caused by a combination of increased ICP (headache, vomiting, confusion, coma) and focal neurologic brain tissue damage (hemiparesis, aphasia). The most frequent presenting symptoms are headache, drowsiness, confusion, seizures, hemiparesis, or speech difficulties. The symptoms depend largely on the specific location within the brain.

Intracerebral Hemorrhage. Hemorrhage may result from trauma such as skull fracture, penetrating injury, contrecoup decelerative forces, and systemic diseases such as hypertension, leukemia, and aplastic anemia. Symptoms are dependent on the location of the hemorrhage but include contralateral paralysis, aphasia (if dominant hemisphere) and slurred speech. Other signs and symptoms include nausea, vomiting, dizziness, and headache. A delayed intracerebral hemorrhage may occur hours to days after a closed head injury.

Subarachnoid Hemorrhage. Symptoms usually include abrupt severe headache, vomiting, dizziness, drowsiness, confusion, nuchal rigidity, and hemiparesis or hemiplegia.

Arteriovenous Malformation (AVM). AVMs are defects of the circulatory system that are believed to arise during fetal development. AVMs can occur in various parts of the body and when occurring in the brain are called cerebral AVMs. AVMs occur due to abnormal configurations of the arterial and venous circulation networks in which capillaries are replaced by larger-sized blood vessels called shunts. The result is that the very high pressure in the arteries is no longer dampened by the capillaries, and the veins now experience the same high pressure as the arteries, resulting in intracerebral bleeding. Symptoms of AVM vary according to the location of the malformation and often include headache, weakness, aphasia, vertigo, or seizures. An AVM is typically treated with surgical repair, radiation, or embolization.

Hydrocephalus. Hydrocephalus results from an abnormal accumulation of CSF in the ventricles, or cavities, of the brain. Hydrocephalus can cause increased ICP, seizures, and mental disability.

There are two main classifications of hydrocephalus: communicating and noncommunicating (obstructive). Both forms can be either congenital or acquired.

Communicating hydrocephalus, also known as nonobstructive hydrocephalus, is caused by impaired CSF reabsorption in the absence of any CSF-flow obstruction between the ventricles and subarachnoid space. Several conditions that may result in communicating hydrocephalus include subarachnoid or intraventricular hemorrhage, meningitis, and scarring or fibrosis of the subarachnoid space following infectious, inflammatory, or hemorrhagic events. Normal-pressure hydrocephalus is a form of communicating hydrocephalus, characterized by enlarged cerebral ventricles, with only intermittently elevated CSF pressure. Noncommunicating hydrocephalus, or obstructive hydrocephalus, is caused by a CSF-flow obstruction that prevents CSF from flowing into the subarachnoid space (either due to external compression or intraventricular mass lesions). Noncommunicating hydrocephalus results in increased ICP. Sustained elevated ICP may result in uncal and/or cerebellar herniation, with resulting life-threatening brain stem compression.

The treatment of hydrocephalus is surgical and involves the placement of a ventriculostomy to drain the excess CSF fluid or a shunt to redirect the CSF into other body cavities, where it can be reabsorbed. Most shunts drain the fluid into the peritoneal cavity (ventriculoperitoneal shunt), but alternative sites include the right atrium or pleural cavity (ventriculopleural shunt).

30.3 INTRACRANIAL PRESSURE MONITORING

Indications

The outcome of many neurologic conditions can be mediated by the early recognition of increasing ICP and appropriate intervention. There are six conditions where ICP monitoring may be indicated:

1. Head injuries. A *Glasgow coma scale (GCS) score of 8 or less* accompanied by an abnormal computed tomography (CT) scan indicates significant neurologic impairment. The parameters and scoring for the GCS are shown in **Table 30-1**. With ICP monitoring, intracranial problems can be identified and treatment initiated *before* clinical signs and symptoms develop. Treatment of increasing ICP can be evaluated for effectiveness.

TABLE 30-1. ADVANTAGES AND DISADVANTAGES OF ICP MONITORING SENSORS AND THEIR PLACEMENT

Type of Sensor	*Placement of Sensor*	*Advantage of Sensor*	*Disadvantage of Sensor*
Epidural	Between the skull and dura	Less invasive Fiberoptic sensor does not require recalibration Intact dura	Easily obstructed or diaphragm can rupture; fragile catheter affected by heat or fevers Inaccurate because of dampened waveform Inserted postoperatively Requires special equipment Unable to drain CSF
Subdural	Below the dura and above the subarachnoid space	No penetration of brain Easy placement—often after completion of surgery	Poor waveform, trend data only; increased baseline drift over time Unable to drain CSF Brain tissue may migrate into device with high pressure/unreliable at high pressures
Subarachnoid	In subarachnoid space via a bolt device	No penetration of brain Easy placement	Unable to drain CSF Brain tissue may migrate into device with high pressure/unreliable at high pressures
Intraparenchymal	Placed approximately 1 cm below the subarachnoid space in parenchymal tissue via a bolt device	Easy placement Accurate reading of ICP and waveform Lower risk of infection than intraventricular	Unable to drain CSF Requires separate monitoring system
Intraventricular	Inserted in the frontal horn of the lateral ventricle of the nondominant hemisphere	The "gold standard"—more reflective of whole brain pressure Excellent waveform New catheters with fiberoptics or microsensors allow accuracy with fiberoptic transducer monitor with second port for drainage of CSF Access for: —Determination of volume pressure curve —CSF for drainage and sampling	If ventricles are small, difficulty locating ventricles Requires separate monitoring system and drainage system Increased risk of infection—is the most invasive ICP monitoring technique Penetrates tissue and may cause additional injury, especially with cerebral trauma, edema, or increased ICP Catheter may become occluded by blood clot or tissue debris

QUICK TIP! A commonly cited rule of thumb if, "GCS less than 8, then intubate" due to likelihood of the patient's inability to protect their own airway.

2. Cerebrovascular disorders such as ischemic stroke with significant edema/mass effect, subarachnoid hemorrhage, intraventricular hemorrhage, and intracerebral hemorrhage.
3. Hydrocephalus.
4. Neuroinfectious processes resulting in significant cerebral edema.
5. Brain tumors or postoperative cerebral edema. Certain brain tumors grow slowly, allowing the cranial contents to compensate for the increasing mass volume. After the tumor is removed, cerebral edema may be severe and life threatening. ICP monitoring will allow early intervention.
6. Preoperative and postoperative monitoring.

Measurement Sites

The ICP can be measured in the lateral ventricles in the brain: the cranial subdural or epidural space, brain parenchyma, or brain subarachnoid space.

Several methods are used to measure the ICP:

- Insertion of an intraventricular catheter, which is threaded into one of the lateral ventricles of the brain; the use of a screw or bolt placed in the subarachnoid space. This approach allows monitoring of the ICP as well as drainage of CSF through the catheter, a measure used to decrease elevated ICP.
- The use of a sensor placed into the epidural or subdural space.
- The use of an intraparenchymal fiberoptic catheter. **Figure 30-1** outlines the major types of ICP monitoring.

Monitoring System Components

ICP monitoring systems include a catheter, sensor, or bolt introduced into the cranium, a transducer, and a monitor or recording instrument. An ICP monitoring system is a closed system. Depending on the transducer system, the connection from patient to monitor/recording instrument will vary. The exact placement and the advantages and disadvantages of ICP monitoring devices are tivin shown in Table 30-1.

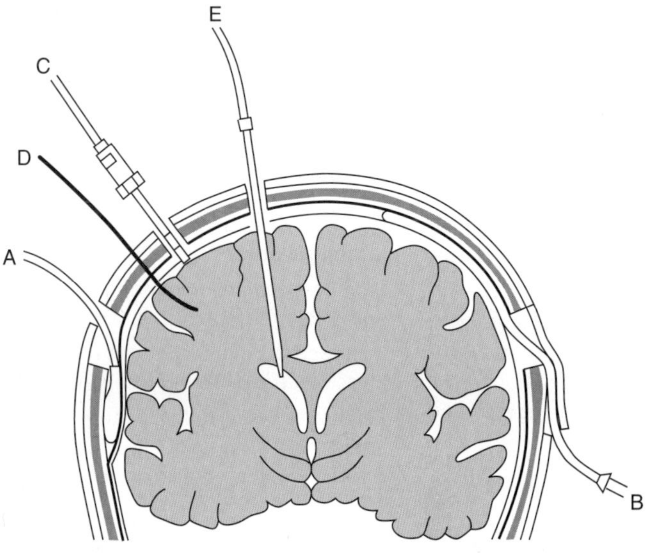

Figure 30-1. Placement of ICP devices. A, epidural; B, subdural; C, subarachnoid; D, intraparenchymal; E, ventricular.

QUICK TIP! The exam will expect you to know the clinical significance of ICP and how to manage it. However, the actual devices and transducer systems for ICP monitoring are not a focus on the exam.

Considerations for Zero Calibrations

See Table 30-1 for the various ICP monitoring and (CSF) drainage methods. When a fluid-filled system is used, the transducer is positioned at the level of the *foramen of Monro.* Zeroing of the system must be done every shift. *Head of bed or patient repositioning requires rechecking the zero reference level.* A fiberoptic system is zeroed upon insertion with the transducer located at the tip of the catheter. The microsensor is zeroed at time of insertion, and the same interface box must be utilized during use. Both the fiberoptic sensor and the microsensor have factory-set calibrations. The air-pouch system rezeros every hour automatically.

Waveforms

Pulse Waveforms. The ICP pulse waveform corresponds to each heartbeat. The waveform arises primarily from pulsations of the intracranial arteries and retrograde venous pulsation. *The ICP pulse waveform consists of three components: P1, P2, and P3.*

The first peak, P1, is the percussion wave and is arterial in origin. The choroid plexus pulsations create a sharp peak, which is consistent in amplitude. The tidal wave forms the P2. The P2 peak varies in size and shape and ends with the dicrotic notch. The P3 wave, also called the dicrotic wave, begins the final tapering of the waveform and is venous in origin. Normally P1, P2, and P3 appear as a descending sawtooth waveform. As the ICP increases, the amplitude of all the waves increases. **When P2 becomes greater in amplitude than P1, this signals a decrease in the adaptive compliance of the brain and possibly impairment of autoregulation.** The loss of compliance represents a situation where the patient is at risk for significant increases in ICP. Patients can still show increases in ICP with normal ICP waveforms.

Occlusion of the monitoring tip causes a flat-line tracing. The flat line may be high or low. As long as a tracing is scalloped in phase with arterial pulsation, the readings are acceptable.

Trend Waveforms. Three trend waveforms (A, B, and C) are seen in ICP monitoring. The shape of the waves is affected by both cardiac pulsations and the respiratory cycle.

"A" waves, or plateau waves, occur when there is a sudden, sustained rise in ICP. "A" waves may be present for 5 to 20 minutes. "A" waves are not normally present and occur if the ICP rises to 50 to 100 mm Hg and is sustained. *"A" waves reflect cerebral ischemia secondary to a decreased arterial blood pressure and intracranial hypertension.*

"B" waves are evident when the ICP is elevated to 20 to 40 mm Hg, but it may rise to approximately 50 mm Hg. These waves are variable in shape and size and usually last for 0.5 to 2 minutes. They can occur with changes in cerebrovascular resistance or pressure and respiratory variations.

"C" waves occur every 4 to 8 minutes and raise ICP up to 20 mm Hg. Their significance has not been established.

QUICK TIP! As a pneumonic to help you remember:

- A waves are "alarming," "abnormal," or "awful."
- B waves are "bad."
- C waves are worth, "consider keeping an eye on it" or "controlled."

With intraventricular monitoring, sharp-peaked waveforms occur. Systolic and diastolic portions of the wave cycle are "dampened."

30.4 IMPLICATIONS AND INTERVENTIONS

ICP monitoring is useful to determine interventions and monitor response.

Cellular hypoxia is most likely to occur if there is sustained increase in ICP. The patient's neurologic status will change in the presence of sustained increased ICP. Signs and symptoms of early neurologic decline occur, including headache, restlessness, agitation, decreasing level of consciousness, **contralateral motor weakness, and ipsilateral pupillary changes**. Changes in vital signs and breathing patterns and the presence of *flexor or extensor posturing represent late signs of neurologic decline*. Identification of the patient with increased ICP allows the team to quickly secure the patient's airway, plan for placing an ICP monitoring system, and implement other interventions geared toward reducing ICP. Evidence-based guidelines for the management of severe traumatic brain injury outline interventions for the management of increased ICP to *keep the ICP less than 20 mm Hg* to minimize secondary injury.

When the patient's neurologic status declines and he or she is unable to protect the airway, endotracheal intubation is performed. The patient is connected to a ventilator and titration of $PaCO_2$ occurs. *Hyperventilation or lowering of the $PaCO_2$ below 35 mm Hg will cause vasoconstriction, which may help to control ICP but may also worsen cerebral hypoxia by reducing the delivery of oxygenated blood.* Therefore, hyperventilation should be employed only with acute neurologic deterioration with adjunctive brain oxygen or cerebral blood flow monitoring to monitor for ischemia. **Bagging and hyperventilating to induce hypocapnia will temporarily induce ICP reduction but should only be used in the initial, acute period and not as a sustained treatment.** Maintaining the $PaCO_2$ at 35 to 40 mm Hg will reduce the chances of cerebral ischemia. It is important to optimize the systemic oxygenation to maintain adequate cerebral oxygenation. ICP monitor placement can help guide primary and secondary interventions aimed at decreasing the ICP to below 20 mm Hg.

Many nursing procedures have an effect on the ICP. Keeping the patient's *head of bed at 30 degrees with the neck at midline provides for optimal venous drainage* from the cranium to the heart. *Turning the patient may increase the ICP. This increase is lessened if the patient is log-rolled with the head in alignment.* In addition, ensure ET tube tape or securement device is not too tight.

In reducing the ICP, it is helpful to optimize the CPP with fluids and vasopressors. *A target CPP of 50 to 70 mm Hg is indicated.* Dehydration and electrolyte imbalances may occur rapidly in conditions that precipitate increased ICP. Careful monitoring of the electrolytes and serum osmolality will allow early interventions to regulate ICP responses.

CSF drainage is used as a primary intervention to reduce ICP when an intraventricular catheter is in place. Infections are a major threat in intraventricular monitoring. The most important step in preventing infection is maintaining a "closed" system. *Sterile technique* is required whenever the system is entered for CSF sampling, and an occlusive dressing is maintained over the catheter insertion site.

The provision of analgesia and sedation will help to decrease agitation and ICP. The addition of a neuromuscular blockade agent is used for those patients whose ventilatory problems or associated pulmonary injuries interfere with optimal ventilation.

Second-tier interventions are used if the primary interventions fail to control elevated ICP. The use of osmotherapy (*osmotic diuretics or hypertonic saline) can help reduce ICP by decreasing brain water.* The serum sodium is monitored to make sure that ICP does not increase dramatically following treatment. It is imperative to monitor the urine output following the administration of osmotic diuretics. Replacement of fluids to maintain euvolemia and maintenance of the serum osmolarity less than 320 mOsm are two important interventions in using these interventions.

QUICK TIP! An easier way to remember the normal range for serum osmolarity is to note that it is approximately double the sodium value. For example: Sodium of 145 × 2 = Osmolarity of 290.

When primary and secondary interventions cannot reduce increased ICP, tertiary interventions with barbiturate-induced coma and/or craniectomy are used. Mild hypothermia (32°C–34°C) can be used for refractory-increased ICP. Pentobarbital is the most common barbiturate used to suppress neuronal activity, decrease CBF and oxygen consumption, and reduce ICP. Dosing includes a loading regimen of 10 mg/kg over 30 minutes followed by 5 mg/kg over 60 minutes for three doses. An infusion of 1 to 3 mg/kg/h is started to maintain the drug-induced coma. Appropriate levels of coma are monitored by such measures as continuous electroencephalography with burst suppression or bi-spectral index monitoring. Craniectomy is a surgical intervention for increased ICP that removes the skull over part of the cranium in an effort to provide room for the swollen brain.

Other Nursing Interventions

The control of body temperature is imperative in neurologic disorders. Optimal temperature is 36°C to 37°C. Temperature elevations above 37°C should be avoided due to increase in oxygen consumption by the brain and worsening neurologic outcomes, especially in patients with head injuries and stroke.

Suctioning is imperative if the patient cannot clear his or her secretions. The increase in ICP may be decreased by preoxygenation with 100% oxygen, limiting suctioning to a maximum of 10 seconds and one or two passes, the use of an appropriate-sized suction catheter, and the use of less than 120 mm Hg negative-pressure suction. The prevention of thick, tenacious secretions will help to limit increases in the ICP with this procedure. Avoid excessive coughing, as this could increase the ICP. Glucocorticoids may be used to decrease cerebral edema in patients with brain tumors. The use of glucocorticoids in patients with head injuries is not indicated.

Nursing activities should be spaced out to ensure adequate rest periods for the patient with increased ICP. Keeping the room quiet with low lighting ensures a decrease in stimulation. The use of familiar touch by family and purposeful touch by team members may decrease ICP.

Patients with intracranial pathology are at risk for or have increased ICP. Nursing activities and interventions can minimize the impact of these pathologies on the brain.

KEY CLINICAL CONCEPT

Nursing interventions should be timed to ensure adequate rest periods for the patient with increased ICP. Measures such a low lighting and noise should be implemented to decrease stimulation.

KEY CONTENT CHECKLIST

- ❒ Remember that decreased LOC may be the earliest and most sensitive indicator of neurologic decline
- ❒ Monro–Kellie doctrine provides the framework for reviewing physiology and treatments for elevated ICP. The hypothesis states that brain tissue, blood volume, and CSF are balanced in a state of dynamic equilibrium. If an increase occurs in the relative volume of one component, such as CSF, the volume of one or more of the other components must decrease or an elevation in ICP will result.
- ❒ Autoregulation maintains a constant CBF by vasodilating or vasoconstricting cerebral arteries normally during MAP of 50 to 150 mm Hg despite increases or decreases in blood pressure.
- ❒ In adults, the normal ICP range is 5 to 15 mm Hg. Increase in ICP greater than 20 mm Hg is considered elevated and treatment measures are generally initiated. Intracranial hypertension is defined as an ICP greater than 20 mm Hg that persists for 5 minutes or longer.
- ❒ CPP is the difference between MAP and CPP = MAP – ICP. Normal CPP is 80 mm Hg. When reducing ICP, a target CPP of 50–70 is indicated.
- ❒ As a refresher, the calculation for MAP: MAP = [SBP + (2 × DBP)]/3. This is because the heart is in diastole two-thirds of the time.
- ❒ When P2 becomes greater in amplitude than P1, this signals a decrease in the adaptive compliance of the brain and possibly impairment of autoregulation.
- ❒ As a pneumonic to help you remember ICP trend waveforms:
  - A waves are "alarming," "abnormal," or "awful."
  - B waves are "bad."
  - C waves are worth, "consider keeping an eye on it" or, "controlled."
- ❒ Nursing interventions should be timed to ensure adequate rest periods for the patient with increased ICP. Measures such as low lighting and noise should be implemented to decrease stimulation.
- ❒ On the exam, increased ICP will appear as obviously high or normal. You will generally not be asked to manage a situation in a question with a "borderline" ICP value.
- ❒ Bagging and hyperventilating to induce hypocapnia will temporarily induce ICP reduction but should only be used in the initial, acute period and not as a sustained treatment.
- ❒ An easier way to remember the normal range for serum osmolarity is to note that it is approximately double the sodium value. For example: Sodium of 145 × 2 = Osmolarity of 290.

Review Questions:

1. The presence of an intracranial pressure (ICP) of 50 indicates which situation?

a. A lower motor neuron lesion
b. Cerebral ischemia
c. Peripheral nerve damage
d. An intact spinal arc

Answer: B. Rationale: ICP represents the ever-changing relationship between the brain, blood, and CSF inside the cranial vault. In adults, the normal ICP range is 5 to 15 mm Hg. Increase in ICP greater than 20 mm Hg is considered elevated and treatment measures are generally initiated at that level. Intracranial hypertension is defined as an ICP greater than 20 mm Hg that persists for 5 minutes or longer. The control of ICP elevations is an important aspect of the management of severe traumatic brain injury and other intracranial pathologies, since sustained increases in ICP can result in decreases in the delivery of oxygenated blood to the brain as well as herniation and compression of the brain and brainstem. Without interventions to reduce the ICP, blood flow to the brain is compromised. The comprehension of blood flow dynamics is essential to managing ICP.

2. A 28-year-old man is admitted to the ICU with a diagnosis of closed head injury. The nurse should be aware of which potential complications?

a. Hypotension
b. Respiratory alkalosis
c. Tremors
d. Cerebral edema

Answer: D. Rationale: Complications include cerebral edema (vasogenic and cytotoxic), hydrocephalus, seizures, increased ICP, diabetes insipidus, and residual neurologic deficits. Metabolic complications include respiratory insufficiency, infection, and systemic dysfunction as a result of associated trauma.

3. Nursing interventions for the patient with an intraventricular ICP monitoring device would include which of the following?

a. Routine flushing of the system with heparinized saline
b. Maintaining the transducer at the level of the heart
c. Administration of prophylactic antibiotics
d. Monitoring the patient for signs and symptoms of infection

Answer: D. Rationale: CSF drainage is used as a primary intervention to reduce ICP when an intraventricular catheter is in place. Infections are a major threat in intraventricular monitoring. The most important step in preventing infection is maintaining a "closed" system. Sterile technique is required whenever the system is entered for CSF sampling and an occlusive dressing is maintained over the catheter insertion site.

31

Acute Head Injuries and Craniotomies

CHAPTER OVERVIEW AND OBJECTIVES

The primary focus of this chapter is head injury and space-occupying lesions (brain tumors). The CCRN exam may include one to three questions on the content covered in this chapter.

After studying this chapter, you should be able to:

- Identify the Glasgow Coma Scale (GCS) associated with mild, moderate, and severe traumatic brain injury (TBI).
- Describe diffuse axonal injury (DAI).
- Describe symptoms of basilar skull fracture.
- Identify nursing interventions to control intracranial pressure (ICP).

31.1 INTRODUCTION TO HEAD INJURIES

Acute traumatic brain injuries (TBI) are caused by blunt, penetrating, or blast mechanisms. They commonly occur because of motor vehicle accidents, falls, assaults, or sports injuries. The incidence of TBI is higher in men than women and higher in persons aged 0 to 4, 15 to 19 years, and those older than 75 years. Adults older than 75 years have the highest rates of TBI-related hospitalizations and deaths.

TBI can be classified by severity using the GCS.

- Mild brain injury refers to patients with a GCS score of 13 to 15.
- Moderate injury indicates a GCS score of 9 to 12.
- Severe brain injury refers to patients with a score of 8 or less.

The damage caused by the event produces a primary injury to the brain, blood vessels, cranial nerves, or supporting structures. Primary injury occurs due to the biomechanical effects of trauma on the brain and skull because of the initial injury. Injuries are categorized as focal and diffuse.

Focal injuries include:

- Cerebral contusions
- Coup–contrecoup injuries where injury occurs both at the side of impact and the contralateral side
- Brain lacerations
- Cranial nerve injuries
- Tearing of arteries/veins in the brain
  - Arterial tears of the middle meningeal artery produce epidural hematomas.
  - Tearing of the bridging cortical veins produces subdural hematomas.
  - Tears of small vessels can produce traumatic subarachnoid hemorrhage

Diffuse injuries are produced by twisting and turning of the brain tissue at the time of injury and can result in axonal damage. Mild diffuse injuries are called cerebral concussions and result in a brief, less than 15 minutes, alteration in consciousness. Severe DAI produces profound coma and severe derangement of the axons, with cerebral swelling and ischemia. The impact to the brain extends beyond the primary event. In addition to the primary source of injury, cytotoxic processes such as release of calcium, excitatory amino acids, and oxygen-free radicals can cause progressive cellular damage for up to 6 hours following the primary injury.

Following the primary event, the brain is susceptible to secondary brain injury, which is defined as any subsequent injury to the brain after the initial insult. Secondary brain injury can result from hypotension, hypoxia, hypocapnea, elevated ICP, infection, anemia, elevated temperature, electrolyte imbalances, or the biochemical changes initiated by the original trauma. The treatment of head injury is directed at recognizing and treating the primary injury produced by the traumatic event. It is also directed at preventing or minimizing secondary brain injury.

A focused neurologic examination establishes the level of consciousness and responses to stimulation or pain.

31.2 CLASSIFICATION OF INJURY

TBI occurs due to the result of blunt trauma (direct blow to the head) or from penetrating trauma (eg, gunshot wound). Blunt injury occurs because of several factors including:

1. Deceleration: the head is moving and strikes a stationary object (eg, stairs).
2. Acceleration: a moving object (eg, hammer) strikes the head.
3. Acceleration–deceleration: the brain moves rapidly within the skull, resulting in a combination of injury-causing forces.
4. Rotation: twisting motion of the brain occurs within the skull, usually due to side impact.
5. Deformation or compression: direct injury to the head changes the shape of the skull, resulting in compression of brain tissue.

Closed Head Injuries

In a closed head injury, the scalp is intact and there is no break in the skull bones. As described above, the injuries produced at the time of the event are classified as diffuse or focal primary injuries.

Diffuse Head Injury

Blunt trauma to the head by an accelerative or decelerative force causes a stretch injury to the axons in the brain. This type of injury occurs along a continuum with DAI on the severe end and concussion on the mild end.

Concussion. It is generally believed that a concussion results from the axons sustaining a stretch injury. Clinically, the duration of unconsciousness may alter the description of the injury, but the primary consideration is that of neurologic deficit. Symptoms of a concussion include difficulty concentrating, amnesia, visual problem, headache, sensitivity to light and/or sound, dizziness, and anxiety or mood changes.

Momentary confusion and disorientation may be seen with posttraumatic amnesia. Two types of amnesia may be seen; antegrade which is the inability to form new memories after the injury and retrograde which is the inability to recall memories prior to the injury.

Although the patient may appear to have recovered, postconcussive syndrome can develop. Postconcussive syndrome presents within weeks to 1 year later. Symptoms include headache, dizziness, irritability, emotional lability, fatigue, poor concentration, decreased attention span, memory difficulties, depression, and intellectual dysfunction.

Brainstem Injury

Brainstem injury is associated with other diffuse cerebral injury. An immediate loss of consciousness (LOC) with pupillary changes and posturing will be seen. On examination, cranial nerve deficits and *changes in vital functions, such as respiratory rate and rhythm, are present.* These injuries are classified as DAIs.

Diffuse Axonal Injury

DAI is also known as diffuse neuronal injury or shearing injury. Damage to nerve fibers is produced by linear and rotational shear strains following high-speed deceleration injuries. The injury disconnects the cerebral hemispheres from the reticular activating system. DAI is characterized by immediate coma. Mild DAI involves LOC lasting 6 to 24 hours. Basal skull fractures are associated with moderate DAI. Severe DAI is seen with primary brainstem injuries. Such patients present with prolonged coma, increased ICP, hypertension, and fever. *Prognosis is poor.*

Focal Head Injury

Contusion. Due to accelerative or decelerative blunt trauma forces to the head, the cerebral cortex may bruise. These forces propel the brain against the rigid cranium (the coup force). With initial impact, the brain is then rotated or thrown back in the opposite direction (the contrecoup force), as shown in **Fig. 31-1**.

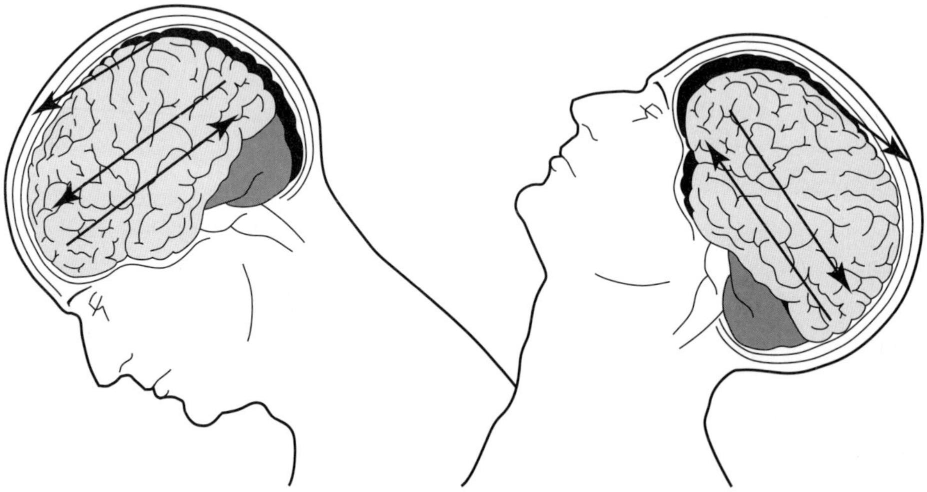

Figure 31-1. Coup and contrecoup forces.

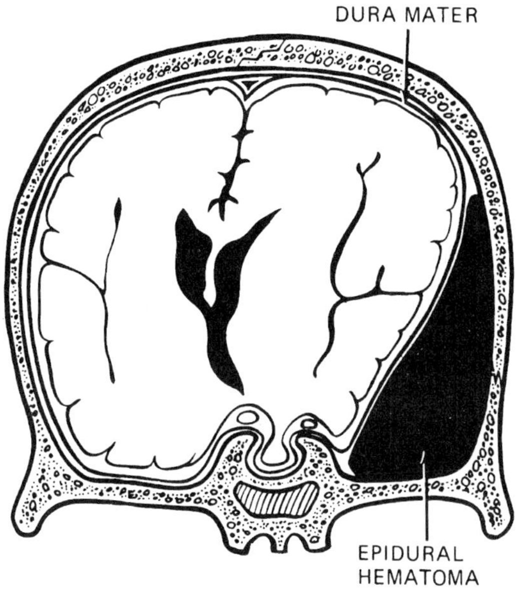

Figure 31-2. Epidural hematoma.

This trauma invariably results in cerebral bruising and edema. Most susceptible to bruising are the inferior frontal and temporal lobes. Contusions are visible on computed tomography (CT) or magnetic resonance imaging (MRI) of the brain. The contusions may not appear for 6 to 24 hours after the event.

If the forces are strong enough, lacerations and scattered intracerebral hemorrhages may occur. These usually occur along the axis line of the coup and contrecoup forces. Mild contusions will clear as the bruising and edema resolve, leaving no neurologic deficit. Temporal lobe contusions carry a great risk of swelling and brain herniation. **Some patients present with a period of lucidity, which is followed by rapid deterioration and death without surgical intervention**. Severe contusions that do not resolve, as indicated by continuing coma, indicate that the original bruising and/or lacerations caused a necrosis of brain tissue (possibly secondary to prolonged cerebral hypoxia at the injury sites).

Acute Epidural Hematoma. Epidural hematomas are true neurosurgical emergencies. They occur at the time of the injury (**Fig. 31-2**) and are usually *associated with a temporal or parietal skull fracture with laceration of the middle meningeal artery (and often vein)*. **There is usually a LOC, which may be followed by a brief period (up to 4–6 h) of lucidity, followed by increasing restlessness, agitation, and confusion progressing to coma** in one-third of patients. During the lucid period, nausea and vomiting often occur. Other signs may include **ipsilateral oculomotor paralysis** and seizures, **contralateral hemiparesis/hemiplegia** and positive Babinski reflexes. As the hematoma increases in size, *uncal herniation* is the most common type to occur.

In one type of epidural hematoma, the linear fracture occurs across the sagittal sinus or the transverse sinus. In this instance, venous blood oozes into the area above the dura mater, producing a venous epidural hematoma. Symptoms may be delayed for several days.

KEY CLINICAL CONCEPT

A history of a brief LOC followed by a brief period of lucidity, followed by restlessness, agitation, and confusion progressing to coma is the classic presentation of an acute epidural hematoma. Epidural hematomas are neurosurgical emergencies and require immediate treatment.

Subdural Hematomas. Subdural hematomas are the most common type and have the highest mortality rate. There are three types of subdural hematomas: acute, subacute, and chronic forms. Subdural hematomas develop from bleeding in the subdural space between the dura mater and the arachnoid.

QUICK TIP! For the purposes of the exam, subdural hematomas are more slowly developing than compared to epidural hematomas

In the acute subdural hematoma (**Fig. 31-3**), symptoms occur usually within hours to several days. Acute subdural hematomas usually present with signs of increasing ICP, decreasing LOC, and **ipsilateral oculomotor paralysis with contralateral hemiparesis.** The signs and symptoms are those of a rapidly expanding mass lesion.

From 48 hours to 2 weeks after the initial injury a subacute subdural hematoma may develop, requiring surgery. *A steady decline in level of responsiveness indicates a potential subacute hematoma.* Symptoms include headaches, slowness in thinking, confusion, and sometimes agitation. These symptoms progressively worsen.

In the chronic subdural hematoma, a period of weeks may follow the low-impact injury before symptoms occur, generally in the elderly. Symptoms include changes in personality, confusion, occasional headaches, problems walking, incontinence, and rarely a seizure. ICP may be normal, elevated, or decreased.

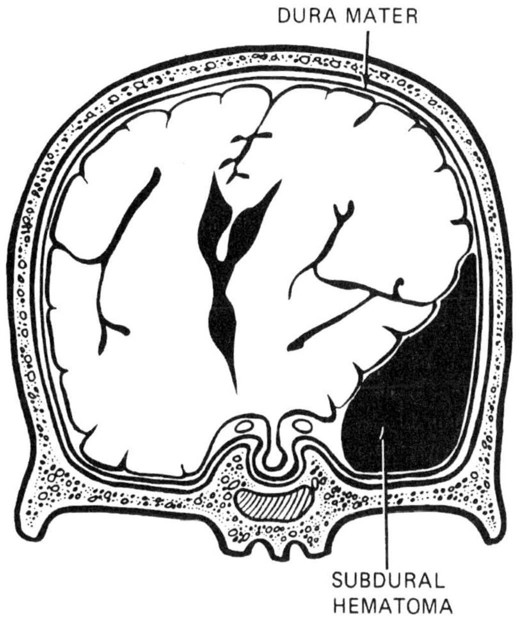

Figure 31-3. Subdural hematoma.

Subdural hematomas may occur spontaneously without any form of injury in patients on anticoagulant therapy or in those with clotting dysfunction. CT will provide a diagnosis. Surgery is the treatment of choice.

KEY CLINICAL CONCEPT

A steady decline in the level of responsiveness post a traumatic brain injury may indicate a subacute subdural hematoma.

Skull Fractures. Skull fractures are usually classified as linear, depressed, or basilar. A linear skull fracture that does not tear the dura mater will heal without treatment. If the linear fracture occurs over the temporal lobe and tears the dura (**Fig. 31-4**), there is a chance that the middle meningeal artery will also be torn. Such an injury constitutes a medical emergency, **since the bleeding is arterial; this is commonly known as an acute epidural hematoma.** The fracture may tear the dura mater over a venous sinus, resulting in slow bleeding that causes a chronic (nonacute) epidural hematoma. A depressed skull fracture that is not depressed more than the thickness of the skull is usually just monitored. However, a depressed skull fracture greater than the thickness of the skull (usually <5–7 mm) requires surgery to relieve the compression. Assessment of the extent of brain injury is essential. If the dura is torn, bone fragments may have entered brain tissue, requiring removal within 24 hours, and the chance of infection is greatly increased.

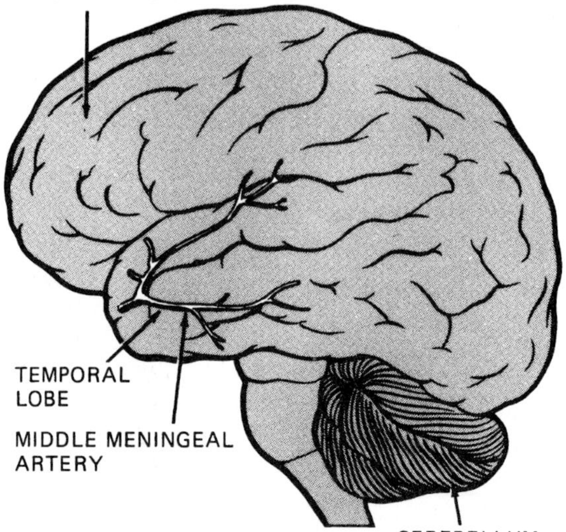

Figure 31-4. Linear skull fracture over the middle meningeal artery.

With a basilar skull fracture, there is a high risk of injury to cranial nerves, infection, and residual neurologic deficits due to coup and contrecoup forces (**Fig. 31-5**). Basilar fractures may

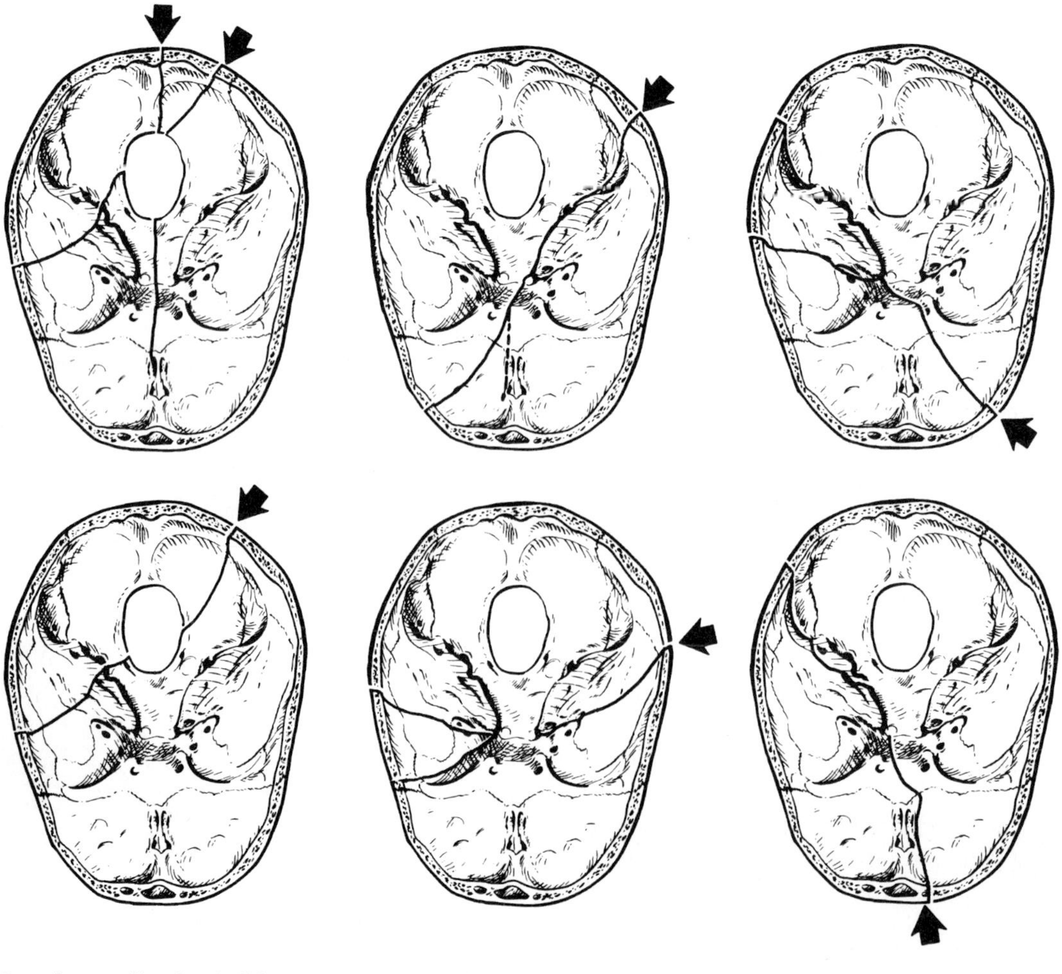

Figure 31-5. Coup forces of basilar skull fractures. Contrecoup forces go in the opposite direction along similar paths.

occur in the anterior, middle, or posterior fossa. **Battle's sign** is a sign of bleeding into the paranasal sinuses and refers to ecchymosis behind the ears and/or developing around the eyes (also called **Racoon's eyes**). Along with cerebrospinal fluid (CSF) draining from the nose (rhinorrhea), these signs indicate a basilar fracture in the anterior fossa. *CSF draining from the ear canal (otorrhea) is a sign of a middle fossa basilar skull fracture.* A temporal or basilar fracture in the posterior fossa is indicated by Battle's sign. Other symptoms of basilar fracture include tinnitus, facial paralysis, hearing difficulty, nystagmus, and conjugate deviation of gaze.

Patients with rhinorrhea will complain of a salty taste as the CSF drains into the pharynx. Caution the patient against blowing the nose, and avoid suctioning or nasal packing if rhinorrhea is present. Otorrhea can be tested for glucose. (Laboratory testing is more accurate than glucose testing sticks.) If glucose is present, the drainage is CSF. The **"halo sign,"** a yellow ring that appears around bloody drainage on a nose or ear pad, is another indication of CSF leakage. The goal is early detection of intracranial fluid leakage and prevention of infection. Severe neurologic deficits are common with basilar fractures.

QUICK TIP! The "halo sign" is a yellow ring that appears around bloody drainage on a nose or ear pad. This can be indicative of a CSF leakage and should be evaluated.

Compound Injuries

Compound injuries involve a laceration of the scalp with a head injury or skull fracture. If there is a laceration with a head injury (depressed fracture), surgery is usually performed immediately because of the threat of infection.

31.3 COMPLICATIONS OF HEAD INJURY

Closed Head Injuries

Complications include cerebral edema (vasogenic and cytotoxic), hydrocephalus, seizures, increased ICP, diabetes insipidus, and residual neurologic deficits. Metabolic complications include respiratory insufficiency, infection, and systemic dysfunction because of associated trauma.

If the hypothalamus and/or pituitary gland is affected, diabetes insipidus will most likely occur. Biochemical stress ulcers are common and are frequently associated with electrolyte disturbances. Depending on the site and degree of injury, seizures may develop. Infections, both cerebrospinal and respiratory, are continuous threats.

31.4 DIAGNOSTIC TESTS AND FINDINGS

CT is the primary diagnostic test in head injuries. A CT scan can reveal if:

1. Air has entered the brain from fractures of the eye, mastoid, or sinuses.
2. Blood is present in brain tissue or in the ventricular system.
3. Blood is on the surface of the brain or in the basal cisterns.
4. Presence of cerebral edema and intracranial shift.
5. Ventricles are of normal size and in normal position.
6. The pineal gland has calcified and is in normal position.

Lumbar puncture is contraindicated in increased ICP and is rarely done in the diagnosis of head injuries.

Cerebral angiography or CT angiography is used if there is a suspicion of arterial dissection or the presence of a ruptured aneurysm or arteriovenous malformation (AVM).

MRI of the brain is obtained in more stable patients. Injuries to the brain parenchyma and the brainstem are more visible with MRI.

Arterial blood gases (ABGs) are helpful in determining the presence of hypoxia, hypocarbia, or hypercarbia. Electrolyte studies are done frequently, especially serum sodium and serum osmolality, to monitor changes. Coagulation studies are done to monitor for the development of coagulopathy, which is detrimental to the brain-injured patient.

KEY CLINICAL CONCEPT

A lumbar puncture is contraindicated in the setting of increased ICP due the risk of uncal herniation. It should rarely be performed on a patient with a head injury.

31.5 EXAMINATION OF THE PATIENT

Patients with acute head injuries may present along the neurologic continuum from awake to comatose. Prior to describing the interventions needed to care for the severe TBI patient, an overview of the neurologic examination applicable to all patients is presented.

Neurologic Examination

Mentation. There are five possible states or levels of consciousness. The definition and/or progression may differ in various institutions. It may be defined as follows:

1. Alert: The patient is oriented to person, place, and time.
2. Lethargic: The patient prefers to sleep and, when aroused, his or her degree of alertness or confusion is variable.
3. Obtunded: The patient can be aroused with minimal stimulation but will drift off to sleep quickly.
4. Stuporous: The patient is aroused only by constant, deep, and usually painful stimuli. The patient may respond by some attempt to withdraw, moaning, or exhibiting decerebrate or decorticate positioning.
5. Coma: The patient cannot be aroused.

The GCS (**Table 31-1**) is one of the standard methods used to identify a patient's level of consciousness (mentation) and

TABLE 31-1. GLASGOW COMA SCALE

Eye Opening (E)	*Best Motor Response (M)*	*Verbal Response (V)*
Spontaneous = 4 To speech = 3 To pain = 2 No response = 1	Obeys = 6 Localizes = 5 Withdraws = 4 Abnormal Flexion = 3 Extension = 2 No response = 1	Oriented = 5 Confused conversation = 4 Inappropriate words = 3 Incomprehensible sounds = 2 No response = 1

determine his or her prognosis. The GCS measures both arousal and awareness. Eye-opening is a measure of arousal. Verbal and best motor responses are measures of awareness. The lower the score, the worse the prognosis.

QUICK TIP! A GCS of less than 8 is considered comatose and requires intubation for airway protection.

Cranial Nerves. Some of the 12 cranial nerves can be checked during routine patient care as well as during neurologic checks:

- II: Optic nerve. Sensory limb of the pupillary light reflex. Visual acuity.
- III: Oculomotor nerve. Motor limb of the pupillary light reflex; causes constriction of the pupil. Eyelid elevation. It controls four of the six eye muscles.
- IV: Trochlear nerve. It turns the eye down and in.
- V: Trigeminal nerve. Corneal sensation. Provides the sensory side of the arc for the corneal reflex. Sensation to the face. Muscles of mastication. *Note*: The seventh nerve (facial) provides the motor side of arc.
- VI: Abducens nerve. It turns the eye out. This is the longest unprotected nerve in the brain.
- VII: Facial nerve. Facial symmetry and movement and eyelid closure.
- X: Vagus nerve. This controls palatal deviation. If the nerve is damaged, the uvula deviates away from the side of paralysis. In vagal nerve paralysis, there is ipsilateral paralysis of the palatal, pharyngeal, and laryngeal muscles. The soft palate at rest is usually lower on the affected side, and if the patient says "ah," it elevates on the intact side.
- XI: (Spinal) Accessory nerve. It turns the head by use of the sternocleidomastoid muscles. It has some association with the upper trapezius muscles.
- XII: Hypoglossal nerve. It controls tongue movement. If it is damaged, the patient cannot move the tongue from side to side, and tongue protrusion results in deviation toward the side of nerve damage.

QUICK TIP! There will always be 1 to 2 questions on cranial nerves. Often one question will refer to the cranial nerve simply by its number. Remember, "On Old Olympus Tiny Tops A Fin and German Viewed Some Hops," or consider writing them down on the scratch paper prior to starting your exam.

Motor Function. Motor function can be determined by assessing the patient's ability to move all extremities voluntarily and equally. Note a one-sided weakness. If muscle weakness is suspected, have the patient close his or her eyes and extend the arms directly in front. If there is a muscle weakness, there will be a drifting downward of the weakened extremity. Motor strength is measured using a scale from 0 to 5. Note any abnormal posturing of the arms or legs. **Flexor posturing** occurs when the arms flex up and inward. **Extensor posturing** occurs when the arms extend down with palms out and the feet extend downward.

QUICK TIP! Remember "flexor" posturing (decorticate) flexes limbs "toward the cord." Think of "Extensor" posturing (decerebrate) as being spelled "d-E-c-E-r-E-brat-E" to emphasize the "E."

Sensation

In patients suffering severe neurological trauma, patients may respond only to pain. In the awake neurologic patient, determine whether the patient has any numbness or tingling in the arms, legs, or face. Test sensation with the light touch of a cotton swab and pinprick with a pin. Additional assessment parameters in the head-injured patient include the following:

Scalp: Check for tears and/or swelling.

Face: Palpate the eye orbits, nose, teeth, maxilla, and mandible for facial fractures. Some facial fractures may cause leakage of CSF, and this would be an entry port for infection.

Ears: Blood in the external canal usually indicates a basal skull fracture.

Neck/Spine: Note any purple bruises over spinous processes. If the patient is awake, palpate the spinous processes to determine whether pain is present. *Note*: This should be done only by the physician with a team present to log-roll the patient to the side, ensuring that the cervical spine is maintained in alignment.

Resuscitation Phase—ABCs: Airway, Breathing, and Circulation

The ABCs of emergency care pertain to any patient presenting with an acute head injury. Multiple assessment and intervention priorities occur simultaneously. Patients presenting with a *GCS of less than 8 are considered comatose and require intubation for airway protection.* Always establish a patent airway, *using extra care to protect the cervical spine (a jaw thrust/chin lift may be indicated over the "sniffing position" to open the airway).* Following endotracheal intubation, confirmation of correct tube placement is done. Cerebral ischemia can be prevented by maintaining a PaO_2 of greater than 60 mm Hg and $PaCO_2$ of approximately 35 mm Hg. Capnography can be useful by providing continuous measurement of end-tidal CO_2. Two large-bore intravenous lines should be placed IV fluids to support blood pressure; this is essential to optimizing perfusion to the brain. Monitor for signs of impending shock. Treatment of shock should include determination of cause and *maintenance of a mean arterial pressure (MAP) of at least 90 mm Hg to prevent a precipitous drop in the central perfusion pressure (CPP) in the patient with increased ICP.* Continually monitor the respiratory and cardiac systems to ensure early intervention in cases of dysfunction. Inadequate function of either system may result in the extension of neurologic impairment.

A brief focused neurologic examination, including level of consciousness, is a key initial assessment in any neurologically impaired patient. The patient's pupils should be assessed and responses to stimulation noted. The secondary survey follows with an assessment of major organ systems.

Foley catheters and orogastric tubes are placed after the secondary survey is completed. *Cervical spine precautions* are paramount during this entire phase and maintained until the spine is cleared.

31.6 NURSING INTERVENTIONS

The primary nursing intervention after assurance of a patent airway and the prevention of hypoxia is frequent neurologic assessment. Signs of increasing ICP may be treated with drainage of CSF via intraventricular cannulas; *maintaining CPP between 50 and 70 mm Hg* with fluids/vasopressors; sedation and analgesia; osmotic diuretics such as mannitol or administration of hypertonic saline; hyperventilation only ($Paco_2$ 30–35 mm Hg) for brief periods of significantly increased ICP, with continual monitoring of cerebral blood flow or brain oxygen; and barbiturate-induced coma. *Nursing interventions include facilitating venous drainage by elevating the head of the bed 30 degrees and maintaining the head in a neutral position; in addition, spacing of suctioning procedures may help to avoid hypoxemia* or hypercarbia/hypocarbia. ICP monitoring may be instituted in patients with GCS score of 3 to 8.

Monitoring of vital signs and the maintenance of fluid balance and accurate intake/output records will help in evaluating treatment modalities aimed at stabilizing the patient. *Hyperthermia in the head-injured patient can increase the brain metabolic rate, the cerebral blood volume, and ICP; therefore, temperature control is an additional area of focus.* Patients should be *kept normothermic with temperatures between 36°C and 37°C.* In the care of the acutely head-injured patient, it may also be advisable to *control environment stimuli as these can have a direct effect on ICP*; in addition, the *spacing of nursing care procedures* such as bathing and linen changes may be wise. Nursing care related to reducing ICP, preventing seizures, and maintaining glucose between 140 and 180 mg/dL are additional considerations. Standard procedures to prevent infections are employed.

KEY CONTENT CHECKLIST

- ❒ A history of a brief LOC followed by a brief period of lucidity, followed by restlessness, agitation, and confusion progressing to coma is the classic presentation of an acute **epidural hematoma. Epidural hematomas** are neurosurgical emergencies and require immediate treatment.
  - **Epidural hematomas** are usually associated with a temporal or parietal skull fracture with laceration of the middle meningeal artery.
- ❒ A steady decline in the level of responsiveness post a traumatic brain injury may indicate a subacute **subdural hematoma.**
- ❒ Battle's sign (ecchymosis behind the ears and/or around the eyes) and CSF leakage from the nose (rhinorrhea) or ears (otorrhea) are signs of a basilar skull fracture. Ecchymosis around the eyes may also be called Racoon's eyes.
- ❒ The "halo sign" is a yellow ring that appears around bloody drainage on a nose or ear pad, this can be indicative of a CSF leakage and should be evaluated.
- ❒ A lumbar puncture is contraindicated in the setting of increased ICP due the risk of uncal herniation. It should rarely be performed in a patient with a head injury.
- ❒ TBI patients with a GCS score of less than 8 require intubation for airway protection.
- ❒ Nursing interventions in the care of the TBI patient include facilitating venous drainage by elevating the head of the bed 30 degrees and maintaining the head in a neutral position. Suctioning procedures should be spaced to avoid hypoxemia or hypercarbia/hypocarbia. Normothermia should be maintained and a low-stimulation environment should be provided.
- ❒ ICP monitoring should be considered in patients with a GCS of less than 8.
- ❒ Remember "flexor" posturing (decorticate) flexes limbs "toward the cord." Think of "Extensor" posturing (decerebrate) as being spelled "d-E-c-E-r-E-brat-E" to emphasize the "E." Decerebrate is associated with a worse prognosis.

Review Questions:

1. Initial assessment of the neurologically impaired patient should include measurement of which of the following?

a. Level of consciousness
b. Pupillary eye movement
c. Deep tendon reflexes
d. Brainstem reflexes

Answer: A. Rationale: There are five possible states or levels of consciousness. The definition and/or progression may differ in various institutions. It may be defined as follows:

1. Alert: The patient is oriented to person, place, and time.
2. Lethargic: The patient prefers to sleep and, when aroused, his or her degree of alertness or confusion is variable.
3. Obtunded: The patient can be aroused with minimal stimulation but will drift off to sleep quickly.
4. Stuporous: The patient is aroused only by constant, deep, and usually painful stimuli. The patient may respond by some attempt to withdraw, moaning, or exhibiting decerebrate or decorticate positioning.
5. Coma: The patient cannot be aroused.

The GCS is one of the standard methods used to identify a patient's level of consciousness (mentation) and determine his or her prognosis. The GCS measures both arousal and awareness. Eye-opening is a measure of arousal. Verbal and best motor responses are measures of awareness. The lowest score received has the worse prognosis.

Use this scenario for questions 2 and 3.

A 45-year-old man is admitted to your unit with a diagnosis of intracranial hypertension due to a severe traumatic brain injury. The current vital signs include a blood pressure (BP) of 110/70 mm Hg, ICP 30, pulse 140, respiratory rate 20.

2. Based on the preceding information, what is the CPP?

a. 83
b. 53
c. 120
d. Not calculable

Answer: B. Rationale: CPP is the difference between the MAP and the mean ICP (CPP = MAP – ICP). Even though the MAP is not included in the information provided, it can be calculated by: [(DBP × 2) + SBP]/3. Therefore, in this case the ICP (30) subtracted from the calculated MAP (83) is equal to 53. Choose B.

3. Which of the following are measures that would improve the CPP?

a. Increase the MAP
b. Decrease the MAP
c. Decrease the heart rate
d. All of the above

Answer: A. Rationale: CPP is the difference between the MAP and the mean ICP (CPP = MAP – ICP). Increasing the MAP in the setting of increased ICP will increase CPP.

32

Stroke

CHAPTER OVERVIEW AND OBJECTIVES

In this chapter, the concept of cerebrovascular disturbance is covered. Common interruptions in cerebrovascular blood flow may be the result of thrombosis, embolus, or hemorrhage. The CCRN exam will most likely have one to three questions on this content.

A stroke is a sudden focal or global neurologic deficit due to cerebrovascular disease. It is the most common cause of cerebral dysfunction in the United States.

After studying this chapter, you should be able to:

- Describe the difference between ischemic and hemorrhagic stroke.
- Identify nursing care priorities that pertain to both ischemic and hemorrhagic stroke.
- Describe the treatments for rupture of intracranial aneurysms
- Identify interventions for treatment of vasospasm in subarachnoid hemorrhage.

32.1 ETIOLOGY

Stroke is a leading cause of disability and is the fifth leading cause of death in the United States. A stroke is a neurologic event resulting from altered cerebral circulation, often due to either cellular ischemia/infarction caused by a blockage of an artery feeding the brain or arterial rupture (intracranial hemorrhage [ICH]). Cerebral ischemia occurs as a result of reduced cerebral blood flow, which can last from several seconds to minutes. The end result of any interruption of oxygen to brain tissue for more than a few minutes is the death of those neurons not being oxygenated. Such a decrease in oxygen may be partial or complete. *Symptoms due to an acute stroke can occur in about 10 seconds, from hypoxia and energy depletion.*

There are two main types of stroke: ischemic and hemorrhagic. Discrimination between the two is important as it dictates the indicated treatment. Ischemic strokes account for 85% to 88% of all strokes. The vascular origin is from (1) a thrombotic or (2) embolic occlusion of a cerebral artery, resulting in an infarction. Hemorrhagic strokes are responsible for 12% to 15% of all strokes. Causes include spontaneous vessel rupture, severe hypertension, uncontrolled anticoagulation, or brain tumor. Risk factors include family history, hypertension, diabetes mellitus, smoking, atherosclerosis, atrial fibrillation and other cardioembolic sources, prior transient ischemic attack (TIA), advanced age, and trauma.

32.2 CLINICAL PRESENTATION

Ischemic stroke results from decreased or disrupted blood flow.

Any patient with sudden changes in neurologic functioning should be evaluated for stroke. Specific symptomatology depends on location of the injury and the hemispheric dominance of the patient. The extent of the deficit is determined by which artery is occluded.

If the ischemic stroke occurs in the **right cerebral hemisphere** (usually the nondominant hemisphere), **left-sided motor and sensory deficits** occur. Autotopagnosia (an inability to determine the position of parts of the body in relation to the rest of the body, constructional apraxia (inability to completed the left half of a figure when drawing), and dressing apraxia (inability to dress oneself properly) are common in right cerebral strokes. Neglect of the paralyzed side; impulsive, quick behavior; and poor judgment of one's abilities and limitations occur with right cerebral strokes.

Left cerebral hemispheric (dominant hemisphere) strokes are associated with **right-sided motor and sensory impairment and aphasia**. *Expressive aphasia* is the inability to express oneself verbally and understandably. *Receptive aphasia* is loss of the ability to understand spoken or written words. Other deficits include dyslexia, acalculia, agraphia, and astereognosis.

Astereognosis occurs when the patient, with eyes closed, is unable to identify a common object placed in his or her hand.

KEY CLINICAL CONCEPT

For the purposes of the exam, strokes will always present with ipsilateral (same-sided) pupillary changes and contralateral (opposite-sided) motor deficits

Regardless of which hemisphere is involved in a stroke, such patients tend to have a reduced memory span, are emotionally labile, and have spasticity of the affected extremities. Some patients will have anosognosia, which is the denial of a neurologic deficit such as hemiplegia. Anosognosia differs from a psychological denial state.

All of the above symptoms can occur with an intracerebral hemorrhage. Additional symptoms include severe headache, nuchal rigidity, hemiparesis to posturing, cranial nerve deficits, stupor, and coma. The severity of symptoms depends on the size and location of the hemorrhage.

QUICK TIP! It is unusual for ischemic stroke patients to present with coma, this is usually an indication of a hemorrhagic stroke.

Diagnosis

The diagnosis of stroke is usually made based on history, clinical symptoms, and diagnostic tests.

To differentiate between the two types of stroke, a **computed tomography (CT) scan should be completed within 25 minutes of the patient's arrival**. Patients presenting within the first hours of ischemic stroke will generally have a negative CT scan of the brain. In some instances, an "MCA" sign, or white clot visible in the middle cerebral artery (MCA), will be seen in MCA occlusions. *Patients presenting 12 to 24 hours after stroke onset will have ischemic changes on CT*, which will reveal decreased density in ischemic and infarcted areas. Hemorrhage on CT shows up as an increased white-appearing density. A magnetic resonance imaging (MRI) study can differentiate between the presence of an infarction, hemorrhage, the presence of a clot, or dissection of a vessel wall. Cerebral angiography may show vessel occlusion, vasospasm, arteriovenous malformations, and aneurysms.

Medical Treatment

Stroke patients presenting to a hospital are considered emergent cases. Rapid identification, triage, and diagnosis are imperative.

If the patient has had an ischemic stroke, treatment options depend on the time from symptom onset as well as a number of other factors. *In patients presenting within 4.5 hours of symptom onset, thrombolytic therapy (with tissue plasminogen activator, or tPA) should be considered as a treatment option if the patient meets inclusion criteria and has no exclusions. If tPA is given, the systolic blood pressure is maintained less than 185 mm Hg and the diastolic less than 110 mm Hg prior to initiation. Once tPA is started systolic blood pressure is maintained less than 180 and the diastolic less than 105.* Patients receiving tPA must be closely monitored with vital signs and neurologic checks every 15 minutes for 2 hours, every 30 minutes for 6 hours, and every hour for 16 hours. These patients are often admitted to the intensive care unit (ICU), where cardiac/respiratory monitoring occurs as well as close neurologic observation. In patients with large vessel occlusion (blood clot in one of the large arteries of the brain including the internal carotid artery, MCA, and posterior cerebral artery), those unable to receive tPA due to time (>4.5 h from symptom onset) or another contraindication mechanical thrombectomy should be performed. Mechanical thrombectomy is the removal of blood clot through an endovascular procedure. *Aspirin therapy used within 48 hours of onset of symptoms* has been demonstrated to reduce risk and mortality. The maintenance of cerebral perfusion pressure (CPP) is an important component of treatment; blood pressure control is usually not instituted unless it is more than 220 mm Hg systolic or more than 120 mm Hg diastolic, as even minor decreases in blood pressure can affect the recovery of the area of ischemic penumbra. The **penumbra** is the area surrounding an ischemic event where blood flow is reduced causing hypoxia of the cells; however, the tissue is still viable and can survive with timely intervention. Drugs of choice for blood pressure management in stroke include labetalol and nicardipine. Anticoagulant therapy (heparin, warfarin, or Factor Xa inhibitors) may be considered dependent on stroke etiology.

KEY CLINICAL CONCEPT

Treatment for ischemic stroke is time-dependent. Patients who present within 4.5 hours and have no exclusion criteria should be treated with IV tPA. Mechanical thrombectomy should be considered for patients with a large vessel occlusion regardless of if IV tPA was administered.

Hemorrhagic stroke patients usually present with an altered level of consciousness. Depending on the location of the bleed, the intensity of care will vary. Treatment options are determined based on the area of hemorrhage, dominant versus nondominant hemisphere, and prior health of the patient.

In patients who are at risk for further immediate decompensation or are unable to protect their airway, endotracheal intubation is performed and ventilatory management is instituted. An intracranial pressure (ICP) monitor, usually a ventriculostomy, may be inserted into the lateral ventricle. *The goal is to keep the ICP less than 20 mm Hg* through various interventions. **Mannitol** or **hypertonic saline** may be ordered. Blood pressure control is based on the needed CPP to maintain perfusion. Barbiturate-induced coma and craniectomy are other options to control ICP.

Nursing Interventions

To some extent nursing interventions (and patient complications) depend on the type and site of a stroke, the patient's age, his or her general health, and the extent of neurologic deficit.

Priorities with regard to the patient with an ischemic stroke include the maintenance or restoration of cerebral perfusion, maintenance of life support, prevention of further injury or escalation of the life-threatening problem, and preservation of motor function, speech, and cognition to the greatest possible extent. *Early dysphagia screening should be performed, to lower the risk of aspiration and resultant pneumonia.* The patient should be NPO (nothing by mouth) until the swallowing screen is done. Accurate systematic monitoring and assessment of neurologic status will identify extensions of deficits that may be treatable. Nursing assessment should include level of consciousness and pupil size and reactivity; change in motor function and/or cranial nerve function; signs and symptoms of increased ICP, seizure, or hydrocephalus; and analysis of arterial blood gases (ABGs) and laboratory studies. Many centers utilize the *National Institute of Health Stroke Scale (NIHSS) to assess the stroke patient.* Communication with the patient is achieved in any way possible—through writing, pictures, gestures, and so on. Different aphasias make this task difficult. Generally, patients with left hemispheric stroke respond to visual images and gestures, while those with right hemispheric stroke respond to verbal cues. The latter patients usually suffer from left-sided neglect, therefore call lights and other important aids should be placed on the right side of the bed.

KEY CLINICAL CONCEPT

Early dysphagia screening should be performed on all patients suspected of stroke to decrease the risk of aspiration pneumonia. Patients should remain NPO until the screening is completed.

Care priorities that apply to both types of stroke patients include glucose and temperature control as well as the prevention of deep venous thrombosis (DVT). Glucose levels are monitored closely. If the blood glucose exceeds 140 mg/dL, an insulin protocol is used to decrease glucose to a normal glycemic level. Normothermia should be maintained, at 36°C to 37°C. An increase in temperature of 1°C should be treated with Tylenol and cooling measures as indicated. It is imperative to prevent DVT through the use of sequential compression devices on the legs and/or the use of low-molecular-weight heparin.

If the patient with ischemic stroke has significant edema or there is a large hemorrhage, the patient may experience increased ICP; interventions are instituted to reduce this. Such interventions will vary and depend on the patient. They include airway control with endotracheal intubation and ventilation, cerebrospinal fluid (CSF) drainage via a ventriculostomy, CPP enhancement with fluids, **vasopressors, mannitol,** or **hypertonic saline,** and barbiturate-induced coma, which must be closely monitored.

Other important measures include turning, positioning, skin care, fluid and nutritional intake, emotional support, and early implementation of rehabilitation.

32.3 INTRACRANIAL ANEURYSMS

An aneurysm is a congenital, developmental, or traumatic defect in the muscle layer of arteries, normally occurring at points of bifurcation. (Recall that there are three layers in the arterial wall: the inner endothelial layer [the intima], a middle smooth muscle layer [the media], and an outer layer of connective tissue [the adventitia].)

Pathophysiology

The congenital weakness of the arterial wall results in a gradual "ballooning out" of that segment of the artery over a period of years. When vascular pressure rises to a sufficient (unknown) pressure, the weakened ballooning segment of the artery bursts.

Location, Incidence, and Etiology

Most cerebral aneurysms develop in the anterior arteries of the circle of Willis. Aneurysms are rare in children and teenagers and most common in middle-aged persons. Slightly more women than men develop aneurysms. Some 10% to 20% of patients with aneurysms have more than one (may be found on same or opposite side).

Etiologic risk factors include family history, hypertension (present in a majority of cases), and smoking. Diseases such as Ehlers–Danlos syndrome, coarctation of the aorta, and polycystic kidneys also put individuals at risk. No specific precipitating factors are present in all patients. Congenital anomalies account for some aneurysms and others occur for unknown reasons.

Clinical Presentation

Aneurysms are commonly asymptomatic until a bleed occurs. The exception is a very large aneurysm, which may cause symptoms related to pressure against surrounding tissues. The signs and symptoms of an unruptured cerebral aneurysm are dependent on its size and rate of growth and can range from no symptoms for a small aneurysm to loss of feeling in the face or visual changes with a larger aneurysm. *Symptoms that may be experienced immediately after an aneurysm ruptures include sudden and unusually severe headache, nausea, vision impairment, vomiting, and loss of consciousness.* **Severe headache (unlike any other headache)** occurs as the aneurysm starts to bleed. Unconsciousness may occur and be transient or sustained secondary to ischemia and/or necrosis of brain tissue. *Nausea and vomiting are common.* Other neurologic deficits include numbness, aphasia, and hemiparesis.

Nuchal rigidity, photophobia, diplopia, **Kernig's sign** (inability to fully extend leg when the thigh is flexed at a 90-degree angle to the abdomen), **Brudzinski's sign** (involuntary adduction and flexion of legs when neck is flexed), and headache are common because of meningeal irritation. All these signs except diplopia are sometimes grouped together under the term "meningismus."

QUICK TIP! Imagine the leg being raised in a supine patient, making the bottom part of a "K" for "Kernig's" sign. Imagine the neck flexing, creating the top curve of a "B" for "Brudzinski's" sign.

Diagnosis

Initial evaluation includes a CT scan of the brain without contrast. *If subarachnoid blood is present on CT, either a CT angiogram or cerebral angiogram is done to identify the presence of aneurysms.* If subarachnoid blood is suspected but not confirmed on a CT scan, a lumbar puncture may be performed. *Elevated CSF pressure, elevated protein levels, elevated red blood cells and oxyhemoglobin, decreased glucose, and grossly bloody CSF indicate hemorrhage in the subarachnoid space.*

Classification of Clinical State Following Aneurysmal Rupture

Aneurysms may be placed in one of five categories (grades). These are summarized in **Tables 32-1** and **32-2**. If patients can be stabilized in grades I through V, they may be candidates for surgical intervention or coiling.

TABLE 32-1. GRADES OF ANEURYSMS

Symptom	*Grade I*	*Grade II*	*Grade III*	*Grade IV*	*Grade V*
Level of consciousness	Alert	Decreased	Confused	Unresponsive	Moribund
Headache	Slight	Mild to severe	Severe	—	—
Nuchal rigidity	Slight	Yes	Yes	—	—
Vasospasm	—	—	—	May be present	May be present
Decerebrate posturing	—	—	—	—	Yes

—, absent.

Prognosis

The prognosis depends on the site and severity of the bleed. Persistent coma beyond 2 days is a poor sign. Rebleeding may occur, the highest risk is in the first 2 to 12 hours. Bleeding may recur as the original clot that formed around the bleed is absorbed (or lysed).

The risk of rebleeding has decreased dramatically with early obliteration of the aneurysm through surgery or coiling. *Cerebral vasospasm results in cerebral ischemia.* Cerebral vasospasm occurs when the arteries become irritated by broken down blood products leading to vasoconstriction. ***Vasospasm is commonly seen on days 7 through 10 postbleed but may occur up to 21 days.*** Marked cerebral edema and/or the development of hydrocephalus places the patient at greater risk for a poor outcome.

Nursing Interventions Preoperatively

Stabilization of the patient is the primary objective of treatment. Preoperative care priorities include rapid identification of the bleed. *The systolic blood pressure is lowered to less than 160 mm Hg to reduce the risk of rebleeding prior to treatment of the aneurysm.* If alert, the patient should *avoid Valsalva maneuvers and any other action that produces straining*, such as forced coughing to clear secretions. These actions will increase ICP and may start a rebleed. Complete *bed rest in a quiet, dark environment promotes stabilization.* Sedating drugs may be used to decrease stress, anxiety, or restlessness and may have the additional side effect of lowering the blood pressure in a hypertensive patient. *The head of the bed may be elevated up to 30 degrees in an attempt to promote cerebral venous return by gravity.* A bedside commode may be used. **The patient is monitored closely for signs of hydrocephalus and increased ICP**. If this occurs before the aneurysm is secured, the patient may need emergent CT to confirm it and a ventriculostomy/ICP monitor is placed. Anticonvulsants (eg, phenytoin or levetiracetam) may be used to prevent or control seizure activity in the immediate posthemorrhage period. **Calcium channel blockers, such as nimodipine,** which cross the blood–brain barrier, should be utilized to reduce the risk of developing vasospasm.

TABLE 32-2. HUNT AND HESS SCALE

Grade 1	Asymptomatic, mild headache, slight nuchal rigidity
Grade 2	Moderate-to-severe headache, nuchal rigidity, no neurologic deficit other than cranial nerve palsy
Grade 3	Drowsiness/confusion, mild focal neurologic deficit
Grade 4	Stupor, moderate-to-severe hemiparesis
Grade 5	Coma, decerebrate posturing

KEY CLINICAL CONCEPT

In patients with a ruptured, untreated aneurysm systolic blood pressure should be less than 160 mm Hg to reduce the risk of rebleeding.

Surgical Intervention and Nursing Implications

If an aneurysm is diagnosed prior to a bleed, surgery may be performed to prevent a bleed, depending on the size and location of the aneurysm. If an aneurysmal bleed has occurred and the patient has stabilized, surgery may be performed, as indicated. Conventional therapy for aneurysms includes clipping or endovascular techniques such as stenting and coil implantation. The decision to surgically clip versus coil is based on site, shape, and condition of the patient.

Surgery may consist of one of several procedures:

1. Aneurysms may be treated with surgical clipping or endovascular coiling. The multidisciplinary team, including the neurosurgeon will determine the best approach based on the characteristics of the patient and the aneurysm.
2. Aneurysm clipping is performed by a neurosurgeon. Endovascular coiling of the aneurysm is done by a physician with neurointerventional training.

If the aneurysm cannot be reached and/or surgical risk of one of the above procedures is extremely high, the common carotid artery may be clamped. Prior to this procedure, angiography must demonstrate that vascular perfusion of the involved hemisphere is adequate from the opposite side.

Postoperative Nursing Interventions

Following occlusion of the aneurysm, nursing priorities include *monitoring for neurologic changes to detect increased ICP or vasospasm,* monitoring and intervening to treat vasospasm, and preventing complications associated with bed rest. After aneurysm repair, the patient needs to be monitored for complications including seizures, cerebral edema, hydrocephalus, vasospasm, and hyponatremia.

The patient must be assessed frequently for any change in neurologic examination. Transcranial Doppler (TCD) ultrasound is performed daily as possible to assess for vasospasm. The patient is also monitored for polyuria and hypernatremia which may signify cerebral salt wasting which often accompanies vasospasm. *Physician-directed interventions to treat vasospasm include blood pressure augmentation and management of cerebral salt wasting with fluid administration.* Interventional treatment may be required for patients that do not improve with medical management. These patients may require intra-arterial verapamil or nicardipine, and/or cerebral angioplasty.

Close monitoring of the neurologic status is essential to detect increased ICP from cerebral edema or hydrocephalus and/or the onset of cerebral vasospasm. If increased ICP is present, interventions include CSF drainage via a ventriculostomy ICP catheter, optimization of CPP, mannitol, and barbiturate-induced coma. *Cerebral vasospasm typically presents as stroke symptoms such as the sudden onset of hemiparesis, word-finding problems or aphasia, neglect, or hemisensory changes.* Laboratory and diagnostic tests indicative of vasospasm include a precipitous drop in serum sodium and/or an increase in blood flow velocities on TCDs. Early detection is vital since treatment must be instituted within 8 hours of symptom onset.

The prevention of vasospasm includes administering nimodipine and IV fluids to maintain euvolemia. Patients may have arterial, central venous, and/or pulmonary artery catheters placed to closely monitor cardiac and vascular pressures. *After the aneurysm is secured and if vasospasm develops, hypertensive therapy may be instituted.* In the event that these maneuvers fail to prevent spasm, interventional procedures can be implemented. The performance of a cerebral angiogram confirms the presence of angiographic spasm.

KEY CLINICAL CONCEPT

Prevention and treatment of vasospasm is imperative to avoiding complications of aneurysm rupture. Prevention includes administering nimodipine and IV fluids to maintain euvolemia. Close neuro checks are important to detect any changes that may indicate vasospasm.

Systemic support is provided, including glycemic control, nutritional support, maintenance of normothermia, and DVT prevention. Skincare and range of motion to all four extremities are important. Consultation with occupational, speech-language, and physical therapists take place following stabilization.

KEY CONTENT CHECKLIST

- ❒ For the purposes of the exam, strokes will always present with ipsilateral (same-sided) pupillary changes and contralateral (opposite-sided) motor deficits.
  - A computed tomography (CT) scan should be completed within 25 minutes of the patient's arrival.
  - In patients presenting within 4.5 hours of symptom onset, thrombolytic therapy (with tissue plasminogen activator, or tPA) should be considered as a treatment option if the patient meets inclusion criteria and has no exclusions.
- ❒ Left cerebral hemispheric (dominant hemisphere) strokes are associated with right-sided motor and sensory impairment and aphasia. *Expressive aphasia* is the inability to express oneself verbally and understandably. *Receptive aphasia* is loss of the ability to understand spoken or written words.
- ❒ It is unusual for ischemic stroke patients to present with coma; this is usually an indication of a hemorrhagic stroke.
- ❒ Early dysphagia screening should be performed on all patients suspected of stroke to decrease the risk of aspiration pneumonia. Patients should remain NPO until the screening is completed.
- ❒ Nuchal rigidity, photophobia, diplopia, **Kernig's sign** (inability to fully extend leg when the thigh is flexed at a 90-degree angle to the abdomen), **Brudzinski's sign** (involuntary adduction and flexion of legs when neck is flexed), and headache are common because of meningeal irritation often present in intracranial aneurysm rupture.
- ❒ Classic presentation with cerebral aneurysm rupture or subarachnoid hemorrhage includes severe headache, often the worst headache the patient has ever experienced.
- ❒ In patients with a ruptured, untreated aneurysm systolic blood pressure should be less than 160 mm Hg to reduce the risk of rebleeding.
- ❒ Prevention and treatment of vasospasm is imperative to avoiding complications of aneurysm rupture. Prevention includes administering nimodipine and IV fluids to maintain euvolemia. Close neuro checks are important to detect any changes that may indicate vasospasm.

Review Questions:

1. **Where are intracranial aneurysms most commonly found?**
   a. External carotid arteries
   b. Anterior cerebral circulation
   c. Common carotid arteries
   d. Posterior cerebral circulation including the vertebrobasilar arteries

Answer: B. Rationale: Most cerebral aneurysms develop in the anterior arteries of the circle of Willis.

2. **Which of the following is a common complication of a ruptured intracranial aneurysm?**
   a. Hypotension due to hypovolemia
   b. Cardiac dysrhythmias
   c. Acid–base disturbances
   d. Vasospasm of cerebral arteries

Answer: D. Rationale: Cerebral vasospasm results in cerebral ischemia. Vasospasm is commonly seen on days 4 and 14 post-bleed.

3. What are the interventions to prevent vasospasm?

a. Administering nimodipine and maintaining hypovolemia
b. Administering labetalol and maintaining euvolemia
c. Administering nimodipine and maintaining euvolemia
d. Administering nicardipine and maintaining euvolemia

Answer: C. Rationale: Administering nimodipine and maintaining euvolemia. Nimodipine has a dilatory effect on arterial smooth muscle, decreasing the risk of vasospasm. Euvolemia ensures the patient is not dehydrated which can cause vasoconstriction.

33

The Vertebrae and Spinal Cord

CHAPTER OVERVIEW AND OBJECTIVES

In this chapter, anatomy, physiology, and concepts of spinal cord dysfunction are reviewed. Usually anatomy and physiology questions are not asked directly on the CCRN exam. Focus your study on the function of the cord and the clinical conditions that stem from cord injury/dysfunction.

After studying this chapter, you should be able to:

- Differentiate between complete and incomplete spinal cord injury.
- Explain neurogenic and spinal shock.
- Describe potential complications of spinal cord injury.
- Identify symptoms of autonomic hyperreflexia and nursing interventions.

33.1 VERTEBRAL COLUMN

The spinal cord is protected and housed by the vertebrae. The vertebral column comprises a total of 33 vertebrae: 7 cervical, 12 thoracic, 5 lumbar, 5 sacral fused, and 4 fused as the coccygeal segment.

The body of a typical vertebra (**Fig. 33-1**) is the solid portion that lies anteriorly. Opposite the vertebral body is the spinous process (the bony segment felt down the back). Projecting laterally from each side of each vertebra are the transverse processes. The lamina is the curved portion of bone joining the transverse processes to the spinous process. The vertebrae may be fractured in the same way that other bones in the body are. The most common fractures of the vertebral column are vertebral body compression fractures. Between the vertebral body and the spinous process is the spinal foramen, the cavity through which the spinal cord passes.

The Cervical Vertebrae

The seven cervical vertebrae are the smallest. Unique to the first six cervical vertebrae is the foramen transversarium. This foramen allows for the passage of the vertebral arteries through the six vertebral bones. **Figure 33-2** shows the atlas (C1), which articulates with the occipital bone and the axis (C2). The axis has an odontoid process (the only vertebra that does), which permits the atlas to articulate directly and provides rotation of the head. Trauma to the odontoid process may result in one of three fracture types and is rarely associated with cord injury.

The Thoracic Vertebrae. The 12 thoracic vertebrae (**Fig. 33-3**) have points of attachment for the ribs to help support the chest musculature.

The Lumbar Vertebrae. The five lumbar vertebrae (**Fig. 33-4**) are the largest; they support the back muscles. Their vertebral disks are the most frequently herniated.

The Sacral Vertebrae. The five sacral vertebrae (**Fig. 33-5**) are fused to form the sacrum, a frequent point of low back pain.

The Coccygeal Vertebrae. Depending on the individual, four vertebrae are fused to form the coccyx (**Fig. 33-5**).

33.2 INTERVERTEBRAL DISKS

Between each of the lumbar, thoracic, and cervical vertebrae excluding the atlas and axis is an intervertebral disk. These fibrocartilaginous disks absorb shock and reduce the pressure between one vertebra and another. The outer portion of the disk is called the annulus fibrosus. The center portion of the disk is a gelatinous material called the nucleus pulposus. Unexpected movement and/or force may "rupture" the disk, forcing the nucleus pulposus out of position. When out of position, the disk may impinge on the spinal canal, the spinal cord, or the emerging spinal nerves.

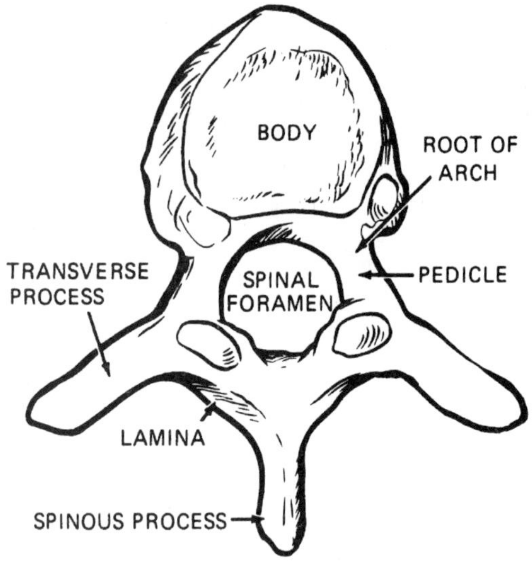

Figure 33-1. Typical vertebra.

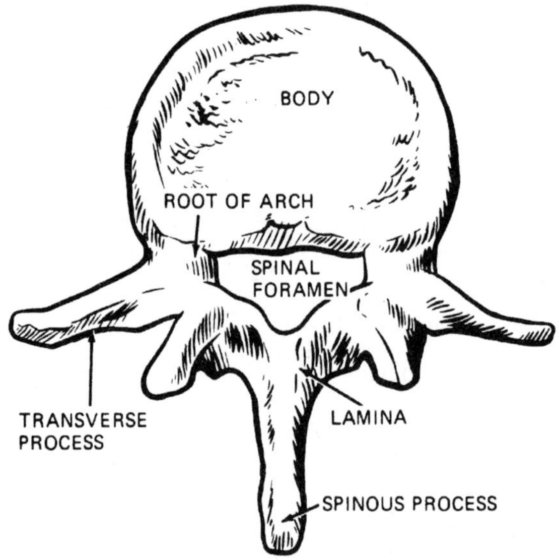

Figure 33-3. Thoracic vertebra.

33.3 LIGAMENTS

A series of ligaments support the vertebral column. The anterior and posterior ligamentous structures support the vertebral column and help support the spinal cord. The series of ligaments that join various segments of the vertebral column give it stability. Disruption of the ligaments can lead to instability and movement of the bony structures of the vertebral column into the spinal cord.

It is very common for the spinal cord to be damaged by extreme hyperextension, hyperflexion, and rotational or axial loading forces (**Fig. 33-6**). Damage may occur with or without fracture of the vertebrae.

33.4 THE SPINAL CORD

The spinal cord is the second major component of the central nervous system (the brain is the other) and is vital for life.

The spinal cord (**Fig. 33-7**) is continuous with the medulla oblongata in the brainstem. It is located in the spinal canal and is protected by the vertebral column. The cord is some 25 cm shorter than the vertebral column. Within the vertebral column, the spinal cord extends from the foramen magnum to the first to second lumbar vertebrae. Its tapered end is called the conus medullaris. The filum terminale is a group of fibers extending from the conus medullaris at the level of L1 to L2 to the first coccygeal vertebra.

Structure of the Spinal Cord

The spinal cord is surrounded by the same meninges that encase the brain. Between the L1 and S2 vertebrae, the arachnoid membrane enlarges to form the space known as the lumbar cistern. This is the space accessed during a lumbar puncture.

The spinal cord has a minute cavity in its center known as the central canal. It is an extension of the fourth ventricle and contains cerebrospinal fluid (CSF).

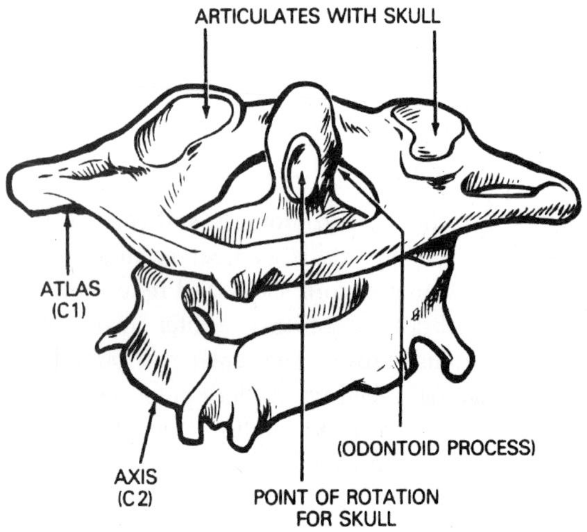

Figure 33-2. Articulation of C1 and C2 vertebrae.

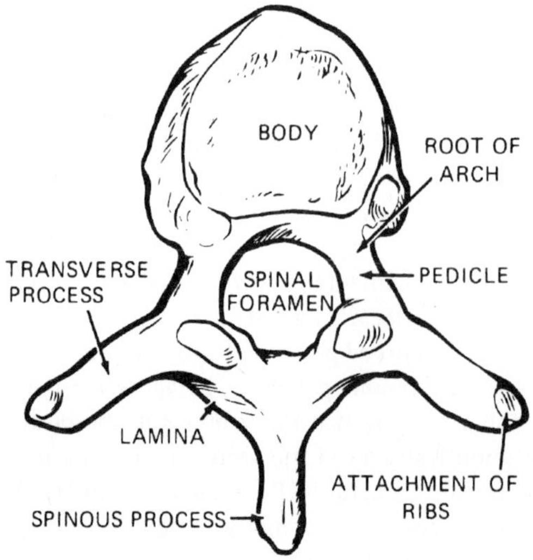

Figure 33-4. Lumbar vertebra.

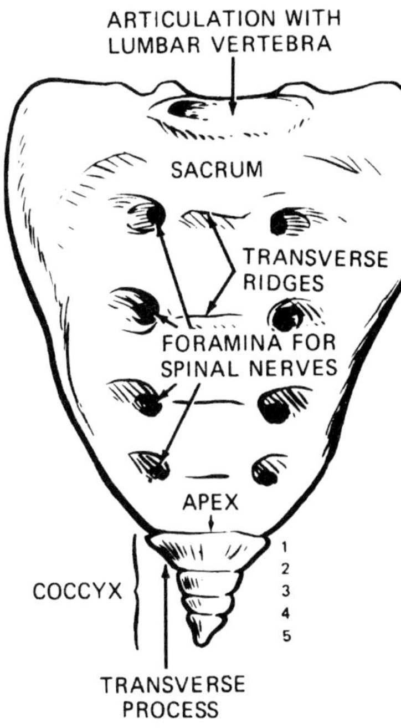

Figure 33-5. Sacral vertebrae and coccyx.

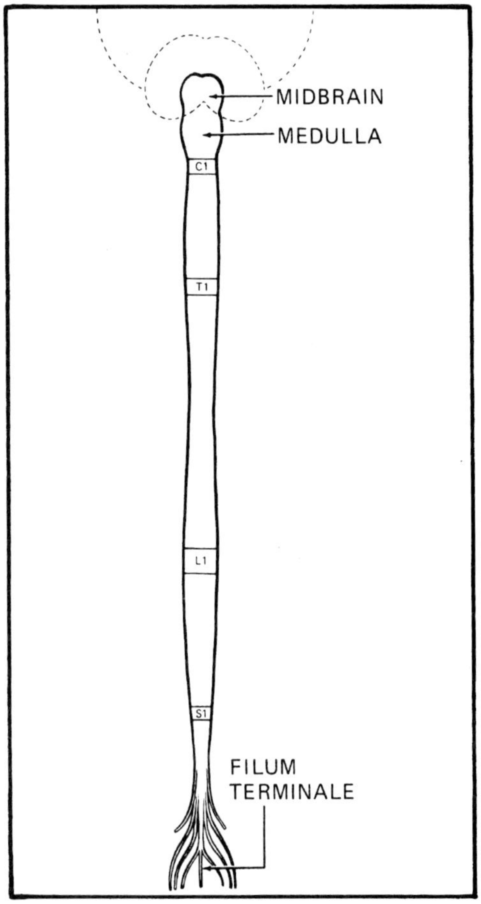

Figure 33-7. Spinal cord.

The spinal cord is composed of both white (myelinated) and gray (unmyelinated) tissue. The gray matter appears to be shaped like an H, which is surrounded by white matter (**Fig. 33-8**). The amount of gray matter varies with its location in the vertebral column.

Gray matter is composed of nerve cells and unmyelinated fibers arranged in three columns (**Fig. 33-9**). The anterior gray columns are also known as the anterior horns. They contain cell bodies of efferent (motor) fibers. The middle gray columns, known as the lateral columns, contain preganglionic fibers of the autonomic nervous system. The lateral columns are largest in the upper cervical, thoracic, and midsacral regions. The posterior columns, also known as the posterior horns, contain cell bodies of afferent (sensory) fibers.

The white matter (myelinated) is arranged in three columns called the anterior, lateral, and posterior funiculi (**Fig. 33-10**). Within these columns are ascending (sensory) and descending (motor) tracts termed fasciculi (**Fig. 33-11**).

The significant ascending tracts are the fasciculus gracilis, fasciculus cuneatus, lateral spinothalamic tract, anterior

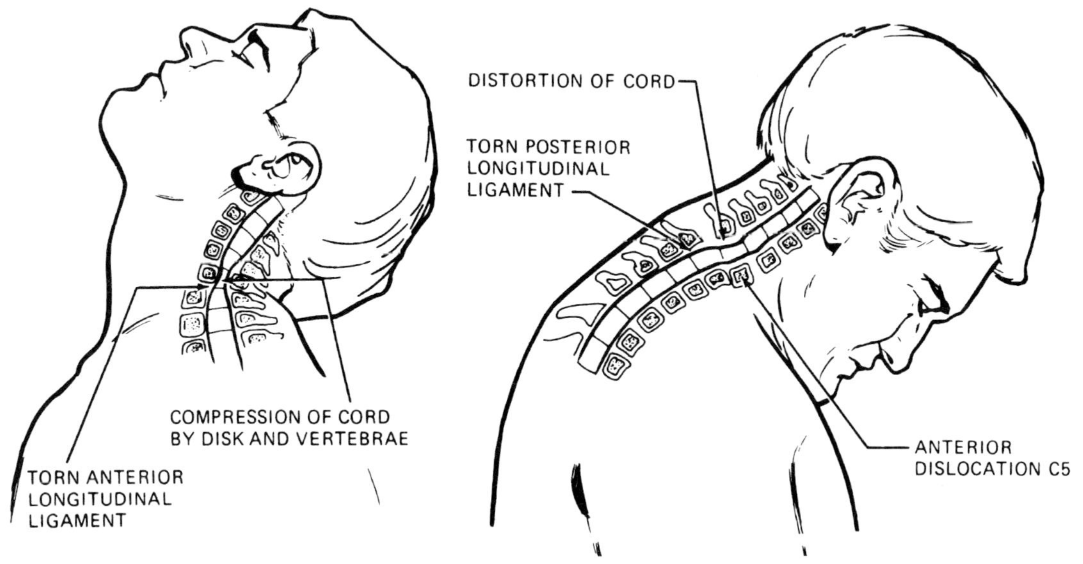

Figure 33-6. Hyperextension and hyperflexion of the spinal cord.

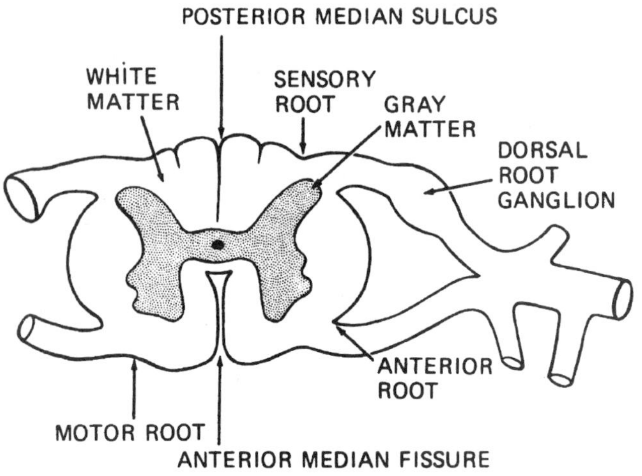

Figure 33-8. Gray and white matter of the spinal cord (cross section).

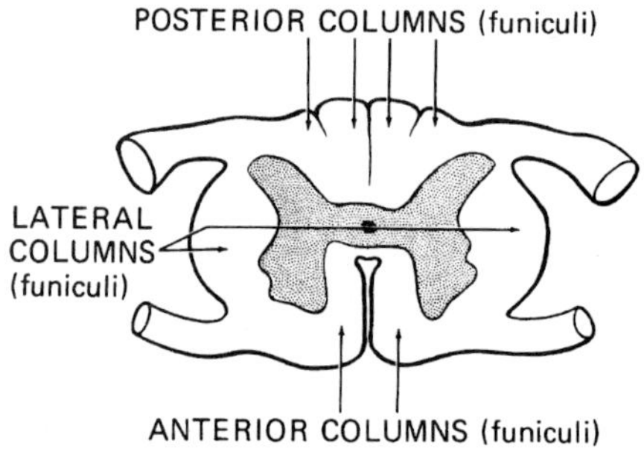

Figure 33-10. Funiculi of white matter in the spinal cord.

spinothalamic tract, dorsal and ventral spinocerebellar tracts, and spinotectal tract. These tracts carry sensory impulses.

The significant descending tracts (**Fig. 33-11**) are the rubrospinal tract, ventral and lateral corticospinal tracts, and tectospinal tract. These carry motor impulses.

Lower motor neurons are spinal and cranial motor neurons that directly innervate muscles. Lesions cause flaccid paralysis, muscular atrophy, and absence of reflex responses. Upper motor neurons in the brain and spinal cord activate lower motor neurons. Lesions cause spastic paralysis and hyperactive reflexes.

33.5 SPINAL CORD INJURIES

Motor vehicle accidents and unintentional falls are the leading mechanisms of spinal cord injury. Injuries also occur due to gunshot wounds, physical violence, and sports-related injuries. About 78% of individuals with spinal cord injuries (SCI) are male and two-thirds of all injuries occur in persons younger than 30 years. However, older adults are more susceptible to spinal injuries related to their increase risk for falls and the presence of underlying conditions. Over 50% of SCI involve the cervical region of the spinal cord. SCI cause varying degrees of motor and sensory loss below the level of injury. Similar to brain injury, deficits are due to both the initial impact (primary injury) and ongoing physiologic changes (secondary injury).

- Hyperflexion injuries usually accompany head-on collisions and result in a sudden deceleration type of force. This type of injury results in flexion of the neck and disruption of the posterior ligaments and compression of the anterior vertebral column.
- Hyperextension injuries are associated with rear-end collisions. Rotational forces produce lateral rotation of the vertebral column, disrupting the ligaments and producing instability of the column.
- Axial loading injuries are associated with diving mishaps where force is exerted onto the spinal column. Burst fractures of the body and disruption of the posterior bony segments of the column occur.

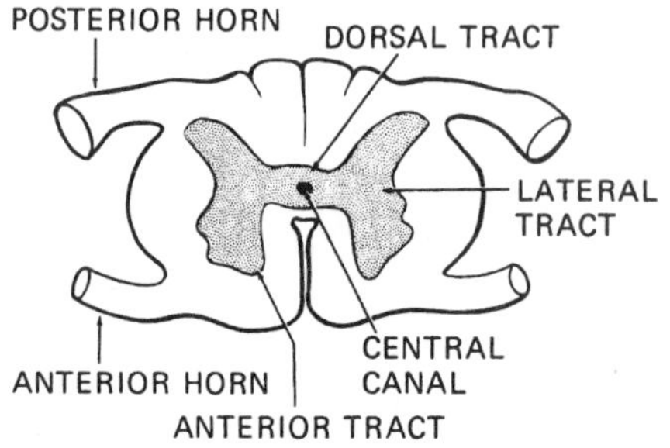

Figure 33-9. Columns (tracts) of gray matter in the spinal cord (cross section).

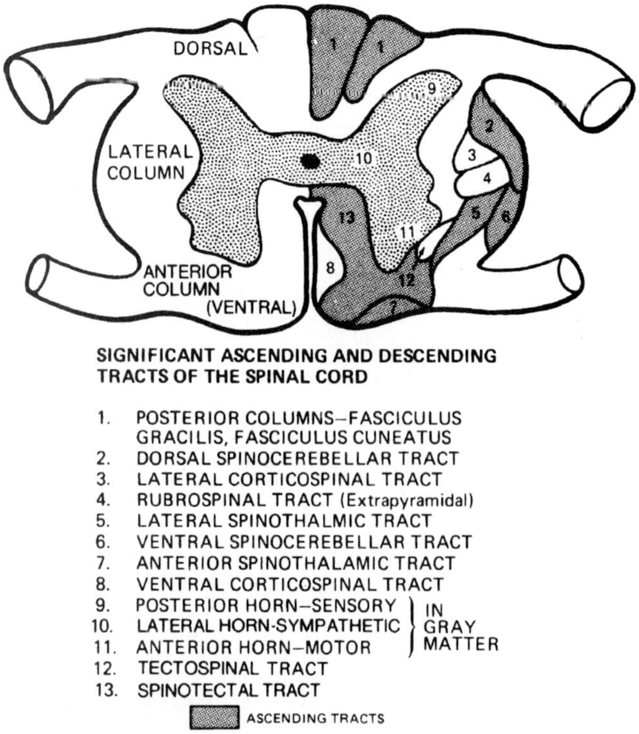

Figure 33-11. Significant ascending and descending tracts of the spinal cord. The left half of the picture is a mirror image of the right half.

- Penetrating forces cause an array of injuries due to penetration through bone, ligaments, meninges, and spinal cord. The end result of these forces is fractures of the bones, disruption of ligaments, and damage to the fragile spinal cord.

Damage to the spinal cord can be characterized as concussion, contusion, laceration, transection, hemorrhage, or damage to the blood vessels supplying the spinal cord.

- Concussion causes temporary loss of function.
- Contusion is bruising of the spinal cord that includes bleeding into the spinal cord, subsequent edema, and possible neuronal death from compression due to edema or tissue damage.
- Laceration occurs when a tear in the spinal cord occurs that results in permanent injury. Contusion, edema, and cord compression can be seen with a laceration.
- Transection is a severing of the spinal cord resulting in complete loss of function below the level of injury.
- Hemorrhage is bleeding that occurs in and around the spinal cord and can result in edema and cord compression.
- Damage to the blood vessels that supply the spinal cord can result in ischemia and infarction.

SCIs can also be categorized as stable (ligaments are intact preventing movement of the vertebral bodies and bones into the spinal canal) or unstable (ligaments are disrupted and allow the vertebral bodies and bones to move, possibly injuring the spinal cord). Injuries may be classified according to the injury to the vertebral column. Such injuries include simple fracture, compression fracture, comminuted fracture, teardrop fracture, dislocation, subluxation, and fracture/dislocation. Injuries may also be classified in relation to the specific level of injury. These injuries are summarized in **Table 33-1**.

Disruption of the ligaments causing vertebral movement into the spinal canal, fractures of the vertebra, and/or disruption of the disks may injure the fragile spinal cord. A SCI often results in fractures and compression of the vertebrae, which then crush and result in axonal injury. SCIs are classified as either complete or incomplete. A *complete injury* involves a total lack of sensory and motor function below the level of injury. In an *incomplete injury*, some motor or sensory function is maintained below the injury.

Additional complications that may result from a SCI are *respiratory impairment* (inability to breathe without a ventilator to diminished thoracic cavity excursion limiting tidal volume and cough reflex), inability to regulate blood pressure (BP), variability in heart rate, reduced control of body temperature, an inability to sweat below the level of injury, skin breakdown due to loss of sensation, deep vein thrombus/pulmonary emboli, increased susceptibility to respiratory disease, sexual dysfunction, urine/bowel dysfunction, hypertrophic ossification, autonomic dysreflexia, and chronic pain. The psychological impact of SCI includes depression, perceived altered body image, anxiety, and lack of independence.

Classification of Spinal Cord Injuries

The severity of an injury depends on the level of the spinal cord that is affected. Tetraplegia (quadriplegia) results from injuries to the spinal cord in the cervical (neck) region, with associated loss of muscle strength in all four extremities. Paraplegia results from injuries to the spinal cord in the thoracic or lumbar areas, resulting in paralysis of the legs and lower body. A **complete SCI** *produces total loss of all motor and sensory functions below the level of injury*. Nearly 50% of all SCIs are complete. The level of injury may be cervical, thoracic, or lumbar.

Incomplete cord lesion involvement (or partial transection) leaves some tracts intact. The degree of sensorimotor loss is variable depending on the level of lesion. There are a number of incomplete lesions.

When the damage is in the cervical central cord, it is termed **central cord syndrome**, which is characterized by microscopic hemorrhage and edema of the central cord (**Fig. 33-12**). There is motor weakness in both the upper and lower extremities, but the *weakness is much greater in the upper extremities than the lower. Sensory dysfunction varies according to the site of injury or lesion but is generally more pronounced in the upper extremities.* Reflexes in the lower extremities may be hyperactive temporarily. This syndrome is frequently due to hyperextension of an

TABLE 33-1. CLASSIFICATION OF INJURY ACCORDING TO SPECIFIC VERTEBRAL LEVEL

Injury Level	*Intact Function*	*Lost Function*
Below L2	Mixed motor/sensory, depending on intact nerve fibers	Mixed motor/sensory; possibly bladder, bowels, and sexual functioning
T1 to L1 or L2	Arm function	Loss of intercostal muscles, leg functions; bladder, bowels, and sexual functioning
C7, C8	Arm movement include deltoids, biceps, and triceps muscles, head rotation, respiration	No intrinsic muscles of hand; no other function retained above
C6, C7	Biceps muscle, head rotation, respiration	No triceps; no other function retained
C5, C6	Gross arm movement, head rotation, diaphragmatic respiration	No other function retained
C4, C5	Head rotation, diaphragmatic respiration	No other function intact
C3, C4	Head rotation	No other function intact (many die)
C1, C2	None	Poor prognosis

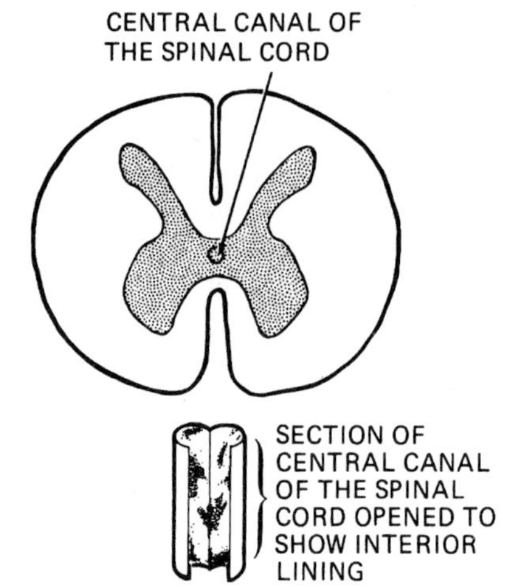

Figure 33-12. Central cord syndrome.

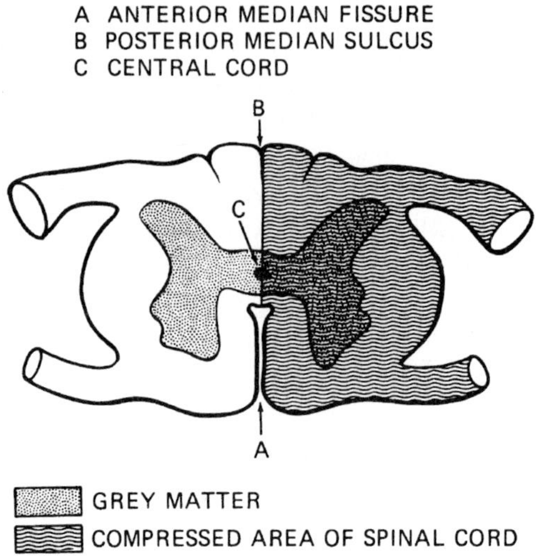

Figure 33-14. The Brown–Séquard syndrome.

osteoarthritic spine. It is the most common type of cord injury when there is no overt fracture or dislocation. The extent of recovery depends on the resolution of edema and the intactness of the spinal cord tracts. As improvement occurs, it proceeds from proximal to distal parts.

Anterior cord syndrome is characterized by injury resulting in an acute compression of the anterior portion of the spinal cord, often a flexion injury (**Fig. 33-13**). Compression is usually caused by a disk or bony fragment. It may also be caused by the actual destruction of the anterior cord by an anterior spinal artery occlusion (thrombus). Symptoms include immediate *anterior paralysis, which is complete from the injury or compression down. Hypesthesia (decreased sensation) and hypalgesia (decreased pain sensation) occur below the level of injury. Since the posterior cord tracts are not injured, there are sensations of touch, position, vibration, proprioception, and motion.* If the syndrome is caused by the compression of the anterior cord from bony fragments, surgical decompression is indicated.

Posterior cord syndrome is extremely rare and is characterized by an isolated loss of proprioception (the ability to sense movement, activity, and location). Motor and sensory function are preserved. This is caused by the dorsal location of the proprioceptive tracts in the spinal cord.

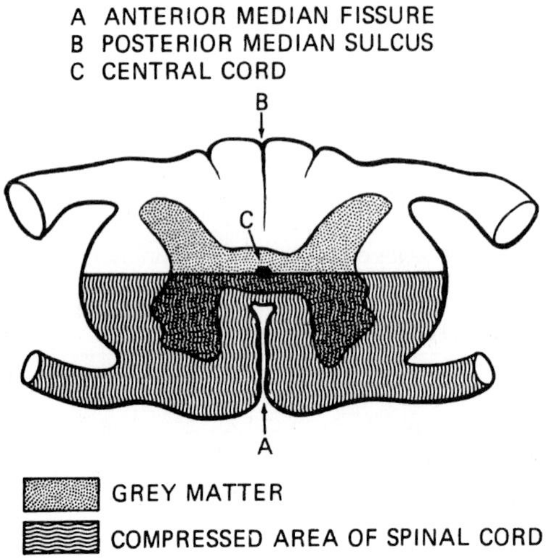

Figure 33-13. Anterior cord syndrome.

Brown–Séquard syndrome is due to transection or lesion of one-half of the spinal cord (**Fig. 33-14**). *There is loss of motor function (paralysis) and position and vibratory sense as well as vasomotor paralysis on the same side (ipsilateral) and below the hemisection. On the opposite (contralateral) side of the hemisection, there is loss of pain and temperature sensation below the level of the lesion or hemisection.*

> **QUICK TIP!** It is highly likely there will be a question in which you will have to distinguish between the different symptom characteristics of the cord syndromes.

Conus medullaris syndrome is compression of the last segment of the spinal cord. There is loss of bowel, bladder, and sexual function.

Cauda equina syndrome is caused by injury to the nerve roots below L1. There is motor loss to the lower extremities, variable sensory loss, and a reflexive bowel and bladder.

When the spinal cord has sustained an injury, various pathophysiologic processes follow the injury. Injury to the spinal cord produces edema and reduction in blood flow to the cord. The ischemia that ensues is followed by a number of intracellular changes leading to cell death. Two other pathologic processes may accompany SCI.

Spinal Shock. Spinal shock is a state where all reflexes as well as motor and sensory impulses are shut down below the level of the injury. Due to spinal shock, prognosis related to permanent loss of function cannot be determined until shock resolves. It generally occurs within hours of the injury and lasts for weeks. The resolution of spinal shock is manifest by return of the bulbocavernosus reflex and a state of hyperreflexia.

Neurogenic Shock. Neurogenic shock results from the *loss of normal sympathetic nervous system response* and commonly occurs following cervical and upper thoracic (above T6) cord injury. Peripheral vasodilation occurs, resulting in *hypotension and bradycardia. The bradycardia is caused by the unopposed parasympathetic tone of the vagus nerve.* The loss of the cardiac acceleration reflex prevents vasoconstriction and tachycardia. There is no sweating below the level of injury and hypothermia may present. Management of *decreased systemic vascular resistance* and decreased cardiac output includes administration of fluids, vasopressors, and other sympathomimetic agents. The choice of vasopressor has significant implications in the care of the patient. **Norepinephrine** has both alpha and beta activity which may improve BP and heart rate. **Phenylephrine** is sometimes chosen when limited to peripheral access but may potentially worsen bradycardia. **Atropine** should be at the bedside if profound bradycardia occurs.

KEY CLINICAL CONCEPT

Neurogenic shock is treated by managing the decreased systemic vascular resistance and cardiac output with fluids and vasopressors such as norepinephrine and phenylephrine.

Nursing Spinal Cord Assessment

Assessment begins with obtaining information on the mechanism of injury. Information is obtained related to any motor movement present at the scene of the accident. On arrival at the hospital, a functional spinal cord assessment is done, including motor, sensation, and reflexes. The motor examination includes assessing each muscle group of the upper and lower extremities. Assessment of diaphragm strength should be done to ensure adequate ventilatory ability. Each muscle group is graded on the 0 to 5 muscle strength scale.

- A 0 score represents the absence of motor strength
- 1 equals slight muscle contraction
- 2 is the movement of the muscle with gravity eliminated
- 3 represents motor movement against gravity
- 4 equals good movement against some resistance
- 5 is normal strength with resistance

The sensory examination includes assessing sharp versus dull in each dermatome, proprioception, and vibration sense in the upper and lower extremities. Reflexes are assessed for presence or absence. Rectal tone is assessed; the absence of tone is a sign of spinal shock and possible SCI. Other elements of the neurologic examination should be done to rule out concurrent head injury. These include the Glasgow Coma Scale, mental examination, cranial nerve examination, and vital signs.

Treatment

Treatment includes the *stabilization of the vertebral column*, prevention of further injury with movement, and monitoring for evidence of spinal or neurologic shock, autonomic dysreflexia, and complications related to the effects of the spinal injury. Early treatment in the initial 60 to 90 minutes is thought to limit or reverse neurologic deficit. Treatment consists of a number of interventions. During the course of treatment, the *cervical spine is immobilized with a cervical collar and in-line stabilization* is done to prevent movement and further injury. A backboard is maintained to prevent movement of the spine. The patient's airway and breathing must be assessed. If the patient is unable to maintain adequate oxygenation or ventilation, endotracheal intubation must be done while maintaining in-line stabilization of the cervical spine. Intravenous access is secured. Heart rate and BP are assessed. Generally, if the patient is hypotensive and bradycardic, **neurogenic shock** is the primary cause. *One way to differentiate neurogenic shock from hypovolemic shock is to feel the patient's knees to assess temperature. In neurogenic shock, the knees are warm due to vasodilation. In the presence of hypovolemic shock, blood loss causes the knees to be cold.* If the patient's mean arterial pressure (MAP) is less than 85 mm Hg, intravenous fluids and/or vasopressors are then administered. The use of steroids following SCI is not definitively recommended and should be balanced against the possible complications.

Other interventions include placement of a Foley catheter, an orogastric tube to decompress the stomach, and keeping the patient normothermic, as *poikilothermia (the inability to regulate core temperature)* can occur, with blankets. Primary and secondary surveys are completed looking for the presence of concurrent injuries. A complete neurologic examination is done to determine the presence of a head injury.

Following cervical spine X-rays, computed tomography (CT) scan, and identification of fractures, vertebral stabilization is secured. The goal is the prevention of secondary injury from the release of endogenous factors stimulated from the hypoxic and ischemic cord. Vertebral stabilization includes external devices such as cervical collars, cervical traction, halo vest, cervicothoracic and thoracolumbar orthoses, as well as surgical intervention. Surgery may be done early in the hospitalization if there is an intrusion into the cord space, or it may be delayed. Timing and the surgical procedure to achieve internal spinal fixation will vary with injury and physician preference.

QUICK TIP! One way to differentiate neurogenic shock from hypovolemic shock is to feel the patient's knees to assess temperature. In neurogenic shock, the knees are warm due to vasodilation. In the presence of hypovolemic shock, blood loss causes the knees to be cold.

Complications

Immediate postinjury problems are (1) maintaining a patent airway, (2) maintaining adequate ventilation, (3) maintaining an adequate circulating blood volume, and (4) preventing the extension of cord damage.

Respiratory System. Cervical injury or fracture may disrupt the diaphragm leading to diminished or absent respiratory function. **Injury or fracture above C5 presents special problems in that total respiratory function is lost. Remember that diaphragmatic function depends on C3 to C5. If this area is injured, artificial ventilation will be required to keep the patient alive.** Injury or fracture of C5 or the lower cervical vertebrae will result in diaphragmatic breathing if the phrenic nerve is functioning. Hypoventilation almost always occurs with diaphragmatic respirations because there is a decrease in vital capacity and tidal volume.

Since cervical fractures or severe injuries cause paralysis of the abdominal and frequently intercostal musculature, the patient is *unable to cough effectively enough to remove secretions; this leads to atelectasis and pneumonia.* Artificial airways provide direct access for pathogens, so bronchial hygiene and chest physiotherapy become extremely important. If multiple trauma is involved, neurogenic pulmonary edema may result from the sudden changes in thoracic pressures at the time of injury. The occurrence of pulmonary edema (as opposed to neurogenic pulmonary edema) is probably due to fluid overload. *Respiratory failure is the leading cause of death in the patient with SCI.*

Cardiovascular System. Any cord transection above the level of T5 abolishes the influence of the sympathetic nervous system. Consequently, the immediate problems will be *bradycardia and hypotension.* If the bradycardia is only slight, close cardiac monitoring may reveal a stable cardiac condition. Junctional escape beats may be observed and a junctional rhythm may become established. If the bradycardia is marked, appropriate medications (**atropine**) to increase the heart rate and avoid hypoxia will be necessary.

With the abolition of the influence of the sympathetic nervous system, vasodilatation occurs, decreasing venous return of blood to the heart. This decreases cardiac output, and hypotension results. Intravenous fluids may resolve the problem, otherwise vasopressor drugs may be required. **Dopamine** is an ideal agent due to its ability to increase BP and heart rate. The goal is to keep the MAP more than 85 to 90 mm Hg for a minimum of 7 days.

Because of the loss of vascular tone, the patient is at risk for deep venous thrombosis (DVT). Sequential compression devices and/or low-molecular-weight heparin are used to reduce the risk of DVT.

Renal System. *Urinary retention* is a common development in acute spinal injuries and spinal shock. The bladder is hyperirritable. There is a loss of inhibition of reflexes from the brain. Consequently, the patient will void small amounts of urine frequently. In spite of this, the bladder becomes distended, since this is actually urinary retention with overflow. Urinary retention increases the chance of infection. In addition, urinary calculi are likely to develop in a distended bladder that is retaining urine. Continuous catheterization is indicated in the early phase. As soon as spinal shock resolves, the indwelling Foley catheter is discontinued and intermittent catheterization every 4 to 6 hours instituted.

Gastrointestinal System. If the cord transection has occurred above T5, the loss of sympathetic innervation may lead to the development of an ileus or gastric distention. Intermittent suctioning by means of a nasogastric or orogastric tube may relieve the gastric distention, and standard treatment may be used for an ileus. A common occurrence in the past has been the development of biochemical stress ulcers due to excessive release of hydrochloric acid in the stomach. An H_2 antagonist is frequently used to prevent the occurrence of these ulcers during the initial extreme body stress. Because of the absence of clinical signs, any intra-abdominal bleeding that occurs will be difficult to diagnose. *There will be no pain, tenderness, guarding, or other signs or symptoms.* Continued hypotension in spite of vigorous treatment is suspicious. Expanding girth of the abdomen may be ascertainable, but not always.

If the rectum is not emptied on a regular basis, the patient may develop *fecal impaction.* Therefore, a bowel regimen is instituted as soon as possible with chemical stimulant agents and digital stimulation on a regular schedule. Nutritional support is instituted parenterally at first, followed by a transition to oral or enteral when peristalsis resumes.

Musculoskeletal System. The integrity of the patient's skin is of primary importance. Denervated skin can deteriorate very quickly, leading to major, life-threatening infection. The use of rotational beds (**Fig. 33-15**) can help to prevent skin breakdown. Turning the patient every 1 to 2 hours will relieve skin pressure points. In addition, meticulous skin care is required with frequent inspection to identify reddened areas or early stage of skin compression. A certain degree of muscle atrophy will occur during the flaccid paralysis stage, whereas contractures tend to occur during the spastic paralysis stage.

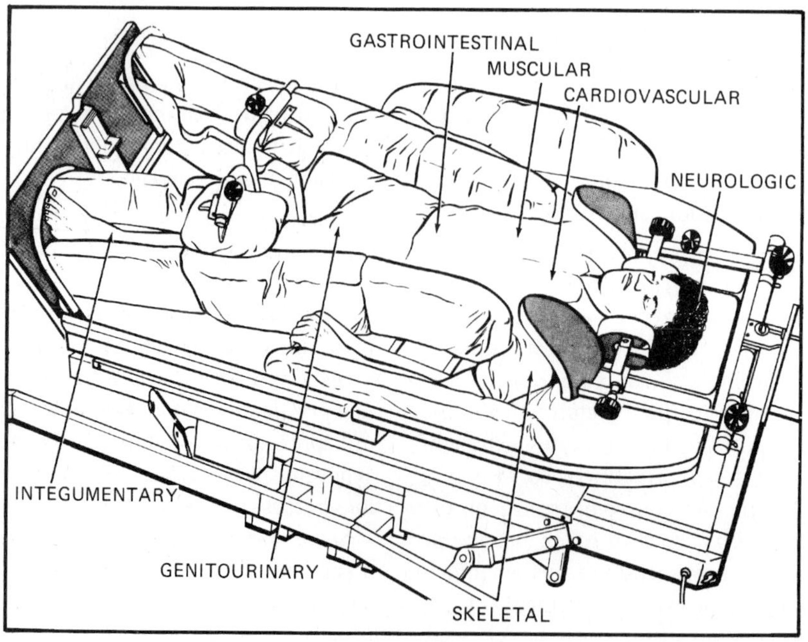

Figure 33-15. Roto-Bed.

Poikilothermy is the adjustment of the body temperature toward room temperature. This occurs in these injuries because the interruption of the sympathetic nervous system prevents its temperature-controlling fibers from sending impulses that will reach the hypothalamus. Keep the patient normothermic.

Metabolic Needs. Correcting an existing acid–base disturbance and maintaining acid–base balance will promote the function of other body systems. Recall that nasogastric suctioning may lead to alkalosis, and decreased perfusion may lead to acidosis. Electrolytes must be monitored until a normal diet is resumed and suctioning has been discontinued. A positive nitrogen balance and a high-protein diet will help to prevent skin breakdown and infections and also to decrease the rate of muscle atrophy.

KEY CLINICAL CONCEPT

With respect to how GI losses affect the pH: Remember that when GI losses *"come up"* (eg, excessive NG suction, vomiting), the *pH also comes up* (metabolic alkalosis). When the GI losses *"go down"* (eg, increased diarrhea), the *pH also goes down* (metabolic acidosis).

Nursing Interventions

The goal of nursing care is to prevent secondary injury and complication postinjury, prevent commonly occurring infections such as pneumonia and urinary tract infection, and begin planning for the patient's return home.

The primary nursing intervention is **ensuring a patent airway at all times** to provide for adequate ventilation. Most patients with cervical fractures will have an endotracheal tube or a tracheostomy. Frequent gentle suctioning of the nasopharynx, oropharynx, and endotracheal tube or tracheostomy is imperative to help prevent hypoxia secondary to retained secretions. *However*, suctioning must not exceed 10 to 15 seconds. It is recommended that Pao_2 be kept more than 80 mm Hg to help prevent the effect of hypoxia on the ischemic cord surrounding the injury.

The "quad-assist" cough should be done frequently to help keep the airway clear. The nurse places a fist or heel of the hand between the patient's umbilicus and xiphoid process and presses inward and upward when the patient coughs. After having been instructed, the patient is asked to take several slow, deep breaths. On the next deep breath, a quad-assist cough is initiated. Aggressive chest physiotherapy protocols should be followed according to neurologic and cardiovascular parameters. The patient's vital capacity, tidal volume, and arterial blood gases (ABGs) should be carefully and frequently monitored until he or she is stable and ventilatory support is no longer needed. Acceptable weaning parameters for a tetraplegic include a vital capacity of more than 15 mL/kg of ideal body weight and a $Paco_2$ up to 50 mm Hg.

Cardiovascular monitoring of dysrhythmias and hypotension is essential. The dysrhythmias that occur may require standard treatment or only continued close monitoring. Hypotension is often controlled with intravenous administration of fluids, which requires that the nurse monitor the patient for the development of pulmonary edema. Minimum MAP is 85 to 90 mm Hg for the first 7 days after the injury.

The prevention of extension of cord injury is the next major nursing responsibility. If traction is employed, the rope knots should be taped, weights hanging freely, and traction lines kept straight or as positioned by the physician. Sensorimotor assessment should be done with monitoring of vital signs.

Renal status is usually monitored hourly in the first few days following injury. The amount of intravenous fluids necessary to prevent hypotension is usually sufficient to prevent renal complications of oliguria or anuria unless there is multiple trauma involving the kidneys. The common renal problem after vertebral and cord injury above the sacral level is *urinary retention*. A Foley catheter is often used in the early stages of the injury. If a Foley catheter is not inserted, intermittent catheterization is needed to ensure that an excessive urinary volume is not retained in the bladder, leading to further problems.

Gastrointestinal interventions include initial drainage of the stomach contents followed by intermittent suction by nasogastric tube, since gastric distention occurs and acid secretions are increased in the first few days. Contents suctioned should be routinely monitored for blood, since biochemical stress ulcers may occur.

The patient's musculoskeletal needs include proper body alignment, support of bony prominences to prevent skin breakdown, and frequent turning (unless rotational bed therapy is used) to promote circulation and induce comfort. During the flaccid paralysis stage, extremities should be maintained in a functional position. During the spastic stage of the paralysis, medications and some physiotherapy may help control the spasms. Assessment should include motor testing every 4 hours. Prevention of thrombus formation is important and may include passive range of motion or use of antithrombotic devices.

The patient's metabolic needs are initially met with intravenous fluids. As soon as he or she is stabilized, tube feedings are often started. Depending on the site of the injury and the residual deficits, the patient may be able to start oral feedings relatively soon after the injury. Rarely is hyperalimentation used unless protracted treatment of multiple trauma is required. The patient should be weighed on admission and then at least weekly.

Autonomic Hyperreflexia

Autonomic hyperreflexia (formerly known as "*autonomic dysreflexia*") is usually seen with injuries to the spinal cord at the level of T6 or higher. The condition is a life-threatening situation requiring immediate attention.

The most common precipitating causes are a distended bladder or a full rectum. Contraction of the bladder or rectum, stimulation of the skin, stimulation of the pain receptors, or sudden change in environmental temperature may also cause autonomic hyperreflexia.

Symptoms include *extreme hypertension*, blurred vision, severe throbbing headache, unusual apprehension, marked diaphoresis, and flushing above the level of the lesion with pallor and coolness below, bradycardia, piloerection (body hair erect) due to pilomotor spasm, nasal congestion, and nausea. *The hypertension can be so severe that the patient may suffer a stroke or myocardial infarction.*

Pathophysiology of this condition involves the stimulation of sensory receptors below the level of cord lesion. The intact autonomic system reacts with a reflex arteriolar spasm, which increases BP. Baroreceptors in the cerebral vessels, carotid sinus, and aorta sense the hypertension and stimulate the parasympathetic system. The heart rate decreases, but the visceral and peripheral vessels do not dilate because efferent impulses cannot pass through the cord lesion. ***The hypertension continues until it is blocked by medication and the source of the stimulation is resolved.*** Ganglionic blocking agents are used to interrupt the hyperreflexia state. Drugs used include hydralazine hydrochloride, nitroprusside, nitroglycerin, prazosin, terazosin, and diazoxide.

Nursing interventions in this very serious emergency include notification of the physician, assessment to ***determine the cause,*** and elevation of the head of the bed or putting the patient into a sitting position if possible. BP should be monitored every 3 to 5 minutes. *Abdominal palpation for a distended bladder* is done very gently to avoid increasing the stimulus. The *urinary catheter should be checked for a kink or irrigation performed* very slowly and gently to open a plugged catheter. A *digital rectal examination* should be done only after application of a local anesthetic ointment (Nupercainal) to decrease rectal stimulation and prevent an increase of symptoms. If signs and symptoms persist after the bladder and bowel have been thoroughly checked, the next step is to check the skin for irritation. Assess the room temperature for sudden change and apply appropriate intervention (blankets or cooling modalities) if necessary. The patient and family should be educated as to how to monitor for, prevent, and treat autonomic hyperreflexia.

QUICK TIP! A recurring theme with exam questions is that correct answers are often associated with being able to identify and/or treat the **underlying cause** of the problem or condition.

KEY CONTENT CHECKLIST

- ❒ Neurogenic shock is treated by managing the decreased systemic vascular resistance and cardiac output with fluids and vasopressors such as norepinephrine and phenylephrine.
- ❒ One way to differentiate neurogenic shock from hypovolemic shock is to feel the patient's knees to assess temperature. In neurogenic shock, the knees are warm due to vasodilation. In the presence of hypovolemic shock, blood loss causes the knees to be cold.
- ❒ Injury or fracture above C5 presents special problems in that total respiratory function is lost. Remember that diaphragmatic function depends on C3 to C5. If this area is injured, artificial ventilation will be required to keep the patient alive.
- ❒ Acceptable ventilator weaning parameters for a tetraplegic include a vital capacity of more than 15 mL/kg of ideal body weight and a $Paco_2$ up to 50 mm Hg.
- ❒ With respect to how GI losses effect the pH: Remember that when GI losses *"come up"* (eg, excessive NG suction, vomiting), the *pH also comes up* (metabolic alkalosis). When the GI losses *"go down"* (eg, increased diarrhea), the *pH also goes down* (metabolic acidosis).
- ❒ Autonomic hyperreflexia is a life-threatening condition with extreme hypertension caused by stimulation of sensory receptors below the level of injury. Treatment includes identifying the cause such as bladder distention, constipation or abrupt temperature change, and administering ganglionic blocking agents to treat hypertension.
- ❒ It is highly likely there will be a question in which you will have to distinguish between the different symptom characteristics of the cord syndromes.

Review Questions:

1. Spinal cord injury above which level results in loss of respiratory function?

a. C3
b. C5
c. C7
d. T2

Answer: B. Rationale: Injury or fracture above C5 presents special problems in that total respiratory function is lost. Remember that diaphragmatic function depends on C3 to C5. If this area is injured, artificial ventilation will be required to keep the patient alive.

2. Anterior gray columns in the spinal cord contain cell bodies of which fiber type?

a. Afferent (sensory)
b. Efferent (motor)
c. Parasympathetic
d. Sympathetic synaptic

Answer: B. Rationale: Gray matter is composed of nerve cells and unmyelinated fibers arranged in three columns. The anterior gray columns are also known as the anterior horns. They contain cell bodies of efferent (motor) fibers. The middle gray columns, known as the lateral columns, contain preganglionic fibers of the autonomic nervous system. The lateral columns are largest in the upper cervical, thoracic, and midsacral regions. The posterior columns, also known as the posterior horns, contain cell bodies of afferent (sensory) fibers.

3. Treatment of autonomic hyperreflexia includes:

a. Identifying and treating cause, administering ganglionic blocking agents
b. administering ganglionic blocking agents
c. Performing bladder, bowel and skin assessment
d. Assessing room temperature for sudden change

Answer: A. Rationale: To treat autonomic hyperreflexia the underlying cause must be removed. Agents such as hydralazine hydrochloride, nitroprusside, nitroglycerin, prazosin, terazosin, and diazoxide are administered to treat the severe hypertension. However, the condition will persist unless the underlying cause is treated.

34

Encephalopathies, Coma, and Brain Herniation

CHAPTER OVERVIEW AND OBJECTIVES

The concepts covered in this chapter address the CCRN exam areas of encephalopathies, coma, and brain herniation. Expect one to three questions on the content of this chapter. After studying this chapter, you should understand the following:

- Identify the three reasons of changes in level of consciousness occur.
- Define the terms used to describe level of consciousness.
- Identify clinical symptoms of herniation.
- Identify clinical exam features consistent with brain death.

34.1 ENCEPHALOPATHIES

Encephalopathy is a term used for any diffuse disease of the brain that alters brain function or structure. It is the result of any disease that changes the structures of the brain or its functions. There are a number of different causes, including infectious diseases (bovine spongiform encephalopathy, Reye syndrome, Lyme disease), thiamine deficiency (Wernicke's encephalopathy), abnormal metabolic or mitochondrial dysfunction, exposure to toxic chemicals, liver dysfunction (cirrhosis), hypertension (hypertensive encephalopathy), and hypoxia ischemia (hypoxic encephalopathy). *The hallmark of encephalopathy is an altered mental state.* Clinical signs usually involve progressive loss of memory, changes in cognition, problems concentrating, depressed level of consciousness to complete loss of consciousness (LOC), myoclonus, tremor, muscle atrophy and weakness, dysphagia, aphasia, and nystagmus. If an infectious agent is the cause, other symptoms include fever and headache. If the infection affects the limbic area of the brain, personality and behavioral changes, delirium, and mental status changes can occur.

34.2 COMA (AROUSAL DEFICIT)

A coma is a profound state of unconsciousness and the severity and mode of onset of coma depends on the underlying cause. Level of consciousness is differentiated into two components: arousal and awareness. Alterations in arousal reflect changes in the state of wakefulness, while alterations in awareness reflect changes in the content and quality of interactions.

Changes in level of consciousness occur for three reasons:

1. Reduction in oxygen delivery
2. Reduction in blood glucose
3. Reduction in cerebral perfusion pressure

A change in the level of consciousness is considered the most important indicator of neurologic alteration. Decreased alertness and responsiveness represent a continuum that ranges from drowsiness to stupor (patient can be awakened only by vigorous stimuli) to coma, a deep sleep-like state from which the patient cannot be aroused. **Table 34-1** outlines the terms used to describe level of consciousness. Two general types of pathologic processes lead to coma: (1) conditions that widely and directly depress the function of the cerebral hemispheres and (2) conditions that depress or destroy brainstem-activating mechanisms. Common to all impairments is a reduction in either cerebral metabolism or cerebral blood flow.

Three categories of disease are important in the aforementioned pathologic processes that lead to coma:

1. A supratentorial mass lesion will encroach on deep diencephalic structures, compressing or destroying the ascending reticular-activating system.

TABLE 34-1. DEFINITIONS FOR TERMS DESCRIBING LEVEL OF CONSCIOUSNESS

Term	*Definition*
Alert	Awake and fully conscious and responsive
Drowsy	Sleepy but easily aroused and maintains alertness for brief periods
Confused	Disoriented to time, place, or person; may also exhibit agitation, restlessness, or irritability
Lethargic	Oriented but has sluggish response time for speech, motor, or cognitive activities
Obtunded	Arousable with stimulation; responds verbally or follows simple commands with stimulation
Stupor	Arousable only with vigorous stimulation
Comatose	Deep sleep-like state from which the patient cannot be aroused even with repeated noxious stimuli

Source: Adapted with permission from Chulay M, Burns S. AACN Essentials of Critical Care Nursing. New York: McGraw-Hill; 2006.

2. A subtentorial mass or destructive lesion may directly damage the central core of the brainstem.
3. Metabolic disorders may lead to generalized interruption of brain function.

Coma does not occur as a result of focal injury or ischemia in a specific lobe; it occurs only when both cerebral hemispheres or brainstem divisions are dysfunctional. The major catastrophe of coma is death due to brain herniation.

34.3 HERNIATION SYNDROMES

Herniation is the result of increased intracranial pressure (ICP) beyond compensatory levels. The rapid increase in size of a hematoma, tumor, or cerebral edema may cause the movement of brain tissue from an area of the cranium where it is normally located. The brain tissue is not evenly distributed, and unless the change is corrected rapidly, the impingement on blood flow and compression of the brain tissue will cause ischemia and permanent damage. This shift of tissue or protrusion through an abnormal opening is called *herniation*; it occurs from an area of greater pressure into an area of lower pressure. The most common type of brain herniation occurs when a portion of the temporal lobe is displaced (uncal herniation), resulting in compression of cranial nerve III, the midbrain, and posterior cerebral artery.

Frequent neurologic assessment and ICP monitoring are important parameters in monitoring for herniation syndrome. *Note:* Herniation can occur without fixed or dilated pupils and increases in ICP may be localized and not reflected by ICP monitoring, *however more classic findings are more likely to appear on the exam (if relevant to the question at hand).*

Herniation

The tentorium cerebelli divides the supratentorial structures (the cerebral hemispheres) from the infratentorial structures (the cerebellum). The tentorium cerebelli has an opening, the incisura or tentorial notch, through which the midbrain passes. As the ICP increases, movement of the brain tissue can occur, forcing the brain tissue from the area of higher pressure to an area of lower pressure. Herniation can occur above supratentorial and/or below infratentorial herniation. Four types of supratentorial herniation can occur: cingulate, central, uncal, and transcalvarial. Two types of infratentorial herniation can occur: tonsillar or downward cerebellar herniation and upward transtentorial herniation. The symptoms differ with the type and location of the herniation.

Supratentorial Herniation

Cingulate herniation or subfalcine herniation is a space-occupying lesion that causes lateral movement of the frontal lobe or unilateral hemisphere and forces the cingulate gyrus under the falx cerebri. The lesion may be a tumor, infarct, hemorrhage, or abscess and may present with accompanying edema. On computed tomography (CT) and magnetic resonance imaging (MRI), a midline shift is noted; contralateral swelling may occur secondary to cerebrospinal fluid (CSF) outflow tract obstruction.

In **central herniation**, increasing ICP forces the cerebral hemispheres and basal nuclei through the tentorial notch, compressing the diencephalon, mesencephalon (midbrain), and pons. Divisions of the basilar artery are also displaced, causing ischemia and brainstem deterioration. The displacement also blocks the aqueduct of Sylvius, effectively preventing the *downward displacement of CSF* (a compensatory mechanism of increasing ICP). This further increases ICP. Effects of central herniation usually *progress in a head-to-tail direction.* Thus, an *alteration in level of consciousness is often a subtle first sign of impending herniation.*

Uncal herniation occurs when the uncus (medial part of the temporal lobe) impacts on the tentorial notch. An expanding temporal lobe lesion and/or increasing middle fossa pressure may force the uncus over the edge of the incisura. This movement of the uncus compresses the mesencephalon (midbrain) against the opposite edge of the incisura. Uncal herniation often presses the oculomotor nerve and posterior cerebral artery against the incisura. The *earliest consistent sign of uncal herniation is a unilaterally dilating pupil accompanied by a change in the level of consciousness.*

Transcalvarial herniation is movement of the brain tissue, which is swollen after cranial trauma or penetrating brain injury with skull fracture, through the cranium. The bone flap can be removed in anticipation of additional swelling.

Infratentorial Herniation

Tonsillar herniation occurs when there is downward displacement of the cerebellar peduncles or tonsils through the foramen magnum. The earliest sign is nuchal rigidity. Changes in heart rate and blood pressure, small pupils, and ataxic respirations can occur. Coma and death follow compression of the brainstem and medulla.

Upward transtentorial herniation is rare. Presenting signs are nuchal rigidity, loss of upward gaze, and LOC. Cranial nerve deficits increase and posturing begins. Drainage of CSF from the ventricle can worsen the herniation syndrome.

Monitoring Parameters. Specific parameters that indicate impending or active herniation can be monitored. Serial CT or MRI can identify pathophysiology; management consists of prevention and control of ICP.

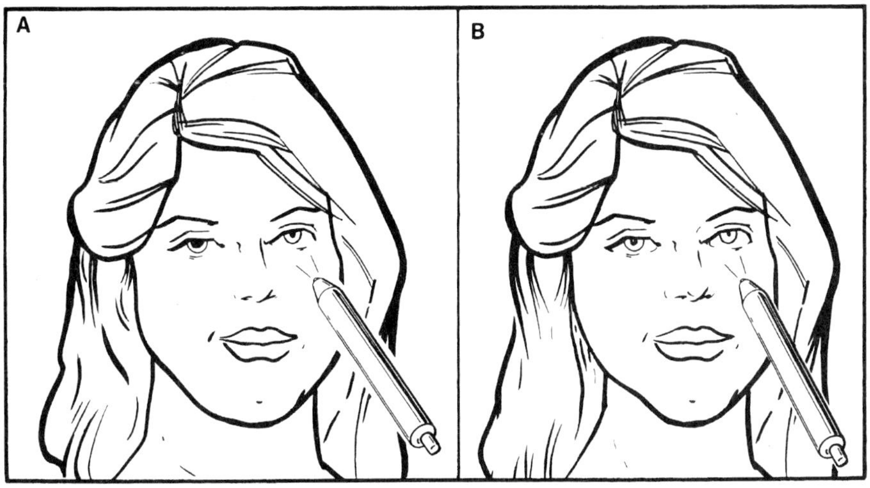

Figure 34-1. Pupillary light reflex **A** and consensual light reflex **B**.

In **central herniation**, the parameters are a decrease in the level of consciousness, pupillary function (small pupils to fixed, nonreactive midposition pupils to dilated, fixed, nonreactive pupils), respiratory pattern (Cheyne–Stokes respirations, central neurogenic hyperventilation, ataxic breathing patterns, and apnea), oculocephalic and oculovestibular responses (intact to disconjugate doll's eyes to no response), motor responses (localizes to pain to flexor/extensor posturing to quadriparesis), loss of cough and gag reflex, and deteriorating vital signs **(bradycardia and widening pulse pressure** on blood pressure monitoring).

In **uncal herniation,** *altered level of consciousness, contralateral hemiparesis, unequal pupillary response, and unilateral third cranial nerve palsy are early important signs.* Late signs include changes in respiration (central neurogenic hyperventilation or Cheyne–Stokes pattern), ipsilateral/nonreactive pupil, disconjugate oculocephalic reflex, and the presence of flexor/extensor posturing.

Parameter Norms and Testing Methods. Level of consciousness is explained in Chapter 32 and is not discussed again here.

Pupillary function is controlled by both sympathetic and parasympathetic tracts. These tracts are not easily affected by metabolic states. Therefore, the presence or absence of an equal pupillary light reflex is the single most important factor in differentiating metabolic from structural (neurologic) coma. The pupillary light reflex (**Fig. 34-1**) is best tested in a darkened room. In a normal state, the pupil will constrict when a light beam is directed into it. Normally, there is also a consensual response; that is, the pupil *not* having a light beam directed into it will constrict with the eye being tested.

KEY CLINICAL CONCEPT

The absence of an equal pupillary light reflex should be considered a sign of herniation in a patient with altered mental status and should be immediately evaluated with a CT scan.

The ciliospinal reflex is tested by pinching the skin on the back edge of the neck (**Fig. 34-2**). Normally, this action causes ipsilateral pupillary dilatation. The key eye movements observed in the comatose patient are (1) the spontaneous motion of each eye, (2) the resting position of each eye, and (3) responses of the eyes to the oculocephalic and oculovestibular tests.

The resting position of the eyes may be conjugate, disconjugate, or skewed. A conjugate position is any resting position with both eyes in the same position. A disconjugate position is a resting position with the eyes in different positions. Right eye midline, midposition, and left eye midline, fixed to the right side is an example of a disconjugate position. "Skewedness" refers to any vertical disconjugate positioning. Skewing indicates a brainstem lesion.

The oculocephalic response (**Fig. 34-3**) **is often called doll's eyes.** Doll's eyes can be tested only in the unconscious patient and is normally recorded as present or absent. To test the oculocephalic response, hold the patient's eyelids open and quickly but gently turn the head to one side. Make sure that the patient's cervical spine has been cleared before undertaking this test. The normal response is for the eyes to deviate conjugately in the contraversive direction of the head turning. Repeat by flexing and extending the head. Again, the *normal response is conjugate (parallel) contraversive movement of the eyes in relation to the*

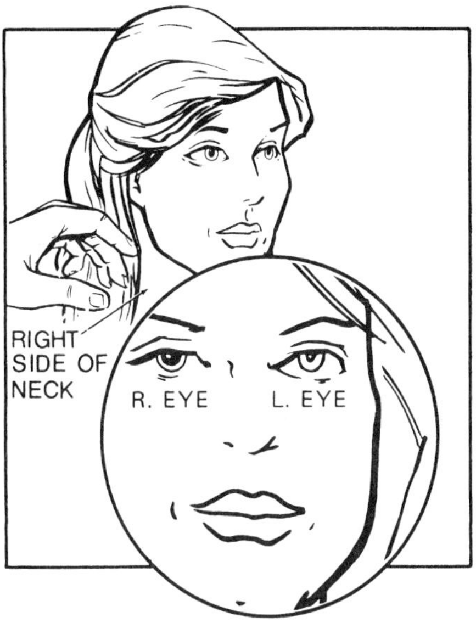

Figure 34-2. Pupillary response in the ciliospinal reflex (depicted in inset).

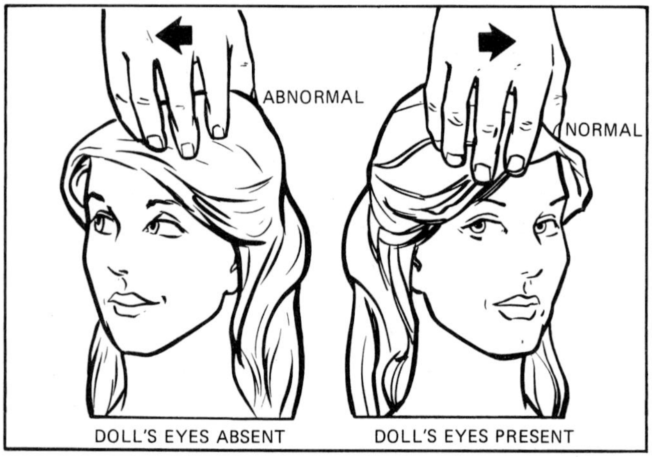

Figure 34-3. Oculocephalic response (doll's eyes phenomenon).

direction of head movement. This is recorded using the phrase **"doll's eyes present."** Abnormal responses are recorded using the phrase **"doll's eyes absent."** *If the eyes move in the same direction as the head is turned (ie, when the head is flexed, the eyes go down, or when the head is turned right, eyes go right or no further than midline), the test is abnormal* **(doll's eyes absent)**. This means that cranial nerves III, VI, and VIII, which are responsible for ocular movements, are *not intact.* Turning the head to both the right and the left will test each pair of these nerves. The oculocephalic reflex must *never* be tested unless injuries of the cervical spinal cord and vertebral have been ruled out.

The **ice-water caloric test,** in which the oculovestibular reflex is examined, is more powerful in eliciting eye movements. An intact tympanic membrane is essential for the test to be accurate. The head of the bed is elevated about 30 degrees. The physician slowly injects ice water until nystagmus (eye deviation) occurs (or until 200 mL of ice water has been used). *In the unconscious patient, the eyes move slowly toward the irrigated ear* and remain there for 2 to 3 min (**Fig. 34-4**). This indicates a supratentorial lesion or a metabolic condition. An extremely abnormal movement (skewing, jerky rotation) usually indicates a cerebellar or brainstem lesion. *The absence of movement indicates no functional connection between cranial nerves III, VI, and VIII.*

Motor responses are not dependent on level of consciousness but they usually correlate with LOC. Motor responses are important sources of information concerning the geographic spread of neurologic dysfunction. *If the patient is awake, ask him or her to hold both arms out in front with palms up and count to 10.* If the arms stay in the same position, there is normal strength. *If a palm rotates and drifts downward, then hemiparesis is present.* In the patients with altered level of consciousness who are unable to follow commands, observe motor movement to a stimulus. Use a central painful stimulus such as pinching on the trunk or pushing on the sternum. Note the motor response to the stimulation. *Localization represents a purposeful response*, and the patient moves to the stimulation site attempting to remove it. *Withdrawal of an extremity or body part away from the stimulus is the next lower response.* The cortex is not working at this level of response; the thalamus controls withdrawal. Lower-level motor responses to painful stimulation include abnormal flexion, abnormal extension, and no response, respectively.

Flexor posturing (decorticate posturing) (**Fig. 34-5**) is characterized by flexion of the arm, wrist, and fingers. Adduction of arms and extension and internal rotation with plantar flexion of the lower extremities complete the motor responses.

Extensor posturing (decerebrate posture) is characterized by opisthotonos (arching of the back so that the head and heels remain on the surface and the remainder of the back is raised) with the arms slightly extended, adducted, and hyperpronated (**Fig. 34-6**). The legs are stiffly extended and the feet are flexed in a plantar position. Respiratory patterns are discussed in Part II (Pulmonary) and are not discussed again here.

QUICK TIP! Remember in flexor posturing (decorticate) the arms flex inward "toward the cord." Extensor posturing (d-E-c-E-r-E-brate) has several "E's" in the name due to the "extensor" nature of the position. Decerebrate posturing is associated with a worse prognosis.

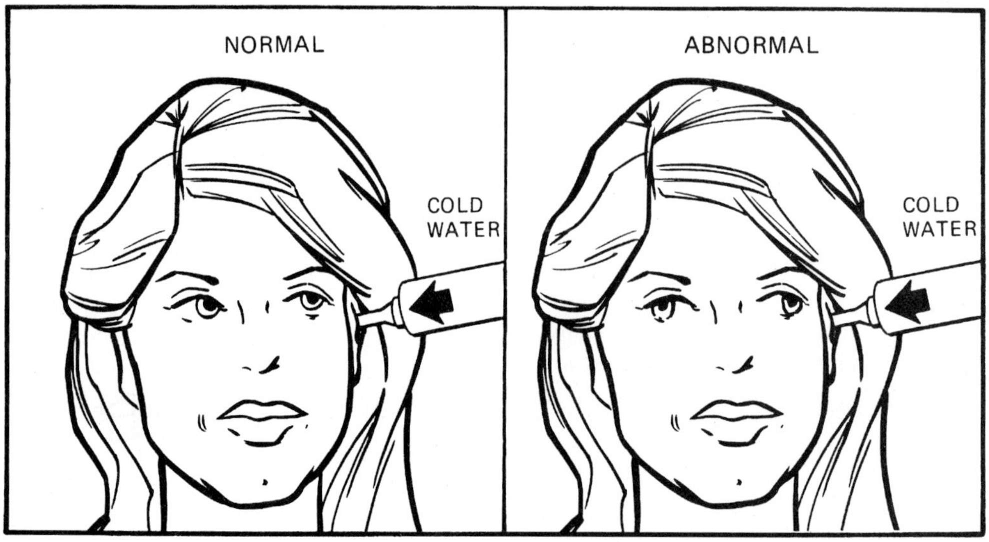

Figure 34-4. Pupillary response in the oculovestibular reflex.

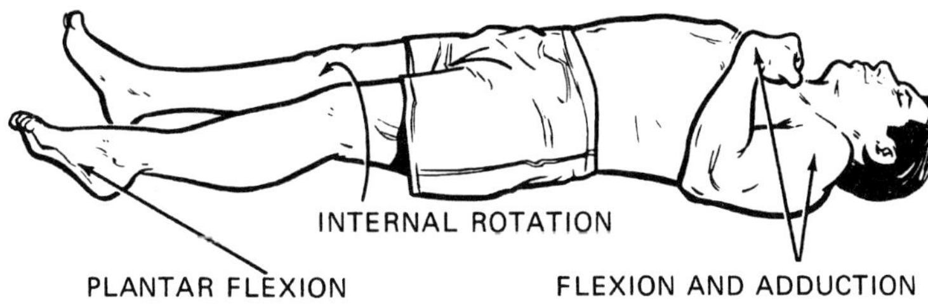

Figure 34-5. Decorticate posturing (abnormal extension response).

Table 34-2 identifies the stages and parameter responses in central herniation. **Table 34-3** identifies the stages and parameter responses in uncal herniation.

Herniation Through the Foramen Magnum

If the ICP rises precipitously, the pressure may be sufficient to compress the cerebellum and medulla oblongata through the foramen magnum. *A lumbar puncture performed in the presence of high ICP may result in brainstem herniation through the foramen magnum as the counterpressure in the spinal canal is lost.* Herniation through the foramen magnum results in death secondary to cardiopulmonary arrest. This form of herniation is not clinically separable from central and uncal herniation.

Brain Death

Brain death is a fatal condition, often following injury or loss of blood flow to the brain. Brain death is fatal regardless of whether life support is continued. Brain death is different from a persistent vegetative state, where essential brainstem activity remains but cortical function is lost or severely impaired.

The clinical evaluation for brain death includes establishing there is an irreversible coma of a known or proximately known cause. Patients must have achieved normal core temperature and normal blood pressure before assessment. Determination of brain death has several guidelines, including coma or unresponsiveness, absence of cerebral motor responses to pain in all extremities, absence of brainstem reflexes, and apnea. *A key part in identifying brain death is the detection of apnea.* Loss of brainstem function clearly results in loss of centrally controlled breathing, leading to apnea. Neurologic tests will show abnormalities consistent with loss of brain and brainstem function. These tests include the following.

Cerebral Motor Responses to Pain

Applying painful stimuli, for example, pressure to the supraorbital ridge and the nail beds, will *elicit motor responses* (no painful stimulus should leave a mark or injure the patient). All cerebrally modulated motor responses are absent in brain death. Some motor responses may occur during apnea testing because spinal cord reflexes remain.

Brainstem Reflexes

Pupillary Response. *The pupillary light response is absent in brain death.*

Ocular Examination. *The oculocephalic ("doll's eye") and vestibuloocular (caloric test) reflexes are absent in brain death.*

Facial Sensory and Motor Responses. *Corneal reflexes are absent in brain death* (tested by lightly touching the eye with a cotton-tipped swab).

Pharyngeal and Tracheal Reflexes. *Both gag and cough reflexes are absent* in patients with brain death (tested by suctioning and attempting to touch the carina). They can also be tested with a tongue blade (for the gag reflex).

Ancillary Neurodiagnostic Tests

Ancillary tests can be used when uncertainty exists, the exam is not considered reliable or the apnea test cannot be performed. However, ancillary tests are not required for the diagnosis of brain death.

Electroencephalography. One of the simplest tests for brain death determination is the electroencephalogram *(EEG). No electrical activity occurs during a period of at least 30 minutes of EEG recording in patients who are brain dead.*

Assessment of Cerebral Blood Flow. On conventional cerebral angiography, no blood flow is present in the brain in brain death (intracerebral filling is absent at the level of the carotid

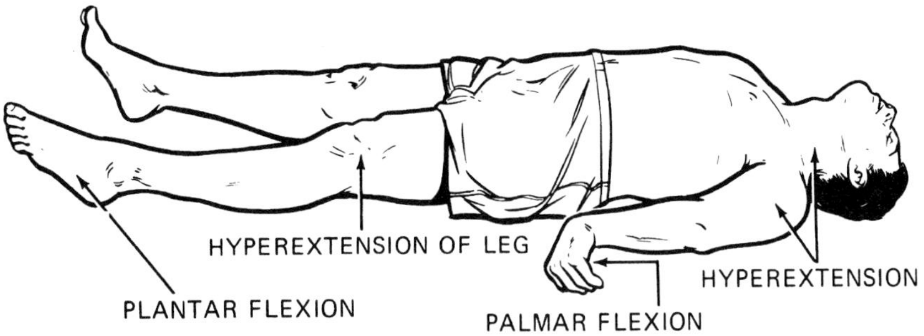

Figure 34-6. Decerebrate posturing (abnormal flexion response).

TABLE 34-2. STAGES AND PARAMETERS OF CENTRAL HERNIATION

	Central–Early Diencephalic	*Central–Late Diencephalic*	*Mesencephalon Upper Pons*	*Lower Pons–Upper Medulla*
Respirations				
Pupillary response				
Consensual light response	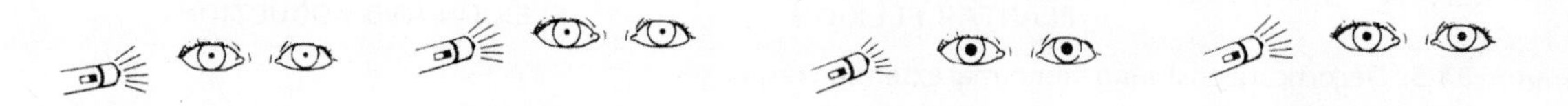			
Ciliospinal reflex	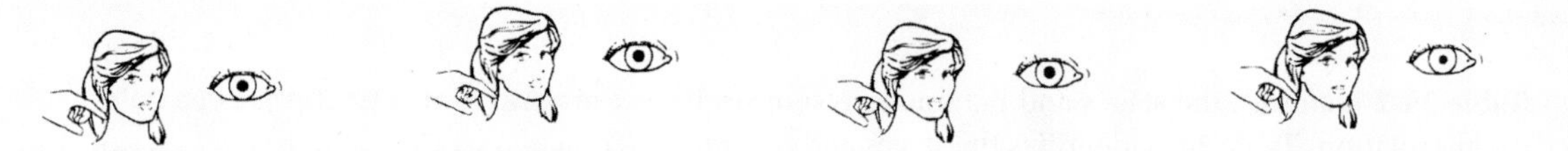			
Oculovestibular response	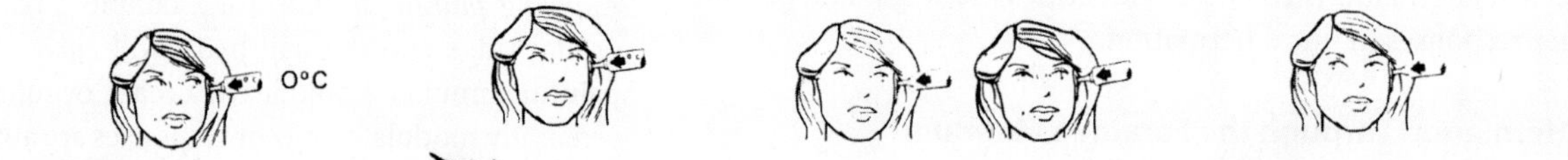			
Doll's eye response	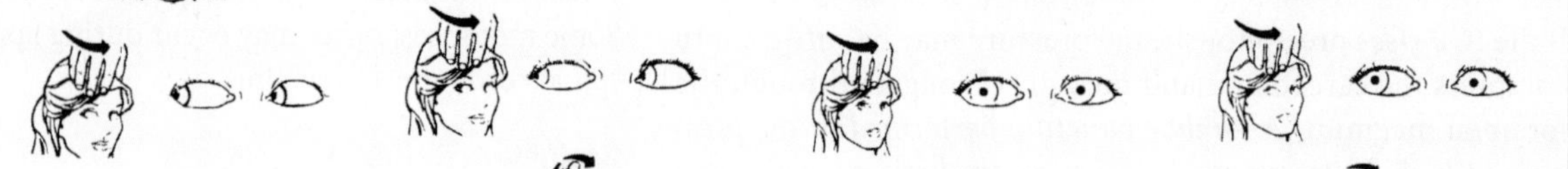			
Babinski response				
Body position response	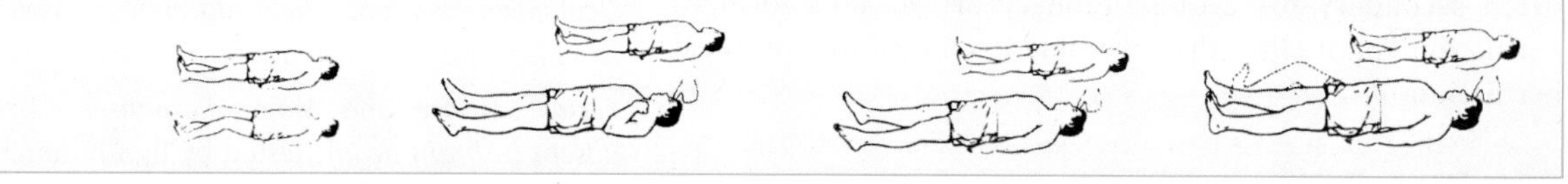			

TABLE 34-3. STAGES AND PARAMETERS OF UNCAL HERNIATION

	Uncal–Early Third Cranial Nerve	*Uncal Mesencephalon–Late Third Cranial Nerve*	*Lower Pons–Upper Medulla*
Respirations	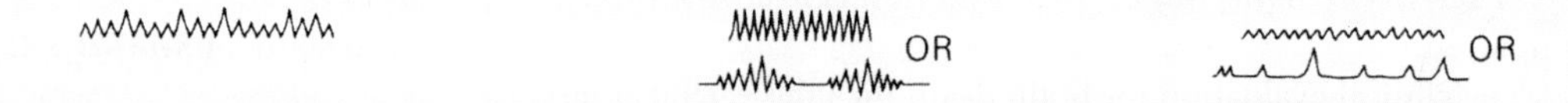		
Pupillary response	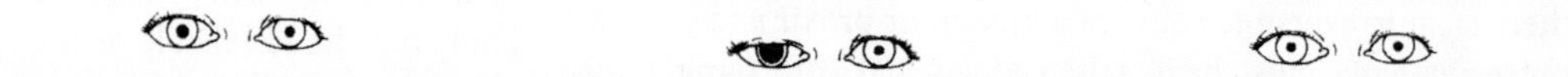		
Consensual light response	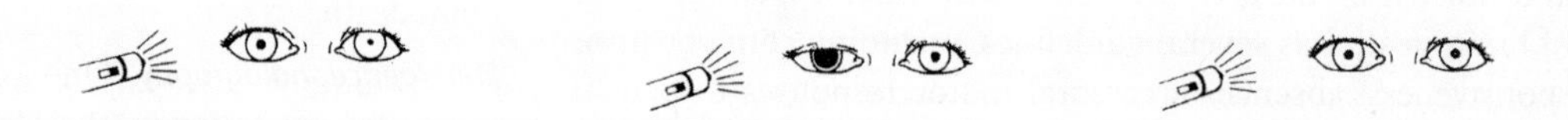		
Ciliospinal reflex	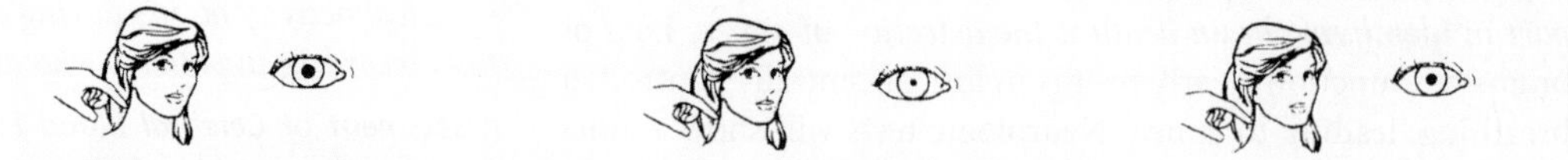		
Oculovestibular response	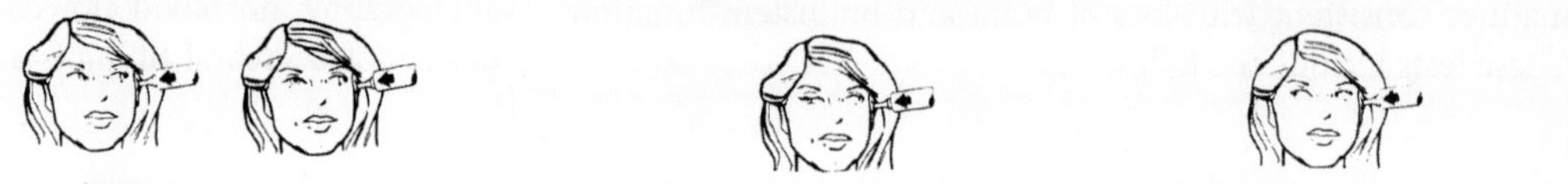		
Doll's eye response	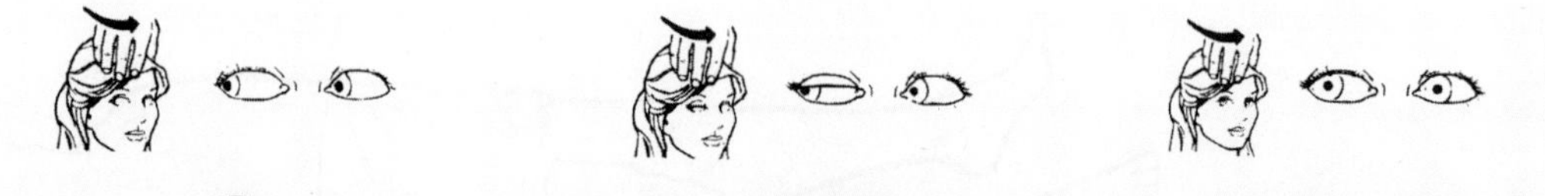		
Babinski response	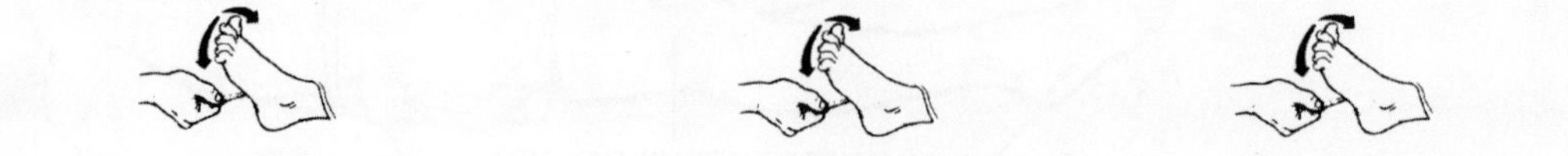		
Body position response	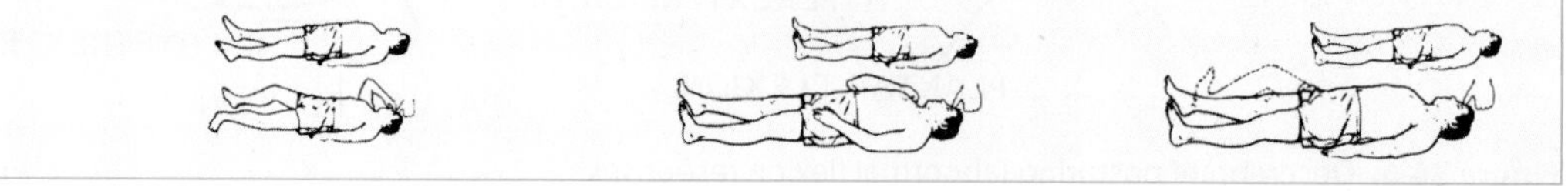		

bifurcation or circle of Willis). This can happen when the ICP is greater than the mean arterial pressure (MAP).

Transcranial Doppler sonography can also be used to assess blood flow. Absence of Doppler signals for blood flow indicates brain death.

MRI can be used to identify nonperfusion in the brain.

Somatosensory and Brainstem Auditory Evoked Potentials. In these tests of bilateral stimulation of median nerves, patients will have no response if they are brain dead. These tests may be less sensitive than perfusion studies or angiography.

KEY CONTENT CHECKLIST

- ❒ A change in the level of consciousness is considered the most important indicator of neurologic alteration.
- ❒ Be familiar with the distinguishing clinical features between the different types of herniation, such as central versus uncal herniation.
- ❒ Cushing's Triad is a set of classic late findings during herniation: (1) Bradycardia, (2) Irregular respirations, and (3) Wide pulse pressure (Remember pulse pressure = SBP – DBP).
- ❒ Know the differences between "Doll's eyes present" versus "Doll's eyes absent." When Doll's eyes are absent, there is a worse prognosis.
- ❒ The absence of an equal pupillary light reflex should be considered a sign of herniation in a patient with altered mental status and should be immediately evaluated with a CT scan.
- ❒ Remember flexor posturing (decorticate) the arms flex inward "toward the cord." Extensor posturing (d-E-c-E-r-E-brate) has several "E's" in the name to due to the "extensor" nature of the position.

Review Questions:

1. Impending uncal herniation is indicated by which of the following?

a. Decreased level of consciousness
b. Positive doll's eyes
c. Unilateral pupil dilation
d. Bilateral pupil dilation

Answer: C. Rationale: Uncal herniation occurs when the uncus (medial part of the temporal lobe) impacts on the tentorial notch. An expanding temporal lobe lesion and/or increasing middle fossa pressure may force the uncus over the edge of the incisura. This movement of the uncus compresses the mesencephalon (midbrain) against the opposite edge of the incisura. Uncal herniation often presses the oculomotor nerve and posterior cerebral artery against the incisura. Although decreased LOC is the most sensitive indicator of a change in neurologic status, the earliest consistent sign of uncal herniation is a unilaterally dilating pupil accompanied by a change in the level of consciousness.

2. Which of the following indicate brain death?

a. Loss of pain response in all extremities
b. Loss of Brainstem reflexes
c. Apnea
d. All of the above

Answer: D. Rationale: Loss of pain response in extremities, loss of brain stem reflexes and apnea must all be present in for the diagnosis of brain death. Any apnea test is performed for confirmation.

35

Meningitis, Guillain–Barré, Muscular Dystrophy, and Myasthenia Gravis

CHAPTER OVERVIEW AND OBJECTIVES

In this chapter, we address the concepts of infectious diseases of the neurologic system that will most likely be covered on the CCRN exam. Meningitis is more likely to be addressed than Guillain–Barré syndrome (GBS) and myasthenia gravis (MG). It is possible that a question or two will address GBS, particularly relating to the acute respiratory failure that develops in the advanced stages of this condition.

As you read this chapter, focus on infectious processes affecting the neurologic system. It will be useful to have a basic understanding of the other conditions, although it is unlikely that they will appear on the CCRN exam. Expect one to three questions on the exam to be based on the content of this chapter.

After studying this chapter, you should be able to:

- Identify clinical signs and symptoms of meningitis and appropriate nursing interventions.
- Identify the most serious complication of GBS and what test should be monitored for identification.
- Identify a major nursing intervention in MG.
- Differentiate between myasthenia crisis and cholinergic crisis

35.1 MENINGITIS

Meningitis is an acute inflammation of the pia and arachnoid membrane surrounding the brain and spinal cord.

Pathophysiology

A bacterial, viral, or fungal pathogenic organism gains access to the pia–subarachnoid space after gaining entrance to the central nervous system through local invasion of tissue or the bloodstream. After crossing the blood–brain barrier, it invades and causes an inflammatory reaction in the pia and arachnoid, in the cerebrospinal fluid (CSF), and in the ventricles of the brain. There is no host defense in the CSF allowing for rapid duplication of the pathogen. An exudate forms and very quickly enlarges, covering the base of the brain and extending through the subarachnoid space and into the sheaths of cranial and spinal nerves. Polymorphonuclear neutrophils (PMNs) attempt to control the invading pathogen. Within a few days, leukocytes and histiocytes increase in number to "wall off" the exudate from the pathogen or its toxins. Toward the end of the second week, the cellular exudate has formed two layers. The outer layer directly under the arachnoid membrane is composed of PMNs and fibrin. The inner layer is composed of lymphocytes, plasma cells, and macrophages and is next to the pia.

With appropriate drug therapy to destroy the pathogen, these two layers begin to resolve. The outer cellular layer against the arachnoid disappears. If the infection is arrested quickly enough, the inner layer will also disappear. However, if the infection lasts for several weeks, the inner layer, which contains fibrin, forms a permanent fibrous structure over the meninges. This produces a thickened, often cloudy arachnoid membrane and causes adhesions between the pia and arachnoid membranes.

The adhesions and prior inflammation result in the congestion of tissues and blood vessels. A degeneration of nerve cells follows, eventually resulting in congestion of adjacent brain tissue. This causes cortical irritation and increased intracranial pressure (ICP). Cerebral edema may lead to hydrocephalus. If uninterrupted, a progression of vasculitis with cortical necrosis, petechial hemorrhage within the brain, hydrocephalus, and cranial nerve damage occurs.

Etiology

Organisms obtain access to the subarachnoid space through penetrating head injuries, basal skull fractures with a torn dura mater, ICP monitoring, cranial surgery, mastoiditis, acute otitis media, lumbar punctures, injury to the paranasal sinuses, septic emboli, and sepsis. The organism may be fungal, viral, or bacterial. Eighty percent of all bacterial meningitis is caused by *Streptococcus pneumoniae, Neisseria meningitidis*, and *Haemophilus influenzae*. Other gram-positive bacteria include *Diplococcus pneumoniae*. Gram-negative bacteria include *Klebsiella, Escherichia coli*, and *Pseudomonas*. After neurologic surgery, *Staphylococcus aureus* or *Staphylococcus epidermidis* are common bacterial contaminants. In children, it is *H. influenzae*, although the incidence continues to decrease due to immunizations. Other bacteria include *Streptococcus, Pneumococcus*, and occasionally *Mycobacterium tuberculosis*. The outcome of bacterial meningitis depends on early and aggressive treatment. Viral causes of meningitis include enteroviruses, arboviruses, and herpes viruses. Viral meningitis is commonly referred to as aseptic meningitis. Fungal meningitis is primarily caused by *Cryptococcus neoformans*.

Clinical Signs and Symptoms

Suspect meningitis if a fever, severe headache, and nuchal rigidity (resistance to flexion of the neck) exist. **Positive Kernig's and Brudzinski's signs**, *photophobia*, decreased sensorium, and signs of increased ICP are common. **Kernig's sign** is the inability to fully extend the leg at the knee when the leg is flexed at the hip. **Brudzinski's sign** is the involuntary adduction and flexion of the legs with attempts to flex the neck. With meningitis, signs of increased ICP can include a progressively worsening headache accompanied by nausea, vomiting, irritability, confusion, and seizures. Dysfunction of cranial nerves II through VIII may be present. Increased ICP is secondary to purulent exudate, cerebral edema, and hydrocephalus. Changes in vital signs may also occur secondary to brain stem pressure. If the causative organism is the meningococcus, a *petechial skin rash* is common in 50% of cases. The rash progresses to purple blotches.

> QUICK TIP! To remember Brudzinski's sign, imagine the neck flexed as if it is forming the curve of the letter, "B." Whereas for Kernig's sign, imagine the leg flexed at the hip, like the leg is forming part of the letter, "K."

Diagnosis

Diagnosis is typically made by analysis of CSF, usually obtained via lumbar puncture. A major diagnostic tool is examination of the CSF. Variations in the CSF depend on the causative organism. CSF protein levels are usually elevated, more so in bacterial than in viral cases (**Table 35-1**). A decreased CSF glucose level is common in bacterial meningitis but may be normal in viral meningitis. In bacterial meningitis, the CSF appears purulent and turbid. It may be the same or clear in viral meningitis. The predominant cell in the CSF is the PMN.

TABLE 35-1. USING CSF CHARACTERISTICS TO DIFFERENTIATE BACTERIAL vs. VIRAL MENINGITIS

	Bacterial Meningitis	*Viral Meningitis*
Clarity	Cloudy/turbid	Clear
Glucose	Low	Normal
Protein	Increased	Normal
Gram Stain	Positive	Negative
Opening LP pressure	Increased	Normal or mildly elevated

Cultures of blood, sputum, and nasopharyngeal secretions are performed to identify the causative organism.

Roentgenograms of the skull may demonstrate infected sinuses. Computed tomography (CT) scans are usually normal in uncomplicated meningitis. In other cases, CT may reveal evidence of increased ICP.

Complications

The most common complication of meningitis is increased ICP and subsequent damage to the brain including residual neurologic dysfunction. Dysfunction of cranial nerves III, IV, VI, or VII often occurs in bacterial meningitis due to increased ICP. Usually this disappears within a few weeks. Hearing loss may be permanent after bacterial meningitis but is not a complication of viral meningitis.

Cranial nerve irritation can have serious sequelae. When cranial nerve II is compressed by increased ICP, papilledema is often present and blindness may occur. When cranial nerves III, IV, and VI are impacted, ocular movements are affected. Ptosis, unequal pupils, and diplopia are common. Irritation of cranial nerve V is evidenced by sensory and corneal changes, and irritation of cranial nerve VII results in facial paresis. Irritation of cranial nerve VIII causes tinnitus, vertigo, and deafness.

Hemiparesis, dysphasia, and hemianopsia may occur. These signs usually resolve within hours. If resolution does not occur, a cerebral abscess, subdural empyema, subdural effusion, or cortical venous thrombophlebitis is implicated and further investigation is warranted.

Acute cerebral edema may occur with bacterial meningitis, causing seizures (occur in one-third of patients), third nerve palsy, bradycardia, hypertension, coma, and death.

A communicating hydrocephalus may occur if the inner layer of the exudate has caused adhesions that prevent the normal flow of CSF from the ventricles. Surgical implantation of a shunt is the only treatment.

Endocrine dysfunction resulting in hyponatremia and excessive release of antidiuretic hormone may increase cerebral edema.

These patients will often present with septic shock. Careful measures should be taken to assure that the source of infection is thoroughly evaluated in these patients. In the pediatric patient, they will be more likely to present with signs of septic shock than with neurologic symptoms.

The most lethal complications are Waterhouse–Friderichsen syndrome and bleeding into the adrenal gland, which occurs as a complication of fulminating meningococcal meningitis and disseminated intravascular coagulation.

Nursing Interventions

Rapid identification of possible meningitis is imperative. Make sure that airway and breathing are adequate. Intravenous lines are started and blood cultures obtained. **Antibiotics** should be started within 30 minutes of the patient's arrival at the hospital. The antibiotic selected is based on the organism. Most often penicillin, ceftriaxone (Rocephin), and vancomycin are initiated until the organism is identified. Administration of antibiotics at scheduled times maintains a therapeutic blood level. Dexamethasone may be used prior to antibiotic therapy in patients with suspected bacterial meningitis in whom the causative organism is not yet known. Respiratory isolation precautions will protect the staff and visitors but need not be continued past 24 to 48 hours after the institution of antibiotic therapy.

Body temperature can be controlled by the administration of antipyretic drugs as indicated, use of a hypothermia blanket, and environmental temperature change.

Headache is usually treated with analgesics. *A darkened, quiet room will help both the headache and photophobia. Avoid sudden quick movements.*

Due to the high prevalence of seizures in patients with meningitis, seizure precautions should be initiated. If seizures occur, anticonvulsant medication is indicated. Documentation of progression, limb involvement, and duration of the seizures will help determine an effective medication regimen.

Supportive care including respiratory and hemodynamic support is imperative for patient survival. Dyspnea and respiratory distress require standard treatment. Severe cases are managed with mechanical ventilation. Profound shock may occur in bacterial meningitis, requiring intense vasopressor support and hemodynamic monitoring. A central venous pressure line or a pulmonary artery catheter may be inserted to monitor fluid balance and cardiovascular status. Monitoring of electrolyte levels, especially sodium, is essential. Standard nursing procedures for these types of complications are followed.

35.2 GUILLAIN–BARRÉ SYNDROME

GBS is a rare acute inflammatory demyelinating polyneuropathy of unknown etiology, which is characterized as an often *rapidly progressing, ascending symmetric paralysis.* Synonyms for GBS include Landry–Guillain–Barré–Strohl syndrome, acute inflammatory polyradiculoneuropathy, and infectious polyneuritis.

Pathophysiology

GBS causes progressive muscle weakness, sensory loss, and areflexia because of peripheral nerve demyelination. *The predominant pattern is weakness starting in the lower extremities and advancing (often very rapidly) to motor paralysis as it progresses up the body.* The progression may stop at any point.

The first pathologic sign of the syndrome is a perivascular lymphocytic infiltration. Following this, characteristic infiltration occurs in the myelin, breaking it down but not damaging the axon. This is called segmental demyelination. If the syndrome progresses, the infiltration becomes more intense and affects the axon, resulting in muscle denervation and atrophy. If the infiltration occurs in the distal segment of the axon, regeneration will occur because the nerve cell body has been spared. If the infiltration occurs at the proximal end of the axon, the nerve cell body may die and regeneration cannot occur. This is known as Wallerian degeneration. Collateral motor fibers may reinnervate the destroyed muscle, restoring the lost function partially or completely. As the infiltration process ends, *recovery of motor function begins proximally and progresses distally.* In the anterior horn cells and the neurons in the dorsal root ganglia, destruction of the Nissl bodies, which synthesize proteins essential for cellular repair and growth, prevents the recovery of function.

Diagnosis

CSF is normal or with low protein initially; however, after approximately a week CSF protein elevates with an otherwise normal cell count. This represents albuminocytologic dissociation (high protein/few cells), which is specific for GBS. Increased antibody titers in serum are seen, in particular IgM. Electromyography (EMG) and nerve conduction studies indicate a slowing or conduction block in motor or sensory nerve conduction velocity.

Etiology

Specific etiologic agents are unknown. Viruses or viral immunizations often precede GBS. Herpes simplex virus (HSV), Cytomegalovirus (CMV), and Epstein–Barr virus (EBV) are some of the potential viruses that may trigger GBS, though culture and seroepidemiologic testing have shown that 20% to 30% of all cases are preceded by *Campylobacter jejuni gastroenteritis.* Recent trauma or surgery may also instigate an immune system response that leads to GBS occurrence. GBS can occur at any age, with a peak incidence between 30 and 40 years. Both sexes are equally affected.

Clinical Presentation

Patients with GBS typically present with an evolving symmetric lower extremity weakness that typically presents on day 14 of the disease course. Distal muscles are the most severely affected. Paresthesia (numbness and tingling) is prominent and is typically followed by paralysis. Hypotonia and areflexia are common and persistent symptoms. Objective sensory loss is variable, with deep sensibility more affected than superficial sensations. Pain is common and may be severe. Agent such as gabapentin (Neurontin) and pregabalin (Lyrica) may be useful for treating this pain. Other patients may require opioids for adequate pain relief.

Autonomic nervous system dysfunction occurs and may require hemodynamic support. This dysfunction occurs because of abnormal vagal stimulation and can manifest as bradycardia, heart block, orthostatic hypotension or hypertension. Bowel or bladder dysfunction may also occur. Some patients may experience syndrome of inappropriate antidiuretic hormone (SIADH). Careful monitoring of volume status is essential in these patients.

As muscle weakness continues to ascend, patients may present with impending respiratory failure. Paradox alternans (paradoxical movement of the chest and abdomen) can occur. These patients also often have poor inspiratory effort and are tachypneic with severely diminished breath sounds.

If cranial nerve involvement occurs, it is most frequent in cranial nerve VII, followed by cranial nerves VI, III, XII, V, and X (most to least frequent). Facial nerve dysfunction includes an inability to smile, frown, whistle, or drink through a straw. Consequently, dysphasia and laryngeal paralysis are common if the paresthesia and paralysis extend to the cranial nerves.

Variations in Clinical Presentation

Ascending paralysis moves from legs to trunk to arms to head. It usually peaks in 10 to 14 days but can last for weeks to months. Fisher's variant is complete ophthalmoplegia (paralysis of the eye muscles), ataxia, and areflexia.

Cases with a steady or stepwise progression over weeks or months may be asymmetrical. Some body parts will be recovering while others are getting worse. There may be relapses, but these are uncommon.

KEY CLINICAL CONCEPT

Ascending paralysis is the classic presentation of Guillan-Barré syndrome.

Complications

GBS is a potentially fatal disease. **The most serious complication is respiratory failure as the paralysis advances upward.** Approximately 30% of patients require mechanical ventilation due to progressive respiratory failure. Frequent reassessment of respiratory status is essential to provide timely intervention. **Patients at risk for impending respiratory failure can be monitored utilizing serial measurements of forced vital capacity (FVC) and peak (or negative) inspiratory effort. Endotracheal intubation is often considered when FVC drops to less than 12 mL/kg body weight and peak negative inspiratory pressures is less than 20 cm H_2O.** Arterial blood gases (ABGs) can demonstrate respiratory acidosis or hypoxemia, also indicating the need for intubation.

QUICK TIP! Questions about GBS are less common (usually no more than 1). However, GBS questions that do appear often ask about respiratory mechanics parameters that may suggest impending respiratory failure.

Other complications include the hemodynamic instability that can occur because of autonomic dysfunction. These patients may require frequent titration of medications to maintain heart rate or blood pressure. Health-care providers should maintain a high suspicion for infection if fever develops. Ileus, venous thrombophlebitis, and pulmonary emboli may occur due to muscle atony and immobility.

Interventions

The objective of therapy is to support body systems until recovery occurs. Respiratory failure represents the most serious immediate concern and infection the most serious threat to recovery. Rigorous bronchial hygiene and chest physiotherapy will help clear secretions and could prevent respiratory deterioration. Vigilant assessment of respiratory status is essential to detect impending respiratory failure and the healthcare team should remain prepared to intervene acutely. If the patient does ultimately require intubation, strict sterile suctioning is needed to prevent infection, whether the patient has an endotracheal tube or a tracheostomy. If fever develops, sputum cultures should be obtained to identify a specific pathogen (if one is present in the respiratory tract) so that appropriate antibiotic therapy may be instituted.

Hemodynamic monitoring, including blood pressure, heart rate and rhythm, and accurate documentation of intake and output, is vital. Continuous telemetry is useful since some cardiac dysrhythmias have been reported. As both hypotension and hypertension may occur, patients may require vasopressors or antihypertensive agents transiently. Lastly, volume overload can contribute to pulmonary deterioration and volume deficit can contribute to hypotension necessitating nurses to keep careful track of intake and output.

A communication system must be established with the patient using whatever muscle action is possible. This is extremely difficult if the disease progresses to involvement of the cranial nerves. At the peak of a severe syndrome, communication from the patient may be impossible. The nurse must explain all procedures before doing them and reassure the patient that muscle function will eventually return to some part of the body, enabling the patient to communicate his or her needs and desires to the nurses. The patient and family need assistance in developing positive coping skills and education regarding the disease process.

Physiotherapy is indicated very early to help counter the hazards of immobility. Passive range of motion and attention to body extremity position help maintain function and prevent contractures. Splints and a continuous passive motion machine may be used for selected joints.

Patients with GBS are at risk for protein-calorie malnutrition and may require tube feeding if the gag reflex is altered. This should be initiated promptly to prevent development of ileus or delayed gastric emptying. *Head-of-bed elevation to 30 degrees may prevent aspiration.* Antacids, sucralfate, and H_2 inhibitors may be used to decrease the risk of gastrointestinal bleeding.

Treatment

Treatment is often multifaceted including organ support as previously described, intravenous immunoglobulin (IVIG) and/or steroid therapy and plasmapheresis in persisting cases. Plasmapheresis is the process of separating blood components to remove specific parts of it. In GBS, plasmapheresis is used to remove autoantibodies in the plasma that are believed to cause the disease. While the role of plasmapheresis is unclear in certain diseases, there is an apparent benefit to its use in diseases such as MG and GBS.

Prognosis

Recovery from GBS is slow, with approximately 85% of patients achieving full functional recovery within several months to a year. About one-third of patients have some residual weakness following the disease. If complications from respiratory failure are avoided, good recovery can be expected with minimal permanent neurologic dysfunction. With critical care, medical treatment, and nursing, specifically the management of respiratory failure, morbidity, and mortality will decrease.

35.3 MUSCULAR DYSTROPHY

Muscular dystrophy refers to a group of genetic, inherited muscle diseases that lead to muscle weakness. Muscular dystrophies are characterized by progressive skeletal muscle weakness, defects in muscle proteins, and the death of muscle cells and tissue.

Main symptoms of muscular dystrophy include progressive muscle weakness, poor balance, frequent falls, calf pain, decreased range of movement, drooping eyelids (ptosis), and difficulty walking. The diagnosis of muscular dystrophy is based on the results of a muscle biopsy. In some cases, a DNA blood test may be all that is needed.

A physical examination and the patient's medical history will help determine the type of muscular dystrophy as specific muscle groups are affected by different types of muscular dystrophy.

There is no specific treatment and no known cure for muscular dystrophy; the goal of treatment is to control symptoms. As inactivity (such as bed rest and even sitting for long periods) can worsen the disease, physical therapy and occupational therapy may be helpful. Physical therapy is aimed at preventing contractures and maintaining muscle tone. Orthopedic appliances such as braces can be used to improve mobility. Surgery on the spine or legs may be indicated in some cases to improve function. The cardiac problems that occur with Emery–Dreifuss muscular dystrophy and myotonic muscular dystrophy may require a pacemaker.

The focus of nursing interventions is on maximizing functional status during acute illness by promoting mobility and activities of daily living.

35.4 MYASTHENIA GRAVIS AND CRISIS

MG is an autoimmune-mediated neuromuscular disorder caused by a decrease in the number of available acetylcholine receptors at the neuromuscular junction. It is a chronic disorder of neuromuscular transmission resulting in weakness with exercise and the improvement of strength with rest.

Pathophysiology

Acetylcholine is released at nerve terminals and combines at the postsynaptic muscle membrane, producing an electrochemical reaction resulting in muscle contraction. In MG, the immune system attacks acetylcholine receptors resulting in a decreased amount of postsynaptic receptor sites. Therefore, acetylcholine released cannot bind at these receptor sites and a full muscular contraction cannot occur.

Etiology

MG is an autoimmune process with a statistically significant number of cases associated with antiacetylcholine receptor antibodies. In patients that do not have these antibodies, other antibodies related to muscle receptors are likely involved. Most MG patients have thymoma, with a small percentage having thymic tumors.

Occurrence

The prevalence of MG is estimated at 14 to 20 cases per 100,000 or about 36,000 to 60,000 cases per year. It may occur at any age but is rarely seen in persons younger than 10 years or those older than 90 years. The most common ages of onset are 20s and 30s for women and 60s to 80s in men.

Clinical Signs, Symptoms, and Course

MG is characterized by fatigability of voluntary muscle groups with repeated use. Pathognomonic signs of MG include uneven drooping of the eyelids (ptosis), a smile that resembles a snarl, a drooping lower jaw that must be supported by the hand, and a partially immobile mouth with the corners turned downward. However, few patients are first seen with these signs. In more than 90% of the cases, the eyebrows and extraocular muscles are involved, accompanied by weakness in eye closure. Ptosis and diplopia are common. The next most commonly affected muscles exhibiting symptoms are those of facial expression, mastication, swallowing, and speaking (dysarthria). Hoarseness occurs after only a few minutes of talking. Neck flexor and extensor muscles, the shoulder girdle, and hip flexors are less frequently involved. There is usually no sensory disturbance.

The course of MG is variable. Remission may occur for no discernible reason in fewer than half the cases and usually does not last longer than 1 to 2 months. The prognosis has improved because of advances in treatment and most myasthenia patients can be successfully managed with proper therapy.

Associated Conditions

Approximately 15% of patients have a tumor of the thymus. There is an increasing incidence of tumors in older men. Thyroiditis, thyrotoxicosis, lupus erythematosus, and rheumatoid arthritis occur more often than statistically expected. A pregnancy may make the disease worse or better or may have no effect. Close to 15% of children born to myasthenia mothers exhibit symptoms of the disease. These symptoms are usually transient and resolve within 1 to 12 weeks.

Diagnosis

A history of an increasing muscular fatigability that improves with rest is a common characteristic of MG. Various laboratory tests can be used to aid in the diagnosis, including fatigue on repetitive electrical stimulation, single-fiber electromyographic testing, elevated serum acetylcholine-R antibody titers, and radiographic evidence of thymus enlargement on CT or magnetic resonance imaging (MRI). However, anticholinesterase tests are considered conclusive.

"The Tensilon test" can aid in diagnosis of MG. **Edrophonium chloride (Tensilon)** is an *anticholinesterase agent that is injected intravenously after the patient's muscle strength has been assessed.* The limit used to test for MG is 10 mg given in 2- to 5-mg doses. The duration of action for Tensilon is about 5 minutes. When injected, it increases the level of acetylcholine at the myoneural junction by blocking cholinesterase (which breaks down acetylcholine). **A clinical increase in muscle strength is positive for MG. No improvement or a deterioration in muscle strength is negative for MG.**

If Tensilon testing is not conclusive, *neostigmine bromide 0.5 mg* intravenously or 1.5 mg intramuscularly may be used. *Atropine sulfate (0.6 mg)* should be given prior to intravenous neostigmine and may be needed with intramuscular injection of neostigmine to counter nausea, vomiting, increased salivation, and sweating. Intravenous *neostigmine* may cause ventricular fibrillation or cardiac arrest. After intramuscular injection, maximum effect will be apparent within 30 minutes, but effects may last 2 to 3 hours. Curare is seldom used because of its paralytic action; if properly administered, however, it is definitive.

Treatment

The most useful treatments include anticholinesterase medications, immunosuppressive agents, thymectomy, and plasmapheresis or IVIG. The major objective of therapy is to improve neuromuscular transmission and prevent complications. Early thymectomy may be employed.

Neuromuscular transmission is improved by administration of anticholinesterase drugs. Pyridostigmine bromide (Mestinon) is a popular choice. If pyridostigmine bromide is not adequate to establish control of neuromuscular transmission, neostigmine (Prostigmin) is used. *Prednisone* has become an adjunctive drug of choice. It is extremely important to medicate the patient on schedule and to document carefully the patient's muscular response. The medication should be taken with a snack to prevent abdominal cramps and diarrhea. The major difference between pyridostigmine bromide and neostigmine is their duration of action. Mestinon has a 4-hour effect; neostigmine, 2 hour. Fasciculation and increased weakness occurring 50 minutes after administration of drug is a sign of toxicity and should be reported immediately. Steroids may decrease the amount of anticholinesterase drug required to control myasthenic symptoms. Immunosuppression using glucocorticoids, azathioprine, and other drugs is effective in nearly all patients with MG. Glucocorticoids and cyclosporine generally produce clinical improvement within a period of 1 to 3 months. The beneficial effects of azathioprine and mycophenolate mofetil usually begin after many months (up to 1 year), and these drugs have advantages for long-term treatment.

Nursing Interventions

A major nursing intervention is to maintain adequate ventilation due to a weak cough, an inability to clear secretions, and an increased likelihood of aspiration. Vital capacity is checked every 2 to 4 hours. Ventilators often are set up and kept available.

Prevention of aspiration, infection from any source, and emotional support of the patient are very important. If the patient is on a ventilator, a communication system should be established. If the patient has had a thymectomy, the monitoring and nursing treatment as for any patient with a thoracotomy must be followed.

Specific drugs that impair neuromuscular transmission must be avoided. The aminoglycoside antibiotics and true mycin drugs are contraindicated. Such drugs include aureomycin, kanamycin, polymyxin, neomycin, streptomycin, and gentamicin.

Quinidine, procainamide, morphine sulfate, and sedatives will also aggravate muscle weakness.

Nursing education concerning the importance of taking prescribed medications on schedule is extremely important since an early or late dosage may immediately affect muscle strength. Regulation of daily living habits to avoid fatigue and provide rest must be tailored to the patient's lifestyle as much as possible. While immunosuppression therapy is gradually reduced, usually treatment for months or years may be needed, and close monitoring for side effects is required.

Postthymectomy Nursing Interventions. Routine postsurgical care is needed, as are the following:

1. Post-thoracic surgical procedures (eg, chest tubes)
2. Ventilatory support with frequent suctioning
3. Anticholinesterase and steroid drugs started slowly
4. Reassurance that positive effects of a thymectomy occur over long periods (even years)
5. Protection from infections (ie, sterile technique for suctioning, intermittent urinary catheterization rather than an indwelling catheter)

Complications: Myasthenic or Cholinergic Crisis?

Myasthenic and cholinergic crises both have an extreme weakness as the predominant symptom. There are important characteristics that help to differentiate these two complications.

Cholinergic crisis is rare and is due to an overdose of drugs. The crisis is signaled by miotic pupils, increased salivation, mucus plugging, diarrhea, and sweating. An impending cholinergic crisis can be detected by noting constricted pupils; 2 mm is the maximum constriction that should be allowed before intervention. To distinguish between these crises, an edrophonium bromide test is performed with a ventilator on standby. If the patient becomes weaker, a cholinergic (overdose) crisis exists. Treatment is to discontinue anticholinesterase drugs. After 72 hours, drug therapy is usually restarted in small increments. Atropine (an anticholinergic drug) may control symptoms but may also block important symptoms of anticholinesterase overdose. *It is imperative to monitor ventilatory function with ABGs.*

Myasthenic crisis is more common and precipitated by stress, infection, steroids, and/or medications. Signs include pupils mydriatic, *diaphragmatic failure,* and absence of diarrhea. This crisis is further established by muscular improvement with the **edrophonium bromide (Tensilon)** test. Anticholinesterase drugs are given and repeated as needed. Steroids are usually avoided during a crisis. Monitoring, assessment, and the documentation of muscular strength and ABGs are continued throughout the crisis. Muscle assessment may include presence of the gag reflex, voice quality, swallowing difficulty, ptosis on upward gaze, diplopia on lateral gaze, and the ability to do deep knee bends, raise arms above head, rise from chair, or lift the head off the bed. Identification of the precipitating cause is important to treat and/or correct the cause. The most common cause of myasthenic crisis is infection. Other causes include heat exposure, emotional upset, surgery, thyroid disease, pregnancy, menses, hypokalemia, and drugs that block the neuromuscular junction. With advances in treatment, however, crisis rarely occurs in properly managed patients.

KEY CLINICAL CONCEPT

Tensilon test is used to differentiate between a cholinergic crisis and a myasthenia crisis. In cholinergic crisis patients will become weaker after the administration of Tensilon. In myasthenia crisis weakness will improve.

KEY CONTENT CHECKLIST

- ❒ Fever, headache, and nuchal rigidity are symptoms of meningitis.
- ❒ Ascending paralysis is a classic presentation of Guillan Barré Syndrome. The most serious complication of Guillan Barré is respiratory failure as the paralysis advances upward.
- ❒ Patients at risk for impending respiratory failure can be monitored utilizing serial measurements of forced vital capacity (FVC) and peak (or negative) inspiratory effort. Endotracheal intubation is often considered when FVC drops to less than 12 mL/kg body weight and peak negative inspiratory pressures is less than 20 cm H_2O.
- ❒ Tensilon testing is used to diagnose Myasthenia Gravis and to differentiate between a cholinergic crisis and a myasthenia crisis. In cholinergic crisis, patients will become weaker after the administration of Tensilon. In myasthenia crisis weakness will improve.
- ❒ Be able to differentiate bacterial versus viral infected CSF characteristics (See Table 35-1).
- ❒ To remember Brudzinski's sign, imagine the neck flexed as if it is forming the curve of the letter, "B." Whereas for Kernig's sign, imagine the leg flexed at the hip, like the leg is forming part of the letter, "K."

Review Questions:

1. Myasthenia gravis is characterized by which of the following?

a. Ascending paralysis
b. Neuromuscular weakness with exercise and improvement with rest
c. Uncoordinated motor control
d. Peripheral sensory deficits

Answer: B. Rationale: A history of an increasing muscular fatigability that improves with rest is a common characteristic of myasthenia gravis.

2. Guillain–Barré syndrome affects which neurologic component?

a. Peripheral nervous system
b. Central nervous system
c. Autonomic nervous system
d. Schwann cells

Answer: A. Rationale: Guillain–Barré syndrome is an acute inflammatory disease, thought to be autoimmune or viral, that affects peripheral nerves, spinal nerves, and sometimes cranial nerves, first with edema and then demyelination.

3. Which of the following organisms is the most common cause of bacterial meningitis in adults?

a. Meningococcus
b. *Haemophilus influenzae*
c. *Diplococcus pneumoniae*
d. Pneumococcus

Answer: B. Rationale: Organisms obtain access to the subarachnoid space through penetrating head injuries, basal skull fractures with a torn dura mater, ICP monitoring, cranial surgery, mastoiditis, acute otitis media, lumbar punctures, injury to the paranasal sinuses, septic emboli, and sepsis. The organism may be fungal, viral, or bacterial. Eighty percent of all bacterial meningitis is caused by *Streptococcus pneumoniae*, *Neisseria meningitidis*, and *Haemophilus influenzae*. Other gram-positive bacteria include *Diplococcus pneumoniae*. Gram-negative bacteria include *Klebsiella*, *Escherichia coli*, and *Pseudomonas*. After neurologic surgery, *Staphylococcus aureus* or *Staphylococcus epidermidis* are common bacterial contaminants. In children, it is *H. influenzae*. Other bacteria include *Streptococcus*, *Pneumococcus*, and occasionally *Mycobacterium tuberculosis*. The outcome of bacterial meningitis depends on early and aggressive treatment. Viral causes of meningitis include enteroviruses, arboviruses, and herpesviruses. Viral meningitis is commonly referred to as aseptic meningitis. Fungal meningitis is primarily caused by *Cryptococcus neoformans*.

36

Seizures and Status Epilepticus

CHAPTER OVERVIEW AND OBJECTIVES

In this chapter, concepts are covered that address the CCRN exam items of seizures and status epilepticus. You can expect between one and three questions on this content.

After studying this chapter, you should understand the following:

- Identify nursing interventions in care of patient having a seizure.
- Describe the variants of clinical presentation in status epilepticus.
- Name the first-line medication for status epilepticus.
- Identify nursing interventions in care of patient in status epilepticus

36.1 SEIZURES

A seizure is a symptom of paroxysmal electrical discharges in the brain, resulting in autonomic, sensory, and/or motor dysfunction. Seizures may be associated with infection, trauma, tumors, cerebrovascular disease, genetic or congenital defects, or metabolic dysfunction. A temporary condition, such as exposure to drugs, withdrawal from certain drugs, or abnormal levels of sodium or glucose in the blood may also cause seizures. Seizures can cause involuntary changes in body movement or function, sensation, awareness, or behavior. A seizure can last from a few seconds to status epilepticus, a continuous seizure that will not stop without intervention. If seizures are recurrent and transient, the condition is classified as epilepsy. The term "convulsion" refers to the musculoskeletal contractions accompanying a seizure. *A seizure lasting longer than* ***5 minutes*** *is considered a medical emergency.*

Classification

Seizures are classified according to where they start in the brain, if awareness is affected and what symptoms are involved. Focal seizures start in and affect one part of the brain. Focal onset seizures are further broken down into awareness or impaired awareness focal seizures. Generalized onset seizures start in and affect both sides of the brain at once. They can cause visible motor movement of no motor movement. Seizures are identified as unknown onset when there is not enough information to determine if it is focal or general.

Focal Onset.

Focal Onset Aware Seizures. In a focal aware seizure, the patient is conscious and will usually know something is happening. There is awareness the seizure occurred. Focal aware seizures are sometimes called "auras" and may progress into another type of seizure. The symptoms depend on the area of the brain that is affected.

Focal Onset Impaired Awareness Seizures. In a focal impaired awareness seizure, the patient may be confused and unable to respond. However, the patient may be able to hear. The patient may appear awake but do not respond to instructions or questions. They may stare into space or demonstrative repetitive movements such as lip smacking or chewing.

Generalized Onset Seizures. Generalized seizures affect both hemispheres of the brain and present with impaired consciousness. The most common type is tonic–clonic seizures. Tonic–clonic movements are noted as the muscles of the arms, legs, chest, and back become stiff and then jerk and twitch. The patient may appear cyanotic. Other types of generalized seizure include absences seizures, clonic seizures, myoclonic seizures, tonic seizures, and atonic seizures.

Unknown Onset Seizures. Unknown seizures include all seizures for which there are insufficient data to classify them as focal or generalize.

Pathophysiology

It is unknown whether seizures occur as a result of increased neuronal excitability or a decreased neuronal inhibitory force. Focal neurons appear to be unusually sensitive to acetylcholine and possibly to deficits in specific neurotransmitters. Altered cell permeability and/or alteration in electrolytes may have a role in seizure activity. It is logical to assume that an electrical threshold for seizures exists in all persons. Factors thought to lower the electrical threshold of neurons include:

- Fever
- Fatigue
- Altered electrolyte–fluid balance
- Stress
- Emotional distress
- Pregnancy

Regardless of these factors, the hyperexcited neurons become hyperactive. As these localized neuronal discharges become more intense, the hyperirritability spreads synaptically to adjacent neurons. In many instances the entire brain is involved. *When only one hemisphere is involved, consciousness is preserved. When both cerebral hemispheres are involved, there is usually a loss of consciousness.*

36.2 EPILEPSY

Etiology

Epilepsy is a characterized by repeated seizures. Multiple causes of epilepsy are known. The most common is the abrupt cessation of antiepileptic drugs or other chronic sedative medications. Other causes include trauma, tumor, injuries (both perinatal and postnatal), central nervous system (CNS) infections, and cerebrovascular disease, including arteriovenous malformations. Metabolic and toxic disorders may cause seizures. The role of genetics and heredity is controversial at this time. In a large number of cases, the cause is unknown. These cases are termed idiopathic epilepsy.

Diagnosis

Epilepsy is a common chronic neurologic disorder characterized by recurrent unprovoked seizures. These seizures are transient signs and/or symptoms of abnormal, excessive or synchronous neuronal activity in the brain. The patient's history of seizure activity (duration, frequency, intensity, and progression) is among the most useful tools in establishing a diagnosis. The family should be asked for their observations and their knowledge of participating factors if the patient is unable to provide them. Past medical history should be closely examined for previous seizures, head injury, or other illness. Physical examination, laboratory studies, radiologic studies, and electroencephalograms (EEGs) may reveal factors supporting a diagnosis of epilepsy, or the studies may all be within normal limits.

Nursing Interventions and Complications

There are five major areas of nursing intervention for the patient having seizures:

1. *Protecting the patient from injury is a priority. Remove objects from the immediate environment that might cause injury. Stay with the patient during the seizure. Bed rails should be up and padded and the bed placed in low position. The patient should not be restrained, but efforts to protect the patient's head from injury* are appropriate (eg, if a seizure occurs with the patient out of bed, a pillow may be placed under the head or a nurse may cradle—*not* restrain—the patient's head to protect it). *Nothing* should ever be used to pry open the patient's mouth, nor should anything be forced into the mouth during a seizure. Damage to the mouth and tongue occurs at the start of a seizure and only more damage will result by forcing objects into the mouth.
2. The observation and recording of seizure patterns with a video camera may help to identify the seizure focus. When surface EEG electrodes are insufficient, an implanted grid for EEG monitoring may be used to locate the lesion. Data collected include precipitating factors, presence and type of aura, duration of unconsciousness, the pattern and progression of seizure activity, body parts involved (generalized or one-sided), incontinence, postictal activity, and, if monitored, EEG data.
3. *Assessment of the respiratory system is extremely important.* The danger in a tonic–clonic seizure is that the patient's *respiratory status will be compromised during the tonic phase.* The respiratory status may be further compromised by *aspiration. Oxygen and suction* should be at the bedside. The patient should be turned to the side to *protect the airway* after the seizure and be allowed to sleep.
4. Administration of medication on a regular basis and the evaluation of its effectiveness in controlling seizures as well as the psychological effects on the patient are important actions and assessments. Teaching the patient the beneficial effects of following the prescribed medication regimen and identifying and overcoming patient objections may result in better patient adherence in the future.
5. The promotion of physical and mental health may sharply curtail the number of seizures. Regular routines for eating, sleeping, and physical activity should be established. Alcohol, stress, and fatigue tend to precipitate seizure activity. Modification of these factors will alter the seizure pattern. The patient should be instructed to take showers and avoid baths owing to the potential for seizure activity.

Treatment of Seizures and Epilepsy

The treatment of a seizure disorder is almost always multimodal and includes treatment of underlying conditions, avoidance of precipitating factors, and suppression of recurrent seizures by prophylactic therapy with antiepileptic medications or surgery. If seizures are the result of tumor, infection, or metabolic dysfunction, correcting the underlying cause is the goal of therapy. In a majority of cases, an underlying cause may not be identifiable or be amenable to curative therapy. Antiepileptic drug therapy is used for the management of recurrent seizures of unknown etiology or a known cause that cannot be reversed. It is preferable to use a single drug to achieve control of seizure activity. Common drugs include phenytoin sodium (Dilantin), phenobarbital, primidone (Mysoline), ethosuximide (Zarontin), clonazepam (Klonopin), carbamazepine (Tegretol), valproic acid (Depakene), and lamotrigine (Lamictal). Adjunctive therapeutic agents include topiramate (Topamax), zonisamide (Zonegran), gabapentin (Neurontin), levetiracetam

(Keppra), and tiagabine (Gabitril). For the therapeutic serum level of these drugs, their affinity for specific types of seizures, and their side effects, the reader is referred to any standard pharmacology text.

If drug therapy is ineffective and seizures are intractable and deny the patient a normal life, surgery may be considered. After identifying the specific epileptic focus and the patient's dominant hemisphere, a temporal lobectomy, extratemporal resection, or hemispherectomy may be done. Seizures may continue for a period after the surgery; therefore, the patient's medication is continued for approximately a year. Palliative surgery to restrict seizure spread includes partial or complete callosotomy. The patient must continue on antiepileptic medication following palliative surgery.

36.3 STATUS EPILEPTICUS

Status epilepticus is described as a seizure or series of seizures lasting longer than 30 minutes. Status epilepticus is a medical emergency and has an overall mortality of 20% to 30%. The state of status epilepticus is present when seizures follow each other so closely that a state of consciousness is not recovered between seizures. Status epilepticus may be partial or generalized in origin. An EEG is necessary to determine the type or, in the patient in coma, the presence of seizures.

Etiology

Inadequate dosage of antiepileptic medication in a known epileptic is a common precipitating factor. Other factors include sudden withdrawal of antiepileptic drugs and other sedative drugs, hyponatremia, fever, intercurrent infection (commonly in the CNS), cerebrovascular disease, and cerebral hypoxia, anoxia, and edema. Progressive neurologic diseases such as brain tumors and subdural hematoma may cause status epilepticus. A common triad of causes consists of alcohol abuse, drug abuse, and sleep deprivation. Head trauma or pregnancy (preeclamptic state) may precipitate status epilepticus. Metabolic causes include hypoglycemia, hyponatremia, hypocalcemia, uremia, and electrolyte imbalances.

Incidence and Prognosis

Approximately 6% of known epileptics will develop status epilepticus. Almost 50% of the cases of status epilepticus occur in known epileptics. Approximately 10% of patients in status epilepticus will die. Death is commonly due to respiratory and metabolic acidosis, hypoxemia, hypoglycemia, hyperthermia, electrolyte disturbances, and/or renal failure.

Pathophysiology

The pathophysiology is the same as that of epilepsy; however, in status epilepticus the seizures are almost continuous. The rapidly repeating tonic–clonic seizures lead to hypoxemia (patients are apneic during such seizures) and *cerebral anoxia*. The increased metabolic activity of the brain causes hypoglycemia and hyperthermia. Hypoxemia, hypoglycemia, and hyperthermia may themselves precipitate seizure activity, resulting in a vicious cycle.

Electrical status occurs in every type of status and is not a distinct type. It is always associated with some clinical abnormality. The EEG shows continuous epileptic activity.

Treatment

The goal of therapy is to restore physiologic homeostasis and to stop the seizures by correcting the underlying cause. *Treatment should occur simultaneously. The priorities for care are to ensure a patent airway, maintain breathing and circulation, administering medications to stop the seizures and identifying the cause.* Blood is drawn for antiepileptic drug levels, toxicology screen, glucose, electrolytes, calcium, magnesium, creatinine, blood urea nitrogen, complete blood count with differential, liver profile, arterial blood gases (ABGs), and creatine phosphokinase and to establish an intravenous line. *Thiamine* 100 mg intravenously is administered prior to *50% glucose* 50 mL intravenously if alcoholism or hypoglycemia is suspected.

Benzodiazepines and lorazepam (Ativan) *given intravenously are often the drugs of choice in spite of their potential for suppressing respirations.* Fast-acting antiepilepsy drugs very quickly enter and quickly leave the brain. But these very properties often make benzodiazepines a poor choice for long-term management of status epilepticus.

Phenytoin is given intravenously. It must be injected slowly (50 mg/min), and cardiac monitoring is essential for early intervention if a dysrhythmia develops. Bradycardia and hypotension are especially common in patients older than 40. Phenytoin requires 15 to 20 minutes to peak in brain tissue, and it remains in brain tissue over a long period.

If seizures persist after 30 minutes, there is a high probability that acute CNS disease is causing them. *Phenobarbital* may be tried in intractable cases. A slow intravenous injection is recommended (50–100 mg/min). Respiratory depression and hypotension may develop. Phenobarbital and diazepam should not be administered concurrently. If benzodiazepines are used to stop seizures, phenytoin is given simultaneously to block recurrence of the seizures. A combination of benzodiazepines and barbiturate may cause respiratory depression and hypotension.

In some medical centers general anesthesia (barbiturate coma) is administered to a depth of EEG silence when other drugs have failed. *Pharmacologic neuromuscular blockade will not stop brain electrical activity but will stop movement.* Surgical excision of epileptic foci that have not responded to medical therapy is being used with increasing effectiveness. Vagal nerve stimulation for intractable partial and secondarily generalizing seizures is also used for selected cases.

Nursing Interventions

An initial priority of seizure management for nursing care is maintaining patient safety. Maintaining a patent airway and providing adequate oxygenation are additionally important. Observation of the seizure type, duration, precipitating factors, along with any focal neurologic deficits, is essential. An intravenous line should be maintained. ECG monitoring, continuous pulse oximetry, and blood pressure monitoring are indicated in patients with prolonged seizures. Cardiac drugs should be available, as cardiac monitoring may reveal dysrhythmias. Hyperthermia is often treated with a hypothermia blanket. Because hypoglycemia can induce seizure activity, a glucose level should be checked. Fluid and electrolyte balance is monitored. Neurologic status is monitored closely.

KEY CONTENT CHECKLIST

- ❒ In general, in seizures, when only one hemisphere is involved, consciousness is preserved. When both cerebral hemispheres are involved, there is usually a loss of consciousness.
- ❒ A seizure lasting greater than 5 minutes is a medical emergency.
- ❒ Nursing interventions for the patient experiencing a seizure are
  - a. Protecting the patient from injury
  - b Recording the seizure
  - c. Assessment and intervention of the respiratory system
  - d. Administration of anti-seizure medications, such as **benzodiazepines**
  - e. Promotion of health practices to prevent seizure
- ❒ Status epilepticus is an emergency. Treatment should occur simultaneously. The priorities for care are to ensure a patent airway, maintain breathing and circulation, administering medications to stop the seizures and identifying the cause.

Review Questions:

1. Nursing interventions for the patient having seizures include all of the following EXCEPT:

a. Protecting the patient from injury
b. Observing and recording seizure patterns
c. Administering anticonvulsive drugs such as phenytoin (Dilantin)
d. Restraining the patient

Answer: D. Rationale: An initial priority of seizure management for nursing care is maintaining patient safety. Maintaining a patent airway and providing adequate oxygenation are additionally important. Observation of the seizure type, duration, precipitating factors, along with any focal neurologic deficits, is essential. An intravenous line should be maintained. Medications to stop seizure activity may be indicated and require administration and monitoring of response.

2. Pathophysiologic consequences of status epilepticus include all of the following except one. Which of the following consequences is NOT associated with status epilepticus?

a. Hypoxemia
b. Hypoglycemia
c. Hyperthermia
d. Hypothermia

Answer: D. Rationale: Hyperthermia is often treated with a hypothermia blanket. Because hypoglycemia can induce seizure activity, a glucose level should be checked.

3. If a patient develops a tonic–clonic seizure, which initial nursing action should take place?

a. Forcing of an airway into the mouth
b. Protecting the patient from injury
c. Starting oxygen therapy
d. Placing a padded tongue blade into the mouth

Answer: B. Rationale: Protecting the patient from injury is a priority. Remove objects from the immediate environment that might cause injury. Stay with the patient during the seizure. Bed rails should be up and padded and the bed placed in low position. The patient should not be restrained, but efforts to protect the patient's head from injury are appropriate (eg, if a seizure occurs with the patient out of bed, a pillow may be placed under the head or a nurse may cradle—*not* restrain—the patient's head to protect it). *Nothing* should ever be used to pry open the patient's mouth, nor should anything be forced into the mouth during a seizure. Damage to the mouth and tongue occurs at the start of a seizure, and only more damage will result by forcing objects into the mouth.

PART V
Neurology Practice Exam

1. **Which meningeal layer lies closest to the brain?**
   (A) pia mater
   (B) dura mater
   (C) arachnoid
   (D) subarachnoid
2. **Which cerebral component is responsible for reabsorbing cerebrospinal fluid (CSF)?**
   (A) lateral ventricle
   (B) dura mater
   (C) arachnoid villi
   (D) subarachnoid cisterns
3. **Which meningeal layer lies closest to the skull?**
   (A) pia mater
   (B) dura mater
   (C) arachnoid
   (D) subarachnoid
4. **Which structure separates the left and right cerebral hemispheres?**
   (A) dura mater
   (B) subarachnoid space
   (C) fissure of Rolando
   (D) falx cerebri
5. **Crossing of impulses between the two hemispheres is made possible by which structure?**
   (A) corpus callosum
   (B) lateral ventricle
   (C) postcentral gyrus
   (D) falx cerebri
6. **An injury to the temporal lobe would cause disturbances in which sensory component?**
   (A) sight
   (B) hearing
   (C) spatial orientation
   (D) taste
7. **A patient in your unit has suffered frontal head injuries from a motor vehicle accident. Which type of impairment may result from injury to the frontal lobe?**
   (A) loss of sensation
   (B) loss of vision
   (C) alterations in hearing
   (D) alterations in personality
8. **Maintenance of an awake and alert status is dependent on the proper functioning of which two cerebral structures?**
   (A) reticular-activating system and both cerebral hemispheres
   (B) parietal and occipital lobes
   (C) pons and basal ganglia
   (D) thalamus and hypothalamus
9. **The thalamus is responsible for integrating all of the following body sensations except one. Which sense does the thalamus NOT integrate?**
   (A) smell
   (B) sight
   (C) hearing
   (D) touch
10. **Neurohumoral control of respiration is located in which structure(s)?**
    (A) pons and medulla
    (B) diencephalon
    (C) reticular-activating system
    (D) basal ganglia
11. **The primary function of the cerebellum includes which of the following?**
    (A) thought integration
    (B) maintenance of personality characteristics
    (C) sight
    (D) maintenance of equilibrium and muscle coordination
12. **The lateral ventricles are connected to the third ventricle via which structure?**
    (A) cerebral aqueduct of Sylvius
    (B) choroid plexus
    (C) foramen of Monro
    (D) foramen of Magendie
13. **Obstruction of the foramen of Monro would produce which condition?**
    (A) ipsilateral dilatation of the pupils
    (B) hydrocephalus
    (C) hemiparesis
    (D) compression of the third cranial nerve
14. **CSF is synthesized by which structure?**
    (A) corticospinal tract
    (B) subarachnoid villi
    (C) lateral ventricle
    (D) choroid plexus
15. **Which of the following corresponds most closely to the primary purpose of the CSF?**
    (A) transport of oxygen to the brain
    (B) manufacture of neurotransmitters
    (C) cushioning the brain and spinal column
    (D) maintenance of cerebral perfusion pressures

16. **Which area of the brain is responsible for voluntary motor function?**
    (A) parietal lobe
    (B) frontal lobe
    (C) occipital lobe
    (D) temporal lobe
17. **The parietal lobe is responsible for which function?**
    (A) temperature regulation
    (B) sensory integration
    (C) motor function
    (D) vision
18. **Which artery or arteries are responsible for anterior circulation to the brain?**
    (A) external carotids
    (B) internal carotids
    (C) basilar
    (D) vertebrals
19. **Adrenergic fibers of the sympathetic nervous system release which of the following neurotransmitters?**
    (A) serotonin and dopamine
    (B) dopamine and acetylcholine
    (C) epinephrine and norepinephrine
    (D) acetylcholine and gamma aminobutyric acid (GABA)
20. **Autoregulation of the cerebral circulatory system is most sensitive to changes in which of the following parameters?**
    (A) mean arterial pressure
    (B) PaO_2
    (C) pH
    (D) glucose level
21. **Which area of the brain is most sensitive to hypoxia?**
    (A) brainstem
    (B) cerebral cortex
    (C) cerebellum
    (D) subarachnoid villi
22. **Which statement most accurately describes the circle of Willis?**
    (A) It is located in the cerebrum.
    (B) It helps provide adequate circulation through its anastomosis.
    (C) It is responsible for sleep and wakefulness.
    (D) It is part of the brainstem.
23. **Hypothalamic disorders would be manifest by disturbances in which function?**
    (A) water balance and temperature control
    (B) sensory processing
    (C) vision
    (D) sensory organization
24. **The gray matter of the spinal cord represents which type of tissue?**
    (A) dendrite
    (B) axon
    (C) unmyelinated tissue
    (D) myelinated tissue
25. **How are the descending tracts within the spinal cord best described?**
    (A) columns
    (B) funiculi
    (C) sensory
    (D) motor

Question 26 refers to the following scenario:
A patient is admitted to the intensive care unit (ICU) after sustaining a knife wound to the back. Assessment findings include loss of pain and temperature sensation on the right side and loss of motor function on the left. Vital signs are stable and he is alert and oriented. No other injuries are noted.

26. **Based on the preceding information, which type of neurologic syndrome is likely to be developing?**
    (A) central cord
    (B) Brown–Séquard
    (C) anterior cord
    (D) Horner
27. **Signs of acute subdural hematoma appear during what time frame after an injury?**
    (A) 2 to 3 days
    (B) 1 week
    (C) up to 2 weeks
    (D) more than 2 weeks
28. **Which of the following is a necessary immediate assessment for an injury of C3–C4?**
    (A) heart rate
    (B) motor ability
    (C) temperature
    (D) ventilation
29. **Which vital sign changes (due to loss of sympathetic nervous stimulation) would occur after a spinal cord lesion above T5?**
    (A) bradycardia and hypotension
    (B) hyperthermia and tachycardia
    (C) tachycardia and hypotension
    (D) hypertension and bradycardia
30. **Which symptoms are present in cases of autonomic hyperreflexia?**
    (A) bradycardia and hypertension
    (B) hyperthermia and tachycardia
    (C) tachycardia and hypotension
    (D) hypertension and hyperthermia
31. **The presence of an intracranial pressure (ICP) of 50 indicates which situation?**
    (A) a lower motor neuron lesion
    (B) cerebral ischemia
    (C) peripheral nerve damage
    (D) an intact spinal arc
32. **All of the following are symptoms of a basilar skull fracture but one. Which symptom is NOT indicative of a basilar skull fracture?**
    (A) rhinorrhea and otorrhea
    (B) Battle's sign, raccoon eyes
    (C) tinnitus, nystagmus, and hearing difficulty
    (D) loss of consciousness and dilated pupils

33. Which of the following corresponds most closely to the range of adequate cerebral perfusion pressures (CPPs)?
(A) more than 30 mm Hg
(B) less than 60 mm Hg
(C) more than 60 mm Hg
(D) any value less than the intracranial pressure

34. Which of the following can cause an epidural hematoma?
(A) skull fracture lacerating the middle meningeal artery
(B) rupture of an intracranial aneurysm
(C) infectious meningitis
(D) cerebral edema

35. Where are intracranial aneurysms most commonly found?
(A) external carotid arteries
(B) anterior cerebral circulation
(C) common carotid arteries
(D) posterior cerebral circulation including the vertebrobasilar arteries

36. A 28-year-old man is admitted to the ICU with a diagnosis of closed head injury. The nurse should be aware of which potential complications?
(A) hypotension
(B) respiratory alkalosis
(C) tremors
(D) cerebral edema

37. The use of hyperventilation ($Paco_2$ 30–35 mm Hg) to treat increased ICP is indicated in which of the following situations?
(A) brief periods of time with signs of significant neurologic deterioration
(B) any time ICP increases
(C) prophylactically to keep control of ICP at all times
(D) never used

38. Which of the following is a common risk factor associated with aneurysmal subarachnoid hemorrhage?
(A) cerebral edema
(B) hypertension
(C) prolonged hypotensive episodes
(D) Valsalva maneuvers

39. CPP is calculated according to which of the following formulas?
(A) mean arterial pressure (MAP) – intracranial pressure (ICP)
(B) systolic blood pressure – ICP
(C) ICP + cerebral blood flow
(D) MAP + ICP

Questions 40 and 41 refer to the following scenario:
A 45-year-old man is admitted to your unit with a diagnosis of intracranial hypertension due to a severe traumatic brain injury. The current vital signs include a blood pressure (BP) of 110/70 mm Hg, ICP 30, pulse 140, respiratory rate 20.

40. Based on the preceding information, what is the CPP?
(A) 83
(B) 53
(C) 120
(D) not calculable

41. Which of the following are measures that would improve the CPP?
(A) increase the MAP
(B) decrease the MAP
(C) decrease the heart rate
(D) all of the above

42. Which of the following corresponds most closely to the range of minimum clinically acceptable CPPs?
(A) 30 to 40 mm Hg
(B) 40 to 50 mm Hg
(C) 50 to 60 mm Hg
(D) more than 60 mm Hg

43. What is normal ICP?
(A) −5 to +5 mm Hg
(B) 0 to 10 mm Hg
(C) 15 to 25 mm Hg
(D) more than 20 mm Hg

44. Nursing interventions for the patient with an intraventricular ICP monitoring device would include which of the following?
(A) routine flushing of the system with heparinized saline
(B) maintaining the transducer at the level of the heart
(C) administration of prophylactic antibiotics
(D) monitoring the patient for signs and symptoms of infection

45. The hypothalamus secretes which hormone to regulate water balance?
(A) aldosterone
(B) renin
(C) antidiuretic hormone (ADH)
(D) oxytocin

46. Approximately two-thirds of the brain's blood supply is transported through which arteries?
(A) internal carotid
(B) anterior communicating
(C) vertebral
(D) middle meningeal

47. What percent of total body oxygen consumption is accounted for by the brain?
(A) 2% to 5%
(B) 5% to 10%
(C) 10% to 15%
(D) 20%

48. How much of a reserve of oxygen exists in the brain?
(A) 100 mL
(B) 225 mL
(C) 450 mL
(D) none

49. Of the following factors, which does NOT play a role in maintaining consciousness?
(A) cerebral perfusion pressure
(B) oxygen transport level
(C) adequate blood glucose level
(D) normal serum potassium level

50. The reticular-activating system is responsible for which of the following functions?
(A) motor control of skeletal muscle
(B) relay of sensory impulses to the parietal lobe
(C) sleep and wakefulness
(D) secretion of all neurotransmitters

Questions 51 and 52 refer to the following scenario:
A 56-year-old factory worker is admitted to your unit following a 20-ft fall from a scaffold. He is unresponsive on admission to the emergency department and is taken to the operating room for a craniotomy. Upon his return to the ICU, you learn that he has had an epidural hematoma evacuated from a depressed skull fracture. He has a ventriculostomy ICP monitor in place. During the first postoperative day, you note waveform pressures of approximately 12 mm Hg on the ICP monitor. The P2 wave is lower than the P1. C waves are evident. His level of consciousness is variable, with a Glasgow Coma Scale (GCS) score of 8 on stimulation.

51. Based on the preceding information, which condition is likely to be developing?
(A) increased ICP
(B) possible rebleeding, as indicated by the lack of an A wave
(C) an obstruction of the catheter due to the presence of C waves
(D) a normal ICP with good compliance

52. Which treatment should be undertaken for this condition?
(A) Level the CSF transducer to the phlebostatic axis.
(B) Increase the frequency of ICP monitoring.
(C) Flush the ICP catheter with normal saline.
(D) No treatment.

53. Neurogenic hyperventilation is associated with damage to which structure?
(A) cerebral cortex
(B) cerebellum
(C) thalamus
(D) brainstem

54. Initial assessment of the neurologically impaired patient should include measurement of which of the following?
(A) level of consciousness
(B) pupillary eye movement
(C) deep tendon reflexes
(D) brainstem reflexes

55. A fixed and dilated pupil indicates compression of which cranial nerve?
(A) I
(B) II
(C) III
(D) IV

Questions 56 through 59 refer to the following scenario:
A 79-year-old woman is in the ICU following a head injury from a fall down a series of steps. On arrival several hours earlier, she was confused but able to open her eyes to voice and localize pain. Currently she is unresponsive, but with painful stimuli opens her eyes, manifests extensor postures, and makes groaning noises. In addition, you note that the left pupil is larger than the right, whereas previous examinations noted pupillary equality.

56. Based on the preceding information, what is the GCS score?
(A) 3
(B) 6
(C) 9
(D) 15

57. What might the change in pupillary size indicate?
(A) decreased cerebral perfusion pressure
(B) loss of upper motor neuron function
(C) loss of cerebellar function
(D) increased ICP

58. Treatment for this condition could include which of the following?
(A) cervical support
(B) spinal tap to relieve increased ICP
(C) mechanical ventilation to augment MAP
(D) intubation to control the airway, placement of an ICP monitor, and administration of osmotic diuretics

59. While monitoring ICP, you note that it is 18 mm Hg and the P2 wave is higher than the P1 and P3 waves. You anticipate that suctioning of the patient will produce what type of reaction?
(A) A wave: increase in ICP from 18 to 28 mm Hg
(B) B wave: no change in ICP
(C) C wave: decrease in ICP from 18 to 10 mm Hg
(D) D wave: decrease in the CO_2, thus decreasing ICP

60. Which structure or structures are a part of the supratentorial space?
(A) cerebellum
(B) pons
(C) cerebral hemispheres
(D) medulla

61. Which of the following is a common complication of a ruptured intracranial aneurysm?
(A) hypotension due to hypovolemia
(B) cardiac dysrhythmias
(C) acid–base disturbances
(D) vasospasm of cerebral arteries

62. Signs and symptoms of meningeal irritation include all of the following EXCEPT:
(A) nuchal rigidity and headache
(B) Kernig's and Brudzinski's signs
(C) aphasia and paresis
(D) photophobia

63. Which of the following is an early sign of increased ICP?
(A) dilated pupils
(B) respiratory depression
(C) papilledema
(D) depressed level of consciousness

64. Which of the following reflexes indicate third cranial nerve involvement?
(A) pupillary light reflexes
(B) oculocephalic responses
(C) oculovestibular responses
(D) spinal reflexes

65. Decerebrate posturing is characterized by which of the following?
(A) abnormal extension response
(B) abnormal flexion response
(C) hyperflexion of the lower extremities
(D) absent motor response

66. Diagnostic procedures usually performed when intracranial hypertension is suspected may include all of the following but one. Which of the following procedures is NOT performed?
(A) CT scan
(B) lumbar puncture
(C) ventriculostomy
(D) cranial nerve examination

67. Nursing interventions for the patient having seizures include all of the following EXCEPT:
(A) protecting the patient from injury
(B) observing and recording seizure patterns
(C) administering anticonvulsive drugs such as phenytoin (Dilantin)
(D) restraining the patient

68. The nurse should be aware of the characteristics of psychomotor seizures. Which of the following statements regarding psychomotor seizures is true?
(A) They are psychological in origin.
(B) The patient usually becomes unconscious.
(C) They involve repetitive behavioral patterns.
(D) They involve acts of random violence.

69. The most important treatment for the patient in status epilepticus is:
(A) maintenance of ventilation or respiratory support
(B) administration of diazepam
(C) administration of glucose
(D) administration of phenytoin

70. Pathophysiologic consequences of status epilepticus include all of the following except one. Which of the following consequences is NOT associated with status epilepticus?
(A) hypoxemia
(B) hypoglycemia
(C) hyperthermia
(D) hypothermia

Questions 71 and 72 refer to the following scenario:
A 71-year-old woman is admitted to your unit with a large intracerebral hemorrhage. She is currently responsive to painful stimuli and has a GCS score of 8. Her BP is 180/110 mm Hg and pulse is 64; she is intubated on mechanical ventilation with a respiratory rate of 10. Her pupils are equal and reactive. During your shift, you note that her level of consciousness suddenly decreases. On examining her eyes, you note that the left pupil is large and not reactive to light. Vital signs are BP 192/114 mm Hg, pulse 56, respiratory rate 10. The patient's blood glucose level is 70.

71. Based on the preceding information, what has most likely occurred?
(A) Decreasing ICP has caused negative-pressure dysfunction of the second (optic) cranial nerve.
(B) Hypoglycemia has occurred.
(C) Increasing MAP has decreased cerebral perfusion.
(D) Increasing ICP has compressed the third (oculomotor) cranial nerve.

72. What is the prognostic implication of herniation through the foramen magnum?
(A) With aggressive treatment, neurologic function can be recovered.
(B) Neurologic function is unlikely to be recovered.
(C) Visual defects are likely to be permanent but other neurologic functions will recover.
(D) No predictions regarding neurologic recovery can be made.

73. Myasthenia gravis is characterized by which of the following?
(A) ascending paralysis
(B) neuromuscular weakness with exercise and improvement with rest
(C) uncoordinated motor control
(D) peripheral sensory deficits

74. Which of the following is the major objective of therapy in myasthenia gravis?
(A) stimulation of synaptic terminals to produce adrenocorticotropic hormone (ACTH)
(B) supportive care for the patient, since the disease is self-limiting
(C) administration of anticholinesterase medications
(D) administration of ACTH

Questions 75 and 76 refer to the following scenario:
A 56-year-old man is admitted to your unit with a decreasing level of consciousness. His primary diagnosis is adenocarcinoma of the lung with possible metastatic spread to the brain. The family wants "everything done," which is why he has been admitted to the unit. His pupils are small but reactive. Respiration is cyclic, increasing in depth and rate and then characterized by short periods of apnea. Later in your shift, the patient's level of consciousness decreases further, his pupils become dilated (3–4 mm) and unresponsive to light, and his respiration increases in frequency and depth.

75. Based on the preceding information, which condition is likely to be developing?
(A) central herniation syndrome
(B) uncal herniation syndrome
(C) unilateral hemispheric compression
(D) pontine angle compression

76. The patient is intubated to protect his airway and has an ICP monitor placed. Which of the following treatments would NOT be indicated in this situation?
(A) CSF drainage via the ventriculostomy
(B) osmotic diuretics
(C) corticosteroids
(D) lumbar puncture

77. Nursing interventions for myasthenia gravis include all of the following EXCEPT:
(A) monitoring ventilation status due to muscle weakness
(B) administration of aminoglycosides
(C) administration of anticholinesterase medications
(D) timing of activities to avoid fatigue

78. Cholinergic crisis in myasthenia gravis is due to which of the following events?
(A) insufficient dose of medication
(B) overdose of medication
(C) fatigue, stress, or infection
(D) worsening of the disease process

79. Guillain–Barré syndrome affects which neurologic component?
(A) peripheral nervous system
(B) central nervous system
(C) autonomic nervous system
(D) Schwann cells

Questions 80 and 81 refer to the following scenario:
A patient of yours has been in a motor vehicle accident and has received cervical and spinal stabilization. He is alert and oriented with no evidence of head injury. He has weakness of the upper extremities but has normal 5/5 strength in the lower extremities.

80. Based on the preceding information, this type of response to spinal injury would be referred to as:
(A) total transection
(B) anterior cord syndrome
(C) central cord syndrome
(D) Brown–Séquard syndrome

81. Treatment for this condition would most likely include:
(A) Lowering the MAP to 70 mm Hg to reduce edema
(B) Immediate surgical spinal fusion
(C) Increasing the MAP to more than 85 mm Hg to enhance perfusion
(D) Keeping the patient cool to reduce swelling

82. A patient is admitted to the ICU with signs and symptoms of ascending paralysis and respiratory failure. The critical care nurse would investigate for a past history of:
(A) trauma to the spinal cord
(B) trauma to the head
(C) postviral, respiratory, or gastrointestinal infection
(D) aspiration

83. Which of the following organisms is the most common cause of bacterial meningitis in adults?
(A) meningococcus
(B) *Haemophilus influenzae*
(C) *Diplococcus pneumoniae*
(D) pneumococcus

84. Clinical signs and symptoms of meningitis include all of the following EXCEPT:
(A) positive Kernig's and Brudzinski's signs
(B) headache and photophobia
(C) hemiparesis and atrophy of muscles
(D) photophobia and seizures

85. Which of the following are treatments for myasthenia gravis?
(A) pyridostigmine (Mestinon)
(B) neostigmine (Prostigmin)
(C) prednisone
(D) all of the above

86. Which of the following surgical treatments may be useful in myasthenia gravis?
(A) splenectomy
(B) thymectomy
(C) nerve transplants
(D) pineal transplants

87. What is the reason that even a nonmalignant brain tumor may have dangerous consequences?
(A) Nonmalignant brain tumors can convert into malignant tumors.
(B) Brain tumors can secrete exogenous catecholamines.
(C) The mass in the brain can distort the ability to sense normal balance.
(D) Any mass will increase the ICP because of the cranial structure's lack of distensibility.

88. Which of the following is NOT considered a neurotransmitter?
(A) dopamine
(B) dobutamine
(C) acetylcholine
(D) norepinephrine

89. Which of the following is the precursor to both epinephrine and norepinephrine?
(A) dopamine
(B) dobutamine
(C) acetylcholine
(D) norepinephrine

90. Which substrate does the brain depend on most heavily for nutritional needs?
(A) fats
(B) proteins
(C) carbohydrates
(D) neurotransmitters

91. Anterior gray columns in the spinal cord contain cell bodies of which fiber type?
(A) afferent (sensory)
(B) efferent (motor)
(C) parasympathetic
(D) sympathetic synaptic

92. **Fracture of which vertebra is termed the "hangman's fracture" because of the loss of spinal stabilization of the head?**
(A) C2
(B) C3
(C) C7
(D) T1

93. **Lesions of the cerebellum cause which type of response?**
(A) spastic muscle activity
(B) changes in level of consciousness
(C) changes in behavior
(D) disturbances of equilibrium

94. **Lesions of the medulla cause which type of response?**
(A) disturbances in heart and respiratory rate or pattern
(B) changes in level of consciousness
(C) changes in behavior
(D) flaccid paralysis

Questions 95 and 96 refer to the following scenario:
A 19-year-old man is admitted to your unit following a motor vehicle accident. He currently is responsive but has no sensation below the upper chest area. Lateral cervical films reveal a possible C6 fracture. A cervical magnetic resonance imaging (MRI) reveals transection of the cord at C6.

95. **Based on the preceding information, what is the likelihood of the patient's recovering the ability to walk?**
(A) good likelihood with rehabilitation
(B) good likelihood with surgery
(C) possible only if stabilization of the injury allows new spinal growth
(D) unlikely

96. **Treatment of this condition would most likely include which of the following measures?**
(A) supportive care, because no treatment would be effective
(B) surgical decompression
(C) bed rest on a spinal board
(D) cervical traction

97. **Which condition characterizes upper and lower extremity weakness with more pronounced upper extremity weakness?**
(A) Guillain–Barré syndrome
(B) Brown–Séquard syndrome
(C) central cord syndrome
(D) anterior cord syndrome

Questions 98 and 99 refer to the following scenario:
A 39-year-old construction worker is admitted to your unit after being crushed between two metal sheets. No head injury occurred and he is alert and oriented. He is able to sense pain and touch, although the sensations are faint. He has no ability to move his legs or abdomen. MRI reveals additional cord compression from bony fragments.

98. **Based on the preceding information, which condition is likely to be present?**
(A) C6 transection
(B) Brown–Séquard syndrome
(C) central cord syndrome
(D) anterior cord syndrome

99. **Which treatment would most likely be indicated for this condition?**
(A) supportive care, since no treatment would be effective
(B) surgical decompression
(C) bed rest on a spinal board
(D) cervical traction

100. **A patient sustains a spinal cord injury at C6. He is conscious and alert. Barring complications, he should be able to perform all of the following actions EXCEPT one. Which action will he have difficulty performing?**
(A) diaphragmatic breathing
(B) picking up objects with his fingers
(C) reaching forward
(D) sitting upright with support

101. **Spinal cord injury above which level results in loss of respiratory function?**
(A) C3
(B) C5
(C) C7
(D) T2

102. **Treatment of autonomic hyperreflexia consists of which of the following?**
(A) identifying and treating cause, administering ganglionic blocking agents
(B) administering ganglionic blocking agents
(C) performing bladder, bowel, and skin assessment
(D) assessing room temperature for sudden change

103. **A patient with cerebrospinal rhinorrhea would benefit most from which of the following?**
(A) assistance with nasal packing to tamponade the leak
(B) insertion of a nasogastric tube to aspirate swallowed CSF
(C) testing of the CSF with litmus paper to determine the origin of the fluid
(D) administration of prophylactic antibiotics

104. **Which of the following types of skull fractures will heal without treatment provided there is no injury to the dura mater?**
(A) basilar
(B) linear
(C) depressed
(D) compound

105. **Which reflex is indicative of an intact seventh nerve?**
(A) sensory component of the spinal reflex
(B) motor component of the corneal reflex
(C) motor component of the anal wink
(D) Hering–Breuer reflex

106. **A normal consensual light reflex indicates proper functioning of which two cranial nerves?**
(A) abducens and acoustic
(B) ophthalmic and hypoglossal
(C) optic and oculomotor
(D) trochlear and vagal

107. What is the highest score on the GCS?
(A) 3
(B) 8
(C) 15
(D) 18

108. Which of the following would NOT cause a decrease in level of consciousness?
(A) right-sided cerebral infarct without cerebral edema
(B) glucose level less than 30
(C) cerebral perfusion pressure of 40
(D) oxygen transport of 400 mL/min

109. Given the following information, what is the CPP in this patient?

Blood pressure	90/60 mm Hg
ICP	15
CVP	12
$Paco_2$	35
Pao_2	88
pH	7.34

(A) 15
(B) 35
(C) 55
(D) 75

110. Which of the following would be least likely to produce a decreased level of consciousness?
(A) acute blunt head trauma
(B) acute intracerebral hemorrhage
(C) ischemic stroke affecting anterior cerebral artery distribution
(D) grade V subarachnoid hemorrhage

Questions 111 and 112 refer to the following scenario:
S.A., a 49-year-old man, was admitted to the ICU 7 days ago with an aneurysm of the left middle cerebral artery. His aneurysm was coiled on day 1. At 0900, he was alert and oriented × 3, motor 5/5 bilaterally, with clear speech. At 1100, he complained of a headache, had a motor drift on his right arm, and was having word-finding problems.

111. You suspect that the patient is having
(A) vasospasm
(B) hydrocephalus
(C) rebleeding
(D) increased ICP

112. In order to treat the problem identified in question 111, you anticipate the following intervention:
(A) Give Lasix to help with fluid overload.
(B) Hyperventilate to reduce ICP.
(C) Give 500 mL of fluid and increase the systolic blood pressure to between 160 and 180 mm Hg.
(D) Give steroids.

113. Assume that a patient has had a severe head injury and does not respond to verbal stimuli. Which of the following supports a possible injury to the brainstem?
(A) hearing deficits
(B) motor responses impairment
(C) hemiparesis
(D) cranial nerve deficits and changes in respiratory rate and rhythm

114. Impending uncal herniation is indicated by which of the following?
(A) decreased level of consciousness
(B) positive doll's eyes
(C) unilateral pupil dilation
(D) bilateral pupil dilation

115. Which of the following are signs of increasing ICP?
(A) bradycardia and hypertension
(B) bradycardia and hypotension
(C) tachycardia and hypertension
(D) tachycardia and hypotension

116. Which of the following best describes the absence of the doll's eyes response?
(A) movement of the eyes in opposition to the movement of the head
(B) dysconjugate eye movements
(C) movement of the eyes in the same direction as movement of the head
(D) eyes remaining stationary, midline, and midposition no matter which direction the head is turned

117. Which of the following indicate(s) brain death?
(A) Loss of pain response in all extremities
(B) Loss of brainstem reflexes
(C) Apnea
(D) All of the above

Question 118 refers to the following scenario:
A patient is admitted with head and chest trauma after a motor vehicle accident. He requires a craniotomy with the insertion of an ICP monitor. On the second postoperative day, he is responsive to stimuli and follows commands. Later in your shift, he becomes responsive only to painful stimuli. The following information is available:

Blood pressure	90/58 mm Hg
Pulse	107
ICP	24
CVP	13
Serum glucose	92
Pao_2	68
$Paco_2$	36

118. Based on the preceding information, what is the likely reason for the loss of responsiveness?
(A) decreased substrate (ie, glucose) availability
(B) decreased PaO_2 levels
(C) reduced ICP
(D) decreased cerebral perfusion pressure

119. Which structure primarily regulates the autonomic nervous system?
(A) cerebellum
(B) thalamus
(C) hypothalamus
(D) frontal lobe of the cerebral cortex

120. Which function is primarily regulated by the occipital lobe?
(A) speech
(B) vision
(C) coordination
(D) respiration

121. Meningeal irritation is indicated by which of the following signs?
(A) nuchal rigidity
(B) Homan sign
(C) positive extensor plantar (Babinski) reflex
(D) flaccid paralysis

Questions 122 and 123 refer to the following scenario:
A 72-year-old woman is admitted to the unit following a fall at home. Her daughter explains that her mother tried to stand after dinner and immediately fell. Currently, she is awake but unable to move her left side. She is able to talk and is alert and oriented. Admission vital signs are as follows:

Blood pressure	176/110 mm Hg
Pulse	62
Respiratory rate	16
Temperature	36.8°C

Pupils are equal and reactive; eye movements are normal. The patient states that she has been healthy and has never "needed to see a doctor."

122. Based on the preceding information, which condition is likely to be developing?
(A) left-sided cerebrovascular accident (CVA)
(B) internal carotid vasospasm
(C) right-sided CVA
(D) external carotid obstruction

123. Which neurologic test would be most helpful in establishing the diagnosis in this patient?
(A) CT scan
(B) cold-water caloric test
(C) oculocephalic testing
(D) electroencephalogram (EEG)

124. Which neurotransmitter is most important for synaptic transmission?
(A) serotonin
(B) acetylcholine
(C) dobutamine
(D) glucose

125. Contrecoup head injuries arise from which of the following mechanisms?
(A) injury to the side opposite the trauma
(B) injury to the side of the trauma
(C) cranial vault fracture due to high torque forces
(D) epidural tears from superficial scalp pressures

Questions 126 and 127 refer to the following scenario:
A 24-year-old woman is admitted to your unit following a fall from a horse. After the fall, the horse kicked her in the temporal region of the head. She is admitted to the unit directly from the emergency department. She is unresponsive except to deep, painful stimuli. Computed tomography (CT) scans of the head reveal a temporal skull fracture. The following data are available:

Blood pressure	170/90 mm Hg
Pulse	56
Respiratory rate	10

126. Based on the preceding information, which condition is likely to be developing?
(A) epidural hematoma
(B) subdural hematoma
(C) obstructive hydrocephalus
(D) contrecoup head injury

127. Which treatment would be indicated based on the preceding data?
(A) increasing the ventilator rate
(B) placement of an ICP monitor
(C) immediate craniotomy
(D) mannitol infusion

128. Which of the following is an indication of a basilar skull fracture?
(A) raccoon eyes
(B) decreasing pulse pressure
(C) spastic paralysis
(D) flaccid paralysis

129. Which of the following is the best description of Battle's sign?
(A) generalized petechial development
(B) bleeding from the paranasal sinus
(C) hyperreflexia
(D) ecchymosis over the mastoid projection

130. Which type of head injury typically produces rapid clinical deterioration?
(A) subdural hematoma
(B) depressed skull fracture without displacement
(C) epidural hematoma
(D) subarachnoid hematoma

131. Which test is the most diagnostic for identifying head injuries?
(A) cranial roentgenogram
(B) lumbar puncture
(C) CT scan
(D) positron emission tomography (PET) scan

Questions 132 and 133 refer to the following scenario:
An 81-year-old man in your unit has a cerebral mass that has compressed the right optic tract. He is alert and oriented with no complaints except for visual disturbances. The physician has described the visual defect as left homonymous hemianopsia.

132. Which visual symptoms would be seen with this lesion?
(A) loss of vision in the right eye
(B) loss of vision in the left eye
(C) loss of vision on the left hemifield of each eye ("left visual field cut")
(D) loss of vision on the right hemifield of each eye ("right visual field cut")

133. What should the nurse do with regard to placing items that might be needed by the patient?
(A) Instruct the patient not to reach for any items without assistance.
(B) No precautions are needed.
(C) Keep objects toward the right.
(D) Keep objects toward the left.

134. Myasthenia gravis is thought to occur due to which mechanism?
(A) loss of myelinated tissue
(B) disturbances in the reticular-activating system
(C) deficient production of phenylephrine
(D) disturbance of acetylcholine utilization

Questions 135 and 136 refer to the following scenario:
A 37-year-old woman is admitted to your unit with possible aspiration pneumonia. She has complained of gradually worsening difficulty in swallowing, which she believes is what precipitated her respiratory difficulties. During the examination, you note that she has ptosis of both eyes and has weak eye closure strength. Muscle weakness is generalized. No sensory deficits exist. She states that she fatigues easily, although she recovers some strength after rest.

135. Based on the preceding information, which condition could be developing?
(A) multiple sclerosis
(B) Guillain–Barré syndrome
(C) temporal lobe tumor
(D) myasthenia gravis

136. Which test would be performed to help identify the disease?
(A) administration of edrophonium chloride (Tensilon)
(B) a 6-min walk
(C) administration of epinephrine
(D) CT scan

137. Which of the following is NOT a treatment for myasthenia gravis?
(A) thymectomy
(B) Mestinon
(C) plasmapheresis
(D) Neo-Synephrine

138. A 69-year-old man has a cardiopulmonary arrest and is brought to your unit. Which of the following medications, if given previously, would interfere with an assessment of pupillary response?
(A) atropine and procainamide
(B) bretylium
(C) lidocaine
(D) atropine and epinephrine

Questions 139 and 140 refer to the following scenario:
A 43-year-old man is admitted to your unit with complaints of severe headache, pain in the neck on flexion, and sensitivity to light. He has no specific muscle weakness or sensory deficits but does have a positive Kernig's sign. Vital signs are as follows:

Blood pressure	142/84 mm Hg
Pulse	118
Respiratory rate	30
Temperature	40°C

139. Based on the preceding information, which condition is likely to be developing?
(A) meningitis
(B) intracerebral bleeding
(C) myasthenia gravis
(D) subarachnoid bleeding

140. Which treatment would most likely be instituted?
(A) craniotomy
(B) administration of anticholinesterase agents
(C) insertion of a ventricular drain to reduce the increased ICP
(D) administration of antibiotics

Questions 141 and 142 refer to the following scenario:
A 36-year-old man is admitted to your unit with rapidly increasing symptoms of generalized weakness following an episode of "flu." He noted that the weakness started in his arms and legs and has progressed to his upper legs, abdomen, and chest. He has difficulty taking a deep breath. Vital signs are normal and he has some complaints of shortness of breath.

141. Based on the preceding symptoms, which condition is likely to be developing?
(A) Guillain–Barré syndrome
(B) myasthenia gravis
(C) multiple sclerosis
(D) amyotrophic lateral sclerosis

142. Which treatment is likely to be given for this condition?
(A) administration of anticholinesterase agents
(B) supportive treatments, particularly of the respiratory system
(C) administration of antibiotics
(D) administration of sympathetic stimulation agents, such as norepinephrine

143. Which of the following best describes Kernig's sign?
(A) muscle spasms in the arm upon occlusion with a blood pressure cuff
(B) twitching of the face upon tapping the cheek
(C) inability to flex the neck
(D) inability to extend the leg when the thigh is flexed to the abdomen

144. Brudzinski's sign is best described by which of the following definitions?
(A) adduction and flexion of the legs with neck flexion
(B) pain in the neck upon raising the arms above shoulder level
(C) temporary flaccid paralysis after neck compression
(D) development of superficial muscle tremors after repetitive reflex testing

145. If a patient develops a tonic–clonic seizure, which initial nursing action should take place?
(A) forcing of an airway into the mouth
(B) protecting the patient from injury
(C) starting oxygen therapy
(D) placing a padded tongue blade into the mouth

PART V
Neurology Practice Exam

Practice Fill-Ins

1. ____________
2. ____________
3. ____________
4. ____________
5. ____________
6. ____________
7. ____________
8. ____________
9. ____________
10. ____________
11. ____________
12. ____________
13. ____________
14. ____________
15. ____________
16. ____________
17. ____________
18. ____________
19. ____________
20. ____________
21. ____________
22. ____________
23. ____________
24. ____________
25. ____________
26. ____________
27. ____________
28. ____________
29. ____________
30. ____________
31. ____________
32. ____________
33. ____________
34. ____________
35. ____________
36. ____________
37. ____________
38. ____________
39. ____________
40. ____________
41. ____________
42. ____________
43. ____________
44. ____________
45. ____________
46. ____________
47. ____________
48. ____________
49. ____________
50. ____________
51. ____________
52. ____________
53. ____________
54. ____________
55. ____________
56. ____________
57. ____________
58. ____________
59. ____________
60. ____________
61. ____________
62. ____________
63. ____________
64. ____________
65. ____________
66. ____________
67. ____________
68. ____________
69. ____________
70. ____________
71. ____________
72. ____________
73. ____________
74. ____________
75. ____________
76. ____________
77. ____________
78. ____________
79. ____________
80. ____________
81. ____________
82. ____________
83. ____________
84. ____________
85. ____________

86. ______
87. ______
88. ______
89. ______
90. ______
91. ______
92. ______
93. ______
94. ______
95. ______
96. ______
97. ______
98. ______
99. ______
100. ______
101. ______
102. ______
103. ______
104. ______
105. ______
106. ______
107. ______
108. ______
109. ______
110. ______
111. ______
112. ______
113. ______
114. ______
115. ______
116. ______
117. ______
118. ______
119. ______
120. ______
121. ______
122. ______
123. ______
124. ______
125. ______
126. ______
127. ______
128. ______
129. ______
130. ______
131. ______
132. ______
133. ______
134. ______
135. ______
136. ______
137. ______
138. ______
139. ______
140. ______
141. ______
142. ______
143. ______
144. ______
145. ______

PART V
Answers

1. **A** Chapter 30 Rationale: The three membranes covering the entire brain surface, the spinal cord, and the spinal canal below the cord are the meninges (Fig. 30-3). The mnemonic "PAD" may help you to remember the meningeal coverings and their purpose: the *p*ia mater, *a*rachnoid, and *d*ura mater are the meningeal layers, and they absorb shocks from sudden movements or trauma; they literally "PAD" the brain. Starting from the brain itself, the first meningeal layer is the pia mater. The pia mater is contiguous with the brain's surface and its convolutions.
2. **C** Chapter 30 Rationale: After circulating (in the subarachnoid space) over the entire brain and spinal cord, the CSF is reabsorbed by the arachnoid villi in dural sinuses and by Pacchionian bodies found in the superior sagittal sinus.
3. **B** Chapter 30 Rationale: The outermost layer of the meninges is the dura mater. It is actually two layers of tough fibrous membrane that protect the underlying cortical matter. The outermost layer forms the periosteum of the cranial cavity. The inner layer is lined with flat cells and contains arteries and veins. Between the two layers are clefts, which form the dural venous sinuses. The inner layer also gives rise to several folds, which divide the cranial cavity into compartments.
4. **D** Chapter 30 Rationale: The cerebrum is contained in the anterior and middle fossae of the cranium. The left and right cerebral hemispheres are incompletely separated by a deep medial longitudinal fissure, called the falx cerebri, formed by the sagittal folds of the dura mater.
5. **A** Chapter 30 Rationale: The two cerebral hemispheres are joined by the corpus callosum (Fig. 30-6). It provides a path for fibers to cross from one hemisphere to the other.
6. **B** Chapter 30 Rationale: The temporal lobes are located under the lateral fissures of Sylvius. The temporal lobes are each divided into a primary auditory receptive area (in the dominant hemisphere), a secondary auditory association area, and a tertiary visual association area.
7. **D** Chapter 30 Rationale: The frontal lobe is responsible for voluntary motor function and higher mental functions such as judgment and foresight, affect, personality, inhibition, abstract thinking, and motor speech (dominant hemisphere).
8. **A** Chapter 30 Rationale: The midbrain is also known as the mesencephalon. Located between the diencephalon and the pons, it contains the major motor nerves for eye movement, carries impulses down from the cerebrum, and controls the wakefulness of the brain through the reticular-activating system (Fig. 30-11). Reticular-activating system fibers connect with the thalamus, cerebral cortex, cerebellum, and spinal cord. They contain nuclei of the third and fourth cranial nerves.
9. **A** Chapter 30 Rationale: The thalamus is the largest structure in the diencephalon; it integrates all body sensations except smell. It is also the major relay area for all neuronal impulses.
10. **A** Chapter 30 Rationale: The pons in conjunction with the medulla controls the rate and length of respirations.
11. **D** Chapter 30 Rationale: Equilibrium, posture, muscle tone, and ultimately muscle coordination are mediated by the cerebellum. Thought integration is associated with the cerebral cortex, and personality with the frontal lobes. The occipital lobe involves sight. Choose D.
12. **C** Chapter 30 Rationale: The lateral ventricles are connected to the third ventricle via the interventricular foramen, or the foramen of Monro.
13. **B** Chapter 30 Rationale: The foramen of Monro allows the CSF to leave the lateral ventricles and flow into the third ventricle. Obstruction at this point will produce hydrocephalus. The most common site of obstructive hydrocephalus occurs in the aqueduct of Sylvius at or above the fourth ventricle, obstruction at the foramen of Monro, or at the outlets of the fourth ventricle. From the third ventricle, CSF flows through the aqueduct of Sylvius into the fourth ventricle. Foramina of Luschka and Magendie direct the CSF from the fourth ventricle into the cisterns and subarachnoid space.
14. **D** Chapter 30 Rationale: CSF is synthesized at approximately 20 mL/h by the choroid plexus. This is an area of modified epithelial cells covering tufts of capillaries found in all ventricles but predominating in the anterior segment of the lateral ventricles. CSF is a clear, colorless liquid having a few cells, some protein, glucose, and a large amount of sodium chloride.
15. **C** Chapter 30 Rationale: The CSF "cushions" the brain and spinal cord to protect them from colliding with the cranium and vertebrae in response to moving forces. The CSF also reduces the gravitational weight of the brain.
16. **B** Chapter 30 Rationale: The frontal lobe (approximately the anterior one-third of the hemisphere) is the portion that is anterior to the central sulcus and above the lateral fissure. The frontal lobe is responsible for voluntary motor function and higher mental functions such as judgment and foresight, affect, personality, inhibition, abstract thinking, and motor speech (dominant hemisphere).

17. **B** Chapter 30 Rationale: The parietal lobe extends from the central sulcus to the parietooccipital fissure. This lobe is responsible for sensory function, sensory association, and higher-level processing of general sensory modalities.
18. **B** Chapter 30 Rationale: The brain is supplied with oxygenated blood from two arterial systems: the anterior circulation, originating with the internal carotid arteries, and the posterior circulation, which originates with the vertebral arteries. The common carotid arteries bifurcate, forming the external (supplying the neck and face) and internal carotid arteries (supplying the anterior circulation).
19. **C** Chapter 30 Rationale: The sympathetic nervous system releases norepinephrine, which stimulates and prepares the body for "fight, fright, or flight." Norepinephrine and epinephrine are categorized as adrenergic chemicals (hormones). Fibers originating in the thoracic and lumbar areas form the peripheral sympathetic nervous system division. Epinephrine and norepinephrine are found in adrenergic fibers of the sympathetic nervous system. In the central nervous system (CNS), norepinephrine cell bodies are confined to the brainstem, but their axons extend to all parts of the CNS. Epinephrine neurons are restricted to the lower brainstem.
20. **A** Chapter 30 Rationale: The brain has its own autoregulatory mechanism, which functions mainly by increasing (constricting arteries) resistance to blood flow or by decreasing (dilatation of arteries) resistance to blood flow, thus altering the diameter of the vessels. Autoregulation maintains constant blood flow over a range of perfusion pressures. The limits of autoregulation are generally thought to be a mean arterial pressure (MAP) between 50 and 150 mm Hg. This system works well until the ICP increases beyond a certain unknown point, when compensatory mechanisms fail. The key words in the question are "autoregulation" and "circulatory".
21. **B** Chapter 30 Rationale: The area of the brain most sensitive to hypoxia is the telencephalon, particularly the hippocampus, which is most likely to be damaged by small amounts of decreased oxygen. Since the cerebral cortex is only six layers (cells) deep (Fig. 30-7), the entire cerebral cortex, especially layer four, is very sensitive to decreases in oxygen. Damage here results in a condition termed laminar cortical necrosis.
22. **B** Chapter 30 Rationale: The brain is supplied with oxygenated blood from two arterial systems: the anterior circulation, originating with the carotid arteries, and the posterior circulation, which originates with the vertebral arteries. The common carotid arteries bifurcate, forming the external and internal carotid arteries. As a reserve to these two systems, the circle of Willis helps to provide adequate circulation through its anastomoses. The circle of Willis anastomoses are between the two vertebral arteries and the two carotid arteries (Fig. 30-14). The internal carotid carries about two-thirds of the blood that flows to the brain. The right and left vertebral arteries branch off the subclavian arteries. They pass through the foramen magnum as they enter the skull.
23. **A** Chapter 30 Rationale: The hypothalamus has neural as well as endocrine functions. It is responsible for the production of antidiuretic hormone (ADH) and oxytocin as well as influencing body temperature, water balance, and the intake of food.
24. **C** Chapter 34 Rationale: Gray matter is composed of nerve cells and unmyelinated fibers arranged in three columns. Myelinated tissue refers to white matter.
25. **D** Chapter 34 Rationale: The significant descending tracts are the rubrospinal tract, ventral and lateral corticospinal tracts, and tectospinal tract. These carry motor impulses. Ascending tracts transmit sensory information
26. **B** Chapter 34 Rationale: Brown–Séquard syndrome is due to transection or lesion of one-half of the spinal cord (Fig. 34-14). There is loss of motor function (paralysis) and position and vibratory sense as well as vasomotor paralysis on the same side (ipsilateral) and below the hemisection. On the opposite (contralateral) side of the hemisection, there is loss of pain and temperature sensation below the level of the lesion or hemisection.
27. **A** Chapter 32 Rationale: In the acute subdural hematoma (Fig. 32-3), symptoms occur usually within hours to several days. Acute subdural hematomas usually present with signs of increasing ICP, decreasing loss of consciousness (LOC), and ipsilateral oculomotor paralysis with contralateral hemiparesis. The signs and symptoms are those of a rapidly expanding mass lesion. The key word is "acute." B refers to acute-on-chronic or "subacute." C & D are associated with a chronic subdural.
28. **D** Chapter 34 Rationale: Cervical injury or fracture may disrupt the diaphragm, leading to diminished or absent respiratory function. Injury or fracture above C5 presents special problems in that total respiratory function is lost. Remember that diaphragmatic function depends on C3 to C5. If this area is injured, artificial ventilation will be required to keep the patient alive. Injury or fracture of C5 or the lower cervical vertebrae will result in diaphragmatic breathing if the phrenic nerve is functioning. Hypoventilation almost always occurs with diaphragmatic respirations because there is a decrease in vital capacity and tidal volume.
29. **A** Chapter 34 Rationale: Any cord transection above the level of T5 abolishes the influence of the sympathetic nervous system. Consequently, the immediate problems will be bradycardia and hypotension. If the bradycardia is only slight, close cardiac monitoring may reveal a stable cardiac condition. Junctional escape beats may be observed and a junctional rhythm may become established. If the bradycardia is marked, appropriate medications (atropine) to increase the heart rate and avoid hypoxia will be necessary.

    With the abolition of the influence of the sympathetic nervous system, vasodilatation occurs, decreasing venous return of blood to the heart. This decreases cardiac output, and hypotension results. Intravenous fluids may resolve the problem, otherwise vasopressor drugs may be required. Dopamine is an ideal agent due to its ability to increase BP and heart rate. The goal is to keep the MAP more than 85 to 90 mm Hg for a minimum of 7 days.

30. **A** Chapter 34 Rationale: Autonomic hyperreflexia (formerly known as autonomic dysreflexia) is usually seen with injuries to the spinal cord at the level of T6 or higher. The condition is a life-threatening situation requiring immediate attention.

    The most common precipitating causes are a distended bladder or a full rectum. Contraction of the bladder or rectum, stimulation of the skin, stimulation of the pain receptors, or sudden change in environmental temperature may also cause autonomic hyperreflexia.

    Symptoms include extreme hypertension, blurred vision, severe throbbing headache, unusual apprehension, marked diaphoresis, and flushing above the level of the lesion with pallor and coolness below, bradycardia, piloerection (body hair erect) due to pilomotor spasm, nasal congestion, and nausea. The hypertension can be so severe that the patient may suffer a stroke or myocardial infarction.

31. **B** Chapter 31 Rationale: ICP represents the ever-changing relationship between the brain, blood, and CSF inside the cranial vault. In adults, the normal ICP range is 5 to 15 mm Hg. Increase in ICP greater than 20 mm Hg is considered elevated and treatment measures are generally initiated at that level. Intracranial hypertension is defined as an ICP greater than 20 mm Hg that persists for 5 minutes or longer. The control of ICP elevations is an important aspect of the management of severe traumatic brain injury and other intracranial pathologies, since sustained increases in ICP can result in decreases in the delivery of oxygenated blood to the brain as well as herniation and compression of the brain and brainstem. Without interventions to reduce the ICP, blood flow to the brain is compromised. The comprehension of blood flow dynamics is essential to managing ICP.

32. **D** Chapter 32 Rationale: With a basilar skull fracture, there is a high risk of injury to cranial nerves, infection, and residual neurologic deficits due to coup and contrecoup forces (Fig. 32-5). Basilar fractures may occur in the anterior, middle, or posterior fossa. "Raccoon eyes" is a sign of bleeding into the paranasal sinuses and refers to ecchymosis developing around the eyes. Along with CSF draining from the nose (rhinorrhea), these signs indicate a basilar fracture in the anterior fossa. CSF draining from the ear canal (otorrhea) is a sign of a middle fossa basilar skull fracture. A temporal or basilar fracture in the posterior fossa is indicated by Battle's sign, an area of ecchymosis over the mastoid projection. Other symptoms of basilar fracture include tinnitus, facial paralysis, hearing difficulty, nystagmus, and conjugate deviation of gaze.

33. **C** Chapter 31 Rationale: Cerebral blood flow (CBF) is calculated by measuring the CPP and dividing it by the cerebrovascular resistance. CPP is used as a primary means to approximate the delivery of blood flow. CPP is the difference between the MAP and the mean ICP (CPP = MAP – ICP). Normal CPP is 80 mm Hg. In severe head injury, the minimal acceptable CPP is 50 to 70 mm Hg. When CPP declines below this threshold, there is a risk that the cerebrovasculature will vasodilate, leading to worsening of ICP. Optimal or target CPP for patients should be individualized.

34. **A** Chapter 32 Rationale: Epidural hematomas are true neurosurgical emergencies. They occur at the time of the injury and are usually associated with a temporal or parietal skull fracture with laceration of the middle meningeal artery (and often vein).

35. **B** Chapter 33 Rationale: Most cerebral aneurysms develop in the anterior arteries of the circle of Willis. To narrow down the choices, external carotids supply the face & neck and common carotids refer to the area before the bifurcation.

36. **D** Chapter 32 Rationale: Complications include cerebral edema (vasogenic and cytotoxic), hydrocephalus, seizures, increased ICP, diabetes insipidus, and residual neurologic deficits. Metabolic complications include respiratory insufficiency, infection, and systemic dysfunction as a result of associated trauma.

37. **A** Chapter 31 Rationale: Hyperventilation or lowering of the $PaCO_2$ below 35 mm Hg will cause vasoconstriction, which may help to control ICP but may also worsen cerebral hypoxia by reducing the delivery of oxygenated blood. Therefore, hyperventilation should be employed only with acute neurologic deterioration with adjunctive brain oxygen or cerebral blood flow monitoring to monitor for ischemia. Maintaining the $Paco_2$ at 35 to 40 mm Hg will reduce the chances of cerebral ischemia. The Fio_2 should be titrated to maintain adequate oxygenation. It is important to optimize the systemic oxygenation so as to maintain adequate cerebral oxygenation.

38. **B** Chapter 33 Rationale: Etiologic risk factors include hypertension (present in a majority of cases) and smoking. Diseases such as Ehlers–Danlos syndrome, coarctation of the aorta, and polycystic kidneys put individuals at risk.

39. **A** Chapter 31 Rationale: CPP is the difference between the MAP and the mean ICP (CPP = MAP – ICP). Normal CPP is 80 mm Hg.

40. **B** Chapter 31 Rationale: CPP is the difference between the MAP and the mean ICP (CPP = MAP – ICP). Even though the MAP is not included in the information provided, it can be calculated by: [(DBP × 2) + SBP]/3. Therefore, in this case the ICP (30) subtracted from the calculated MAP (83) is equal to 53. Choose B.

41. **A** Chapter 31 Rationale: CPP is the difference between the MAP and the mean ICP (CPP = MAP – ICP). Increasing the MAP in the setting of increased ICP will increase CPP.

42. **C** Chapter 31 Rationale: In severe head injury, the minimal acceptable CPP is 50 to 70 mm Hg. When CPP declines below this threshold, there is a risk that the

cerebrovasculature will vasodilate, leading to worsening of ICP.

43. **B** Chapter 31 Rationale: In adults, the normal ICP range is 5 to 15 mm Hg. Increase in ICP greater than 20 mm Hg is considered elevated and treatment measures are generally initiated at that level. Intracranial hypertension is defined as an ICP greater than 20 mm Hg that persists for 5 min or longer.

44. **D** Chapter 31 Rationale: CSF drainage is used as a primary intervention to reduce ICP when an intraventricular catheter is in place. Infections are a major threat in intraventricular monitoring. The most important step in preventing infection is maintaining a "closed" system. Sterile technique is required whenever the system is entered for CSF sampling and an occlusive dressing is maintained over the catheter insertion site.

45. **C** Chapter 30 Rationale: The hypothalamus has neural as well as endocrine functions. It is responsible for the production of ADH and oxytocin as well as influencing body temperature, water balance, and the intake of food.

46. **A** Chapter 30 Rationale: The internal carotid carries about two-thirds of the blood that flows to the brain.

47. **D** Chapter 30 Rationale: The cerebral need for oxygen does not decrease in a resting state. Even though it weighs only about 3 lbs (2% of the body weight), brain tissue requires about 20% of the body's oxygen supply.

48. **D** Chapter 30 Rationale: The brain needs a constant supply of oxygen and is unable to store oxygen for future use.

49. **D** Chapter 35 Rationale: Changes in level of consciousness occur for three reasons:

1. Reduction in oxygen delivery
2. Reduction in blood glucose
3. Reduction in CPP

50. **C** Chapter 30 Rationale: Reticular-activating system fibers connect with the thalamus, cerebral cortex, cerebellum, and spinal cord to control sleep and wakefulness.

51. **D** Chapter 31 Rationale: Normally P1, P2, and P3 appear as a descending sawtooth waveform. As the ICP increases, the amplitude of all the waves increases. When P2 becomes greater in amplitude than P1, this signals a decrease in the adaptive compliance of the brain and possibly impairment of autoregulation. The loss of compliance represents a situation where the patient is at risk for significant increases in ICP.

52. **D** Chapter 31 Rationale: No treatment is necessary, as ICP is within normal range and ICP indicates a normal descending sawtooth waveform. Continue to monitor patient.

53. **D** Chapter 30 Rationale: Collectively, the mesencephalon, pons, and medulla oblongata constitute the brainstem. Regulation of respiratory rhythm, rate, and strength of heartbeat and blood vessel diameter are controlled by the medulla. The nuclei for reflex activities such as coughing, sneezing, swallowing, and vomiting and the ninth to twelfth cranial nerves are found here.

54. **A** Chapter 32 Rationale: There are five possible states or levels of consciousness. The definition and/or progression may differ in various institutions. It may be defined as follows:

1. Alert: The patient is oriented to person, place, and time.
2. Lethargic: The patient prefers to sleep and, when aroused, their degree of alertness or confusion is variable.
3. Obtunded: The patient can be aroused with minimal stimulation but will drift off to sleep quickly.
4. Stuporous: The patient is aroused only by constant, deep, and usually painful stimuli. The patient may respond by some attempt to withdraw, moaning, or exhibiting decerebrate or decorticate positioning.
5. Coma: The patient cannot be aroused.

The GCS is one of the standard methods used to identify a patient's level of consciousness (mentation) and determine their prognosis. The GCS measures both arousal and awareness. Eye opening is a measure of arousal. Verbal and best motor response are measures of awareness. The lowest score received has the worse prognosis.

55. **C** Chapter 32 Rationale:

I: Olfactory nerve. Sense of smell

II: Optic nerve. Sensory limb of the pupillary light reflex. Visual acuity.

III: Oculomotor nerve. Motor limb of the pupillary light reflex; causes constriction of the pupil. Eyelid elevation. It controls four of the six eye muscles.

IV: Trochlear nerve. It turns the eye down and in.

56. **B** Chapter 32 Rationale:

Eye opening = 2

Best motor response = 2

Verbal response = 2

57. **D** Chapter 32 Rationale: Compression of cranial nerve III from increased ICP.

58. **D** Chapter 32 Rationale: Patients presenting with a GCS of 3 to 8 require aggressive support of their ABCs. Always establish a patent airway, using extra care to protect the cervical spine; placement of an ICP monitor and administration of osmotic diuretics to decrease cerebral edema and control ICP should be done.

59. **A** Chapter 31 Rationale: As the ICP increases, the amplitude of all the waves increases. When P2 becomes greater in amplitude than P1, this signals a decrease in the adaptive compliance of the brain and possibly impairment of autoregulation. The loss of compliance represents a situation where the patient is at risk for significant increases in ICP. "A" waves, or plateau waves, occur when there is a sudden, sustained rise in ICP. "A" waves may be present for 5 to 20 minutes. "A" waves are not normally present and occur if the ICP rises to 50 to 100 mm Hg and is sustained. "A" waves reflect cerebral ischemia secondary to a decreased arterial BP and intracranial hypertension. Remember, "A" waves are "awful".

60. **C** Chapter 35 Rationale: The tentorium cerebelli divides the supratentorial structures (the cerebral hemispheres) from the infratentorial structures (the cerebellum).

61. **D** Chapter 33 Rationale: Cerebral vasospasm results in cerebral ischemia. Vasospasm is commonly seen on days 4 and 14 post-bleed.

62. **C** Chapter 36 Rationale: Suspect meningitis if a fever, severe headache, and nuchal rigidity (resistance to flexion of the neck) exist. Positive Kernig's and Brudzinski's signs, photophobia, decreased sensorium, and signs of increased ICP are common. Kernig's sign is the inability to fully extend the leg at the knee when the leg is flexed at the hip. Brudzinski's sign is the involuntary adduction and flexion of the legs with attempts to flex the neck. With meningitis, a headache becomes progressively worse and is accompanied by nausea, vomiting, irritability, confusion, and seizures. Dysfunction of cranial nerves II through VIII may be present.

63. **D** Chapter 35 Rationale: In central herniation, increasing ICP forces the cerebral hemispheres and basal nuclei through the tentorial notch, compressing the diencephalon, mesencephalon (midbrain), and pons. Divisions of the basilar artery are also displaced, causing ischemia and brainstem deterioration. The displacement also blocks the aqueduct of Sylvius, effectively preventing the downward displacement of CSF (a compensatory mechanism of increasing ICP). This further increases ICP. Effects of central herniation usually progress in a head-to-tail direction. Thus, an alteration in level of consciousness is often a subtle first sign of impending herniation.

64. **A** Chapter 35 Rationale: III: Oculomotor nerve. Motor limb of the pupillary light reflex; causes constriction of the pupil. Eyelid elevation. It controls four of the six eye muscles.

65. **A** Chapter 35 Rationale: Motor responses are not dependent on level of consciousness but they usually correlate with LOC. Motor responses are important sources of information concerning the geographic spread of neurologic dysfunction. If the patient is awake, ask them to hold both arms out in front with palms up and count to 10. If the arms stay in the same position, there is normal strength. If a palm rotates and drifts downward, then hemiparesis is present. In the patients with altered level of consciousness who are unable to follow commands, observe motor movement to a stimulus. Use a central painful stimulus such as pinching on the trunk or pushing on the sternum. Note the motor response to the stimulation. Localization represents a purposeful response, and the patient moves to the stimulation site attempting to remove it. Withdrawal of an extremity or body part away from the stimulus is the next lower response. The cortex is not working at this level of response; the thalamus controls withdrawal. Lower-level motor responses to painful stimulation include abnormal flexion, abnormal extension, and no response, respectively.

Flexor posturing (decorticate posturing) is characterized by flexion of the arm, wrist, and fingers. Adduction of arms and extension and internal rotation with plantar flexion of the lower extremities complete the motor responses.

Extensor posturing (decerebrate posture) is characterized by opisthotonos (arching of the back so that the head and heels remain on the surface and the remainder of the back is raised) with the arms slightly extended, adducted, and hyperpronated. The legs are stiffly extended and the feet are flexed in a plantar position.

66. **B** Chapter 35 Rationale: If the ICP rises precipitously, the pressure may be sufficient to compress the cerebellum and medulla oblongata through the foramen magnum. A lumbar puncture performed in the presence of high ICP may result in brainstem herniation through the foramen magnum as the counterpressure in the spinal canal is lost. Herniation through the foramen magnum results in death secondary to cardiopulmonary arrest. This form of herniation is not clinically separable from central and uncal herniation.

67. **D** Chapter 37 Rationale: An initial priority of seizure management for nursing care is maintaining patient safety. Maintaining a patent airway and providing adequate oxygenation are additionally important. Observation of the seizure type, duration, precipitating factors, along with any focal neurologic deficits, is essential. An intravenous line should be maintained. Medications to stop seizure activity may be indicated and require administration and monitoring of response.

68. **C** Chapter 37 Rationale: The patient appears to be awake but is in an unresponsive state. Simple or elaborate behavior patterns known as automatisms may be carried out during the seizure. These robot-like behavior patterns can include such behaviors as lip smacking, blinking, or picking at clothes.

69. **A** Chapter 37 Rationale: The goal of therapy is to restore physiologic homeostasis and to stop the seizures by correcting the underlying cause. The first step in treatment is to ensure a patent airway and maintain breathing and circulation.

70. **D** Chapter 37 Rationale: Hyperthermia is often treated with a hypothermia blanket. Because hypoglycemia can induce seizure activity, a glucose level should be checked.

71. **D** Chapter 35 Rationale: Herniation is the result of increased ICP beyond compensatory levels. The rapid increase in size of a hematoma, tumor, or cerebral edema may cause the movement of brain tissue from an area of the cranium where it is normally located. The brain tissue is not evenly distributed and unless the change is corrected rapidly, the impingement on blood flow and compression of brain tissue will cause ischemia and permanent damage. This shift of tissue or protrusion through an abnormal opening is called herniation; it occurs from an area of greater pressure into an area of lower pressure. The most common type of brain herniation occurs when a portion of the temporal lobe

is displaced (uncal herniation), resulting in compression of cranial nerve III, the midbrain, and posterior cerebral artery.

72. **B** Chapter 35 Rationale: If the ICP rises precipitously, the pressure may be sufficient to compress the cerebellum and medulla oblongata through the foramen magnum. Herniation through the foramen magnum results in death secondary to cardiopulmonary arrest. This form of herniation is not clinically separable from central and uncal herniation.
73. **B** Chapter 36 Rationale: A history of an increasing muscular fatigability that improves with rest is a common characteristic of myasthenia gravis.
74. **C** Chapter 36 Rationale: The most useful treatments include anticholinesterase medications, immunosuppressive agents, thymectomy, and plasmapheresis or intravenous immunoglobulin. The major objective of therapy is to improve neuromuscular transmission and prevent complications. There is no cure for myasthenia gravis, eliminating B. ACTH is secreted from the pituitary and acts on the adrenal glands, eliminating A and D. Choose C.
75. **A** Chapter 35 Rationale: In central herniation, increasing ICP forces the cerebral hemispheres and basal nuclei through the tentorial notch, compressing the diencephalon, mesencephalon (midbrain), and pons. Divisions of the basilar artery are also displaced, causing ischemia and brainstem deterioration. The displacement also blocks the aqueduct of Sylvius, effectively preventing the downward displacement of CSF (a compensatory mechanism of increasing ICP). This further increases ICP. Effects of central herniation usually progress in a head-to-tail direction. Thus, an alteration in level of consciousness is often a subtle first sign of impending herniation.
76. **D** Chapter 35 Rationale: A lumbar puncture performed in the presence of high ICP may result in brainstem herniation through the foramen magnum as the counterpressure in the spinal canal is lost.
77. **B** Chapter 36 Rationale: A major nursing intervention is to maintain adequate ventilation in spite of a weak cough, an inability to clear secretions, and an increased likelihood of aspiration. Specific drugs that impair neuromuscular transmission must be avoided. The aminoglycoside antibiotics and true mycin drugs are contraindicated.
78. **B** Chapter 36 Rationale: Cholinergic crisis is due to an overdose of drugs and is signaled by increased salivation and sweating. An impending cholinergic crisis can be detected by noting constricted pupils; 2 mm is the maximum constriction that should be allowed before intervention.
79. **A** Chapter 36 Rationale: Guillain–Barré syndrome is an acute inflammatory disease, thought to be autoimmune or viral, that affects peripheral nerves, spinal nerves, and sometimes cranial nerves, first with edema and then demyelination.
80. **C** Chapter 34 Rationale: Central Cord Syndrome is the only disorder listed where the upper extremities are comparitively more affected than the lower extremities. Not enough detail is given to associate the symptoms with B or D. Choose C.
81. **C** Chapter 34 Rationale: With the abolition of the influence of the sympathetic nervous system, vasodilatation occurs, decreasing venous return of blood to the heart. This decreases cardiac output, and hypotension results. Intravenous fluids may resolve the problem, otherwise vasopressor drugs may be required. Dopamine is an ideal agent due to its ability to increase BP and heart rate. The goal is to keep the MAP more than 85 to 90 mm Hg for a minimum of 7 days.
82. **C** Chapter 36 Rationale: Guillain–Barré syndrome causes progressive muscle weakness, sensory loss, and areflexia as a result of peripheral nerve demyelination. It is often preceded by a virus. The predominant pattern is weakness starting in the lower extremities and advancing (often very rapidly) to motor paralysis as it progresses up the body.
83. **B** Chapter 36 Rationale: Organisms obtain access to the subarachnoid space through penetrating head injuries, basal skull fractures with a torn dura mater, ICP monitoring, cranial surgery, mastoiditis, acute otitis media, lumbar punctures, injury to the paranasal sinuses, septic emboli, and sepsis. The organism may be fungal, viral, or bacterial. Eighty percent of all bacterial meningitis is caused by *Streptococcus pneumoniae*, *Neisseria meningitidis*, and *Haemophilus influenzae*. Other Gram-positive bacteria include *Diplococcus pneumoniae*. Gram-negative bacteria include *Klebsiella*, *Escherichia coli*, and *Pseudomonas*. After neurologic surgery, *Staphylococcus aureus* or *Staphylococcus epidermidis* are common bacterial contaminants. In children, it is *H. influenzae*. Other bacteria include *Streptococcus*, *Pneumococcus*, and occasionally *Mycobacterium tuberculosis*. The outcome of bacterial meningitis depends on early and aggressive treatment. Viral causes of meningitis include enteroviruses, arboviruses, and herpesviruses. Viral meningitis is commonly referred to as aseptic meningitis. Fungal meningitis is primarily caused by *Cryptococcus neoformans*.
84. **C** Chapter 36 Rationale: Suspect meningitis if a fever, severe headache, and nuchal rigidity (resistance to flexion of the neck) exist. Positive Kernig's and Brudzinski's signs, photophobia, decreased sensorium, and signs of increased ICP are common. Kernig's sign is the inability to fully extend the leg at the knee when the leg is flexed at the hip. Brudzinski's sign is the involuntary adduction and flexion of the legs with attempts to flex the neck. With meningitis, a headache becomes progressively worse and is accompanied by nausea, vomiting, irritability, confusion, and seizures.
85. **D** Chapter 36 Rationale: Neuromuscular transmission is improved by administration of anticholinesterase drugs. Pyridostigmine bromide (Mestinon) is a popular choice.

If pyridostigmine bromide is not adequate to establish control of neuromuscular transmission, neostigmine (Prostigmin) is used. Prednisone has become an adjunctive drug of choice.

86. **B** Chapter 36 Rationale: The major objective of therapy is to improve neuromuscular transmission and prevent complications. Early thymectomy may be employed.

87. **D** Chapter 35 Rationale: Three categories of non-malignant brain tumors are important in the aforementioned pathologic processes that lead to coma:
    1. A supratentorial mass lesion will encroach on deep diencephalic structures, compressing or destroying the ascending reticular-activating system.
    2. A subtentorial mass or destructive lesion may directly damage the central core of the brainstem.
    3. Metabolic disorders may lead to generalized interruption of brain function.

88. **B** Chapter 30 Rationale: Neurotransmitters include dopamine, acetylcholine, epinephrine, norepinephrine, serotonin, and gamma aminobutyric acid (GABA).

89. **A** Chapter 30 Rationale: Dopamine is a precursor of epinephrine and norepinephrine. Dopamine acts as an inhibitory chemical transmitter and is among the most important chemicals involved in basal ganglionic functions (acetylcholine is the other important transmitter in basal ganglionic functions). Dopamine is decreased in the brains of patients with parkinsonism. It may play a role in eating, drinking, and sexual behavior.

90. **C** Chapter 30 Rationale: The extensive, continuous activity of the brain results in very high metabolic energy needs. Glucose, a carbohydrate, is the main source of energy (adenosine triphosphate, or ATP) for cellular activity. Glucose and oxygen are essential for reestablishing electrochemical gradients for impulse transmission, for the synthesis of neurotransmitters, and for maintaining cellular integrity.

91. **B** Chapter 34 Rationale: Gray matter is composed of nerve cells and unmyelinated fibers arranged in three columns. The anterior gray columns are also known as the anterior horns. They contain cell bodies of efferent (motor) fibers. The middle gray columns, known as the lateral columns, contain preganglionic fibers of the autonomic nervous system. The lateral columns are largest in the upper cervical, thoracic, and midsacral regions. The posterior columns, also known as the posterior horns, contain cell bodies of afferent (sensory) fibers.

92. **A** Chapter 34 Rationale: Trauma to the odontoid process may result in one of three fracture types and is rarely associated with cord injury. Hangman's fracture occurs when there has been a bilateral pedicle fracture of C2. The fracture causes separation of C2, C3, and their respective posterior elements. A common fracture to C1 is a Jefferson fracture, where there is disruption of the posterior and anterior arches; this rarely causes a neurologic deficit.

93. **D** Chapter 30 Rationale: Gray and white matter compose the cerebellum. The cerebellum receives input from the brainstem and spinal cord nuclei, whose axons project to the cerebellar cortex. These tracts carry excitatory impulses to cerebellar cortex. Equilibrium, posture, muscle tone, and ultimately muscle coordination are mediated by the cerebellum.

94. **A** Chapter 30 Rationale: Collectively, the mesencephalon, pons, and medulla oblongata constitute the brainstem. Regulation of respiratory rhythm, rate, and strength of heartbeat and blood vessel diameter are controlled by the medulla. The nuclei for reflex activities such as coughing, sneezing, swallowing, and vomiting and the ninth to twelfth cranial nerves are found here.

95. **D** Chapter 34 Rationale: MRI in the scenario reveals a transection, and right-hand column of the table below suggests the likely associated loss of function.

TABLE 34-1. CLASSIFICATION OF INJURY ACCORDING TO SPECIFIC VERTEBRAL LEVEL

Injury Level	*Intact Function*	*Lost Function*
Below L2	Mixed motor/sensory, depending on intact nerve fibers	Mixed motor/sensory; possibly bladder, bowels, and sexual functioning
T1 to L1 or L2	Arm function	Loss of intercostal muscles, leg functions; bladder, bowels, and sexual functioning
C7, C8	Arm movement include deltoids, biceps, and triceps muscles, head rotation, respiration	No intrinsic muscles of hand; no other function retained + above
C6, C7	Biceps muscle, head rotation, respiration	No triceps; no other function retained
C5, C6	Gross arm movement, head rotation, diaphragmatic respiration	No other function retained
C4, C5	Head rotation, diaphragmatic respiration	No other function intact
C3, C4	Head rotation	No other function intact (many die)
C1, C2	None	Poor prognosis

96. **D** Chapter 34 Rationale: The goal is the prevention of secondary injury from the release of endogenous factors stimulated from the hypoxic and ischemic cord. Vertebral stabilization includes external devices such as cervical collars, cervical traction, halo vest, cervicothoracic and thoracolumbar orthoses, as well as surgical intervention.

97. **C** Chapter 34 Rationale: When the damage is in the cervical central cord, it is termed central cord syndrome, which is characterized by microscopic hemorrhage and edema of the central cord (Fig. 34-12). There is motor weakness in both the upper and lower extremities, but the weakness is much greater in the upper extremities than the lower. Sensory dysfunction varies according to the site of injury or lesion but is generally more pronounced in the upper extremities. Reflexes in the lower extremities may be hyperactive temporarily.

98. **D** Chapter 34 Rationale: Anterior cord syndrome is characterized by injury resulting in an acute compression of the anterior portion of the spinal cord, often a flexion injury (Fig. 34-13). Compression is usually caused by a disk or bony fragment. It may also be caused by the actual destruction of the anterior cord by an anterior spinal artery occlusion (thrombus). Symptoms include immediate anterior paralysis, which is complete from the injury or compression down. Hypesthesia (decreased sensation) and hypalgesia (decreased pain sensation) occur below the level of injury. Since the posterior cord tracts are not injured, there are sensations of touch, position, vibration, proprioception, and motion.

99. **B** Chapter 34 Rationale: If the syndrome is caused by the compression of the anterior cord from bony fragments, surgical decompression is indicated.

100. **B** Chapter 34 Rationale:

TABLE 34-1. CLASSIFICATION OF INJURY ACCORDING TO SPECIFIC VERTEBRAL LEVEL

Injury Level	*Intact Function*	*Lost Function*
Below L2	Mixed motor/sensory, depending on intact nerve fibers	Mixed motor/sensory; possibly bladder, bowels, and sexual functioning
T1 to L1 or L2	Arm function	Loss of intercostal muscles, leg functions; bladder, bowels, and sexual functioning
C7, C8	Arm movement include deltoids, biceps, and triceps muscles, head rotation, respiration	No intrinsic muscles of hand; no other function retained + above
C6, C7	Biceps muscle, head rotation, respiration	No triceps; no other function retained
C5, C6	Gross arm movement, head rotation, diaphragmatic respiration	No other function retained
C4, C5	Head rotation, diaphragmatic respiration	No other function intact
C3, C4	Head rotation	No other function intact (many die)
C1, C2	None	Poor prognosis

Injuries below C6 may leave gross arm movement, but fine motor movement will be affected.

101. **B** Chapter 34 Rationale: Injury or fracture above C5 presents special problems in that total respiratory function is lost. Remember that diaphragmatic function depends on C3 to C5. If this area is injured, artificial ventilation will be required to keep the patient alive.

102. **A** Chapter 34 Rationale: To treat autonomic hyperreflexia, the underlying cause must be removed. Agents such as hydralazine hydrochloride, nitroprusside, nitroglycerin, prazosin, terazosin, and diazoxide are administered to treat the severe hypertension. However, the condition will persist unless the underlying cause is treated.

103. **D** Chapter 32 Rationale: Patients with rhinorrhea will complain of a salty taste as the CSF drains into the pharynx. Caution the patient against blowing the nose, and avoid suctioning or nasal packing if rhinorrhea is present. Otorrhea can be tested for glucose. (Laboratory testing is more accurate than glucose testing sticks.) If glucose is present, the drainage is CSF. The "halo sign," a yellow ring that appears around bloody drainage on a nose, gauze or ear pad, is another indication of CSF leakage. The goal is early detection of intracranial fluid leakage and prevention of infection.

104. **B** Chapter 32 Rationale: A linear skull fracture that does not tear the dura mater will heal without treatment. If the linear fracture occurs over the temporal lobe and tears the dura (Fig. 32-4), there is a chance that the middle meningeal artery will also be torn. Such an injury constitutes a medical emergency, since the bleeding is arterial; this is commonly known as an acute epidural hematoma.

105. **B** Chapters 30 and 35 Rationale: Cranial nerve VII is the facial nerve. It is responsible for closing the eyelid, the muscles of facial expression, secretion by glands of mouth and eyes, and taste on the anterior two-thirds of the tongue.

106. **C** Chapters 30 and 35 Rationale: Cranial nerves II and III are the optic and oculomotor nerves. The optic nerve is responsible for central and peripheral vision. The oculomotor nerve is responsible for eye movement, elevation of the upper eyelid, and pupil constriction.

107. **C** Chapters 32 and 35 Rationale: The GCS (Table 32-1) is one of the standard methods used to identify a patient's level of consciousness (mentation) and determine his or her prognosis. The GCS measures both arousal and awareness. Eye opening is a measure of arousal. Verbal and best motor response are measures of awareness. The lowest score received has the worst prognosis.

TABLE 32-1. GLASGOW COMA SCALE

Eye Opening (E)	*Best Motor Response (M)*	*Verbal Response (V)*
Spontaneous = 4	Obeys = 6	Oriented = 5
To speech = 3	Localizes = 5	Confused conversation = 4
To pain = 2	Withdraws = 4	Inappropriate words = 3
No response = 1	Abnormal	Incomprehensible sounds = 2
	Flexion = 3	No response = 1
	Extension = 2	
	No response = 1	

108. **A** Chapter 35 Rationale: A right-sided cerebral infarct without edema is a focal injury and would not affect level of consciousness. A low glucose level, decreased oxygen transport (< 500 mL/min), and decreased CPP affect global cerebral perfusion, which will cause decreased level of consciousness.

109. **C** Chapter 31 Rationale: In this question the MAP needs to be calculated. MAP can be calculated by doubling the diastolic BP and adding it to the systolic BP then divide by 3. In this case the MAP is 70. CPP = MAP – ICP, 70 – 15 = 55.

110. **C** Chapter 35 Rationale: A stroke in the anterior cerebral artery distribution does not affect wakefulness or arousal. Those centers, including the reticular-activating system, are found in the diencephalon.

111. **A** Chapter 33 Rationale: The sudden onset of a hemiparesis, word-finding problems or aphasia, neglect, or hemisensory changes represent signs of cerebral vasospasm and should be looked for.

112. **C** Chapter 33 Rationale: Physician-directed interventions to treat vasospasm include hypertensive therapy, maintaining euvolemia, and interventional treatment with intra-arterial verapamil or nicardipine, and/or cerebral angioplasty.

113. **D** Chapter 32 Rationale: Brainstem injury is associated with other diffuse cerebral injury. An immediate LOC with pupillary changes and posturing will be seen. On examination, cranial nerve deficits and changes in vital functions, such as respiratory rate and rhythm, are present. These injuries are classified as diffuse axonal injuries.

114. **C** Chapter 35 Rationale: Uncal herniation occurs when the uncus (medial part of the temporal lobe) impacts on the tentorial notch. An expanding temporal lobe lesion and/or increasing middle fossa pressure may force the uncus over the edge of the incisura. This movement of the uncus compresses the mesencephalon (midbrain) against the opposite edge of the incisura. Uncal herniation often presses the oculomotor nerve and posterior cerebral artery against the incisura. Although decreased LOC is the most sensitive indicator of a change in neurologic status, the earliest consistent sign of uncal herniation is a unilaterally dilating pupil accompanied by a change in the level of consciousness.

115. **A** Chapter 31 Rationale: Bradycardia and hypertension occur as part of Cushing's reflex when increased ICP leads to herniation.

116. **C** Chapter 35 Rationale: The oculocephalic response (Fig. 35-3) is often called doll's eyes. Doll's eyes can be tested only in the unconscious patient and is normally recorded as present or absent. The normal response is for the eyes to deviate conjugately in the contraversive direction of the head turning. This is recorded using the phrase "doll's eyes present." Abnormal responses are recorded using the phrase "doll's eyes absent." If the eyes move in the same direction as the head is turned (ie, when the head is flexed, the eyes go down, or when the head is turned right, eyes go right or no further than midline), the test is abnormal (doll's eyes absent). This means that cranial nerves III, VI, and VIII, which are responsible for ocular movements, are not intact.

117. **D** Chapter 35 Rationale: Loss of pain response in extremities, loss of brain stem reflexes and apnea must all be present in for the diagnosis of brain death. An apnea test is performed for confirmation.

118. **D** Chapters 31 and 35 Rationale: In this scenario MAP is calculated by adding diastolic twice, adding to systolic, and dividing by 3. MAP is 68. CPP = MAP – ICP. Here CPP is 44, below goal of 50 to 70, leading to decreased level of consciousness.

119. **C** Chapter 30 Rationale: The hypothalamus regulates the autonomic nervous system, stress response, sleep, appetite, body temperature, water balance, and emotions.

120. **B** Chapter 30 Rationale: The function of the occipital lobe is visual reception and visual association.

121. **A** Chapter 36 Rationale: Suspect meningitis if a fever, severe headache, and nuchal rigidity (resistance to flexion of the neck) exist.

122. **C** Chapter 33 Rationale: If the ischemic stroke occurs in the right cerebral hemisphere (usually the nondominant hemisphere), left-sided motor and sensory deficits occur such as autotopagnosia, and spatial-perceptual deficits resulting in apraxia can occur.

123. **A** Chapter 33 Rationale: To differentiate between the two types of stroke, it will help to obtain a rapid CT scan within 25 minutes of the patient's arrival. Patients presenting within the first hours of ischemic stroke will generally have a negative CT scan of the brain. In some instances, an "MCA" sign, or white clot visible in the middle cerebral artery (MCA), will be seen in MCA occlusions. Patients presenting 12 to 24 hours after stroke onset will have ischemic changes on CT, which will reveal decreased density in ischemic and infarcted areas. Hemorrhage on CT shows up as an increased white-appearing density.

124. **B** Chapter 30 Rationale: Acetylcholine is the primary neurotransmitter of the peripheral nervous system. As the action potential in the axon reaches the neuromuscular junction, the neuromuscular junction is stimulated to release the chemical in its vesicles. The chemical diffuses across the synaptic cleft, coming in contact with receptors on the postsynaptic membrane.

125. **A** Chapter 32 Rationale: Due to accelerative or decelerative blunt trauma forces to the head, the cerebral cortex may bruise. These forces propel the brain against the rigid cranium (the coup force). With initial impact, the brain is then rotated or thrown back in the opposite direction (the contrecoup force).

126. **A** Chapter 32 Rationale: Epidural hematomas are true neurosurgical emergencies. They occur at the time of the injury and are usually associated with a temporal or parietal skull fracture with laceration of the middle meningeal artery (and often vein). There is usually a LOC, which may be followed by a brief period (up to 4–6 h) of lucidity, followed by increasing restlessness, agitation, and confusion progressing to coma in one-third of patients. During the lucid period, nausea and vomiting often occur. Other signs may include ipsilateral oculomotor paralysis and seizures, contralateral hemiparesis/hemiplegia, and positive Babinski reflexes. As the hematoma increases in size, uncal herniation is the most common type to occur.

127. **C** Chapter 32 Rationale: Epidural hematoma is a neurosurgical emergency and requires immediate surgical decompression with craniotomy. Consider what treatment definitively addresses the underlying cause.

128. **A** Chapter 32 Rationale: "Raccoon eyes" is a sign of bleeding into the paranasal sinuses and refers to ecchymosis developing around the eyes. Along with CSF draining from the nose (rhinorrhea), these signs indicate a basilar fracture in the anterior fossa.

129. **D** Chapter 32 Rationale: A temporal or basilar fracture in the posterior fossa is indicated by Battle's sign, an area of ecchymosis over the mastoid projection.

130. **C** Chapter 32 Rationale: In epidural hematoma, there is usually a change in LOC, which may be followed by a brief period (up to 4–6 h) of lucidity, followed by increasing restlessness, agitation, and confusion progressing to coma in one-third of patients. During the lucid period, nausea and vomiting often occur. Other signs may include ipsilateral oculomotor paralysis and seizures, contralateral hemiparesis/hemiplegia, and positive Babinski reflexes. As the hematoma increases in size, uncal herniation is the most common type to occur.

131. **C** Chapter 32 Rationale: CT is the primary diagnostic test in head injuries. It will reveal whether

1. Air has entered the brain from fractures of the eye, mastoid, or sinuses.
2. Blood is present in brain tissue or in the ventricular system.
3. Blood is on the surface of the brain or in the basal cisterns.
4. There is presence of cerebral edema and intracranial shift.
5. Ventricles are of normal size and in normal position.
6. The pineal gland has calcified and is in normal position.

132. **C** Chapter 30 Rationale: Homonymous hemianopsia is defined as visual field loss on the left or right side of the vertical midline. It occurs because the right half of the brain has visual pathways for the left hemifield of both eyes and the left half of the brain has visual pathways for the right hemifield of both eyes.

133. **C** Chapter 30 Rationale: The patient will be unable to see in the peripheral field on the left. Keeping items to the right will ensure they are visible.

134. **D** Chapter 36 Rationale: Myasthenia gravis is an autoimmune process. A majority of patients with myasthenia gravis have antiacetycholine receptor (AChR) antibodies. In the patients who do not have these antibodies, other autoantibodies related to muscle receptors are likely involved.

135. **D** Chapter 36 Rationale: Myasthenia gravis is characterized by fatigability of voluntary muscle groups with repeated use. Pathognomonic signs of myasthenia gravis include uneven drooping of the eyelids, a smile that resembles a snarl, a drooping lower jaw that must be supported by the hand, and a partially immobile mouth with the corners turned downward. However, few patients are first seen with these signs. In more than 90% of the cases, the eyebrows and extraocular muscles are involved, accompanied by weakness in eye closure. Ptosis and diplopia are common. The next most commonly affected muscles exhibiting symptoms are those of facial expression, mastication, swallowing, and speaking (dysarthria). Hoarseness occurs after only a few minutes of talking. Neck flexor and extensor muscles, the shoulder girdle, and hip flexors are less frequently involved. There is usually no sensory disturbance.

136. **A** Chapter 36 Rationale: Edrophonium chloride (Tensilon) is injected intravenously after the patient's muscle strength has been assessed. The limit used to test for myasthenia gravis is 10 mg given in 2- to 5-mg doses. The duration of action for edrophonium chloride is about 5 min.

137. **D** Chapter 36 Rationale: The most useful treatments include anticholinesterase medications, immunosuppressive agents, thymectomy, and plasmapheresis or intravenous immunoglobulin. The major objective of therapy is to improve neuromuscular transmission and prevent complications. Early thymectomy may be employed.

138. **D** Chapter 30 Rationale: Both atropine and epinephrine cause pupillary dilation via different mechanisms of action due to their action on the autonomic nervous system (ANS). Epineprhine is a sympathetic stimulant, facilitating a "fight or flight" reaction that causes dilated pupils. Conversely, atropine is a parasympathetic blocker, which blocks the "rest and digest" part of the ANS, allowing the "flight or flight" effects to be up-regulated.

139. **A** Chapter 36 Rationale: Suspect meningitis if a fever, severe headache, and nuchal rigidity (resistance to flexion of the neck) exist. Positive Kernig's and Brudzinski's signs, photophobia, decreased sensorium, and signs of increased ICP are common. Kernig's sign is the inability to fully extend the leg at the knee when the leg is flexed at the hip.

140. **D** Chapter 36 Rationale: Antibiotics should be started within 30 min of the patient's arrival at the hospital.

The antibiotic selected is based on the organism. Most often penicillin, ceftriaxone (Rocephin), and vancomycin are begun until the organism is identified. Administration of antibiotics at scheduled times maintains a therapeutic blood level.

141. **A** Chapter 36 Rationale: Guillain–Barré syndrome causes progressive muscle weakness, sensory loss, and areflexia as a result of peripheral nerve demyelination. In the normal course of the disease, the patient usually has had an upper respiratory or gastrointestinal infection 1 to 2 weeks prior to the development of Guillain–Barré syndrome. The predominant pattern is weakness starting in the lower extremities and advancing (often very rapidly) to motor paralysis as it progresses up the body.

142. **B** Chapter 36 Rationale: The objective of therapy for Guillain-Barré syndrome is to support body systems until recovery occurs. Respiratory failure and infection are serious threats to recovery. It is essential to monitor the vital capacity and arterial blood gases (ABGs). If the vital capacity drops to less than 12 to 15 mL/kg body weight, the peak negative pressure is less than −20 cm H_2O, and the respiratory rate is more than 30, there is paradoxical movement of the chest and abdomen (paradox alternans); if the ABGs reflect the development of a respiratory acidosis, intubation or tracheostomy may be done so that the patient can be mechanically ventilated. Treatment may also include IVIG or plasmapheresis.

143. **D** Chapter 36 Rationale: Kernig's sign is the inability to fully extend the leg at the knee when the leg is flexed at the hip. A refers to Trousseau's sign, B is Chvostek's sign, and C suggests nuchal rigidity. Choose D.

144. **A** Chapter 36 Rationale: Brudzinski's sign is the involuntary adduction and flexion of the legs with attempts to flex the neck.

145. **B** Chapter 37 Rationale: Protecting the patient from injury is a priority. Remove objects from the immediate environment that might cause injury. Stay with the patient during the seizure. Bed rails should be up and padded and the bed placed in low position. The patient should not be restrained, but efforts to protect the patient's head from injury are appropriate (eg, if a seizure occurs with the patient out of bed, a pillow may be placed under the head or a nurse may cradle—*not* restrain—the patient's head to protect it). *Nothing* should ever be used to pry open the patient's mouth, nor should anything be forced into the mouth during a seizure. Damage to the mouth and tongue occurs at the start of a seizure and only more damage will result by forcing objects into the mouth.

PART VI

GASTROENTEROLOGY

Kelly A. Thompson-Brazill

Section Overview

This chapter covers the anatomy and physiology of the gastrointestinal system along with the nursing management of gastrointestinal disturbances commonly seen in critical care and covered on the CCRN exam, including

- Upper and lower GI bleeding
- Acute and chronic liver failure, hepatic encephalopathy, hepatitis, portal hypertension, and esophageal varices
- Intestinal disorders due to hypoperfusion (eg, mesenteric ischemia), adhesive disease (obstruction), perforation, and traumatic injuries

37

Anatomy and Physiology of the Gastrointestinal System

CHAPTER OVERVIEW AND OBJECTIVES

This chapter provides a good review of the general anatomy and physiology of gastrointestinal (GI) function. Few if any questions from this chapter will be included on the CCRN exam. Use this chapter as a reference as needed to strengthen your overall understanding of GI anatomy and physiology. However, there is essentially no basic, "normal" anatomy and physiology on the CCRN exam.

After studying this chapter, you should understand the following:

- The basic anatomy and physiology of the GI system including the accessory organs.
- Describe the process of digestion with clear knowledge acquisition related to digestive properties, chemical digestion, and the impact of gastric dysfunction on digestion.
- Appreciate the impact of the accessory organs' relationship with the GI tract and hemodynamics.

The process of digestion and absorption of nutrients requires an intact, healthy epithelial lining in the GI tract that can resist the effects of its own digestive secretions. In this system, enzymes and hormones are produced, vitamins are synthesized and stored, food is broken down, and waste products are eliminated. Nutrients, vitamins, minerals, electrolytes, and water enter the body through the GI tract. The two main functions of the GI tract can be summarized as the absorption of nutritional elements and the elimination of waste products.

37.1 UPPER GASTROINTESTINAL SYSTEM

Oral Cavity and Oropharynx

The oral cavity is the beginning of the GI tract. It contains the lips, cheeks, teeth, gums, tongue, palate, salivary glands, and palatine tonsils. Its main functions include ingestion, mastication, salivation, and the initiation of swallowing (deglutition).

The major salivary glands are the parotid, submandibular, and sublingual glands. Saliva performs several functions:

- It hydrates and protects the oral mucosa from trauma and desiccation.
- It softens and lubricates food as it passes through the oropharynx.
- It initiates starch digestion by amylase and fat digestion by lipase.
- It defends against bacteria by secreting immunoglobulin A (IgA) and lysozymes.

The oropharynx extends inferiorly from the soft palate to just above the epiglottis. It connects the oral cavity to the esophagus.

Esophagus

At the level of the sixth cervical vertebra (CVI), the oropharynx transitions into the esophagus. It lies posterior to the trachea. The esophagus is divided into three portions: cervical, thoracic, and abdominal with each part of the esophagus having a different blood supply.

- The inferior thyroid artery supplies the cervical portion.
- The bronchial and esophageal branches of the thoracic aorta feed the thoracic segment.
- The ascending branches of the left phrenic and left gastric arteries supply the abdominal section.

A submucosal venous plexus drains blood from the esophagus into the periesophageal plexus. In the abdomen, this plexus blood drains into the left gastric vein, part of the portal venous system.

A complex network of nerves supplies the esophagus. The recurrent laryngeal branches of the vagus nerve innervated the upper third of the esophagus. These branches become part of the Meissner (submucosal) plexus and Auerbach (myenteric) plexus.

Gastroesophageal reflux disease (GERD) may occur because of inadequate esophageal motility, lower esophageal sphincter dysfunction, or delayed gastric emptying due to a variety of conditions that increase intra-abdominal pressure, such as pregnancy or obesity.

KEY CLINICAL CONCEPT

- Common **cardiovascular medications** such as nitrates and calcium channel blockers may also relax the lower esophageal sphincter.
- Common symptoms include pyrosis, hoarseness, **noncardiac chest pain,** and bronchospasm or asthma.

Stomach

The stomach is a hollow, distensible organ that can expand from 75 mL, when empty, to hold about 1 L of solid or liquid food. It is located between the esophagus and the beginning of the small intestine. The stomach is divided into four sections: the cardia, the fundus, the body, and the pylorus (**Fig. 37-1**).

The stomach contains two sphincters. The esophageal sphincter is located just above the gastric cardia and helps prevent reflux of food and gastric acid into the esophagus. The pyloric sphincter is located at the distal portion of the stomach. When it is open, chyme (partially digested food) passes into the duodenum.

Layers. The stomach wall is composed of three muscular layers: the outer layer, consisting of longitudinal muscle fibers; the middle layer, consisting of circular fibers; and the innermost third layer, consisting of transverse (oblique) fibers.

The interior mucosa of the stomach has a layer called the *submucosa*, which is composed of blood and lymph vessels and connective and fibrous tissue.

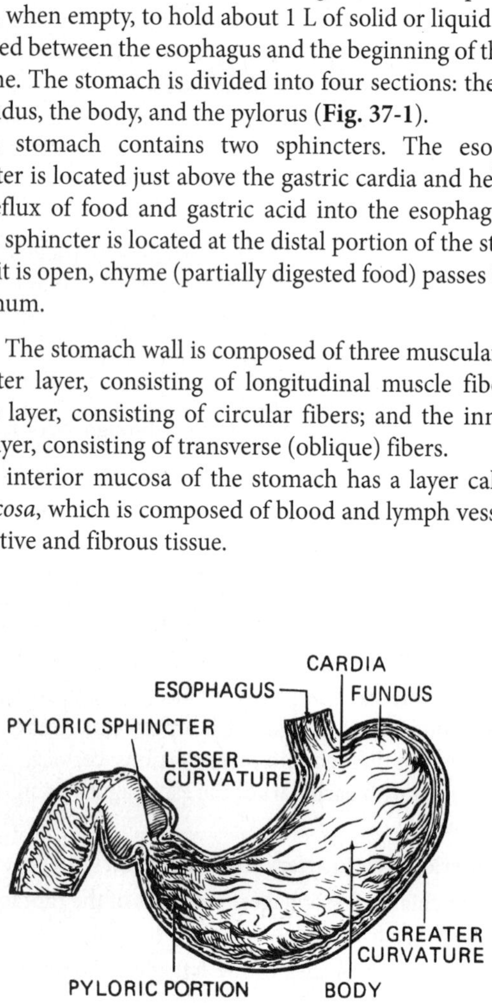

Figure 37-1. Divisions and curvatures of the stomach.

KEY CLINICAL CONCEPT

The vascular interior layer of the stomach is noteworthy as a source of GI bleeding occurs when there is a disruption in the mucosal barrier and vascular epithelium.

Gastric Glands. Glands are present throughout the GI tract to secrete chemicals that mix with the food and digest it. These secretions are of two types:

- Mucus, which protects the wall of the GI tract and liquefies the stomach contents.
- Enzymes and allied substances, which break the large chemical compounds of the food into simple compounds.

Mucus is secreted by every portion of the GI tract. It contains a large amount of mucoprotein that is resistant to almost all digestive juices. Mucus also lubricates the passage of food along the mucosa, and it forms a thin film everywhere to prevent the food and hydrochloric acid from excoriating the mucosa.

Many substances—such as nonsteroid anti-inflammatory drugs (NSAIDs), bile salts, ethyl alcohol, and acetic acid—have been shown to alter ion influxes and potential differences across gastric mucosa; these changes have been interpreted as a reflection of damage to the gastric mucosa. How these substances disrupt the gastric mucosa and lead to ulcer formation is unknown.

The proximal portion of the stomach, the cardia, receives the bolus of food from the esophagus. This stimulates gastric glands to secrete lipase, pepsin, the intrinsic factor (IF), mucus, hydrochloric acid. These substances are collectively known as gastric juice. The mucosa of the stomach contains few gastric glands at the fundus, many glands in the body, and fewer glands at the antral (pyloric) portion of the body.

Control of Gastric Secretions. Gastric secretions may be controlled through ANS functions, by hormonal alterations, and/or through baroreceptors. *These secretions and hormones maintain the stomach pH range from 1 to 3.*

The control of the gastric secretions, specifically hydrochloric acid, may be broken down into three phases: cephalic, gastric, and intestinal. When the stomach is at rest, normal secretion occurs at a rate of about 0.5 mL/min. With food in the stomach, the rate of secretion increases to about 3.0 mL/min.

Cephalic Phase. The first phase of gastric secretion occurs in response to the sight or smell or food and is controlled by the parasympathetic nervous system (PNS). ACh is released by the vagus nerve leading to hydrogen ions (H^+) accumulation, while histamine increases H^+ proliferation and the G cells produce gastrin. In turn, approximately one-third of the hydrochloric (HCl^-) acid required for food digestion is released prior to the arrival of food into the stomach.

QUICK TIP! A "vagotomy" is a dissection of the vagus nerve (near stomach) that can be performed to limit gastric acid secretion for peptic ulcer disease.

Gastric Phase. This second phase of gastric secretion begins when food enters the stomach. The oxyntic cells release gastrin when they are stimulated by antral distention, secretion pepsinogen secretion, and an alkaline pH in the stomach. This leads to hydrochloric acid secretion that acidifies the stomach contents. Hydrogen ions (+) are released until the gastric juices are sufficiently acidic. When the stomach pH reaches 2.0, SST is released, decreasing gastrin secretion as part of a negative feedback loop.

Intestinal Phase. This phase begins when chyme enters the duodenum. Chyme entering the duodenum is more acid than that in the body of the stomach, because as polypeptide fragments move from the body of the stomach to the antrum, they stimulate acid secretion by an unknown mechanism (but to a lesser extent than in the stomach).

Gastric Digestion. Gastric digestion includes carbohydrates, proteins, and fats. The stomach is a poor absorptive area of the GI tract. Only a few highly lipid-soluble substances, such as alcohol, can be absorbed in small quantities.

Carbohydrates. Digestion of starches begins in the mouth with action of ptyalin and continues in the stomach by hydrolyzing carbohydrates into oligosaccharides.

Protein. The first stage of protein breakdown by proteolytic enzymes occurs in the stomach.

Fats. Digestion of fats in the stomach is minimal. The only action the stomach has on fats is by gastric peristalsis, which reduces the size of triglyceride droplets and facilitates contact with a lipase secreted by von Ebner's glands.

- Upper GI system anatomy consists of oral cavity, oropharynx, esophagus, and stomach.
- Dysfunction of the stomach can include
  - GERD that may mimic cardiac conditions and result in the prescription of cardiac medications such as nitrates or calcium channel blockers.
  - GI bleeding occurs with dysfunction of the structural layers of the stomach.
- Gastric glands not only aide digestion but serve as a protective mechanism.

37.2 LOWER GASTROINTESTINAL SYSTEM

The Small Intestine

The small intestine extends from the pyloric sphincter to the cecum. This 18- to 20-ft tube is divided into three segments:

- The first segment is the duodenum, arising at the pyloric sphincter. It is a C-shaped segment about 10 in. long and ends at the ligament of Treitz.
- The middle segment, the jejunum, extends about 8 ft from the ligament of Treitz and has an alkaline pH (7.8).
- The third segment is the ileum, which is about 12 ft long. There is no distinct change from the jejunum to the ileum.

Ileocecal Valve

The ileocecal valve is located at the junction of the ileum and the cecum (beginning of large intestine). This valve controls the flow of contents into the cecum and prevents regurgitation of cecal contents into the ileum.

Villi. Villi (singular, villus) are the distinguishing characteristics of the small intestine (**Fig. 37-2**). These finger-like projections into the lumen provide an extensive surface area.

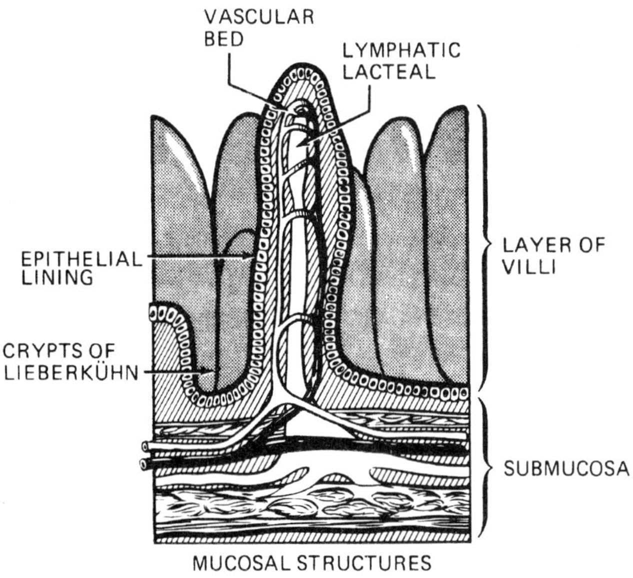

Figure 37-2. Structure of a villus (a lacteal).

The villi and microvilli increase in absorptive capacity 600-fold, for a total surface area of about 250 m^2. Carbohydrates, fats, proteins, vitamins, and minerals are absorbed into the small bowel through the villi.

Glands of the Small Intestine. The intestinal lumen is lined with simple, cuboidal, and columnar epithelial cells interspersed with goblet cells. The many goblet cells secrete mucus to protect the mucosa. The goblet cells decrease in numbers markedly toward the end of the ileum. Crypts of Lieberkühn (**Fig. 37-3**) are tubular glands found between the villi in the submucosa of the duodenum.

Brunner's glands are mucus-secreting glands that are concentrated in the first portion of the duodenum, between the pylorus and the ampulla of Vater. The function of Brunner's glands is inhibited by the SNS. Lack of sufficient mucus may be related to the development site of peptic ulcers. Brunner's glands are thought to protect the duodenum from digestion by the gastric juices.

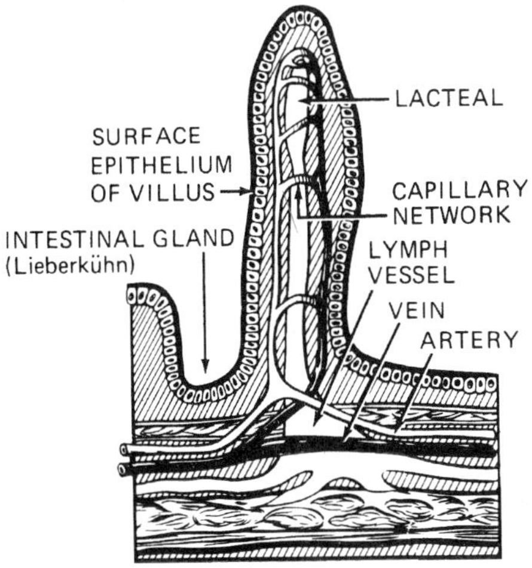

Figure 37-3. Crypts of Lieberkühn.

Peyer's patches are lymphoid follicles that lie in the mucosa and submucosa of the ileum. They participate in antibody synthesis and the body's immune responses.

Absorption Mechanisms in the Small Intestine. Normally, absorption from the small intestine each day consists of several hundred grams of carbohydrates, 100 g or more of fat, 50 to 100 g of amino acids, 50 to 100 g of ions, and 8 or 9 L of water. Its absorptive capacity is much greater than this. There are five basic mechanisms for absorption in the small intestine: hydrolysis, nonionic movement, passive diffusion, facilitated diffusion, and active transport.

Hydrolysis. Hydrolysis is the chemical action of uniting compounds with water to split the compounds into simpler compounds. Enzymes and hormones act as catalysts in the process of hydrolysis.

Nonionic Movement. Nonionic transport allows substances to move freely in and out of cells with no need for energy or carrier substances. Such molecules include drugs and unconjugated bile salts.

Passive Diffusion. In passive diffusion, there is free movement of molecules based on a concentration gradient, primarily from an area of high concentration to an area of low concentration. Free fatty acids and water are molecules that move by passive diffusion.

Facilitated Diffusion. Facilitated diffusion may be defined as a process by which a carrier picks up an ion, crosses the cell membrane, liberates the ion inside the cell, and then returns outside to pick up another molecule (ion). This diffusion does not require energy, and ions cannot move alone against an electrochemical gradient.

Active Transport. For nutrients to be absorbed by active transport, energy (adenosine triphosphate [ATP]) is required. Ions such as Na^+ and K^+ and molecules such as proteins and glucose require active transport.

Nutrient Digestion and Absorption. Some 90% of nutrients and 50% of water and electrolytes are absorbed in the jejunum. Meticulous nutritional counseling and follow-up are important for patients who have undergone resection of the small bowel.

Carbohydrates. Carbohydrates enter the duodenum in the forms of starch, polysaccharides (complex sugars), disaccharides, and monosaccharides. The starch and polysaccharides are hydrolyzed under the influence of amylase to form maltose. Maltose and directly ingested disaccharides such as sucrose, lactose, and maltose are hydrolyzed by intestinal enzymes into simple sugars of monosaccharides, which are then absorbed into the bloodstream via the intestinal mucosa.

Approximately 350 g of carbohydrates are absorbed daily (60% starch, 30% sucrose, and 10% lactose). The three basic sugars are fructose, glucose, and galactose. Each of these basic sugars yields 4 kcal/g. Glucose and galactose are actively transported across the small intestinal wall into the blood. Fructose is transported by facilitated diffusion.

Proteins. Dietary proteins are first acted upon by enzymes called proteases. The principal *proteases* are pepsin (in the gastric secretion) and trypsin (in the pancreatic secretion). These enzymes catalyze the hydrolysis of the very large protein molecules into intermediate compounds (proteoses and peptones) and subsequently into amino acids. In the digestive sequence, protein is broken down into proteoses and peptones in the stomach. These simpler compounds are next broken down into polypeptides and then into amino acids in the small intestine.

Approximately 70 to 90 g of protein are absorbed daily, yielding 4 kcal/g. Of the amino acids, eight (isoleucine, leucine, lysine, methionine, phenylalanine, threonine, tryptophan, and valine) are essential. Amino acids are absorbed (primarily from the duodenum and jejunum) by active transport into the blood of the intestinal villi.

Fats. Before fats can be digested, they must be emulsified. This function is performed in the small intestine by bile, which is secreted by the liver and stored in the gallbladder.

The bile salts aggregate to form micelles. These micelles have a fatty core but are still stable in the intestines because the surfaces of the micelles are ionized, which is a property that promotes water solubility. The fatty acids and the glycerides become absorbed in the fatty portions of these micelles as they are split away from fat globules and are then carried from the fat globules to the intestinal epithelium, where absorption occurs.

The emulsification of ingested fat globules provides a greater contact area between the fat molecules and pancreatic lipase, which is the principal fat-digestive enzyme. The end products of fat digestion are glycerides, fatty acids, and glycerol. Most fatty acids and glycerides are absorbed into the lymphatic system via the lacteals of the intestinal villi.

Approximately 60 to 100 g of fat are absorbed daily, providing 9 kcal/g.

Electrolytes. Electrolytes are absorbed in all parts of the intestine by active transport.

Water. Approximately 8 to 9 L of water are absorbed from the intestine each day by both diffusion and osmosis.

Water-Soluble Vitamins. The water-soluble vitamins, vitamin C and B complex, are absorbed in all parts of the intestine through passive diffusion directly into the blood.

Fat-Soluble Vitamins. The fat-soluble vitamins, A, D, E, and K, are absorbed from the GI tract (mainly the jejunum) in the same way as lipids are. Once in the bloodstream, these vitamins are escorted by protein carriers because they are insoluble in water.

Calcium. The top portion of the duodenum is specialized for the absorption of calcium.

Iron. In the intestines, only about 10% of dietary iron is normally absorbed, but if the body's supply is diminished or if the need increases for any reason, absorption increases. This regulation is provided by a blood protein, transferrin, which captures iron from food and carries it to tissues throughout the body by active transport.

Large Intestine

The large intestine (colon) is approximately 5 ft long and extends from the ileum to the anus. It is significantly different from the small intestine in that it contains no villi. The colon is 2.5 in.

in diameter (larger than the small intestine) and has many sacculations (sac-like segmentations) called haustra. The colon has three segments: the cecum, large intestine, and rectum. The colon is further subdivided into four sections: the ascending, transverse, descending, and sigmoid colons. The large intestine is mainly responsible for the absorption of water and some electrolytes and the elimination of waste products.

Cecum. The cecum the beginning of the large intestine. It is located in the right lower quadrant of the abdomen (**Fig. 37-4**). The vermiform appendix is attached to the base of the cecum. The appendix is a blind pouch that has no physiologic function.

Colon. Immediately above the cecum is the ascending colon. It extends superiorly forming hepatic flexure at the level of the liver. The hepatic flexure gives rise to the transverse colon, which extends from the right side of the abdomen to the left until it turns into the splenic flexure. The descending colon is located between the splenic flexure and the sigmoid colon. At the iliac crest, the descending colon arches backward to form the sigmoid colon (Fig. 37-4). The sigmoid colon is the portion of the colon that crosses from the left side to the midline to become the rectum (Fig. 37-4), which follows the curvature of the lower sacrum and coccyx.

Rectum and Anus. The rectum is about 7 in. long. The distal 1 to 2 in. are the anal canal. Mucous membrane lines the rectum and is arranged in vertical rows called rectal columns. Each rectal column contains an artery and a vein. These veins frequently enlarge to form hemorrhoids. Two sphincters control the anus (the exterior opening of the rectum). The internal sphincter is composed of involuntary smooth muscle. The external sphincter is voluntary striated muscle.

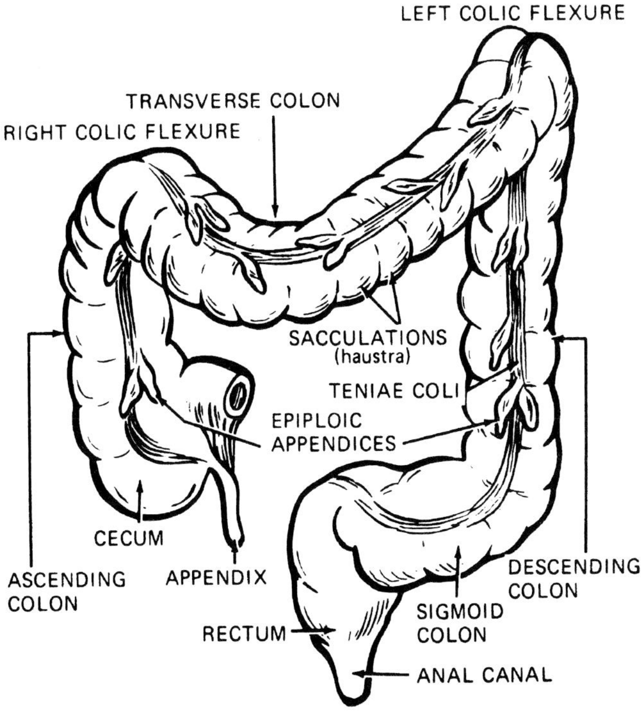

Figure 37-4. Large intestine (anterior view).

Propulsive Movements in the Colon. The propulsive movements in the colon result from the haustral contractions, but they are insufficient to provide for the necessary expulsion of waste products. A mass movement occurs in response to an irritation or distention, usually in the transverse colon. These contractions, as a unit, force the entire mass of fecal material forward. A series of mass movements usually occur for up to 30 minutes and may then occur again in one-half to one full day.

Mass movements can cause colonic motility because of intense PNS stimulation, irritation secondary to conditions such as ulcerative colitis, osmotic overload or simply distention, the use of drugs such as **morphine sulfate** or magnesium sulfate, an increase in bile salts, bacterial endotoxins, and high-residual diets. Hypermotility results in diarrhea and may cause severe fluid loss and electrolyte imbalance.

Mass movements are inhibited by all the *anticholinergic* drugs and by diets deficient in bulk. This may result in constipation, since the extra length of time in the large intestine allows for more fluid absorption.

KEY CLINICAL CONCEPT

The impact of narcotics and other drugs used in the care of a critically ill patient should be considered in relationship to their impact on the motility of the digestive system—specifically noting when motility is reduced and the preventative measures that should be taken to support the patient.

Colonic Absorption. The colon may increase its absorption rate by threefold if threatened with large amounts of fluid. Most absorption in the colon occurs in its proximal half (the ascending and transverse colon). The distal colon functions principally for storage.

The mucosa of the large intestine has a very high capacity for active absorption of sodium, and the electrical potential created by the absorption of the sodium causes passive chloride absorption. The mucosa of the colon actively secretes both bicarbonate and potassium.

Bacteria. Bacterial action in the colon causes the formation of gases, which provide bulk and help to propel the feces. Bacteria are capable of digesting small amounts of cellulose, in this way providing a few calories of nutrition to the body each day. These organisms also synthesize some important nutritional factors such as vitamin K, thiamine, riboflavin, vitamin B_{12}, folic acid, biotin, and nicotinic acid. The main anaerobic bacterium in the colon is *Bacteroides fragilis*. The main aerobic bacterium is *Escherichia coli*.

37.3 BLOOD SUPPLY OF THE GASTROINTESTINAL TRACT

Arterial Blood Supply

Several branches of the abdominal aorta supply blood to the GI tract. Most arterial blood is supplied by the celiac artery, the superior mesenteric arteries (SMAs), and the inferior mesenteric arteries (IMAs). **Figure 37-5** shows the arterial vascularization of the GI tract.

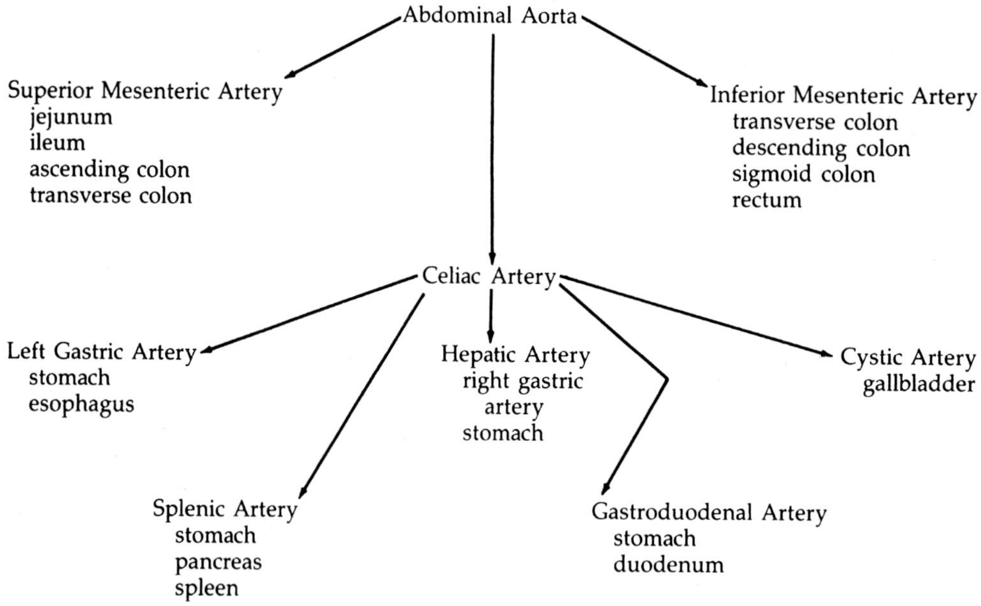

Figure 37-5. Arterial vascularization of the GI tract.

The arterial blood supply with the GI tract is notable when considering a patient's hemodynamic status especially if patient has experienced recent trauma including surgery to the abdominal cavity and/or related structures.

Venous Blood Return

The venous circulation of the GI system is unique in that the venous blood enters the portal vein system (**Fig. 37-6**). All blood from the GI tract enters the portal vein system, which empties into the liver sinusoids. Not surprisingly, the portal vein supplies 75% of the blood to the liver, while the hepatic artery supplies only 25%. The liver sinusoids join branches of the hepatic artery to form the hepatic vein. In turn, the hepatic veins drain blood from the portal vein and hepatic artery into the inferior vena cava.

37.4 INNERVATION OF THE GASTROINTESTINAL SYSTEM

In comparison with the other body systems, the GI tract is unique with its own separate intrinsic nervous system, which is influenced by the both the *parasympathetic (PNS) and sympathetic (SNS) portions of the ANS*. The intrinsic nervous system

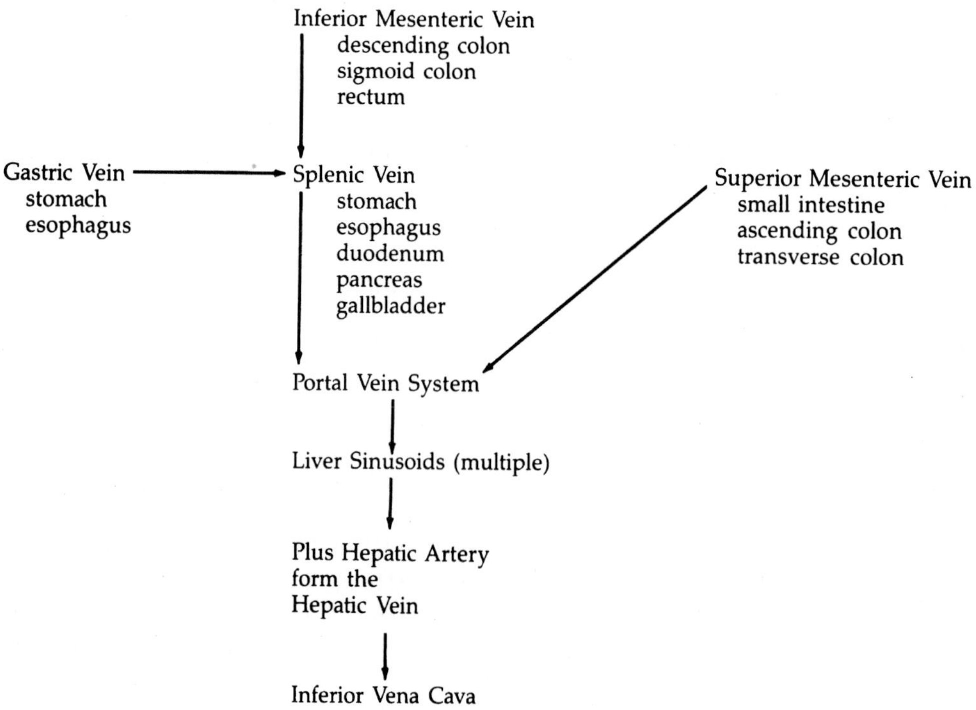

Figure 37-6. Venous return of the GI tract.

has two layers of neurons connected by specific fibers. The outer layer of neurons is called the *myenteric plexus* or *Auerbach's plexus*. It is located between the longitudinal and circular muscle layers. The inner layer of neurons, called the *submucosal plexus* or *Meissner's plexus*, is in the submucosa.

Generally, the myenteric plexus controls movement of the GI tract and the submucosal plexus (Meissner's plexus) controls the secretions of the GI tract and sensory function through impulses received by stretch receptors in both the GI wall and GI epithelium.

Stimulation of the myenteric plexus results in increasing motor tone of the GI wall and increasing intensity, rate, and speed of peristaltic waves. Increase in Meissner's plexus activity results in increasing mucosal secretions.

The extrinsic nerves of the ANS can alter the effects of the GI system at specific points or from the mouth to the stomach and then from the distal end of the colon to the anus. *Parasympathetic* supply for the gut is from the 10th cranial (vagus) and sacral nerves. ACh is the primary parasympathetic neurotransmitter. A few cranial parasympathetic fibers innervate the mouth and pharynx. Extensive *parasympathetic* innervation exists in the esophagus, stomach, pancreas, and first half of the large intestine. The sacral parasympathetic fibers innervate the distal half of the large intestine, especially the sigmoidal, rectal, and anal portions.

The SNS fibers flow along blood vessels of the entire gut. The *sympathetic* fibers to the GI tract originate in the spinal cord between segments T8 and L3. The SNS neurotransmitter, norepinephrine, inhibits GI tract activity. This causes effects opposite those of ACh.

The liver synthesizes vitamin K–dependent clotting factors of the blood-clotting factors II, VII, IX, and X.

37.5 ACCESSORY ORGANS OF DIGESTION

Salivary Glands

There are three salivary glands: the parotid, the submandibular, and the sublingual (**Fig. 37-7**). All the salivary glands are paired.

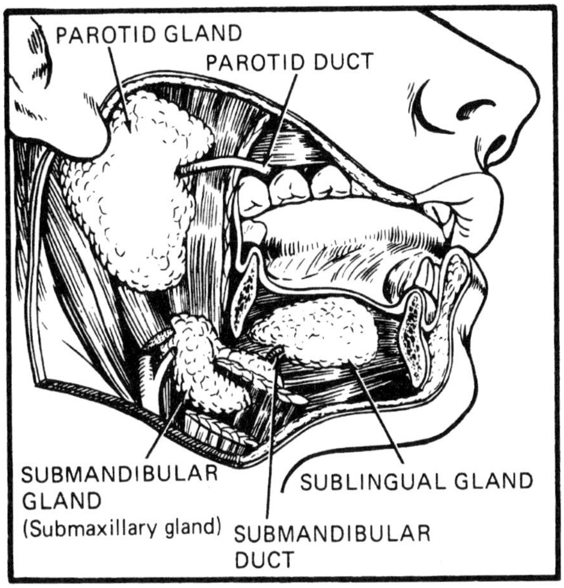

Figure 37-7. Salivary glands.

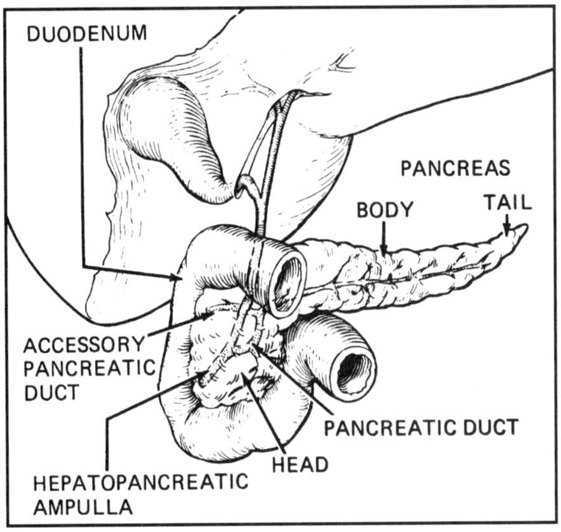

Figure 37-8. Pancreas.

Salivary secretion is controlled by the superior and inferior salivatory nuclei located in the brainstem. Nervous stimuli of the glands occur from the thought, sight, and smell of food.

Pancreas

The pancreas is a soft, fish-shaped lobulated gland lying behind the stomach in the retroperitoneum (**Fig. 37-8**). It is composed of three segments: the head, the body, and the tail. The main pancreatic duct is the duct of Wirsung, which runs the whole length of the pancreas from left to right and joins the common bile duct on the right.

The pancreas is both an endocrine and exocrine organ. The endocrine portion includes the secretion of insulin from the beta cells, the secretion of glucagon from the alpha cells, and the secretion of SST from the delta cells (See Table 37-1). The exocrine function of the pancreas occurs in the acinar glands. These cells are arranged around a small central lumen into which the cells drain the exocrine enzymes that they have synthesized. The central lumens drain into multiple ducts, which eventually drain into the main pancreatic duct. The ampulla of Vater (**Fig. 37-9**) is the short segment just before the common bile duct enters the duodenum.

In addition to the digestive enzymes, pancreatic secretions contain large amounts of bicarbonate, which reacts with the hydrochloric acid emptied into the duodenum in the chyme from the stomach to form sodium chloride and carbonic acid. The carbonic acid is absorbed into the blood and eliminated through the lungs as carbon dioxide. The net result is an increase in the quantity of sodium chloride, a neutral salt, in the intestine. Thus, pancreatic secretions neutralize the acidity of the chyme coming from the stomach. This is one of the most important functions of pancreatic secretion.

Two other important pancreatic enzymes are nuclease and deoxyribonuclease. These enzymes degrade nucleotides within DNA and RNA molecules into free mononucleotides.

Regulation of Pancreatic Secretions. The cells lining the acinar glands contain large amounts of carbonic anhydrase.

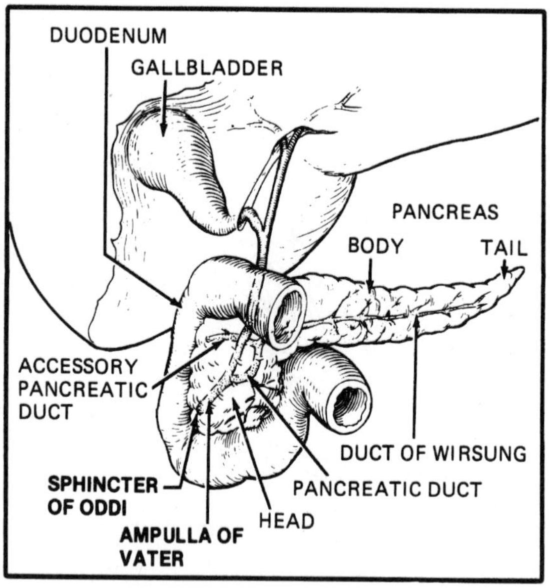

Figure 37-9. Ampulla of Vater and sphincter of Oddi.

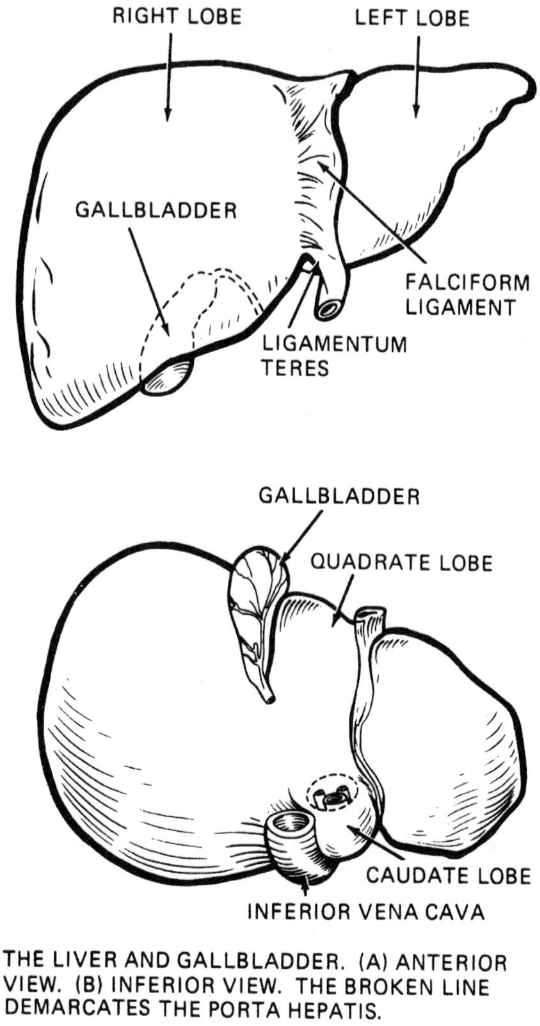

Figure 37-10. Divisions of the liver.

The alkaline secretions (HCO_3^-) of the duct cells (cells lining the acinar glands) mix with the amylolytic, lipolytic, and proteolytic enzymes prior to reaching the major pancreatic duct, the duct of Wirsung.

Secretions of the pancreas are controlled by hormonal and neural factors. There are three phases of secretion: cephalic, gastric, and intestinal. The cephalic phase is activated by the same factors as in the cephalic state of the stomach and is mainly controlled by the vagus nerve (*parasympathetic* impulses). Stimulation of the **vagus** nerve (by thought, smell, taste, chewing, and swallowing of food) causes the secretory cells of the pancreas to secrete highly concentrated enzymes with minimal amounts of HCO_3^-.

The gastric and intestinal phases are interrelated and controlled by two hormones, secretin and cholecystokinin. When the chyme is predominantly undigested proteins and fats, the pancreatic juice will be rich in enzymes. When the chyme is mainly acidic (low pH), the pancreatic juice will be rich in HCO_3^-. The secretion of cholecystokinin stimulates the enzyme-rich secretion of pancreatic juices; secretin stimulates the release of HCO_3^- and water-rich pancreatic juice. The pancreatic juices enter the duodenum along with the biliary system secretions at the sphincter of Oddi.

KEY CLINICAL CONCEPT

The acid-base balance along with the function of the vagus nerve are often referenced on the CCRN exam, and it is recommended to focus on this understanding this physiology. For example, the pH of the stomach is approximately 1.5 to 3.5, whereas the pH of the blood is normally 7.35 to 7.45.

Biliary System

The biliary system is composed of the liver and gallbladder.

Liver. The liver is the single largest organ in the body, weighing 3 to 4 lb. It is in the right upper quadrant of the abdomen, lying up against the right inferior diaphragm.

Gross Structure. The liver is divided into right and left lobes by the falciform ligament (**Fig. 37-10**).

Functional Unit. Each of the hepatic lobes is further divided into numerous lobules. The hepatic lobule is the functioning unit of the liver (**Fig. 37-11**). Each lobule has a hepatic artery, a portal vein, and a bile duct; these are known collectively as the portal triad.

Blood Supply. Each sinusoid receives oxygenated blood from the hepatic arterioles and blood rich in metabolic precursors from the hepatic vein. Products removed from the blood include amino acids, nutrients, sugars, and bacterial debris. Blood leaves the sinusoid by entering the vein of the central lobule. It then enters the hepatic veins and follows the normal venous circuit.

Function. The role of the liver in digestion is to synthesize and transport bile pigments and bile salts for fat digestion. The liver cell, the hepatocyte, synthesizes bile (approximately 600 mL/day), which aids in the metabolism of carbohydrates, fats, and proteins.

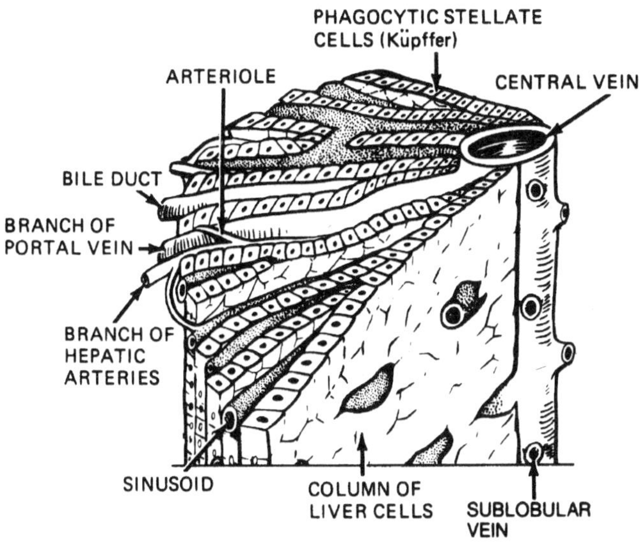

Figure 37-11. Liver lobule.

The bile is secreted into bile canaliculi (ducts), which branch and combine, eventually forming the right and left hepatic ducts. Immediately after leaving the liver, the right and left hepatic ducts merge to form the common hepatic duct. The hepatic ducts drain bile salts and the products of hemoglobin and drug metabolism.

The cystic duct of the gallbladder joins the common hepatic duct to form the common bile duct. The common bile duct joins the major pancreatic duct to form the ampulla of Vater just prior to entering the duodenum at the sphincter of Oddi.

The Kupffer cells of the liver sinusoids are typical reticuloendothelial cells. They are tissue macrophages that are capable of removing and phagocytizing old and defective blood cells, bacteria, and other foreign material from the portal blood as it flows through the sinusoid. This phagocytic action removes the colon bacilli and detoxifies harmful substances that filter into the blood from the intestine.

The liver eliminates bilirubin (by-product of the breakdown of hemoglobin) from the blood through urine and feces. Failure to eliminate bilirubin causes jaundice.

The liver is involved in the metabolism of many hormones by its role in hormone biotransformation, activation, and excretion. It is particularly involved in the metabolism of steroid hormones, such as the estrogens and progesterone, testosterone, glucocorticoids, and aldosterone. Steroid hormones are taken up from the circulation by the liver and then metabolized by hepatic enzymes. The steroid hormones directly influence many of the liver's biochemical and physiologic functions.

A major biochemical function of the liver is the detoxification and metabolism of drugs, vitamins, and hormones. Some compounds are metabolically converted to relatively inactive forms (steroid hormones), whereas others become more biologically active (vitamin D). Of prime importance in maintaining homeostasis and protecting the body against ingested toxins is the ability of the liver to metabolize and detoxify a wide variety of absorbed substances that reach it directly in the portal blood.

The liver is essential in the regulation of carbohydrate metabolism, since it directly receives from the portal circulation most of the ingested carbohydrates and then, by hormonal regulation, controls the concentration of blood glucose in the fed and fasting states. The liver stores glycogen through glycogenesis (glucose to glycogen) and breaks it down in a process called glycogenolysis (glycogen to glucose) as needed. It also synthesizes glucose from amino acids (gluconeogenesis), lactic acid, and glycerol.

The liver is involved in many aspects of lipid synthesis and metabolism. It is a major site of triglyceride, cholesterol, and phospholipid synthesis. It is involved in the formation of lipoproteins, the conversion of carbohydrates and proteins to fats, and the formation of ketones from fatty acids.

The liver's role in protein metabolism includes the deamination of proteins for glucose availability, the formation of urea from ammonia so it may be eliminated from the blood, and the synthesis of plasma proteins such as albumin, haptoglobin, transferrin, and alpha and beta globulins.

The liver synthesizes vitamin K–dependent clotting factors of the blood-clotting fibrinogen (factor I), prothrombin (factor II), and factors V, VII, and X. It also stores the fat-soluble vitamins (A, D, E, and K), as well as vitamin B_{12}, iron, and copper.

KEY CLINICAL CONTENT

- Understanding the anatomy and physiology of the liver is foundational in correlating the clinical significance of portal HTN and cirrhosis later in the GI section.
- Noteworthy for CCRN questions:
  - The hepatic ducts drain bile salts and the products of hemoglobin and drug metabolism.
  - Failure to eliminate bilirubin causes jaundice.
  - A major biochemical function of the liver is the detoxification and metabolism of drugs, vitamins, and hormones.
  - The liver synthesizes vitamin K–dependent clotting factors of the blood-clotting fibrinogen (factor I), prothrombin (factor II), and factors V, VII, and X.
  - There are usually several questions on the CCRN exam related to blood glucose, it is important to understand the liver's role in the processing and release of blood glucose.

Gallbladder. The gallbladder (**Fig. 37-12**) is a sac-like storage structure for bile.

Function. Bile is manufactured by the parenchymal cells (hepatocytes) of the liver and secreted by them into the bile canaliculi. The bile then travels to the hepatic duct, to the cystic duct, and then to the gallbladder for concentration (by as much as 12-fold) and storage. Upon stimulation, the gallbladder forces bile into the cystic duct, the common bile duct, and the duodenum.

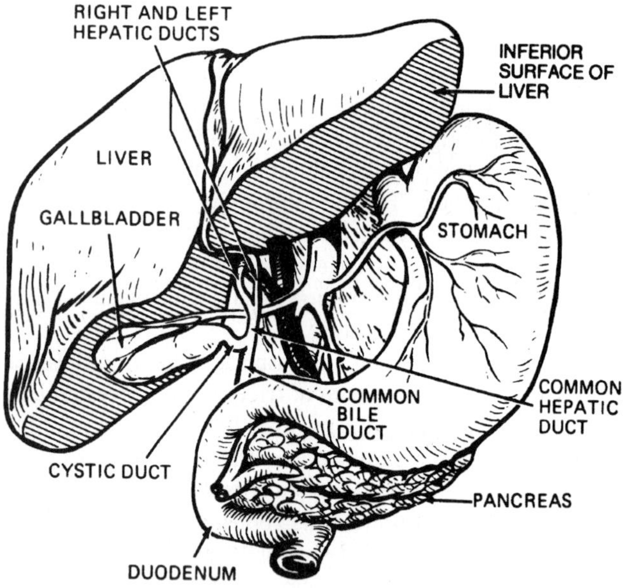

Figure 37-12. Location of the gallbladder.

Bile is responsible for the emulsification of fats and micelle formation. Inside the gallbladder, bile salts react with water, leaving a fat-soluble end to mix with cholesterol and/or lecithin. These formed particles are called micelles. Gallstones may form when the micelles become supersaturated with cholesterol. If bile salts are absent or diminished in the small intestine, normal fat digestion and absorption cannot occur. This results in fat malabsorption and steatorrhea (fatty stools).

Bile pigments result from the degradation of hemoglobin. These pigments give the feces its brown color. Absence of bile pigments, as with obstructive jaundice, produces whitish-gray feces.

Normally bile pigments do not form stones. However, in some diseases, there is an overconcentration of bile pigments, resulting in precipitation of bilirubinate stones. Most of gallstones (approximately 90%) are composed essentially of cholesterol.

Bilirubin is the main bile pigment. Once red blood cells have completed their 120-day sojourn through the circulatory system, they become fragile and rupture, releasing hemoglobin. The hemoglobin is phagocytized by cells of the reticuloendothelial system and split into heme and globin. It is from the heme ring that bile pigments are made. Bilirubin is the first pigment to be formed; however, it is soon reduced to free bilirubin and released into the plasma. Once in the plasma, free bilirubin combines quickly with plasma albumin and becomes protein-bound free (fat-soluble) bilirubin. It is also known as unconjugated or indirect bilirubin. Free bilirubin becomes conjugated (or direct) once it is absorbed into the hepatic ducts and combines with other substances. Conjugated bilirubin is now water-soluble.

Normally the total plasma concentration of both the free and conjugated forms of bilirubin is approximately 0.5 mg/100 mL plasma. The concentration of bilirubin in the plasma represents a balance between the rate of entry of the pigment into the plasma and the hepatic clearance of bilirubin.

With jaundice, plasma levels of both unconjugated (indirect) and conjugated (direct) bilirubin are measured.

Stimulation of the Gallbladder. *The sphincter of Oddi opens upon vagal and hormonal stimulation. Vagal stimulation increases bile secretions through the sphincter of Oddi.* The sphincter of Oddi in a normal state remains slightly opened, providing for a constant but minuscule amount of bile to enter the small intestine.

During normal digestion, the gallbladder contracts in response to the hormone cholecystokinin, pushing increasing amounts of bile through the sphincter of Oddi into the duodenum. The gallbladder does not contract without CCK (eg, between meals or during starvation diets).

37.6 GUIDE TO GASTROINTESTINAL ELEMENTS AND DIAGNOSTIC TESTS

Table 37-1 provides a quick reference to key chemical elements in the GI system. **Tables 37-2** to **37-5** provide quick references to common GI diagnostic tests presented in the next several chapters.

TABLE 37-1. CHEMICAL ELEMENTS IN THE GASTROINTESTINAL TRACT

Chemical Messenger	*Origin*	*Stimulus*	*Inhibitors*	*Action*
Gastrin (endocrine)	G-cells of gastric antrum, duodenal mucosa	Distention of stomach from food Presence of products from protein digestion, vagal stimulation, elevated blood levels of calcium and epinephrine	Acid in stomach	Stimulates secretion of HCl and pepsin, growth of gastric mucosa, relaxes ileocecal sphincter. Promotes antral activity. Stimulates parietal cells and chief cells.

(*Continued*)

TABLE 37-1. CHEMICAL ELEMENTS IN THE GASTROINTESTINAL TRACT *(CONTINUED)*

Chemical Messenger	*Origin*	*Stimulus*	*Inhibitors*	*Action*
Secretin (endocrine)	Duodenal mucosa	Acidic duodenal pH; digested proteins in the upper small intestine	None known	Regulates duodenal pH by preventing gastric acid secretion. Stimulates pancreatic HCO_3^- production and augments the action of cholecystokinin. Increases insulin release from the pancreas.
Cholecystokinin (neuroendocrine)	Duodenal mucosa	Products of protein and fat digestion entering the duodenum	Lack of stimulus	Stimulation of pancreatic enzyme secretion, stimulates gallbladder contraction caused by fat in the intestine, relaxation of the sphincter of Oddi, stimulation of pancreatic growth, inhibits gastric emptying, enhances insulin release, stimulates pepsin secretion, may weakly and selectively stimulate gastric acid secretion, stimulates motility of small bowel, augments secretion in stimulating secretion of alkaline pancreatic juice.
Vasoactive intestinal peptide	Produced in the intestines, pancreas, and brain	Esophageal distention, intestinal distention, electrical vagal stimulation, intraduodenal fat or acid, serotonin, oxytocin, by intestinal ischemia	None known	Stimulates pancreatic HCO_3^- secretion and intestinal secretion. It induces glycogenolysis. Improves GI motility by relaxing smooth muscle with the GI tract and stimulating intestinal secretion of electrolytes and water, while inhibiting gastric acid secretion. Improves cardiac contractility, dilates peripheral blood vessels and lowers blood pressure.
Gastric inhibitory polypeptide (endocrine)	Duodenal and jejunal mucosa	Presence of glucose in the duodenum	Lack of stimulus	Enhances insulin release and fatty acid metabolism.
Insulin (endocrine)	Beta cells of the islets of Langerhans in the pancreas	Presence of glucose in the gut and blood	Low glucose levels	Controls glucose metabolism in the body by controlling the entry of glucose into the fat and muscle cells, increases the quantities of amino acids available in the cells for synthesizing proteins, stimulates the formation of proteins by ribosomes, stimulates the formation of RNA in cells. The presence of insulin causes the body to use carbohydrates as fuel. In the absence of insulin, fatty acids are mobilized and used in place of carbohydrates.
Glucagon (endocrine)	Alpha cells of the islets of Langerhans in the pancreas	Low glucose concentrations (as low as 60 mg/100 mL of blood), intense exercise, and/or starvation	Normal-to-high glucose concentrations (>60 mg/100 mL of blood)	Regulates blood glucose level, mobilizes glucose from the liver by glycogenolysis (breakdown of the glycogen to glucose), increases gluconeogenesis (conversion of proteins to glucose) by the liver—does this by mobilizing proteins from the tissues of the body and then promotes the uptake of amino acids into the liver as well as conversion of amino acids into glucose.

TABLE 37-2. LIVER TESTS BASED ON DETOXIFICATION AND EXCRETORY FUNCTIONS

Type of Test	*Associated Pathologies*
Serum bilirubin (direct and indirect)	Increased indirect (unconjugated) bilirubin is associated with hemolysis of red blood cells (RBCs) or decreased RBC production in the bone marrow (ie, anemia). Increased direct (conjugated) bilirubin is associated with biliary tract obstruction (ie, acute pancreatitis, choledocholithiasis, etc), liver disease, liver injuries, sepsis, and Gilbert disease.
Urine bilirubin	Indicates increased direct serum bilirubin and implies liver disease.
Urine urobilinogen	Elevations can occur from liver disease or increased RBC hemolysis. Decreases can signal biliary or hepatic obstruction.
Blood ammonia	Increased levels indicate hepatocellular disease and portal hypertension. Useful for diagnosis and treating hepatic encephalopathy.
Serum bile acids	Elevated fasting levels are associated with liver disease. Postprandial elevations are seen in a variety of liver diseases. If there are no changes in the levels after eating, it can represent malabsorption or disordered hepatic metabolism (ie, Gilbert disease).

TABLE 37-3. TESTS THAT MEASURE BIOSYNTHETIC FUNCTION OF THE LIVER

Type of Test	*Associated Pathologies*
Albumin	Decreased levels may indicate chronic hepatocellular disorders, malnutrition, protein-losing enteropathy, inflammatory bowel disease, and nephrotic syndrome.
Serum protein electrophoresis (SPEP)	Separates blood proteins into five groups. Used to diagnose protein disorders. Diseases that increase the level one protein are called monoclonal gammopathies. These include multiple myeloma, plasma cell leukemia, and amyloidosis. Polyclonal gammopathies are increases in more than one protein and are typically associated with inflammation.
Coagulation factors Prothrombin time Partial thromboplastin time Fibrinogen	Elevated in end-stage liver disease, hepatitis, cirrhosis, vitamin K deficiencies, malabsorption, obstructive jaundice, and treatment with broad-spectrum antibiotics. Decreased in chronic malnutrition, end-stage liver disease, large volume blood transfusions (acute). Elevated by any type of acute inflammatory condition such as trauma, sepsis, acute coronary syndromes, and malignancies.
Ceruloplasmin	Elevated in Wilson disease. May also be increased during sepsis, inflammation, and certain malignancies.
Ferritin	Elevated in diseases that cause iron overload such as hemochromatosis. Increases are also common during infection, and with hepatic cirrhosis or fibrosis. Decreased in iron deficiency.
Alpha$_1$-fetoprotein	Elevated in hepatocellular, testicular, and ovarian cancer.
Serum Enzymes	
Aminotransferases	Elevated levels indicate either acute or chronic hepatocellular diseases or injuries caused by medications, ethanol, hepatitis, or biliary obstruction.
ALT (alanine transaminase)	
AST (aspartate transaminase)	
Alkaline phosphatase	Elevated in cholestasis, liver disease, and bone disease.
5′-Nucleotidase	Elevated in cholestasis.
Gamma-glutamyltranspeptidase (GGT)	Elevated in cholestasis, ethanol use, and hyperthyroidism.

TABLE 37-4. TESTS USEFUL IN THE DIAGNOSIS OF MALABSORPTION

Type of Test	*Associated Pathologies*
Stool fat	Steatorrhea.
Xylose absorption	Evaluate nutrient absorption for patients with malnutrition, diarrhea, or unexplained weight loss.
Small intestinal biopsy	Value of the differential diagnosis of malabsorption.
Secretin stimulation test	Evaluate pancreatic secretion for patients with suspected pancreatic insufficiency such as those with chronic pancreatitis, pancreatic cancer, or cystic fibrosis.
Serum calcium, albumin, cholesterol, magnesium, and iron	Low level may be indicative of malabsorption.
Serum carotenes, vitamin A, and prothrombin time	May indicate malabsorption of the fat-soluble vitamins.
Breath tests (hydrogen and bile acid)	Abnormal hydrogen breath test results indicate lactose, fructose, or sucrose intolerance. Abnormal bile acid breath test indicates bacterial overgrowth in the small intestine.

TABLE 37-5. GASTROINTESTINAL AND RADIOLOGIC STUDIES

Upper GI series	Barium and/or gas is taken orally to show structural or functional problems of the esophagus and stomach. Barium is usually followed through the small bowel with roentgenograms to determine its rate of passage and look for structural abnormalities.
Lower GI series (barium enema)	The large colon is studied with barium and/or gas given per rectum. Sufficient barium and/or gas is given to distend the bowel and show any abnormalities in structure or a tumor.
Cholangiography	Oral cholangiography is based on the ability of the liver to extract from the blood a radiopaque dye that has been absorbed from the intestinal tract and then secrete it into bile. Indicates gallbladder disease. Intravenous cholangiography is based on the slow intravenous injection of a radiopaque dye, its extraction from blood by the liver, and then its rapid excretion into bile. Indicates cystic duct obstruction, most likely from gallstones.
Endoscopy (upper GI endoscopy, colonoscopy, proctosigmoidoscopy, and fiberoptic sigmoidoscopy)	Endoscopy is the visualization of the inside of a body cavity by means of a lighted tube. Useful in diagnosing mass lesions, ulcers, strictures, dyspepsia, heartburn, bleeding, or cancers. Also, used for biopsies and removal of foreign objects. Being used widely therapeutically for sclerosing, polyp removal, heater probe therapy, and removal of gallstones from the common bile duct.
Endoscopic retrograde cholangiopancreatography (ERCP)	The ampulla of Vater is cannulated through a side-viewing endoscope. A radiopaque dye is injected, and both the pancreatic and bile ducts can be visualized. Allows for diagnosing obstruction, malignancy, and inflammation. Endoscopic sphincterotomy and extraction of gallstones may also be performed.
Percutaneous liver biopsy	Puncture of the liver to diagnose hepatocellular disease, prolonged hepatitis, hepatomegaly, hepatic filling defects, fever, and staging of lymphoma.
Angiography	The femoral artery is entered with a large needle that is then exchanged with a catheter that is passed into the celiac artery or one of its branches (superior mesenteric or hepatic). The contrast medium is injected, and films are taken. This procedure allows visualization of the visceral vessels to identify abnormalities of vascular structure and function, visualize masses, and note sites of bleeding.
Computed tomography	Noninvasive procedure used in identifying masses. Provides a three-dimensional image.
Ultrasound	Noninvasive procedure using sound waves to outline the pancreas, liver, gallbladder, and spleen. It will distinguish fluid from solid structures and will show an abscess or the volume of fluid present in ascites.
Esophageal manometry	Contractions generated by the esophageal wall are measured as luminal pressures. Useful in the evaluation of achalasia, diffuse spasm, scleroderma, and other motility disorders.
Hepatobiliary imaging	Noninvasive nuclear medicine scan allowing visualization of extra hepatic biliary system and hepatic takeup and excretion of isotope.
Tagged RBC scan	Noninvasive nuclear medicine scan used to gauge leakage of isotope-tagged RBCs in acute GI hemorrhage.

KEY CONTENT CHECKLIST

- ❒ Venous drainage of GI tract → portal vein → liver → hepatic vein → inferior vena cava
- ❒ pH of gastric secretions = 1–3.
- ❒ Inspection, auscultation, percussion, palpation (remember in this order).
  - Unable to palpate normal spleen (unless enlarged ×3).
  - Peritonitis = decreased bowel sounds
- ❒ Vagotomy is the dissection of the vagus nerve (near stomach) for stomach ulcer.
- ❒ Morphine causes spasms of sphincter of Oddi.
- ❒ Pain from GERD can mimic cardiac chest pain.
- ❒ The vascular interior layer of the stomach is noteworthy as a source of GI bleeding when there is a disruption in the mucosal barrier and vascular epithelium.
- ❒ The arterial blood supply with the GI tract is notable when considering a patient's hemodynamic status especially if patient has experienced recent trauma including surgery to the abdominal cavity and/or related structures.
- ❒ The impact of narcotics and other drugs used in the care of a critically ill patient should be considered in relationship to their impact on the motility of the digestive system—specifically noting when motility is reduced and the preventative measures that should be taken to support the patient.
- ❒ Understanding the anatomy and physiology of the liver is foundational in correlating the clinical significance of portal HTN and cirrhosis later in the GI section.

Review Questions:

1. **Which substance will increase the production of hydrochloric acid?**
   a. Histamine
   b. Atropine
   c. Bicarbonate
   d. Potassium salts

Answer: A. Rationale: Histamine is released during the cephalic phase of digestion. Approximately 30% of gastric acid is produced during this phase. Atropine, bicarbonate, and potassium do not affect the production of hydrochloric acid, eliminating answers B, C, and D.

2. **The normal pH of the stomach falls within which of the following ranges?**
   a. 0
   b. 1–2
   c. 6
   d. More than 7

Answer: B. Rationale: Normal gastric pH is acidic, with a normal range of 1 to 3. It is usually not higher than 5. Higher pH levels (>6) are associated with fluid from the small intestine or the lungs.

3. **All venous blood from the intestines eventually drains into which vein?**
   a. Inferior vena cava
   b. Superior vena cava
   c. Portal vein
   d. Iliac vein

Answer: A. Rationale: The inferior vena cava drains all venous blood from organs below the thorax and brings the blood to the right atrium. The superior vena cava is not correct, as it drains the head, neck, and thorax. The portal vein supplies 75% of blood to the liver. The iliac veins drain the portions of the pelvis. Therefore, options B, C, and D are incorrect.

38

Gastrointestinal Hemorrhage and Esophageal Varices

CHAPTER OVERVIEW AND OBJECTIVES

This chapter addresses the CCRN exam items of acute gastrointestinal (GI) hemorrhage and portal hypertension. Expect two to four questions on the exam in this content area.

After studying this chapter, you should be able to:

- Identify the key clinical presentation of both gastrointestinal hemorrhage and esophageal varices.
- Describe key nursing intervention supporting the care of the patient experiencing gastrointestinal hemorrhage and esophageal varices.

There are many sources of GI bleeding. The location and appearance of blood help clinicians determine the bleeding source.

- Bloody emesis (hematemesis) is associated with more acute bleeding from a proximal source such as the stomach or esophagus.
- Coffee-grounds emesis or nasogastric tube (NGT) drainage is characteristic of older blood mixed with gastric acid.
- Blood from the upper GI tract appears as dark, tarry stool (melena).
- Maroon feces are associated with right (ascending) colon bleeding. Bright red blood from the rectum (hematochezia) is typically the result of left (descending) colon or rectal hemorrhage; however, it can also be seen with brisk right colon hemorrhage.

38.1 GASTROINTESTINAL HEMORRHAGE

GI hemorrhage can occur in any portion of the GI tract. Bleeding sources are categorized as either nonvariceal or variceal. Nonvariceal bleeding occurs more frequently and has a mortality rate of approximately 10%. Frequent etiologies associated with nonvariceal bleeding include the use of nonsteroidal anti-inflammatory drugs (NSAIDs) or infection with *Helicobacter pylori*. Mallory–Weiss tears, lacerations of the mucosal tissue at the gastroesophageal junction, account for 10% to 15% of upper GI bleeds (UGIB). They are caused by sudden elevations in esophageal pressure due to retching. The bleeding is self-limiting.

Other etiologies may include

- Inherited or acquired (connective tissue or autoimmune related) arteriovenous malformations or other vascular abnormalities are the source of 5% to 10% of GI hemorrhage.
- Dieulafoy lesion is a small vessel, protruding from damaged mucosa. It causes less than 5% of cases of upper GI bleeds.
- Tumors, whether benign or malignant, also cause less than 5% of upper GI bleeding.
- Rarely, patients with a previous history of surgical repair of the abdominal aorta may develop an aortoenteric fistula. It is usually first signaled by a "herald bleed" that occurs when a small fistula forms. The herald bleed is usually self-limited and stops when a blood clot forms. It is followed by a catastrophic bleed that can occur hours, days, or weeks later.
- Lower GI bleeds (LGIBs) may be acute or chronic. Most LGIBs are caused by diverticula (40%), angiodysplasia (37%), and ischemic colitis (19%). Other etiologies include inflammatory bowel disease (IBD), radiation, hemorrhoids, anorectal fissures, proctitis, and tumors.

Pathophysiology

Disruption of the mucous membranes of either the stomach or duodenum can extend in to the muscularis mucosa. The epithelial cells secrete mucus to decrease acidic destruction of the tissues. This erosion of the mucosa layer may extend into the innermost layer of muscle (muscularis mucosa) or into the underlying vasculature, resulting in blood loss.

Etiology

Upper GI bleeding can result from gastritis, peptic ulcers, acute mucosal tears, or esophageal varices. The most prevalent causes of upper GI bleeding are peptic and duodenal ulcers. The duodenal bulb is the most frequent site.

There are multiple causes of peptic ulcer disease (PUD) including:

- *Helicobacter pylori* (*H. pylori*) infection.
- Excessive acid production by gastrin secreting tumors as seen in Zollinger–Ellison syndrome.
- Medications (eg, **NSAIDs** and **corticosteroids**).
- Stress-related mucosal disease (SRMD) refers to the development of gastritis or ulcers in the stomach caused by disruption in the intramucosal blood flow. Physiologic stress from critical illness that lasts greater than 48 hours puts patients at risk due to increased catecholamine production (eg, **norepinephrine, epinephrine**) leading to vasoconstriction and lowering splanchnic blood flow.

Risks associated with prolonged critical care illness include the following chain of events:

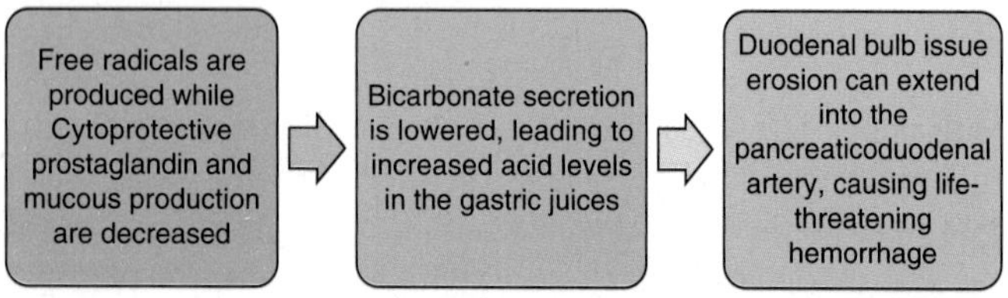

Patients who are coagulopathic (platelet count <50,000/mL, international normalized ratio [INR] >1.5, or partial thromboplastin time [PTT]) greater than two time the control are at high risk of bleeding. Anticoagulant and antiplatelet drugs are held and may require administration of a reversal agent during an acute UGIB.

KEY CLINICAL CONCEPT

- Patients who are coagulopathic (platelet count <50,000/mL, INR >1.5, or PTT) greater than two time the control are at high risk of bleeding.
- Anticoagulant and antiplatelet drugs are held and may require administration of a reversal agent during an acute UGIB.

Clinical Presentation

Many patients with gastric or duodenal ulcers present with epigastric pain. Gastric ulcer pain occurs immediately after eating. Duodenal ulcer pain typically appears 2 to 3 hours later. Hematemesis points to bleeding from an upper GI source. Melena occurs when more than 50 mL blood is lost from the stomach or proximal small intestine. Seemingly minor mental status changes such as slight to moderate anxiety and mild tachypnea (respiratory rate >20) are early signs of shock. Hypotension and significantly elevated heart rate (>120 bpm) do not occur until class III shock (**Table 38-1**). Early identification and treatment of hemorrhagic shock improves patient outcomes.

KEY CLINICAL CONCEPT

- Seemingly minor mental status changes such as slight to moderate anxiety and mild tachypnea (respiratory rate >20) are early signs of shock.
- Hypotension and significantly elevated heart rate (>120 bpm) do not occur until class III shock (Table 38-1).
- Early identification and treatment of hemorrhagic shock improves patient outcomes.

Diagnosis

Esophagogastroduodenoscopy (EGD) is the preferred method for diagnosing UGIB. Endoscopy is highly sensitive and specific for locating and identifying bleeding lesions in the upper GI tract. In addition, once a bleeding lesion has been identified, therapeutic endoscopy can achieve acute hemostasis and prevent recurrent bleeding in most patients. Endoscopy involves passage of a long, flexible tube into the esophagus, stomach, and duodenum through which the physician can see the inside lining of the GI tract. Unfortunately, massive bleeding can prevent adequate endoscopic evaluation and treatment. In such cases, angiography or a nuclear medicine tagged red blood cell (RBC) scan may locate the source of bleeding.

Colonoscopy is the primary diagnostic modality for lower GI bleeding. Radiologic tests are used to locate bleeding sources when endoscopy fails. Radionucleotide scanning is done by labeling RBCs with technetium-99. It is often called a red-tag study. It is noninvasive diagnostic test that can detect

TABLE 38-1. CLASSIFICATION OF HEMORRHAGIC SHOCK

	Class I	*Class II*	*Class III*	*Class IV*
Blood Loss	<750 mL	750–1500 mL	1.5–2 L	>2 L
% Blood Vol	<15%	15–30%	30–40%	>40%
HR	<100	>100	>120	>140
BP	Normal	Normal	Decreased	Decreased
Pulse Press	Normal	Decreased	Decreased	Decreased
Resp Rate	14–20	20–30	30–40	>40
UOP/hour	>30 mL	20–30 mL	5–15 mL	Negligible
Mental Status	Slight anxiety	Moderate anxiety	Confused	Lethargic
Fluid	Crystalloid	Crystalloid	Blood	Blood

Reproduced with permission from Parrillo JE, Dellinger RP. Critical Care Medicine: Principles of Diagnosis and Management in the Adult. *3rd ed. Philadelphia, PA: Mosby-Elsevier; 2008.*

bleeding rates as low as 0.05 to 0.1 mL/min. Scoring scales such as Glasgow-Blatchford Bleeding Score (GBS), pre-endoscopic Rockall score (PRS), complete Rockall score (CRS), and Cedars–Sinai Medical Center Predictive Index (CSMCPI) help predict which patients require urgent endoscopy, in addition to calculating risk of rebleeding and death.

Hemodynamics

The hemodynamic profile of hemorrhagic shock is related to significantly low circulatory volume and reflect the intravascular volume depletion.

- Systolic blood pressure (SBP) may be less than 90 mm Hg or lower than 40 mm Hg from baseline.
- Pulse pressure (SBP–DBP) is narrowed.
- Low filling pressures.
- CVP (central venous pressure) less than 2 mm Hg.
- Pulmonary artery occlusion pressure (PAOP) less than 8 mm Hg.
- Catecholamines such as **epinephrine** and **norepinephrine** respond by vasoconstriction and increasing **afterload**.

KEY CLINICAL CONCEPT

- Remember to compare the patient's current SBP with their baseline. Patients with a history of hypertension may have BPs that appear normal but are actually significantly lower than their baseline. Hypotension in these patients is a considered an SBP 40 mm Hg or lower than baseline.
- In hypovolemic shock, since the root cause of the shock is volume depletion, choose interventions that restore volume over vasopressors in borderline hypotensive patients on the exam.

Complications

Ongoing hypotension and tissue hypoxia can lead to multiple organ failure that may cause watershed-pattern strokes and ischemic pancreatitis. Prolonged shock can also lead to intestinal ischemia and infarction. Patients with decreased levels of consciousness are at risk for poor airway protection and may aspirate during emesis. Aspiration can lead to aspiration pneumonitis and/or aspiration pneumonia.

Treatment

In all cases of PUD, **NSAIDs** or other causative agents should be discontinued. Unstable patients and those with a significant risk of clinical deterioration benefit from management in a critical care setting. Immediately obtain vascular access with two large-bore (14 or 16 Fr) peripheral intravenous (IV) lines with a treatment focusing on replacing circulating blood volume and maintaining adequate hemodynamics.

Initially, IV boluses of isotonic fluids (**lactated Ringers or 0.9% saline** are preferred). Blood administration is necessary in patients with ongoing blood loss as **packed red blood cells (PRBCs)** improves both circulating volume and tissue oxygenation. For patients with *coagulopathy* or those requiring massive transfusion, administering blood products, such as **fresh frozen plasma (FFP), platelets, and/or cryoprecipitate,** is paramount in preventing ongoing blood loss. Goals of resuscitation of the acutely bleeding patient include

- Restoration of mental status
- Urine output ≥0.5 mL/kg/h (or 30 mL/h)
- Mean arterial pressure (MAP) ≥60 mm Hg
- Resolution of tachycardia
- Increased hemoglobin and hematocrit (H&H) with a target Hgb ≥8.0 g/dL
- Normalization of lactic acid less than 2.0 mEq/L.

In patients undergoing invasive or less invasive hemodynamic monitoring, the goal includes restoring normal filling pressures: CVP 2 to 6 mm Hg or PAOP 8 to 12 mm Hg. The increased in **preload** will improve myocardial contractility, **stroke volume (SV), and cardiac output (CO)**. Appropriate resuscitation will lower afterload and bring it into a normal range: SVR 900 to 1200 dynes/s/cm^5 or SVRI 1970 to 2390 dynes/s/cm^5. Decreasing **afterload** reduces the workload of the left ventricle, augmenting SV and CO. Together, the normalization of preload and afterload results in higher CO 4 to 8 L/min and CI 2.5 to 4.3 L/min/m^2.

Endoscopy is the preferred diagnostic and treatment modality for upper GI bleeding due to its versatility and low complication risk. In addition to endoscopy, there are several different types of therapeutic options that can be employed alone or in combination. These interventions may include:

- Thermal or argon plasma coagulation.
- Hemostatic clips.
- Thrombin or fibrin sealants.
- Injection therapy can include the use of normal saline to tamponade bleeding or epinephrine for vasoconstriction.
- Emergent endoscopy is indicated for patients in hemorrhagic shock and those who cannot be stabilized with fluid volume or blood product resuscitation.

Interventions, such as surgery or angiography, are indicated in patients who have active bleeding not stopped or slowed down with endoscopic therapy. Interventional radiology is sometimes needed to manage GI bleeding. Angiography can control GI bleeding can by local arterial infusion of vasoconstrictive drugs and/or by embolizing particulate matter into the bleeding artery. Complications can include intestinal ischemia and infarction. General surgery consultation is indicated in for control of bleeding, refractory to above mentioned modalities.

Preventing acid production is important in treating acute UGIB. **Proton pump inhibitors (PPIs)** not only raise gastric pH, but they also improve platelet function, stabilize blood clots, and inhibit pepsin, as well as promote ulcer healing. IV PPIs are preferred over H_2 receptor blockers for acute bleeding due to their higher degree of acid suppression. They are typically administered as an IV bolus then as a continuous infusion.

The following outlines supportive interventions aiding in the management of the patient:

- Sucralfate is an oral agent that binds to the gastric mucosa. It creates a barrier preventing hydrochloric acid (HCl) from degrading mucosa and eroding the mucosa. It is used to prevent peptic ulcers without changing the gastric pH. *Sucralfate is not used as frequently since the advent of antisecretory therapy.*

- *Acid suppression*, with histamine (H_2) receptor blockers (eg, **famotidine**) or PPIs (eg, **pantoprazole**), is a mainstay of medical therapy for gastroesophageal reflux and PUD.
- The above agents are also used in combination with antibiotics to treat *Helicobacter pylori* infection.
- **Octreotide (Sandostatin)** was previously shown to decrease the risk of rebleeding in patients without varices, but its routine use is no longer recommended for UGIB.

Nursing Interventions

The most important role for the nurse is to monitor the patient's hemodynamic status and observe for signs of continued bleeding.

- Insertion of at least two large-bore (14- to 16-gauge) IV lines is imperative for rapid fluid replacement and blood product administration. In cases where peripheral access is unattainable, large-bore central venous catheters (introducer sheath) should be placed by a physician or another qualified provider (NP or PA).
- Carefully monitor vital signs and both cardiac and pulmonary status during fluid and blood replacement to prevent over- or under-resuscitation and to provide early detection of pulmonary edema.
- Additionally, when large volumes of fluids or blood products are being infused, the nurse should be carefully monitoring the patient for signs of hypothermia.
- **The Trendelenburg position is no longer recommended to raise BP in shock patients. It is associated with risk of aspiration, facial/laryngeal edema, hypoventilation, cardiac arrhythmias, and decreased lower extremity arterial blood flow.**

KEY CLINICAL CONCEPT

- Carefully monitor vital signs and both cardiac and pulmonary status during fluid and blood replacement to prevent over- or under-resuscitation and to provide early detection of pulmonary edema.
- The Trendelenburg position is no longer recommended to raise BP in shock patients. It is associated with risk of aspiration, facial/laryngeal edema, hypoventilation, cardiac arrhythmias, and decreased lower extremity arterial blood flow.

Laboratory studies should include a complete blood count (CBC), basic metabolic panel (BMP), liver (hepatic) function test (LFTs), prothrombin time (PT), and activated partial thromboplastin time (aPTT), as well as blood type and cross matching. Key considerations when monitoring the patient and lab values include:

- H&H may appear within normal limits at the onset of bleeding, due to equal losses of both RBCs and plasma volume. This can be falsely reassuring.
- A combination of hemodilution from isotonic fluid administration and ongoing blood loss will cause the H&H to fall over a period of several hours.
- Ongoing management for the risk of dilutional thrombocytopenia due to extreme replacement of fluid loss or preexisting disseminated intravascular coagulation.

Commonly seen electrolyte anomalies include hypernatremia (sodium >145 mEq/dL) due to intravascular volume depletion. Hypokalemia (potassium <3.5 mEq/dL) may occur in patients with severe vomiting or large amounts of NGT output. Hypovolemia may also lead to elevations in blood urea nitrogen (BUN >20 mg/dL) and creatinine (>1.5 mg/dL), as well as prerenal acute kidney injury (AKI). *In prerenal causes of AKI, the BUN/creatinine ratio is typically more than 20:1.* UGIB also raises BUN due to the large amount of protein released. If hemorrhagic shock is present, serum lactic acid levels will rise (>4 mg/dL).

Blood transfusions can cause hyperkalemia, due to blood cell lysis. Monitor for hyperkalemia and hypocalcemia in patients who receive large amounts of transfused blood. Patients undergoing massive transfusion, especially those with impaired liver function, may require IV calcium administration. While transfusions are often lifesaving, they are associated with the development of transfusion-related acute lung injury (TRALI), transfusion acquired circulatory overload (TACO), and may predispose patients to bacterial infections through transfusion-related immunomodulation (TRIM).

Nursing care of the patient with either an orogastric tube (OGT) or NGT includes monitoring the tube's output and its characteristics. Maintaining patency of the OGT or NGT is important.

Emotional support for the patient and family reduces stress and facilitates understanding of the medical interventions necessary to stabilize the patient. Reassuring the patient during resuscitation and therapeutic interventions will help allay the patient's fears.

38.2 ESOPHAGEAL AND GASTRIC VARICES

Varices are abnormally dilated collateral veins. Although they are most frequent in patients with cirrhosis, those without cirrhosis that have portal vein thrombosis, superior vena cava (SVC) obstruction, Budd–Chiari syndrome, or constrictive pericarditis develop these collateral veins allowing venous blood return to the inferior vena cava (IVC) and right heart when portal vein or SVC become obstructed.

Normal hepatic portal venous system pressure gradients (HVPGs) range from 3 to 5 mm Hg. When the HVPG increases to greater than 10 to 12 mm Hg, varices form. Varices are chronically dilated veins that shunt blood away from the liver. They occur in various parts of the GI system but are most prevalent in the esophagus and at the gastroesophageal junction. The risk of developing varices increases as liver disease progresses.

Forty percent of variceal bleeding is self-limited. The larger the varices, the more likely they are to bleed. Patients with HVPG greater than 20 mm Hg are at highest risk for hemorrhage and rebleeding within 1 week (early). These patients have a 64% risk of mortality within 1 year after the initial bleeding episode. Varices are more common in the esophagus than the stomach—with those located at the gastroesophageal junction the most rupture-prone. Ongoing alcohol intake, bacterial infections, and increased intra-abdominal pressure can propagate bleeding. Other factors such as postprandial increases in splanchnic (gut, liver, pancreas, and spleen) blood flow, or processes that cause acute increases in portal pressure also increase the bleeding risk.

Clinical Presentation

Most patients with bleeding esophageal varices have signs of cirrhosis such as jaundice, icteric sclera, and ascites. Other common signs of liver disease include gynecomastia, splenomegaly, spider angiomas, and some patients may develop abdominal wall varices, called *caput medusae*.

These patients also often have elevated LFTs, such as bilirubin, lactic dehydrogenase (LDH), transaminases (aspartate transaminase [AST] and alanine transaminase [ALT]), alkaline phosphatase, and PT. One-third of cirrhotics may develop hyponatremia due to decreased free water excretion. This may contribute to ascites, risk of falling, and cognitive changes. Patients may present with signs of shock due to massive and painless bleeding. This can lead to confusion or lead to coma due to bleeding and underlying cirrhosis.

Diagnosis

Endoscopy is the preferred modality for detecting gastroesophageal varices, determining their size, and predicting their risk of rupture. Varices with red wheals represent tense, dilated veins that are at higher risk of rupture. Other tests such as computed tomography (CT) with IV contrast or magnetic resonance imaging (MRI), angiography, or portal venography scans, or endoscopic ultrasound (EUS) can provide important about portal hypertension and the extent of variceal formation outside of the gastroesophageal mucosa. In patients who have contraindications to endoscopy, barium swallow may detect esophageal varices.

Treatment

The goal of therapy for variceal hemorrhage is to stop the acute bleeding and prevent future bleeding. Volume resuscitation and hemodynamic stabilization are paramount in ensuring patient survival. Some patients may need endotracheal intubation for airway protection.

Medical Therapy

Primary prophylaxis of variceal bleeding includes the use of nonselective beta blockers (eg, **propranolol, nadolol**) to lower CO and unopposed splanchnic vasoconstriction. Moreover, carvedilol, a nonspecific beta blocker with alpha-blocking effects, has also been shown to decrease resistance in the intrahepatic and collateral portal veins.

Prophylactic antibiotic administration is part of the standard of care in patients with bleeding varices. Up to 50% of these patients develop infections during hospitalization and the use of quinolones, cephalosporins, and other antibiotic classes decreases mortality.

Due to the efficacy of endoscopic treatment, **vasopressin (Pitressin)** infusions are not commonly used. **Vasopressin** reduces portal pressure by increasing splanchnic vasoconstriction. **Vasopressin** can achieve initial hemostasis in 60% to 80% of patients, but it has only marginal effects on early rebleeding episodes and does not improve survival from active variceal hemorrhage. **Vasopressin** also induces systemic vasoconstriction which can cause strokes, myocardial infarctions and mesenteric ischemia and should be used with caution in patients with coronary artery disease (CAD). Frequently checking vital signs and cardiac rhythm in addition to assessing neurologic status are necessary for safely administering **vasopressin**. **Nitroglycerin** infusions are sometimes given with vasopressin to attenuate the risk of cardiac ischemic. **Nitroglycerin** is a venodilator that also decreases pressure in the intrahepatic venous system.

Somatostatin is a peptide that reduces portal pressure induces splanchnic vasoconstriction, thereby lowering portal venous pressure. And unlike vasopressin, it does not affect the systemic circulation. **Octreotide (Sandostatin)** a long-acting somatostatin analogue. It inhibits numerous hormones including glucagon, insulin, and growth hormone (GH). It is typically used as an adjunct to endoscopy.

Endoscopic Therapy

Endoscopic therapy is the definitive treatment for active variceal bleeding. Two forms of endoscopic treatment are available: sclerotherapy and variceal band ligation. Sclerosants, including ethyl alcohol, phenol, ethanolamine, polidocanol, or hypertonic dextrose, are used to cause endothelial cell injury and vessel thrombosis. In the United States, variceal banding has essentially replaced sclerotherapy, due to its lower risk of complications. Band ligation involves placing small elastic bands around varices. Esophageal stricture is the most frequent long-term complication of endoscopic therapy. Other adverse events such as odynophagia, perforation, deep ulcers, rebleeding, and bacteremia can occur.

Transjugular Intrahepatic Portosystemic Shunt

Transjugular intrahepatic portosystemic shunt (TIPS) is an interventional radiology procedure, where a covered stent is placed between the intrahepatic portal and hepatic veins using ultrasound and angiographic guidance. It is performed to alleviate portal hypertension, prevent variceal bleeding, treat acute variceal hemorrhage, and/or treat ascites (**Fig. 38-1**). Once jugular venous access is obtained, a hepatic vein sheath is placed, and the portal vein is identified. A tract is made through the liver parenchyma between the hepatic and portal veins. This immediately drains blood from the portal vein into the hepatic vein allowing for the blood to drain from the hepatic vein into the IVC and back to the right heart. This results in lower portal vein pressures and typically controls bleeding in 90% of patients.

Acute complications include hematoma at jugular access site, bleeding, biliary system puncture, liver ischemia, hepatic vein obstruction, heart failure, shunt mispositioning or migration, shunt-related hepatic encephalopathy, sepsis, and death. The mortality rate is heavily dependent on whether or not the patient was actively bleeding throughout the procedure ranging from 3% to 30% with increasing rates associated with bleeding during the procedure.

Ultrasonic Doppler shunt monitoring is first done within 48 to 72 hours of the procedure to establish baseline shunt velocities. Subsequent shunt monitoring is performed at 1, 3, and 6 months, and every 6 months thereafter or when symptoms such as rebleeding or ascites develop. Potential long-term complications related to decreased blood flow through the liver include severe portal vein thrombosis, hyperbilirubinemia and encephalopathy. Hemolytic anemia or rebleeding can also occur.

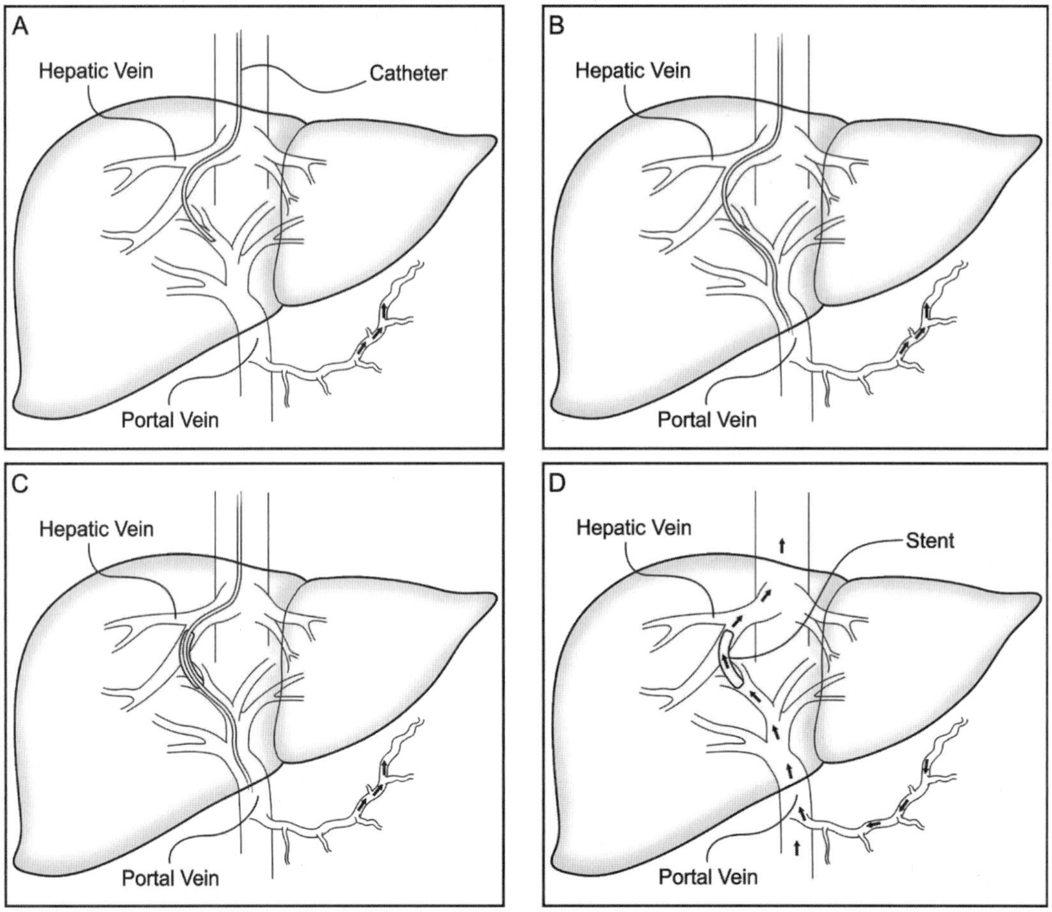

Figure 38-1. Transjugular intrahepatic portosystemic shunt (TIPS) procedure. **(A)** Needle directed through liver parenchyma to portal vein. **(B)** Guidewire passage. **(C)** Balloon dilatation. **(D)** Placement of stent.

The rebleeding rate is less than 20%. Rebleeding may be caused by stent stenosis or occlusion. These blockages are treated with angioplasty or shunt replacement.

Surgical Therapy

Portosystemic (portocaval) shunt surgery is indicated in patients who fail both endoscopic and medical therapy, or if TIPS and/or balloon-occluded retrograde transvenous obliteration (BRTO) is not available. It treats and prevents variceal bleeding by diverting blood flow from the liver by connecting the portal vein to the IVC. This lowers portal venous pressure and stops variceal bleeding. Emergency portosystemic shunts are more likely to cause encephalopathy and are associated with higher mortality rates.

Esophageal/Gastric Balloon Tamponade Therapy

Since the advent of endoscopy and other therapies, such as TIPS, the use of balloon tamponade therapy is increasingly rare. It is currently used as a last resort to control variceal bleeding in those who have failed or are unable to undergo endoscopy. They are primarily used in areas where more definitive variceal treatments are not available. They are placed either nasally or orally into the stomach. There are three types of tubes available:

- The Linton–Nachlas tube has a single gastric balloon.
- The *Sengstaken–Blakemore tube* (**Fig. 38-2**) has three parts: an esophageal balloon, a gastric balloon, and a gastric suction port.

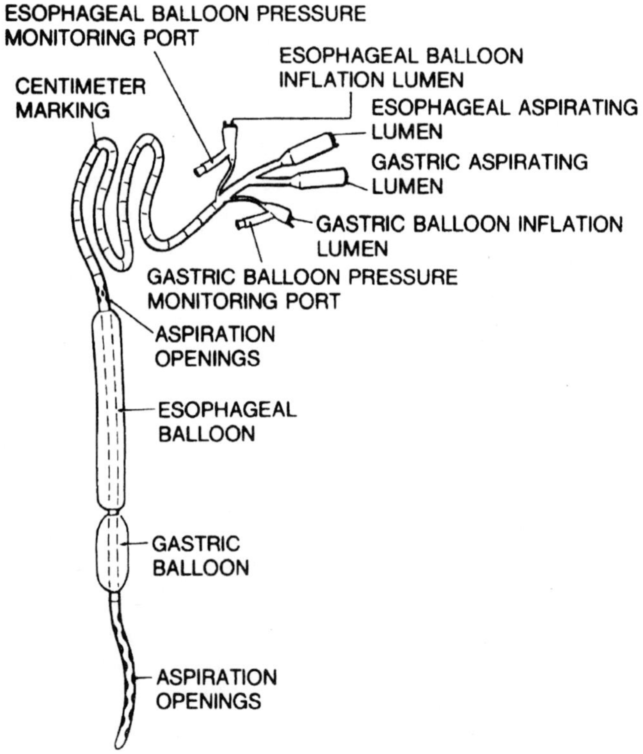

Figure 38-2. Sengstaken–Blakemore tube.

- *Minnesota tubes* are like the Sengstaken–Blakemore tube, except this type contains an esophageal suction port. The Minnesota tube is preferred because of its ability to suction above the esophageal balloon.

Since these tubes can cause esophageal necrosis and/or perforation, they are contraindicated in patients with recent esophageal surgery and in those with esophageal strictures. Carefully monitoring balloon pressure as air volume is inserted into the gastric balloon may help prevent esophageal necrosis or perforation. The maximum recommended air volume is 500 mL. Maintaining intermittent gastric and esophageal suction aids in avoiding aspiration. *Securing the proximal end of the tube with a traction device will help prevent dislodgement. Patients may require sedation and/or soft-wrist restraints, in addition to analgesia.* Properly positioned tubes typically are left in place for 24 hours after hemostasis occurs. The gastric balloon is always inflated before the esophageal balloon. *There is a high incidence of rebleeding once the balloons are deflated or mispositioned. A major risk of using these tubes is migration of the gastric balloon into the esophagus leading to airway compromise.* Keep scissors at the bedside at all times. If airway obstruction occurs, cut across the entire tube below the bifurcation of the suction and inflation ports. Clinicians may prefer to endotracheal intubate patients for airway protection.

KEY CLINICAL CONCEPT

- A major risk of using these balloon tamponade tubes is migration of the gastric balloon into the esophagus leading to airway compromise.
- Keep scissors at the bedside at all times. If airway obstruction occurs, cut across the entire tube below the bifurcation of the suction and inflation ports.

Nursing Interventions

The intervention goals for patients with variceal bleeding:

- Controlling hemorrhage
- Repleting intravascular volume losses
- Preventing or reversing hypovolemic shock.

Nursing care of the patient with acute variceal bleeding is similar to that of other types of acute upper GI blood loss. Monitoring vital signs and assessing the patient's hemodynamic status are paramount. Closely monitoring H&H and transfusing blood and blood products as ordered will improve the patient's hemodynamics and tissue oxygenation. Observing for and treating fluid, electrolyte, and acid–base anomalies are necessary for optimal patient outcomes.

38.3 LOWER GASTROINTESTINAL BLEEDING

Etiology

Approximately 40% of acute lower GI bleeding is caused by diverticular disease. Other etiologies include colitis (eg, ischemic, infectious, radiation), angiodysplasia, and colonic polyps or tumors.

Diverticulosis, Diverticulitis, and Diverticular Bleeding

Diverticulosis is the presence of multiple sac-like protrusions of vascular structures called vasa recta through the circular muscle in weaker areas of the bowel wall. These areas may be prone to bleeding since there is only one layer of mucosa protecting the vasa recta. Diverticulosis can occur anywhere in the small and large intestines but is most prevalent in the sigmoid colon. The risk of developing the disorder increases with age, with the majority of cases occurring in those older than age 60. Diverticulosis is thought to result from alterations in intestinal peristalsis such as intestinal spasms, slow transit constipation, low-fiber diets, and higher pressures within the bowel lumen. It is most prevalent in the countries that eat a Western diet, such as the United States, Europe, and Australia. Although it usually asymptomatic, some people will experience bloating, change in bowel habits, or cramping lower abdominal pain, or painless rectal bleeding.

Etiology. Diverticulitis occurs when diverticula become infected or inflamed. In simple cases, patients may be febrile, have an elevated white blood cell (WBC), and have left lower quadrant pain. It is associated with nausea, vomiting, and anorexia. Some patients will have right lower quadrant tenderness that mimics appendicitis. Peritonitis and abscesses may form in cases of diverticular perforation. Diverticular bleeding is more common in the right side of the colon and is bright red or maroon with gelatinous clots.

Diagnosis and Treatment. CT of the abdomen and pelvis with oral contrast is the preferred diagnostic test in acute cases, due to the risk of colonic perforation with colonoscopy or barium enema. For severe cases, hospitalization and treatment with IV antibiotics are indicated. CBC and BMP are drawn to assess for leukocytosis, as well as drops in H&H and electrolyte abnormalities. Emergent intervention for bleeding diverticula focuses on supporting the patient's hemodynamic status via fluid and blood product administration. Rapid bowel preparation with polyethylene glycol solution and urgent colonoscopy within 12 to 48 hours are recommended. Colonoscopy allows both diagnosis and therapeutic intervention. Angiography also allows for diagnosis and embolization of actively bleeding diverticula. Nuclear medicine tagged red cell scans are useful for detecting active bleeding but are not therapeutic. Video capsule endoscopy (VCE) is used to detect obscure GI bleeding (OGIB) in the small intestine. Surgical intervention is indicated in patients with intra-abdominal free air, peritonitis, and uncontrolled sepsis. It is sometimes necessary to control diverticular hemorrhage.

Acute Ischemic Colitis

Acute ischemic colitis is responsible for approximately 19% of LGIBs. *It is caused by hypoperfusion of the colon because of hypotension, prolonged shock, the use of vasopressor infusions, vascular occlusion, emboli, hypercoagulability, or trauma.* It is associated with the *sudden onset of abdominal pain* that is out of proportion to the patient's abdominal exam. GI bleeding occurs late in the disease process. Ischemic colitis and mesenteric ischemia are discussed in more detail in Chapter 40.

Presentation. The intestinal (splanchnic) circulation consists of three major arterial trunks that include the celiac axis, the superior mesenteric artery (SMA), and the inferior mesenteric artery (IMA). The locations most often affected are the "watershed" regions that are supplied by the distal ends of two major arteries. During hypoperfusion, watershed areas are susceptible to ischemia. The abrupt decrease in blood flow to these portions of the large intestine leads to abdominal pain, which may be located in the left side. Tenderness is common over the affected areas of the colon. Although many patients will not have guaiac positive stool or GI bleeding, hematochezia can occur.

Diagnosis. In patients with ischemic colitis, the following laboratory findings are common:

- Elevated WBC counts
- Metabolic acidosis (pH <7.35 with a bicarbonate level of <22 mEq/L) may occur.
- Lactic acidosis (>4 mEq/L) can occur from bowel hypoperfusion.

Colonoscopy is the preferred test for diagnosing ischemic colitis. It not only shows ischemic mucosal damage but also allows for tissue biopsies. CT scan of the abdomen and pelvis are frequently performed to evaluate the extent and severity of the ischemia.

Treatment. Treatment involves supportive care measures such as analgesia, bowel rest, and maintaining adequate CO, tissue oxygenation, and blood pressure (BP) through IV fluids are administration. It is important to monitor for fever, increasing leukocytosis, and worsening abdominal pain. Cases that involve gangrenous tissue or the full thickness of the intestine (transmural) require surgical resection. In these severe cases, even with operative intervention, mortality is more than 50%.

Angiodysplasia

Angiodysplasia is the most common cause of OGIB in adults. It is implicated in up to 20% to 30% of LGIBs in patients with end-stage renal disease (ESRD). It is also common in patients with von Willebrand disease, aortic stenosis, and those with left ventricular assist devices (LVAD). It involves development of ectatic blood vessels in the right colon. They receive blood flow from a central feeder vessel. They are diagnosed by colonoscopy and appear as flat, red lesions. Bleeding is brisk and typically stops spontaneously. In severe cases, hemodynamic stabilization is key, along with either endoscopic or angiographic therapy.

Less Common Etiologies of GI Bleeding. Up to 6% of patients who undergo removal of precancerous colon polyps will experience post procedure bleeding. Intestinal tumors, hemorrhoids, and anorectal fissures can also cause lower GI bleeding.

KEY CONTENT CHECKLIST

- ❒ Seemingly minor mental status changes such as slight to moderate anxiety and mild tachypnea (respiratory rate >20) are early signs of shock.
- ❒ Hypotension and significantly elevated heart rate (>120 bpm) do not occur until class III shock (Table 38-1).
- ❒ Early identification and treatment of hemorrhagic shock improves patient outcomes.
- ❒ Compare the patient's current SBP with their baseline. Patients with a history of hypertension may have BPs that appear normal but are actually significantly lower than their baseline. Hypotension in these patients is a considered an SBP 40 mm Hg or lower than baseline.
- ❒ Carefully monitor vital signs and both cardiac and pulmonary status during fluid and blood replacement to prevent over- or under-resuscitation and to provide early detection of pulmonary edema.
- ❒ The Trendelenburg position is no longer recommended to raise BP in shock patients. It is associated with risk of aspiration, facial/laryngeal edema, hypoventilation, cardiac arrhythmias, and decreased lower extremity arterial blood flow.
- ❒ A major risk of using these balloon tamponade tubes is migration of the gastric balloon into the esophagus leading to airway compromise.
- ❒ Keep scissors at the bedside at all times. If airway obstruction occurs, cut across the entire tube below the bifurcation of the suction and inflation ports.
- ❒ Patients who are coagulopathic (platelet count <50,000/mL, INR >1.5, or PTT) greater than two time the control are at high risk of bleeding.
- ❒ Anticoagulant and antiplatelet drugs are held and may require administration of a reversal agent during an acute UGIB.
- ❒ In hypovolemic shock, since the root cause of the shock is volume depletion, choose interventions that restore volume over vasopressors in borderline hypotensive patients on the exam.
- ❒ Remember that the gold standard for NGT placement confirmation is x-ray.
- ❒ UGIB patients are more likely to demonstrate vomiting and bright red blood. LGIB patients tend to have distention, less vomiting, and dark stools (since the enzymatic activity of the digestive system has been allowed enough time to act on the blood, making it dark in color).

Review Question:

1. A patient who admitted for anticoagulation and direct current cardioversion for new-onset atrial fibrillation is increasingly confused and tachycardic. A large amount of melanotic feces is noted in the bed. In addition to drawing stat labs and intravenously administering a crystalloid bolus, which intervention should the nurse anticipate?

a. Continuing the heparin drip to prevent embolic stroke
b. Placing the patient in the Trendelenburg position to raise BP
c. Stopping the heparin drip and administering protamine sulfate
d. Transfusing packed RBCs for a goal hemoglobin of 7

Answer: C. Rationale: In acute UGIB, anticoagulation is held, and a reversal agent administered is indicated. Protamine sulfate reverses unfractionated heparin. Answer A is not correct since the risks of ongoing blood loss out weight the risk of a stroke. The use of the Trendelenburg positioning in hypovolemic shock is no longer recommended. Answer D is not correct since it is recommended to transfuse to a hemoglobin goal of >8.0 g/dL in patients with acute GIB.

REFERENCES

Bala M, Kashuk J, Moore EM, et al. Acute mesenteric ischemia: guidelines of the World Society of Emergency Surgery. *World J Emerg Surg*. 2017;12:38. doi: 10.1186/s13017-017-0150-5.

Choi JY, Jo YW, Lee SS, et al. Outcomes of patients treated with Sengstaken-Blakemore tube for uncontrolled variceal hemorrhage. *Korean J Intern Med*. 2018;33(4):696–704. doi: 10.3904/kjim.2016.339.

Ellison DL Acute diverticulitis management. *Crit Care Nurs Clin North Am*. 2018;30(1):67–74. doi: 10.1016/j.cnc.2017.10.006.

Fehrenbach U, Gul-Klein S, de Sousa Mendes M, et al. Portosystemic shunt surgery in the era of TIPS: imaging-based planning of the surgical approach. *Abdom Radiol (NY)*. 2020;45(9):2726–2735. doi: 10.1007/s00261-020-02599-z.

Gnanapandithan K, Feuerstadt P. Review article: mesenteric ischemia. *Curr Gastroenterol Rep*. 2020;22(4):17. doi: 10.1007/s11894-020-0754-x.

Rajesh S, George T, Philips CA, et al. Transjugular intrahepatic portosystemic shunt in cirrhosis: an exhaustive critical update. *World J Gastroenterol*. 2020;26(37): 5561–5596. doi: 10.3748/wjg.v26.i37.5561.

Rich K. Trendelenburg position in hypovolemic shock: a review. *J Vasc Nurs*. 2019;37(1):71–73. doi: 10.1016/j.jvn.2019.01.002.

Sakai E, Ohata K, Nakajima A, Matsuhashi N. Diagnosis and therapeutic strategies for small bowel vascular lesions. *World J Gastroenterol*. 2019;25(22):2720–2733. doi: 10.3748/wjg.v25.i22.2720.

Stolow E, Moreau C, Sayana H, Patel S. Management of non-variceal upper GI bleeding in the geriatric population: an update. *Curr Gastroenterol Rep*. 2021;23(4):5. doi: 10.1007/s11894-021-00805-6.

Tuncer H, Yardan T, Akdemir HU, Ayyildiz T. Comparison of four scoring systems for risk stratification of upper gastrointestinal bleeding. *Pak J Med Sci*. 2018;34(3):649–654. doi: 10.12669/pjms.343.14956

Wan D, Krisko T. Diverticulosis, diverticulitis, and diverticular bleeding. *Clin Geriatr Med*. 2021;37(1):141–154. doi: 10.1016/j.cger.2020.08.011.

39

Acute and Chronic Hepatic Failure, Cirrhosis, Hepatitis, and Acute Pancreatitis

CHAPTER OVERVIEW AND OBJECTIVES

The content of this chapter addresses the CCRN exam test area that includes hepatic failure, hepatitis, cirrhosis, and acute pancreatitis. Expect two to three questions in this content area.

After studying this chapter, you should be able to:

- Identify the key clinical presentation of acute and chronic hepatic failure, cirrhosis, hepatitis, and acute pancreatitis.
- Appreciate how hepatitis affects the immune system and impacts patient presentation.
- Describe key nursing interventions when clinical compromise arises including implications related to drug metabolism. Liver disease (LD) is responsible for over 700,000 hospitalizations in the United States each year. Over half of these cases are related to ethyl alcohol (EtOH) abuse. Other common etiologies include hepatitis and drug-induced acute liver failure.

39.1 ACUTE AND CHRONIC LIVER FAILURE

Acute Liver Failure Overview

Acute liver failure (ALF) is rare life-threatening emergency affecting patients *without* chronic LD. ALF affects approximately 2000 to 2500 people per year in the United States (Thomas and Lewis, 2018). Major causes of ALF are included in **Table 39-1**. ALF results from hepatocyte necrosis or programmed cell death (apoptosis). It is categorized according to symptom development from the time of onset. Hyperacute LF occurs within 7 days. ALF occurs within 1 to 4 weeks. Subacute LF develops within 5 to 12 weeks. In the United States, 50% of ALF cases are drug-induced (DI-ALF) (**Table 39-2**). (Thomas and Lewis, 2018). In developing countries, there is a higher incidence of ALF due to hepatitis B and E (Montrief et al, 2019). ALF is diagnosed when a patient without a history of LD meets the following American Association for the Study of Liver Diseases' (AASLD) criteria: neurologic dysfunction due to any degree of hepatic encephalopathy (HE), an international normalized ratio (INR) $\geq$1.5, and a disease process lasting $\leq$26 weeks (Montrief et al, 2019).

Acute-on-Chronic Liver Failure

Acute-on-chronic liver failure (ACLF) is the acute decompensation of a patient with chronic liver failure (CLF) due to a precipitating event, such as hepatitis (viral, drug-induced, alcohol-related), surgery, ischemia, or infection (Bajaja et al, 2022). ACLF may be irreversible. It has a poor prognosis and a high mortality rate. Scoring systems such as the EASL-CLIF and NACSELD score evaluate the likelihood of sequential organ failure, 28-day prognosis, and futility of medical treatment, respectively.

Pathophysiology

During liver failure, albumin production decreases, which can lead to ascites and pedal edema. Compounding the complex physiology

TABLE 39-1. COMMON CAUSES OF ACUTE LIVER FAILURE IN THE UNITED STATES		
Drug-induced (50%)	Heart or respiratory failure	Metabolic (Wilson disease)
Viral hepatitis	Shock states (sepsis)	Acute venous or arterial thrombosis in hepatic vessels
Idiopathic Ethyl alcohol	Neoplasm	Pregnancy-induced

is the production of potentially toxic metabolic byproducts including, ammonia ($NH_{3)}$. Increased levels of NH_3 contribute to mental status changes and could be indicative of HE. Patients with ALF may not be able to synthesize vitamin K–dependent clotting factors causing a high INR. However, most patients require venous thromboembolism (VTE) prophylaxis due to coagulation changes that predispose them to clot formation.

Etiology

- Vascular causes of ALF include portal vein thrombosis, hepatic vein thrombosis (Budd–Chiari syndrome), veno-occulsive disease, and ischemic hepatitis.
- Metabolic causes include Wilson disease, acute fatty liver of pregnancy, and Reye syndrome.

Establishing the underlying cause of ALF is important since it will direct the treatment and determine the prognosis.

ACLF Clinical Presentation

Decompensated cirrhosis presents with ascites, GIB, HE, and potentially hepatorenal syndrome (HRS). HE is associated with elevated NH_3 levels that lead to increased glutamine within the astrocyte cells of the brain. Glutamine increases the osmolality within the astrocytes causing fluid absorption leading to both astrocyte and cerebral edema with mental status changes can range from subtle to severe.

> **QUICK TIP!** Expect a question on the exam related to the identification of HE in relationship to elevated blood levels of ammonia ($NH_{3)}$. Normal ammonia levels are usually <45 μg/dL (reference ranges may vary per institution).

TABLE 39-2. COMMON ETIOLOGIES OF DRUG-INDUCED LIVER FAILURE	
Analgesics	Acetaminophen and combination medications that contain narcotics and acetaminophen
Anesthetics	Enflurane, isoflurane, halothane
Antiarrhythmics	Amiodarone
Antituberculosis drugs	Isoniazid, rifampin, ethambutol, pyrazinamide
Antiepileptics	Carbamazepine, phenytoin, valproic acid
Nonsteroidal anti-inflammatory drugs (NSAIDs)	Diclofenac, etodolac, sulindac, ibuprofen, indomethacin, meloxicam, nabumetone, naproxen

Diagnosis

ACLF is diagnosed when a patient with CLD develops altered mental status, and abnormal liver function tests (See **Table 39-3**) such as hyperammonemia, alanine aminotransferase (ALT), aspartate aminotransferase (AST), alkaline phosphatase, albumin, with or without coagulopathy.

Key considerations related to associated lab values:

- There are two types of bilirubin that may be elevated in LD: unconjugated and conjugated.
  - Unconjugated (indirect) bilirubin is bound to albumin in the bloodstream.
  - Conjugated (direct) bilirubin has been processed by the liver. The majority of it travels to the small intestine and a small amount to the kidneys for excretion.
- Check hepatitis serologies to exclude a viral etiology.
- Decreasing hemoglobin and hematocrit may signal gastrointestinal (GI) bleeding.
- White blood cell (WBC) counts are generally low in patients with ACLF. A normal WBC may be a clue to the presence of infection or sepsis.
- *ALF and ACLF patients may develop hyperglycemia or hypoglycemia. Most patients with CLF are insulin resistant, and approximately 30% are diabetic. They may require insulin infusions to maintain euglycemia. Hypoglycemia can occur in patients who have lost the ability to produce glucose from amino acids (gluconeogenesis) and/or breakdown glucose stores (glycogenolysis).*

> **QUICK TIP!** Jaundice is a yellowish discoloration of the skin and/sclera associated with impaired bilirubin excretion occurring when total serum bilirubin levels (direct and indirect) are more than 3.0 mg/dL. In patients with darker skin tones, the development of jaundice may be initially seen as yellow (icteric) sclera.

A computed tomography (CT) scan of the brain is indicated in patients with overt HE. This will rule out other clinical findings that may be the cause of the mental status changes (such as a subdural hematoma from trauma) and may demonstrate cerebral edema (**Table 39-4**).

Treatment

The initial goals of treatment in ALF are restoring hemodynamic stability, correcting fluid and electrolyte imbalances, and addressing the underlying cause.

- Shock or hypovolemia: administration of isotonic fluids replete intravascular (IV) volume and may improve hepatic perfusion. *Avoid using hypotonic solutions since they may precipitate hyponatremia and cerebral edema.*
- Protein Supplementation: Many ALF patients are catabolic and require patients to be given 1.2 to 1.5 g of protein per kilogram per day.
- Plasma exchange improves survival in ALF patients, however, its effects on those with ACLF is unknown (Bajaj et al, 2022; Tan et al, 2020).
- Extracorporeal liver assist devices are available at some quaternary care institutions. Currently, there is no survival benefit in using this technology based on randomized clinical trial (RCT) data.

TABLE 39-3. LIVER FUNCTION TESTS

Test	Normal Range	Causes of Increased Levels
Transaminases: (ALT and AST) Enzymes located in the liver	ALT Male: 10–55 international unit/L Female: 7–30 international unit/L AST Male: 10–40 international unit/L Female: 9–32 international unit/L	Acute or chronic liver diseases, or injuries caused by medications, ethanol, hepatitis, trauma, or biliary obstruction
Gamma-glutamyl transferase (GGT) More concentrated in the liver, but can also be found in bone, intestines, and placenta.	Male: 8–61 international unit/L Female: 5–36 international unit/L	Cholestasis Intrahepatic disease processes Parenteral nutrition
Alkaline phosphatase Located in bone, intestines, liver, and placenta	Male: 45–115 international unit/L Female: 30–100 international unit/L	Cholestasis Liver disease Bone disease Parenteral nutrition
Indirect (unconjugated) bilirubin Byproduct of hemoglobin metabolism. NOT water-soluble	0.0–0.6 mg/dL	Red blood cell (RBC) hemolysis Decreased bone marrow production of RBCs (anemia)
Direct (conjugated) bilirubin Unconjugated bilirubin binds with glucuronide in the liver to form water-soluble bilirubin that is excreted in bile	0.0–0.4 mg/dL	Bile duct obstruction (acute pancreatitis; choledocholithiasis) Cirrhosis Cholangitis Gilbert disease Hepatic disease Hepatic injury Medications Sepsis
Total bilirubin Consists of unconjugated and conjugated bilirubin	0.0–1.0 mg/dL	
Albumin 3.3–5.0 g/dL Prothrombin time (PT): 11.0–13.7 s		

Patients with ALF are susceptible to a wide variety of complications in addition to encephalopathy. These include cerebral edema, renal failure, hypoglycemia, metabolic acidosis, sepsis, coagulopathy, and multiorgan failure. All patients with FHF should be managed in an intensive care unit at a facility capable of performing liver transplantation.

Nursing Intervention

- Frequent assessment of the patient's neurologic status provides an index of response to therapy.
- Administer medications as ordered, avoiding sedatives and hepatotoxic drugs.
- Monitor intake and output, fluid status, and electrolyte status. Signs of anemia, infection, alkalosis, melena, or hematemesis should be reported to the physician to provide an opportunity to prevent complications.
- Monitor glucose levels with bedside glucose measurements, as acute hypoglycemia can occur.
- Monitor respiratory status closely, especially during times of decreasing mental status.
- Maintain a patent airway and administer oxygen as needed. Patients with advanced encephalopathy who may not be able to protect their airway may need intubation.
- Monitor all side effects of medications and decrease dosages as needed. Some 80% of patients will respond to lactulose therapy with improved mental status. Continuous

TABLE 39-4. LABORATORY TESTS FOR CIRRHOSIS

Decreased Levels	Increased Levels
WBC Hemoglobin Hematocrit Albumin Serum sodium Serum potassium Serum chloride Serum magnesium Folic acid	Globulin Total bilirubin Alkaline phosphatase Transaminase Lactate dehydrogenase Urine bilirubin Fecal urobilinogen Urine urobilinogen Prothrombin time International normalized ratio

administration of lactulose in patients with recurrent or subclinical encephalopathy is recommended.

- Preventing infection and monitoring for signs of infection are essential in the care of patients with liver failure. Meticulously following bundles for preventing central venous line associate blood stream infections (CLABSI).
- Prophylactic use of antibiotics is not recommended. Antibiotics may be considered if there is rapid progression of encephalopathy, refractory hypotension, and the presence of systemic inflammatory response syndrome (SIRS).

Emotional support of the patient and family with realistic reports of the patient's condition is appropriate and essential, since the expected outcome is poor. Honest and open discussion of the end of life should take place.

39.2 CHRONIC LIVER FAILURE

CLF can result from a variety of etiologies. Some of the more common causes are alcohol, cirrhosis, and hepatitis.

Alcohol-Induced Liver Failure

EtOH damages hepatocytes both acutely and chronically. Long-term heavy alcohol intake permanently changes the structure of the hepatocytes by allowing fat to replace healthy tissue. If cessation occurs, the damage is potentially reversible. Overtime, hepatocytes and fat cells (lipocytes) are replaced with fibrous (scar) tissue. Liver damage occurs more quickly in patients with concomitant hepatitis B or C. Acute alcoholic hepatitis due to heavy EtOH ingestion can present with symptoms such as right upper quadrant tenderness, fever, and/or jaundice which can occur with biliary tree disorders such as cholecystitis, cholelithiasis, or choledocholithiasis. Leukocytosis and severely elevated bilirubin levels are common.

Cirrhosis

Cirrhosis occurs from many types of diseases that affect the liver. Diffuse hepatic fibrosis alters the normal structure and function of the liver. As the liver tissue becomes more fibrotic, blood flow through the portal vein diminishes and can lead to portal hypertension and varices. Depending on the cause and severity, the disease progresses over weeks to years toward end-stage liver disease (ESLD). *ESLD manifestations often include HE, ascites, immune system compromise, and coagulation deficits due to decreased production of vitamin K–dependent clotting factors.*

Cirrhosis is divided into two major categories based on nodule size: micronodular and macronodular. Different disorders can cause either micro or macronodular disease. Cirrhosis usually results in increased resistance to blood flow through the liver and failure of the hepatic cells to function properly.

Micronodular cirrhosis is the most common type with alcoholism being the most common cause; however, for unexplained reasons, only a minority of alcoholics develop cirrhosis. Cirrhosis is very unusual with less than 5 years of alcohol abuse, demonstrating that chronic injury is usually necessary for cirrhosis to develop. Alcohol itself injures liver cells directly, but other factors influence the development of cirrhosis. Micronodular cirrhosis is also seen with cholestatic causes of cirrhosis and obstruction of hepatic venous outflow.

Macronodular cirrhosis results from a variety of causes. Chronic viral hepatitis is the most common cause of this type of cirrhosis worldwide. Other causes include other types of infection, biliary cirrhosis, iron or copper overload, autoimmune diseases, and idiopathic or cryptogenic cirrhosis. All types of cirrhosis generally produce a firm, shrunken liver, although at times the liver can be enlarged. Fibrosis, or scarring, is prominent. The scarring causes resistance to normal blood flow through the liver. Loss of hepatocytes can result in hepatic failure. Splenomegaly may occur.

Etiology

- Hepatitis
- Alcohol abuse
- Autoimmune disorders
- Nonalcoholic fatty liver disease (NAFLD)
- Hepatitis
- Inherited disorders: alpha 1-antitrypsin deficiency, cystic fibrosis, glycogen storage disorders, Wilson disease (copper accumulation), hemochromatosis (iron accumulation)
- Bile duct obstruction (primary biliary cirrhosis)
- Budd–Chiari syndrome: obstruction of blood flow out of the liver
- Right heart failure (HF)
- Medications including **amiodarone, antibiotics, and statins**, among many others

Clinical Presentation

Early symptoms of cirrhosis include fatigue, pruritus, and right upper quadrant pain may occur early on. Anorexia is commonly seen with disease progression.

As liver failure progresses, the patient's physical examination findings change dramatically to include the following:

- Dry eyes.
- Dry mouth.
- Skin hyperpigmentation may develop.
- Other stigmata of LD include hepatomegaly, splenomegaly, muscle wasting (advanced disease), spider veins, and palmar erythema.
- Third-spacing of fluid leads to ascites and peripheral edema.
- Jaundice generally occurs when bilirubin levels are >3 mg/dL. Bilirubin accumulation causes yellow skin discoloration. In patients with darker skin tones, the development of jaundice may be initially seen as yellow (icteric) sclera.
- Endocrine changes such as gynecomastia and testicular atrophy resulting from reduced testosterone levels are often seen in those with male reproductive organs, and menstrual irregularities are seen in those with the capacity to become pregnant. Axillary and pubic hair loss may occur, regardless of sex.

Other findings include a decreased or abnormal mentation, termed *hepatic encephalopathy* (HE). This is often seen with an increased serum NH_3 level and/or accumulation of toxins that would normally be filtered by the liver. Clinical exam findings may include, *asterixis* (an abnormal flapping of the hands), a hyperkinetic circulation, cyanosis, fetor hepaticus (musty, sweet breath odor), renal failure, and easy bruising, in addition anemia, thrombocytopenia, and leukopenia (low WBC count) (**Fig. 39-1**).

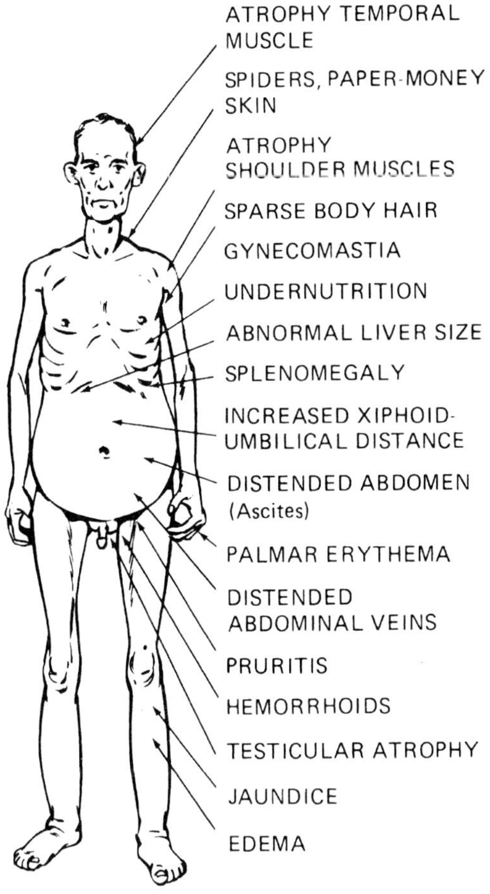

Figure 39-1. Signs of advanced cirrhosis.

Diagnosis

Abnormalities in the patient's physical examination and laboratory data (Table 39-4) suggest the diagnosis.

Laboratory:

- Patients may have anemia due to anemia of chronic disease, low levels of folate, splenic enlargement, or hemolysis.
- Abnormal liver functions tests, including elevated alkaline phosphatase, gamma-glutamyl transpeptidase (GGPT).
- Transaminitis: elevated aminotransferases (ALT and AST).
- Elevated cholesterol levels.
- Increased erythrocyte sedimentation rate (ESR).
- Thrombocytopenia due to splenic enlargement (hypersplenism).

Diagnostics:

- Ultrasonography (US) is routinely used during the evaluation of the cirrhotic patient, as well as a screening test for hepatocellular carcinoma (HCC) and portal hypertension.
- A liver biopsy may be necessary to confirm the presence and cause of cirrhosis.
- Cirrhosis prognosis and treatment depend on its etiology.

Treatment

At present, advanced cirrhosis is irreversible.

- Treatment is aimed at decreasing any further liver damage, through the cessation of alcohol use, symptom management, preventing complications, and evaluation for and timing of liver transplantation.

TABLE 39-5. CHILDS–PUGH CLASSIFICATION OF SEVERITY OF LIVER DISEASE

Parameter	*Points Assigned*		
	1	2	3
Ascites	Absent	Mild	Moderate
Bilirubin (mg/dL)	<2	2–3	>3
Albumin (g/dL)	>3.5	2.8–3.5	<2.8
Prothrombin time Seconds over control	1–3	4–6	>6
INR	<1.7	1.8–2.3	>2.3
Encephalopathy	None	Grade 1–2	Grade 3–4
Total score/grade	5–6/grade A	7–9/grade B	10–15/grade C
	Grade A	Grade B	Grade C
1–2-year survival	100/85%	80/60%	45/35%

- Non-selective beta-blockers, such as **propranolol (Inderal)**, are used to prevent variceal bleeding in cirrhotic patients with portal hypertension.
- Management of ascites consists of a low-sodium diet, **spironolactone, diuretics,** and paracentesis for ascites.
- **Vitamin K therapy** may be used for the treatment of coagulation abnormalities associated with decreased hepatic synthesis of vitamin K–dependent clotting factors (INR >1.5).
- Prevention of hepatitis B by immunizing high-risk populations is one of the most important ways to decrease the prevalence of cirrhosis worldwide.

Orthotopic liver transplantation, although costly and involving lifelong intense medical care, is the only long-term treatment option for those with irreversible liver failure. Although the 5-year-survival rate is approximately 70%, the demand for donor livers is greater than the supply. As a result, death may occur while awaiting transplantation. Survival in patients with cirrhosis is improving. The predicting prognosis is difficult due to the multiple variables involved. There are models used to help predict survival. One helpful method of classification is the Childs–Pugh system (**Table 39-5**). A newer method, the Model for End-Stage Liver Disease (MELD) was updated in 2016. It uses the patient's values for serum sodium, bilirubin, creatinine, and INR in combination with the need for hemodialysis at least twice in the past week to predict survival (**Table 39-6**).

TABLE 39-6. MELD

Three-Month Mortality in Hospitalized Patients	
MELD Score	*Mortality (%)*
≥40	100
30–39	83
20–29	76
10–19	27
<10	4

KEY CLINICAL CONCEPT

Orthotopic liver transplantation is the only long-term treatment option for those with irreversible liver failure.

39.3 COMPLICATIONS OF LIVER FAILURE

Ascites

Ascites is common in advanced LD. The 1-year mortality rate for patients with recurrent ascites is 50%. Ascites is a consequence of portal hypertension, hypoalbuminemia, and elevated volumes of lymphatic fluid within the liver. Low albumin levels decrease plasma oncotic pressure, allowing for the third-spacing of fluid into the peritoneal cavity. When lymphatic ducts, such as the thoracic duct or cisterna chyli, are not able to effectively drain lymph fluid, it can enter the peritoneal space. *Physiologic stressors induce the renin–angiotensin–aldosterone (RAAS) system, resulting in fluid and sodium retention.* Mesenteric venous thrombosis (MVT) can worsen ascites due to decreased venous blood return to the right heart. On exam, ascites may manifest as a tense, distended abdomen with or without an "abdominal fluid wave."

Severe ascites leads to intra-abdominal hypertension (IAH), decreasing venous blood return to the heart, and inducing hypotension. Ultrasound-guided paracentesis is indicated for the relief of tense ascites. Volume expansion with IV albumin is recommended to prevent subsequent IV fluid volume depletion and hypotension. Post-paracentesis, patients may have continuous leakage of ascitic fluid from the puncture site.

Spontaneous Bacterial Peritonitis

The diseased liver is unable to produce sufficient quantities of antibodies (immunoglobulin). Immunoglobulin (Ig) is released by plasma cells (B-lymphocytes) as part of the humoral immune system response to infections. Without adequate Ig levels, the body's ability to respond to infections is decreased. This immunosuppression places patients with LD at risk for developing spontaneous bacterial peritonitis (SBP). The suspected etiology of SBP is bacterial translocation from the intestines to the peritoneal cavity. SBP occurs in up to 26% of patients hospitalized with decompensated liver failure. The mortality rate for SBP ranges from 20% to 30% without prompt identification and adequate treatment.

Patients with SBP often present with fever, altered levels of consciousness, and worsening abdominal pain. Increased ascites, fatigue, and myalgia may occur. Paracentesis is performed. The presence of bacteria in the peritoneal fluid on gram stain is diagnostic. Empiric IV antibiotic therapy should cover gram negative and anaerobic bacteria, which are found in the GI tract. Antibiotics are deescalated based on culture and sensitivity results.

Hepatic Encephalopathy

HE is a complication of cirrhosis that results in over 100,000 hospital admissions in the United States per year. The 1-year risk of mortality in patients with HE is roughly 50%. Its course fluctuates between stable and acute exacerbations that lead to hospitalization. There are multiple factors associated with the development and progression of HE, including systemic inflammation, oxidative stress, genetic factors, and the bacterial flora of the gut.

TABLE 39-7. Conn's (Westhaven) Score for Hepatic Encephalopathy

Grade	*Symptoms*
0	Lack of detectable changes in personality or behavior
1	Short attention span. Mood changes such as euphoria, depression, or irritability
2	Lethargic, apathetic, disoriented, personality changes. May be intermittently disoriented or display inappropriate behaviors. Asterixis may be present.
3	Somnolent, but arousable. Disoriented to place or time. May have angry outbursts
4	Comatose; may or may not respond to noxious stimuli

Ammonia (NH_3) is produced by bacterial flora in the gut by bacterial degradation of amines, amino acids, purines, and urea which is normally detoxified by the liver. NH_3 levels are elevated in liver failure due to nonfunctioning hepatocytes. Congenital or surgically creating portosystemic shunts patients without cirrhosis increase NH_3 levels since they bypass the hepatic circulation NH_3 is a neurotoxin that can cause edema within brain astrocytes. Suspect cerebral edema in patients with mental status change and/or nausea and vomiting. These patients require immediate treatment with medications that decrease serum NH_3 levels (e.g., **lactulose**). Patients with grade 3–4 HE should be intubated for airway protection. *Patients with or at high risk for cerebral edema may require intracranial pressure (ICP) monitoring and administration of hypertonic saline or osmotic diuretics* (**Table 39-7**).

KEY CLINICAL CONCEPT

Patients with grade 3–4 HE require intubation for airway protection and prevention of aspiration.

Malnutrition

Malnutrition affects 20% to 50% of patients with cirrhosis. As it progresses, the body uses fat instead of glucose for energy. Glucogenesis decreases and less protein is produced. The breakdown of protein (proteolysis) and fat reduce muscle mass (sarcopenia) and body fat. Malnourished patients have a poorer prognosis and are at risk for complications such as ascites, HE, and infection. In addition to nutritional screening tools and dietitian consultation, the European Society of Parenteral and Enteral Nutrition (ESPEN) guidelines for malnutrition recommend daily protein intake of 1.2 to 1.5 g/kg of body weight (Bischoff et al, 2020). This prevents protein breakdown and helps synthesize new proteins. Research has shown that normal to high protein intake does not worsen HE. Contrary to previously held beliefs, this level of protein intake may improve mental status in those with HE. Cirrhotic patients should eat three to five meals per day and a bedtime snack to improve protein reserves.

KEY CLINICAL CONCEPT

Research has shown that normal to high protein intake benefits cirrhotic patients. Current guidelines support administering 1.2 to 1.5 g of protein/kg/day in patients with ALF.

TABLE 39-8. PRECIPITATING FACTORS FOR DECOMPENSATED HEPATIC ENCEPHALOPATHY

Intravascular Volume Depletion	*GI Disturbances*	*Electrolyte and Acid–Base Abnormalities*	*Other*
Diuretics	Constipation	Hyponatremia	Infection
Vomiting	Diarrhea	Hypokalemia	Benzodiazepines
Diarrhea	GI bleeding	Hyperkalemia Alkalosis	Increased protein loads: GI bleeding or increased protein intake

Treatment

Reducing serum NH_3 levels improves symptoms but doesn't affect survival. **Lactulose** is a standard treatment for HE. It is a nonabsorbable disaccharide which aids in the conversion of NH_3 into NH_4, which is unable to be absorbed by the gut, thereby lowering serum NH_3 levels. Rifaximin (Xifaxan) is a broad-spectrum antibiotic with poor oral absorption, which can be used by itself of in conjunction with lactulose reduce blood NH_3 levels. For patients on antimicrobial therapy, monitor for the development of *Clostridium difficile*–associated diarrhea (**Table 39-8**).

Coagulation Issues

In CLF, the liver is unable to synthesize certain proteins such as albumin or vitamin K–dependent clotting factors (II, VII, IX, X). There is an increased occurrence of fibrinolysis (fibrin clot breakdown). In theory, this puts ESLD patients at risk for excessive bleeding. New research is dispelling this age-old notion by demonstrating imbalances in both anticoagulation and procoagulation factors. Interestingly, ESLD is associated with low levels of natural anticoagulants protein C and antithrombin, which can lead to clot formation. Other studies have demonstrated increased levels of the procoagulants, Factor VIII and von Willebrand factor, as well as thrombin production. Thrombocytopenia (platelet count <100,000) is common in patients with cirrhosis and other advanced LDs, as a result of portal hypertension and hypersplenism. Platelets not only aggregate to form clots, but they also promote thrombin (factor II) generation, leading to blood clotting. The increase in certain procoagulants may not only lessen the bleeding risks associated with ESLD but may also lead to thrombus formation.

Hepatorenal Syndrome

HRS is a severe complication or ALF or CLF. Neurohormones and cytokines systemically vasodilate and decrease renal perfusion pressure. Compensatory mechanisms such as the sympathetic nervous system (SNS), RAAS system, and vasopressin release produce renal vasoconstriction. The associated acute kidney injury (AKI) results from vasoconstriction and hypoperfusion and is not associated with proteinuria or evidence of structural kidney disease. Common precipitating factors include hepatitis (viral, alcoholic, etc), hypotension, infection, *intra-abdominal hypertension (IAP >12 mm Hg)*, and large volume paracentesis (4–5 L), and SBP.

HRS is characterized by oliguria, a very low rate of sodium excretion, and a progressive rise in serum creatinine. There is no specific test to diagnose HRS. The diagnosis is based on clinical presentation. The renal dysfunction does not respond to the withdrawal of diuretics or reverse with administration of 1 g/kg of 25% albumin IV over 2 days (Simonetto et al, 2020).

Early treatment of the underlying cause and preventing complications may improve outcomes. Maintain adequate systemic blood pressure with vasopressors such as **norepinephrine**. Identify and treat infections. Avoid nephrotoxic medications. Patients may require renal replacement therapy. Although a small percentage of patients recover with medical management, HRS carries a poor prognosis; however, it does reverse over time after successful liver transplantation.

Surgical Issues Related to Liver Disease

Patients with LD are at high risk for surgery and anesthesia-related complications due to altered drug metabolism, the potential for coagulopathy, and poor tissue perfusion. The risk is highest during emergent procedures. During the first 30 minutes after induction, general anesthesia is associated with a 35% decrease in hepatic blood flow. Some inhaled anesthetics lower hepatic artery blood flow. Elevations in CO_2 lead to SNS activation, which lowers portal venous blood flow. Neuromuscular blocking agents with short half-lives that are not metabolized by the liver, such as cisatracurium (Nimbex), are preferred. **Fentanyl** is frequently ordered for postoperative pain relief due to its shorter half-life and decreased risk of hypotension.

Nursing Interventions

Safety

- Monitor the neurologic status for behavior changes, increasing lethargy, and neuromuscular dysfunction such as *asterixis*.
- Provide a safe environment (three side rails up, bed in low position, low lighting) for patients who are not completely lucid.
- Avoid pharmacologic sedation despite restlessness and irritable states because of decreased drug clearance. Use verbal reassurance and family involvement.
- Serum NH_3 levels do not correlate to the degree of encephalopathy in most patients, but in individual patient's, the levels can be trended to gauge their response to treatment.
- **Lactulose,** a poorly absorbed sugar, prevents intestinal reabsorption of NH_3.
- Rifaximin (Xifaxan) is a broad-spectrum antibiotic with poor oral absorption, which can be used by itself of in conjunction with **lactulose** reduce blood NH_3 levels.
- Nutritional intervention is mandatory since poor nutrition is influential in the development and progression of cirrhosis. Percutaneous endoscopic gastrostomy (PEG) tubes are not placed in cirrhotic patients due to the potential for injury and bleeding from enlarged veins on the abdominal wall (caput medusae).

- Tube feedings or parenteral nutrition (PN) may be necessary. In non-obese patients, recommended daily caloric intake is 35 cal/kg. Vitamin supplements are usually necessary due to micronutrient depletion.
- In patients elevated INR or clinical bleeding, check the skin, gums, emesis, and stools for bleeding and apply pressure to bleeding sites. Notify a provider of the development of bleeding dyscrasias or an increase in bleeding. Minimize bleeding risk by educating the patient on avoiding the use of harsh toothbrushes, forceful nose blowing, and bodily injury.
- Monitor fluid retention by weighing the patient daily. Check for dependent edema and maintain accurate intake and output records. *Fluid and sodium restrictions may be necessary.* Administer diuretics as ordered. Monitor for the development of intravascular dehydration and hypovolemic shock.
- **Spironolactone (Aldactone)** is frequently referred to as a potassium-sparing diuretic. It is an *aldosterone antagonist,* which prevents aldosterone release and subsequent sodium and water retention, and *decreases urinary potassium excretion. Monitor for hyperkalemia.*
- Paracentesis may be indicated in the patient with marked ascites refractory to medical therapy. If paracentesis is performed, note the amount of fluid removed, make sure that a specimen is sent for appropriate laboratory and microbiology tests. Fluid shifts can cause hypotension and hemodynamic instability. Closely monitor the patient for signs of shock. If the patient does not have an indwelling bladder catheter, encourage voiding prior to undergoing paracentesis to prevent bladder injury.
- Monitor respiratory status for signs of ineffective breathing patterns. Pressure on the diaphragm due to ascites causes reduced lung volumes, and hypoxemia may occur. Semi-Fowler's or High-Fowler's positions may be necessary. Auscultate lung sounds and turn the patient every 2 hours; also, have the patient breathe deeply and change his or her position at the same intervals. Monitor include arterial blood gases (ABGs), as indicated.
- Skin breakdown may result from edema and pruritus. Bathe the patient with moisturizing lotion, not soap. Turn the patient regularly (at least every 2 hours), elevate heels, and ensure rest to prevent fatigue.
- Educate the patient and family on the importance of proper diet, avoiding alcohol, moderate exercise, and avoidance of any drugs (including over-the-counter medications), especially **aspirin** and **acetaminophen,** unless a provider approves their use.

KEY CLINICAL CONCEPT

- Measuring and trending NH_3 levels are key to identifying and trending response to treatment for hepatic failure. Ammonia is a toxin normally processed and eliminated by the liver.
- Asterixis is flappy tremoring and jerking movements of outstretched hands. NH_3 interferes with neurotransmitter function in the nervous system.

QUICK TIP! Nutritional questions are rare on the CCRN (perhaps only 1 question at most).

39.4 HEPATITIS

Viral hepatitis is an inflammatory insult to the liver hepatocytes. Scar tissues results and surrounds the injured areas, leading to irreversible fibrosis. Over time, the accumulation of fibrotic tissue leads to liver cirrhosis. The four major types of hepatitis are A, B, C, and D.

Hepatitis A

Hepatitis A virus (HAV) is an RNA picornavirus that is a common cause of acute hepatitis world-wide. It is primarily spread through the fecal-oral (contamination of water or produce) route and close contact with infected persons. Those who use illicit intravenous drugs or are men who have sex with men (MSM) are at risk for contracting HAV. It is endemic in many developing countries. Hand hygiene, washing fruit and vegetables prevent HAV transmission. HAV vaccination and drinking bottled water are recommended for those traveling to endemic regions.

Hepatitis A's presentation varies from asymptomatic to fulminant hepatitis. It is mild and has an excellent prognosis in most cases. Common symptoms include fatigue, fever, nausea, vomiting, anorexia, right upper quadrant discomfort or pain. Jaundice, pruritus, and clay-colored stools can occur in more severe cases. HAV elicits both IgM and IgG antibody responses. HAV is diagnosed by serologic testing. It is diagnosed by the presence of HAV-specific IgM antibiotics. The IgM antibodies indicate HAV infection within the last 6 months. IgG is produced later and may remain in an infected person for life (Abutaleb and Kottilil, 2020).

Patients with acute hepatitis A should be placed on universal precautions. Treatment is supportive since the disease is self-limiting in most individuals.

HAV vaccines have decreased the occurrence of hepatis A. It is also used for post-exposure prophylaxis. HAV vaccination is recommended for patients with CLD due to their risk of increased morbidity and mortality if they develop acute hepatitis A. IV HAV IgG may be indicated for close personal contacts of an infected person and those exposed to the food and water in an identified epidemic.

QUICK TIP! There is often at least one question on the exam focused on the differences between IgM and IgG—more information can be found in the immunology chapter.

Hepatitis B

Hepatitis B is a global health problem. In the United States approximately 60,000 people are diagnosed with hepatitis B. It transmitted by blood, saliva, semen, and vaginal secretions. Maternal-fetal transmission can also occur. The hepatitis B virus (HBV) can survive outside the human body for a prolonged period, allowing it to spread via contaminated household articles such as toothbrushes and utensils. Risk factors for HBV include working in health care immunosuppression, and living in areas where HBV is endemic. Those with high-risk behaviors such as illicit intravenous drug use, MSM, multiple sexual partners are more likely to become infected.

HBV is a small DNA virus consisting of a protein coat (known as the surface antigen [HBsAg]), the e antigen (HBeAg), the core antigen (HBcAg), and the DNA polymerase. Each of these can be detected either in the liver itself or the circulating blood, and various antigens and antibodies have clinical relevance. HBsAg in the blood indicates either an acute or chronic continuing infection. The presence of the surface antibody (HBsAb) indicates prior HBV vaccination or chronic infection. Those who test positive for HBeAg are synthesizing the virus and are highly infectious. E antibody (HBeAb) persists for a few months after the acute infection resolves. IgM HBcAb indicates either acute or chronic infection, and IgG HBcAb is usually a marker for a previous, nonactive infection.

The incubation period for HBV infection is generally 6 to 9 weeks. A person is usually infectious 1 to 2 weeks before symptoms appear. The clinical course can vary between asymptomatic to mild. Initial symptoms and lab tests are similar to those of HAV. Patients with acute hepatitis B infections may present with or without scleral icterus. The most severe cases can result in FHF and/or death. Patients who survive are at risk of developing chronic HBV. Chronic HBV can lead to cirrhosis, portal hypertension, FHF, and HCC. Over two-thirds of those with chronic HBV are asymptomatic carriers. Immunocompromised individuals are more likely to develop chronic HBV. Alcohol use in the presence of HBV has been associated with worsening LD and an increased risk of HCC.

Therapy for acute HBV is supportive. Currently there is no cure for HBV; however, INF and antivirals such as entecavir (Baraclude) and tenofovir (Vemlidy) decrease viral replication and prevent cirrhosis (Almeida et al, 2021). Research toward a cure is ongoing, Prevention focuses on vaccination and avoiding high-risk behaviors. Those exposed to HBV should undergo screening. Hepatitis B immune globulin (HBIG) and the HBV vaccine are administered to patients who are positive for HBsAg- and negative for HBsAb. For full immunity, the HBV vaccine requires doses is 1 and 6 months after the initial administration. If the HBsAb is positive, the person exposed is already immune, and neither HBIG nor the vaccine need be given. If the HBsAg is positive, the individual is already infected and should be evaluated for acute or chronic hepatitis. Follow standard precautions to prevent exposure to blood and body fluid precautions infected individuals.

Hepatitis D

Hepatitis D virus (HDV) is an RNA virus that only infects patients with preexisting HBV infection. Acute HDV infection increased this risk of ALF. It doubles the risk of developing decompensated cirrhosis and triples the risk of HCC.

At present, there is no vaccine for HDV. HBV immunization prevents the development of hepatitis B and subsequently hepatitis D. Although newer drugs have been approved for use in Europe, PEG interferon alpha (IFN-α) is only approved treatment in the United States (Almeida et al, 2021). It tends to be poorly tolerated and is contraindicated in those with certain psychiatric disorders, autoimmune diseases, and cirrhosis (Almeida et al, 2021).

Hepatitis C

Approximately 3.7 million people in the United States are infected with the hepatitis C virus (HCV). HCV, an RNA virus, is a common reason for liver transplant and is a leading cause of death from LF. HCV risk factors include intravenous drug use, chronic, long-term hemodialysis, health-care workers with needle stick or mucosal exposure to HCV-positive blood, MSM, people with multiple sexual partners and/or HIV. Perinatal transmission accounts for 0% to 4% of cases. Lastly, patients who received blood or blood products before 1992, when HCV screening tests became widely available. Currently, there is no vaccine against HCV. Prevention focuses on avoiding high-risk behaviors and using standard precautions when exposed to the risk of blood or body fluid exposure.

HCV has an incubation period of approximately 7 weeks. Many of people with HCV are asymptomatic and unaware they have the disease. The clinical manifestations are the same as for a mild case of HBV such as malaise, nausea, and RUQ pain. It can later cause jaundice and dark urine. Without treatment, HCV may lead to liver fibrosis or cirrhosis, fibrosis, portal hypertension, esophageal varices, and HCC. Unfortunately for those exposed to HVC, immune globulin is not effective as postexposure prophylaxis.

HCV is diagnosed when antibodies to HCV are detected on blood testing. If the antibody test is positive, a reflex PCR test is performed to confirm the diagnosis. Newer medications called direct-acting antivirals (DAAs) such as glecaprevir/pibrentasvir (Mavyret) and sofosbuvir/velpatasvir (Epclusa) have HCV cure rates >90%. There are a number of other regimens may be prescribed based on HCV genotype. These drugs are taken by mouth over a period of 8 to 12 weeks and are well-tolerated. Treatment failures are associated with medication nonadherence and drug resistance. Success of treatment is determined largely by the achievement of a sustained virologic response (SVR), defined as undetectable HCV RNA level in the blood at the end of the treatment period and at 6 months after treatment ends. Patients with decompensated cirrhosis should be referred for consideration of liver transplantation.

Hepatitis E

Hepatitis E virus (HEV) is a single-stranded RNA virus that causes a self-limited, acute viral hepatitis. Transmission occurs via the oral-fecal route. Contaminated water sources have been associated with large outbreaks. The clinical features of acute HEV are similar to those of HAV. ALF is more likely in pregnant patients and those with preexisting LD. Diagnosis is based on detection of HEV in serum or feces by PCR or by the detection of IgM antibodies to HEV. Treatment is largely supportive. Ribavirin is used in immunocompromised patients with acute HEV (Almeida et al, 2021). HEV vaccines are being developed.

Nursing Interventions

Nursing priorities are aimed at reducing demands on the liver while promoting patient well-being, minimizing disturbance in self-concept due to communicability of disease, relieving symptoms and increasing patient comfort, promoting patient understanding of the disease process and rationale of treatment, and stressing the patient's awareness of potential complications such as hemorrhage, hepatic coma, and permanent liver damage.

- Good skin care, providing a quiet environment, pacing activities, and increasing activity as tolerated can help to prevent decreased mobility due to the lowered energy metabolism of the liver, activity restrictions, pain, and depression.
- Nutritional monitoring is important because of anorexia, nausea, and vomiting from visceral reflexes that may reduce peristalsis. Bile stasis as well as altered absorption and metabolism of ingested foods may also produce these symptoms. Diet is ordered according to the patient's need and tolerance. A low-fat, high-carbohydrate diet is most palatable to the anorexic patient. Protein intake should not be restricted, except in special cases. Counsel the patient to avoid alcoholic beverages.
- Accurate records of intake and output may be necessary because of severe continuing vomiting and diarrhea. Adequate hydration with intravenous fluids may be necessary. Serum electrolytes must also be monitored.
- Attention must be paid to the patient's self-concept. Annoying symptoms, confinement, isolation, and length of illness may lead to feelings of depression.
- Universal precautions should be observed by health-care workers with any patient contact. In addition, members of the health-care team should be aware of those patients with acute hepatitis.
- Allow times with the patient for listening. Offer diversional activities based on energy levels.
- Discuss the side effects of and dangers of taking over-the-counter drugs as well as prescribed medications.
- Emphasis should be placed on the importance of follow-up physical examination and laboratory evaluation.
- Repeat ultrasound examination is recommended every 6 months to screen for the development of hepatic malignancy since it occurs in up to 25% of cirrhosis patients.

Assess the patient's level of understanding of the disease process and provide specific information regarding prevention and transmission of the disease. Transmission considerations should include:

- Exposed contacts may receive gamma globulin.
- Personal items should not be shared.
- Strict handwashing and sanitizing of clothes, dishes, and toilet facilities are necessary.
- While liver enzymes are elevated, avoid mucous membrane contact.
- Avoid high-risk behaviors.
- Blood donations should be discouraged.

39.5 ACUTE PANCREATITIS

Acute pancreatitis is an inflammatory process that leads to a spectrum of physiologic abnormalities, not only in the pancreas and surrounding fat but in distant organs as well. Its incidence is 13 to 45 cases per 100,000 persons per year. Each year in the United States, approximately 270,000 people are hospitalized with the disorder.

Pathophysiology

Acute pancreatitis results from early activation of digestive enzymes within the pancreas, which leads to local or systemic pathology. Typically, the enzymes are released in an inactivated form into the duodenum and activation occurs when the enzymes combine with duodenal fluid. Blockages prevent the enzymes from leaving the pancreatic duct. Acinar cells then decrease exocrine secretions and the paracellular barrier in the pancreatic duct is disrupted. Later, secretions are redirected to the basolateral areas of the acinar cells. Trypsinogen converts to trypsin. This leads activation of other digestive enzymes, including elastase and phospholipase, and to local tissue damage. Proinflammatory cytokines and digestive enzymes are released into the systemic circulation. In 10% to 15% of patients, a SIRS may lead to hypoperfusion and multisystem organ failure (MSOF). Protease stimulation, within the organ, can cause cellular injury and death. Necrosis can occur within the pancreas itself, as well as in surrounding fat and other tissues.

Severe acute pancreatitis progresses through two pathologic phases. The first phase lasts approximately 7 to 14 days and consists of local inflammation due to duct obstruction from trauma, infectious, or toxic causes. The second phase involving pancreatic necrosis typically appears later in the disease process, approximately 2 to 3 weeks after onset. It occurs when pancreatic enzymes extravasate into the fatty tissues of the retroperitoneum. It is characterized by both parenchymal tissue and vascular necrosis, which may result in hemorrhage. Small, loculated fluid collections occur and can induce pseudocyst formation. A pseudocyst is a walled-off area of both solid and liquid necrotic pancreatic tissue. Hypocalcemia results from calcium salts bind to areas of necrotic fat. Physiology stress increases adrenal cortisol production and leads to hyperglycemia.

Infection is responsible for 80% of deaths from acute pancreatitis. During acute pancreatitis, the intestinal mucosal barrier is interrupted and there is increased permeability. This allows for bacteria and other microbes to translocate to ascitic fluid, the lymphatics, and the blood stream. This translocation is linked to the development of infected pancreatic necrosis and bacteremia. Investigate the presence of infection in those patients whose clinical course initially improves then wanes, those who do not improve, and in those who deteriorate. The ensuing anaerobic metabolism and lactic acidosis propagate organ dysfunction and increase the body's metabolic oxygen demands. A hypercatabolic state results and decreases levels of total protein and albumin.

KEY CLINICAL CONCEPT

Extravasation of pancreatic enzymes can interrupt the intestinal barrier, allowing bacterial translocation from the intestinal lumen into to the bloodstream. Sepsis results.

Etiology

Approximately 70% to 80% of cases of acute pancreatitis are related to gallstones or excessive EtOH consumption. Methyl alcohol has also been implicated in the development of the disorder. Alcohol impairs pancreatic microcirculation and encourages calcium deposition, in addition to damaging acinar cells and accelerating pancreatic duct narrowing. Protein plugs may form in the main pancreatic duct leading to ductal obstruction. The sphincter of Oddi may spasm, increasing pressure in the ducts. Interestingly, smoking is an independent risk factor for developing both acute and chronic pancreatitis.

There are a multitude of other acute pancreatitis etiologies, including pancreatic duct obstruction due to strictures or tumors (benign or malignant). Additionally, blunt or penetrating abdominal trauma causing pancreatic transection or crush injury. Iatrogenic duct injury during endoscopic retrograde cholangiopancreatography (ERCP) may occur in 3.5% of cases. Acute pancreatitis can result from ischemia postcardiopulmonary bypass during open heart surgery, shock states, or from vasculitis.

Over 120 medications have been implicated in the development of acute pancreatitis. Some of the more commonly associated drugs include azathioprine, sulfonamides, thiazide diuretics, estrogens, and valproic acid. Infectious etiologies including cytomegalovirus, coxsackie B virus, mumps, rubella, histoplasmosis, and *Candida*. Toxins such as scorpion venom and organophosphate-based insecticides are less common etiologies. Metabolic issues such as severe hypertriglyceridemia (triglyceride level >1000 mg/dL) and hypercalcemia. Many of cases each have no identifiable cause and are deemed idiopathic.

Clinical Presentation

Most patients with severe pancreatitis will complain of epigastric or upper abdominal pain radiating to the back. Nausea and vomiting are common.

Physical findings are often caused by massive systemic inflammation. Many patients with severe pancreatitis develop SIRS. There are four criteria necessary for diagnosing SIRS:

- Temperature more than 38.0°C or less than 36.0°C
- Heart rate more than 90 bpm.
- Respiratory rate more than 20 breaths/min or $P\text{CO}_2$ <32 mm Hg.
- WBC more than 12,000/mm^3 or less than 4000/mm^3.

Additional Clinical Findings

- Mental status may range from normal to confused or obtunded, depending on the severity of the illness.
- Lung auscultation may reveal basilar crackles (typically on the left) due to the presence of a pleural effusion, or breath sounds may be diminished due to atelectasis.
- The abdomen is usually distended. Some patients may develop peritoneal signs such as guarding or rebound tenderness. Bowel sounds may be normoactive, hypoactive, or absent depending on if an ileus is present.
- **Cullen sign** is periumbilical ecchymosis. **Grey Turner sign** is flank ecchymosis. Both are signs of hemorrhagic pancreatitis and retroperitoneal bleeding.
- Muscle spasms and tetany can occur with hypocalcemia. A thorough examination may demonstrate positive **Chvostek's** (same-sided lip raising and facial muscle twitching with tapping on the mandible) or **Trousseau's sign** (carpal spasm of the hand when a blood pressure cuff is maximally inflated for 3 minutes).
- Electrocardiographic (ECG) changes vary depending on the presence of electrolyte deficiencies. Hypocalcemia may include the development of *U waves*, ventricular ectopy, prolonged ST segments that cause prolonged QT intervals Hypokalemia may lead to ectopy, flattened or inverted T waves, diffuse ST depression, U waves, bradycardia, first-degree heart block, supraventricular tachycardia, atrial fibrillation, or ventricular tachycardia and cardiac arrest.

QUICK TIP! Both **Chvostek** and **Trousseau sign** are key signs of hypocalcemia to know for the CCRN exam.

KEY CLINICAL CONCEPT

- **Cullen sign** is key to know for the exam, periumbilical ecchymosis suggestive of hemorrhagic pancreatitis.
- **Grey Turner sign** is ecchymosis of the flanks, which can be a late, but severe sign of retroperitoneal bleeding.

Diagnosis

Acute pancreatitis is diagnosed when two of the following three conditions are met:

1. Abdominal pain.
2. Elevated lipase or amylase more than three times the upper limit of normal.
3. CT, MRI, or US findings consistent with pancreatitis.

Laboratory Findings:

- Hypocalcemia: Serum calcium <8.5 mg/dL.
- Hyperglycemia occurs due to stress response, decreased insulin secretion, and increased glucagon activity.
- Elevated blood urea nitrogen (BUN) and creatinine if prerenal azotemia (failure) is present.
- Triglyceride levels more than 500 mg/dL.
- Elevated liver functions tests may be seen in patients with gallstone-induced pancreatitis or other causes of common bile duct obstruction.
- WBC may be elevated.
- Elevated lactic acid.
- Elevated C-reactive protein (CRP), elevated Westergren ESR

QUICK TIP! Expect one question regarding common lab abnormalities seen in acute pancreatitis on the CCRN exam.

Diagnostic Studies

- US is usually the first imaging study ordered, especially if gallbladder pathology is suspected.
- CT scan with intravenous contrast is the gold standard for evaluating pancreatic edema and necrosis.
- Balthazar's scale grades pancreatitis severity based on CT scan findings (**Table 39-9**). Monitor creatinine and urine output since third-spacing of fluid and vasodilatation put the patient at increased risk of contrast nephropathy from the iodinated IV contrast.
- Magnetic resonance cholangiopancreatography (MRCP) is a noninvasive modality for diagnosing the presence of gallstones, but it is not therapeutic. ERCP, on the other hand, allows for both diagnosis and therapeutic interventions.

TABLE 39-9. BALTHAZAR'S GRADING OF CT FINDINGS IN ACUTE PANCREATITIS (Balthazar, 1989)

Grade	*Findings*
A	Normal pancreas
B	Pancreatic enlargement
C	Pancreatic or peripancreatic inflammation
D	Single peripancreatic fluid collection
E	Two or more peripancreatic fluid collections and/or retroperitoneal air

Atlanta Classification System

The Atlanta Classification System determines if acute pancreatitis is mild, moderate, or severe based on its duration and systemic effects.

- Mild: No organ failure or systemic complications.
- Moderate: Transient organ failure that resolves within 48 hours and/or local or systemic complications without ongoing organ failure.
- Severe: Single or multiple organ failure lasting >48 hours.

Treatment

- Severe acute pancreatitis treatment focuses on fluid administration, control of pain, and resting the pancreas.
- This condition requires intensive care unit admission and prompt fluid resuscitation to decrease the risk of mortality.
- Hypovolemic shock during acute pancreatitis is multifactorial and primarily related to vasodilation and third-spacing of fluid. Nausea and vomiting in addition to poor oral intake can worsen fluid-volume deficits.
- The American Pancreatic Association guidelines recommend lactated Ringer's (LR) for initial goal-direct fluid resuscitation, as studies showed decreased inflammation with LR.
- Patients with severe pancreatitis who develop SIRS may require high volume resuscitation.
- Unstable patients may require invasive or noninvasive hemodynamic and tissue oxygenation monitoring, in addition to monitoring traditional endpoints of resuscitation such as *mean arterial pressure (MAP) ≥65 mm Hg, urine output ≥0.5 mL/kg/h, and normalization of lactic acid.*
- Guidelines recommend 5 to 10 mL/kg/h of crystalloid IV fluid until resuscitation goals are met.
- It is important to monitor for clinical signs of fluid volume overload in patients with a history of HF or end-stage renal disease (ESRD).
- Vasopressors such as **norepinephrine** are indicated for hypotension that is refractory to fluid administration.
- Excessive procoagulant factors can lead to thrombosis of the splenic, superior mesenteric, or portal vessels. If it is not contraindicated, administer anticoagulants such as **unfractionated (UFH) or low-molecular-weight heparin (LMWH)** prevent ongoing thrombosis.
- Control pain with intravenous narcotic medications such as **hydromorphone (Dilaudid)** or **fentanyl (Sublimaze)**. Using **morphine** is controversial since it may induce sphincter of Oddi spasm.
- Prohibiting oral intake promotes pancreatic rest in severe acute pancreatitis. There is no benefit to preventing oral intake in patients with mild to moderate pancreatitis. Nasogastric (NG) or orogastric suction is indicated for patients with an ileus or intractable vomiting. Enteral feeding is initially done via fluoroscopically placed nasoenteric tubes. Oral feeding may start once the ileus, severe signs of inflammation, or distal organ hypoperfusion have resolved.
- **Octreotide (Sandostatin)** is a somatostatin analogue which decreases pancreatic enzyme secretion. Research shows **octreotide** decreases organ failure has no effect on mortality.
- Institute stress mucosal prophylaxis with either an H_2 receptor blocker or proton pump inhibitor (PPI). Pharmacologic or mechanical deep venous thrombosis (DVT) prophylaxis is imperative given the risk of hypercoagulable events in this population.
- Antibiotics are only used if there is evidence of infection.

KEY CLINICAL CONCEPT

Patients with severe acute pancreatitis are at high risk for hypovolemic shock due to vasodilation and third spacing of fluid. They require aggressive fluid resuscitation to restore circulating blood volume.

Surgical Intervention

Complications

Prognosis. Ranson's criteria

- Hematologic: Circulating proteases may stimulate the clotting cascade and lead to a hypercoagulable state.
- GI: Splenic, portal, superior mesenteric vessel thrombosis, intestinal ischemia due to low flow states. Pancreatic necrosis, pseudocyst, abscess, or fistula formation. Bleeding may occur if erosion extends into the splenic, gastroduodenal, or pancreatic duodenal arteries. Treatment for this is angiography with embolization.

QUICK TIP! Be familiar with Ranson's criteria. One question may appear on the CCRN that asks if you can determine if pancreatitis is severe based on Ranson's criteria (See Table 39-11).

Chronic Complications

Long-term complications include the development of chronic pancreatitis, food and nutrient malabsorption, and diabetes mellitus (**Table 39-10**).

TABLE 39-10. LABORATORY TESTS TO DIAGNOSE PANCREATITIS

Markedly elevated serum amylase levels, often >500 units.

Characteristically, amylase levels return to normal 3–5 days after the onset of pancreatitis.

Supportive laboratory values include the following:

1. Increased serum lipase levels
2. Low serum calcium (hypocalcemia)
3. WBC counts ranging from 8000 to 20,000/mm^3, with increased polymorphonuclear cells
4. Elevated glucose levels may be as high as 500–900 mg/100 mL
5. Serum amylase to serum lipase ratio >2:1 (alcohol-induced pancreatitis)

TABLE 39-11. RANSON'S CRITERIA FOR PANCREATITIS[a]

Zero Hour (Onset)	
Age	>55 years
White blood cell (WBC) count	>16,000/mm^3
Serum glucose	>200 mg/dL
Lactate dehydrogenase (LDH)	>350
Aspartate aminotransferase (AST)	>250
48 h	
Hematocrit	Fall by ≥10%
Blood urea nitrogen despite fluids	Increase by ≥5 mg/dL
Serum calcium	<8 mg/dL
Pao_2	<60 mm Hg
Base deficit	>4 mEq/L
Fluid sequestration	>6000 mL

[a]The presence of 1–3 criteria is associated with mild pancreatitis and <1% mortality. The mortality increases with 4 (6%), 5–6 (40%), and >6 (100%).

Other diseases that can be confused with pancreatitis include cholecystitis, ulcers, and myocardial infarction. The measurement of amylase usually leads to the correct diagnosis.

Ranson's criteria can be used as a prognostic tool to identify patients at risk for complications, guide early therapy, and predict prognosis. This is done at hospital admission and at 48 hours (**Table 39-11**). A rising CRP at 48 hours can be another marker of severe pancreatitis.

Pain management a high priority. Often, intravenous analgesia is required to control the pain. If the patient is awake enough, a patient-controlled analgesia may be considered.

The pancreas is placed at rest by strict adherence to an NPO regimen and often by NG suction (in the presence of ileus). **Somatostatin** inhibits release of pancreatic polypeptides. Its use is controversial since it has been reported to worsen pancreatitis in some patients. Nutritional support is important to counteract catabolism. Jejunal EN prevents both pancreatic stimulation and bacterial translocation. PN is used in patients who fail a trial of enteral feeding. Closely evaluate glycemic control. H_2 blockers or PPIs are indicated for prevention of stress-related mucosal damage.

Image-guided drainage of peripancreatic and intra-abdominal fluid collections is indicated at times to guide antibiotic therapy. Antibiotic prophylaxis should be restricted to patients with substantial pancreatic necrosis. Drainage of fluid is the mainstay of therapy.

Patients who have severe acute pancreatitis and signs of biliary obstruction require further investigation of the cause of the obstruction. MRCP is useful in assessing for ductal blockages but lacks an interventional capacity. ERCP should be done within 72 hours of diagnosis. ERCP allows for both diagnosis and treatment of ductal obstruction.

Surgery is indicated in acutely necrotizing pancreatitis with documented infection where there is solid or semisolid material that cannot be drained percutaneously. Among the techniques used are surgical drainage of abscesses, pancreatic lavage, and subtotal or total pancreatectomy. These procedures carry high morbidity and mortality.

QUICK TIP! Generally speaking, often at least one question appears on the CCRN when "anticipate and prepare for surgery" is the best answer. This may seem counterintuitive on a nursing exam but will occur when medical therapy seems to have been maximized.

Nursing Intervention

Patients with severe acute pancreatitis are at risks for multiple complications including ARDS, abdominal compartment syndrome (ACS), ileus, and VTE.

In acute cases, pancreatitis is life threatening and requires both vigorous treatment and nursing care.

- All vital signs are checked at least hourly.
- Intake and output should be documented carefully. Insensible losses should be taken into account.
- Monitor laboratory values such as hematocrit and hemoglobin, BUN, total serum protein, creatinine, blood glucose, and electrolytes.
- Frequent fingerstick glucose monitoring is necessary to monitor insulin therapy and maintain glycemic control.
- Observe for muscular twitching, jerking, irritability, or tetany related to hypocalcemia. Frequent vomiting and/or gastric suctioning may cause loss of potassium.
- Respiratory status is monitored by levels of arterial oxygen saturation and ABGs as well as hourly auscultation of lungs for crackles, wheezes, and diminished breath sounds.
- Cardiac monitoring detects dysrhythmias, which are frequent with acidosis, shock, and/or electrolyte imbalances.

QUICK TIP! On the CCRN, consider pancreatitis as a leading cause of ARDS.

An NGT is inserted and placed to low-intermittent wall suction to evacuate stomach contents and decrease pancreatic stimulation and/or reduce the risk of gastric aspiration if an ileus is present. Observe and record color, amount, and nature of NG drainage as well as pH and the presence of blood. Mouth and nose care should be given hourly, especially if anticholinergic drugs, which cause dry oral mucous membranes, are administered.

Nutritional support is very important. Placement of a feeding tube will be necessary so that post-duodenal enteral feeds can begin as soon as possible. Increases in serum amylase and lipase levels after feeding indicate EN intolerance. PN may be required. PN is indicated in severe cases acute pancreatitis to prevent GI tract stimulation. Small amounts of clear liquids are allowed when the patient can tolerate NGT clamping. The diet is often advanced a bland, high-protein, high-carbohydrate, low-fat diet with frequent small meals, as tolerated.

Medicate the patient to alleviate pain. Use a pain scale to guide therapy. Observe for side effects of all medications.

- Monitor frequent vital signs.

Both vasodilatation and hypovolemia predispose patients to AKI. If prolonged, this prerenal kidney injury can progress to acute intrinsic renal failure.

- Monitor I/O—*UOP more than 0.5 mL/kg/h*, renal function tests
- VTE and stress mucosal prophylaxis
- Monitor Hgb/Hct, WBC
- Counsel regarding alcohol and tobacco cessation.

KEY CONTENT CHECKLIST

- ❒ Know signs and symptoms of end-stage liver failure (ESLF).
- ❒ Elevated NH_3 levels cause HE >45 μg/dL.
- ❒ Asterixis is the flappy tremor seen in liver failure.
- ❒ Grade 3–4 HE patients require intubation for airway protection and prevention of aspiration.
- ❒ Research has shown that normal to high protein intake benefits cirrhotic patients. Current guidelines support administering 1.2 to 1.5 g of protein/kg/day in patients with ALF.
- ❒ Nutritional questions are rare on the CCRN (perhaps only 1 question at most).
- ❒ Extravasation of pancreatic enzymes can interrupt the intestinal barrier, allowing bacterial translocation from the intestinal lumen into to the bloodstream. Sepsis results.
- ❒ Patients with severe acute pancreatitis are at high risk for hypovolemic shock due to vasodilation and third spacing of fluid. They require aggressive fluid resuscitation to restore circulating blood volume.
- ❒ Pancreatitis is a lesser known but a significant etiology of ARDS.
- ❒ Cullen sign: Periumbilical ecchymosis indicative of hemorrhagic pancreatitis.
- ❒ Grey Turner sign: Ecchymosis of flanks, often a late sign of retroperitoneal bleeding.
- ❒ Be familiar with Ranson's criteria. One question may appear on the CCRN that asks if you can determine if pancreatitis is severe based on Ranson's criteria.

Review Questions:

1. Which lab results are most likely in a patient with acute pancreatitis?

a. Elevated alkaline phosphatase, elevated bilirubin, decreased glucose
b. Decreased serum amylase, elevated calcium, elevated glucose
c. Elevated amylase, decreased total protein, decreased calcium
d. Elevated total protein, decreased calcium, decreased INR

Answer: C. Rationale: Acute pancreatitis requires amylase or lipase levels more than three times the upper limit of normal. Total protein is decreased due to catabolism. Hypocalcemia is common. Answer A is not correct as acute pancreatitis typically causes hyperglycemia. Answers B and D are incorrect based on the above rationales.

2. A patient with a history of severe LD is admitted to the intensive care unit with pneumonia and septic shock. He becomes increasingly tachycardic, cold, and clammy. Blood glucose is 35. Based on this information, which interventions should the nurse anticipate?

a. Administer 50 mL of dextrose 50% intravenously and check blood glucose levels every 4 hours.
b. Administer glucagon 1mg intramuscularly ×1 then repeat in 15 minutes if blood glucose is less than 70.
c. Administer glucagon 1 mg intramuscularly ×1 and start a D10 infusion with frequent glucose checks.
d. Administer 50 mL of dextrose 50% intravenously ×1 and start a dextrose 10% infusion with frequent glucose monitoring.

Answer: D. Rationale: Patients with LF-associated hypoglycemia require fluids with high dextrose concentrations (≥ 10%) to maintain normoglycemia. IV dextrose is a primary treatment of hypoglycemia in hospitals. Answers B and C are incorrect since glucagon breaks down glycogen (glycogenolysis) to raise blood glucose levels. Glucagon may not be effective in LF-associated hypoglycemia as patients may have depleted glycogen stores. Moreover, glucagon is used most frequently in the outpatient setting.

3. A patient with a history of hepatitis C and evidence of liver dysfunction is admitted after being found unresponsive by relatives. The patient is now lethargic. Skin is jaundiced and sclera are icteric. Abdomen is diffusely tender, ascites is present, with hypoactive bowel sounds. Vital signs: T 102.5F, BP 155/90, RR 18, HR 97, WBC 17,000 mm³. Which immediate interventions should the nurse anticipate:

a. Paracentesis, fluid culture, blood cultures, and administration of third-generation cephalosporin.
b. Toxicology screen and referral to drug and alcohol counseling.
c. Obtain blood, urine, and sputum cultures, and start empiric vancomycin and piperacillin-tazobactam.
d. Make the patient NPO and obtain a CT of abdomen and pelvis.

Answer: A. Rationale: The patient in this scenario is experiencing classic signs of SBP. Paracentesis is performed with fluid sent for gram stain, culture, and sensitivities. Blood cultures are also performed to evaluate for the presence of bacteremia. Unless contraindicated, SBP is empirically treated with 3rd generation cephalosporins, pending culture and sensitivity reports. Answer B is incorrect as the patient presentation does not correlate with EtOH intoxication. Answer C is not correct, as there is nothing in the presentation to suggest pneumonia or bronchitis. Answer D is not correct because it does not include empirically treating the infection.

REFERENCES

Abutaleb A, Kottilil S. Hepatitis A: epidemiology, natural history, unusual clinical manifestations, and prevention. *Gastroenterol Clin North Am.* 2020;49: 191–199. doi: 10.1016/j.gtc.2020.01.002.

Almeida PH, Matielo CEL, Curvelo LA, et al. Update on the management and treatment of viral hepatitis. *World J Gastroenterol.* 2021;27(23):3249–3261. doi: 10.3748/wjg.v27.i23.3249.

Balthazar EJ. CT diagnosis and staging of acute pancreatitis. *Radiol Clin North Am.* 1989;27:19–37.

Bajaj JS, O'Leary JG, Lai JC, et al. Acute-on-chronic liver failure clinical guidelines. *Am J Gastroenterol.* 2022;117(2):225–252. doi: 10.14309/ajg.0000000000001595.

Bernal W, Karvellas C, Saliba F, Saner FH, Meersseman P. Intensive care management of acute-on-chronic liver failure. *J Hepatol.* 2021;75(Suppl 1):S163–S177. doi: 10.1016/j.jhep.2020.10.024.

Bischoff S, Bernal W, Dasarathy S, et al. ESPEN practical guideline: clinical nutrition in liver disease. *Clin Nutr.* 2020;39(12):3533–3562. doi: 10.1016/j.clnu.2020.09.001.

de-Madaria E, Buxbaum JL, Maisonneuve P. et al. Aggressive or moderate fluid resuscitation in acute pancreatitis. *N Engl J Med.* 2022;387(11):989–1000. doi: 10.1056/NEJMoa2202884.

Gogia P, Doukas S, Porcelli M, Gilbert T. Acute liver failure masquerading an occult malignancy. *BMJ Case Rep.* 2020;13(9):e235935. doi: 10.1136/bcr-2020-235935.

Hines OJ, Pandol SJ. Management of severe acute pancreatitis. *BMJ.* 2019;367:l6227.doi: 10.1136/bmj.l6227.

Mederos MA, Reber HA, Girgis MD. Acute pancreatitis: a review. *JAMA.* 2021;325(4):382–390. doi: 10.1001/jama.2020.20317.

Montrief T, Koyfman A, Long B. Acute liver failure: a review for emergency physicians. *Am J Emerg Med.* 2019;37(2):329–337. doi: 10.1016/j.ajem.2018.10.032.

Simonetto DA, Gines P, Kamath PS. Hepatorenal syndrome: pathophysiology, diagnosis, and management. *BMJ.* 2020;14(370):m2687. doi: 10.1136/bmj.m2687.

Tan EXX, Wang MX, Pang J, Lee GH. Plasma exchange in patients with acute and acute-on-chronic liver failure: a systematic review. *World J Gastroenterol.* 2020;26(2):219–245. doi: 10.3748/wjg.v26.i2.219.

Thomas AM, Lewis JH. Nonacetaminophen drug-induced acute liver failure. Clin Liver Dis. 2018;22(2):301–324. doi: 10.1016/j.cld.2018.01.006.

Thome J, Byon D. Addressing hypoglycemic emergencies. *US Pharmacist*, 2019. https://www.uspharmacist.com/article/addressing-hypoglycemic-emergencies.

40

Intestinal Infarction, Obstruction, Perforation, and Trauma

CHAPTER OVERVIEW AND OBJECTIVES

This chapter addresses the areas of the CCRN exam on bowel infarction, obstruction, perforation, and trauma. Expect one to three questions on the exam in these areas.

After studying this chapter, you should understand the following:

- Identify key clinical indications related to gastrointestinal (GI conditions) that require medical or surgical intervention.
- Define critical hemodynamic changes arising from GI conditions and the supporting clinical interventions.

40.1 GASTROINTESTINAL INFARCTION

The intestinal tract receives blood from three major vascular trunks that arise from the aorta.

- The celiac axis supplies oxygenated blood to the first and second portions of the duodenum, part of the pancreas, liver, and spleen. This is often referred to as splanchnic circulation and includes many vessels providing collateral blood flow to the gut, which help maintain blood flow during periods of poor arterial inflow.
- The superior mesenteric artery (SMA) is the primary source of blood flow to the small intestine. The SMA distributes blood to the distal duodenum, jejunum, ileum, ascending colon, and proximal transverse colon.
- The inferior mesenteric artery (IMA) distributes blood to the distal portion of transverse, descending, and sigmoid portions of the colon, and the proximal rectum.

Mesenteric ischemia is an uncommon, yet potentially fatal cause of abdominal pain. It results from decreased blood to the splanchnic circulation. It is categorized as either acute or chronic. Acute ischemia requires prompt diagnosis and treatment.

Acute Mesenteric Ischemia (Occlusive and Nonocclusive)

Pathophysiology. Although acute mesenteric ischemia (AMI) occurs in approximately 2% of patients, *its mortality rates range from 40% to 70%*. AMI results from rapid decreases in intestinal blood flow occurring with any type of shock or other causes of significant hypoperfusion. Risk increases with age and atherosclerosis. Patients who are elderly and those with heart failure (HF), peripheral arterial disease (PAD), coronary artery disease (CAD), or cardiac dysrhythmias have the highest chance of developing AMI (Balas et al, 2017).

Occlusive Mesenteric Ischemia. Acute occlusive mesenteric ischemia (OMI) often results from acute occlusion of the SMA. Approximately 50% of cases are caused by cardiac emboli. Cardiac emboli arise from blood clots in the left atria or left ventricle that form from blood pooling in atrial fibrillation or cardiomyopathy, respectively. Heart valve vegetations caused by infective endocarditis can dislodge, forming septic cardiac emboli. OMI can also occur from procedures requiring aortic cannulation, such as left heart catheterization and cerebral angiography. Other etiologies include type B aortic dissections or localized dissections that involve the SMA (Gnanapandithan and Feuerstadt, 2020).

Mesenteric venous thrombosis (MVT) accounts for 5% to 10% of AMI cases. MVT is the most frequently seen in patients who are hypercoagulable, such as those with genetic clotting disorders (eg, antiphospholipid syndrome factor V Leiden, Protein C and S deficiency, antithrombin III deficiency, etc), persons using estrogen-containing contraception, and those with malignancies. Tobacco use, recent surgery, or trauma increase the risk of clot formation. Other etiologies include abdominal trauma, abdominal compartment syndrome, vasculitis, pancreatitis, cirrhosis, and inflammatory bowel disease (IBD) (Gnanapandithan and Feuerstadt, 2020).

Additionally, some patients may develop AMI due to occluded vessels by intestinal torsion occurring with a strangulated hernia or an intestinal volvulus (intestinal twisting of the cecum, splenic flexure of the large intestine [rarely], sigmoid colon, or small intestine)

Nonocclusive Mesenteric Ischemia. Nonocclusive mesenteric ischemia (NOMI) occurs from decreased splanchnic blood flow. It can result from acute HF, any type of shock, or after heart or thoracic aortic surgery. It is more common in older adults with histories of myocardial infarction, renal insufficiency, and liver disease. *Hypovolemia, the use of vasopressors, and the presence of abdominal compartment syndrome contribute to intestinal hypoperfusion.*

Presentation. Regardless of the etiology, AMI requires prompt identification and treatment to prevent infarction. The intestines can withstand approximately 75% decrease in blood flow for up to 12 hours. Tissue damage is caused by both hypoperfusion and reperfusion. AMI is associated with the sudden onset of severe abdominal pain that is out of proportion to the patient's abdominal exam. The pain is typically located on the left side, the periumbilical area, or epigastrium. Patients may complain of significant pain, but on examination may only have diffuse, nonspecific tenderness without peritoneal signs, such as guarding or rebound tenderness.

The locations most often affected by AMI are the "watershed" regions. Watershed regions are supplied by the distal ends of two major arteries. In the colon, this includes the rectum, rectosigmoid junction, splenic flexure, and left colon, which are supplied by both the SMA and IMA. During hypovolemia or hypoperfusion, watershed areas are susceptible to ischemia. The abrupt decrease in blood flow to these portions of the large intestine leads to abdominal pain. Gastrointestinal (GI) bleeding occurs late in the disease process. If the entire thickness of the bowel wall is involved, bowel perforation and peritonitis can occur.

KEY CLINICAL CONCEPT

- AMI is associated with the sudden onset of severe abdominal pain that is out of proportion to the patient's abdominal exam. The pain is typically located on the left side, periumbilical area, or epigastrium.
- Regardless of the etiology, AMI requires prompt identification and treatment to prevent infarction.

Diagnosis. Laboratory tests should include

- Basic metabolic panel (BMP)
- Liver function tests (LFTs)
- Complete blood count (CBC)
- Prothrombin time (PT)
- Activated partial thromboplastin time (aPTT)
- Lactic acid
- Lactate dehydrogenase (LDH)

Although there is no definitive lab test for AMI, patients often have leukocytosis and **elevated lactic acid levels** and are at risk for electrolyte imbalances such as hyperkalemia (Bala et al, 2017). However, these values may be normal during the onset of an acute episode.

Invasive angiography is considered the gold standard for diagnosing mesenteric ischemia since it can diagnose the disorder earlier in its course than computed tomography angiography (CTA). However, CTA of the abdomen and pelvis without oral contrast is the initial imaging of choice for many clinicians. The IV contrast helps assess for emboli, thrombi, and other forms of vascular occlusion such as vessel compromise due to a small bowel obstruction (SBO) (Bala et al, 2017; Gnanapandithan and Feuerstadt, 2020; Huber et al, 2021). Oral contrast is not needed to diagnose intestinal ischemia, and patients with AMI may not tolerate it. CT scans can assess for bowel wall edema or intramural hemorrhage. Reperfusion events are associated with bowel wall thickening and mesenteric fat stranding on CT. Free fluid within the abdominal cavity is commonly found in patients with NOMI, but free air is rarely seen.

KEY CLINICAL CONCEPT

- Patients with AMI often have leukocytosis and elevated lactic acid levels and are at risk for electrolyte imbalances such as hyperkalemia. However, these lab values may be normal during the onset an acute episode.
- CTA of the abdomen and pelvis are often preferred when evaluating patients for AMI as they not only assess for vascular occlusion but can also diagnose other signs of ischemia including bowel wall edema or intramural hemorrhage.

Initial Treatment. Patients with suspected AMI should be made NPO and have nasogastric tubes (NGTs) inserted for gastric decompression. They require IV fluids to provide oxygenated blood to the tissues and improve organ perfusion (Bala et al, 2017; Gnanapandithan and Feuerstadt, 2020).

- Reestablish blood flow as quickly as possible by administering IV fluids to prevent worsening ischemia.
- Correct acid-base and electrolyte imbalances.
- *Providers may discontinue vasopressors in* AMI patients without signs of peritoneal irritation, such as guarding or rebound tenderness, to improve tissue perfusion.
- Inotropic therapy with **dobutamine** or **milrinone** may improve hemodynamics by increasing **stroke volume (SV)** resulting in increased **cardiac output (CO)**.
- *Administering empiric broad-spectrum antibiotics helps prevent sepsis* in cases of necrotic bowel perforation and bacterial contamination of the peritoneal cavity.
- *Controlling pain by administering IV opioid medications will help decrease sympathetic nervous system (SNS) responses,* decreased peripheral vasoconstriction, which may improve splanchnic blood flow.

Definitive Treatment. Revascularization is the definitive treatment for AMI. In patients without evidence of perforation or peritoneal signs, catheter-based interventions such as stenting, embolectomy, thrombectomy with or without intra-arterial vasodilator infusions, for example, **nitroglycerin** or papaverine, are performed for embolic or thrombotic AMI (Gnanapandithan and Feuerstadt, 2020). Additionally, intra-arterial thrombolytics may be administered to in patients without any absolute contraindications within 8 hours of the onset of abdominal pain to restore blood flow.

Surgery is warranted in patients with acute occlusion who present with acute abdominal pain, signs of peritoneal irritation, evidence of necrosis, and/or clinical deterioration. Exploratory laparotomy with surgical embolectomy or mesenteric bypass with bowel resection may be necessary depending on size of the clot(s) and the extent of the intestinal ischemia (Gnanapandithan and Feuerstadt, 2020). Postoperative management includes treating the underlying cause, which may include dual-antiplatelet therapy for 3 to 12 months or systemic anticoagulation with low molecular weight or unfractionated **heparin** to prevent new embolic events.

Nursing Interventions. Astute assessment of patients with unexplained abdominal pain is the key to recognizing intestinal infarction. Monitor the type of pain and relieving factors.

Supportive management of patients with intestinal infarction include:

- General nursing care includes NPO, NGT decompression, bowel rest, appropriate fluid and electrolyte replacement, and *monitoring for signs of abdominal compartment syndrome.*
- *In patients with elevated lactic acid levels or signs of shock, intravenous (IV) fluid resuscitation with isotonic fluids such as normal saline (NS) or lactated Ringer's (LR) increases intravascular volume, blood pressure (BP), and may improve intestinal circulation.*
- Positive inotropic agents such as **dobutamine** or **milrinone** may be used to augment low CO.
- Prepare the patient for urgent catheter-based or surgical revascularization to prevent complications such as intestinal infarction and perforation.

Key considerations for ongoing stabilization and supportive care after revascularization include:

- Monitor for bleeding, hypovolemia, and postoperative ileus.
- Take measures to prevent infection, deep venous thrombosis (DVT), and stress ulcers.
- Pain is controlled with IV opioids, either as intermittent IV push or patient-controlled analgesia (PCA).
- Patients who have extensive small bowel resections are at risk for developing short bowel syndrome, for example, chronic malabsorption of nutrients, diarrhea, and may require long-term parenteral nutrition (PN).

Chronic Mesenteric Ischemia

Pathophysiology. Chronic mesenteric ischemia (CMI) is caused by atherosclerosis and progressively worsens. Patients with CMI often have wide-spread atherosclerotic disease, including CAD and PAD. CMI risk factors are similar to those associated with atherosclerosis, such as smoking, diabetes mellitus (DM), hypertension (HTN), and dyslipidemia. Symptoms of CMI usually occur when two of the three major arteries are affected. As CMI progresses, pain occurs between 30 minutes to 6 hours after eating, due to the increased need for blood flow after food ingestion. The pain is typically described as dull or cramping and located in the mid-abdomen (Huber et al, 2021).

Presentation. Patients with CMI present with chronic postprandial abdominal pain, sitophobia (fear of eating), and weight loss. Others may have non-specific symptoms such as nausea, vomiting, abdominal discomfort, constipation, or diarrhea (Huber et al, 2021). Physical exam findings may include abdominal bruits as well as decreased lower extremity hair growth and poor pulses.

Diagnosis. Primary care providers (PCPs) begin the initial assessment of symptomatic patients. The PCP may refer them to gastroenterology to exclude non-vascular etiologies. Vascular surgeon evaluation is, and CTA scans are imperative for definitive diagnosis and determining whether medical management and/or revascularization are indicated (Huber et al, 2021).

Treatment. Since the majority of CMI cases are caused by atherosclerosis, medical management focuses on controlling comorbidities such as hyperlipidemia (HLD), HTN, DM, and lifestyle changes such as exercise and tobacco cessation to prevent disease progression (Huber et al, 2021). Patients are instructed to eat smaller, low-fat meals throughout the day to prevent the blood flow and oxygen demand associated with large meals. They may benefit from dietary counseling and supplemental vitamins (Gnanapandithan and Feuerstadt, 2020). Patients who undergo stenting require dual-antiplatelet therapy (DAPT) for 3 to 12 months to prevent stent stenosis. Patients with mesenteric stents need routine imaging with CT or duplex scans plus regular physician follow-up. Signs of stent restenosis are similar to those patients have pretreatment, including postprandial abdominal pain.

KEY CLINICAL CONCEPT

- Weight loss, pain after eating, and fear of food are common signs of CMI.
- Controlling comorbidities such as HLD, HTN, and DM, and lifestyle modifications such as diet, exercise, and tobacco cessation are key to preventing CMI progression.
- Patients who undergo stenting require dual-antiplatelet therapy (DAPT) for 3 to 12 months to prevent stent stenosis.

40.2 GASTROINTESTINAL OBSTRUCTION

Intestinal obstruction can occur anywhere in the tract; however, obstruction occurs more frequently in the small bowel. Obstruction is characterized as either complete or incomplete. Blood supply to affected area can either be normal (simple obstruction) or occluded (strangulated obstruction). The patient usually presents with cramps accompanied by abdominal pain, vomiting, and decreased passage of stool or flatus. Intestinal obstruction is classified as gastroduodenal, proximal or distal small intestinal, and colonic.

Etiology and Pathophysiology

Up to 75% of SBOs result from adhesions which are bands of scar tissue that form in the abdominal cavity after surgical procedures. The adhesions can be thick or thin and generally lead to either partial or complete obstruction. Less common causes are small intestinal tumors and incarcerated hernias (Catena et al, 2019).

Obstruction leads to intestinal dilatation above the blockage, resulting in decreased blood flow and risk of perforation. Lymph ducts in the intestine are compressed and if this is not promptly corrected, hydrostatic forces within the bowel wall increase, resulting in third-spacing of intravascular fluid and decreasing circulating fluid volume.

Clinical Presentation

Many patients with SBO will have a nonspecific presentation consisting of diffuse abdominal pain, fever, nausea, or vomiting. The pain is described as crampy and worsens overtime as the intestines increased peristalsis to overcome the blockage (Catena et al, 2019). Emesis can range from bilious (green) to dark with a feculent odor. *Tachycardia and hypotension are common in severely dehydrated.* Visual examination typically reveals abdominal distention. Bowel sounds are usually high-pitched and tinkling. Upon palpation, the abdomen may be diffusely tender, with or without guarding or rebound tenderness. The abdomen is usually tympanic upon percussion.

Diagnosis

Abdominal radiographs are done first. They may show dilated small bowel loops with air–fluid levels, along with decreased air in the colon. CT scans with oral contrast provide information about the location and severity (partial obstruction vs complete obstruction) of the obstruction. It can also identify areas of intestinal strangulation. CT scans may also reveal etiologies of SBOs, such as tumors. In some cases, surgery is needed to definitively diagnosis the cause. Laboratory studies may reveal fluid and electrolyte imbalances. Leukocytosis may be present depending on the cause of the SBO.

Treatment

Approximately 80% of SBO resolve with conservative management. It is done for 72 hours, except in cases of ischemia or perforation, and consists of the following clinical interventions:

- Bowel rest (making the patient NPO)
- Inserting an NGT decompresses the stomach and prevents vomiting, decreases distention, and may alleviate abdominal discomfort.
- Administering antiemetics, such as **ondansetron (Zofran)**, can alleviate nausea.

Strangulated SBOs require emergency surgery to restore intestinal blood flow. If it is not promptly treated, the intestine will become ischemic and perforate, leading to septic shock, and death. In cases of complete obstruction or malignancy, surgery is indicated.

Nursing Intervention

Nursing interventions are aimed at ensuring hemodynamic stability and maintaining fluid and electrolyte balance.

- Monitor vital signs for the presence of fever, hypotension, tachypnea, and tachycardia.
- Strictly record intake, NGT output (volume, characteristics), urine output, and daily weights.
- *Monitor labs for signs of intravascular volume depletion: Hypernatremia, elevated blood urea nitrogen (BUN), elevated serum osmolality, and hemoconcentration (elevated hemoglobin and hematocrit levels).*
- For patients with prolonged NPO status, PN may be indicated.
- Monitor postoperative patients for signs of wound infection (erythema, drainage, warmth) and dehiscence.
- *Monitor for signs of sepsis and peritonitis, which may indicate a leak at the surgical anastomosis site.*

KEY CLINICAL CONCEPT

- Know the difference between an SBO and a Large Bowel Obstruction (LBO).
- SBO patients suffer from nausea, vomiting (sometimes fecal matter), less likely to have distention, and are treated with IV fluids and decompression.
- LBO patients are LESS likely to have nausea, less vomiting, more distention, and treatment usually does NOT require an NGT. This patient often does not appear as ill (compared to SBO patient).
- As a result, the difference between SBO vs. LBO may be remembered by thinking that the LBO is less labor-intensive from a nursing care standpoint.

40.3 GASTROINTESTINAL PERFORATION

Visceral organ perforation (perforated viscus) is a potentially catastrophic event associated with a 30% to 50% mortality. The appendix is the most commonly perforated site, followed by the stomach, duodenum, small bowel, and large bowel. Depending on its location, GI tract perforation results in leakage of gastric or intestinal contents into either the peritoneal or retroperitoneal. Without prompt diagnosis and treatment, peritonitis, sepsis, and death may occur.

Etiology

IBDs, such as Crohn disease and ulcerative colitis, are the most common causes of nontraumatic GI perforation. Approximately 10% to 15% of patients with diverticulitis will develop perforations. Intestinal obstruction, ischemia, or infection (eg, tuberculosis or *Clostridioides difficile*), as well as ingestion of foreign bodies (eg, fish bones, razor blades, toothpicks), and malignancies can also lead to GI perforation. Traumatic perforation can occur from either blunt or penetrating trauma, or due to iatrogenic injury during procedures such as endoscopy.

Peritonitis develops either from chemical irritation from gastric acid or from bacterial spillage from gram-negative and anaerobic organisms in the GI tract, such as *Escherichia coli* and *Bacteroides fragilis*, into the peritoneal cavity. Patients with distal colonic perforations are at the highest risk of developing peritonitis, septic shock, and intra-abdominal abscesses.

Clinical Presentation

GI perforation is associated with the onset of severe, unrelenting abdominal pain. Associated symptoms include fever, nausea, and vomiting. Peritoneal signs such as guarding, rigidity, tenderness, and rebound tenderness are common. Tachycardia can occur because of pain and/or intravascular volume depletion.

Diagnosis

CBC with differential, BMP, and *lactic acid levels* are commonly ordered. Leukocytosis with bandemia (bands > 10%) and electrolyte disturbances are common. Hemoglobin and hematocrit may appear elevated in patients with low intravascular volumes and hemoconcentration.

Abdominal radiographs may reveal free air underneath the diaphragm (pneumoperitoneum). A CT of the abdomen and pelvis may be performed to locate and evaluate the perforation prior to surgery. In patients with suspected GI perforation, a water-soluble contrast agent such as diatrizoate (Gastrografin) is used. Barium contrast is avoided due to its potential for peritoneal inflammation and granuloma formation (Shin et al, 2020).

Treatment

Isotonic crystalloid IV fluid resuscitation improves intravascular volume and raises BP. Broad-spectrum IV antibiotics decrease the risk of intra-abdominal infections and sepsis. Making the patient NPO assists with bowel rest and prepares the patient for possible surgical intervention. Nasogastric suction decompresses the stomach and prevents vomiting. Most patients with GI perforation require prompt intervention with either laparoscopy or laparotomy to repair the affected areas. However, If the CT scan reveals that the perforation is encapsulated or walled-off from the rest of the peritoneum, surgery is not acutely warranted. Management of these patients is conservative and may include image-guided percutaneous drainage in addition to antibiotics.

Nursing Interventions

Nursing interventions are similar to those for intestinal infarction and obstruction. Please refer to those sections of this chapter for more information.

KEY CLINICAL CONCEPT

Free air under the diaphragm on abdominal x-ray is very suspicious for GI tract perforation. A CT of the abdomen and pelvis may be performed to locate and evaluate the perforation prior to surgery.

40.4 GASTROINTESTINAL SURGERY

Esophageal Surgery

The most common esophageal surgical procedures treat gastroesophageal reflux disease (GERD), achalasia, esophageal diverticula, esophageal perforation, and precancerous and cancerous lesions of the esophagus. Barrett esophagus is considered a precursor to esophageal cancer and occurs when abnormal columnar epithelium replaces the stratified squamous epithelium normally lining the distal esophagus. Barrett esophagus is generally a consequence of chronic GERD. Treatment is focused on suppressing acid release with **PPIs** and H_2 blockers, as well as preventing acid reflux by nonmedical interventions for GERD. Patients with severe GERD or hiatal hernias may benefit from Nissen fundoplication. The laparoscopic Nissen procedure involves wrapping the fundus of the stomach around the lower esophagus, closing the esophageal sphincter, and preventing further reflux of gastric acid.

Esophageal cancer is the fifth most common type of cancer in the United States with roughly 17,000 new cases each year. Five-year survival ranges from 12% to 20% (Kelly, 2019). There are two types of esophageal cancer: adenocarcinoma and squamous cell carcinoma. This disease most frequently occurs in men 60 years or older. Barrett's esophagus is a risk factor. The majority cases are associated with cigarette smoking, alcohol use, GERD, high body mass index (BMI), and diets low in fruits and vegetables (Kumar et al, 2022a). Patients usually have progressive dysphagia, epigastric pain, and recent unexplained weight loss. Others may experience bleeding, a persistent cough, or hoarse voice. Flexible endoscopy is performed to identify the location and extent of the tumor and provide a tissue sample for biopsy. Positron emission tomography (PET) scan evaluates for the presence of hypermetabolic (PET avid) tissue throughout the body. Inflammation, primary tumors, and metastatic cancer uptake the glucose-based tracer and appear as PET avid. Since the brain utilizes glucose, a PET scans cannot exclude brain metastasis. Magnetic resonance imaging (MRI) of the brain is performed instead. CT scans are used for staging. At the time of diagnosis, the great majority of tumors have spread beyond the esophagus to the mediastinum, lymph nodes, liver, or pulmonary system. Depending on the severity of the tumor, and degree of malnutrition, patients may have an esophageal stent placed to alleviate dysphagia or a surgically placed jejunostomy tube (J-tube) performed for enteral feeding access (Watkins et al, 2020). In cases of locally advanced disease, neoadjuvant chemotherapy and radiation therapy are administered for an average of four months to shrink the tumor and prevent metastasis prior to surgical resection. Surgery is not recommended for patients with metastatic disease or tumor invasion of nearby structures (trachea, laryngeal nerve, etc). Consider palliative care consults for goals of care discussions in those with a low likelihood of survival.

A number of patients may benefit from surgical removal of the esophagus (esophagectomy) Esophagectomy surgery involves tabularizing the stomach to create a neo-esophagus. The affected portion of the esophagus is removed. The remaining portion of the esophagus is anastomosed to the neo esophagus. The mortality rate associated with this procedure is anywhere from 2.8% to 17%. Surgical complications such as surgical site infection, bleeding, and anastomotic leakage are seen in occur in 26% to 41% of patients (Brown et al, 2028). Pneumonia is a common postoperative pulmonary complication.

Esophageal Surgery Nursing Interventions.

- In esophagectomy patients, hypotension is treated with fluid volume resuscitation. Vasopressors are avoided due to the risk causing ischemia in the neo esophagus.

- A nasoenteric tube is placed at the time of surgery to prevent distention of the neo esophagus. It may be fastened to the nose with sutures. Do not move or reposition the tube. The tube is placed to low-intermittent wall suction. Flush the tube to maintain patency if ordered by the thoracic surgeon.
- Chest tubes are placed during surgery. Monitor the amount, color, and consistency of drainage to assess for blood loss or purulence, which may indicate an anastomotic leak. Chest tubes are continued until the patient undergoes a Gastrografin or barium swallow test that is negative for an anastomotic leak.
- Keep the head of bed elevated to prevent esophageal bile reflux and aspiration pneumonia.
- Esophageal surgery patients are strictly NPO for 10 to 14 days depending on surgeon preference.
- Monitor for leukocytosis, fever, and other signs of sepsis.
- Maintain adequate fluid and electrolyte balance.
- Educate the patient and family regarding J-tube care and safe administration of enteral feeds.

KEY CLINICAL CONCEPT

Esophageal surgery patients are at high risk for pulmonary and GI complications. Monitor for leukocytosis, fever, and other signs of sepsis.

Bariatric Surgery

Morbid obesity is a complex disease with associated comorbidities, e.g., DM, obstructive sleep apnea, HDL, and HTN, that requires special management. Bariatric surgery is increasingly performed for weight loss in patients with a BMI > 40 kg/m^2 and no associated comorbidities, and those whose BMI is >35 kg/m^2 who have obesity-associated conditions such as DM, HTN, HDL, nonalcoholic fatty liver disease (NAFLD), and obstructive sleep apnea. The most commonly performed procedures are laparoscopic Roux-en-Y gastric bypass (LRYGB), laparoscopic sleeve gastrectomy (LSG), and laparoscopic adjustable gastric banding (LAGB), and vertical banding gastroplasty (VBG). Patients benefit psychosocial support and lifestyle modifications, including weight loss and exercise, both before and after surgery. Administration of vitamins B1, B_{12}, A, D, E, and K, along with calcium, copper, folate, iron, and zinc supplementation, is indicated to prevent postoperative nutritional deficiencies (Tabesh et al, 2019).

Bariatric patients are at risk for complications and require close surgical, medical, and dietitian follow-up. Immediate complications include bleeding is associated with immediate postoperative complications include bleeding, vomiting, and ileus. Early complications including surgical site infections, anastomotic leaks occur within the first few weeks. Anastomotic ulceration, dilatation, and stenosis, choledocholithiasis, reflux esophagitis, band slippage, and band necrosis are seen months to years after post-operatively. Complications such as bowel obstruction and fistula formation can happen any time after surgery (Schulman and Thompson, 2017).

Patients with LRYGB may experience dumping syndrome. Dumping syndrome occurs within 15 minutes of eating foods high in refined sugar. These foods are hyperosmolar and cause fluid shifts from the blood stream into the small bowel. This results in symptoms such as abdominal pain, bloating, nausea, diarrhea, flushing, and diaphoresis. Cardiovascular changes such as tachycardia, hypotension, and syncope follow (Schulman and Thompson, 2017). Subsequent hypoglycemia can cause confusion, perspiration, palpitations, tremors, and syncope. Nursing interventions focus on counseling patients to avoid food high in simple sugars.

KEY CLINICAL CONCEPT

- Bariatric surgery patients require vitamin and mineral supplementation to prevent deficiencies.
- LRYGB patients are at risk of dumping syndrome from ingestion of simple sugars. Dumping syndrome results in GI symptoms, tachycardia, hypotension, and late hypoglycemia.

Gastric Surgery for Treatment of Peptic Ulcer Disease

Vagotomy and pyloroplasty is a gastric surgical option in the treatment of peptic ulcer disease (PUD).

- The vagotomy (severing of the vagus nerve) results in decreased acid production because of the loss of vagally mediated gastric secretion.
- Pyloroplasty, or widening of the pyloric channel, is necessary to prevent gastric stasis. This surgery is generally associated with a low rate of ulcer recurrence, but a combination of vagotomy and antrectomy has an even lower recurrence rate.
- In this more complicated combined vagotomy and antrectomy surgery, the distal half of the stomach is removed to decrease gastrin production, another stimulus to acid production.
- Another surgical treatment for ulcers is a highly selective vagotomy, also called the parietal cell or proximal gastric vagotomy. In this operation, the vagal branches to the proximal stomach, the fundus, and the body are severed. Because this is where acid secretion occurs, this surgery decreases acid production without affecting the motor activity of the distal stomach. This surgery, however, is technically more difficult to perform than the other two.

Gastric (Stomach) Cancer Surgery

Adenocarcinoma is the most common stomach malignancy, with approximately 27,000 cases per year in the United States (Hoshi, 2020). Symptoms often appear late, after metastasis has already occurred. Patients commonly present with weight loss, abdominal pain, nausea, early satiety (feeling full after eating small amounts of food), indigestion, dysphagia, and hematemesis (Kumar et al, 2022b). It is diagnosed by endoscopy with biopsy. Staging with brain MRI and PET-CT determines the needs for neoadjuvant therapy and/or surgical intervention. Tumors near or invading major vascular structures are likely not resectable. If lesions have not spread, a subtotal gastrectomy, which removes over half of the stomach is usually performed. However, some tumors are large enough to require a total gastrectomy. Patients tend to have significant weight loss after surgery and may experience nausea, vomiting, nutrient malabsorption, and dumping syndrome (Hoshi, 2020).

Pancreatic Surgery

Pancreatic carcinoma accounts for only 3% of cancers but is the fourth leading cause of cancer deaths in the United States. Pancreatic metastasizes quickly. Most tumors are advanced-stage and unresectable at the time of diagnosis (Tempero, 2019). Risk factors for pancreatic cancer include cigarette smoking, age > 55, high BMI, sedentary lifestyle, DM, chronic pancreatitis, and family history (Zhang et al, 2018).

Most patients with pancreatic cancer present with dyspepsia, nausea, weight loss, and abdominal pain. If the bile duct is obstructed, gallbladder distends, jaundice, pruritus, and clay-colored or greasy stools can result. Hepatomegaly can occur in patients with liver metastases. The tumor can spread to the duodenum, liver, lymph nodes, and lungs and can impinge on the stomach. Other symptoms vary with the sites of metastases.

Pancreatic cancer is diagnosed by CT or MRI of the pancreas, followed by either endoscopic ultrasound (EUS) fine needle aspirate (FNA), image-guided fine needle biopsy (FNB). Depending on the location and severity of the tumor, elevated pancreatic and liver enzymes can occur. Two tumor markers carbohydrate antigen (CA) 19-9 and carcinoembryonic antigen (CEA) may be elevated. CA 9-19 can be falsely positive so is not used as a screening tool. However, it is good for evaluating pancreatic cancer prognosis and recurrence (Zhang et al, 2018).

Pancreatic cancer is often fatal. In patients who are not candidates for surgery, survival rates range from 18% at 1 year to 4% at 5 years, worldwide. Patients with resectable tumors and no metastases at time of surgery have a 5-year survival rate of approximately 20%. Patients with resectable cancer require 4 to 6 months of neoadjuvant chemotherapy prior to an extensive, complicated surgery for attempted cure. The two major procedures undertaken are pancreaticoduodenectomy (Whipple's procedure) and total pancreatectomy. Whipple's procedure involves resection of the head of the pancreas along with contiguous structures including the gastric antrum, duodenal C loop, gallbladder, and lymph nodes are removed. A loop of jejunum is anastomosed to the tail of the pancreas, the stomach, and the common bile duct. The procedure is difficult, and surgical mortality (death within 30 days of surgery) is 5%. Major complications of the procedure have been leakage or hemorrhage at the site of pancreatojejunostomy.

Total pancreatectomy is another option in pancreatic cancer. In this procedure, the same organs are removed as for Whipple's procedure, but a pancreatojejunostomy is not necessary since the whole pancreas is removed. This procedure is technically simpler to perform than Whipple's procedure. Metabolic management, however, is much more difficult.

Most surgical procedures for pancreatic cancer are palliative rather than curative. The aim is to treat or prevent obstruction of the common bile duct and gastric outlet. Therefore, anastomosis of the jejunum to either the gallbladder or common bile duct as well as gastrojejunostomy is most often done.

Appendicitis

Appendicitis is a major cause of acute abdominal pain, and a leading indication for acute abdominal surgery. Appendicitis arises from appendiceal outlet obstruction by stones, feces, infection, lymphoid hyperplasia, and benign or malignant tumors. In early appendicitis, the appendix becomes inflamed and distended. Small vessels thrombose, which prevents lymph drainage and decreases venous blood return. Over time, the appendix may perforate or become gangrenous.

Severe pain is the reason most patients with appendicitis seek medical attention. The pain is typically located in the right lower quadrant, epigastrium, or periumbilical areas. Patients often present with fever, leukocytosis, nausea, vomiting. The primary presenting symptom is abdominal pain. Patients may develop peritoneal signs including guarding or rebound tenderness. CT scan of the abdomen and pelvis is the most accurate way of diagnosing acute appendicitis.

Uncomplicated cases of appendicitis caused by infection may be treated conservatively with IV antibiotics tailored to cover GI flora and may not require surgery. Perforated appendicitis is treated with antibiotics and surgery. Surgical appendectomy (either laparoscopic or open), fluid resuscitation, and addressing electrolyte abnormalities are the mainstays of therapy (Moris et al, 2021).

Small and Large Intestine Surgery

Surgery of the large intestine is performed a variety of reasons, including appendicitis, colon cancer, IBD, diverticulitis, or lower GI bleeding. Surgery of the small intestine is generally performed for removal of tumors, treatment of hemorrhage, or correction of intestinal herniation. Tumors of the small intestine are rare, and treatment usually involves simple resection of the tumor itself plus a limited margin of normal intestine on either end.

- Hemorrhage in intestine surgery is also uncommon and usually results from arteriovenous malformations, which in most cases form in the colon and not the small intestine.
- Small intestinal herniation can be either internal or external.
  - External herniation involves trapping of an intestinal loop outside the peritoneal cavity, as in inguinal, femoral, or ventral hernias.
  - Surgical therapy involves freeing the trapped loop of intestine and attempting to prevent its recurrence.

Colon Carcinoma

Colon carcinoma is the second leading cause of cancer deaths in the United States. Unfortunately, symptoms often appear late in the disease course and patients may ignore the symptoms or attribute them to other causes. Common symptoms include abdominal pain, changes in bowel habits (diarrhea or constipation), melena, bloody stools, anemia, unexplained weight loss, or fatigue. Ninety percent of colon cancers are found in patients >50 years old. However, there is an increasing incidence in those younger than 50. Patients over age 50 and those with significant risk factors such as family or personal history of colon cancer or history of IBD are encouraged to undergo routine screening colonoscopies. Other risk factors for colon cancer include tobacco use, alcohol use, and diets high in fats or processed meats.

The earlier colon cancer is detected, the higher the likelihood of cure with surgical excision. Patients with locally advanced disease may undergo neo adjuvant chemotherapy and/or radiation therapy. Surgical excision involves removal of the tumor with wide margins of uninvolved intestine surrounding the mass. A temporary or permanent colostomy may be created depending on the tumor location and other factors. Regional lymph nodes are also removed for pathological examination. Colon cancer staging, treatment decisions, and prognosis are determined by the characteristics of the tumor, lymphatic or surrounding structure involvement, and metastasis (Vogel et al, 2022). The lymph nodes, lungs, liver, peritoneum, and brain are common sites of metastasis.

Diverticulitis

Diverticulosis is a common cause of abdominal discomfort in patients older than age 50. It is becoming more common in the developed world due to constipation and a lack of dietary fiber intake. The left colon is more frequently affected. Diverticular disease occurs when the intestinal mucosa protrudes through the muscular layer leading to outpouchings of the colon. Most patients with diverticulosis never experience any symptoms. Patients may have anywhere from mild abdominal pain and tenderness to diffuse peritonitis from colonic perforation. CT scans of the abdomen and pelvis are the gold standard for diagnosing diverticulitis. Colonoscopy is not recommended during acute flares due to the increased risk of perforation. Therapy is usually with antibiotics and bowel rest. However, perforation is a surgical emergency. Surgical resection includes creation of a temporary diverting colostomy.

Nursing Interventions

Nursing priorities for patients undergoing GI surgery include maintaining hemodynamics, promoting adequate fluid and electrolyte balance, alleviating psychosocial concerns, meeting nutritional needs, promoting proper GI functioning postoperatively, and preventing complications.

Postoperatively, the primary goal of therapy is ensuring hemodynamic and respiratory stability.

- Maintaining a patent airway and providing by ventilation or oxygen therapy as indicated are quintessential for surgical recovery.
- In extubated patients, encourage coughing and incentive spirometry every 2 hours. Instruct the patient on splinting the incision to prevent wound complications and to decrease discomfort.
- Assess vital signs at least every 15 minutes initially after surgery and progress to longer intervals as the patient's stability allows. Assess vital signs for hypotension, tachypnea, tachycardia, and hypoxia.
- Assess intake and output every hour.
- Assess urine output and intervene to maintain at least 30 mL/h.
- Monitor serum electrolytes and correct abnormalities.
- Monitor for signs of infection such as fever, leukocytosis, and erythema, drainage, or warmth at the incision site.
- Assess the type and amount of drainage from the nasogastric and drainage tubes. Note the color, consistency, and the presence of foul odor from any drainage.
- Monitor for signs of bleeding and decreases in hemoglobin and hematocrit.

Maintain nutritional status by PN if the patient will not tolerate oral or enteral intake within the first week after surgery. If enteral feeding is contraindicated, maintain the patency of the NGT and record the characteristics of any drainage. Once bowel sounds are present, clear liquids—progressing to full liquids and then to diets low in residue and high in protein, carbohydrates, and calories—may be initiated.

Maintain skin integrity by providing pressure relief and turning the patient at least every 2 hours. Assess for the presence of hyperglycemia in all patients. *Hyperglycemia results from the body's stress response.* Patients who have had pancreatic resections are at increased risk for hyperglycemia. A continuous insulin infusion and hourly blood glucose checks may be needed for adequate glycemic control.

Emotional support of the postoperative patient is important to both the patient and the family. This is particularly important for patients who have had ostomies placed. Maintain a reassuring, accepting environment and give the patient opportunities to express fears and anxieties regarding the patient's altered self-concept.

40.5 GASTROINTESTINAL TRAUMA

Blunt or Penetrating Abdominal Trauma

Blunt abdominal trauma (BAT) often occurs due to motor vehicle crashes, falls from height, sports injuries, or assaults. These injuries may occur even though the abdominal wall is still intact. Blunt trauma can cause organ lacerations (tearing), hematomas, or ruptures.

- Blunt injuries typically involve the liver, spleen, and to a lesser degree, kidneys.
- Penetrating abdominal trauma can occur from stabbings, gunshot wounds, or even impalement. Wounds can range from superficial to deep, with or without organ involvement.
- Injuries to solid organs and vascular structures can lead to hypovolemic shock.
- Noting locations and patterns of bruising, lacerations, or abrasions are helpful in recognizing patients at risk for intra-abdominal injuries. **Kehr sign** can be seen in BAT. It is left shoulder pain that is referred from either splenic rupture or hemidiaphragm injury.

KEY CLINICAL CONCEPT

Kehr sign is left shoulder pain that is referred from either splenic rupture or hemidiaphragm injury.

Diagnosis

- Physical exam alone is usually inadequate in diagnosing BAT injuries. Focused abdominal sonography for trauma (FAST) exam is commonly used in the trauma bay to look for free fluid in the abdominal cavity to exclude hemoperitoneum. The downside of using the FAST exam is that it cannot detect injuries that do not cause bleeding into the peritoneal cavity. CT scans are primarily used to diagnose organ injury in patients who are undergoing nonoperative management and correcting fluid and electrolyte imbalances and are also used for surgical planning.

Treatment

Initial treatment is aimed at maintenance of the patient's hemodynamic status and prevention of shock by addressing airway, breathing, and circulation.

- Rapid IV isotonic fluid administration is indicated for patients in shock.
- Blood and blood products may be needed in patients with ongoing blood loss and those who are refractory to crystalloid fluid boluses.
- Antibiotics may be necessary to prevent peritonitis and wound infections, especially for open, penetrating wounds.
- Monitor the CBC for decreases in hemoglobin and hematocrit and increases in WBC measurements.

In hemodynamically stable patients, conservative management of low-grade spleen or liver injuries begins bedrest and making the patient NPO. Serial CBCs are drawn to evaluate for ongoing blood loss or worsening leukocytosis. Serial abdominal exams are performed to evaluate the patient for development of peritoneal signs including tenderness, guarding, and rigidity. Patients declining hemoglobin and hematocrit (H&H) may require blood transfusion, arterial embolization, or surgical intervention to treat the source of blood loss. Placement of a resuscitative endovascular balloon occlusion of the aorta (REBOA) catheter may be indicated for hemorrhage below the diaphragm (Brenner and Hicks, 2018), *Immediate surgery is indicated in patients with abdominal compartment syndrome (ACS), perforated or ischemic bowel, or hemodynamic instability or severe bleeding not amenable to other interventions.*

KEY CLINICAL CONCEPT

- Rapid IV isotonic fluid administration is indicated for patients in shock.
- Blood and blood products may be needed in patients with ongoing blood loss and those who are refractory to crystalloid fluid boluses.

Abdominal Compartment Syndrome

ACS results from intra-abdominal hypertension (IAH). Common causes include abdominal trauma, intestinal edema, ruptured abdominal aortic aneurysm, severe pancreatitis, ascites, and conditions requiring large volume fluid resuscitation (>3 L) and/or blood/blood product administration. *Normal intra-abdominal pressure (IAP) is 0 to 5 mm Hg in healthy people. IAH occurs when IAP is sustained >12 mm Hg.* Ventilated patients with ACS may present with a triad of signs including increased peak inspiratory pressures (PIPs) due to intra-abdominal contents pressing up on the hemidiaphragms, decreased urine output secondary to decreased renal perfusion, and hypotension due to impaired venous blood return to the heart. This elevated IAP decreases organ perfusion and leads to multiorgan failure if left untreated (Kimball, 2021).

Accurate diagnosis requires a high index of suspicion in any patient with a recent history of abdominal surgery, abdominal trauma, or high-volume resuscitation who has a firm, distended abdomen, and exhibits signs of the ACS triad. Bladder pressure measurements are used to confirm a diagnosis of ACS. Bladder pressure measurement is easily performed using aseptic technique with commercially available devices or by using an arterial pressure line attached to an indwelling bladder catheter. To obtain the most precise pressures, clamp the bladder catheter, zero the transducer at the symphysis pubis prior tor to instillation of 25 mL of fluid, and measure pressure at end-expiration. *For patients with abdominal surgery, postoperative IAP may be 10-15 mm Hg. IAP pressures more than 25 mm Hg are suspicious for ACS and require frequent monitoring.* As IAP increases, the patient may become more physiologically unstable. Interventions aimed at lowering IAP are indicated when pressures are increasing or if the patient develops clinically relevant manifestations.

Nonoperative interventions revolve around decreasing intra-abdominal contents to lower IAP. Routine measures include nasogastric and bladder decompression, evacuating stool, draining an intra-abdominal abscess or other fluid collections, fluid volume removal via diuretics or continuous renal replacement therapy (CRRT) as well as maximizing organ perfusion via the administration of vasoactive medications and judicious use of IV fluids (Jacobs et al, 2022).

Improving abdominal wall compliance by placing the patient in reverse Trendelenburg, administering analgesics or neuromuscular blocking agents can also reduce IAP. *Patients with sustained IAH > 25 mm Hg may require operative decompression via decompressive laparotomy.* Visceral herniation through the abdominal incision is diagnostic of ACS. Once the abdomen is opened, IAP decreases, and symptoms dramatically improve. After the end of procedure, temporary abdominal closure with a commercially available negative pressure wound therapy (NPWT) system may be indicated. Within 5 to 7 days, many open abdomens are surgically closed. For those who are unable to undergo closure, mesh placement with subsequent skin grafting is required. After an acceptable period (6–12 months), patients can undergo component separation and abdominal wall reconstruction to remove the large ventral hernia.

KEY CLINICAL CONCEPT

- Ventilated patients with ACS may develop a clinical triad of high PIPs, low urine output, and hypotension.
- Interventions to decompress the stomach and bladder, promote bowel movements, remove excess fluid, promote abdominal wall relaxation, and drain space-occupying lesions such as abscesses should be performed.
- Trend bladder pressures in patients at risk of ACS. Sustained pressures >25 mm Hg may require decompressive laparotomy.

Nursing Intervention

Multiple injured patients are at risk for numerous complications requiring diligent attention to detail to provide excellent nursing care.

- Patients with abdominal injury must be carefully observed for coexisting cardiac and pulmonary injury.

- Signs of pneumothorax, cardiac tamponade, cardiac rupture, and injuries to the aortic or pulmonary vasculature must be assessed.
- Continually assess the patient's hemodynamic and respiratory status. Supplemental oxygen and ventilatory support may be necessary.
- In nonventilated patients, incentive spirometry helps treat atelectasis and prevents pneumonia.
- Replace intravascular fluid to counteract third-spacing and hypovolemic shock. Correct electrolyte abnormalities.
- Bladder pressures measurements are contraindicated in patients with bladder injuries or pelvic hematomas.

A careful abdominal assessment is performed to evaluate injuries. The nurse must assess for rebound tenderness, muscle rigidity, anorexia, nausea, vomiting, abdominal distention, presence of bowel sounds, and pain. Monitor wounds and incisions for erythema, drainage, and other signs of infection. In cases of gross fecal contamination from intestinal injury, midline abdominal incisions are at risk for fascial dehiscence and possible evisceration. Notify the surgical team immediately if wound drainage or tissue separation occurs.

Unless contraindicated, early mobility protocols help critically injured patients recover sooner. Emotional support is important for the patient and family, since GI trauma is usually quite unexpected and coping mechanisms are not readily available.

Toxic Ingestion and Gastrointestinal Tract Injury

Caustic injury to the GI tract is usually produced by strong alkaline (pH >12) or acidic (pH <2) agents. The ingestion of caustic agents can initiate a progressive and devastating injury to the esophagus and stomach. Accidental ingestions are seen in patients who are very young. Teens and adults with suicidal ideations may ingest these substances during suicide attempts.

Acidic solutions usually cause immediate pain and are rapidly expelled. The alkali liquid solutions are often tasteless and odorless. They are swallowed before protective reflexes can be elicited. Alkali solutions penetrate tissue more rapidly than acid solutions do and are more difficult to treat. Caustic injuries to the GI mucosa are classified pathologically in the same manner as skin burns.

Symptoms may be present rapidly after the ingestion. Edema, ulceration, or a white membrane may be present over the palate, uvula, and pharynx. Hoarseness, stridor, dysphagia, epigastric pain, emesis of tissue or blood, tachypnea, and shock may be present. Late symptoms include perforation of the stomach or esophagus, mediastinitis, and peritonitis. Toxic ingestion patients are at high risk for losing their aways. Those with voice changes or an inability to control oral secretions will likely require intubation.

Resuscitation focuses on establishment of an airway, breathing, and maintain circulatory volume. Early treatment includes neutralization of the caustic agent. Consult with your local poison control agency regarding the treatment of unfamiliar toxins. Once the patient is stable, endoscopy should be done within 24–48 hours evaluate the extent of tissue damage and assess the risk of esophageal perforation. If there is perforation, a thoracotomy or laparotomy may be necessary to repair organ injury. Patients may require prolonged PN. The mortality rate after caustic ingestion is 1% to 3%. However, if the patient survives the acute effects of caustic ingestion, the reparative response can result in esophageal and gastric stenosis and an increased incidence of esophageal cancer.

KEY CLINICAL CONCEPT

Toxic ingestion patients are at high risk for losing their airways. Those with voice changes or an inability to control oral secretions will likely require intubation.

Esophageal Perforation

Esophageal perforation is relatively rare, but morbidity and mortality can be as high due to sepsis. Those who present more than 24 hours after the perforation occurs are at highest risk. Full-thickness esophageal perforations can occur from increased pressure in the esophagus that results from forceful vomiting (Boerhaave syndrome), ruptured esophageal diverticula, necrotizing infections, ingestion of caustic agents, and either blunt, penetrating, or iatrogenic esophageal trauma. Esophageal perforation allows GI tract secretions and flora (bacteria and fungi) to enter the mediastinum and/or pleural spaces in the chest cavity. Emergency stenting or surgery with drainage of the affected spaces prevents sepsis, multiorgan failure, and death (Aiolfi et al, 2020).

Symptoms of esophageal perforation vary depending on the location of the perforation. Pain is the most common complaint. If the perforation occurs in the cervical portion of the esophagus, presentation may also include dysphagia. Those that occur in the thoracic esophagus often cause back, chest, or epigastric pain. Odynophagia and/or subcutaneous emphysema may be present.

Diagnosis is made via flexible endoscopy or with water-soluble contrast (Gastrografin) swallowing test. CT scans may not identify all esophageal perforations; however, they are often used to evaluate inflammatory changes and surrounding structures. NGTs should only be inserted during flexible endoscopy. Blindly inserting an NGT may worsen the esophageal injury.

Immediate treatment with fluid volume resuscitation and administration of IV broad-spectrum antibiotics are necessary to prevent septic shock. IV antifungals, such as fluconazole are indicated for distal esophageal injuries. Management of the perforation itself depends on its size and location, as well as the severity of patient symptoms. For micro-perforations, management can include conservative treatment by making the patient NPO and providing total PN. Endoscopic insertion of covered esophageal stents (esophageal exclusion) may be indicated for distal perforations. Esophageal clip placement via endoscopy can be used for smaller perforations. Surgical resection is necessary in cases of full-thickness esophageal perforation, necrosis, or malignancy. Patients with large amounts of contaminated fluid in the mediastinum require either surgical drainage via a thoracotomy, or image-guided insertion of a drainage tube by interventional radiology.

Patients with esophageal perforations may be NPO for a protracted period of type while the perforated area heals. Nutrition is delivered by either PN or jejunal EN. Nursing care includes maintaining adequate fluid volume status, providing wound care, and monitoring for resolution of fever, leukocytosis, and other signs of sepsis.

KEY CLINICAL CONCEPT

Patients with esophageal perforations require immediate treatment with fluid volume resuscitation and administration of IV broad-spectrum antibiotics to prevent septic shock.

KEY CONTENT CHECKLIST

- ❒ AMI is associated with the sudden onset of severe abdominal pain that is out of proportion to the patient's abdominal exam. The pain is typically located on the left side, periumbilical area, or epigastrium.
- ❒ Regardless of the etiology, AMI requires prompt identification and treatment to prevent infarction.
- ❒ Generally, patients with AMI have leukocytosis, metabolic acidosis, and elevated lactic acid levels. However, these lab values may be normal early during an acute episode.
- ❒ CTA of the abdomen and pelvis are often preferred when evaluating patients for AMI as they not only assess for vascular occlusion but can also diagnose other signs of ischemia including bowel wall edema or intramural hemorrhage.
- ❒ Weight loss, pain after eating, and fear of food are common signs of CMI.
- ❒ Controlling comorbidities such as HLD, HTN, and DM, and lifestyle modifications such as diet, exercise, and tobacco cessation are key to preventing CMI progression.
- ❒ Patients who undergo stenting require dual-antiplatelet therapy (DAPT) for 3 to 12 months to prevent stent stenosis.
- ❒ Free air under the diaphragm on abdominal x-ray is very suspicious for GI tract perforation. A CT of the abdomen and pelvis may be performed to locate and evaluate the perforation prior to surgery.
- ❒ Esophageal surgery patients are at high risk for pulmonary and GI complications. Monitor for leukocytosis, fever, and other signs of sepsis.
- ❒ Bariatric surgery patients require vitamin and mineral supplementation to prevent deficiencies.
- ❒ LRYGB patients are at risk of dumping syndrome from ingestion of simple sugars. Dumping syndrome results in GI symptoms, tachycardia, hypotension, and late hypoglycemia.
- ❒ Rapid IV isotonic fluid administration is indicated for abdominal trauma patients in shock.
- ❒ Blood and blood products may be needed in patients with ongoing blood loss and those who are refractory to crystalloid fluid boluses.
- ❒ Ventilated patients with ACS may develop a clinical triad of high PIPs, low urine output, and hypotension.
- ❒ Interventions to decompress the stomach and bladder, promote bowel movements, remove excess fluid, promote abdominal wall relaxation, and drain space-occupying lesions such as abscesses should be performed when IAP >12 mm Hg.
- ❒ Trend bladder pressures in patients at risk of ACS. Sustained pressures >25 mm Hg may require decompressive laparotomy.
- ❒ Toxic ingestion patients are at high risk for losing their aways. Those with voice changes or an inability to control oral secretions will likely require intubation.
- ❒ Patients with esophageal perforations require immediate treatment with fluid volume resuscitation and administration of IV broad-spectrum antibiotics to prevent septic shock.
- ❒ Know the difference between an SBO and a Large Bowel Obstruction (LBO).
- ❒ SBO patients suffer from nausea, vomiting (sometimes fecal matter), less likely to have distention, and are treated with IV fluids and decompression.
- ❒ LBO patients are LESS likely to have nausea, less vomiting, more distention, and treatment usually does NOT require an NGT. This patient often does not appear as ill (compared to SBO patient).
- ❒ As a result, the difference between SBO vs. LBO may be remembered by thinking that the LBO is less labor-intensive from a nursing care standpoint.
- ❒ Kehr sign is left shoulder pain that is referred from either splenic rupture or hemidiaphragm injury.

Review Questions:

1. A patient who underwent endoscopy for evaluation of a suspected upper GI bleed a few hours ago is reporting dysphagia and odynophagia. Vital signs are T 101.8, HR 125, BP 89/46 mm Hg, RR 26. Oxygen saturations are 90% on room air. After assessing the air way and notifying the medical team, the nurse should anticipate which of the following interventions?

a. Intubation and antibiotics for pneumonia
b. Fluid resuscitation, antibiotics, and CT scan
c. Pain control, NPO, and swallow evaluation
d. Blood transfusion and repeat endoscopy

Answer: B. Rationale: The patient in this scenario has likely experienced an iatrogenic esophageal perforation during endoscopy. Fluid resuscitation and broad-spectrum antibiotics are indicated to prevent septic shock. CT chest/abdomen/pelvis is needed to diagnose the perforation and help with surgical planning. A is incorrect, as the patient does not have symptoms of pneumonia such as cough or shortness of breath and has an oxygen saturation of 90% without supplemental oxygen. C is incorrect as a swallow evaluation is contraindicated in cases of expected esophageal perforation.

2. **A patient with a history of IBD and colon resection is post-op day 2 s/p hip surgery. The patient developed severe, diffuse abdominal pain with guarding and rebound tenderness. Vital signs are T 98.7, HR 102, BP 110/65 mm Hg, RR 21. Oxygen saturations are 98% on room air. A stat abdominal radiograph demonstrates free air under the diaphragm. Which of the following interventions should the nurse anticipate?**
   a. Prepare the patient for surgery to repair a perforated viscus.
   b. Insert an NGT to treat a small bowel obstruction.
   c. Insert an NGT and measure bladder pressure.
   d. Make the patient NPO and administer IV antiemetics.

Answer: A. Rationale:. The patient in this scenario has peritoneal signs and free air under the diaphragm on abdominal imaging, which indicates a perforated viscus. B is not correct as the patient's symptoms and exam findings aren't consistent with a bowel obstruction. C is not correct as the patient doesn't have risk factors or physical exam findings of abdominal compartment syndrome. Although making the patient NPO is part of preparing for surgery, the patient didn't have nausea or vomiting, making an antiemetic unnecessary.

REFERENCES

Aiolfi A, Micheletto G, Guerrazzi G, et al. Minimally invasive surgical management of Boerhaave's syndrome: a narrative literature review. *J Thorac Dis.* 2020;12(8):4411–4417. doi: 10.21037/jtd-20-1020.

Bala M, Kashuk J, Moore EM, et al. Acute mesenteric ischemia: guidelines of the World Society of Emergency Surgery. *World J Emerg Surg.* 2017;12:38. doi: 10.1186/s13017-017-0150-5.

Brenner M, & Hicks C. Major abdominal trauma: critical decisions and new frontiers in management. *Emerg Med Clin North Am.* 2018;36(1):149–160. doi: 10.1016/j.emc.2017.08.012.

Brown AM, Pucci MJ, Berger AC, et al. A standardized comparison of peri-operative complications after minimally invasive esophagectomy: Ivor Lewis versus McKeown. *Surg Endosc.* 2018;32(1):204–211. doi: 10.1007/s00464-017-5660-4.

Catena F, De Simone B, Coccolini F, Di Saverio S, Sartelli M, Ansaloni L. Bowel obstruction: a narrative review for all physicians. *World J Emerg Surg.* 2019;14(20). doi: 10.1186/s13017-019-0240-7.

Gnanapandithan K, & Feuerstadt P. Review article: mesenteric ischemia. *Curr Gastroenterol Rep.* 2020;22(4):17. doi: 10.1007/s11894-020-0754-x.

Hoshi H. Management of gastric adenocarcinoma for general surgeons. *Surg Clin North Am.* (2020);100(3):523–534. doi: 10.1016/j.suc.2020.02.004.

Hoffman RS, Burns MM, Gosselin S. Ingestion of caustic substances. *N Engl J Med.* 2020;382(18):1739 1748. doi: 10.1056/NEJMra1810769.

Huber TS, Bjorck M, Chandra A, et al. Chronic mesenteric ischemia: clinical practice guidelines for the Society for Vascular Surgery. *J Vasc Surg.* 2021;73(1S):87S–115S. doi: 10.1016/j.jvs.2020.10.029.

Jacobs R, Wise RD, Myatchin I, et al. Fluid management, intra-abdominal hypertension and the abdominal compartment syndrome: a narrative review. Life (Basel). 2022;12(9):1390. doi: 10.3390/life12091390.

Kelly RJ. Emerging multimodality approaches to treat localized esophageal cancer. *J Natl Compr Canc Netw.* 2019;17(8):1009–1014. doi: 10.6004/jnccn.2019.7337.

Kimball EJ. Intra-abdominal hypertension and abdominal compartment syndrome: a current review. *Curr Opin Crit Care.* 2021;27(2):164–168. doi: 10.1097/MCC.0000000000000797.

Kumar S, Mukkamalla R, Recio-Boiles A, Babkiker HM. Esophageal cancer. StatPearls [Internet]. 2022a. https://www.ncbi.nlm.nih.gov/books/NBK459267/.

Kumar S, Mukkamalla R, Recio-Boiles A, Babkiker HM. Gastric cancer. StatPearls [Internet]. 2022b. https://www.ncbi.nlm.nih.gov/books/NBK459142/.

Moris D, Paulson EK, Pappas TN. Diagnosis and management of acute appendicitis in adults: a review. *JAMA.* 2021;326(22):2299–2311. doi: 10.1001/jama.2021.20502.

Shin D, Rahimi H, Haroon S, et al. Imaging of gastrointestinal tract perforation. *Radiol Clin North Am.* 2020;58(1):19–44. doi: 10.1016/j.rcl.2019.08.004.

Schulman AR, Thompson CC. Complications of bariatric surgery: what you can expect to see in your GI practice. *Am J Gastroenterol.* 2017;112(11):1640–1655. doi: 10.1038/ajg.2017.241.

Tabesh MR, Maleklou F, Ejtehadi F, Alizadeh Z. Nutrition, physical activity, and prescription of supplements in pre- and post-bariatric surgery patients: a practical guideline. *Obes Surg.* 2019;29(10):3385–3400. doi: 10.1007/s11695-019-04112-y.

Tempero MA. NCCN guidelines updates: pancreatic cancer. *J Natl Compr Canc Netw.* 2019;17(5.5):603–605. doi: 10.6004/jnccn.2019.5007.

Vogel JD, Felder SI, Bhama AR, et al. The American Society of Colon and Rectal Surgeons Clinical Practice Guidelines for the Management of Colon Cancer. *Dis Colon Rectum.* 2022;5(2):148–177. doi: 10.1097/DCR.0000000000002323.

Watkins AA, Kent MS, Wilson JL. Surgical adjuncts during esophagectomy. *Thorac Surg Clin.* 2020;30(3):315–320. doi: 10.1016/j.thorsurg.2020.04.009.

Zhang L, Sanagapalli S, Stoita A. Challenges in diagnosis of pancreatic cancer. *World J Gastroenterol.* 2018;24(19):2047–2060. doi: 10.3748/wjg.v24.i19.2047.

41

Management of the Patient with a Gastrointestinal Disturbance

CHAPTER OVERVIEW AND OBJECTIVES

This chapter provides an overview of general nursing interventions for patients with any type of gastrointestinal (GI) disturbance, including the conditions previously discussed in Chapters 38 through 40. Priority interventions include measures to maintain fluid and electrolyte balance, ensure adequate nutritional intake, maintain bowel elimination, maintain comfort, and prevent infection. The chapter concludes with a summary of physical assessment steps in assessing the GI system.

After studying this chapter, you should understand the following:

- Risk factors for and nursing management of fluid and electrolyte imbalance in patients requiring enteral or parenteral nutrition.
- Safe initiation of enteral nutrition, assessment of nutritional status, and evaluation for potential complications.
- Interventions to prevent infection in patients receiving enteral or parenteral nutrition.

41.1 INTERVENTIONS TO MAINTAIN FLUID AND ELECTROLYTE BALANCE

Fluid and electrolyte balance are necessary for normal organ function and recovery from acute and critical illness. Common issues such as emesis, gastrointestinal decompression, and diarrhea often contribute to hypovolemia, electrolyte disturbances, and metabolic acidosis or alkalosis, depending on the amount and source of the fluid loss.

1. Maintenance of accurate intake and output. Include number, character, amount, and site of GI fluid losses.
2. Monitoring of serum electrolytes per laboratory data. Excessive GI fluid losses through tube suction, ostomy drainage, diarrhea, and vomiting can lead to metabolic acidosis, alkalosis (loss of H^+ and Cl^-) and hypokalemia.
3. Correct use of GI tubes for decompression and diagnosis. No matter which type of tube is used, it is important to place the suction port to low, intermittent wall suction to prevent gastric injury. Frequently monitor for blockages in the tubing. Assess volume, color, and consistency of evacuated fluid.
   a. Short tubes, used for the stomach and duodenum. Example: nasogastric tubes.
      i. Levin (single-lumen tube): This single-lumen tube is approximately 4-ft long and has openings at various points to allow for passage of diagnostic equipment. It is often used for gastric lavage, but can also be used for enteral feeding.
      ii. Salem sump (double-lumen tube): This is the most widely used type because the second lumen is open to air and acts as a vent. This provides continuous irrigation of the drainage tube with air.
   b. Long tubes. These are intended to extend the length of the small bowel.
      i. Miller–Abbott: This is a double-lumen tube that has a balloon near the tip. It is used for removing intestinal contents and decompressing small bowel obstructions.
      ii. Cantor: This is a 10-ft long, single-lumen tube with mercury in its tip. It is used for intestinal decompression.

4. Administer antiemetics to relieve nausea and vomiting.
   a. Monitor for abdominal distention. Nasogastric tube decompression may be indicated for worsening distention associated with an ileus or small bowel obstruction.
   b. Monitor emesis for amount, color, frequency, and the presence of blood.
   c. If patient is vomiting, place the patient in a side-lying position to prevent aspiration.

41.2 ASSESSING AND MAINTAINING NUTRITIONAL STATUS

Patients in the intensive care unit who are unable to eat must be fed enterally or parenterally. The number of calories and protein required vary depending on the underlying condition. For instance, burn and polytrauma patients often have higher protein-calorie requirements due to catabolism. Patients with preexisting poor nutrition may also have different nutritional needs. Assessing the patient's nutritional status prior to the hospitalization is important in determining the type of nutrition needed. Clinicians commonly order laboratory indicators of protein malnutrition, such as prealbumin and transferrin levels. Unfortunately, these are not useful in patients with critical illness or liver disease. The European Society of Parenteral and Enteral Nutrition (ESPEN) recommends using updated indirect calorimetry (IC) every 3 to 5 days to accurately identify nutritional needs in critically ill patients receiving enteral nutrition (EN) (Singer et al, 2019) (**Table 41-1**).

Enteral Nutrition

A person who has a functioning GI tract but has dysphagia or is unable to eat (eg, endotracheal intubation), or who is not eating adequate amounts of food may be a candidate for EN. **EN is preferred over PN, since it is associated with less non-infectious complications and shorter hospital length of stays.** EN should routinely be administered into the stomach (gastric feeds). Post-pyloric feeds are used when medically necessary (eg, post-esophagectomy, etc), and in cases concerning for aspiration. ESPEN recommends 1.5 to 2 g of protein/kg/day for critically ill adults who are candidates for full-dose (also known as goal rate) feeds (Singer et al, 2019).

TABLE 41-1. DEFINITIONS

Early enteral nutrition (EEN): Enteral nutrition started within 48 hours of intensive care unit admission.

Energy expenditure (EE): The amount of energy required for the body to function. EE is produced from the metabolism of protein, fats, and carbohydrates. This process consumes O_2 and produces CO_2.

Full-dose: Enteral nutrition administered at the calculated goal rate.

Gastric: Enteral nutrition delivered to stomach. This is the standard route for enteral nutrition, unless contraindicated.

Hypocaloric enteral nutrition: EN providing <70% of goal caloric intake.

Indirect calorimetry (IC): Method of assessing nutritional needs in critically ill patients via exhaled respiratory gases via a metabolic cart machine. IC measures energy expenditure by evaluating the amount of O_2 consumed or CO_2 produced.

Post-pyloric: Enteral nutrition delivered to either the duodenum or jejunum.

Trophic: Enteral nutrition administered between 10–20 mL/h.

Enteral feeding intolerance (EFI): May occur from delayed gastric emptying or ileus resulting in emesis, gastric residual volume (GRV) >500 mL/6 h, or abdominal pain or distention. Diarrhea signals decreased EN absorption.

Enteral Feed Formulations

Polymeric formulas are the most commonly used. They contain higher molecular weight proteins, carbohydrates, and fats. A person must be able to digest and absorb nutrients without difficulty using this type of formula. Standard formulas are typically isotonic solutions that contain 1 kcal/mL. They are typically well-tolerated when administered into the stomach. These formulas have about 75% free water. Most patients may require the administration of additional free water to maintain adequate fluid balance. Energy-dense formulas (>1 kcal/mL) have less volume and are typically prescribed for patients who can't tolerate full-dose isotonic feeds and those on fluid restrictions (Preiser et al, 2021).

Monomeric formulas are used infrequently. They contain smaller molecules of protein, fat, and carbohydrates. These were previously referred to as semi-elemental or elemental. However, the preferred term is "predigested." Instead of protein molecules, these formulas are comprised of peptides. They are typically prescribed for patients who have issues with nutrient malabsorption or enteral feeding intolerance (EFI).

Insertion of Oro or Nasoenteric Feeding Tubes

The American Association of Critical Care Nurses (AACN) recommends using two of the following methods of clinical assessment of feeding tube location during insertion: Observing for signs of respiratory distress, use capnography to assess for color changes, evaluate the characteristics of the aspirated fluid and/or test the fluid's pH, if test strips are available. **Auscultation of an air bolus is unreliable for determining location of enteral tubes. Once the tube is inserted, an abdominal radiograph should be done prior to initiating parenteral feeding. Abdominal X-ray is the only 100% accurate, "gold standard" method of assessing feeding tube placement (AACN, 2020).**

Initiating Enteral Nutrition

Historically, EN has been thought to increase gut oxygen demand potentially leading to bowel ischemia in shock patients. *Recent studies have shown that it is safe to begin early EN (EEN) [within 48-hours] on shock patients* who have been adequately resuscitated, including those requiring low (<0.1 μg/kg/min) or moderate (0.1–0.3 μg/kg/min) of norepinephrine. EEN significantly decreased 28-day mortality compared to late EN (LEN) in the low and moderate norepinephrine groups. Unfortunately, there was no difference in mortality in patients receiving EEN or LEN while on high doses of norepinephrine (>0.3 mg/kg/min) (Singer et al, 2019; Preiser et al, 2021).

For resuscitated shock patients and those with vasopressor requirements, ESPEN recommends using trophic feeds at 10 to 20 mL/h to decrease the risk of tube feeding intolerance. The NUTRIREA-2 trial showed that aggressive EEN (titration to goal rate within 24 hours) lead to increases in bowel ischemia and acute colonic pseudo-obstruction. To prevent these complications, feeds should be titrated to full dose over 48 hours for hemodynamically stable patients. ESPEN recommends starting full-dose EN by 7 days in all critically ill patients (Singer et al, 2019).

Refeeding syndrome (RFS) is a potentially fatal complication of EN that can occur within the first 5 days of EN. Malnourished patients are at higher risk of developing it. RFS develops when the body stops using fat and protein for energy (catabolism) and starts metabolizing the carbohydrates supplied by the EN (anabolism). Carbohydrate ingestion increases the amount of insulin secreted by the pancreas, which subsequently lowers serum levels of thiamine, magnesium, potassium, and phosphorous by moving them into cells (Ponzo et al, 2021). Employing hypocaloric (<500 kcal/day) feedings, administering thiamine, and monitoring and repleting phosphorous levels in the first 3 days of EN decreases the risk of developing RFS (Preiser et al, 2021).

KEY CLINICAL CONCEPT

- Although it is important to clinically assess a patient during naso or orogastric tube insertion, an abdominal X-ray confirming tube placement is necessary to safely initiate enteral feeds.
- Hypocaloric EN combined with thiamine administration and correcting hypophosphatemia may prevent the development of refeeding syndrome.

Nursing Care of Patients Receiving Enteral Nutrition

For patients receiving enteral nutrition, follow hospital policy and manufacturer recommendations. Change feeding containers (or bag) and tubing, at least daily. Flush tube with 50 to 100 mL of water before and after each feeding to maintain patency. Minimize feeding interruptions to ensure adequate caloric intake. Monitor intake and output in addition to laboratory data, such as serum electrolytes and glucose.

Potential Complications of Enteral Feeding. Although EN is beneficial, it is not without potential complications. Monitor for signs of EFI such as abdominal distention or pain, nausea, passage of stool or flatus. Check residual amounts of feeds in stomach. Follow hospital policy regarding high tube feed residuals. *ESPEN does not recommend routinely holding feeds for gastric residual volumes (GRVs) less than 500 mL in patients who do not have any other signs of feeding intolerance* (Singer et al, 2019). *Patients with GRV's >500 mL/6 h may benefit from a lower volume of EN and/or the use of laxatives or promotility agents to promote gastric emptying* (Preiser et al, 2021).

Diarrhea is common with EN. Its potential etiologies include bacterial contamination of the product and lactose intolerance in patients receiving lactose-containing formulas. Hypertonic, energy-dense formulas cause diarrhea by drawing increased fluid into the intestinal lumen. Nurses should monitor for signs of infectious diarrhea and notify providers for further investigation and treatment. Intravascular volume depletion occurs because of diarrhea, inadequate fluid administration, or third-spacing of intravascular fluid.

Patients receiving EN are at risk for "*micro aspirating*" stomach contents and developing aspiration pneumonitis or aspiration pneumonia. **Preventative measures include keeping the head of bed (HOB) elevated 30 to 45 degrees**, frequently checking tube placement, and assessing and promptly intervening for EFI. Hyperglycemia is common with enteral nutrition formulas high in carbohydrates. Blood glucose checks every 4 to 6 h along with the administration of long- or short-acting insulin will help restore normoglycemia.

KEY CLINICAL CONCEPT

Patients receiving EN should have the HOB elevated 30 to 45 degrees and be assessed for enteral EFI (GRV > 500 mL/6 h) to prevent aspiration pneumonitis and aspiration pneumonia.

Parenteral Nutrition

Parenteral nutrition (PN) is a hypertonic mixture of dextrose, amino acids, electrolytes, vitamins, and trace minerals. PN is administered to patients who are unable to take oral or enteral feeds due to trauma, surgery, protracted ileus, difficulty with intestinal nutrient absorption, intestinal fistula, and those who need additional nutritional support (Katoue, 2018). Due to the risk of infectious complications, ESPEN recommends starting PN within 3 to 5 days for patients at risk of nutritional deficiencies and who are unexpected to achieve >60% of their goal caloric intake from EN. A recent study showed supplemental use of early PN (post-op day 3) decreased nosocomial infections compared to late supplemental PN (post-op day 8) in abdominal surgery patients (Gao et al, 2022). Lipid emulsions are often given in conjunction with dextrose-based PN solutions 2 to 3 days per week to prevent essential fatty acid deficiencies. *Thiamine administration prevents Wernicke's encephalopathy* (Katoue, 2018).

Peripheral administration of PN is not recommended since it can lead to venous thrombosis. Only administer PN with dextrose concentrations ≥20% through central venous access. When initiating PN in malnourished patients, evaluate for signs of RFS (Katoue, 2018). In patients who are on PN, monitor intake and output, serum electrolytes, hepatic function tests, triglycerides, and white blood cell (WBC) counts. Assess for signs of complications from PN, including bacteremia, acalculous *cholecystitis,* fluid-volume overload intravascular volume depletion, and glucose or electrolyte imbalances. Acalculous cholecystitis can occur in patients who are *nil per os* (NPO) due to lack of gallbladder contraction and emptying. *Signs and symptoms may include right upper quadrant pain, nausea, vomiting, fever, and leukocytosis.* Fluid volume overload is another potential adverse effect of PN. Evaluate for signs of fluid volume overload such as rapid weight gain, peripheral edema, crackles or rales during lung auscultation, and jugular venous distention (JVD). Check serum glucose at least every 4 h. It may be necessary to administer subcutaneous or IV insulin depending on the blood sugar levels and if the patient has diabetes mellitus. *Monitor serum glucose every 1 h if patient is on an insulin infusion. Hypoglycemia can occur from excessive insulin administration or if PN therapy is interrupted.* Electrolyte disturbances: Monitor electrolytes frequently for patients on IV fluids, total parenteral nutrition (TPN), enteral nutrition, and those with naso or orogastric tube drainage. Maintain appropriate concentrations.

KEY CLINICAL CONCEPT

- Assess for signs of complications from PN, including refeeding syndrome, bacteremia, acalculous cholecystitis, fluid-volume overload, intravascular volume depletion, and glucose or electrolyte imbalances.

41.3 INTERVENTIONS TO MAINTAIN BOWEL ELIMINATION STATUS

1. Diarrhea
   a. Identify causative factors.
   b. Record color, amount, and frequency of stools.
   c. Maintain intake and output to prevent dehydration.
   d. Monitor serum electrolytes.
   e. Check for blood in stools.
   f. Administer antidiarrheal medications to decrease intestinal motility if there are no contraindications, such as in untreated *Clostridium difficile*-associated diarrhea.
   g. Begin nutritional supplement.
   h. Protect skin with barrier creams or use a stool collection system.
2. Constipation
   a. Increase fluid intake if not contraindicated.
   b. Monitor frequency and consistency of stools.
   c. Administer laxatives orally, per tube, or rectally if not contraindicated.

41.4 INTERVENTIONS TO MAINTAIN COMFORT STATUS

1. Pain: Onset, aggravating factors, alleviating factors, severity, characteristics, radiation.
   a. Observe for signs and location of pain.
   b. Administer analgesics and monitor their effectiveness.

41.5 INTERVENTIONS TO PREVENT INFECTION

1. Monitor temperature and WBC counts to detect the presence of infection.
2. Use aseptic technique when changing central venous access device dressings and make sure that dressings remain intact.
3. Use standard precautions prior to potential exposure to blood and body fluids.
4. Assess sources of contamination. Culture infected drainage and blood.
5. Use good handwashing techniques to prevent cross contamination.
6. *Elevate head of bed 30 degrees to 45 degrees, if not contraindicated to prevent aspiration.*
7. In patients who are intubated or who have a tracheostomy, brush the patient's teeth every 12 h and use chlorhexidine oral swabs or rinse twice daily, in addition to routine oral care to prevent pneumonia.

KEY CLINICAL CONCEPTS

- Wash hands before patient and contact to prevent infection.
- Use aseptic technique when changing central venous access device dressings and make sure that dressings remain intact to prevent catheter-associated bloodstream infections.
- Oral care with chlorhexidine gluconate and twice daily teeth brushing helps prevent pneumonia in patients who are intubated or have tracheostomies.

41.6 PHYSICAL ASSESSMENT

Physical assessment of the GI system can be briefly summarized by following steps listed below:

1. Begin the assessment with inspection of the abdomen. Do not begin palpation, particularly deep palpation, until the last phase of assessment. This will avoid any stimulation of the GI system and the initiation of painful stimuli.
2. Auscultation is the second phase of assessment. Bowel sounds are usually heard in all four abdominal quadrants. Observe for a change in sounds or bowel sound intensity and character. Bowel sounds are heard during intestinal contraction; however, they are not always reliable in assessing intestinal function.
3. Percussion is the third step in assessment. Usually, the GI tract has air present and will result in hearing a resonant or hyperresonant sound. Tympanic sounds are normal over the gastric air bubble. However, the presence of a diffusely tympanic abdomen may signal an ileus or bowel obstruction.
4. Palpation, both superficial and deep, is the last phase of assessment. The goals of palpation are to detect masses, assess for abnormal organ size, such as liver or spleen enlargement, and to determine whether pain, tenderness, rebound, or guarding are present.

KEY CONTENT CHECKLIST

- ❐ Although it is important to clinically assess a patient during naso or orogastric tube insertion, an abdominal x-ray confirming tube placement is necessary to safely initiate enteral feeds (**"gold standard" method of assessing feeding tube placement)**
- ❐ Hypocaloric EN combined with thiamine administration and correcting hypophosphatemia may prevent the development of refeeding syndrome.
- ❐ Patients receiving enteral nutrition should have the HOB elevated 30 to 45 degrees and be assessed for enteral feeding intolerance (GRV > 500 mL/6 h) to prevent aspiration pneumonitis and aspiration pneumonia.
- ❐ Assess for signs of complications from PN, including refeeding syndrome, bacteremia, acalculous cholecystitis, fluid-volume overload, intravascular volume depletion, and glucose or electrolyte imbalances.
- ❐ Wash hands before patient and after patient contact to prevent infection.
- ❐ Use aseptic technique when changing central venous access device dressings and make sure that dressings remain intact to prevent catheter-associated bloodstream infections.
- ❐ Oral care with chlorhexidine gluconate and twice daily teeth brushing helps prevent pneumonia in patients who are intubated or have tracheostomies.
- ❐ Begin the abdominal assessment with inspection of the abdomen. Do not begin palpation, particularly deep palpation, until the last phase of assessment. This will avoid any stimulation of the GI system and the initiation of painful stimuli (the correct order is Inspection, Auscultation, Percussion, and then Palpation).
- ❐ EN is preferred over PN, since it is associated with less noninfectious complications and shorter hospital length of stays.

Review Question:

1. A patient has bleeding esophageal and gastric varies that continued bleeding despite catheter-based interventions. A Sengstaken–Blakemore tube was placed. The patient's oxygen saturation has decreased to 75% on 2 L nasal cannula. Which of the following is the most urgent intervention?

a. Checking pressure in the esophageal and gastric balloons
b. Assessing airway patency
c. Ensuring that the tube has enough traction
d. Assessing for aspiration pneumonitis

Answer: B. Rationale: Assessing airway patency should occur prior to checking balloon pressures.

REFERENCES

American Association of Critical Care Nurses. (2020). Initial and Ongoing Verification of Feeding Tube Placement in Adults, 2020 update. Available at: https://www.aacn.org/clinical-resources/practice-alerts/initial-and-ongoing-verification-of-feeding-tube-placement-in-adults. Accessed October 7, 2022.

Gao X, Liu Y, Zhang L, et al. Effect of early vs late supplemental parenteral nutrition in patients undergoing abdominal surgery: a randomized clinical trial. *JAMA Surg.* 2022;157(5):384–393. doi:10.1001/jamasurg.2022.0269.

Katoue MG. Role of pharmacists in providing parenteral nutrition support: current insights and future directions. *Integr Pharm Res Pract.* 2018;7:125–140. doi: 10.2147/IPRP.S117118.

Mealie CA, Ali R, Manthey DE. *Abdominal Exam.* StatPearls [Internet]. Treasure Island (FL): StatPearls Publishing; 2021. Available at: https://pubmed.ncbi.nlm.nih.gov/29083767/

Methany NA. Monitoring adult patients for intolerance to gastric tube feedings. *Am J Nurs.* 2021;121(8):35–43. doi: 10.1097/01.NAJ.0000767356.16777.f1.

Ponzo V, Pellegrini M, Cioffi I, Scaglione L, Bo S. The refeeding syndrome: a neglected but potentially serious condition for inpatients. A narrative review. *Inter Emerg Med.* 2021;16(1):49–60. doi: 10.1007/s11739-020-02525-7.

Preiser JC, Arabi YM, Berger MM, et al. A guide to enteral nutrition in intensive care units: 10 expert tips for the daily practice. *Crit Care.* 2021;25:424. doi: 10.1186/s13054-021-03847-4.

Singer P, Blaser AR, Berger MM, et al. ESPEN guideline on clinical nutrition in the intensive care unit. *Clin Nutr.* 2019;38:48–79. doi: 10.1016/j.clnu.2018.08.037.

Wischmeyer P. Overcoming challenges to enteral nutrition delivery in critical care. *Curr Opin Crit Care.* 2021;27(2):169–176.doi: 10.1097/MCC.0000000000000801.

PART VI
Gastroenterology Practice Exam

1. **Atropine, an anticholinergic agent, would cause which of the following physical symptoms by blocking the effects of acetylcholine?**
   (A) increased salivary flow
   (B) hypothermia
   (C) increased heart rate
   (D) decreased respiratory rate
2. **Kehr's sign in a patient with blunt abdominal trauma mostly likely indicates a:**
   (A) bowel injury
   (B) ruptured kidney
   (C) ruptured bladder
   (D) diaphragm injury
3. **Which lab results are most likely in a patient with acute pancreatitis?**
   (A) elevated alkaline phosphatase, elevated bilirubin, decreased glucose
   (B) decreased serum amylase, elevated calcium, elevated glucose
   (C) elevated amylase, decreased total protein, decreased calcium
   (D) elevated total protein, decreased calcium, decreased INR
4. **A patient has an acute GI bleed. Gastroenterology consult is pending. BP is 81/49, HR 125 sinus tachycardia. They have +1 pulses and skin is cool and clammy. Based on this information, the RN should prepare to *initially* administer:**
   (A) 5% dextrose in water at 100 mL/h
   (B) 0.9% saline 20 mL/kg IV bolus
   (C) phenylephrine (Neo-Synephrine) infusion
   (D) vasopressin infusion
5. **A patient is in hemorrhagic shock after a penetrating liver injury. Which of the following is a compensatory mechanism for hemorrhage?**
   (A) fluid shift from the intravascular space to the extracellular space
   (B) peripheral vasodilatation
   (C) increased reabsorption of sodium and water
   (D) decreased stroke volume
6. **Which of the following signs are associated with hemorrhagic pancreatitis?**
   (A) Cullen's sign
   (B) livedo reticularis
   (C) cutis marmorata
   (D) Roth spots
7. **Total gastrectomy would cause the patient to lose which function?**
   (A) ability to secrete glucagon
   (B) bile production
   (C) vitamin B_{12} synthesis
   (D) regulation of chloride and bicarbonate
8. **A patient is discharged with a percutaneous gastric (PEG) tube in place. Several weeks later, he is admitted to your unit with confusion. Labs reveal hypochloremia and hypokalemia. The family states that they have been checking the tube feed residuals frequently but not reinstilling the residual into the G tube. Given this information, which of the following acid–base disorders would you expect?**
   (A) metabolic acidosis
   (B) metabolic alkalosis
   (C) respiratory alkalosis
   (D) respiratory acidosis
9. **Which substance will increase the production of hydrochloric acid?**
   (A) histamine
   (B) atropine
   (C) bicarbonate
   (D) potassium salts
10. **Ranitidine acts to reduce acid secretion by inhibiting the production of which substance?**
   (A) histamine
   (B) gastrin
   (C) acetylcholine
   (D) calcium
11. **What is the purpose of the intrinsic factor, produced by parietal cells in the stomach?**
   (A) promotes absorption of vitamin K
   (B) promotes absorption of vitamin B_{12}
   (C) increases utilization of vitamin C
   (D) synthesizes vitamin D with calcium
12. **The normal pH of the stomach falls within which of the following ranges?**
   (A) 0
   (B) 1 to 3
   (C) 6
   (D) more than 7
13. **In which part of the GI system is pepsinogen initially produced?**
   (A) mouth
   (B) esophagus
   (C) stomach
   (D) small intestine

14. Which of the following is the most accurate definition of chyme?
(A) a lipoprotein secreted in the stomach that aids in fat digestion
(B) gastric cells responsible for negating excessive hydrochloric acid secretion
(C) a hormone necessary for reducing the desire to eat
(D) a semiliquid mass of food

15. Gastrin secretion causes which of the following effects?
(A) increased desire to eat
(B) inhibited desire to eat
(C) production of vitamin B_{12}
(D) increased production of hydrochloric acid

16. Which of the following is a function of cholecystokinin?
(A) breaks down protein
(B) stimulates gastric emptying
(C) stimulates duodenal catabolism of carbohydrates
(D) stimulates release of bile from the gallbladder

17. Which of the following is a nonselective beta blocker that may decrease portal pressure in patients with cirrhosis?
(A) metoprolol (Lopressor)
(B) bisoprolol (Zebeta)
(C) nebivolol (Bystolic)
(D) propranolol (Inderal)

18. A patient presents with "gnawing" right upper quadrant pain × 4 h. The pain started after they ate a large fatty meal. Over-the-counter analgesics and simethicone have not helped. Physical exam reveals tenderness, rebound tenderness, and guarding in the right upper quadrant. Which of the following is likely the cause of the patient's pain?
(A) acute pancreatitis
(B) right hemidiaphragm injury
(C) acute cholecystitis
(D) chronic mesenteric ischemia

19. A patient has a small bowel obstruction, which is being treated medically. The nasogastric tube output has been 2400 mL over the last 24 h. Which electrolyte disturbances can occur in a patient with excessive nasogastric tube output?
(A) hyperkalemia
(B) hypokalemia
(C) hyponatremia
(D) hypermagnesemia

20. Besides mental status change, which of the following is the earliest clinical sign of impending hypovolemic shock?
(A) urine output of less than 0.5 mL/kg/h
(B) urine output more than 3 mL/kg/h
(C) sinus tachycardia more than 130 bpm
(D) systolic blood pressure less than 85 mm Hg

21. Which of the following enzymes is NOT secreted by the pancreas?
(A) pepsinogen
(B) trypsinogen
(C) lipase
(D) amylase

22. A stroke patient is aphasic and hemiplegic. The physician orders a small-bore feeding tube placed. What is the most accurate way to verify the position of the tube before initiating enteral feeds?
(A) auscultation
(B) abdominal radiograph
(C) gastric pH is more than 6
(D) aspirated gastric content appears light brown

23. Which of the following enzymes is active in the digestion of proteins?
(A) amylase
(B) maltose
(C) lipase
(D) trypsin

24. A septic patient on norepinephrine and vasopressin infusions is complaining of severe abdominal pain around the umbilicus. On exam, the abdomen is soft, mildly tender in all quadrants, nondistended, and hypoactive bowel sounds are present. Which of the following conditions is most likely to be present?
(A) acute mesenteric ischemia
(B) acute cholecystitis
(C) acute pancreatitis
(D) perforated viscous

25. Which of the following enzymes is active in the digestion of carbohydrates?
(A) amylase
(B) pepsin
(C) lipase
(D) trypsin

26. Emulsification (dispersion into small droplets) of fat occurs because of which substance?
(A) chyme
(B) amylase
(C) bile
(D) cholecystokinin

27. A patient with colorectal cancer undergoes exploratory laparotomy, right hemicolectomy, and colostomy creation. Which nursing measure is a priority?
(A) administering proteolytic enzymes
(B) monitoring fluid volume status
(C) administration of methylcellulose
(D) monitoring hemoglobin and hematocrit

28. What is the primary function of the small intestine?
(A) absorption of nutrients
(B) reabsorption of water
(C) reabsorption of carbon dioxide
(D) acting as a reservoir for food

29. Increased colonic motility is produced by which of the following?
(A) parasympathetic stimulation
(B) sympathetic stimulation
(C) central nervous system stimulation
(D) increased fat content in the diet

30. Which drug would potentially decrease colonic motility?
(A) loperamide
(B) atropine
(C) digoxin
(D) gentamicin

31. All venous blood from the intestines eventually drains into which vein?
(A) inferior vena cava
(B) superior vena cava
(C) portal vein
(D) iliac vein

32. The portal vein carries blood to which structure?
(A) inferior vena cava
(B) liver
(C) large intestine
(D) gallbladder

33. Which of the following is NOT a function of the pancreas?
(A) secretion of glucagon
(B) secretion of insulin
(C) secretion of bile
(D) secretion of digestive enzymes

34. A patient with a history of severe liver disease is admitted to the intensive care unit with pneumonia and septic shock. He becomes increasingly tachycardic, cold, and clammy. Blood glucose is 35. Based on this information, the RN anticipates the following interventions:
(A) administer 50 mL of dextrose 50% intravenously and check blood glucose levels every 4 h
(B) administer glucagon 1 mg intramuscularly × 1, then repeat in 15 min if BG less than 70
(C) administer glucagon 1 mg intramuscularly × 1 and start a D_{10} infusion with frequent glucose monitoring
(D) administer 50 mL of dextrose 50% intravenously × 1 and start a dextrose 10% infusion with frequent glucose monitoring

35. All of the following can cause intestinal perforation. Which is the most common infectious cause of hollow viscous organ perforation?
(A) bowel obstruction
(B) appendicitis
(C) colonic ulcers
(D) gastric ulcers

36. A patient is admitted to your unit with complaint of generalized abdominal pain. The pain started on the previous day and then improved slightly. It is now rated 8/10. The pain is diffuse abdominal. An abdominal examination reveals diffuse tenderness, with guarding and rigidity. An upright chest radiograph reveals free air under the diaphragm. Laboratory data reveal the following:

Na^+	141
K^+	4.2
Cl^-	99
HCO_3^-	25
Amylase	50
WBC	13,000

Based on the preceding information, which condition is likely to be present?
(A) pancreatitis
(B) bowel obstruction
(C) perforated viscous
(D) cholecystitis

37. Which of the following treatments is the definitive treatment of a perforated viscous?
(A) A placement on a nil per os (NPO) regimen with GI suction
(B) analgesia with narcotics while waiting for the pain to subside
(C) upper and lower endoscopy to search for the perforation
(D) exploratory laparotomy

38. What is the function of hepatic Kupffer cells?
(A) production of bilirubin
(B) production of pancreatic lipase
(C) production of bile
(D) production of albumin

39. Which of the following are major functions of the liver?
(A) production of bile and synthesis of amino acids
(B) production of bile and gluconeogenesis
(C) synthesis of amino acids and gluconeogenesis
(D) production of bile, synthesis of amino acids, and gluconeogenesis

40. A patient with a history of hepatitis C and evidence of liver dysfunction is admitted after being found unresponsive by relatives. The patient is lethargic. Skin is jaundiced and sclera are icteric. Abdomen is diffusely tender, ascites is present, with hypoactive bowel sounds. Vital signs: T 102.5°F, BP 155/90, RR 18, HR 97, WBC 17,000 mm^3. Which immediate interventions do you anticipate?
(A) paracentesis, fluid culture, blood cultures, and administration of a third-generation cephalosporin
(B) toxicology screen and referral to drug and alcohol counseling
(C) obtain blood, urine, and sputum cultures and start empiric vancomycin and piperacillin–tazobactam
(D) make the patient NPO and obtain a CT of the abdomen and pelvis

41. A patient underwent exploratory laparotomy and a partial colectomy after being stabbed in the right lower quadrant. On postoperative day 6, the patient's wound starts draining brown fluid. He has a temperature of 101.5°F and a white blood cell (WBC) count of 18,000. His abdomen is soft, with hypoactive bowel sounds × 4 quadrants. The incision site is tender. There is no guarding or rebound tenderness. He denies nausea and vomiting. The RN suspects the patient has developed:
(A) sepsis due to intra-abdominal abscess
(B) peritonitis
(C) perforated appendicitis
(D) sepsis and dehiscence of the fascia

42. A primary concern when caring for a patient with acute gallstone pancreatitis is to monitor fluids and electrolytes closely, because:
(A) dehydration is a common in patients with acute abdominal pain
(B) hypoglycemia occurs due to glucagon release
(C) intravascular fluid is depleted as pancreatic enzymes increase vascular permeability
(D) hypercalcemia is common

43. A patient with a grade 3 liver laceration is being treated conservatively. The patient is NPO and has every 6 h hemoglobin and hematocrit levels ordered, in addition to the trauma service performing serial abdominal exams. Which of the following would most likely prompt the trauma service to take the patient for operative or endovascular intervention?
(A) development of nausea and absent bowel sounds
(B) drop in hemoglobin from 14.7 g/dL to 13.0 g/dL
(C) development of rebound tenderness and rigidity on abdominal exam
(D) AST is twice the upper limit of normal

44. A patient who was stabbed in the abdomen had an exploratory laparotomy and repair of liver and intestinal injuries. Between the trauma bay and the operating room, the patient received 10 units of packed red blood cells, along with platelets, plasma, and cryoprecipitate transfusions. Which lab abnormalities should the RN expect?
(A) hypokalemia and hypochloremia
(B) hyperkalemia and hypocalcemia
(C) hypernatremia and hyperphosphatemia
(D) hyponatremia and hypophosphatemia

45. Vomiting of blood from the GI system is denoted by which of the following terms?
(A) hemoptysis
(B) hematemesis
(C) hematopoiesis
(D) hematochezia

46. At which anatomic location do most ulcers occur?
(A) stomach
(B) duodenum
(C) esophagus
(D) jejunum

47. Which of the following is thought to be the most common cause of stress ulcers?
(A) ischemia
(B) excessive acid production
(C) mechanical injury
(D) infections

48. A patient is admitted to the trauma ICU 12 h ago after a motor vehicle crash. The patient has bruising that follows a seatbelt pattern across his chest and abdomen. His abdomen is becoming firm and distended. The high-pressure alarm on the ventilator is sounding. What are the other two physical findings that would prompt the RN to obtain an order for bladder pressure measurements?
(A) hypotension and scrotal contusions
(B) hypotension and oliguria
(C) hypertension and tachycardia
(D) tachycardia and tachypnea

49. Which of the following treatments is NOT routinely indicated in the treatment of upper GI bleeding?
(A) endoscopy with coagulation of bleeding site
(B) fluid replacement with crystalloids
(C) blood transfusions
(D) iced lavage of the stomach

50. Esophageal varices are the result of increases in which of the following vascular parameters?
(A) increased hepatic arterial pressure
(B) decreased hepatic arterial pressure
(C) increased portal venous pressure
(D) decreased portal venous pressure

51. Transjugular intrahepatic portosystemic shunt (TIPS) works to decrease bleeding from esophageal varices by which mechanism?
(A) decreasing portal venous pressure
(B) improving vena caval blood flow
(C) improving production of clotting factors
(D) decreasing blood return to the liver

52. A patient with a history of alcohol use disorder and prior GI bleeding is admitted to your unit with the diagnosis of upper GI bleeding. On exam, the abdomen is distended and liver enlarged. The patient denies pain despite having active hematemesis.

Based on the preceding information, which condition is most likely to be present?
(A) diverticulosis
(B) esophageal variceal bleeding
(C) duodenal ulcers
(D) bile duct obstruction

53. The physician elects to place an esophageal balloon (Sengstaken–Blakemore) to aid bleeding control. Which of the following is a potentially life-threatening complication of the esophageal balloon tamponade?
(A) airway compromise
(B) esophageal necrosis
(C) pain
(D) hypercoagulability

54. Which of the following is NOT a common cause of lower GI bleeding?
(A) diverticulitis
(B) hemorrhoids
(C) arteriovenous malformations
(D) Mallory–Weiss tears

55. Which of the following is NOT a treatment for an upper GI tract bleeding?
(A) octreotide
(B) endoscopy
(C) phenylephrine
(D) proton-pump inhibitor infusion

56. A patient on anticoagulation for atrial fibrillation develops bright red blood per rectum. Which of the following is the immediately indicated nursing intervention?
(A) check the vital signs and perform a focused assessment
(B) make the patient NPO
(C) give 1 L normal saline bolus
(D) give the patient ice chips and consult gastroenterology

57. A patient fell from a height of 20 feet and landed on their right side. In addition to rib fractures and pulmonary contusions, which injury is most likely?
(A) splenic laceration
(B) cardiac herniation
(C) liver laceration
(D) bladder rupture

Questions 58 and 59 refer to the following scenario:
A patient is admitted to your unit after being found unresponsive by paramedics. They have visible needle marks on both arms. After starting an intravenous drip, the RN accidentally sticks themself with the same needle used for the venipuncture.

58. Based on the preceding information, to what type of hepatitis would the RN most likely be exposed?
(A) hepatitis A
(B) hepatitis C
(C) hepatitis D
(D) no risk of hepatitis acquisition

59. Initial treatment for the RN, assuming no prior exposure to hepatitis exists, would include administration of which of the following (after appropriate serologic studies of the RN and the patient had been performed)?
(A) hepatitis B immune globulin (HBIG) and vaccine if not HbsAb-positive
(B) hepatitis C immune globulin (HAIG)
(C) interferon
(D) hepatitis C vaccine

60. For which type of hepatitis does an effective vaccine exist?
(A) hepatitis A
(B) hepatitis B
(C) both hepatitis A and B
(D) hepatitis C

Questions 61 and 62 refer to the following scenario:
A patient is admitted with complaints of shortness of breath, generalized fatigue, and weakness. Abdomen is distended and ascites is present. The liver is firm but not enlarged. Spider angiomas are noted on the chest, and skeletal muscles are atrophied. Sclerae have an icteric appearance. Vital signs are blood pressure 96/60 mm Hg, pulse 110, and respiratory rate 28.

61. Based on the preceding information, which condition is likely to be responsible for the symptoms?
(A) acute hepatitis
(B) cirrhosis
(C) esophageal varices
(D) hepatorenal syndrome

62. A patient with a history of hepatitis C presents to the hospital for respiratory distress. ABG demonstrates hypoxia and uncompensated respiratory acidosis. The patient is jaundiced and has ascites. They are transferred to the ICU for further management. In addition to oxygen and noninvasive positive pressure ventilation, which treatment would be indicated to help relieve the respiratory distress from the ascites?
(A) placing the patient in a supine position
(B) interferon administration
(C) protein restriction in the diet
(D) administration of diuretics

63. A patient has bleeding esophageal and gastric varices that continued bleeding despite catheter-based interventions. A Sengstaken–Blakemore tube was placed. The patient's oxygen saturation has decreased to 75% on 2 L nasal cannula. Which of the following is the most urgent intervention?
(A) checking pressure in the esophageal and gastric balloons
(B) assessing airway patency
(C) ensuring that the tube has enough traction
(D) assessing for aspiration pneumonitis

64. Asterixis is regarded as a sign of the development of which condition?
(A) left ventricular failure
(B) acute calcium disturbance
(C) hepatic encephalopathy
(D) seizures

Questions 65 and 66 refer to the following scenario:
A patient is admitted to the unit with the diagnosis of cirrhosis. The patient is confused and disoriented. "Flapping" movement of both hands and jaundiced skin are noted. Laboratory values are as follows:

SGOT/AST	100
SGPT/ALT	88
Lactate dehydrogenase	250
Alkaline phosphatase	165
Ammonia	78
BUN	10
Creatinine	0.8

65. Based on the preceding information, which condition is likely to be developing and causing the behavioral changes?
(A) acute renal failure
(B) loss of cerebral perfusion pressure
(C) loss of cerebral glucose from hepatic failure
(D) hepatic encephalopathy

66. Which treatment would be utilized in the treatment of this patient?
(A) lactulose
(B) high-protein diet
(C) glucose bolus
(D) vitamin D administration

67. Pancreatitis is partially monitored by means of which parameters?

(A) pepsinogen levels
(B) lipase values
(C) glucagon values
(D) trypsin levels

68. Which of the following is a common cause of acute pancreatitis?

(A) liver failure
(B) diabetes
(C) gallstones
(D) infection

Questions 69 and 70 refer to the following scenario:

A patient with a history of alcohol use disorder is admitted with severe abdominal pain that radiates to the back. The abdomen is tender, although rebound tenderness is not present. The patient is nauseated and has vomited once. Bowel sounds are diminished. Vital signs are blood pressure 98/58 mm Hg, pulse 116, and respiratory rate 34. Laboratory data are as follows:

Na^+	142
K^+	3.8
Cl^-	106
HCO_3^-	22
Ca^{2+}	6.5
Lipase	600
Albumin	4.0

69. Based on the preceding information, which condition is likely to be developing?

(A) superior mesenteric obstruction
(B) cholecystitis
(C) pancreatitis
(D) bowel obstruction

70. A patient with a history of repair of a stab injury to the small intestine develops severe abdominal pain and projectile vomiting. On exam the abdomen is distended and diffusely tender, and there are high-pitched tinkling bowel sounds. All of the following interventions are a priority EXCEPT:

(A) placement on NPO regimen
(B) stat complete blood count, chemistry panel, and coagulation panel
(C) acute abdominal radiograph series
(D) cholecystectomy

71. Which of the following serum electrolytes is frequently depleted with pancreatitis?

(A) sodium
(B) potassium
(C) chloride
(D) calcium

72. A patient is admitted for excruciating periumbilical pain. Abdomen is not tender to palpation, but the patient does have rebound tenderness. All of the laboratory values are normal except for a white blood cell count of 14,000 and a lactic acid level of 5.6. Vital signs are blood pressure 168/92 mm Hg, pulse 113, and respiratory rate 28.

Based on the preceding information, which condition is most likely to be developing?

(A) ischemic bowel
(B) cholecystitis
(C) pancreatitis
(D) bowel obstruction

73. Which treatment, aside from pain relief, would be indicated for this patient?

(A) placement on an NPO regimen with GI suction
(B) upper endoscopy with cauterization
(C) laparotomy with bowel resection and possible mesenteric embolectomy
(D) decompressive colonoscopy with rectal tube placement

74. A patient is admitted with vomiting, nausea, and diffuse abdominal pain. The vomitus has a fecal odor. They had a cholecystectomy in the past but has been in good health until the development of abdominal pain 2 days earlier. The abdomen has a hyperresonant sound on percussion, with the patient complaining of tenderness to palpation. Laboratory data are normal.

Based on the preceding information, which condition is likely to be developing?

(A) bowel obstruction
(B) mesenteric artery occlusion
(C) pyloric stenosis
(D) obstruction of the pancreatic duct

75. The primary treatment for a complete bowel obstruction in a patient with previous abdominal surgery is:

(A) endoscopy for colonic decompression
(B) endoscopy with placement of a rectal tube
(C) nonoperative treatment with bowel rest and nasogastric decompression
(D) laparotomy for with lysis of adhesions

PART VI
Gastroenterology Practice Exam

Practice Fill-Ins

1. __________
2. __________
3. __________
4. __________
5. __________
6. __________
7. __________
8. __________
9. __________
10. __________
11. __________
12. __________
13. __________
14. __________
15. __________
16. __________
17. __________
18. __________
19. __________
20. __________
21. __________
22. __________
23. __________
24. __________
25. __________
26. __________
27. __________
28. __________
29. __________
30. __________
31. __________
32. __________
33. __________
34. __________
35. __________
36. __________
37. __________
38. __________
39. __________
40. __________
41. __________
42. __________
43. __________
44. __________
45. __________
46. __________
47. __________
48. __________
49. __________
50. __________
51. __________
52. __________
53. __________
54. __________
55. __________
56. __________
57. __________
58. __________
59. __________
60. __________
61. __________
62. __________
63. __________
64. __________
65. __________
66. __________
67. __________
68. __________
69. __________
70. __________
71. __________
72. __________
73. __________
74. __________
75. __________

PART VI
Answers

1. **C** Chapter 38 Rationale: Atropine increases heart rate by blocking the effects of acetylcholine. B is incorrect since atropine decreases saliva. Atropine has no effect on respiratory rate. It can also raise body temperature, so both B and C are incorrect.
2. **D** Chapter 41 Rationale: Kehr's sign is radiating left shoulder pain that results from either left hemidiaphragm or splenic injury due to blunt abdominal trauma.
3. **C** Chapter 40 Rationale: Option C is the best answer. In pancreatitis, pancreatic enzymes such as amylase and lipase are elevated. Total protein stores are depleted due to increase in protein catabolism. Calcium levels decrease as calcium binds to necrotic pancreatic fat. Pancreatitis typically causes elevated glucose levels. It should not primarily affect liver function tests or INR, so options A, B, and D are incorrect.
4. **B** Chapter 39 Rationale: The patient's intravascular volume is becoming depleted (the underlying cause of the hypotension). The most correct choice is to administer isotonic fluid bolus to restore intravascular volume. Both C and D are vasopressors and can be eliminated. D5W is hypotonic, elminating A. Choose B.
5. **C** Chapter 39 Rationale: Aldosterone compensates for shock by causing fluid and sodium retention. This increases intravascular volume. Decreased stroke volume (option D) is a result of intravascular volume depletion, not a compensatory mechanism. Shifting of fluid from the intravascular space to the extracellular space and peripheral vasodilation occur during distributive shock, such as sepsis, in addition to systemic inflammatory response syndrome (SIRS), eliminating options A and B.
6. **A** Chapter 40 Rationale: Both Cullen's and Grey Turner's signs are indicative of hemorrhagic pancreatitis. Livedo reticularis is seen with peripheral arterial disease. Cutis marmorata is commonly associated with hypoperfused, mottled skin seen in shock states. Roth spots can occur as a result of endocarditis, thus eliminating options B, C, and D.
7. **C** Chapter 38 Rationale: Cobalamin (vitamin B_{12}) requires the stomach for two reasons: 1. To transform it from dietary protein. 2. Digested, cobalamin binds with intrinsic factor, which is produced by the parietal cells in the stomach. Without intrinsic factor, B_{12} would be further digested in the GI tract, and cobalamin deficiency occurs. Glucagon secretion and bile production occur in the liver, so options A and B are incorrect. Regulation of chloride and bicarbonate is primarily controlled by the kidneys, so option D is incorrect.
8. **B** Chapter 42 Rationale: Excessive removal of gastric contents (hydrochloric acid, potassium) leads to metabolic alkalosis. In alkalosis, serum chloride and potassium levels are lower.
9. **A** Chapter 38 Rationale: Histamine is released during the cephalic phase of digestion. Approximately 30% of gastric acid is produced during this phase. Atropine, bicarbonate, and potassium do not affect the production of hydrochloric acid, eliminating answers B, C, and D.
10. **A** Chapter 38 Rationale: Ranitidine is a histamine-2 receptor blocker. Gastrin and acetylcholine induce digestion. Calcium only neutralizes gastric acid when combined with another ingredient such as carbonate. This eliminates options B, C, and D.
11. **B** Chapter 38 Rationale: Without intrinsic factor, vitamin B_{12} would be metabolized into a nonfunctional state leading to pernicious anemia, peripheral neuropathy, and other manifestations of vitamin B_{12} deficiency. Intrinsic factor is not involved with vitamin K absorption, vitamin C utilization, or vitamin D synthesis, eliminating options A, C, and D.
12. **B** Chapter 38 Rationale: Normal gastric pH is acidic, with a normal range of 1 to 3. It is usually not higher than 5. Higher pH levels (>6) are associated with fluid from the small intestine or the lungs.
13. **C** Chapter 38 Rationale: Pepsinogen is produced in the stomach, eliminating answers A, B, and D.
14. **D** Chapter 38 Rationale: Chyme is a semiliquid mass of food.
15. **D** Chapter 38 Rationale: Gastrin is involved in hydrochloric acid production. It does not affect desire to eat or vitamin B_{12}, eliminating options A, B, and C.
16. **D** Chapter 38 Rationale: Cholecystokinin (CCK) is secreted in the duodenum in response to ingested food. It has several functions, including increasing bile production and secretion, increasing pancreatic enzyme release, and inhibiting gastric emptying. This eliminates options B and C. Bile is used to break down fats, eliminating option A.
17. **D** Chapter 39 Rationale: Propranolol is the only nonselective beta blocker listed. Nonselective beta blockers may decrease portal pressure in patients with cirrhosis, eliminating answers A, B, and C.
18. **C** Chapter 40 Rationale: Cholecystitis commonly presents with pain after eating fatty foods. Pancreatitis pain is typically epigastric and described as a "twisting or stabbing" pain, eliminating option A. There is no mention of trauma in this scenario, so hemidiaphragm injury is highly unlikely, eliminating option B. Chronic mesenteric ischemia presents with patient after eating regardless of the type of food ingested. These patients are also likely to have a history of peripheral vascular disease. The patient's younger age and the acute onset of the pain make option D very unlikely.

19. **B** Chapter 42 Rationale: Potassium and chloride are lost during nasogastric suctioning. Hyponatremia is associated with fluid volume overload and is uncommon in patients who are NPO and on bowel rest. Hypermagnesemia is most often seen in end-stage renal disease patients and is uncommon in patients with nasogastric suction. Therefore, answers, A, C, and D are incorrect.

20. **A** Chapter 39 Rationale: Mental status change is the earliest sign of shock. It is seen during class I hypovolemic/hemorrhagic shock. Decreased urine output (<0.5 mL/kg/h or <30 mL/h) and tachypnea (respiratory rate > 20) are seen in class II hypovolemic/hemorrhagic shock. Hypotension and significant tachycardia (HR > 120) do not occur until class III hypovolemic/hemorrhagic shock.

21. **A** Chapter 38 Rationale: Pepsinogen is not secreted by the pancreas. It is secreted by the stomach, making options B, C, and D incorrect.

22. **B** Chapter 42 Rationale: According to the American Association of Critical Care Nursing's (AACN) Practice Alert, abdominal radiograph is the only 100% reliable method of assessing for feeding tube placement. Auscultation is not reliable and should not be used. Gastric pH sampling (when done in combination with abdominal x-ray) will have a pH <5 and the appearance of bile, eliminating options A, C, and D.

23. **D** Chapter 38 Rationale: Trypsinogen is a proenzyme produced by the pancreas. It travels from down the pancreatic duct to the duodenum where it converts to trypsin. Trypsin breaks down protein into smaller peptides. Maltose is a sugar molecule (disaccharide) that is produced when amylase breaks down carbohydrates (starches). Lipase breaks down fat. Therefore, options A, B, and C are incorrect.

24. **A** Chapter 41 Rationale: The patient is most likely experiencing mesenteric ischemia. The patient has periumbilical pain, and the pain is out of proportion to the abdominal exam findings, which is the classic presentation. The patient is on two vasopressors, which puts them at risk for developing intestinal hypoperfusion. Acute cholecystitis presents with right upper quadrant pain, eliminating option B. Acute pancreatitis presents with stabbing or twisting epigastric pain, eliminating option C. Perforated viscous is associated with abdominal distention and would cause significant peritoneal irritation leading to rebound tenderness and guarding, eliminating option D.

25. **A** Chapter 38 Rationale: Amylase breaks down carbohydrates. Lipase breaks down fat. Pepsin is a gastric enzyme that breaks proteins down into smaller peptides for easier absorption in the small intestine. Trypsin is formed in the small intestine when the pancreas produces trypsinogen (a proenzyme). Trypsin breaks down protein into smaller peptides. Therefore options B, C, and D are incorrect.

26. **C** Chapter 38 Rationale: Bile is involved in fat digestion. Chyme is a semisolid mass of food, making option A incorrect. Amylase breaks down starches, making option B incorrect. Cholecystokinin causes secretion of bile, but it does not break down fat, making option D incorrect.

27. **B** Chapter 42 Rationale: Maintaining adequate intravascular volume is paramount in the postsurgical patient. These patients often have intravascular volume depletion due to blood loss during surgery and third spacing of fluids. Monitoring hemoglobin and hematocrit is important but is not the main priority unless there is active bleeding. In this scenario, there is no mention of active bleeding, making option D incorrect. Immediately postcolectomy, patients are NPO and on bowel rest, so administration of methylcellulose is not indicated at this time. Administering proteolytic enzymes is not indicated for this patient population.

28. **A** Chapter 38 Rationale: The primary function of the small intestines is nutrient absorption. Water reabsorption primarily occurs in the large intestine. The large intestine also absorbs any remaining nutrients before nondigestible matter becomes fecal matter and is stored in the rectum. Options C and D are incorrect as carbon dioxide is not reabsorbed in the small intestine, and the small intestine is not a reservoir for food.

29. **A** Chapter 38 Rationale: The parasympathetic nervous system is the "rest and digest" nervous system. The sympathetic nervous system is the "fight or flight" nervous system and primarily responds to stressors. Options C and D do not readily contribute to colonic motility. Therefore, options B, C, and D are incorrect.

30. **B** Chapter 38 Rationale: Atropine is an anticholinergic that counteracts the effects of acetylcholine and the sympathetic nervous system. It is combined with diphenoxylate to form Lomotil, a commonly used antidiarrheal. Loperamide (Imodium) is used to treat diarrhea, making option A incorrect. Gentamicin and other antibiotics can cause diarrhea, rendering option D incorrect. Digoxin is not associated with diarrhea, making option C incorrect.

31. **A** Chapter 41 Rationale: The inferior vena cava drains all venous blood from organs below the thorax and brings the blood to the right atrium. The superior vena cava is not correct, as it drains the head, neck, and thorax. The portal vein supplies 75% of blood to the liver. The iliac veins drain the portions of the pelvis. Therefore, options B, C, and D are incorrect.

32. **B** Chapter 38 Rationale: The portal vein supplies 75% of blood flow to the liver. The other 25% is supplied by the hepatic artery. The inferior vena cava is a large vein that brings venous blood below the thorax back to the right heart. The large intestine is primarily fed by branches of the superior mesenteric artery. The gallbladder is supplied by branches of the right hepatic artery. Therefore, choice B is the most correct answer.

33. **C** Chapter 38 Rationale: The pancreas secretes glucagon to increase blood glucose levels during hypoglycemia. It also produces insulin in the beta cells. It secretes digestive enzymes including amylase and lipase. It does not secrete bile.

34. **D** Chapter 40 Rationale: The patient in this scenario has a dangerously low blood sugar that needs to be treated immediately. Fifty percent dextrose IV will help raise the blood glucose quickly. Glucagon will not improve blood glucose levels in a patient with severe or end-stage liver disease since the diseased liver is unable to store glycogen or produce glucose. To maintain an adequate blood glucose level, the patient should be started on a 10% dextrose infusion. Frequent blood glucose checks are imperative to assess for hypo- or hyperglycemia in this patient.

35. **B** Chapter 41 Rationale: Perforated appendicitis is the most common infectious cause of hollow viscous perforation. Severe gastric ulcers can also lead to viscous perforation, but they are not infectious. Bowel obstructions and colonic ulcers are uncommonly causes of viscous perforation, so answers A, C, and D are incorrect.

36. **C** Chapter 41 Rationale: Diffuse tenderness, guarding, and rigidity can occur with several causes of an acute abdomen. The finding of free air under the diaphragm is a key finding in patients with perforated viscous, making options A, B, and D incorrect.

37. **D** Chapter 41 Rationale: Patients with viscous perforations require emergent exploratory laparotomy to find and correct the opening in the GI tract. Although making these patients NPO is important, placement of an NGT is not a priority in these cases, eliminating option A. Option B is incorrect because the pain will become septic if surgery is delayed. Option C is incorrect because it requires bowel prep (a slow process) and it does not allow for surgical repair of the defect once found.

38. **A** Chapter 38 Rationale: Kupffer cells are macrophages. They are primarily located in the hepatic sinusoids. In the liver, the Kupffer cells play a role in bilirubin production. They do not play a role in producing lipase, bile, or albumin, eliminating options B, C, and D.

39. **D** Chapter 38 Rationale: The liver produces glucose via gluconeogenesis, it synthesizes amino acids, and it produces bile.

40. **A** Chapter 40 Rationale: The patient in this scenario has chronic liver disease and presents with the classic signs of spontaneous bacterial peritonitis. The treatment of spontaneous bacterial peritonitis involves performing a paracentesis, sending ascites fluid for culture, and starting either a third-generation cephalosporin or alternative agent that covers anaerobic bacteria. Option C is incorrect since obtaining urine and sputum cultures is not necessary given the presentation. Empiric administration of vancomycin is not indicated based on the presentation. The patient in this scenario has an obvious infection, so antibiotic administration is paramount. Although making the patient NPO is important, there is no indication for a CT abdomen and pelvis at this time, eliminating option D.

41. **D** Chapter 41 Rationale: All of these conditions could potentially lead to peritonitis. In general, patients with peritonitis have abdominal guarding, rigidity, and rebound tenderness. The patient does meet these criteria, eliminating option B. Perforated appendicitis is unlikely since the patient was stabbed in the right lower quadrant (where the appendix is located) and had a partial colectomy. Nausea is present in more than 60% and vomiting is present in 50% of patients with appendicitis, eliminating option C. The patient meets at least two SIRS criteria ($T > 101.2°F$ and $WBC > 12,000$), which make both A and D attractive options. Intra-abdominal abscesses typically do not drain spontaneously. When they are drained surgically or percutaneously, the fluid is typically purulent white to tan or yellow and foul smelling. The brown drainage from the incision is a sign of fascial dehiscence, making option D the most correct.

42. **C** Chapter 40 Rationale: Pancreatitis leads to vasodilation and third-spacing of fluid leading to intravascular dehydration. Option A is incorrect as abdominal pain by itself does not cause dehydration. Option B is incorrect as increased glucagon could lead to hyperglycemia. Option D is incorrect since hypocalcemia commonly occurs in pancreatitis.

43. **C** Chapter 41 Rationale: The exam in option C is consistent with the development of peritonitis, which requires immediate intervention—either surgically or endovascularly. The development of nausea and absent bowel sounds is not commonly seen in this scenario, eliminating option A. The drop in hemoglobin and the increase in AST are not clinically significant, eliminating options B and D.

44. **B** Chapter 39 Rationale: The classic electrolyte abnormalities that occur after massive blood transfusion are hyperkalemia (due to lysis of red blood cells) and hypocalcemia (due to chelation of calcium in the liver by citrate). Hypernatremia can occur due to intravascular volume contraction, eliminating option D. In trauma, hypochloremia is uncommon. Hyperchloremia is more commonly seen due to the higher amounts of chloride in isotonic solutions used for volume resuscitation, compared to hypotonic fluids, making option A incorrect. Hypophosphatemia is common in polytrauma patients, but it is not caused by massive transfusion, eliminating option C.

45. **B** Chapter 39 Rationale: Hematemesis is vomiting bright red blood. Hemoptysis is coughing up bright red blood. Hematopoiesis refers to bone marrow production of red blood cells. Hematochezia refers to bright red blood from the rectum. Therefore, options A, C, and D are incorrect.

46. **B** Chapter 39 Rationale: The duodenum is the most common site for ulceration due to the combination of lower blood flow and high amounts of gastric acid. Although peptic ulcers can occur in the stomach, they are not as common as duodenal ulcers since the stomach has a better blood supply. Ulcers of the esophagus and jejunum are much less common. Therefore, options A, C, and D are incorrect.

47. **B** Chapter 39 Rationale: Excessive acid secretion lowers gastric pH, leading to ulcer formation. It can occur from a variety of stressors and diseases. Infections like *H. pylori* can cause ulcers but are less common, making option D

less desirable. GI ischemia and mechanical injury are uncommon, making options A and C incorrect.

48. **B** Chapter 41 Rationale: The patient in this scenario is at high risk for abdominal compartment syndrome as a result of blunt abdominal trauma. The triad of abdominal compartment syndrome is elevated peak inspiratory pressures (on the ventilator), hypotension due to decreased venous return to the heart, and oliguria due to decreased renal perfusion. Option C is incorrect since hypertension is not seen in abdominal compartment syndrome. While tachycardia and tachypnea will likely be seen, they are not part of the triad, eliminating options C and D.

49. **D** Chapter 39 Rationale: Iced lavage of the stomach is not routinely used anymore in the treatment of upper GI bleeding since the advent of modern interventional endoscopy. Volume replacements with crystalloid and blood transfusions are often indicated to treat hypovolemia in patients with GI bleeding.

50. **C** Chapter 39 Rationale: Esophageal varices form as a result of cirrhosis, when the portal venous pressure is greater than 12 mm Hg. The hepatic artery has no involvement in the development of varices. Options A, B, and D are incorrect.

51. **A** Chapter 39 Rationale: TIPS works to decrease portal venous pressure by shunting blood into the hepatic vein so it can flow into the inferior vena cava, allowing it to travel back to the right heart. Although TIPS increases blood flow in the vena cava, it is not how it decreases variceal bleeding, making option B incorrect. Options C and D are incorrect since decreasing portal pressure does not improve production or clotting factors, and TIPS could increase venous blood return to the liver by decreasing liver congestion.

52. **B** Chapter 39 Rationale: Variceal bleeding is usually painless. Bile duct obstruction is associated with right upper quadrant pain. Diverticulosis is not commonly associated with pain. Duodenal ulcers are generally associated with postprandial pain.

53. **A** Chapter 39 Rationale: Airway compromise is life-threatening and can occur if the gastric balloon migrates upward and occludes the trachea. While esophageal necrosis is a serious complication, it is usually not immediately life-threatening, eliminating option B. Pain is not a life-threatening complication, making option C incorrect. The Blakemore tube should not make the patient hypercoagulable, making option D incorrect.

54. **D** Chapter 39 Rationale: Mallory–Weiss tears are tears in the gastroesophageal junction that can cause hematemesis. Diverticulitis, hemorrhoids, and arteriovenous malformations can all cause lower GI bleeding, eliminating options A, B, and C.

55. **C** Chapter 39 Rationale: All of the above, except for Neo-Synephrine, are indicated in the treatment of GI bleeds. In patients with bleeding varices, vasopressin can be used to decrease portal venous pressure. Neosynephrine is an alpha agonist that raises blood pressure but is not specifically indicated for treating upper GI bleeds.

56. **A** Chapter 39 Rationale: Whenever there is a change in patient condition, it is most appropriate to reassess the patient and check vital signs prior to any other intervention. The patient will likely need to be made NPO and a gastroenterology consult will likely be ordered, but they would not occur first. Vital signs and an assessment should be performed before a fluid bolus is administered.

57. **C** Chapter 41 Rationale: The major intra-abdominal organ on the right side is the liver. Splenic laceration would be unlikely, as the spleen is on the left side of the abdomen. It is unlikely that the patient would have a cardiac herniation since the injury occurred on the right side. There is no mechanism to support the presence of a bladder injury.

58. **B** Chapter 40 Rationale: In this question, the presence of puncture marks in the arms should alert the nurse to possible intravenous drug abuse. According to the CDC, most cases of hepatitis C occur from sharing needles. Hepatitis A is unlikely in this patient since it is spread by ingesting contaminated food or water. Hepatitis D only occurs in those already infected with hepatitis B and is fatal in 20% of cases.

59. **C** Chapter 40 Rationale: Interferon is more effective than immunoglobulin for postexposure prophylaxis. Treatment of hepatitis C can include interferon, antiretroviral medications, or direct-acting antivirals. There is no vaccine for preventing hepatitis C, eliminating option A & D.

60. **C** Chapter 40 Rationale: Vaccines are available for both hepatitis A and B. There is no hepatitis C vaccine available at this time.

61. **B** Chapter 40 Rationale: A firm liver without enlargement is often seen with cirrhosis. The spider angiomas are often seen as a result of portal hypertension that can occur with cirrhosis. The patient may have esophageal varies, but the presence of varices is not the cause of the liver failure. Option D is not the correct choice since there is no mention of renal dysfunction in the question's stem. We can eliminate option A since this patient presents with signs of chronic liver disease, and most cases of acute hepatitis occur in patients without chronic liver disease. Additionally, acute hepatitis often presents with nausea, vomiting, and myalgias.

62. **D** Chapter 40 Rationale: The treatment for this patient should focus on alleviating his respiratory distress. Out of all of the options, administering diuretics should help decrease fluid volume overload and improve the patient's respiratory status.

63. **B** Chapter 39 Rationale: In patients with Sengstaken–Blakemore tubes, the priority is assessing airway patency since the gastric balloon may migrate superiorly into the esophagus, leading to airway compromise. If the airway is compromised, cut across the entire tube below the bifurcation of the suction and inflation ports. Although the patient may be at risk for aspiration pneumonitis from suspected hematemesis prior to tube placement, it is not the main priority. Answers A and C are incorrect because they do not place the airway as a priority.

64. **C** Chapter 40 Rationale: Asterixis is seen in grade 2 hepatic encephalopathy. Asterixis is not associated with left ventricular failure, calcium abnormalities, or seizures, eliminating options A, B and D.

65. **D** Chapter 40 Rationale: The patient is presenting with signs of grade 2 hepatic encephalopathy. Option D is the best available answer. Hepatic encephalopathy is thought to occur when ammonia levels are elevated (may be >45 mcg/dL depending on the reference range for the lab assay used). However, patients respond differently to elevated ammonia levels, which decreases the test's sensitivity and specificity for hepatic encephalopathy. Option A is incorrect since the renal function is normal. Option B is incorrect since there is nothing in the stem that deals with cerebral perfusion. Option C is incorrect because although hepatic failure can lead to decreased gluconeogenesis, is does not cause glucose to be "lost" from the cerebral tissue.

66. **A** Chapter 40 Rationale: Administration of lactulose is the mainstay of treatment for patients with hepatic encephalopathy. It raises the pH of stool and traps ammonia (NH_4^+). This decreases the absorption of ammonia from the GI tract.

67. **B** Chapter 40 Rationale: Amylase and lipase are the two most common enzymes utilized to evaluate presence and severity of pancreatitis as well as response to treatment.

68. **C** Chapter 40 Rationale: The two most common causes of pancreatitis in the United States are gallstones and alcohol abuse. Infectious pancreatitis is uncommon, eliminating option D. Liver failure and diabetes are not involved with the development of acute pancreatitis.

69. **C** Chapter 40 Rationale: The patient is presenting with classic symptoms of pancreatitis. Pancreatitis is associated with elevated lipase and hypocalcemia, eliminating bowel obstruction and cholecystitis as causes for abdominal tenderness. Nausea and vomiting are not seen with superior mesenteric occlusion.

70. **D** Chapter 41 Rationale: The patient in the above scenario has the features of an acute small bowel obstruction—for example, history of emesis, abdominal surgery, abdominal pain, with high-pitched tinkling bowel sounds. In patients with suspected bowel obstruction, making the patient NPO starts to promote bowel rest. Diagnostic tests include stat labs to evaluate WBC and electrolyte levels. Coagulation tests such as PT/INR and PTT are useful if the patient may undergo surgery. The history and diffuse abdominal pain are not consistent with cholecystitis, making option D the best answer.

71. **D** Chapter 40 Rationale: Hypocalcemia is common in severe pancreatitis since calcium binds to areas of necrotic pancreatic fat. Hypokalemia, hyponatremia, and hypochloremia can occur as a result of treatment or acid–base imbalances, but are not primarily caused by pancreatitis, making options A, B, and C incorrect.

72. **A** Chapter 41 Rationale: Pain out of proportion to examination, leukocytosis, and lactic acidosis are consistent with a diagnosis of intestinal ischemia. Cholecystitis typically presents with right upper quadrant pain, nausea, and vomiting, making option B incorrect. Pancreatitis typically presents with epigastric pain, making option C unlikely. Bowel obstruction presents with diffuse abdominal pain, nausea, and vomiting, making option D incorrect.

73. **C** Chapter 41 Rationale: Exploratory laparotomy with resection of necrotic bowel and possible mesenteric embolectomy are the definitive treatments for severe mesenteric ischemia. Options A and B are incorrect because they do not address the underlying hypoperfusion. Option D is not the best choice since rectal tube placement may damage the already hypoperfused colon.

74. **A** Chapter 41 Rationale: The most common cause of bowel obstruction in the United States is adhesions from previous abdominal surgery. The patient's symptoms are also consistent with bowel obstruction. Option B is incorrect since mesenteric artery occlusion causes pain out of proportion to exam findings. Option D is incorrect since pancreatic duct obstruction presents with symptoms of pancreatitis. Pyloric stenosis is a more frequent cause of gastric outlet obstruction in children than adults, making option C an inappropriate choice.

75. **D** Chapter 41 Rationale: The treatment of choice for high-grade bowel obstruction. Partial bowel obstructions are treated with bowel rest and nasogastric decompression, eliminating option C. Severe colonic ileus is typically treated with decompressive colonoscopy with or without rectal tube insertion, making options A and B incorrect.

PART VII

RENAL

Bryan Boling

42

Anatomy and Physiology of the Renal System

42.1 Anatomy

42.2 Physiology

Key Content Checklist/Review Questions

CHAPTER OVERVIEW AND OBJECTIVES

Although knowledge of renal anatomy and physiology is not directly assessed on the CCRN exam, understanding the contents of this chapter will prepare you to better appreciate the clinical situations addressed by the CCRN exam. As you review this chapter, concentrate on general anatomic features relevant to renal concepts that might be addressed in clinical practice.

After studying this chapter, you should be able to:

- Describe key components of renal function relevant to the exam.
- Discuss risk factors for renal failure and renal dysfunction.
- Identify key guiding principles for renal function monitoring and treatment.

42.1 ANATOMY

Kidney

Location. The kidneys lie in the retroperitoneal space on each side of the vertebrae, with the upper border between T11 on the right and T12 on the left. This difference in position results from the natural displacement of the right kidney by the liver.

Protective Coverings. The kidneys are protected by coverings that prevent massive blood loss from trauma:

- The outermost protective covering is pararenal fat that completely surrounds the three coverings of the kidneys.
- The next layer is the renal fascia, a membrane sheet that surrounds a layer of perirenal fat.
- This perirenal fat is a dense layer of adipose tissue surrounding the innermost covering of the kidney, the fibrous renal capsule.
- The fibrous renal capsule is a thin, resistant membrane that is contiguous with the kidney tissue itself.

Shape and Size. The kidneys are bean-shaped organs with an indentation on their medial surfaces. The indented area, called the hilum, is the entry site for the renal artery, lymphatics, and nerves and is also the exit site for the renal vein, ureters, lymphatics, and nerves. The average kidney is 10 to 12 cm long and 5 to 6 cm wide.

Gross Anatomy. The kidney is divided into two main layers, the outer one-third called the cortex and the inner two-thirds called the medulla (**Fig. 42-1**).

Nephron. The nephron is the functional unit of the kidney. Each kidney has more than a million nephrons. Up to 75% of the kidney's nephrons can be destroyed before the remaining nephrons are unable to compensate.

About 85% of the kidney's nephrons are cortical nephrons (**Fig. 42-2**) which have glomeruli that lie close to the cortical surface and include thin, short segments of the loops of Henle. As the loops of Henle in the cortical nephrons are short and do not extend into the inner medulla, they do not participate in the concentration of urine.

The juxtamedullary nephrons (**Fig. 42-3**) are found in the inner one-third of the cortex. They have long loops of Henle that dip deep into the medulla and are surrounded by the peritubular network, the vasa recta. These nephrons have a great capacity to retain sodium and concentrate urine because of the long loops of Henle. In hypovolemic and hypotensive patients, a large portion of the renal blood flow is shunted from the cortical nephrons to the juxtamedullary nephrons to maintain urine formation.

Structural Anatomy. The nephron is composed of the glomerulus, the proximal convoluted tubule, the loop of Henle, the distal convoluted tubule, and the collecting ducts. The glomerulus is a spherical network of capillaries (**Fig. 42-4**) enclosed by an epithelium-lined membrane called Bowman's capsule. The afferent arterioles carry blood into Bowman's capsule and divide between two and eight subdivisions to form the glomerulus.

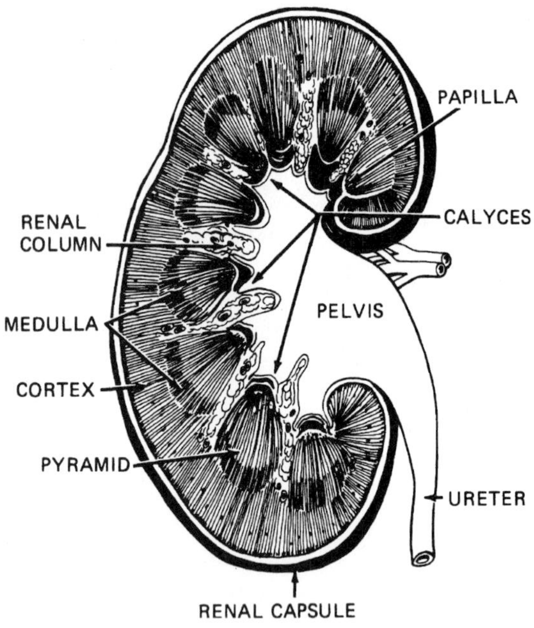

Figure 42-1. Gross anatomy of the kidney.

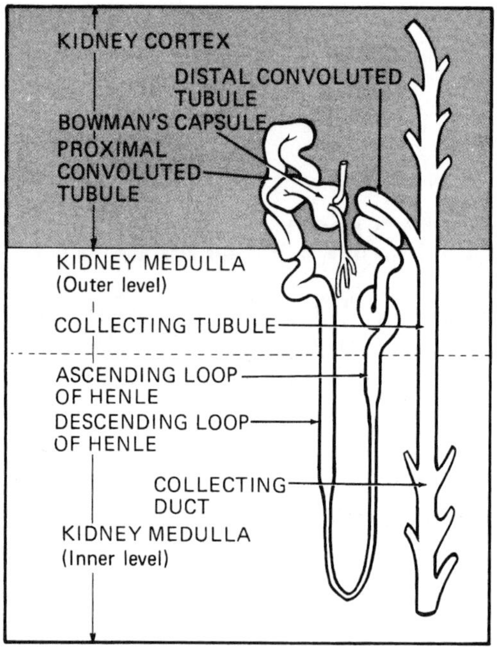

Figure 42-3. Juxtaglomerular nephron.

The efferent arteriole then carries the blood out of the glomerulus and into the proximal convoluted tubule.

The lumen of the proximal convoluted tubule contains tiny thread-like projections that form a brush border that increases the resorptive surface area to help resorb the glomerular filtrate. The proximal convoluted tubule begins in the renal cortex and ends in the medulla of the kidney, becoming the descending limb of the loop of Henle.

The loop of Henle has three distinct portions: a thick descending limb, a thin connecting segment, and a thick ascending limb. The loops of Henle in the cortical nephron extend just inside the medulla while those of the juxtamedullary nephron travel deeper, reaching almost to the tips of the pyramids (the papillae). The loops of the cortical nephrons are surrounded by the peritubular capillary network. The loops of juxtamedullary nephrons are surrounded by the vasa recta.

The distal convoluted tubule begins where the ascending limb of the loop of Henle starts twisting. It closely passes its own glomerulus and may even touch it. The distal convoluted tubule continues without convolutions to become the collecting tubule.

The collecting tubule extends to become the collecting duct, which empties into a common collecting duct; it, in turn, empties into the renal pelvis.

Juxtaglomerular Apparatus. All nephrons have a juxtaglomerular apparatus (JGA) containing three specific components. As the distal convoluted tubule passes between the afferent and efferent arterioles, it encounters specialized cells (**Fig. 42-5**), the macula densa, that are tightly packed together.

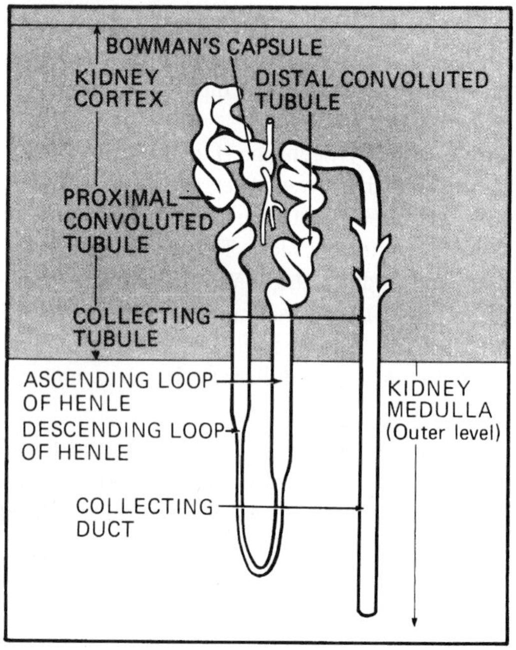

Figure 42-2. Cortical nephron.

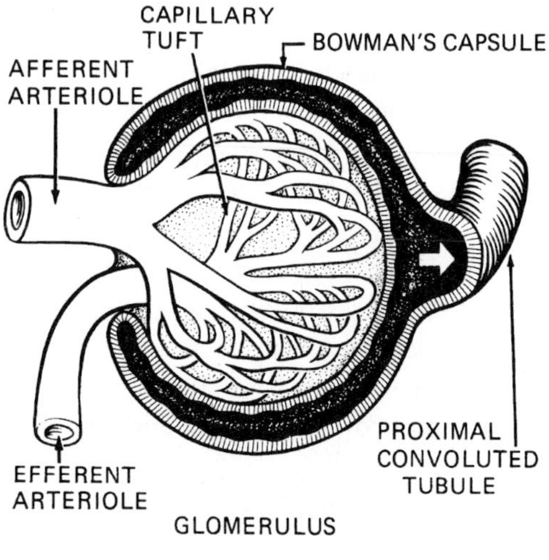

Figure 42-4. Schematic view of the glomerulus.

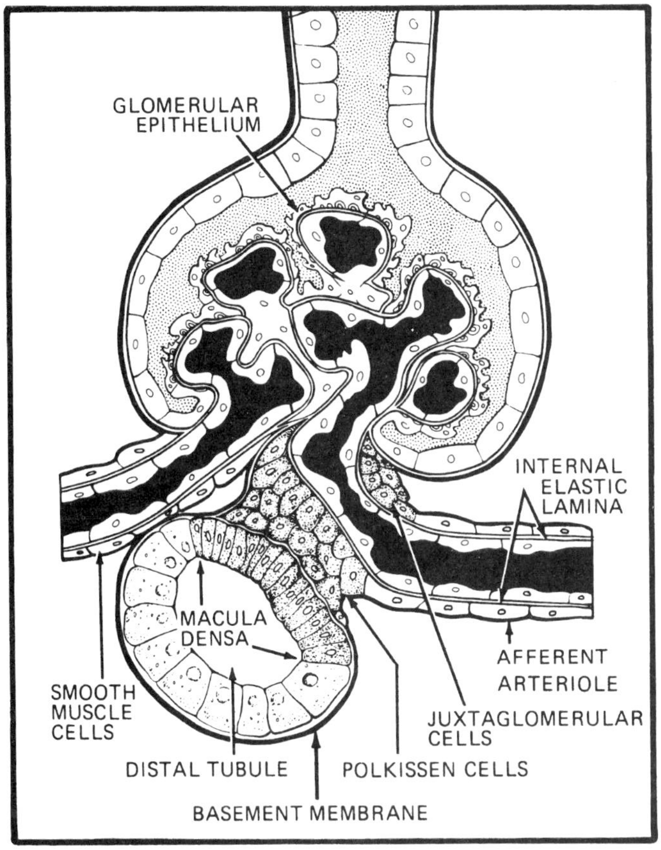

Figure 42-5. Juxtaglomerular apparatus.

There are also specialized cells, called juxtaglomerular cells, on the outside of the afferent and efferent arterioles near their entry point into the glomerulus. These cells secrete granules of inactive renin.

The third type of cell in the JGA, extraglomerular mesangial (lacis) cells, are located in the area where the distal convoluted tubule passes by or touches the efferent arterioles. *Erythropoietin* is synthesized in the mesangial cells but the complete function of these cells is unclear.

Vascular System. A pair of arteries branch off the aorta to supply blood to the left and right kidney. Each renal artery enters their kidney at the hilum and bifurcates immediately at the kidney pelvis (**Fig. 42-6**). After this first splitting at the kidney pelvis, the renal arteries develop many branches called interlobar arteries. These arteries, as their name implies, travel between lobes of the renal parenchyma inside the renal columns toward the point where the cortex and medulla meet.

At the interface of the cortex and medulla, the interlobar arteries branch to form the arcuate arteries. These arteries form arcs between the lobes of the parenchyma.

From each arcuate artery, multiple intralobular arteries spread into the cortex. These intralobular arteries form short muscular afferent arterioles that supply the glomeruli. Efferent arterioles drain the blood from the glomerulus and flow through the peritubular capillary network that surrounds the cortical portions of the tubules. The small amount of remaining arterial blood flows into straight capillary loops called vasa recta, which extend down into the medulla to provide arterial blood to the lower parts of the thin segments of the loop of Henle before looping upward to enter the intralobular veins. From the intralobular veins, the blood enters the arcuate veins, the interlobar veins, the renal veins, and the inferior vena cava.

Nerve Supply. *The sympathetic nervous system controls the constriction of renal arteries.* These nerves follow the same course as the arterioles to maintain the vasoactive tone of the arterioles. The *parasympathetic nervous system* innervates the kidney through the *vagus nerve* fibers arising from the celiac plexus.

Ureter, Urinary Bladder, and Urethra

As the urine leaves the kidney pelvis, it enters the ureter. The ureter moves the urine along by peristaltic action to the urinary bladder, a hollow, muscular organ. It has a normal capacity of 250 to 500 mL. At the bottom of the bladder is the urethra. It is about 6 to 8 in. long in men and 1 to 1.25 in. long in women (**Fig. 42-7**).

42.2 PHYSIOLOGY

Physiologic processes of the kidney include the formation of urine, the regulation of body water and electrolytes, the excretion of metabolic waste products, the regulation of acid–base balance and blood pressure, and the secretion of *erythropoietin*.

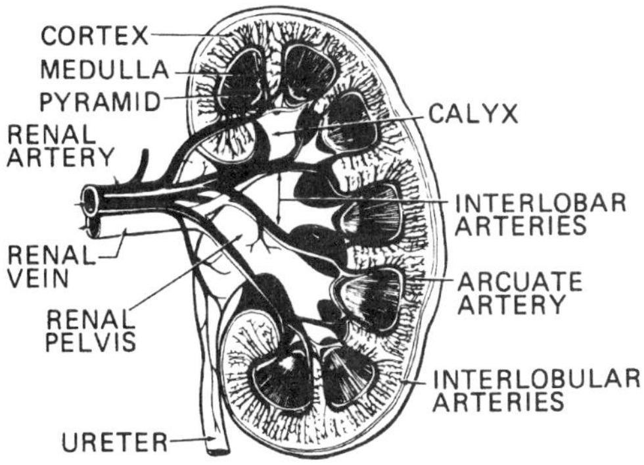

Figure 42-6. Vascular system of the kidney.

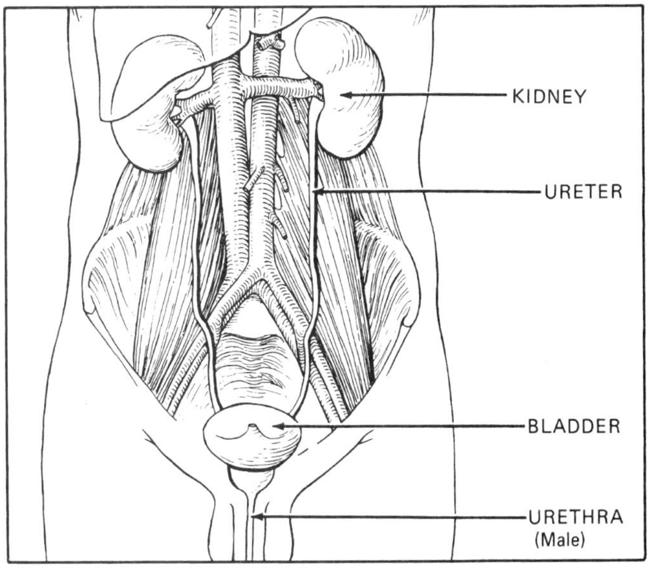

Figure 42-7. Ureter, urinary bladder, and urethra.

Formation of Urine

Three processes are involved in the formation of urine: glomerular filtration, tubular reabsorption, and tubular secretion.

Glomerular Filtration. The kidneys receive 20% to 25% of the cardiac output. Ninety-five percent of this quantity of blood will go through the glomerulus, where some solutes will be filtered out. An *autoregulatory system* exists to protect the glomerulus. The afferent and efferent renal arterioles constrict or dilate in response to systemic blood pressure. If systemic blood pressure increases, the afferent arteriole will constrict. This effectively reduces the pressure of the blood entering the glomerulus. In the same way, if systemic blood pressure decreases, the afferent arteriole will dilate to allow more blood to enter the glomerulus.

When the afferent arteriole constricts to reduce the pressure of blood in the glomerulus, the efferent arteriole relaxes (dilates) to allow the blood to leave more rapidly. This helps to control glomerular pressure. Conversely, when systemic pressure drops, the afferent arteriole dilates to let more blood into the glomerulus and the efferent arteriole constricts to help maintain the glomerular pressure. **Below a mean arterial blood pressure of about 60 mm Hg, this autoregulatory system fails and the glomerulus suffers the effects of hypotension.**

Glomerular filtration is influenced by two factors: filtration pressure and glomerular permeability.

Filtration pressure is determined in part by the anatomic blood flow through the nephron. Each nephron is actually perfused by two capillary beds (**Fig. 42-8**). *The glomerular capillary bed is perfused by the afferent arteriole with an average hydrostatic pressure of about 60 mm Hg.* The peritubular capillary bed is perfused by the efferent arteriole, which resists blood flow. Because of this, the glomerular capillary bed has a high pressure (which may be termed glomerular hydrostatic pressure). The peritubular capillary bed has a low pressure of about 13 mm Hg.

The high pressure in the glomerulus tends to filter fluid out of the glomerulus and into Bowman's capsule. At the same time and following the same principles, the low pressure in the peritubular capillary bed tends to draw fluid from the interstitial spaces into the peritubular capillaries. The high pressures in the glomerulus cause a rapid filtration of fluid. The low pressure of the capillary bed of the peritubular system facilitates

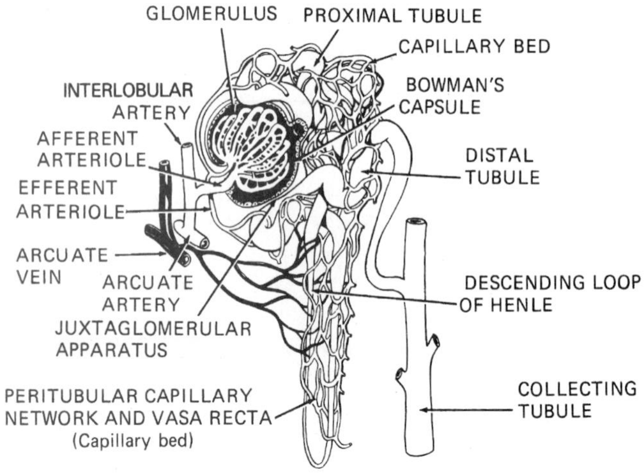

Figure 42-8. Capillary beds of a nephron.

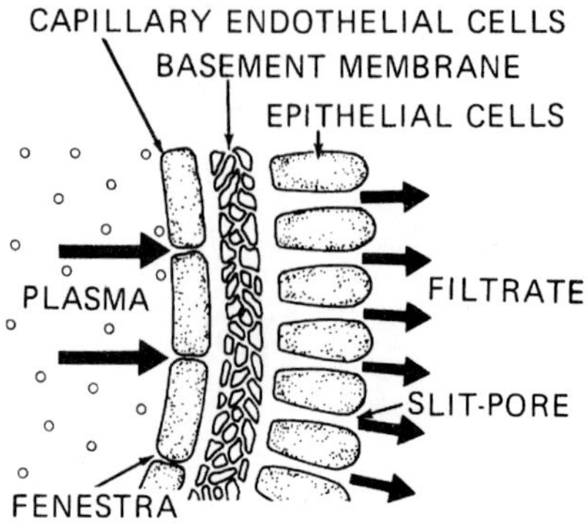

Figure 42-9. Three layers of the glomerular membrane.

rapid uptake of the excreted tubular fluids by the peritubular capillaries.

Blood is brought into the glomerulus by the afferent arteriole. The pressure is close to 60 mm Hg, so fluid is forced from the glomerular capillaries into Bowman's capsule. This fluid is now called the glomerular ultrafiltrate. The fluid is called an ultrafiltrate because protein-sized (and larger) molecules cannot filter out of the glomerular capillaries. Those proteins remain in the blood entering the peritubular capillaries from the efferent arteriole. The retained protein molecules cause an increase in the plasma osmotic pressure, which, in turn, causes the rapid reabsorption of fluid from the peritubular interstitial spaces.

Glomerular permeability is the second influence on glomerular filtration. The glomerular membrane is different from other capillary membranes in the body. It has three layers: the endothelial layer of the capillary, a basement membrane, and a layer of epithelial cells on the other surface of the capillary (**Fig. 42-9**). The endothelial cells lining the glomerular capillary are full of thousands of tiny holes called fenestrae. Outside the capillary endothelium is a basement membrane similar to a mesh of fibers. The epithelial cells of the outer layer do not touch each other. The space between the cells is called a slit pore. Any particle more than 7 nm cannot penetrate the slit pore.

Composition of Glomerular Ultrafiltrate. Normally, the ultrafiltrate is free of protein and red blood cells, as they are too large to pass through the slit pores. The semipermeable membrane of the glomerular capillary allows water, nutrients, electrolytes, and wastes to filter into Bowman's capsule.

Glomerular Filtration Rate. In the healthy kidney, *the average glomerular filtration rate (GFR) is 125 mL/min.* The total quantity of glomerular filtrate per day is about 180 L. More than 99% of this filtrate is reabsorbed in the tubules. The equation for calculating the GFR is the urine concentration of a substance times the urine flow rate divided by the plasma concentration of the same substance. The substance must be freely filtered and not affected by the tubules (**Fig. 42-10**). The normal adult urine volume is 1 to 2 L/day. The Cockcroft-Gault Formula is a commonly used equation for calculating GFR:

$$\mathbf{CCr = \{((140 - age) \times weight)/(72 \times SCr)\} \times 0.85\ (if\ female)}$$

Factors Affecting the Glomerular Filtration Rate. Any change in the glomerular hydrostatic pressure will alter the GFR. The

$$GFR = \frac{(U_x \cdot V)}{P_x}$$

$$GFR = \frac{\text{URINE CONCENTRATION OF A FREELY FILTERED SUBSTANCE} \times \text{URINE FLOW RATE}}{\text{PLASMA CONCENTRATION OF SUBSTANCE IN } U_x}$$

Figure 42-10. Equation for calculating the glomerular filtration rate.

most common cause of change in the hydrostatic pressure is a change in the systemic blood pressure. A change in systemic blood pressure changes the actual flow of blood into the glomerulus. Alterations in the afferent and efferent arteriole tone (constriction–dilation) will also affect the glomerular pressure and hence the GFR.

Any alteration in the composition of the plasma, such as an increase in oncotic pressure (the osmotic pressure due to the presence of colloids in a solution), will alter the GFR. Such conditions as hyperproteinemia, hypoproteinemia, hypovolemia, or hypervolemia will also alter the composition of plasma because of alterations in the extracellular fluid (ECF) and intracellular fluid. Thus, these states will alter the GFR.

The GFR will automatically be altered by any abnormality of structure, presence of disease, or ingestion of nephrotoxic substances.

Tubular Absorption and Secretion

The tubular function of the nephron is responsible (in part) for determining urinary output.

The nephron uses two processes, absorption and secretion, to convert 180 L of ultrafiltrate to 1 to 2 L of urine. These processes may be active or passive and are influenced by hormones, electrochemical gradients, and Starling's law. The following definitions are useful in understanding renal function.

QUICK TIP! Remember that the minimum threshold for urine output can be considered to be at least 0.5 mL/kg/h (this is 35 mL/h in a 70 kg patient).

1. Diffusion is the movement of solutes from an area of high concentration to an area of low concentration.
2. Osmosis is the movement of water from an area of high water concentration to an area of low water concentration.
3. Absorption, as discussed here, is the movement of solutes and water from the tubule into the peritubular network (ie, from the filtrate back into the bloodstream).
4. Secretion, as discussed here, is the movement of solutes and water from the peritubular network into the tubule (ie, from the bloodstream back into the filtrate).
5. Passive transport is the movement of solutes by diffusion following concentration gradients and electrical gradients.
6. Active transport is the movement of any substance against an electrical or concentration gradient. Active transport requires energy, usually supplied by adenosine triphosphate (ATP).

A mnemonic may help unravel the maze of the movement of solutes in the various tubules. Cations are carried by active transport (CAT = carried active transport); anions are passively transported (ANI = a negative ion). *Na^+, K^+, and H^+ are the most common cations in the body; Cl^- and HCO_3^- are the most common anions.*

As with most rules, there is always an exception. In the collecting duct, chloride (anion) is actively absorbed and the cations are passively absorbed. **Table 42-1** traces the formation of urine, starting with the ultrafiltrate and ending with urine after passage through both convoluted tubules, the loop of Henle, and the collecting ducts.

The major function of the loop of Henle is to concentrate or dilute urine as necessary. This is accomplished by the countercurrent mechanism that maintains the hyperosmolar concentration in the renal medulla.

Regulation of Body Water. Throughout the discussion of body regulation, the terms "osmolarity" and "osmolality" will be used interchangeably. Osmolarity is the concentration of particles in solution. Osmolality is the amount of solvent in relation to the particles. The volume and concentration of body water content are maintained by the thirst–neurohypophyseal–renal axis. Approximately 60% of ideal body weight is water in men, and 50% to 55% in women. **Figure 42-11** shows the distribution of water throughout the body. There are three mechanisms that help regulate body fluid: thirst, *antidiuretic hormone (ADH)*, and the countercurrent mechanism of the kidney.

Thirst. Thirst is the major force in our awareness of a need for water. The thirst center is located in the hypothalamus. Intracellular dehydration causes the sensation of thirst. The most common cause of intracellular dehydration is an increase in osmolar concentration of the ECF. Increased sodium concentration of the ECF causes osmosis of fluid from the neuronal cells of the thirst center. *Other important and frequent causes of thirst are excessive angiotensin II in the blood, hemorrhage, and low cardiac output.*

The role of the thirst center is to maintain a conscious desire to drink the exact amount of fluid needed to maintain the body in a normal hydrated state or return a dehydrated state to the normal state of hydration.

Antidiuretic Hormone. ADH works closely with the thirst mechanism. The plasma protein and ECF sodium concentrations determine the osmolality of the ECF. **Normal serum osmolality is 280 to 320 mOsm/L.** Acid–base control mechanisms of the kidney adjust the negative ion in relation to the extracellular concentration (osmolality) to equal the positive ions in the body. ADH is synthesized in the supraoptic nuclei of the hypothalamus and then drips down the supraoptic-hypophyseal tracts to the posterior pituitary (neurohypophysis), where it is stored. The supraoptic area of the hypothalamus is so close to the thirst center that there is an integration of the thirst mechanism, osmolality detection, and ADH release.

QUICK TIP! An easy way to remember the reference range for serum osmolality is that it is approximately twice the serum sodium. For example, 2 × sodium of 145 = 290 osmolality.

TABLE 42-1. URINE FORMATION[a–c]

Start	*Proximal Convoluted Tubule*	*Loop of Henle (Three Parts)*	*Distal Convoluted Tubule*	*Collecting Duct*	*Finish*
Ultrafiltrate	60%–80% of ultrafiltrate absorbed	I. Descending Limb	**Absorbed**	**Absorbed**	**Urine flows into renal pelvis, ureters, bladder**
		H_2O absorbed (highly permeable to H_2O)	HCO_3^-	Na^+	
			H_2O if ADH is present	**H_2O if ADH is present**	
	Absorbed	Ultrafiltrate fluid becomes increasingly hypertonic			
	Na^+		**Na^+ actively if aldosterone is present**		
	Cl^-			**Secreted**	
	Glucose			H^+	
	Amino acids	II. Thin segment loop		K^+	
	All K^+	Permeable to H_2O	**Secreted**	NH_3	
	HCO_3^-		K^+		
	H_2O passively absorbed	III. Ascending limb	H^+		
		Cl^- absorbed actively; Na^+ absorbed			
	Secreted	Impermeable to H_2O			
	H^+	Ultrafiltrate is hypotonic			
	Urea				
	Drugs				
	Organic acids				
	HCO_3^+ and H^+ (regulates acid–base balance)				
	Ultrafiltrate isotonic to plasma				

[a] *Sulfates, nitrates, and phosphates are absorbed only in amounts sufficient to maintain the ECF concentration.*
[b] *All K^+ from the filtrate are absorbed in the proximal tubule.*
[c] *The K^+ secreted in the distal convoluted tubule equals about 12% of the K^+ in the original filtrate. Under certain circumstances, secretion may exceed the original filtered load.*

The osmosodium receptors respond to changes in osmolality (sodium concentration) in the ECF. An increase in osmolality excites the osmoreceptors. They signal the neurohypophyseal tract that ADH is needed. The posterior pituitary (neurohypophysis) releases the ADH that it has stored. *In the presence of ADH, the distal convoluted tubules and collecting ducts reabsorb water. The reabsorption of the water leaves a hypertonic urine.* This cycle continues until the concentration of the ECF compartment and fluid homeostasis are returned to normal.

If osmolality of the ECF decreases, ADH release is inhibited because the osmoreceptors are not stimulated. Without ADH, the distal tubules and collecting ducts are impermeable to water. Urine will be very dilute because the water cannot be reabsorbed. The urine will continue to be diluted until the loss of water has raised the concentration of the ECF solutes to normal.

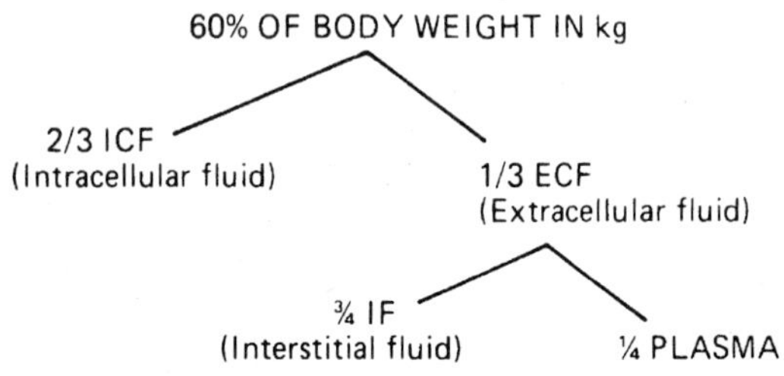

Figure 42-11. Distribution of water throughout the body.

Countercurrent Mechanism. The countercurrent mechanism serves to concentrate urine and excrete excessive solutes. Excreting dilute urine is not a problem for the kidney unless there is a neurologic dysfunction, an endocrine dysfunction, or traumatic injury. These conditions may result in an inappropriate release and affect normal kidney function of ADH, aldosterone, and/or cortisol. Concentrating urine to excrete waste solutes is a complex interaction between the long loops of Henle, the peritubular capillaries, and the vasa recta.

The countercurrent multiplier mechanism functions constantly in a loop cycle, with fresh filtrate continuously entering the loop of Henle. At the entry to the loop, the filtrate has a concentration of 300 mOsm/L. The medulla increases this concentration so that, at the tips of the papillae in the pelvic tip of the medulla, the concentration of the filtrate is 1200 to 1400 mOsm/L.

It is essential for the medullary interstitium to be hyperosmolar. There are four steps in concentrating the solutes to produce this hyperosmolality (**Fig. 42-12**).

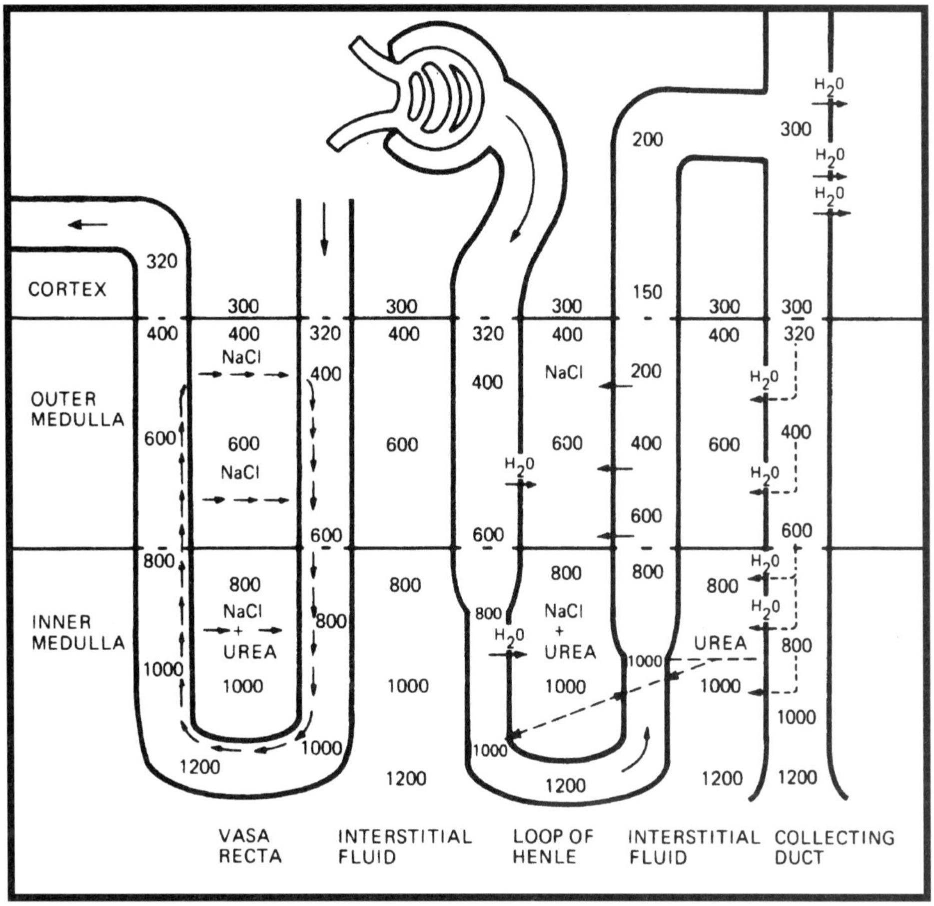

Figure 42-12. Countercurrent multiplier mechanism for maintaining medullary interstitial hyperosmolality and concentrating urine.

1. Chloride ions are actively transported from the thick portion of the ascending limb of the loop of Henle into the upper medullary interstitial fluid, pulling sodium and some potassium, magnesium, and calcium also.
2. Collecting ducts actively transport sodium into the medullary interstitial fluid. Chloride follows along passively. Steps 1 and 2 increase medullary interstitial fluid hyperosmolality by about 500 mOsm.
3. Collecting duct yields urea to the lower medullary interstitial fluid if ADH is present. ADH makes the collecting duct mildly permeable to urea and very permeable to water. Water leaves the collecting duct to enter the medullary interstitium, resulting in a high concentration of urea in the collecting duct. Urea, following concentration gradients, then diffuses out into the medullary interstitial fluid. This increases the medullary osmolarity by about another 200 to 400 mOsm.
4. Water osmosis occurs from the thin (descending) segment of the loop of Henle because of the high urea concentration in the lower medullary interstitial fluid. As the water moves from the loop of Henle, sodium ion concentration in the thin limb increases. Because of the high concentration, sodium and chloride diffuse passively out of the collecting duct into the lower medullary interstitium. This increases the osmolarity of the medullary interstitial fluid to between 1000 and 1200 mOsm.

Excess solutes concentrated in the medullary interstitium must not be allowed to reenter the bloodstream via the peritubular capillary network. This is prevented by sluggish blood flow in these capillaries and a very small amount of blood being present (<2% of the total renal blood supply), keeping ion movement to a minimum. Throughout the countercurrent multiplier activity, ion movement from the loop of Henle into the medullary interstitium has been by ionic secretion (ions moving from the tubule lumen) either actively or passively and by diffusion or osmosis.

The ion solutes present in the medullary interstitial fluid must move into the ascending limb of the loop of Henle so that they can be excreted with the urine. This is accomplished by the countercurrent exchange mechanism. The vasa recta are essentially straight tubes forming a long, slender, U-shaped blood vessel. Because both sides of the U are highly permeable, fluids and solutes readily exchange places in the high-concentration gradients of the lower medullary interstitium.

As the blood in the vasa recta flows back up the ascending loop of Henle, excess sodium and urea diffuse out of the blood in exchange for water diffusing into the blood. The blood leaves the medulla with almost the same osmolarity as when it entered the descending loop.

The fluid in the loop of Henle becomes more concentrated in the presence of ADH since water has diffused out. In the ascending thick limb of the loop of Henle and the diluting segment of the distal convoluted tubule, the osmolarity of the filtrate drops. *In the distal convoluted tubules and the collecting ducts, the osmolarity depends on the presence of ADH and aldosterone.* If these hormones are present, sodium and water will be absorbed and the tubule fluid will remain concentrated as it passes through the collecting ducts to the renal pelvis to enter the ureter. If the hormones are not present, water will be secreted and a more dilute urine will enter the ureter. Only juxtamedullary nephrons have long loops of Henle; they are responsible for concentrating and diluting the filtrate as urine is formed.

Many diuretics influence the reabsorption of sodium, potassium chloride, and water in the nephron. **Table 42-2** presents categories of diuretics.

Excretion of Metabolic Waste Products

The metabolic waste products handled by the kidneys are estimated to be in excess of 200 different substances. These waste products are classified as threshold substances, nonthreshold substances, electrolytes, water, and other substances that may be reabsorbed or excreted by the kidneys according to individual fluctuating needs.

Threshold substances are those that are entirely reabsorbed by the kidneys unless the substances are present in excessive concentration in the blood. Glucose is the most common threshold substance. Nonthreshold substances are not reabsorbed by the kidney tubules. Creatinine is the most abundant nonthreshold substance. Urea is included in this category even though urea passively diffuses back into the kidney bloodstream. Proteins and acids of disease processes (lactic acid, ketones) are nonthreshold substances. Water and most electrolytes will be absorbed or secreted according to individual needs.

There are two commonly used tests to determine efficiency of kidney function in handling waste products: *blood urea nitrogen (BUN) and creatinine.*

The **BUN** measures the level of urea, a nitrogen waste product of protein metabolism. The BUN is an unreliable test of renal function because the BUN level is affected by many factors. In the presence of liver disease, the BUN will remain low because the liver cannot synthesize urea at a normal rate. Conversely, with normal kidney function, dehydration, gastrointestinal bleeding, sepsis, trauma, drugs, diet, and changes in catabolism may elevate the BUN markedly, to as much as 50 mg/100 mL. Food in the digestive tract may also falsely elevate the BUN.

Serum creatinine is a more reliable index of kidney function. Creatinine is a waste product of muscle metabolism and is freely filtered. The normally functioning kidney filters creatinine from the blood at a rate equal to the GFR. As the amount of creatinine produced each day is constant and is proportional to the body's muscle mass, serial serum creatinines are valuable indices of kidney function except in septic patients and patients with muscle-wasting diseases.

TABLE 42-2. CATEGORIES OF DIURETICS

Category of Diuretic	*Drug*	*Mechanism of Action*	*Side Effects*
Loop diuretics	Furosemide (Lasix) Bumetanide (Bumex) Ethacrynic acid (Edecrin) Torsemide (Demadex)	Inhibits sodium chloride reabsorption in thick ascending limb of loop of Henle	Hypovolemia, thrombocytopenia, hypokalemia, hyperglycemia, hypochloremic alkalosis, transient deafness, hypocalcemia, hypomagnesemia, Ototoxicity (deafness, tinnitus), angioedema
Osmotic diuretics	Metolazone (Diulo, Zaroxolyn) Mannitol (Osmitrol) Glycerin (Osmoglyn) urea (Ureaphil)	Inhibits sodium and water reabsorption by increasing the osmolality of the tubular fluid	Blurred vision, rhinitis, rebound hypervolemia, thirst, urinary retention, electrolyte imbalances
Thiazide diuretics	Hydrochlorothiazide (HydroDiuril, Esidrix)	Inhibits sodium reabsorption in proximal and distal tubules	Skin photosensitivity, hypokalemia, hypomagnesemia, hypercalcemia, hyponatremia, Gout/hyperuricemia, ocular effects/glaucoma Rash, leukopenia, acute pancreatitis, thrombocytopenia Sulfonamide ("sulfa") allergy—Hypersensitivity
Potassium-sparing diuretics	Spironolactone (Aldactone) Triamterene (Dyazide, Dyrenium, Maxzide) amiloride (Midamor)	Inhibits aldosterone Promotes sodium excretion and potassium reabsorption in distal tubule causing a mild diuresis	Spironolactone: Gynecomastia Hyperkalemia, headache, hyponatremia, nausea, diarrhea, urticaria, menstrual disturbances, hypocalcemia, hypomagnesemia, hydrogen excretion
Carbonic anhydrase inhibitors	Acetazolamide (Diamox)	Inhibits the enzyme carbonic anhydrase in the proximal tubule preventing bicarbonate and sodium reabsorption	Hyperchloremic acidosis, renal calculi, rash, nausea, vomiting, anorexia Aplastic anemia, growth retardation, hypersensitivity, metabolic acidosis, paresthesia

Normally, a BUN-to-creatinine ratio of 10:1 is present in serum. A ratio of 20:1 or more is indicative of prerenal insufficiency (water and salt depletion), a high protein catabolism, or low renal perfusion pressures.

An elevation of both BUN and creatinine above the normal ratio indicates renal disease. In these patients, creatinine clearance is usually performed. Creatinine clearance is probably the most reliable index of kidney function available. Normal creatinine clearance is 125 mL/min. Urine is collected for 12 or 24 h or for a specified period of time and a blood serum sample is drawn halfway through the urine collection. If the BUN, creatinine, and creatinine clearance tests are normal, the kidneys are functioning adequately in excreting metabolic waste products from the body.

Regulation of Acid–Base Balance

The body's acid–base balance is maintained by the lungs, blood buffers, and kidneys. *The kidneys regulate acid–base balance by controlling the bicarbonate ion (HCO_3^-)* and, in much lesser quantity, the hydrogen ion (H^+). A normal diet contains some acids (phosphates and sulfates) that must be excreted. In addition, protein catabolism is markedly increased in the critically ill, which adds to the acid load of the body. Products of protein catabolism are eliminated by the kidneys.

Regulation of Blood Pressure

The kidneys participate in the regulation of blood pressure through four different mechanisms: by maintaining ECF volume and composition, by regulating aldosterone, through the renin–angiotensin mechanism, and by regulating prostaglandin synthesis.

Maintenance of Extracellular Fluid Volume and Composition. The *autoregulatory system* of the afferent and efferent arterioles responds to change in blood pressure to maintain consistent perfusion of the glomerulus. When this system fails, plasma flow may increase by two mechanisms. Vasoconstriction will maintain or elevate the blood pressure for a short period of time. If no more defense mechanisms exist, then only intravenous fluids (crystalloids or colloids) will alter the volume flow or composition of the plasma and the ECF. As the flow of plasma decreases, the patient becomes hypotensive, hypoxic, and hypoperfused. As the plasma flow deficit and the extracellular deficits are corrected, the patient becomes more closely normotensive.

Effect of Aldosterone on Blood Pressure. *The main effect of aldosterone is to maintain normal sodium concentration in the ECF.* Because sodium is the most abundant cation in the ECF, all other cations and anions will be present in varying ratios to the sodium. *Aldosterone promotes reabsorption of sodium* in both the distal convoluted tubule and the collecting ducts of the kidneys. Sodium will "drag along" water, bicarbonate, chloride, and other ions as it is reabsorbed. This mechanism helps to restore ECF and intracellular fluid volumes, alter the composition of the compartments as needed, and subsequently, in a normal healthy kidney, maintain the blood pressure.

Renin–Angiotensin Mechanism. *Any factor that decreases the GFR will activate the renin–angiotensin system. The most potent effect is upon systemic blood pressure.*

Once activated, the JGA, located adjacent to the glomeruli, releases inactive renin. Factors triggering the release of inactive renin (eg, decreased blood pressure and decreased sodium content in the distal tubule) reflect a diminished GFR. Once released, the inactive renin acts on angiotensinogen to split away the vasoactive peptide angiotensin I. Angiotensin I is split into angiotensin II in the presence of a converting enzyme found primarily in the lung and liver but also located in the kidney and all blood vessels.

Angiotensin II is a potent vasoconstricting agent. Angiotensin II in the circulatory system causes a severe constriction of peripheral arterioles and a milder constriction in the venous system. *It also causes a constriction of renal arterioles. This results in the kidneys reabsorbing sodium and water and expanding the ECF volume.*

Angiotensin II *also stimulates the release of* ***aldosterone*** *to enhance sodium and water reabsorption, thus supporting an increase in circulating volume.* This increase in sodium stimulates the thirst mechanism in an effort to reestablish circulating blood volume.

On rare occasions, some factors initiate the release of renin, and the release is never turned off. *The continuous presence of renin may maintain an active system known as malignant hypertension.* The key to treating malignant hypertension is to cut off the release of renin.

Prostaglandins. It was once thought that prostaglandins were originally located in the seminal vesicles and produced by the prostate gland (thus their name). Prostaglandins are unsaturated fatty acids found in most cells but highly concentrated in the kidneys, brain, and gonads. Prostaglandins or their precursors are synthesized in the medullary interstitial cells and the collecting tubules of the kidneys. Prostaglandins promote a vasodilation of the renal medulla to maintain renal perfusion during severe or prolonged systemic hypoperfusion.

Red Blood Cell Synthesis and Maturation

Renal erythropoietic factor is an enzyme released by a hypoxic kidney as a result of decreased oxygen supply. After being released into the bloodstream, the erythropoietic factor reacts with a glycoprotein to break away as erythropoietin. Erythropoietin circulates in the blood for about 24 hours. During this time, it *stimulates red blood cell production by the bone marrow.* After 5 or more days, a maximum rate of red blood cell production is achieved. The life of the red blood cell is approximately 120 days.

Either the kidney itself or some other factor that is the precursor of erythropoietin synthesizes the erythropoietic factor by releasing an enzyme called renal erythropoietin factor. Bone marrow by itself does not respond to hypoxia by producing new red blood cells.

Patients with chronic renal failure usually have hemoglobins between 5 and 6 g. The diseased kidneys are unable to respond to hypoxia and cannot produce erythropoietin factor. It is believed that possibly 10% of erythropoietin is formed in some place other than the kidney. Diagnostic studies used in evaluating renal function are presented in **Tables 42-3** and **42-4**.

TABLE 42-3. BLOOD AND URINARY DIAGNOSTIC STUDIES FOR THE EVALUATION OF RENAL FUNCTION

Study	*Significance*
Blood	
Hematocrit/hemoglobin	Reflects bleeding or low erythropoietin
Creatinine	Reflects renal disease
Blood urea nitrogen (BUN)	Normal BUN-to-creatinine ratio is 10:1; Ratio in excess of 20:1, suspect dehydration, catabolic state; Elevation in both BUN and creatinine results from decreased GFR
Electrolytes	
Arterial blood gases	
Clotting profile	
Osmolality	
Protein, albumin, glucose, cholesterol	
Urine	
Specific gravity (normal 1.003–1.030)	Less than 1.010, suspect DI, overhydration, or CHF Greater than 1.030, suspect proteinuria, glycosuria, X-ray contrast media, or severe dehydration
Creatinine clearance (24-h urine collection)	Estimates percentage of functioning nephrons
Culture and sensitivity	Presence or absence of infection
pH (normal, 4–8)	Alkaline urine seen with infection
Glucose	Present when renal threshold for glucose exceeded
Acetone	Present during starvation and DKA
Protein	Present in nephrotic syndrome and renal failure caused by myeloma proteins
Spot electrolytes (sodium, potassium, and chloride)	Assesses ability of renal tubules to conserve sodium and concentrate urine
Urinary sediment	
Casts	Protein that takes on the shape of the tubule in which it is formed
Hyaline casts	Present in large amounts in proteinuria
Erythrocyte casts	Diagnostic for active glomerulonephritis
Leukocyte casts	Diagnostic for infection
Granular casts	Result from degenerating erythrocyte or leukocyte casts
Fatty casts	Present in large amounts in lipoid nephrosis and nephrotic syndrome
Renal tubular casts	Present in acute renal failure
Renal epithelial cells	Present in large amounts during ATN and nephrotic injury
Erythrocytes	Present in large amounts in active glomerulonephritis, interstitial nephritis, infections
Bacteria	Presence determined by Gram stain
Leukocytes	Present in infection and interstitial nephritis
Crystals	Present in diseases of stone formation or following ethylene glycol intoxication
Eosinophils	Present during an allergic reaction in kidney

ATN, acute tubular necrosis; CHF, congestive heart failure; DI, diabetes insipidus; DKA, diabetic ketoacidosis.

TABLE 42-4. RADIOLOGIC STUDIES USED IN EVALUATING RENAL FUNCTION

Study	*Significance*
Abdominal radiograph	Determines position, shape, and size of kidney
Intravenous pyelogram (IVP)	Visualizes urinary tract to diagnose partial obstruction, renovascular hypertension, tumor, cysts, and congenital abnormalities
Renal scan	Determines renal perfusion, function, and presence of obstruction and masses
Retrograde pyelography	Determines presence of obstruction in upper region of urinary collecting system
Retrograde urethrography	Evaluates urethra
Cystoscopy	Detects bladder or urethral pathologic processes
Renal arteriography	Identifies tumors and status of renovascular disease
Ultrasonography	Identifies hydronephrosis and fluid collections
Computed tomography (CT)	Identifies tumors and other pathologic conditions that create variations in body density
Magnetic resonance imaging (MRI)	Provides direct imaging in several planes conducive to detecting renal cystic disease, inflammatory processes, and renal cell carcinoma
Kidney biopsy	Determines cause and extent of lesions

KEY CONTENT CHECKLIST

- ❒ Remember that the minimum threshold for urine output can be considered to be at least 0.5 mL/kg/h (this is 35 mL/h in a 70 kg patient).
- ❒ An easy way to remember the reference range for serum osmolality is that it is approximately twice the serum sodium. For example, 2 × sodium of 145 = 290 osmolality.
- ❒ Below a mean arterial blood pressure of about 60 mm Hg, this autoregulatory system fails and the glomerulus suffers the effects of hypotension.
- ❒ Normally, a BUN-to-creatinine ratio of 10:1 is present in serum. A ratio of 20:1 or more is indicative of pre-renal insufficiency (water and salt depletion), a high protein catabolism, or low renal perfusion pressures.
- ❒ Renal erythropoietic factor is an enzyme released by a hypoxic kidney as a result of decreased oxygen supply. It stimulates red blood cell production by the bone marrow.
- ❒ Any factor that decreases the GFR will activate the renin–angiotensin system. The most potent effect is upon systemic blood pressure.
- ❒ **Angiotensin II** also stimulates the release of **aldosterone** to enhance sodium and water reabsorption, thus supporting an increase in circulating volume.

Review Questions:

1. The right kidney is slightly lower than the left. What is the reason for this difference?

a. The right kidney is larger because of the presence of more nephric structures.
b. The left kidney is displaced upward by the spleen.
c. The right kidney is displaced downward by the liver.
d. The left kidney is drawn upward by the diaphragm.

Answer: C. Rationale: The majority of the liver is in the right upper quadrant, displacing the right kidney downward, making option C the best answer. The spleen is a small organ in the left upper quadrant, too small to displace the left kidney, eliminating B. The diaphragm is not in close proximity to the kidneys and does not influence one kidney's position relative to the other, eliminating D as well. Choose C.

2. Which of the following elements is NOT filtered during glomerular filtration?

a. Sodium
b. Potassium
c. Proteins
d. Creatinine

Answer: C. Rationale: Because protein-sized (and larger) molecules cannot filter out of the glomerular capillaries, those proteins remain in the blood entering the peritubular capillaries from the efferent arteriole. Creatinine and all electrolytes are filtered. Note that sodium and potassium are both electrolytes, which helps eliminate options A and B quickly.

3. Fluid is forced from the glomerulus, forming an ultrafiltrate. Into which compartment is the fluid forced?

a. Bowman's capsule
b. Proximal tubule
c. Collecting ducts
d. Distal tubule

Answer: A. Rationale: The high pressure in the glomerulus tends to filter fluid out of the glomerulus and into Bowman's capsule.

43

Renal Regulation of Electrolytes

CHAPTER OVERVIEW AND OBJECTIVES

This chapter contains information from the CCRN section on life-threatening electrolyte imbalances. Expect two to four questions from this chapter on the exam.

After studying this chapter, you should understand the following:

- Recognition of electrolyte disturbances in the critically ill patient.
- Replacement of low electrolyte levels in the critically ill patient.
- Treatment of elevated electrolyte levels in the critically ill patient.

This chapter contains information from the CCRN section on life-threatening electrolyte imbalances. You will find more detail in this chapter than the exam requires. However, understanding this detail is helpful in answering the questions presented on the exam. Expect two to four questions from this chapter on the exam.

Dysfunction of the normal physiologic processes of the kidney can result in abnormalities in both fluid and electrolyte balance. Frequent monitoring is essential to recognize imbalances early, prevent generalized deterioration, and help the kidneys to reestablish homeostasis. Prompt recognition of altered renal status and institution of indicated interventions can prevent the progression of renal and nephron damage.

The electrolytes of major concern are sodium, potassium, calcium, phosphate, magnesium, and chloride. Electrolyte imbalances are a result of (1) excessive ingestion or reabsorption of an electrolyte or (2) the lack of ingestion or excessive excretion of an electrolyte. Most body fluid imbalances are caused by a dysfunction in the regulation of electrolytes and water by the kidney.

43.1 SODIUM

Sodium Regulation

Sodium (Na^+) is the most prevalent cation in the extracellular fluid compartment and exists in the body in combination with an anion, usually chloride. It is important in maintaining extracellular fluid osmotic pressure, serum osmolarity, total body water balance, and acid–base balance. Intracellularly, it plays a major role in a number of chemical pathways and in the control of muscle contraction. The normal serum sodium level ranges between 135 and 145 mEq/L. To maintain this level, sodium is excreted or reabsorbed by the kidney. Reabsorption of sodium increases with a decreased glomerular filtration rate (GFR), as seen with hypoperfusion states (shock, myocardial infarction).

QUICK TIP! Remembering reference ranges such as sodium 135 to 145 may be helpful, however, the exam also often just says "increased" or "decreased." An easy way to remember this reference range is that "35-45" also shows up in the pH range (7.35–7.45) and the pCO_2 range (35–45).

Aldosterone has the greatest influence on sodium excretion. Aldosterone is a mineralocorticoid secreted by the adrenal cortex. *It is the most potent natural inhibitor of sodium excretion.* Aldosterone production and release is stimulated by high potassium levels, steroids (adrenocorticotropic hormone [ACTH]), and angiotensin II. **Aldosterone** acts on the distal convoluted tubule and the collecting duct to **promote reabsorption of**

sodium and excretion of potassium. Without aldosterone present, the distal tubule and collecting ducts cannot closely regulate the amount of sodium reabsorbed. The increased reabsorption of sodium in the presence of aldosterone also **results in the reabsorption of water.**

Diuretic therapy is usually thought of in relation to potassium. However, the loop diuretics (furosemide [Lasix], ethacrynic acid [Edecrin], and bumetanide [Bumex]) block the chloride pump in the thick portion of the ascending limb of the loop of Henle. When chloride reabsorption is blocked, sodium cannot diffuse out of the ascending limb. Other factors that can increase the excretion of sodium include an increased GFR, decreased aldosterone secretion, and increased antidiuretic hormone (ADH) levels.

Hypernatremia

A serum sodium level above 145 mEq/L is termed hypernatremia. Most cases of hypernatremia are due not to Na^+ disturbances but to fluid disturbances. Treatment is centered on giving fluid, not removing sodium. If a pure water loss or decreased intake is causing the hypernatremia, the hematocrit will be elevated, serum chloride will be above 106 mEq/L, *urine-specific gravity will be greater than 1.025, and urine sodium levels will be low.* Hypernatremia may also be associated with fluid volume excess with a gain of both sodium and water but a relatively greater gain of sodium. It is a significant electrolyte disturbance because of the neurologic and endocrine disturbances that result. Hypernatremia may also cause some depression of cardiac function.

Etiology. Hypernatremia typically results from excessive water loss. The most common cause is *insufficient secretion of antidiuretic hormone (eg, diabetes insipidus).* Increased insensible water loss (eg, from severe burn injuries) and inadequate intake of free water may also lead to hypernatremia. This places comatose patients or patients with neurological dysfunction at increased risk as they are not able to drink as needed and may be unable to self-regulate due to impaired sense of thirst. Potassium depletion (eg, from vomiting, diarrhea, or nasogastric suction) and uncontrolled diabetes mellitus with osmotic diuresis secondary to hyperglycemia are additional causes of hypernatremia.

In addition to excess water loss, hypernatremia may result from excessive sodium administration. This rarely occurs through dietary sodium intake but may be iatrogenic. Administration of hypertonic IV fluids or enteric tube feeding formulations may result in the intentional or unintentional increase in serum sodium levels. Medications such as sodium bicarbonate, and high sodium-containing laxatives and antacids may also precipitate a hypernatremia. Lastly, renal dysfunction can result in hypernatremia if the kidneys are too damaged to filter and excrete sodium, resulting in sodium and fluid retention.

Clinical Presentation. Because hypernatremia generally occurs with dehydration, signs include dry, sticky mucous membranes, thirst, oliguria, fever, tachycardia, and agitation. In addition, patients may demonstrate behavior changes, hypotension, decreased cardiac output, convulsion, or coma. Death may result in extreme cases; however, this is rare if renal function is intact. Patients with hypernatremia associated with an excess of sodium and fluid volume present with edema, increased blood pressure, dyspnea, and weight gain.

Treatment. Treatment is going to be dictated somewhat by the etiology of the hypernatremia. *Fluid administration with free water (nonelectrolyte solutions like D_5W) in a dehydrated patient is the key to diluting the sodium and halting the progression toward hypovolemic shock.* In the case of hypernatremia from fluid and sodium retention, identification and treatment of the underlying cause is the key to successful treatment. Any at-risk medications or hypertonic fluids should be stopped. Diuretics and fluid restriction are indicated.

Hyponatremia

Hyponatremia is present when the serum sodium level is less than 130 mEq/L. Usually, the plasma chloride will be less than 98 mEq/L. *Hematocrit may be decreased due to water excess.*

Etiology. Hyponatremia is due to either (1) an excessive amount of water or (2) sodium depletion. Excessive amounts of water can build up in many situations. The patient who has undergone gastric or intestinal surgery, who has nasogastric suction in use, and is receiving intravenous (IV) D_5W may become hyponatremic in only 2 or 3 days. Repeated tap water enemas may result in hyponatremia. Rarely, hyponatremia may result from over ingestion of free water.

The **syndrome of inappropriate ADH (SIADH)** release may precipitate a hyponatremia. In this instance, the stimulus that activated ADH release is never turned off. *The presence of ADH causes the kidneys to reabsorb water* continuously, thus diluting the body's sodium levels. Water retention that dilutes serum sodium levels may also occur with heart failure, cirrhosis of the liver, or nephrotic syndrome. A low cardiac output precipitates water retention by the kidneys.

Hypovolemic hyponatremia due to sodium depletion or loss is commonly caused by the overuse of the **thiazide diuretics, furosemide (Lasix)**, and **mannitol (Osmitrol)**. Diarrhea, Addison's disease, gastric suction, hyperglycemia (with a glucose-induced diuresis), vomiting, and extreme diaphoresis without IV replacement of sodium may also cause hypovolemic hyponatremia. Most causes of hyponatremia are associated with a low plasma osmolality; however, hypertonic hyponatremia due to hyperglycemia or IV administration of mannitol can occur.

Clinical Presentation. The clinical presentation of hyponatremia depends on its magnitude, rapidity of onset, and cause. *In general, the faster the serum sodium drops and the lower the serum sodium level, the more likely that symptoms will be severe.*

Hyponatremia with Water Retention. In hyponatremia with water excess, signs of water intoxication are usually present. They include apathy, coma, confusion, headache, generalized weakness, hyporeflexia, convulsions, and death. Increased blood pressure and edema are usually present.

Hyponatremia with Dehydration. If the hyponatremia is associated with decreased extracellular fluid, the symptoms are essentially the same as for heat prostration. Apprehension and anxiety are followed by a feeling of impending doom. The patient is weak, confused or stuporous, and may have abdominal cramps and nausea. Mucous membranes are dry. Azotemia develops and progresses to oliguria. In severe cases, vasomotor collapse occurs, with hypotension, tachycardia, and shock.

An interesting clinical presentation exists in cases of hyponatremia associated with dehydration. As dehydration progresses, fluid moves from the extracellular to the intracellular compartment. A finger pressed over the sternum will result in a fingerprint. This "fingerprinting of the sternum" indicates that much extracellular fluid has been excreted and plasma fluid has moved into the intracellular spaces from the vascular system. Without appropriate intervention, the patient may die very quickly. In less severe cases, symptoms may include lassitude, apathy, headache, anorexia, nausea, vomiting, diarrhea, muscle spasms, and cramps.

Treatment. The goals of treatment are aimed at reestablishing normal serum sodium levels and correcting the underlying cause. Acute or severe hyponatremia (plasma Na^+ level <110–115 mmol/L) often presents with altered mental status and/or seizures and requires rapid correction with hypertonic saline to raise the plasma Na^+ level by 1 to 2 mmol/L/h for the first 3 to 4 h or until the seizures subside. The plasma Na^+ concentration should not be raised by more than 12 mmol/L during the first 24 h. Fluid restriction or low-dose diuretic therapy is the treatment of choice if the hyponatremia is due to excess vascular fluid. Diuretics, if used, are given cautiously to avoid cerebral injury. *Cerebral injury can occur from the overly rapid expansion of brain cells due to water removal.* In instances other than SIADH, replacement of sodium with normal or hypertonic saline may also be indicated. Close monitoring of all body systems, along with monitoring of serial serum sodium levels, is essential during this period.

In SIADH, the treatment is to restrict water intake while attempting to help the kidneys excrete water normally. In susceptible SIADH patients, the administration of hypertonic saline may induce heart failure.

43.2 POTASSIUM

Potassium Regulation

Potassium (K^+) is the most prevalent intracellular cation in the body. The normal serum potassium level is 3.5 to 5.0 mEq/L. Potassium maintains osmolarity and electrical neutrality inside the cell and helps maintain acid–base balance. Intracellular homeostasis is needed for converting carbohydrates into energy and for reassembling amino acids into proteins. Transmission of nerve impulses is dependent on potassium. The muscles of the heart, lungs, intestines, and skeleton cannot function normally without potassium.

All the potassium filtered by the glomeruli is reabsorbed in the proximal convoluted tubule. Potassium that is excreted is secreted from the interstitial medullary space into the distal convoluted tubules. It amounts to about 10% to 12% of the original potassium volume of the ultrafiltrate in the proximal convoluted tubules. The amount of potassium excreted depends largely on the volume of urine. About 85% of the potassium is excreted in the urine and about 15% in the intestines. Even in hypokalemia (decreased potassium), a large urine volume will contain potassium, further compounding the problems. Sodium and potassium will compete for reabsorption. The normal ratio of potassium to sodium ion reabsorption is 1:35.

Sodium and potassium are intimately related, and factors that affect sodium reabsorption and excretion also affect the potassium level. Potassium levels are commonly raised by IV fluids containing potassium chloride. Although the kidneys act readily to conserve sodium, potassium is poorly conserved, especially in patients who are critically ill.

Factors that enhance the excretion of potassium include an elevated intracellular potassium level, which may be caused by an acute metabolic or respiratory alkalosis that forces potassium into the cells and hydrogen out of the cells. Diuretics and other factors resulting in high-volume flow rates in the distal convoluted tubule result in increased excretion of potassium. **Aldosterone** functions as a feedback mechanism on the distal convoluted tubule and collecting ducts to reabsorb sodium and excrete potassium when the potassium level in the extracellular fluid is increased. The enhancement of sodium reabsorption may force potassium excretion.

Potassium maintains an extracellular-to-intracellular fluid gradient. This gradient is affected by the adrenal steroids, hyponatremia, glycogen formation, testosterone, and pH changes. *The most significant of these influences is the pH. Serum potassium moves inversely to the pH. If the pH falls, potassium concentration increases. If the pH rises, potassium concentration decreases, in part because of the ionic charge of potassium and hydrogen.* Serum potassium must be evaluated with the arterial blood gases (ABGs) to avoid compounding problems of potassium therapy. Metabolic alkalosis is often associated with hypokalemia and occurs because of redistribution of potassium as well as excessive renal potassium loss.

KEY CLINICAL CONCEPT

Remember that alkalosis and hypokalemia are associated with an oxyhemoglobin curve **shift to the left** and acidosis and hyperkalemia are associated with a **shift to the right.** These types of questions about the oxyhemoglobin curve often appear on the test.

Hyperkalemia

Hyperkalemia is a potassium level greater than 5.5 mEq/L. It is due to an inability of the kidney tubules to excrete potassium ions. Tubular damage or increased potassium load that exceeds the kidney's ability to handle the quantity of potassium results in hyperkalemia.

Etiology. Hyperkalemia may be due to acute or chronic renal disease, low cardiac output states, acidosis, sodium depletion, or large muscle mass injury. Any factor that destroys cells (eg, burns, trauma, or crush injuries) will release the intracellular potassium, causing hyperkalemia. Excessive ingestion of potassium chloride (found in antacids and salt substitutes), adrenal cortical insufficiency, and the *hemolysis of banked blood may also cause hyperkalemia.*

QUICK TIP! Banked packed RBCs (PRBCs) contain potassium and transfusions can contribute to hyperkalemia.

Clinical Presentation. The membrane potential is related to the ratio of intracellular and extracellular potassium concentration, and a hyperkalemia partially depolarizes the cell membrane.

TABLE 43-1. POTENTIAL PHYSIOLOGIC EFFECTS OF HIGH AND LOW ELECTROLYTES

	High Levels ("Flaccidity")	*Low Levels ("Irritability")*
Sodium	Lethargy, weakness, coma	Seizures, altered LOC, irritability, muscle twitching
Potassium	Bradycardia/asystole	Ventricular dysrhythmias
Magnesium	Smooth muscle relaxation (eg, hypotension, decreased deep tendon reflexes, muscle weakness)	Tetany, Torsades de Pointes
Calcium	Decreased LOC, AV blocks	Cramps, tetany

LOC, level of consciousness.

Prolonged depolarization impairs membrane excitability and is manifest as muscle weakness (**Table 43-1**). Generalized muscle irritability or flaccidity, which may be severe enough to be a flaccid paralysis, and numbness of extremities are present. There may be abdominal cramping, nausea, and diarrhea. Generally, the patient is apathetic and may be confused.

The most serious effect of hyperkalemia is cardiac toxicity, which does not often correlate well with the plasma potassium concentration. The earliest changes in the electrocardiographic (ECG) tracing show a tall, peaked, or tent-shaped T wave with potassium levels of 5.5 to 7.5 mEq/L. In marked hyperkalemia (potassium of 7.5–9 mEq/L), there is a flattening and widening of the P wave, a prolonged PR interval, and usually depression of the ST segment. In severely advanced hyperkalemia (potassium of 8–9 mEq/L and often >10 mEq/L), the P waves disappear and intraventricular conduction disturbances occur, producing intraventricular and supraventricular dysrhythmias progressing to ventricular tachycardia, ventricular standstill, or asystole and death.

Treatment. A serum potassium level above 5.5 mEq/L requires immediate intervention. Because cardiac toxicity does not correlate well with potassium levels, and due to the not insignificant chance of falsely elevated potassium (eg, from hemolysis), an ECG should be obtained immediately. Treatment is initiated to prevent increasing bradycardia and cardiac arrest. *The objective of treatment is to reduce the serum potassium to a safe level as rapidly as possible.* Cardiac monitoring is essential.

Treatment can be broadly categorized into therapies that reduce extracellular potassium by driving it intracellularly, therapies that increase excretion of potassium, and therapies designed to stabilize the cardiac membrane potential. **Administration of IV insulin w ill temporarily drive potassium into the cell. Coadministration of IV D10 will prevent hypoglycemia from the insulin. IV sodium bicarbonate will also allow for intracellular movement of potassium by buffering hydrogen. Nebulized albuterol shifts potassium into the cell by stimulating Na+/K+-ATPase.**

Sodium polystyrene **(Kayexalate)** is given orally or as an enema and binds potassium, resulting in its excretion in the stool. **Kayexalate's** slow mechanism of action (2–24 hours) makes it better suited for chronic conditions and provides limited use for acute hyperkalemia. Its associated risk for bowel necrosis and other adverse GI effects, especially when administered with sorbitol has led to a decline in use.

> QUICK TIP! Although administration of sodium polystyrene (Kayexalate) is not recommended in the treatment of acute hyperkalemia, standardized tests like the CCRN may continue to include it in test questions.

In patients with normal renal function, diuresis with a combination of loop and thiazide diuretics may result in a net loss of potassium. Hemodialysis is the preferred treatment modality for removal of potassium in cases of hyperkalemia. However, a number of factors including availability of a hemodialysis machine, specialized nursing, and dialysis access may limit its effectiveness in the emergency setting.

Therapies designed to stabilize cardiac membrane potential do not actually affect the potassium level at all. Rather, they reduce the cardiotoxic effects of the potassium. Calcium affects the threshold potential and the speed of impulse propagation. Either IV calcium chloride or gluconate may be used, recognizing that calcium chloride contains three times the amount of calcium. **Calcium chloride will oppose the cardiotoxic effects of hyperkalemia.** *Calcium therapy is contraindicated in patients on digoxin.*

Hypokalemia

Hypokalemia is a serum potassium level of less than 3.5 mEq/L. It can result from one or more of the following: decreased net intake, shift into cells, or increased net loss.

Etiology. *Hypokalemia may be due to alkalosis*, which stimulates hydrogen ion retention and potassium ion secretion in the distal convoluted tubules of the kidney. Diuretic therapy without potassium replacement, endocrine dysfunction (increased ACTH, thyroid storm), and renal dysfunction (tubular acidosis) may all cause hypokalemia.

High potassium losses, gastric and intestinal surgery, nasogastric suctioning, diarrhea, prolonged vomiting, and intestinal diseases predispose the patient to hypokalemia unless replacement therapy is maintained.

Clinical Presentation. The clinical signs and symptoms of hypokalemia vary greatly between individual patients; their severity depends on the degree of hypokalemia, with symptoms usually not occurring unless the potassium level is less than 3 mmol/L. Hypokalemia has many of the same signs as hyperkalemia. There is a general malaise and muscle weakness, which may progress to a flaccid paralysis. Anorexia, nausea, and vomiting may accompany a paralytic ileus. Mental status may range from drowsiness to coma. Hypotension may be present and may lead to cardiac arrest. If the patient is on digitalis, *signs of digitalis toxicity may be present because hypokalemia potentiates the effect of digitalis.*

Cardiac dysrhythmias are most commonly atrial unless the hypokalemia is profound, in which case premature ventricular beats are seen. Other ventricular dysrhythmias are rare unless digitalis toxicity is present. ECG tracings most commonly show a prominent *U wave*. Depression or flattening of the ST segment or inversion of the T wave may be apparent. An inverted T wave may fuse with the U wave, giving the appearance of a prolonged QT interval. *There is a generalized cardiac irritability in hypokalemic states.*

Muscle weakness results in shallow respiration that may progress to apnea. In hypokalemia, death may occur due to respiratory arrest, ventricular fibrillation, or ventricular tachycardia.

Treatment. Emergency treatment of severe hypokalemia is the slow IV administration of potassium chloride (approximately 10–20 mEq/h) while the patient's ECG patterns are monitored for dysrhythmias due to hyperkalemia. Monitoring of symptoms, serum potassium levels, and ABGs is imperative to prevent an iatrogenic hyperkalemia.

Nonemergency treatment is to replace potassium with IV fluids containing potassium chloride or with oral potassium supplements. Oral supplements should be diluted to prevent gastrointestinal irritation and facilitate absorption. The patient is monitored for adequate intake and output, cardiac status, potassium levels, and signs of alkalosis or impending digitalis toxicity.

43.3 CALCIUM

Calcium Regulation

The normal serum calcium (Ca^{2+}) concentration is 8.5 to 10.5 mg/dL. Calcium, with phosphorus, makes bones and teeth rigid and strong. It is integral to determining the strength and thickness of cell membranes. Calcium exerts a quieting action on nerve cells, thus maintaining normal transmission of nerve impulses. It also activates specific enzymes of the blood clotting process and those involved in the contraction of the myocardium.

Ninety-eight percent of calcium filtered by the kidneys is reabsorbed along the same pathways as sodium. There are four major factors influencing calcium reabsorption: parathyroid hormone (PTH), vitamin D, corticosteroids, and diuretics.

Parathyroid Hormone. If the serum PTH level is increased, there is increased reabsorption of ionized calcium from renal tubules. Reciprocally, the PTH increases phosphate excretion as well as calcium absorption from the gastrointestinal tract. PTH will mobilize calcium from the bones when the kidneys cannot or do not reabsorb sufficient calcium.

Vitamin D. Vitamin D must be present in an activated form to promote the absorption of calcium from the small intestine. Vitamin D is ingested in food, especially milk and then must be activated by ultraviolet (sun) light, which changes a chemical in the skin. This vitamin is additionally changed in the liver. Finally, the kidneys convert the vitamin to 1,25-dihydroxycholecalciferol, also known as activated vitamin D. The activated vitamin D promotes absorption of calcium from the small intestine. PTH stimulates this activation process, since a low serum level of calcium precludes an increase of calcium absorption in the kidney without PTH.

Corticosteroids. Corticosteroids are suspected of interfering with the activation of vitamin D, possibly in the liver, and decreasing the amount of calcium absorbed from the small intestine.

Diuretics. Diuretics can cause increased excretion of calcium and other electrolytes. If a loss of fluid volume results in a decreased volume of total body fluid, there will be a decreased GFR, resulting in reduced calcium excretion.

Hypercalcemia

Etiology. Hypercalcemia exists when the serum calcium level is above 10.5 mg/dL. Increased renal reabsorption of calcium may cause hypercalcemia. It may also be the result of increased intestinal absorption of calcium due to excessive dietary calcium intake or excessive vitamin D ingestion.

Hyperparathyroidism caused by parathyroid adenoma will lead to hypercalcemia by increasing the release of calcium from bone and by continuously stimulating the kidneys to reabsorb calcium. This also occurs in carcinoma of the parathyroid glands. Calcium–alkali syndrome can occur in patients with peptic ulcer disease, postmenopausal women, and others who ingest calcium-containing supplements or antacids. Multiple myeloma and metastatic carcinoma of the bone cause hypercalcemia secondary to the release of calcium from bone into the serum. Prolonged bed rest or immobilization potentiates the movement of calcium from the bones, teeth, and intestines. This process is more conspicuous in patients with Paget disease. Frequently, the calcium is deposited in joints, in muscle tissue close to joints, and in the kidneys as calcium stones.

Drugs, especially thiazide diuretics, inhibit calcium excretion, thus causing hypercalcemia in susceptible patients. Renal tubular acidosis, thyrotoxicosis, and hypophosphatemia may all cause hypercalcemia in those who are susceptible.

KEY CLINICAL CONCEPT

Serum phosphate and serum calcium have an inverse, or "teeter-totter"-type relationship. When calcium is increased, phosphate is decreased. When phosphate is increased, calcium is decreased (**Fig. 43-1**).

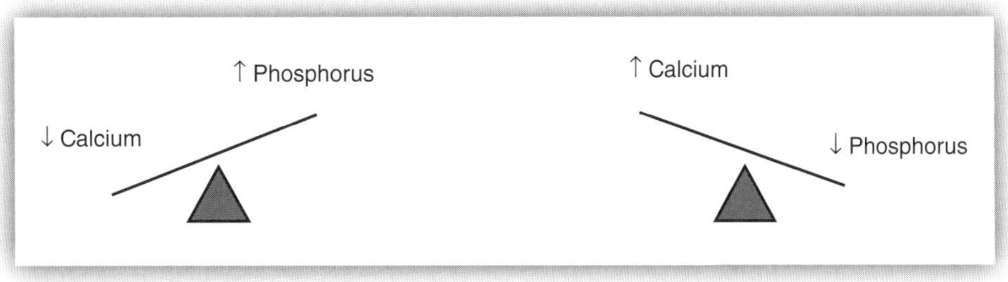

Figure 43-1. "See-saw" relationship of calcium and phosphorus. Hypocalcemia presents with similar signs and symptoms as hyperphosphatemia, and vice-versa.

Clinical Presentation. Neurologic signs include subtle personality changes in early and mild hypercalcemia; this progresses to lethargy, confusion, and coma as the severity of the hypercalcemia increases. Neuromuscular changes progress from weakness and hypotonicity to flaccidity.

The renal system may be affected by the formation of calcium calculi with varying amounts of urine output; depending on their location, such calculi may cause thigh or flank pain. Polyuria and polydipsia are often present because the increased calcium inhibits the action of ADH on the distal tubules and the collecting ducts.

Gastrointestinal symptoms include anorexia, nausea, vomiting, and constipation. Hypercalcemia stimulates the secretion of gastric acid and may lead to peptic ulcers. The hypotonicity caused by hypercalcemia results in decreased intestinal motility and constipation.

Cardiac changes are less common in hypercalcemia than in hyperkalemia. The earliest ECG change is a shortening of the QT interval due to shortening of the ST segment. *Digitalis and calcium are synergistic.* Sudden death in hypercalcemia is often attributed to ventricular fibrillation stemming from this synergism.

An ocular abnormality known as band keratopathy may occur because of the deposition of calcium crystals in the cornea. Calcium is deposited at the lateral borders of the cornea in the shape of parentheses. If the calcification is extensive, calcium will be deposited in semilunar bands across the cornea, connecting the parentheses. This band keratopathy may be seen by the naked eye.

Treatment. The objective of treatment is to reduce the serum calcium level. Normal saline IV solutions and diuretics will increase the GFR and thus the excretion of calcium provided that there are no obstructive calculi. These treatments require accurate monitoring of intake and output.

Contemporary management includes the use of IV bisphosphonates such as pamidronate (which prevent loss of bone mass), furosemide plus fluid administration (to promote renal excretion), corticosteroids (which antagonize vitamin D and decrease gastrointestinal absorption of calcium), mithramycin (which depresses mobilization of calcium from the bones), calcitonin (which reduces bone resorption and increases urinary excretion of calcium), and phosphates (which will bind to calcium in the intestines and precipitate calcium when administered intravenously).

Neurologic and cardiac monitoring is essential in assessing the efficacy of treatment. Some underlying conditions (such as multiple myeloma) will tend to make hypercalcemia refractory to treatment. In such cases, the goal of therapy becomes keeping the calcium level as low as possible.

Hypocalcemia

Etiology. Hypocalcemia is a clinical condition in which the serum calcium level is below 8.5 mg/dL. It usually develops from an excessive loss of calcium because of, for example, diarrhea, use of diuretics, malabsorption syndromes, massive blood transfusion, or hypoparathyroidism. Chronic renal failure is probably the most common cause of hypocalcemia. *If calcium is lost in peritoneal dialysis or hemodialysis, hyperphosphatemia may occur.* This enhances a peripheral deposition of calcium. Calcium deposits prevent calcium from being available to raise serum levels. Furthermore, the patient with chronic renal failure is unable to absorb calcium from the intestines secondary to a lack of activated vitamin D. Alkalosis can cause hypocalcemia because the calcium becomes bound to albumin and thus remains inactive in the serum.

> **QUICK TIP!** As a general rule of thumb, it is indicated to administer 1 g of calcium chloride for approximately every 3 units of PRBCs transfused.

Chronic malabsorption syndromes may cause hypocalcemia. These syndromes are found following gastrectomies, in diseases of the small bowel, in patients with a high-fat diet (fat impairs calcium absorption), and in those with a magnesium deficiency (magnesium inhibits PTH).

Malignancies may also cause hypocalcemia. These include osteoblastic metastases (whereby calcium is used for abnormal bone synthesis) and medullary carcinoma of the thyroid (causing an increased secretion of thyrocalcitonin, which in turn stimulates osteoblasts and prevents calcium from entering the serum).

Hypoparathyroidism of any cause results in hypocalcemia, since the secretion of PTH is decreased. The most common causes are surgical removal of the parathyroid glands, adenoma of the parathyroid glands, depleted magnesium levels (inhibits PTH), and idiopathic hypoparathyroidism.

A vitamin D-deficient state (or state of nonactivated vitamin D) is often seen in chronic renal failure, liver failure, and rickets. Without activated vitamin D, calcium is not absorbed from the intestines. *Acute pancreatitis causes a precipitation of calcium in the inflamed pancreas* and in intra-abdominal lipids.

In hyperphosphatemia, phosphates and calcium bind together and precipitate in tissues. This is commonly found in chronic renal failure because of decreased excretion of phosphates. Increased oral intake of phosphates rarely causes hyperphosphatemia if renal function is normal.

Clinical Presentation. Neuromuscular irritability is the overwhelming symptom present and the most dangerous. Muscle tremors and cramps are present in mild hypocalcemia. As the calcium level drops, tetany and generalized tonic–clonic seizures occur. Neuromuscular irritability causes labored, shallow respirations. Wheezing will be present if bronchospasm has occurred. Bronchospasm may lead to laryngospasm and tetany of the respiratory muscles, resulting in respiratory arrest. The presence of **Chvostek's and Trousseau's signs may be assessed.**

To test for **Chvostek's sign,** tap your finger over the supramandibular portion of the parotid gland, which is located in the subcutaneous tissue of the cheek. If the upper lip twitches on the side of stimulation, the test is positive.

To test for **Trousseau's sign**, apply a blood pressure cuff to the arm and inflate it until a carpopedal spasm occurs. If no spasm appears in 3 minutes, the test is negative. To test this result, remove the blood pressure cuff and have the patient hyperventilate (>30 breaths per min). The respiratory alkalosis that develops may produce a carpopedal spasm. This indicates a positive test.

Neuromuscular irritability frequently causes a decreased cardiac contractility, leading to a cardiac arrest. *The earliest ECG change is a lengthening of the QT interval due to a lengthening of the ST segment.* Patients are predisposed to life-threatening ventricular arrhythmias with hypocalcemia. Neuromuscular irritability may also cause biliary colic and paralytic ileus.

An *alteration in blood clotting* may be seen in hypocalcemia. Since calcium is necessary for normal blood clotting, hypocalcemia is often accompanied by bleeding dyscrasias.

Treatment. The aim of treatment is to raise the calcium level to normal as rapidly as possible to halt or prevent tetany.

In cases of tetany or impending tetany, IV **10% calcium gluconate or calcium chloride** is administered. The patient must be on a cardiac monitor because a rapid infusion may cause cardiac arrest, may enhance digitalis toxicity and because hypocalcemic patients are often also hyperkalemic. Vitamin D supplements are administered if a deficiency is present.

The efficacy of treatment is evaluated by monitoring serum calcium, phosphate, and potassium levels along with the ECG and neurologic status (using **Chvostek's** and **Trousseau's** signs).

43.4 PHOSPHATE

The normal serum level of phosphate (PO_4) is 3.0 to 4.5 mg/dL. The phosphate ion is found in bones and is a major factor in the intracellular production of ATP (energy). Phosphate combines with proteins and lipids to form important intracellular molecules. Intracellular phosphate ions may react with DNA and RNA molecules. Phosphate acts as a buffering agent for urine, is responsible for bone growth, promotes the phagocytic action of white blood cells (WBCs), and is important in platelet structure and function.

Phosphate Regulation

Phosphate levels are influenced by two major factors: PTH secretion (increases renal excretion of phosphate ions) and calcium concentration. **Calcium and phosphate have a reciprocal relationship.** *If calcium levels increase, phosphate levels decrease; conversely, if calcium levels decrease, phosphate levels increase.*

Reabsorption of phosphates occurs actively in the proximal convoluted tubule in the presence of sodium. Without sodium, phosphates will not be reabsorbed. Excretion of phosphates is regulated by PTH and the GFR. PTH inhibits reabsorption of phosphates in the proximal tubule, so phosphates will be excreted. With a decrease in the GFR, phosphate excretion will decrease; with an increase in the GFR, phosphates excretion will increase.

Hyperphosphatemia

Etiology. A serum phosphate level above 4.5 mg/dL constitutes hyperphosphatemia. Inability to excrete phosphates or excessive ingestion of phosphates are the two pathologic processes of hyperphosphatemia. The inability to excrete phosphates may be due to a decreased GFR or to renal failure.

Excessive ingestion of phosphates may be due to routine use (or abuse) of phosphate-containing laxatives and enemas or use of cytotoxic agents for the treatment of leukemias and lymphomas. Hypoparathyroidism causes hyperphosphatemia secondary to the effects of PTH on the kidney. Occasionally, over administration of IV or oral phosphates will induce hyperphosphatemia.

Clinical Presentation. *The clinical presentation of hyperphosphatemia is the same as that of hypocalcemia.* Elevated phosphate levels enhance the movement of calcium into bone. *If seizures occur, they are due to hypocalcemia caused by hyperphosphatemia. Remember that calcium and phosphate have a reciprocal relationship.*

Metastatic calcification occurs when calcium and phosphates combine chemically to form calcium phosphate, which then precipitates in arteries, soft tissue, and joints.

Treatment. The objective of therapy is to decrease the serum phosphate level. This is accomplished by giving aluminum hydroxide gels or calcium antacids that combine with phosphate, thus limiting the amount of phosphate available for absorption in the intestines. Dialysis may be needed if patient is symptomatic. Long-term management of hyperphosphatemia includes the use of oral phosphate binders such as calcium carbonate or calcium acetate, sevelamer, or lanthanum.

Hypophosphatemia

Etiology. Hypophosphatemia is a serum phosphate level below 3 mg/dL. Any factor that increases the cellular uptake to form sugar phosphates will decrease serum levels of phosphate. For example, prolonged intense hyperventilation can depress serum phosphate by inducing respiratory alkalosis. Sepsis and diabetic ketoacidosis also contribute to hypophosphatemia. Decreased phosphate absorption from the intestines (malabsorption syndromes), severe diarrhea, loss of proximal convoluted tubular function with renal phosphate wasting as seen in Fanconi syndrome, rickets, and conditions that are vitamin D resistant may also cause hypophosphatemia.

Chronic alcoholism results in a dietary deficiency of phosphates and may interfere with the absorption of any phosphates present. Abuse (including overuse) of phosphate binding gels such as Maalox or Amphojel causes hypophosphatemia, as does hyperparathyroidism (causing renal phosphaturia).

Long-term hyperalimentation may contribute to hypophosphatemia if phosphates are not included in the solution in adequate amounts. Use of hyperalimentation solutions with high glucose content requires phosphates. This is no longer a common etiology.

Clinical Presentation. Complaints of general malaise, anorexia, and vague muscle weakness may be of chronic or acute onset. With chronic onset, muscle wasting is apparent. With acute onset, rhabdomyolysis (a diffuse muscle-wasting necrosis) is due to a depletion of intracellular ATP and a concurrent decrease in all ATP-mediated processes. Hypercalcemia and hypercalciuria, with associated symptoms, are indicators of acute phosphate depletion due to hyperparathyroidism (PTH increases serum calcium by removing it from bone and decreases serum phosphate by excretion in the urine).

Hypoxia occurs because of a deficit in the red blood cell (RBC) phosphate content necessary for the formation of 2,3-diphosphoglycerate (2,3-DPG). *With a decrease in 2,3-DPG, a decrease in the dissociation of oxygen from hemoglobin is seen and tissue hypoxia results.*

QUICK TIP! The longer banked PRBCs are stored, the more PRBC erythrocyte concentration of 2,3 DPG decreases. When transfused, this creates a shift to the left on the oxyhemoglobin dissociation curve.

Complicating hypophosphatemia may be osteomalacia, severe metabolic acidosis, and insulin resistance resulting in hyperglycemia. This syndrome is rare and is usually seen in chronic alcoholism. It is a severe intravascular hemolysis caused by phosphate depletion, which results in a decrease of 2,3-DPG in RBCs.

Treatment. The objective of therapy is to replace the phosphates, first by IV administration and then orally. Use of phosphate-binding gels is discontinued and then treatment of the underlying cause of hypophosphatemia is begun.

43.5 MAGNESIUM

The normal serum level of magnesium (Mg^{2+}) is 1.5 to 2.5 mEq/L. The magnesium ion is the second major intracellular cation. Magnesium acts as a coenzyme in the metabolism of carbohydrates and proteins. It regulates neuromuscular excitability and phosphate levels. It is stored in bone, muscle, and soft tissue. Cardiovascular effects include peripheral vasodilation and cardiac contraction.

Magnesium Regulation

Renal reabsorption of magnesium is essentially the same as for calcium. The presence of sodium directly affects reabsorption in the proximal tubules. Without sodium, there is no reabsorption of magnesium. PTH appears to have a minimal effect on reabsorption. Reabsorption processes of calcium and magnesium are mutually suppressive.

Hypermagnesemia

Etiology. Hypermagnesemia is a serum magnesium level above 2.5 mEq/L. This is extremely rare. Reabsorption is similar to the calcium process. Absorption of excessive sodium (for any reason) in the renal tubules may "drag" an excessive amount of magnesium back into the blood.

Chronic renal disease and untreated diabetic acidosis are the usual causes. Addison disease, hyperparathyroidism, excessive magnesium administration, and overuse of magnesium-containing antacids or laxatives are other causes of hypermagnesemia.

Clinical Presentation. Lethargy, coma, depressed respirations, hyporeflexia, and hypotension are the usual symptoms. *All the symptoms of hyperkalemia may be present.* ECG changes consist first of prolonged PR intervals followed by widening of the QRS complex as the magnesium concentration rises. Death usually occurs with a concentration of 6 mEq/L or more.

Treatment. Attempts to lower magnesium levels by hemodialysis with a hypomagnesium dialysate have been successful. Administration of normal saline and diuretics will increase the excretion of magnesium. In the presence of life-threatening symptoms such as depressed respirations or cardiac arrhythmias, administer IV calcium gluconate.

Hypomagnesemia

Etiology. A magnesium level below 1.5 mEq/L is a state of hypomagnesemia. Any inhibition of absorption of magnesium from the gastrointestinal tract or of reabsorption from the renal system may account for hypomagnesemia. Severe malabsorption syndromes, acute pancreatitis, chronic alcoholism, primary aldosteronism, diabetic ketoacidosis, diuretic therapy, and renal disease are the usual causes. *Hypomagnesemia is often associated with hypokalemia and hypocalcemia.*

Clinical Presentation. *Neuromuscular and central nervous system hyperirritability characterize hypomagnesemia.* Muscle tremors, delirium, convulsion, and coma are seen. Positive Chvostek's and Trousseau's signs, tachycardia, increased blood pressure, depressed ST segments, and prolonged QT intervals are also seen. Hypomagnesemia may result in dysrhythmias such as **torsades de pointes**, ventricular fibrillation and supraventricular tachycardia. Digitalis toxicity is more likely with hypomagnesemia.

Treatment. The objective of treatment is simply to provide sufficient magnesium to raise the serum level. Low magnesium levels have been implicated in the development of ventricular dysrhythmias and have been treated more aggressively in recent years. Usually 1 to 2 g of magnesium can be given by IV administration.

43.6 CHLORIDE

Chloride Regulation

The normal serum chloride (Cl) level is 98 to 106 mg/dL. Chloride is reabsorbed by the kidney at all the sites for sodium reabsorption. Chloride moves freely with the gastric and intestinal fluids and is reabsorbed accordingly. Chloride is important in acid–base balance, serum osmolality, and water balance.

Anion Gap

Excretion of chloride is influenced by the acid–base balance. In acidosis, chloride is excreted while bicarbonate is reabsorbed. In alkalosis, chloride is reabsorbed while bicarbonate is excreted. Chloride can be used in combination with bicarbonate and sodium to obtain an estimated *"anion gap."* Although an anion gap never really exists, since cations and anions must be in balance to maintain electrochemical neutrality, an anion gap appears to be present if only sodium, bicarbonate, and chloride are measured. *A normal anion gap is less than 15 mEq and is obtained by subtracting bicarbonate and chloride from sodium.* For example, a patient with a sodium of 140, bicarbonate of 25, and chloride of 100 would have an anion gap of 15 ($140 - [100 + 25] = 15$).

The value of computing an anion gap is simple. If an anion gap exceeds 15, a specific type of metabolic acidosis, either a lactic, keto, or chronic renal failure acidosis exists. The anion gap appears to increase because bicarbonate to buffer the acidosis is lost without a simultaneous increase in chloride. In lactic, keto-, and chronic renal failure acidosis, anions other than chloride increase to offset the loss of bicarbonate.

Hyperchloremia

Etiology. Hyperchloremia is a serum chloride level above 106 mg/dL. An excessive ingestion of chloride (such as with infusion of large amounts of 0.9% normal saline, or 0.45% saline or lactated ringers) or kidney reabsorption of chloride ions (and excretion of bicarbonate) create hyperchloremic metabolic acidosis.

Clinical Presentation. The symptoms are the same as (or very similar to) those of metabolic acidosis such as hypernatremia, hypervolemia, tachypnea, hypertension.

Treatment. The objectives of treatment are to reduce the underlying cause of the elevated chloride level, which is most often achieved by the treatment of metabolic acidosis. Administer hypotonic IV fluids and electrolytes as needed and IV sodium bicarbonate or diuretics to increase excretion of chloride ions.

Hypochloremia

Etiology. Hypochloremia is a serum chloride below 98 mg/dL. Chloride ions are lost through excessive urination, vomiting, or gastric suction without replacement of electrolytes. This causes a physiologic metabolic alkalosis. The bicarbonate ion and chloride ion normally balance each other in kidney function.

Clinical Presentation. Symptoms of hypochloremia include changes in the sensorium, possible neuromuscular irritability, and usually slow, shallow respirations.

Treatment. The objective of treatment is to replace the lost chloride ions either orally or intravenously and to treat the cause of metabolic alkalosis to reestablish an acid–base balance.

KEY CONTENT CHECKLIST

- ❐ Remembering reference ranges such as sodium 135–145 may be helpful; however, the exam also often just says "increased" or "decreased." An easy way to remember this reference range is that "35–45" also shows up in the pH range (7.35–7.45) and the pCO_2 range (35–45).
- ❐ **Calcium and phosphate have a reciprocal relationship.** *If calcium levels increase, phosphate levels decrease; conversely, if calcium levels decrease, phosphate levels increase.*
- ❐ *With a decrease in 2,3-DPG, an increase in the affinity of oxygen from hemoglobin is seen and tissue hypoxia results.*
- ❐ Banked PRBCs contain potassium and transfusions can contribute to hyperkalemia.
- ❐ Remember that alkalosis and hypokalemia are associated with an oxyhemoglobin curve **shift to the left** and acidosis and hyperkalemia are associated with a **shift to the right.** These types of questions about the oxyhemoglobin curve often appear on the test.
- ❐ The longer banked PRBCs are stored, the more PRBC erythrocyte concentration of 2,3 DPG decreases. When transfused, this creates a shift to the left on the oxyhemoglobin dissociation curve.
- ❐ Hypomagnesemia may result in dysrhythmias such as **torsades de pointes.**
- ❐ A normal anion gap is less than 15 mEq and is obtained by subtracting bicarbonate and chloride from sodium.
- ❐ As a general rule of thumb, it is indicated to administer 1 g of calcium chloride for approximately every 3 units of PRBCs transfused.
- ❐ *Hyperkalemia* may promote an increase in **aldosterone**, which results in *potassium excretion* and *sodium reabsorption.*
- ❐ *Hypokalemia* may promote a decrease in **aldosterone**, which results in *reabsorption of potassium and excretion of sodium.*
- ❐ The **syndrome of inappropriate ADH (SIADH)** too much ADH release may precipitate a hyponatremia. *The presence of ADH causes the kidneys to reabsorb water* continuously, thus diluting the body's sodium levels. Treatment usually includes fluid restriction.
- ❐ Be familiar with the signs and symptoms of high and low electrolyte levels (see Table 43-1).
- ❐ To test for **Chvostek's sign**, tap your finger over the supramandibular portion of the parotid gland, which is located in the subcutaneous tissue of the cheek. If the upper lip twitches on the side of stimulation, the test is positive.
- ❐ To test for **Trousseau's sign**, apply a blood pressure cuff to the arm and inflate it until a carpopedal spasm occurs. If no spasm appears in 3 minutes, the test is negative.

Review Questions:

1. Which of the following corresponds most closely to the range of normal serum sodium values?

a. 40 to 60 mEq/L
b. 60 to 75 mEq/L
c. 80 to 120 mEq/L
d. 135 to 145 mEq/L

Answer: D. Rationale: This question pertains straight to the serum sodium reference range in a chemistry panel blood test. The serum sodium reference range is 135 to 145 mEq/L. An easy way to remember this is that the $PaCO_2$ reference range is somewhat similar, 35 to 45 mm Hg.

2. An 81-year-old man has been in the ICU for 45 days because of surgical complications from a ruptured bowel. The physician suspects that he may have nutritional impairment despite total parenteral nutrition. Laboratory tests reveal the following serum electrolyte information:

Na^+ 141 mEq/L
K^+ 3.9 mEq/L
Cl^- 102 mEq/L
HCO_3^- 25 mEq/L
Ca^{2+} 8.9 mg/dL
Mg^{2+} 4.3 mg/dL

Which of the preceding laboratory values is/are abnormal?

a. Mg^{2+}
b. Ca^{2+}
c. Cl^- and Na^+
d. K^+ and HCO_3^-

Answer: A. Rationale: The laboratory value that is most abnormal of the options available is magnesium. The reference range for magnesium is 1.7 to 2.2 mg/dL.

3. **Administration of which of the following is a normal initial treatment for hypernatremia?**
   a. Diuretics and fluid restriction
   b. Nonelectrolyte (free water) solutions
   c. Normal saline
   d. Potassium salts

Answer: B. Rationale: Fluid administration with free water (nonelectrolyte solutions like D_5W) in a dehydrated patient is the key to diluting the sodium and halting the progression toward hypovolemic shock. Diuretics and fluid restriction would worsen dehydration, eliminating A. The sodium content in normal saline and potassium salts may also exacerbate existing hypernatremia, eliminating C and D as well. Choose B.

REFERENCES

Ahmed AR, Obilana A, Lappin D. Renal replacement therapy in the critical care setting. *Crit Care Res Pract.* 2019;2019:6948710. Published 2019 Jul 16. doi:10.1155/2019/6948710.

Alvarez G, Chrusch C, Hulme T, Posadas-Calleja JG. Renal replacement therapy: a practical update. Traitement substitutif de l'insuffisance rénale : une mise à jour pratique. *Can J Anaesth.* 2019;66(5):593–604. doi:10.1007/s12630-019-01306-x.

Coccolini F, Moore EE, Kluger Y, et al. Kidney and uro-trauma: WSES-AAST guidelines. *World J Emerg Surg.* 2019;14:54. Published 2019 Dec 2. doi:10.1186/s13017-019-0274-x.

Emory MR, Jabaley CS. The Renal System. In: Boling B, Hatton K, Hatjes T (eds.) *Concepts in Surgical Critical Care.* Burlington, MA: Jones & Bartlett Learning; 2021:73–88.

Goyal A, Daneshpajouhnejad P, Hashmi MF, et al. Acute Kidney Injury. [Updated 2022 Jun 21]. In: StatPearls [Internet]. Treasure Island (FL): StatPearls Publishing; 2022 Jan. Available from: https://www.ncbi.nlm.nih.gov/books/NBK441896/

Griffin BR, Liu KD, Teixeira JP. Critical Care Nephrology: Core Curriculum 2020. *Am J Kidney Dis.* 2020;75(3):435–452. doi:10.1053/j.ajkd.2019.10.010.

Kellum JA, Romagnani P, Ashuntantang G, Ronco C, Zarbock A, Anders HJ. Acute kidney injury. *Nat Rev Dis Primers.* 2021;7(1):52. Published 2021 Jul 15. doi:10.1038/s41572-021-00284-z.

Palmer BF, Carrero JJ, Clegg DJ, et al. Clinical management of hyperkalemia. *Mayo Clin Proc.* 2021;96(3):744–762. doi:10.1016/j.mayocp.2020.06.014.

Pickkers P, Darmon M, Hoste E, et al. Acute kidney injury in the critically ill: an updated review on pathophysiology and management. *Intensive Care Med.* 2021;47(8):835–850. doi:10.1007/s00134-021-06454-7.

Rodriguez M, Hernandez M, Cheungpasitporn W, et al. Hyponatremia in heart failure: pathogenesis and management. *Curr Cardiol Rev.* 2019;15(4):252–261. doi:10.2174/1573403X15666190306111812.

Ronco C, Bellomo R, Kellum JA. Acute kidney injury. *Lancet.* 2019;394(10212):1949–1964. doi:10.1016/S0140-6736(19)32563-2.

Saunders H, Sanghavi D. Continuous Renal Replacement Therapy. [Updated 2022 May 29]. In: StatPearls [Internet]. Treasure Island (FL): StatPearls Publishing; 2022 Jan. Available from: https://www.ncbi.nlm.nih.gov/books/NBK556028/

Bellomo R, Ronco C, Kellum J, et al. Acute renal failure–definition, outcome measures, animal models, fluid therapy and information technology needs: The second international consensus conference of the acute dialysis quality initiative (ADQI) group. *Crit Care.* 2004;8:R204–R212.

Brunton LL, Lazo JS, Parker LK, et al. Diuretics. In: *Goodman & Gillman's The Pharmacological Basis of Therapeutics.* Online. Accessed 8/10/09.

Dirkes S, Hodge K. Continuous renal replacement therapy in the adult intensive care unit: History and current trends. *Crit Care Nurs.* 2007;27:61–80.

Geechan DM, Santucci, RA. Renal trauma. Available at: http://emedicine.medscape.com/article/440811-overview. Accessed 8/20/09.

Gunnerson KJ, Kellum JA. Acid–base and electrolyte analysis in critically ill patients: Are we ready for the new millennium? *Curr Opin Crit Care.* 2003;9:468–473. Harrison's Online. Acute renal failure, 2005. Accessed 8/10/09.

Harrison's Online. Dialysis in the treatment of renal failure. Accessed 8/10/09.

Harrison's Online. Fluid and electrolyte disturbances. Accessed 8/10/09.

Hinkle C. Renal system. In: Chulay M, Burns SM, eds. *AACN Essentials of Critical Care Nursing.* New York: McGraw-Hill; 2005:341–355.

Kellum JAM, Levin N, Bouman C, Lameire N. Developing a consensus classification system for acute renal failure. *Curr Opin Crit Care.* 2002;8:509–514.

Lameire N, Hoste E. Reflections on the definition, classification and diagnostic evaluation of acute renal failure. *Curr Opin Crit Care.* 2004;10:486–475.

Martin RI. Continuous renal replacement therapies. In: Lynn-McHale JD, Wiegand DJ, Carlson KK, eds. *AACN Procedure Manual for Critical Care.* 5th ed. St. Louis, MO: Mosby; 2005:937–960.

McGraw-Hill's Access Medicine Online. Acute renal failure. Accessed 8/2/09.

Rempher KJ. Continuous renal replacement therapy for management of overhydration in heart failure. *AACN Clin Issues.* 2003;14(4):512–519.

Ronco C, Bellomo R, Kellum JA. Continuous renal replacement therapy: Opinions and evidence. *Adv Renal Replace Ther.* 2002;9:229–244.

Salinitri F, Berlie H, Desai H. Pharmacotherapeutic blood pressure management in chronic kidney disease. *AACN Adv Crit Care.* 2009;20(3):205–213.

Tonelli M, Manns B, Wiebe N, et al. Continuous renal replacement therapy in adult patients with acute renal failure: Systematic review and economic evaluation. Technologic Report No. 88. Ottawa: Canadian Agency for Drugs and Technologies in Health. 2007. Accessed 8/22/09.

44

Diagnosis and Treatment of Acute Kidney Injury

CHAPTER OVERVIEW AND OBJECTIVES

The content of this chapter is designed to address CCRN exam questions on acute renal failure (eg, acute tubular necrosis [ATN]). Expect about two to four questions on the exam regarding material covered in this chapter.

After studying this chapter, you should understand the following:

- The signs and symptoms of AKI in the critically ill patient.
- Differentiation of prerenal, intrarenal, and postrenal causes of AKI.
- Indications for the use of renal replacement therapy in the critically ill patient.

Acute kidney injury (AKI) is a sudden loss of renal function with decreased glomerular filtration rate (GFR) that may or may not produce oliguria or anuria with a concurrent increase in plasma creatinine and blood urea nitrogen (BUN). AKI is a common complication of critical illness, occurring in up to 25% of patients in the intensive care unit (ICU). Mortality rates range from 40% to 70% depending on the amount of renal nephron damage, extent and duration of the AKI, and development of organ system dysfunction occurring as a result of AKI.

44.1 PATHOPHYSIOLOGY

Acute renal failure can be classified as prerenal, intrarenal, or postrenal.

- *Prerenal AKI* is caused by a decreased renal perfusion, typically associated with hypotension, hypovolemia, or decreased cardiac output. Prerenal AKI comprises 30% to 60% of all cases of AKI. Decreased renal perfusion causes a decrease in renal artery pressure, leading to a reduced afferent arteriolar pressure.
- *Intrarenal AKI* is caused by disease or injuries of the nephron from the glomerulus to the collecting duct. The most common cause of intrarenal failure is acute tubular necrosis (ATN). Consequently, these intrarenal conditions can be cortical or medullary in nature.
    - Cortical conditions involve swelling of the renal capillaries and cellular proliferation. Infectious, vascular, and/or immunologic processes cause edema and some resultant cellular debris that obstructs the glomeruli, resulting in a fall in urine output.
- Medullary involvement specifically affects the tubular portions of the nephron, causing necrosis. The extent of medullary damage differs depending on the cause of the necrosis: nephrotoxic injury or ischemic injury. Nephrotoxic injury affects the epithelial cells, which can regenerate after the nephrotoxic injury is resolved. Ischemic injury extends to the tubular basement membrane and may involve peritubular

capillaries and other parts of the nephron. *Postrenal AKI* is caused by an intra- or extrarenal obstruction at or below the level of the collecting ducts. If the obstruction is below the level of the bladder outlet, the blockage and subsequent backup of urine flow involves both kidneys. Eventually, urine output is decreased as a result of decreased glomerular filtration. Postrenal AKI is much less frequently encountered (1%–10% of hospital-acquired AKI) and is almost always amenable to treatment.

44.2 ETIOLOGY

Prerenal failure is the result of any condition that decreases perfusion of the kidney. Hypotension will result in preferential shunting of blood flow toward the most vital organs and at low enough pressures. This may result in decreased renal perfusion. Any condition that can cause hypotension, particularly conditions associated with hypovolemia, can lead to prerenal failure. Common causes in the ICU include hemorrhage, sepsis, third-spacing from burns, dehydration, excessive diuresis, and gastrointestinal fluid loss.

In addition to hypovolemic causes, renal perfusion can be decreased by poor forward flow due to an acute decrease in cardiac output, as is seen in cardiogenic shock. This may occur after an acute myocardial infarction or with acute decompensated heart failure.

The causes of *intrarenal failure* can be fairly well categorized as either cortical or medullary. **Table 44-1** summarizes the multiple causes of cortical and medullary intrarenal failure.

TABLE 44-1. CAUSES OF INTRARENAL FAILURE

Cortical Nephron Failure	*Medullary Nephron Failure*
Infections Poststreptococcal glomerulonephritis Acute pyelonephritis	Nephrotoxic causes Heavy metals Pesticides Fungicides
Goodpasture syndrome	Hemoglobinuria
Systemic lupus erythematosus	Myoglobinuria Hypercalcemia
Malignant hypertension	Antibiotics Aminoglycosides Cephalosporins Tetracyclines Penicillins Amphotericin B Ischemic causes Crush injuries Burns Sepsis Cardiogenic shock Postsurgical hypotension Hemorrhage with multiple trauma
Prerenal AKI: NSAIDs, ACE-I, ARBs, cyclosporine, tacrolimus	Contrast agents

Causes of *postrenal AKI* are obstructive in nature and include prostatic hypertrophy; bladder, pelvic, or retroperitoneal tumors; renal calculi; ureteral blockage (after surgery or instrumentation); urethral obstruction; bladder infections; and neurogenic bladder.

44.3 PHASES

There are four phases in the cycle of AKI: onset, oliguric, diuretic, and recovery.

1. **Onset or initial phase**
   The onset or initial phase precedes the actual necrotic injury and is associated with decreased cardiac output, renal blood flow, and GFR. **If mean arterial blood pressure falls below 60 mm Hg for more than 40 minutes, the risk of AKI is high.** An increase in cardiac output will produce an increase in renal blood flow and protect the patient from AKI.
2. **Oliguric phase**
   The oliguric phase reflects obstruction of tubules from edema, tubular casts, and cellular debris. Damage to the tubules makes absorption and secretion of solutes variable. If the obstruction and damage are severe enough, a back leak of filtrate through the epithelium may occur, returning the filtrate into the circulation.
   During the oliguric phase, laboratory reports will indicate rising levels of urea, creatinine, and potassium. Serum and urine osmolality are increased. Hypervolemia and electrolyte imbalances caused by retention of the metabolic waste products are the greatest dangers to the patient. This phase may last days to weeks.
3. **Diuretic phase**
   The diuretic phase indicates the beginning of the return of tubular function. It lasts about 10 days. The greatest danger to the patient in this phase is excessive loss of water and electrolytes. Extreme diuresis is due to the osmotic diuretic effect produced by the elevated BUN and the inability of the tubules to conserve sodium and water, resulting in an output of 3000 mL or more of urine per 24 hours. Hypokalemia is usually present.
4. **Recovery phase**
   The recovery phase begins when the diuresis is no longer excessive. There is a gradual improvement in kidney function, which may continue for 3 to 12 months. The result may be a permanent reduction in the GFR, which may or may not be sufficient to maintain adequate renal function without dialysis. AKI may progress to chronic renal failure, but this is uncommon unless the patient has an underlying kidney disease or is advanced in age.

44.4 CLINICAL PRESENTATION

As stated previously, oliguria may or may not be present in AKI with fifty percent of AKI patients being anuric. ***Therefore urine volume alone is not an adequate guide to renal function.*** Progressive azotemia (an excess of urea or other nitrogenous bodies in the blood) occurs as a result of decreased GFR despite apparently adequate urine output. AKI should be diagnosed before uremic signs are present. **Table 44-2** summarizes the clinical presentation of uremia.

TABLE 44-2. UREMIC SIGNS OF ACUTE RENAL FAILURE

Respiratory	*Metabolic*
Deep or rapid respiratory rate (metabolic acidosis) Bilateral rales Pulmonary edema	Electrolyte imbalance
Cardiovascular Tachycardia Dysrhythmias Pericarditis Friction rub	Integument Dry skin Uremic frost (excretion of urea) Pruritus Increased susceptibility to infection Edema
Neurologic Decreased level of consciousness Confusion Lethargy Stupor	Hematologic Anemias Uremic coagulopathies Bruising
Gastrointestinal Nausea Vomiting Anorexia Constipation or diarrhea Abdominal distention	

44.5 DIAGNOSIS

Diagnosing AKI or ATN may be difficult, especially in the nonoliguric patient. Factors that should be considered in a diagnosis include urinary volume, urinary sediment, BUN levels, serial serum creatinine, creatinine clearance, acid–base balance, trauma, and postsurgical status.

Urinary Volume

Normal urinary output is about 0.5 mL/kg/h. In prerenal failure, urine volume is decreased. In ATN, daily urine output may be constant or may gradually increase or decrease. Complete anuria suggests obstruction or cortical necrosis. It may occur in acute glomerulonephritis and complete postrenal obstruction but is rare otherwise. Different degrees of obstruction are suggested by large, irregular daily urine volumes. Partial obstruction can cause progressive azotemia, even though there may be normal or increased urine volume.

> QUICK TIP! It is helpful to know the reference ranges for urine sodium, specific gravity, and urine osmolality. However, it is also likely that they may only be described as, "increased" or, "decreased" in a scenario on the exam. Know when to anticipate increased or decreased values.

Laboratory Data

In prerenal failure, urinary sodium (Na^+) is less than 20 mEq/L as the kidneys attempt to conserve sodium and water. Urinary osmolality, which reflects the concentrating ability of the kidney, is elevated. Urinary osmolality is usually greater than 500 mOsm (normal level is 300–900 mOsm). *Specific gravity,* a less sensitive indicator of concentrating power than osmolality, is also elevated. Specific gravity is greater than 1.020. There is minimal or no proteinuria and normal urinary sediment. *The BUN increase is greater than the creatinine increase (20:1*; normal ratio is 10:1). Normal serum creatinine is about 0.8 to 1.3 mg/dL and normal BUN is about 10 to 20 mg/dL.

In cortical intrarenal failure, urinary sodium is less than 10 mEq/L. Specific gravity will vary with moderate to heavy proteinuria. Serum BUN and creatinine will be elevated (10–15:1). Hematuria is present with erythrocyte casts and leukocytes. *In medullary intrarenal failure or ATN, urinary sodium is greater than 20 mEq/L,* an abnormal sign when urine output is low. Normally the kidneys conserve sodium in an attempt to maintain extravascular water. In ATN, when urine output is low, the expected conservation of sodium fails to occur, resulting in a normal urinary sodium level (40–220 mEq/L). *Urinary osmolality decreases (<500 mOsm), reflecting the inability of the kidneys to concentrate the urine.* Simultaneously, the *specific gravity also decreases,* usually between 1.008 and 1.012. Minimal to moderate proteinuria is present with an elevated serum BUN and creatinine.

In *postrenal failure* there is scant sediment as well as rare white cells, red cells, hyaline casts, and fine granular (>40 mEq/L) casts. *Urinary sodium is elevated, specific gravity varies, and BUN and creatinine are elevated (10–15:1).*

44.6 MANAGEMENT OF PATIENT CARE PROBLEMS

There are four major problems of patient care in renal failure: an increase in the products of catabolism, severe electrolyte imbalance with associated acidosis, fluid overload, and infection.

1. **Increase in the products of catabolism**
   Protein catabolism increases in the critically ill, stressed patient. A decrease in proteins available for catabolism will retard the rate of azotemia, decrease the incidence and severity of acidosis, and decrease the occurrence and levels of hyperkalemia in the serum. The patient's caloric requirements must be met mainly through an adequate intake of carbohydrates in the diet.
2. **Serum electrolyte imbalance and acidosis**
   Sodium intake is restricted unless there is a serum sodium deficit. No salt substitutes are used because of their potassium content. Careful management of fluids and sodium intake will prevent overhydration, heart failure, hyponatremia, and water intoxication.

   Hyperkalemia is a significant imbalance seen in AKI. It is further compounded as a result of catabolism associated with fever and also occurs as a result of decreased potassium excretion caused by volume depletion or drugs. *Metabolic acidosis can also cause hyperkalemia.* The fall of the pH forces hydrogen ions into the cells and potassium into the extracellular fluid.
3. **Fluid overload**
   It is essential to determine and monitor the patient's volume status. Indicators of overhydration include weight gain, edema, anasarca, ascites, increased blood pressure, jugular

vein distention (JVD), and dyspnea. Indicators for dehydration include weight loss, decreased blood pressure, poor skin turgor, no evidence of JVD, and decreased central venous pressure.

Fluids are restricted to amounts equal to urine output plus 400 mL for insensible fluid loss. It is important that accurate daily weights be taken using the same scales. *It is also important to remember that 1000 mL of fluid weighs about 2.2 lb (1 kg).*

4. **Infection**

   Because proper kidney function affects all body systems, the chance of infection is increased in patients with renal failure. The body's defense systems do not function properly, and the patient is predisposed to urinary tract infections, septicemia, pneumonia, and wound or skin infections (due to the severe pruritus that some patients experience). Good nutritional intake by the patient and proper hygiene will help prevent infections. If fever develops, culture and sensitivities of blood, urine, sputum, or any wound should be performed to identify the invading organism. Once the organism is identified, appropriate antibiotic therapy is started with antibiotic doses adjusted to renal function.

44.7 RENAL REPLACEMENT THERAPY

As renal failure worsens, there may be need for renal replacement therapy (RRT). The purposes of RRT include

1. Removal of the by-products of protein metabolism, including urea, creatinine, and uric acid
2. Removal of excess water
3. Maintenance or restoration of the body's buffer system
4. Maintenance or restoration of the body's concentration of electrolytes

RRT involves the diffusion of dissolved particles from one fluid compartment to another across a semipermeable membrane. Three principles are utilized in dialysis: osmosis, diffusion, and filtration. Osmosis is the movement of fluid across a semipermeable membrane from a less concentrated solution to a more concentrated solution. Diffusion is the movement of particles (or solutes) across a semipermeable membrane from a more concentrated solution to a less concentrated solution. Filtration is the movement of particles or solutes across a semipermeable membrane through the utilization of hydrostatic pressure.

A number of different RRT modalities exist, but the most commonly used in the ICU include peritoneal dialysis, intermittent hemodialysis, and continuous renal replacement therapies (CRRT).

Peritoneal Dialysis

Peritoneal dialysis (PD) uses the peritoneum as the semipermeable membrane. The peritoneum is a strong, smooth, colorless serous membrane that lines the abdominal cavity with a parietal layer and wraps the abdominal organs with a visceral layer (**Fig. 44-1**).

The dialysate is instilled into the abdominal cavity between these two layers of peritoneum through a catheter. The visceral peritoneum is contiguous with the intestinal wall and the capillary beds of the intestines. The dialysate is instilled into the peritoneal space, bathing the intestines. Osmosis, diffusion, and filtration occur readily after "dwelling" in the abdomen.

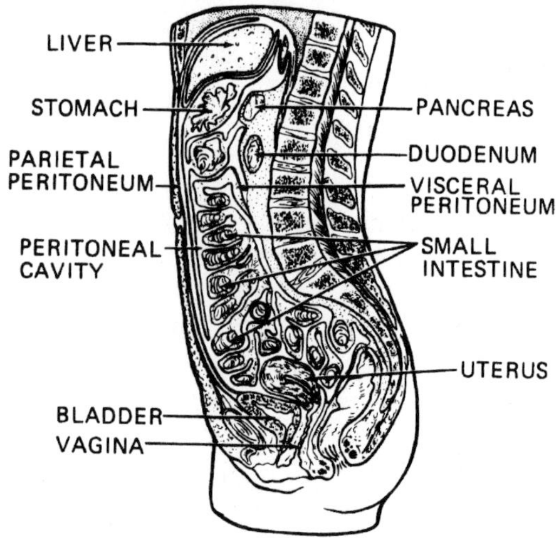

Figure 44-1. The peritoneal space (female).

Indications. PD is less common in treatment of AKI because of the requirement for surgical placement of a PD catheter. However, it is often used in the ICU to dialyze patients who are already undergoing PD as an outpatient.

The use of PD in peritonitis is a controversial topic. Some nephrologists advocate adding antibiotics to the dialysate in addition to using oral or intravenous antibiotics to bathe the infected area itself with antibiotics. Other nephrologists believe that peritonitis is a justification for stopping PD. The rationale here is to treat the patient with intravenous antibiotics to prevent septic shock from developing or to prevent weakening (to the actual point of rupture) of an inflamed, infected visceral peritoneum, and the contiguous intestinal wall.

Contraindications. Contraindications to the use of PD are largely related to the safety of placement of the PD catheter. Active bleeding or clotting disorders may predispose the patient to life-threatening hemorrhage. Patients with fresh postoperative vascular prostheses, such as a fresh femoral-popliteal bypass, are not candidates for PD because the procedure may result in graft failure at the site of anastomosis, leading to exsanguination. Recent abdominal surgery involving placement of drains or disruption of the peritoneum is another contraindication to PD. The peritoneum may not be strong enough to hold the dialysate without rupture or tearing of the peritoneum, and abdominal drains preclude any dwell time since the dialysate would flow out of the drains. Abdominal adhesions or any other condition where a danger of puncturing viscera exists is a contraindication to PD. Pregnant women should not undergo PD because of the increased risk of fetal distress.

Advantages. PD can be performed at the bedside by the ICU nurse without the requirements of specialized dialysis nurses or dialysis machines. Because it takes more time to effectively remove metabolic wastes and restore electrolyte and fluid balance, it is less stressful for pediatric and elderly patients and can be initiated quickly. There is also no need for systemic anticoagulation.

Disadvantages. PD is slower to rid the body of waste products than hemodialysis. Exchanges of 2000 mL performed every 3 hours achieve approximately the same solute clearance as a 4-hour hemodialysis treatment performed every other day. Prolonged PD results in protein depletion and may cause ascites, poor wound healing, and decreased resistance to infection. Peritonitis, usually resulting from staphylococci or Gram-negative organisms, may develop with repeated treatments.

Dialysate. The concentration of the dialysate solution is selected by the provider. The more concentrated the solute concentration, the greater the osmotic forces exerted to remove fluid and waste products. Osmotic forces are determined by the concentration of glucose in the dialysate, usually ranging from 1.5% to 4.25%. During the administration of 4.25% dialysate, the serum glucose must be monitored because glucose can diffuse into the serum.

The temperature of the dialysate influences the effectiveness of PD; urea clearance is 35% greater at body temperature (98.6°F) than at room temperature (75°F). Body-temperature dialysate will also enhance patient comfort.

The volume of the dialysate influences effectiveness. An exchange volume of 3 L of dialysate in 1 hour almost doubles the urea clearance achieved with 1 L/h. Most adults are comfortable with 2 L per exchange, and a few can tolerate 3 L.

Procedure and Nursing Care. To help obtain the patient's cooperation, the nurse should explain the procedure, making the patient aware of the discomforts of the procedure, limited mobility during it, and its duration. *The patient is weighed before the procedure and then either daily or after the last exchange.*

When catheter patency is confirmed, the warmed dialysate is infused, allowed to dwell in the abdomen, usually for 20 to 45 min, and then allowed to drain via gravity as completely as possible. One exchange usually takes about an hour. Turning the patient side to side may enhance the drainage of dialysate.

At the end of the dwell time, the dialysate is assessed for color. Normally, it is a clear pale yellow. *If the drainage is cloudy, suspect infection or peritonitis. If it is brownish, suspect bowel perforation.* Blood-tinged dialysate during the first four exchanges is normal. However, if after four exchanges the dialysate is still bloody, discontinue and notify the provider. The patient may have abdominal bleeding or a uremic coagulopathy.

Monitoring vital signs every 15 minutes during the first hour and then every 1 to 2 hours is the usual procedure if the vital signs are stable. The outflow period is the most likely time for abnormal or changing vital signs. Signs of impending shock, fluid overload, and pulmonary edema will be most apparent in this outflow period.

One of the most important aspects of peritoneal dialysis is the *intake–output record* maintained by the nurse. Hospital policies vary as to the format for recording peritoneal dialysis intake and output. Information needed includes the time the exchange was started, the number of the exchange, the amount of fluid infused, the dwell time, the amount of fluid drained, and the fluid balance.

Fluid balance is crucial. A running total should be maintained over all exchanges. For example, if 2000 mL is instilled and only 1750 mL drains out, the patient's fluid balance would be +250 mL. If the next exchange instills 2000 mL and drains 1900 mL, the patient's fluid balance for the exchange would be +100 mL, but the running balance is now +350 mL. During the third exchange, if 2000 mL was instilled and the output drainage was 2275 mL, the patient's balance for this exchange is −275 mL. However, in the continuous fluid balance columns, the patient is still at a fluid balance of +75 mL. Intake–output records are maintained for each exchange and overall for total exchanges.

Complications. *Infection is among the most common complications of peritoneal dialysis.* Insertion of the catheter under sterile technique and closed sterile instillation and drainage of dialysate will help reduce infection. Daily sterile changes of the dressing over the tube insertion site help decrease the chance of infection. Perhaps the most effective way to prevent infection is to keep the procedure time to 36 hours or less. Other common complications include volume overload, excess volume depletion, and electrolyte disturbances. Respiratory insufficiency may occur as the 2 L of dialysate is infused into the abdomen and push the abdominal viscera against the diaphragm, resulting in decreased depth of respirations.

Intermittent Hemodialysis

Hemodialysis uses extracorporeal circulation to remove fluid and metabolic waste products from the body. Blood is transferred by tubing from the patient to a machine that functions like a kidney to filter out waste products and then returns the filtered blood to the patient by another tube. Hemodialysis uses the same principles of osmosis, diffusion, and filtration that are used in peritoneal dialysis.

Indications. Hemodialysis has the same indications as peritoneal dialysis. Other reasons for performing hemodialysis include AKI due to trauma or infection, chronic renal failure no longer controlled by medication and diet, when rapid removal of toxins, poisons, and drugs is essential, and when peritoneal dialysis is contraindicated.

Contraindications. Labile cardiovascular states that would deteriorate with rapid changes in extravascular fluid volume are the major contraindications to hemodialysis.

In the past, patients who could not tolerate systemic heparinization could not be hemodialyzed. Today, however, the heparin is infused into the dialysis machine to keep blood anticoagulated within the machine. Before the blood is returned to the patient, protamine is infused to neutralize the heparin. This process is called regional heparinization (**Fig. 44-2**).

For the patient without a condition that would be worsened by heparin, intermittent heparinization is used. In these cases, 2000 to 5000 units of heparin are infused at the start of hemodialysis and 1000 to 2000 units of heparin are added for each hour that the patient is on the machine. These patients must be monitored closely for signs of bleeding.

There are three ways to access a patient's blood for hemodialysis: an arteriovenous (AV) shunt, single- or double-lumen catheters, and an AV fistula. The AV shunt (**Fig. 44-3**) consists of two Silastic catheters; one is inserted into an artery and the other is inserted into a nearby vein. Blood is channeled from the artery to the dialysis machine and back to the vein. Part of the shunt lies subcutaneously, and part lies outside the skin.

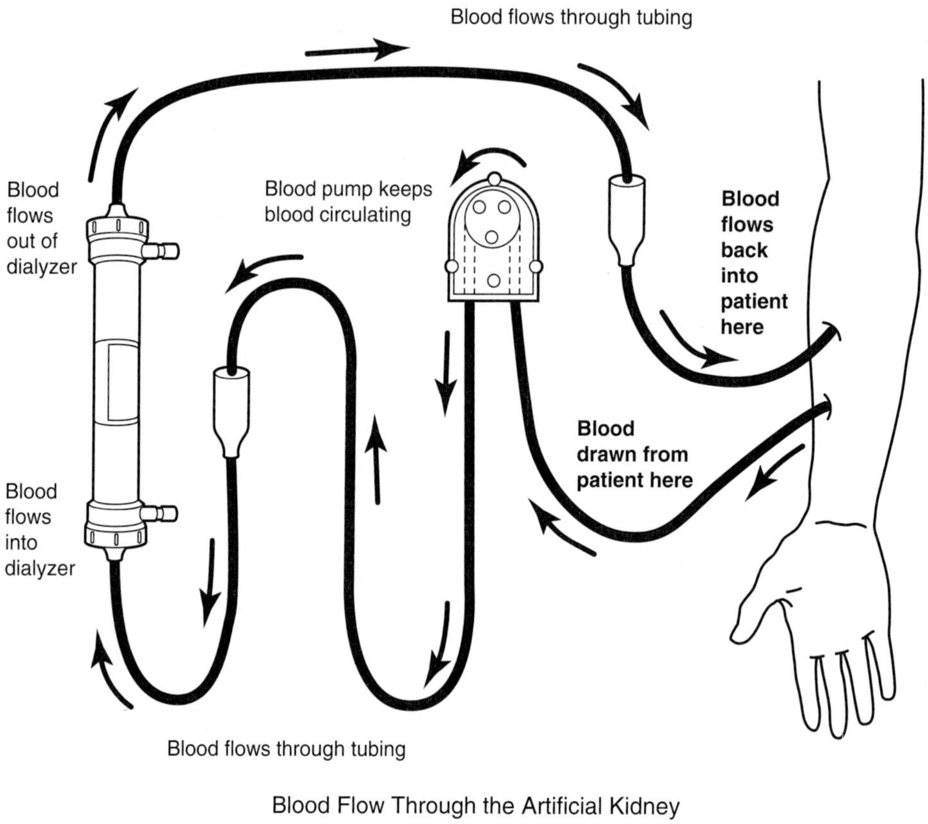

Figure 44-2. Dialysis machine.

When the patient is not undergoing hemodialysis, blood flows directly from the artery through the shunt and into the vein. Shunts are inserted under local anesthesia. The favored sites are the arm, wrist, legs, and ankles. In the upper extremity, the preferred vessels are from the radial artery to the cephalic vein. In the lower extremity, the preferred vessels are from the posterior tibial artery to the great saphenous vein.

Dialysis catheters (**Fig. 44-4**) are dual-lumen (some catheters may have a third lumen that serves solely as vascular access) catheters that function essentially as short-term shunts. They can be placed in the internal jugular, femoral, or subclavian veins. The right internal jugular vein is the preferred site due to the ease of placement and reduced rates of complications. During dialysis, one lumen is used to channel blood to the dialysis

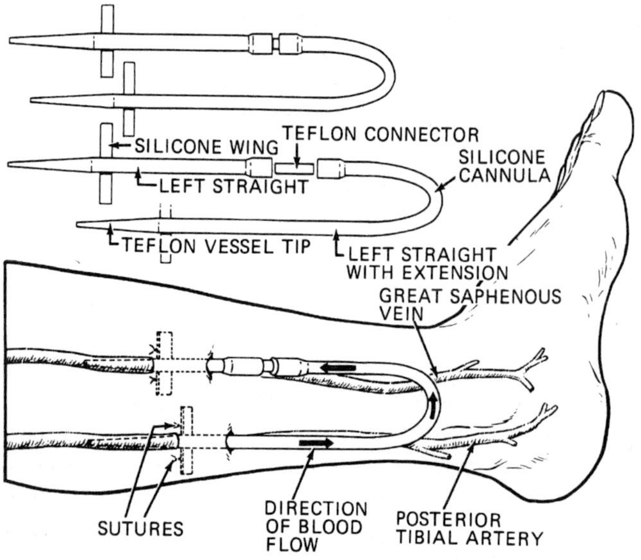

Figure 44-3. Arteriovenous shunt.

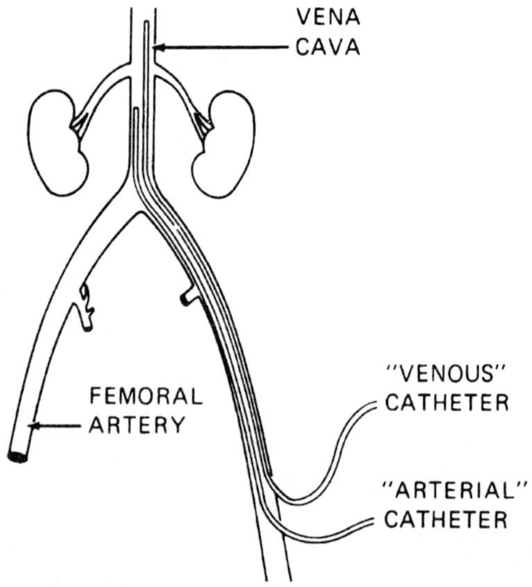

Figure 44-4. Dialysis catheters.

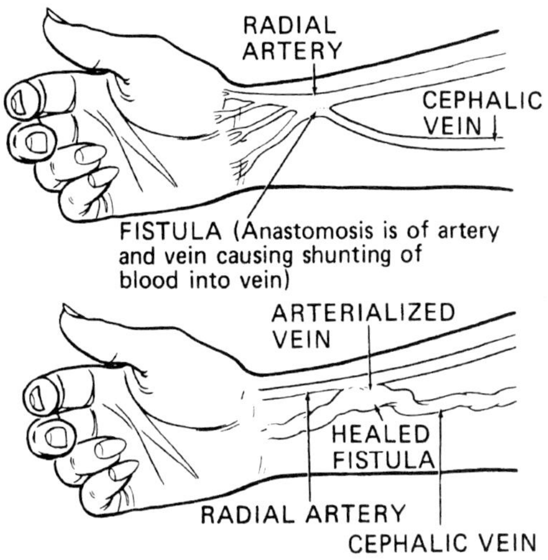

Figure 44-5. Anastomosis to form an arteriovenous fistula.

machine and the other is used to channel blood from the dialysis machine back to the patient. Assessment for signs of bleeding or hematoma formation is done frequently. If the catheter(s) is to remain after dialysis, low-dose heparin is utilized to maintain catheter patency.

AV fistulas are the gold standard; they have a longer life span than do AV shunts and tend to preserve the blood vessels in which they are placed. Fistulas are less restrictive than other forms of vascular access and therefore offer greater freedom to the patient. The fistula can be formed by the patient's vessels or by a graft (**Fig. 44-5**). Examples of graft materials are bovine carotid, woven Dacron, and umbilical vein. If grafts are used, they are tunneled under the skin in a U shape (**Fig. 44-6**). The surgical procedure involves anastomosis of the artery directly to the vein, most often utilizing a side-to-side technique. Fistulas must mature over a 4- to 6-week period. During this time, the vein adapts to the high pressure of the arterial blood by dilatation and thickening of the venous wall. When the fistula matures, the vein will be able to withstand the insertion of a large-bore needle (14–16 gauge). The insertion of needles in the arterial and venous arms of the fistula permits attachments to the dialysis machine.

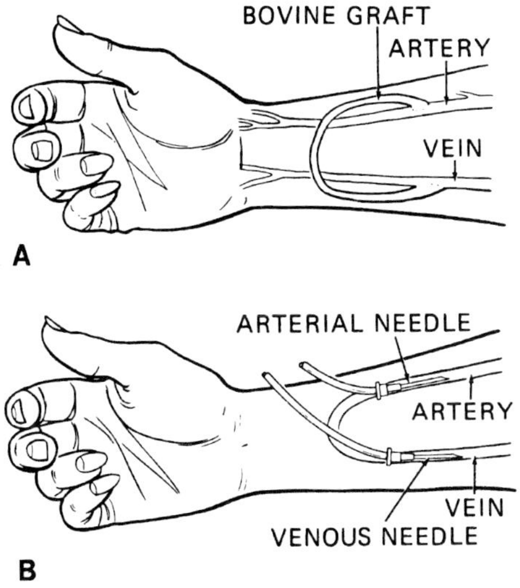

Figure 44-6. **A.** A graft in place and **B.** placement of needles in a graft for hemodialysis.

Complications associated with the AV fistula are infection, clotting, venous hypertension, and steal syndrome. Infection at the fistula site has direct access to systemic circulation and can precipitate septicemia. Localized infections present as reddened, tender, warm areas over the fistula, particularly at the anastomosis or needle puncture sites. Clotting sometimes causes severe pain and numbness in the affected arm; this can be confirmed by the absence of the *bruit and thrill* at the fistula site.

In venous hypertension, there is too much blood in the extremity distal to the fistula. This may cause ulcerations and may necessitate a fistula revision. In the steal syndrome, there is insufficient blood flow to the extremity because of excessive diversion of arterial blood to the vein at the anastomosis. Symptoms include coldness and poor function of the extremity. In severe cases, gangrene with necrosis of the extremity tips may develop. The steal syndrome is corrected by revising the fistula.

Once an access site is available, an evaluation of the patient's most recent electrolytes is made to determine what adjustments in the dialysate bath are to be made. An accurate predialysis weight of the patient is determined daily. By weighing the patient post dialysis, it is possible to calculate exactly how much fluid was removed or added.

Nursing Care. Infection is prevented by cleaning the shunt site daily using sterile technique and also by cleaning the fistula site until the incision is healed. If the shunt or fistula becomes infected, culture and sensitivity tests are done to identify the infecting organism. Once the organism is identified, intravenous antibiotics are started. If the shunt or fistula remains infected, it is removed, and a new shunt or fistula is created.

The prevention of thrombosis is always a challenge. Anything that decreases blood flow increases the chance of thrombosis. Some examples are hypotension, hypovolemia, tourniquets, blood pressure cuffs, tight clothing and jewelry, heavy handbags and packages, and dehydration.

If the shunt is patent, one can see bright red blood flowing freely through it and it feels warm to touch. There should not be any layering of the blood components (cells at the bottom, clear serum at the top). Proximal to the insertion site, one should feel a *thrill* (the turbulence of the arterial blood). With a stethoscope, one should hear a *bruit* (arterial blood turbulence). *If either the thrill or bruit is absent, notify the physician immediately.*

If the shunt becomes clotted, the physician may insert a catheter to remove the clot. After patency has been established, routine use of **heparin** will maintain patency.

To prevent hemorrhage due to shunt disconnection, clamps are attached to the dressing to ensure immediate availability. If the catheter becomes unconnected, the arterial cannula is clamped first to control excessive blood loss from the arterial system, and then the venous cannula is clamped.

The precautions taken for shunts are also taken for fistulas. *A thrill and bruit should be present.* The arm with a fistula is not used for intravenous fluids, blood pressure monitoring, venipuncture, or injections. The fistula is cleansed daily using sterile technique. Bleeding, skin discoloration, or drainage is reported to the physician.

Complications. Problems associated with hemodialysis occur most often during the initial stages or during a procedure lasting more than 4 hours. *Hypotension is caused by dehydration,* sepsis, or blood loss. *The patient may already be hypotensive or may rapidly become hypotensive when dialysis is initiated.* This is treated by reducing the blood flow, discontinuing ultrafiltration (fluid removal), and giving fluids. If the patient does not respond to this method of treatment, dialysis is discontinued.

Cardiac dysrhythmias may be caused by potassium intoxication, but usually no specific electrolyte derangement can be identified. In some instances, dysrhythmias may be related to the development of transient myocardial ischemia as evidenced by premature ventricular contractions. Treatment consists of decreasing the blood flow and using appropriate medication as indicated. The dialysis procedure must be stopped if the dysrhythmia is severe or does not respond to treatment. Heart failure in most instances is secondary to fluid overload, which can be reversed by ultrafiltration.

Disequilibrium syndrome may occur in reaction to the slowed clearance of urea from the cerebrospinal fluid during dialysis. Fluid shifts that occur to restore equilibrium result in cerebral swelling. Symptoms include headache, nausea, vomiting, restlessness progressing to disorientation, twitching, and seizures. Treatment focuses on prevention.

Air embolism may occur through an arterial or venous site as a result of a leak in the dialysis tubing, a loose connection, or the disconnection of dialysis tubing. With arterial air embolism, air travels the arterial system to a point distal to the entry site. In the head, the emboli enter the small vessels of the brain. Seizures may occur, followed by rapid brain cell damage. Death will ensue if critical areas of the brain are destroyed.

Venous emboli migrate back to the lungs and may cause *pulmonary emboli.* In the sitting patient with dialysis access in the lower extremities, air enters the venous system of the leg and travels to the inferior vena cava, then up through the right atrium to the superior vena cava, and finally to the head. In this case, the symptoms are the same as for arterial emboli in the brain.

If the patient is lying flat when air is introduced, the air enters the right atrium and moves into the right ventricle. Essentially, the air is trapped in the right ventricle and cannot be propelled from the heart. Blood cannot enter the pulmonary system. The lack of pulmonary blood return to the left atrium quickly stops the pumping of blood into the systemic circulation.

KEY CLINICAL CONCEPT

If the patient is lying flat when air is introduced into the venous circulation, the air enters the right atrium and moves into the right ventricle. Essentially, the air is trapped in the right ventricle and cannot be propelled from the heart. Blood cannot enter the pulmonary system. The patient must be placed in Trendelenburg position and turned on the left side. Once resuscitated, the patient must be kept in the Trendelenburg left-side position until the air is absorbed. This will prevent movement of the air into the cerebral tissues.

Symptoms of air embolism include deep respirations, coughing, cyanosis, unconsciousness, and cessation of breathing. Auscultation over the heart reveals a "mill wheel" sound during both phases of contraction. This is the sound of air turbulence in the heart.

Once air embolism has occurred, rapid corrective action is imperative. There are several important differences in the resuscitation of a patient with an air embolism as compared with the usual cardiopulmonary resuscitation. *The patient must be placed in Trendelenburg position and turned on the left side. Once resuscitated, the patient must be kept in the Trendelenburg left side position until the air is absorbed. This will prevent movement of the air into the cerebral tissues and heart* and promote movement toward the feet (air will be higher than fluid). The absorption time will vary, but it usually takes from days to weeks; the mortality rate is extremely high.

Continuous Renal Replacement Therapy

CRRT is essentially identical to intermittent hemodialysis, except that it is performed continuously over 24 hours. Because it accomplishes in 24 hours what intermediate hemodialysis accomplishes over 4 hours, CRRT is usually better tolerated hemodynamically and it facilitates gradual correction of metabolic and electrolyte abnormalities. In addition, it is highly effective in removing fluid, and it is technically simple to perform, not requiring the use of a specialized dialysis nurse. CRRT may utilize all the same methods as intermittent hemodialysis.

Indications. The principal indication for CRRT is the treatment of patients with acute oliguric renal failure. Because fluid volume alteration and electrolyte removal are slow processes, CRRT is especially beneficial in treating acute volume overload in patients with unstable cardiovascular systems unresponsive to diuretic therapy, as occurs in acute pulmonary edema, congestive heart failure, post-cardiac surgery, and recent myocardial infarction.

CRRT is also indicated in patients who require large quantities of parenteral fluid, as in hyperalimentation, intravenous antibiotic administration, and the continuous administration of vasopressors. CRRT is also considered when other forms of dialysis are contraindicated, and it may also be used to treat hyperkalemia, azotemia, and drug or poison intoxication. However, the critical care literature currently suggests that no difference in outcomes exists when comparing CRRT versus daily or every other day hemodialysis.

Contraindications. Contraindications to CRRT are an inability to tolerate anticoagulation and a hematocrit greater than 45%. Both of these problems precipitate clotting in the hemofilter. Lack of vascular access is also a contraindication of CRRT.

QUICK TIP! No CRRT questions will appear on the exam.

Advantages. CRRT has distinct advantages over hemodialysis. It allows the elimination of large amounts of fluid without the osmolar changes associated with hemodialysis, thus maintaining extracellular fluid status. During hemodialysis, rapid water removal causes the extracellular fluid to become hypotonic in relation to the hypertonic environment of the cell. Extracellular fluid is drawn into the cell, creating a depleted or hypovolemic state. The slow, consistent process of CRRT maintains osmolality and cardiovascular stability. Another problem occurring

TABLE 44-3. CONTINUOUS RENAL REPLACEMENT THERAPIES

Type of Therapy	*Acronym*	*Description*
Continuous venovenous hemofiltration	CVVH	Uses the principles of convection to promote slow continuous removal of solute and fluids through a permeable membrane filter that is driven by an external extracorporeal pump
Continuous venovenous hemodialysis	CVVHD	Uses the principles of diffusion with limited convection to promote slow continuous removal of solute and fluid facilitated by the addition of dialysate which promotes diffusion of solutes
Continuous venovenous hemodiafiltration	CVVHDF	Uses the principles of diffusion and convection to promote slow continuous removal of solute and fluids

Source: *Data from Villa G, Neri M, Bellomo R, et al: Nomenclature for renal replacement therapy and blood purification techniques in critically ill patients: practical applications, Crit Care. 2016 Oct 10;20(1):283.*

with hemodialysis but absent with CRRT is the reduction in the platelet and white blood cell count as the patient's blood comes into contact with cuprophane, cellulose acetate, or regenerated cellulose membrane. CRRT can be managed by the critical care nurse at the bedside rather than by hemodialysis staff.

Disadvantages. The main disadvantage of CRRT is its limited ability to remove waste products and excess solutes with minimal volume replacement.

Hemofiltration Process. Several modes of CRRT are readily available in the acute care setting: slow continuous ultrafiltration (SCUF), continuous venovenous hemofiltration (CVVH), and continuous venovenous hemodialysis (CVVHD), and continuous venovenous hemodiafiltration (CVVHDF) (**Table 44-3**). All modes use the same equipment: a highly porous hemofilter, venous blood lines, and a fluid collection device (**Fig. 44-7**). A blood pump on the CRRT system propels the blood through the filter at the desired rate to facilitate removal of fluid and solutes.

Cannulation of a large vein is performed by the physician, at the internal jugular, subclavian or femoral site. Venovenous access is established using a dual-lumen catheter. AV access (much less common and will not be discussed here) is achieved with cannulation of an artery and a vein. A hemofilter and blood lines are primed with saline. Venous blood is circulated through the blood line to the hemofilter. The hemofilter separates plasma water and certain solutes from the blood and passes the ultrafiltrate to a graduated measuring device. Blood, minus the ultrafiltrate, is then returned through the venous blood line to the venous site.

Slow Continuous Ultrafiltration. In SCUF, the removal of molecules dissolved in plasma, is based on the principle of convection. Some elements in the plasma water are conveyed across the semipermeable hemofilter as a result of the differences in hydrostatic pressure. Albumin and protein-bound substances are retained in the plasma and returned to the patient. SCUF removes filterable solutes in proportion to plasma water: large amounts of plasma water removed result in large amounts of filterable solutes removed (ultrafiltration). SCUF, therefore, does not alter the concentration of solutes in the blood.

Continuous Venovenous Hemofiltration. CVVH uses the principles of convection and replacement. Large volumes of fluid/ultrafiltrate are removed, pulling a greater variety of solutes with it. A balanced electrolyte replacement solution is used to restore blood volume. The infusion rate of this replacement fluid is determined by the ultrafiltration rate, intake, output, and desired fluid removal. CVVH can filter up to 20 L/24 h.

Continuous Venovenous Hemodialysis. CVVHD uses the principles of convection *and* diffusion. A dialysate bath solution is infused countercurrent through the filter (outside the blood filled semipermeable membranes) to create a diffusion gradient, enhancing the removal of urea and creatinine into the dialysate solution and out of the hemofilter into the ultrafiltrate. It provides more solute (urea, creatinine) clearance; therefore it is used in uremic patients with high catabolic rates (acidosis, hyperkalemia). Urea clearance is approximately twice that of CVVH. The higher the glucose concentration in the dialysate solution (1.5%, 2.5%, and 4.25%), the greater the solute and fluid removal.

Continuous Venovenous Hemodiafiltration. CVVHDF combines CVVH and CVVHD properties. The combination of convection and diffusion to produce maximal fluid and solute removal.

Nursing Care. Access sites are cleansed and inspected daily for signs of infection. Maintain an occlusive dressing at the venous catheter site. *Hypothermia is common; monitor the patient's temperature hourly and provide warming blanket to maintain normothermia.* Monitor the pressures and fluid rates on the dialysis machine to anticipate the clotting and clogging of the filter. Return blood before filter is completely obstructed. Laboratory values, daily weights, and hourly records of intake and output are performed.

Complications. The insertion site is inspected frequently for signs of infection, infiltration, and bleeding. If any of these occur, the access will be changed, and appropriate antibiotic therapy instituted. The tubing and catheter are kept free of kinks. A kinked catheter will decrease blood flow and greatly increase the risk of clotting as blood stagnates in the hemofilter.

Disconnection of the system from the hemofilter, blood lines, or access catheter may result in exsanguination. The system must be reconnected under sterile conditions. The circuit is clamped off to prevent air from entering the system. If air has entered the system, it is allowed to pass through the filter and must be removed through the blood infusion port so that it is not delivered to the patient.

The large doses of heparin required for CRRT place the patient at risk for bleeding. This danger can be minimized by monitoring clotting profiles.

Problems with the ultrafiltration rate may develop from problems with the patient or circuit. If the patient is hypovolemic or hypotensive, the circulation of blood from the patient into the filter/circuit may be reduced. This will decrease the amount of

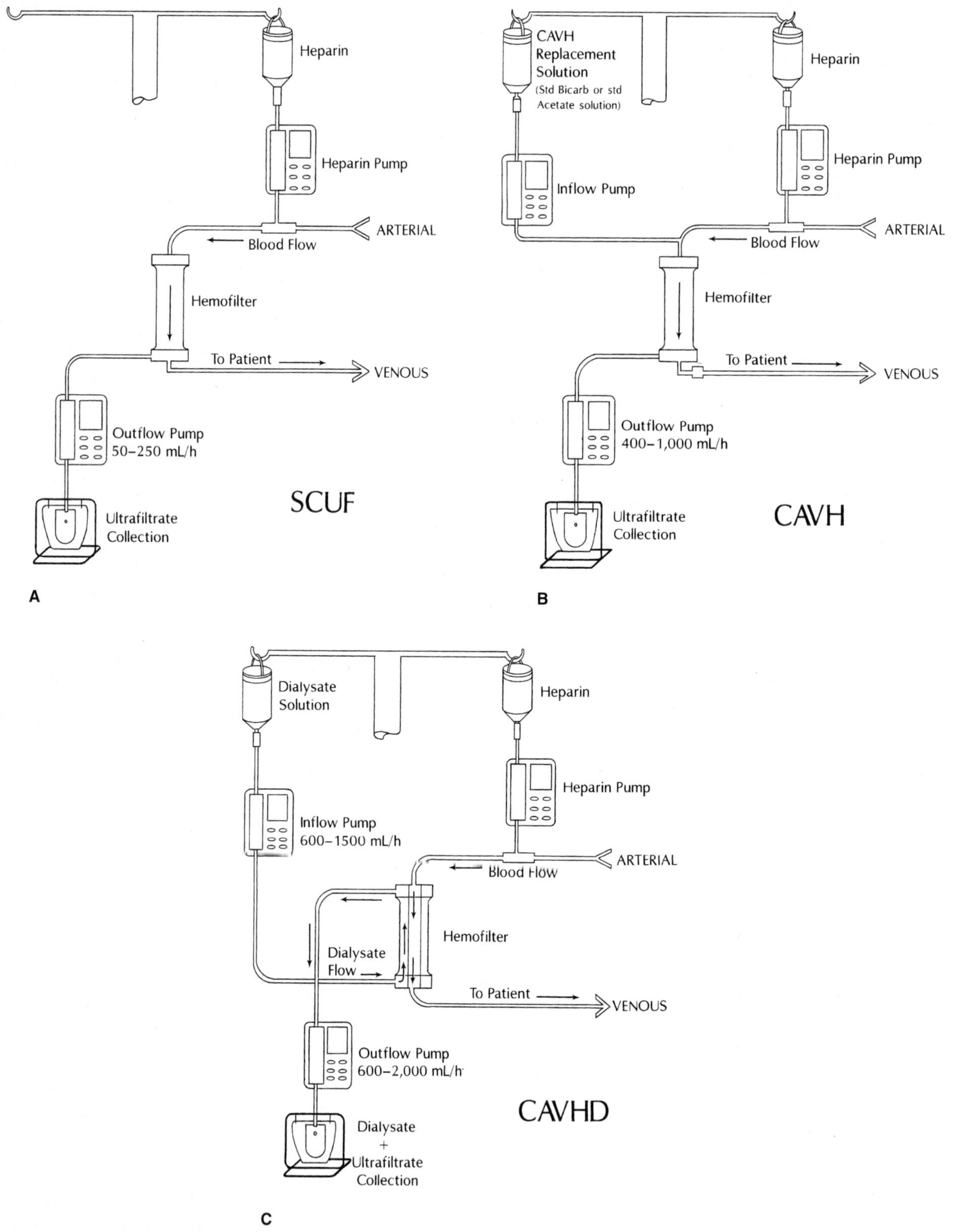

Figure 44-7. Modes of continuous renal replacement therapy (CRRT). **A.** Slow continuous ultrafiltration (SCUF). **B.** Continuous arteriovenous hemofiltration (CAVH). **C.** Continuous arteriovenous hemodialysis (CAVHD).

ultrafiltrate generated. It also contributes to clot formation in the hemofilter, resulting in slower filtration and less ultrafiltrate production. Filter clotting alarms warn of impending necessity to change the filter/circuit.

KEY CONTENT CHECKLIST

- ❒ If mean arterial blood pressure falls below 60 mm Hg for more than 40 minutes, the risk of AKI is high.
- ❒ Normal urinary output is about 0.5 mL/kg/h.
- ❒ The BUN increase is greater than the creatinine increase (20:1; normal ratio is 10:1) in pre-renal failure.
- ❒ In peritoneal dialysis patients, if the drainage is cloudy, suspect infection or peritonitis. If it is brownish, suspect bowel perforation.
- ❒ There will be no CRRT questions on the exam.
- ❒ *Disequilibrium syndrome* may occur in reaction to the slowed clearance of urea from the cerebrospinal fluid during dialysis. Fluid shifts that occur to restore equilibrium result in cerebral swelling. Symptoms include headache, nausea, vomiting, restlessness progressing to disorientation, twitching, and seizures. Treatment focuses on prevention.
- ❒ It is helpful to know the reference ranges for urine sodium, specific gravity, and urine osmolality. However, it is also likely that they may only be described as, "increased" or, "decreased" in a scenario on the exam. Know when to anticipate increased or decreased values.
- ❒ If the patient is lying flat when air is introduced into the venous circulation, the air enters the right atrium and moves into the right ventricle. Essentially, the air is trapped in the right ventricle and cannot be propelled from the heart. Blood cannot enter the pulmonary system. The patient must be placed in Trendelenburg position and turned on the left side. Once resuscitated, the patient must be kept in the Trendelenburg left-side position until the air is absorbed. This will prevent movement of the air into the cerebral tissues.

Review Questions:

1. As you are orienting a preceptor, she asks you about the treatment your patient is receiving for an infection. She tells you she remembers being taught that aminoglycosides (your patient is receiving gentamicin) can cause renal injury. Yet your patient has a normal urine output (2100 mL/day) and the following laboratory values:

Na^+ 142
K^+ 4.6
Cl^- 103
HCO_3^- 21
Creatinine 3.2
BUN 54
Osmolality 278
Urinary osmolality 297
Urinary Na^+ 49

She asks if this patient is at any risk for developing renal injury. Based on the preceding information, what would you answer?

a. As long as the urine output is greater than 30 mL/h she is not in danger of renal injury.
b. As long as her creatinine level is no greater than 2.5 mg/dL she is not at risk for acute renal injury.
c. Based on the information, she already has signs of acute renal injury.
d. Although she may be at risk for renal injury, a renal ultrasound scan would be required to make a definitive diagnosis.

Answer: C. Rationale: Oliguria may or may not be present in AKI. Fifty percent of AKI patients and many ATN patients are anuric. Therefore, urine volume alone is not an adequate guide to renal function. Progressive azotemia (an excess of urea or other nitrogenous bodies in the blood) occurs as a result of decreased GFR in spite of apparently adequate urine output.

2. During the care of a patient undergoing peritoneal dialysis, the infusate has not completely drained. Which method would be acceptable to help facilitate drainage?

a. Applying continuous low-pressure suction
b. Turning the patient from side to side
c. Manipulating the peritoneal catheter
d. Applying manual pressure to the abdomen

Answer: B. Rationale: When catheter patency is confirmed, the warmed dialysate is infused, allowed to dwell in the abdomen, usually for 20 to 45 minutes, and then allowed to drain via gravity as completely as possible. One exchange usually takes about an hour. Turning the patient side to side may enhance the drainage of dialysate.

3. Which of the following will continuous venovenous hemofiltration NOT remove?

a. Fluid
b. Albumin
c. Sodium
d. Potassium

Answer: B. Rationale: The purposes of dialysis are to (1) remove the by-products of protein metabolism, including urea, creatinine, and uric acid; (2) remove excess water; (3) maintain or restore the body's buffer system; and (4) maintain or restore the body's concentration of electrolytes.

45

Renal Trauma

CHAPTER OVERVIEW AND OBJECTIVES

Renal trauma is no longer included in the updated CCRN test plan but the content is provided here for supplemental information to provide a comprehensive overview of critical care conditions.

Trauma or injury to the kidney is frequently seen with colon, spleen, liver, and pancreatic injuries. Renal trauma accounts for approximately 3% of all trauma admissions and is present in approximately 10% of all abdominal injuries. Although the vast majority (90%) is due to blunt trauma, penetrating trauma more commonly causes major injury. The mortality rate is approximately 6% to 12%, with the greatest risk to those who are elderly, who have preexisting renal disease, or who abuse drugs and alcohol.

45.1 ETIOLOGY

Blunt trauma from motor vehicle collisions is the most common cause of renal injury. Acceleration–deceleration forces occur as the victim contacts the steering wheel or dashboard as the vehicle stops and the kidney continues to move forward, tearing blood vessels. Additional mechanisms of blunt trauma are falls, accidents during contact sports, and physical assaults leading to renal injury. Penetrating injuries are associated with a high incidence of intraperitoneal visceral injury, hemorrhage, fistulas, and infections.

45.2 ASSESSMENT

Any trauma to the flank, lower thorax, or abdomen should arouse suspicion of possible renal injury. The mechanism of injury provides the framework for the clinical assessment. Particular attention should be paid to complaints of pain or tenderness in the flank, upper abdomen, or back. It may radiate to the groin or shoulder and may be accompanied by nausea. The lower rib area, flanks, lumbar spine, and abdomen are inspected for ecchymoses, abrasions, contusions, or lacerations. *Ecchymosis over the flank and lower back area,* **Turner's sign**, *is indicative of retroperitoneal hematoma.* Entry and exit sites of any penetrating injuries are noted because they provide clues to potential internal organ injuries.

KEY CLINICAL CONCEPT

Ecchymosis over the flank and lower back area, **Turner's sign,** is indicative of retroperitoneal hematoma.

The external genitalia, perineum, and urethral meatus are inspected for blood or ecchymosis. *If blood is found surrounding the urinary meatus, insertion of a urinary catheter is contraindicated until urethral damage is ruled out.* If a urinary catheter has been inserted, the urine is inspected for clots or blood. Gross hematuria indicates genitourinary injury and requires further investigation. The presence of gross or microscopic hematuria suggests renal injury; however, there is no correlation between the degree of hematuria and the extent of injury. Some renal injuries can occur without producing hematuria.

Auscultation of the abdomen is performed in all four quadrants before palpation is done to avoid stimulating any abdominal sounds or inducing pain. The absence of bowel sounds in the setting of recent trauma may indicate extravasation of blood. Dullness on percussion may indicate the accumulation of blood, urine, or other fluid in the abdominal cavity. *Dullness over the flank may be related to a* **retroperitoneal hematoma**.

Any abdominal rigidity, pain, or tenderness during palpation in the setting of recent trauma is concerning for inflammation or injury to the abdominal wall. Pain on rapid withdrawal of the examiner's hands (*rebound tenderness*) occurs with intra-abdominal inflammation. *Costovertebral angle (CVA) tenderness* is assessed with the patient in a sitting or lateral decubitus position. The palm of one hand is placed over each CVA and struck with the ulnar surface of the opposite fist. CVA tenderness is suspicious for a kidney infection or injury.

45.3 DIAGNOSTIC PROCEDURES

Table 45-1 presents an overview of common diagnostic studies performed to further evaluate renal trauma.

Computed tomography (CT) is the gold standard for assessing hemodynamically stable patients with blunt or penetrating abdominal trauma. Intravenous contrast helps to identify and evaluate hematoma, laceration, vascular injury, and urinary extravasation.

45.4 CLASSIFICATION OF RENAL TRAUMA

A grading system (**Table 45-2**) developed by the American Association for the Surgery of Trauma (AAST) is used to classify renal injury into five categories based on depth of injury and involvement of vessels or the collecting system.

Renal trauma can be further categorized as renal contusion, renal laceration, and renal vascular injury. Renal contusions account for 60% to 80% of all renal injuries. They result from blunt trauma and present with hematuria, ecchymosis over the flank (**Turner's Sign**) or lower thorax, subcapsular hematoma, and *CVA pain with palpation*. Management for this minor injury includes bed rest, increased fluid intake, monitoring of urinary volume, concentration, urinalysis results, hematology results, and vital signs.

A laceration is a disruption in renal tissue that may involve only the cortical layer or may extend into the renal collecting system (calyces). Patients present with flank trauma, hematuria, and may have other injuries. Management is often conservative, with close monitoring for complications and allowing for normal healing; however, uncontrolled bleeding or increased urinary extravasation may require intervention.

A complete renal tear or fracture involves diffuse rupture of both poles and the midportion of the kidney. These patients may present in hemorrhagic shock due to massive bleeding. Trauma is present in the flank area, with an expanding flank mass. Multiple system injuries are usually present on CT scan. Emergent surgery is often performed to remove all or part of the damaged kidney and obtain hemostasis.

Renal vascular injuries include a tear or laceration in the renal vasculature or a thrombosis of the renal artery. Lacerations of the renal vasculature result from penetrating trauma and are considered life-threatening. Since the kidneys receive 20% to 25% of the cardiac output, *massive hemorrhage into the retroperitoneal space may occur*. Persistent hemodynamic instability, unresponsive to trauma resuscitation, indicates the need for emergency intervention or surgery to embolize the vessel,

TABLE 45-1. DIAGNOSTIC PROCEDURES

Type	*Comments*
Hematologic	
Blood urea nitrogen	Elevation of BUN indicates catabolism and/or hypovolemia
(BUN)/creatinine	Elevation of BUN and creatinine indicates poor renal function
Hematocrit/hemoglobin	Decrease indicates hemorrhage
Leukocytes	Elevated slightly with increased polymorphonuclear leukocytes (neutrophils, eosinophils, basophils) from local renal tissue injury
Electrolytes	Vary
Urologic	
Volume	May be decreased in renal trauma or obstruction Decreased in hypovolemia
Urinalysis	Blood and protein may be present or absent in renal trauma
Radiologic	
Intravenous pyelogram (IVP)	The kidneys are compared by the injection of contrast media
Renal angiography	Provides more information on the integrity of the renal vasculature
Computed tomography (CT)	Determines the extent of injury in three dimensions Gold standard for assessment of abdominal and renal injury
Kidneys, ureter, and bladder (KUB) films	Visualizes renal outline rib fractures
Renal scan	Determines status of renal blood flow and presence of parenchymal injury
Ultrasonography	Noninvasive method of defining anatomy of injury
Operative diagnosis	Surgical exploration for repair of renal lacerations, renal pelvis, or ureteral injuries

TABLE 45-2. RENAL TRAUMA GRADING SYSTEM TO CLASSIFY RENAL INJURY BY SEVERITY

Grade 1	Hematuria with normal imaging studies, contusions, nonexpanding subcapsular hematomas
Grade 2	Nonexpanding perinephric hematomas confined to the retroperitoneum, superficial cortical lacerations less than 1 cm in depth without collecting system injury
Grade 3	Renal lacerations greater than 1 cm in depth that do not involve the collecting system
Grade 4	Renal lacerations extending through the kidney into the collecting system, injuries involving the main renal artery or vein with contained hemorrhage, segmental infarctions without associated lacerations, expanding subcapsular hematomas compressing the kidney
Grade 5	Shattered or devascularized kidney, ureteropelvic avulsions, complete laceration or thrombus of the main renal artery or vein

repair or remove the kidney. The goals of interventional therapy for renal laceration are to control hemorrhage and preserve renal tissue. For uncontrolled hemorrhage, multiple concurrent injuries, or a shattered kidney, a nephrectomy may be indicated. A partial nephrectomy may be performed to repair avulsed fragments, penetrating injury, or damage to the collecting system.

Thrombosis of the renal artery occurs when the intima is torn, forcing blood between the intima and the intact media. A thrombus forms, occluding the blood vessel. This usually results from a deceleration injury. The patient presents with flank pain with or without hematuria. On auscultation, bruits in the upper abdominal quadrants may be found. Renal artery thrombosis may not be apparent for several days or weeks following injury, when hypertension secondary to the release of excessive angiotensin appears. Renal arteriography reveals the vascular defect, which is then repaired surgically.

45.5 TREATMENT AND NURSING INTERVENTION

Patients with renal injuries should be managed with initial attention to basic advanced trauma life-support protocols. Initial management following renal trauma is the same for all types of injuries, including maintaining a patent airway, providing oxygenation, controlling hemorrhage, establishing intravenous access, correcting blood losses, and monitoring vital signs and laboratory results. If the patient is unable to void, a urinary catheter is placed. If a catheter cannot be passed because of resistance, radiologic examination of the urinary tract is indicated. *Catheters should never be forced, since obstruction may be indicative of injury or hematoma.*

Most blunt renal injuries are low grade and are usually amenable to treatment with observation and bed rest alone. Minor renal trauma is managed with monitoring of hematocrit, hemoglobin, hematuria, urinalysis, urine concentration, and vital signs; provision of analgesics; and administration of antibiotics. Ambulation begins once gross hematuria clears. Healing takes 4 to 6 weeks.

Major renal trauma with hemodynamic instability is often managed surgically. Nonsurgical intervention, such as angiography and renal embolization, has successfully treated the hemodynamically stable as well as hemodynamically unstable patients. Postoperative care includes maintaining fluid and electrolyte balance, ensuring patency of any drains or tubes, and monitoring for signs of hemorrhage. Urine is monitored for amount, color, clarity, and specific gravity. Hematuria is common except following a nephrectomy. Daily weights and monitoring of intake and output from indwelling catheters and nephrostomy tubes are also performed. All tubes and drains must be kept patent to prevent abscess formation or increased intracalyceal pressure, which can result in tissue damage. Signs of hemorrhage include flank pain or mass, increased bloody drainage from tubes, decreased hematocrit and hemoglobin, and clinical signs of shock.

45.6 COMPLICATIONS

The most common complications of renal trauma are hemorrhage and hypertension. Renal injury causes scarring of the renal parenchyma, which may result in narrowing of the renal vasculature and a decrease in renal blood flow. *The renin–angiotensin mechanism is then activated, causing increased blood pressure.*

Hemorrhage/hypovolemia decreases renal blood flow and contributes to oliguria or anuria. Patients presenting with hemodynamic instability, continuous gross hematuria, expanding hematomas, or active hemorrhage will need invasive nonsurgical intervention or surgical exploration.

Extravasation of urine increases the risk of infection. Signs of extravasation include midline bulging from a distended bladder, abdominal distention, a swollen thigh due to the collection of fluid, abdominal pain, rebound tenderness, and hematuria (not always present).

Other complications include infection, secondary hemorrhage, and acute tubular necrosis (ATN). Massive muscle breakdown from crush injuries may contribute to **rhabdomyolysis**, which obstructs the renal tubules and causes ATN.

KEY CLINICAL CONCEPT

Rhabdomyolysis may be identified by an elevated creatinine kinase (CK) level and brownish or tea-colored urine (suggesting myoglobinuria). Treatment includes fluid resuscitation and alkalinizing the urine with sodium bicarbonate to mitigate the likelihood of ATN.

KEY CONTENT CHECKLIST

- ❐ Ecchymosis over the flank and lower back area, **Turner's sign,** is indicative of retroperitoneal hematoma.
- ❐ Auscultation of the abdomen is performed in all four quadrants before palpation is done to avoid stimulating any abdominal sounds or inducing pain.
- ❐ Computed tomography (CT) is the gold standard for assessing hemodynamically stable patients with blunt or penetrating abdominal trauma.
- ❐ The renin–angiotensin mechanism is then activated, causing increased blood pressure.

Review Questions:

1. **Which of the following is a contraindication for placement of a Foley catheter following suspected renal trauma?**
   a. Ecchymosis of the perineum
   b. Bleeding at the urethral meatus
   c. Ecchymosis of the flank
   d. Costovertebral angle tenderness

Answer: B. Rationale: Bleeding from the urethral meatus may indicate urethral trauma. Insertion of a Foley catheter is contraindicated until trauma has been ruled out. Ecchymosis of the perineum is suggestive of renal trauma but is not a contraindication for catheterization. Flank ecchymosis, also known as Grey Turner's sign, is suggestive of retroperitoneal hemorrhage. Costovertebral angle tenderness is suggestive of kidney infection or injury.

2. **Which of the following signs and symptoms, if present, would raise concern for rhabdomyolysis?**
   a. Abdominal bruising
   b. Swelling of the thigh
   c. Abdominal distension
   d. Dark urine

Answer: D. Rationale: Urine myoglobin is released in rhabdomyolysis and colors the urine dark or tea colored. Abdominal bruising, thigh swelling, and abdominal distension are all nonspecific signs of bleeding or extravasation of urine.

PART VII
Renal Practice Exam

1. A 51-year-old man is in your unit after a fall from a 15-ft ladder. He landed on his back and has complaint of pain between T7 and T12. Neurologic tests, including a computed tomography (CT) scan of the head, are negative. Abdominal CT shows no fracture or active bleeding. He is alert and oriented and has no difficulty in breathing. The following information is available:

Urine and Stool	Blood
Increased RBCs	Hb 13
Stool guaiac-negative	Hct 39
	WBC 7900
	Amylase 50

Based on the preceding information, which organ is most likely to have been injured?

(A) spleen
(B) kidney
(C) pancreas
(D) descending colon

2. Which intervention is most likely to occur?

(A) oxygen therapy and SpO_2 monitoring
(B) urinary catheter
(C) nasogastric tube to suction
(D) head CT

3. A 64-year-old woman is in the intensive care unit (ICU) with the diagnosis of possible sepsis secondary to a urinary tract infection. Upon admission she was markedly short of breath with an a/A ratio of 0.14, an FIO_2 of 80%, and a PaO_2 of 72. She was intubated due to increased work of breathing. Shortly after admission, she became hypotensive and had a pulmonary artery catheter inserted to aid in her management. Over the next 2 days, she was aggressively treated with normal saline fluid bolus (with a subsequent 10-kg weight gain), antibiotics, and dobutamine. Based on the information below, what has happened in terms of her electrolytes?

Na	121
K	4.9
Cl	94
HCO_3	25

(A) Not enough chloride has been given.
(B) She has received too much fluid.
(C) She has become dehydrated.
(D) She needs more sodium in her IV fluids.

4. A 78-year-old man is in your unit with a diagnosis of congestive heart failure (CHF). He has received increasing amounts of furosemide (Lasix) over the past 3 days because of his low urine output. Based on the information below, the physician believes that a contraction alkalosis has developed. Do the following electrolytes agree with this observation?

Na	144
K	4.3
Cl	90
HCO_3	39

(A) yes, based on the increased sodium level
(B) yes, based on the decreased chloride and increased bicarbonate levels
(C) no, based on the high potassium
(D) no, since the key electrolyte, magnesium, is not given

5. The right kidney is slightly lower than the left. What is the reason for this difference?

(A) The right kidney is larger because of the presence of more nephric structures.
(B) The left kidney is displaced upward by the spleen.
(C) The right kidney is displaced downward by the liver.
(D) The left kidney is drawn upward by the diaphragm.

6. The kidneys have the ability to regulate blood flow partially via local regulatory mechanisms. If the systemic blood pressure falls, how do the kidneys maintain perfusion?

(A) decreasing nephronal resistance to glomerular filtrate
(B) afferent arteriolar dilation and efferent arteriolar constriction
(C) efferent arteriolar dilation and afferent arteriolar constriction
(D) decreasing glomerular filtration rate and increase active secretion levels

7. Fluid is forced from the glomerulus, forming an ultrafiltrate. Into which compartment is the fluid forced?

(A) Bowman's capsule
(B) proximal tubule
(C) collecting ducts
(D) distal tubule

8. Which of the following elements is NOT filtered during glomerular filtration?

(A) sodium
(B) potassium
(C) proteins
(D) creatinine

9. **From a renal perspective, secretion can be defined by which of the following descriptions?**
   (A) movement of solutes and water from the peritubular network into the tubule
   (B) movement of solutes and water from the tubule into the peritubular network
   (C) movement of high-molecular-weight particles into the urine
   (D) acceleration of electrolyte elimination at the glomerulus
10. **Glomerular filtration is affected by all of the following factors. Which has the most significant effect on glomerular filtration rate?**
    (A) osmotic pressure of the blood
    (B) hydrostatic pressure of the blood
    (C) dilation of the afferent arteriole
    (D) constriction of the efferent arteriole

Questions 11 and 12 refer to the following scenario:
A 37-year-old man is in your unit following a motor vehicle accident. During the initial 24 h, he was hypotensive and developed acute renal failure (ARF). His current laboratory data reveal the following information:

	Serum	Urine
Na^+	126 mEq/L	59 mEq/L
K^+	3.9 mEq/L	
Osmolality	290 mOsm	485 mOsm
Creatinine	3.0 mEq/L	

11. **Based on the preceding information, which condition is likely to be present?**
    (A) dehydration
    (B) fluid overload
    (C) acute renal failure
    (D) glomerulonephritis
12. **Which laboratory data are abnormal?**
    (A) serum creatinine
    (B) urinary osmolality
    (C) serum osmolality
    (D) urinary Na^+
13. **Which of the following corresponds most closely to normal serum osmolality?**
    (A) 50 to 100 mOsm
    (B) 100 to 250 mOsm
    (C) 280 to 320 mOsm
    (D) 320 to 410 mOsm
14. **Which of the following corresponds most closely to the range of normal serum sodium values?**
    (A) 40 to 60 mEq/L
    (B) 60 to 75 mEq/L
    (C) 80 to 120 mEq/L
    (D) 135 to 145 mEq/L
15. **Which of the following corresponds most closely to the range of normal serum potassium values?**
    (A) 1 to 2 mEq/L
    (B) 2.5 to 3.5 mEq/L
    (C) 3.5 to 5 mEq/L
    (D) 5 to 6.5 mEq/L
16. **Which of the following corresponds most closely to the range of normal urine sodium values?**
    (A) 40 to 220 mEq/L
    (B) 220 to 320 mEq/L
    (C) 335 to 445 mEq/L
    (D) 455 to 470 mEq/L
17. **Which of the following corresponds most closely to the range of normal serum calcium levels?**
    (A) 1 to 3 mg/dL
    (B) 4.5 to 6.5 mg/dL
    (C) 6 to 8 mg/dL
    (D) 8.5 to 10.5 mg/dL
18. **An 81-year-old man has been in the ICU for 45 days because of surgical complications from a ruptured bowel. The physician suspects that he may have nutritional impairment despite total parenteral nutrition. Laboratory tests reveal the following serum electrolyte information:**

Na^+	141 mEq/L
K^+	3.9 mEq/L
Cl^-	102 mEq/L
HCO_3^-	25 mEq/L
Ca^{2+}	8.9 mg/dL
Mg^{2+}	4.3 mg/dL

Which of the preceding laboratory values is/are abnormal?
    (A) Mg^{2+}
    (B) Ca^{2+}
    (C) Cl^- and Na^+
    (D) K^+ and HCO_3^-
19. **Which of the following corresponds most closely to the range of normal phosphate levels?**
    (A) 3 to 4.5 mg/dL
    (B) 4.5 to 6.5 mg/dL
    (C) 6 to 8 mg/dL
    (D) 8.5 to 10.5 mg/dL
20. **Creatinine level is a valuable indicator of glomerular filtration rate for which reason?**
    (A) Once filtered in the glomerulus, creatinine is not reabsorbed in the tubular system.
    (B) Creatinine enters the glomerulus only when glomerular filtration pressures exceed 60 mm Hg.
    (C) Creatinine filtration is unaffected by renal disease.
    (D) Creatinine is formed in the glomerulus and decreases only in filtration, causing creatinine levels to change.
21. **What is the effect of antidiuretic hormone (ADH) on renal function?**
    (A) It inhibits water reabsorption in the distal tubules and collecting ducts.
    (B) It increases water reabsorption in the distal tubules and collecting ducts.
    (C) It increases fluid excretion from the glomerulus.
    (D) It blocks the effect of loop diuretics, such as furosemide (Lasix).

22. Which of the following would stimulate the release of ADH?
(A) decreased serum osmolality
(B) increased serum osmolality
(C) increased serum creatinine
(D) decreased urine sodium

23. The countercurrent mechanism in the nephron is designed to accomplish which purpose?
(A) retaining creatinine
(B) eliminating hydrogen ions
(C) concentrating urine
(D) increasing water loss

24. Most water reabsorption occurs in which part of the nephron?
(A) proximal tubules
(B) loop of Henle
(C) distal tubules
(D) collecting ducts

25. A 46-year-old man is in your unit following an episode of acute respiratory distress syndrome (ARDS) after radiation therapy for large cell lung cancer. On day 3 of his ICU stay, his urine output decreases to 20 mL/h. The physician asks you to call him if the patient's blood urea nitrogen (BUN)/creatinine ratio becomes abnormal. The following laboratory data are available:

Serum BUN	64
Serum creatinine	2
Urine Na^+	76

Based on this information, is the BUN/creatinine ratio abnormal and should you contact the physician?
(A) The BUN/creatinine level is normal; do not call the physician.
(B) The BUN/creatinine level is low; call the physician.
(C) The BUN/creatinine level is high; call the physician.
(D) BUN/creatinine ratios cannot be calculated without urinary creatinine and BUN values.

26. Which of the following corresponds most closely to the range of normal serum creatinine levels?
(A) 0.8 to 1.8
(B) 2 to 2.9
(C) 3.2 to 4
(D) 4.5 to 5

27. Which of the following corresponds most closely to the range of normal serum BUN levels?
(A) 10 to 20 mg/dL
(B) 20 to 30 mg/dL
(C) 30 to 40 mg/dL
(D) 40 to 50 mg/dL

28. The presence of oliguria, a BUN/creatinine ratio greater than normal, suggests that which condition has developed?
(A) prerenal failure
(B) renal failure
(C) postrenal failure
(D) acute tubular necrosis

29. Aldosterone exerts an effect on renal function at which anatomic site?
(A) proximal tubule
(B) loop of Henle
(C) distal tubule
(D) glomerulus

30. The juxtaglomerular system is responsible for releasing which substance?
(A) erythropoietin
(B) aldosterone
(C) secretin
(D) angiotensin

31. Angiotensin II exerts which of the following physiologic actions?
(A) vasoconstriction
(B) vasodilation
(C) increases glomerular filtration rate
(D) promotes secretion of ADH

32. A 34-year-old man with chronic renal failure has a hemoglobin level of 7.4 g/dL and a hematocrit of 23%. His blood pressure is 160/92 mm Hg and his heart rate is 98. What is the most likely explanation for the hemoglobin and hematocrit values?
(A) The values are abnormally elevated because of hemoconcentration.
(B) The values are abnormally low because of a reduced cardiac output.
(C) The values are normal.
(D) The values are decreased because of loss of erythropoietin.

33. Which substance has the most significant effect on sodium regulation?
(A) renin level
(B) aldosterone level
(C) glomerular filtration rate
(D) serum pH

34. What is the primary action of aldosterone?
(A) inhibits sodium excretion
(B) promotes sodium excretion
(C) blocks water reabsorption
(D) stimulates vasoconstriction

35. What is the primary cause of hypernatremia?
(A) vascular water deficits
(B) excessive vascular free water
(C) excessive serum sodium levels
(D) loss of serum chloride

36. **The lack of ADH causes which effect on serum electrolytes?**
   (A) increase in sodium levels
   (B) decrease in sodium levels
   (C) decrease in hydrogen ion levels
   (D) increase in serum bicarbonate levels

37. **Which of the following is NOT a common sign of hypernatremia?**
   (A) tachycardia
   (B) dry mucous membranes
   (C) poor skin turgor
   (D) distended neck veins

38. **Administration of which of the following is a normal initial treatment for hypernatremia?**
   (A) diuretics and fluid restriction
   (B) nonelectrolyte (free water) solutions
   (C) normal saline
   (D) potassium salts

39. **Hypovolemic hyponatremia is most often caused by which of the following?**
   (A) excessive sodium levels
   (B) decreased sodium levels
   (C) excessive vascular volume
   (D) decreased vascular volume

40. **The most dangerous symptoms of hyponatremia center on which organ system?**
   (A) central nervous system
   (B) cardiac system
   (C) renal system
   (D) respiratory system

41. **Excessive secretion of ADH could produce which of the following electrolyte changes?**
   (A) increased serum osmolality
   (B) increased serum sodium
   (C) decreased serum sodium
   (D) decreased hydrogen

42. **Treatment of severe hypervolemic hyponatremia (<120 mEq/L) consists of administration of which of the following?**
   (A) diuretics
   (B) nonelectrolyte (free water) solutions
   (C) normal saline
   (D) potassium salts

43. **Hypokalemia is associated with which acid–base disturbance?**
   (A) metabolic acidosis
   (B) metabolic alkalosis
   (C) respiratory acidosis
   (D) systemic acidosis

44. **Which of the following electrocardiographic (ECG) changes is NOT associated with hyperkalemia?**
   (A) peaked T waves
   (B) depressed P waves
   (C) premature ventricular contractions (PVCs)
   (D) widening QRS complex

45. **Which of the following is NOT recommended for the treatment of hyperkalemia?**
   (A) sodium polystyrene sulfonate (Kayexalate)
   (B) glucose/insulin infusion
   (C) dialysis
   (D) ammonium chloride

46. **Hypokalemia is associated with which of the following ECG changes?**
   (A) peaked T waves
   (B) depressed P waves
   (C) premature ventricular contractions (PVCs)
   (D) widening QRS complex

47. **The concentration of which electrolyte is inversely related to that of calcium?**
   (A) sodium
   (B) potassium
   (C) phosphate
   (D) magnesium

48. **Which mechanism is calcium NOT involved in regulating?**
   (A) coagulation
   (B) formation of bone
   (C) transmission of electrical impulses
   (D) absorption of vitamin D

49. **A 51-year-old man with a history of alcoholism has marked muscle irritability. The following laboratory data are available:**

Na^+	135 mEq/L
K^+	4.8 mEq/L
Ca^{2+}	3.7 mg/dL
Mg^{2+}	1.8 mg/dL

Which of the following electrolytes is most likely to be the source of the muscle hyperirritability?
   (A) sodium
   (B) calcium
   (C) potassium
   (D) magnesium

50. **Chvostek's sign is tested by which maneuver?**
   (A) tapping the flexor tendon over the knee
   (B) tapping the supramandibular area
   (C) stroking the sole of the foot
   (D) measuring clotting times after venipuncture

51. **Trousseau's sign is a test for which electrolyte deficiency?**
   (A) hypophosphatemia
   (B) hypercalcemia
   (C) hypocalcemia
   (D) hypokalemia

52. **Which organ or organ system is involved in the regulation of phosphate elimination?**
   (A) liver
   (B) respiratory system
   (C) renal system
   (D) spleen

53. A 75-year-old woman is admitted to your unit with pneumonia and malnutrition. Her chief complaint currently is weakness and inability to perform her normal "chores." She has stated that she has not eaten well for the past several months. The following information is available:

Na^+	150 mEq/L
K^+	3.6 mEq/L
Cl^-	110 mEq/L
Mg^{2+}	2.1 mg/dL
Ca^{2+}	9.2 mg/dL
PO_4^{3-}	2.3 mg/dL

Which of the preceding levels is a likely source of her weakness?

(A) low phosphate
(B) high sodium and chloride
(C) low magnesium
(D) high calcium

54. Which electrolyte is directly related to the reabsorption of magnesium?

(A) potassium
(B) calcium
(C) sodium
(D) phosphate

55. Which of the following is a primary treatment to reduce magnesium levels?

(A) normal saline bolus
(B) dialysis
(C) mechanical ventilation
(D) calcium carbonate administration

56. Hypomagnesemia is manifested clinically by which of the following symptoms?

(A) muscle irritability
(B) muscle fatigue
(C) nausea
(D) positive Turner's sign

57. A 61-year-old man admitted with the diagnosis of chronic obstructive pulmonary disease (COPD) has the following set of laboratory data for arterial blood gases and electrolytes:

PO_2	63 mm Hg
Pco_2	71 mm Hg
pH	7.37
HCO_3^-	39 mEq/L
Na^+	146 mEq/L
Cl^-	87 mEq/L

The COPD-induced blood gas changes have altered the electrolytes as well. Based on the preceding information, which electrolyte change occurred because of the Pco_2 elevation?

(A) decrease in pH
(B) chloride increased
(C) sodium increased
(D) increased HCO_3^-

58. Elevated chloride levels are associated with which condition?

(A) alkalosis
(B) acidosis
(C) hyponatremia
(D) hypercalcemia

59. Left ventricular failure will cause which effect on the BUN/creatinine ratio?

(A) It will cause the ratio to rise. (BUN rises faster than creatinine.)
(B) It will cause the ratio to fall. (BUN rises more slowly than creatinine.)
(C) It will have no effect on the ratio but will elevate creatinine levels.
(D) It will reverse the ratio.

60. A 74-year-old woman is admitted to your unit with possible sepsis and renal failure. The following laboratory information is available:

Urinary Na^+	13
Urinary osmolarity	1000
Urine output	15 mL/h

Based on these data, what is likely to be occurring?

(A) prerenal azotemia
(B) acute tubular necrosis
(C) postrenal obstruction
(D) vasomotor nephropathy

61. A 61-year-old woman is in your unit after being admitted from a nursing home. At the time of admission, it was noted that she seemed confused, although she is currently alert and oriented. She has had a "cold" for the past several days. Her laboratory data are as follows:

Na^+	155
K^+	3.6
Cl^-	122
HCO_3^-	24

What is the most likely reason for the abnormal sodium level?

(A) excess total sodium
(B) decreased total potassium
(C) dehydration
(D) fluid excess

62. Which of the following patients has an increased anion gap?

	1	**2**	**3**	**4**
Na^+	132	142	121	153
K^+	3.2	4.8	4.1	3.5
Cl^-	93	108	89	113
HCO_3^-	25	17	19	26

(A) patient 1
(B) patient 2
(C) patient 3
(D) patient 4

63. What is the clinical value in establishing whether or not an anion gap exists?

(A) The finding permits determination of a metabolic alkalosis.
(B) The finding permits determination of a metabolic acidosis.
(C) The finding permits identification of respiratory acidosis.
(D) The anion gap acts as a marker of acute renal failure.

Questions 64 and 65 refer to the following scenario:
A 61-year-old man has a 2-day history of abdominal pain with nausea and vomiting. He has intermittent chest pain, which is unrelieved by nitrates, changes in position, or rest. He has a history of CHF and underwent a coronary artery bypass graft (CABG) procedure 2 years earlier. Currently, he has a urine output of 15 mL/h. He has had a urine output of 200 mL over the past 24 h. Currently, he has the following vital signs:

Blood pressure	88/56 mm Hg
Pulse	114
Respiratory rate	32

He has a pulmonary artery catheter in place, from which the following information is available:

Cardiac output	3.7
Cardiac index	2.4
Arterial pressure	20/8
PCWP	6
CVP	2

The following laboratory data are also available:

SMA-6

Na^+	153
K^+	3.6
Cl^-	120
HCO_3^-	19
Creatinine	2.2
Glucose	154
BUN	35
Osmolality	320

He has the following blood gas values:

Pao_2	82
$Paco_2$	28
pH	7.30
HCO_3^-	20
SvO_2	52%
Pvo_2	32

Urinary electrolyte values are as follows:

Na^+	35
Osmolality	845
Creatinine	48

Other laboratory data include the following:

Albumin	3.6
Hemoglobin	15.6
Lactate	2.2

64. **Based on the preceding information, what is the potential problem and the likely reason for the decrease in urine output?**
    (A) prerenal azotemia from hypovolemia
    (B) prerenal azotemia from left ventricular failure
    (C) acute tubular necrosis
    (D) ATN from hypovolemia

65. **What would be the most effective therapy to improve this patient's renal function?**
    (A) fluid bolus
    (B) dobutamine therapy
    (C) diuretics
    (D) renal dose dopamine

66. **A 31-year-old woman is in the ICU following multiple gunshot wounds to her face and abdomen. She has been in the unit for 4 days, and during the fourth day her urine output decreased to 200 mL for the entire day. She is alert and oriented yet cannot communicate because of an endotracheal tube. The following information is available to you:**

Na^+	132
K^+	4.1
Cl^-	99
HCO_3^-	20
Creatinine	2.5
BUN	43
Osmolality	295
Urinary creatinine	50
Urinary osmolality	343

Based on the preceding information, what is the most likely cause of her decreased urine output?
    (A) prerenal azotemia from hypovolemia
    (B) prerenal azotemia from rhabdomyolysis
    (C) acute tubular necrosis
    (D) ureter obstruction

67. **As you are orienting a preceptor, she asks you about the treatment your patient is receiving for an infection. She tells you she remembers being taught that aminoglycosides (your patient is receiving gentamicin) can cause renal injury. Yet your patient has a normal urine output (2100 mL/day) and the following laboratory values:**

Na^+	142
K^+	4.6
Cl^-	103
HCO_3^-	21
Creatinine	3.2
BUN	54
Osmolality	278
Urinary osmolality	297
Urinary Na^+	49

She asks if this patient is at any risk for developing renal injury. Based on the preceding information, what would you answer?
    (A) As long as the urine output is greater than 30 mL/h she is not in danger of renal injury.
    (B) As long as her creatinine level is no greater than 2.5 mg/dL she is not at risk for acute renal injury.
    (C) Based on the information, she already has signs of acute renal injury.
    (D) Although she may be at risk for renal injury, a renal ultrasound scan would be required to make a definitive diagnosis.

68. A 65-year-old man is in the ICU for a traumatic blunt force trauma from a motor vehicle accident (MVA). He is currently intubated after developing a respiratory acidosis in the emergency department. During the second day in the unit, he begins to put out over 2000 mL of urine on your shift. The following laboratory information is available:

Na^+	158
K^+	3.4
Cl^-	112
HCO_3^-	23
Creatinine	1.8
BUN	29
Osmolality	341
Urinary osmolality	343
Urinary Na^+	28

Based on the preceding information, what condition is likely to be developing?
(A) prerenal azotemia
(B) ARF
(C) diabetes insipidus
(D) SIADH (syndrome of inappropriate antidiuretic hormone secretion)

69. Measurement of which of the following is helpful in differentiating ARF from prerenal azotemia (PRA)?
(A) FeNa
(B) BUN
(C) urinary osmolality
(D) serum Na^+

70. During the care of a patient undergoing peritoneal dialysis, the infusate has not completely drained. Which method would be acceptable to help facilitate drainage?
(A) applying continuous low-pressure suction
(B) turning the patient from side to side
(C) manipulating the peritoneal catheter
(D) applying manual pressure to the abdomen

71. Which of the following is NOT considered an indication for continuous venovenous hemofiltration?
(A) treating acute volume overload in CHF
(B) fluid removal when diuretic therapy has failed
(C) acute hyperkalemia
(D) as a replacement for hemodialysis in the nonuniversity hospital setting

72. Which of the following will continuous venovenous hemofiltration NOT remove?
(A) fluid
(B) albumin
(C) sodium
(D) potassium

PART VII
Renal Practice Exam

Practice Fill-Ins

1. ____________________
2. ____________________
3. ____________________
4. ____________________
5. ____________________
6. ____________________
7. ____________________
8. ____________________
9. ____________________
10. ____________________
11. ____________________
12. ____________________
13. ____________________
14. ____________________
15. ____________________
16. ____________________
17. ____________________
18. ____________________
19. ____________________
20. ____________________
21. ____________________
22. ____________________
23. ____________________
24. ____________________
25. ____________________
26. ____________________
27. ____________________
28. ____________________
29. ____________________
30. ____________________
31. ____________________
32. ____________________
33. ____________________
34. ____________________
35. ____________________
36. ____________________
37. ____________________
38. ____________________
39. ____________________
40. ____________________
41. ____________________
42. ____________________
43. ____________________
44. ____________________
45. ____________________
46. ____________________
47. ____________________
48. ____________________
49. ____________________
50. ____________________
51. ____________________
52. ____________________
53. ____________________
54. ____________________
55. ____________________
56. ____________________
57. ____________________
58. ____________________
59. ____________________
60. ____________________
61. ____________________
62. ____________________
63. ____________________
64. ____________________
65. ____________________
66. ____________________
67. ____________________
68. ____________________
69. ____________________
70. ____________________
71. ____________________
72. ____________________

PART VII
Answers

1. **B** Chapter 46 Rationale: Falls, accidents during contact sports, and physical assaults may also cause renal injury due to blunt force trauma. Due to RBCs detected in the urine, priorities for nursing care should include monitoring for rhabdomyolysis.
2. **B** Chapter 46 Rationale: Accurate intake and output, monitoring for urine color and amount, and risk of developing rhabdomyolysis may be indicated. If the patient is unable to void, a urinary catheter is placed. If a catheter cannot be passed because of resistance, radiologic examination of the urinary tract is indicated. Catheters should never be forced, since obstruction is indicative of injury or hematoma.
3. **B** Chapter 45 Rationale: The 10-kg weight gain over 2 days in this patient suggests a hypervolemic hyponatremia has occurred and that too much fluid has been administered with respect to the urine output observed, making option B the best possible answer. Since sodium chloride was the fluid of choice, plenty of sodium and chloride have been administered, eliminating options A and D. The weight gain helps rule out option C. Choose B.
4. **B** Chapter 44 Rationale: Excretion of chloride is influenced by the acid–base balance. Chloride ions are lost through excessive urination, vomiting, or gastric suction without replacement of electrolytes. This causes a physiologic metabolic alkalosis. The bicarbonate ion and chloride ion normally balance each other in kidney function (in this case, chloride has decreased and bicarbonate has increased). Large doses of furosemide precipitated chloride loss and the retainment of bicarbonate, creating contraction alkalosis.
5. **C** Chapter 43 Rationale: The majority of the liver is in the right upper quadrant, displacing the right kidney downward, making option C the best answer. The spleen is a small organ in the left upper quadrant, too small to displace the left kidney, eliminating B. The diaphragm is not in close proximity to the kidneys and does not influence one kidney's position relative to the other, eliminating D as well. Choose C.
6. **B** Chapter 43 Rationale: An autoregulatory system exists to protect the glomerulus. The afferent and efferent renal arterioles constrict or dilate in response to systemic blood pressure. If systemic blood pressure increases, the afferent arteriole will constrict. This effectively reduces the pressure of the blood entering the glomerulus. In the same way, if systemic blood pressure decreases, the afferent arteriole will dilate to allow more blood to enter the glomerulus.
7. **A** Chapter 43 Rationale: The high pressure in the glomerulus tends to filter fluid out of the glomerulus and into Bowman's capsule.
8. **C** Chapter 43 Rationale: Because protein-sized (and larger) molecules cannot filter out of the glomerular capillaries, those proteins remain in the blood entering the peritubular capillaries from the efferent arteriole. Creatinine and all electrolytes are filtered. Note that sodium and potassium are both electrolytes, which helps eliminate options A and B quickly.
9. **A** Chapter 43 Rationale: Secretion is the movement of solutes and water from the peritubular network into the tubule (ie, from the bloodstream back into the filtrate).
10. **B** Chapter 43 Rationale: The high pressure in the glomerulus tends to filter fluid out of the glomerulus and into Bowman's capsule. The arteriole physiology described in options C and D is actually dependent the degree of hydrostatic pressure, which helps eliminate them. Osmotic pressure of the blood is just the pulling power of the blood proteins. Choose B.
11. **C** Chapter 45 Rationale: In ATN, when urine output is low, the expected conservation of sodium fails to occur, resulting in a normal urinary sodium level (40–220 mEq/L). Urinary osmolality decreases (<500 mOsm), reflecting the inability of the kidneys to concentrate the urine. Simultaneously, the specific gravity also decreases, usually between 1.008 and 1.012. In medullary intrarenal failure or ATN, urinary sodium is greater than 20 mEq/L, serum BUN and creatinine will be elevated (10–15:1).
12. **A** Chapter 45 Rationale: Even though several laboratory findings are abnormal in this case, the finding most indicative of acute kidney injury is the serum creatinine.
13. **C** Chapter 43 Rationale: The plasma protein and ECF sodium concentrations determine the osmolality of the ECF. Normal serum osmolality is 280 to 320 mOsm/L. An easy way to remember the serum osmolality reference range is that it is approximately the serum sodium (135–145 mEq/L) multiplied by two.
14. **D** Chapter 44 Rationale: This question pertains straight to the serum sodium reference range in a chemistry panel blood test. The serum sodium reference range is 135 to 145 mEq/L. An easy way to remember this is that the PaCO2 reference range is somewhat similar, 35 to 45 mm Hg.
15. **C** Chapter 44 Rationale: Since potassium is largely an intracellular cation, the serum reference range (3.5–5 mEq/L) is much smaller than the reference range for serum sodium (135–145 mEq/L), which is largely extracellular.

16. **A** Chapter 44 Rationale: The 24-h urine sodium reference range is 40 to 220 mEq/L. The normal value for a random sodium spot urine sample is approximately 20 mEq/L.

17. **D** Chapter 44 Rationale: The reference range for serum calcium is approximately 8.5 to 10.5 mg/dL. This is not to be confused with the serum ionized calcium level, which has a reference range of approximately 1 to 2 mmol/L.

18. **A** Chapter 44 Rationale: The laboratory value that is most abnormal of the options available is magnesium. The reference range for magnesium is 1.7 to 2.2 mg/dL.

19. **A** Chapter 44 Rationale: Option A is the closest to the normal phosphate reference range.

20. **A** Chapter 43 Rationale: Serum creatinine is a more reliable index of kidney function. Creatinine is a waste product of muscle metabolism and is freely filtered. The nephron tubules neither reabsorb nor secrete creatinine. The normally functioning kidney filters creatinine from the blood at a rate equal to the GFR. As the amount of creatinine produced each day is constant and is proportional to the body's muscle mass, serial serum creatinines are valuable indices of kidney function except in septic patients and patients with muscle-wasting diseases.

21. **B** Chapter 43 Rationale: In the presence of ADH, the distal convoluted tubules and collecting ducts reabsorb water. The reabsorption of the water leaves a hypertonic urine. This cycle continues until the concentration of the ECF compartment and fluid homeostasis are returned to normal. If osmolality of the ECF decreases, ADH release is inhibited because the osmoreceptors are not stimulated. Without ADH, the distal tubules and collecting ducts are impermeable to water. Urine will be very dilute because the water cannot be reabsorbed. The urine will continue to be diluted until the loss of water has raised the concentration of the ECF solutes to normal.

22. **B** Chapter 43 Rationale: An increase in osmolality (ie, increase in blood concentration) excites the osmoreceptors. They signal the neurohypophyseal tract that ADH is needed in order to increase water reabsorption to achieve a more normal osmolality (ie, hemoconcentration) level.

23. **C** Chapter 43 Rationale: The countercurrent mechanism serves to concentrate urine and excrete excessive solutes.

24. **A** Chapter 43 Rationale: In the proximal convoluted tubule, 60% to 80% of the ultrafiltrate is absorbed. See Table 43-1.

25. **C** Chapter 45 Rationale: The BUN/creatinine ratio is considered elevated when it exceeds 20:1, and in this case it is 32:1. The only option available listing an elevated ratio is option C.

26. **A** Chapter 45 Rationale: The range most closely associated with a normal serum creatinine range is option A. An easier range to remember may be 0.5 to 1.5.

27. **A** Chapter 45 Rationale: Remember that a normal BUN/creatinine ratio is approximately 20:1. Therefore, if a normal BUN is approximately 20, a normal creatinine should be approximately 1. Choose A.

28. **A** Chapter 45 Rationale: Without more information available, an increased BUN/creatinine ratio and oliguria suggest prerenal failure. In intrarenal and postrenal failure, the BUN/creatinine ratio is usually less than 20:1. Acute tubular necrosis is difficult to determine without a creatinine value. Choose A.

29. **C** Chapter 43 Rationale: In the presence of aldosterone, the distal convoluted tubules and collecting ducts reabsorb water.

30. **D** Chapter 43 Rationale: Once activated, the juxtaglomerular apparatus (JGA), located adjacent to the glomeruli, releases inactive renin. Factors triggering the release of inactive renin (eg, decreased blood pressure and decreased sodium content in the distal tubule) reflect a diminished GFR. Once released, the inactive renin acts on angiotensinogen to split away the vasoactive peptide angiotensin I.

31. **A** Chapter 43 Rationale: Angiotensin II is a potent vasoconstricting agent. Angiotensin II in the circulatory system causes a severe constriction of peripheral arterioles and a milder constriction in the venous system. It also causes a constriction of renal arterioles. This results in the kidneys reabsorbing sodium and water and expanding the ECF volume.

32. **D** Chapter 43 Rationale: Patients with chronic renal failure usually have hemoglobins of 5 and 6 g. The diseased kidneys are unable to respond to hypoxia and cannot produce erythropoietin factor. It is believed that possibly 10% of erythropoietin is formed in some place other than the kidney.

33. **B** Chapter 44 Rationale: Aldosterone has the greatest influence on sodium excretion. Aldosterone is a mineralocorticoid secreted by the adrenal cortex. It is the most potent natural inhibitor of sodium excretion.

34. **A** Chapter 44 Rationale: Aldosterone has the greatest influence on sodium excretion. Aldosterone is a mineralocorticoid secreted by the adrenal cortex. It is the most potent natural inhibitor of sodium excretion.

35. **A** Chapter 44 Rationale: Most cases of hypernatremia are due not to Na^+ disturbances but to fluid disturbances. Hypernatremia may be seen with dehydration.

36. **A** Chapter 43 Rationale: Without ADH, the distal tubules and collecting ducts are impermeable to water. Urine will be very dilute because the water cannot be reabsorbed. With increased urine output, the osmolality of the ECF will increase, as will the sodium level.

37. **D** Chapter 44 Rationale: Most cases of hypernatremia are due not to Na^+ disturbances but to fluid disturbances. Hypernatremia may be seen with dehydration. Options A, B, and C are all associated with dehydration and volume depletion. Distended neck veins are associated with fluid overload; choose D.

38. **B** Chapter 44 Rationale: Fluid administration with free water (nonelectrolyte solutions like D_5W) in a dehydrated patient is the key to diluting the sodium and halting the progression toward hypovolemic shock. Diuretics and

fluid restriction would worsen dehydration, eliminating A. The sodium content in normal saline and potassium salts may also exacerbate existing hypernatremia, eliminating C and D as well. Choose B.

39. **B** Chapter 44 Rationale: Hypovolemic hyponatremia due to sodium depletion or loss is commonly caused by the overuse of the thiazide diuretics, furosemide (Lasix), and mannitol (Osmitrol). Diarrhea, Addison disease, gastric suction, hyperglycemia (with a glucose-induced diuresis), vomiting, and extreme diaphoresis without intravenous replacement of sodium may also cause hypovolemic hyponatremia.

40. **A** Chapter 44 Rationale: Acute or severe hyponatremia (plasma Na^+ level <110–115 mmol/L) often presents with altered mental status and/or seizures and requires rapid correction with hypertonic saline to raise the plasma Na^+ level by 1 to 2 mmol/L/h for the first 3 to 4 h or until the seizures subside. Cerebral injury can occur from the overly rapid expansion of brain cells due to water removal.

41. **C** Chapter 43 Rationale: In the presence of ADH, the distal convoluted tubules and collecting ducts reabsorb water. The reabsorption of the water leaves a hypertonic urine and creates hypotonic plasma and ECF resulting in decreased serum sodium levels.

42. **A** Chapter 44 Rationale: Fluid restriction or low-dose diuretic therapy is the treatment of choice if the hyponatremia is due to excess vascular fluid.

43. **B** Chapter 44 Rationale: Serum potassium moves inversely to the pH. If the pH falls, potassium concentration increases. If the pH rises, potassium concentration decreases, in part because of the ionic charge of potassium and hydrogen.

44. **C** Chapter 44 Rationale: In marked hyperkalemia (potassium of 7.5–9 mEq/L), there is a flattening and widening of the P wave, a prolonged PR interval, and usually depression of the ST segment. In severely advanced hyperkalemia (potassium of 8–9 mEq/L and often more than 10 mEq/L), the P waves disappear and if untreated, may lead to a progressive overall "widening," "flattening," and "over-relaxation" of the EKG tracing that may ultimately lead to ventricular standstill, asystole, and death. Hypokalemia is associated more with "irritability" (i.e., PVCs,) than relaxation, so choose C.

45. **D** Chapter 44 Rationale: Calcium chloride will oppose the cardiotoxic effects of hyperkalemia. However, calcium therapy is contraindicated in patients on digoxin. Kayexalate is given orally or as an enema to rid the body of potassium. Kayexalate forces a one-for-one exchange of sodium for potassium in the intestinal cell wall; however, the patient must be monitored for sodium retention. Sorbitol is used to induce an osmotic diarrhea through semiliquid stools. Ammonium chloride is a substance used in cough medicine, so choose D.

46. **C** Chapter 44 Rationale: ECG tracings most commonly show a prominent U wave. Depression or flattening of the ST segment or inversion of the T wave may be apparent. An inverted T wave may fuse with the U wave, giving the appearance of a prolonged QT interval. There is a generalized cardiac irritability in hypokalemic states which may be associated with PVCs, so choose C.

47. **C** Chapter 44 Rationale: Phosphate levels are influenced by two major factors: PTH secretion (increases renal excretion of phosphate ions) and calcium concentration. Calcium and phosphate have a reciprocal relationship. If calcium levels increase, phosphate levels decrease; conversely, if calcium levels decrease, phosphate levels increase.

48. **D** Chapter 44 Rationale: Calcium, with phosphorus, makes bones and teeth rigid and strong. Calcium is integral to determining the strength and thickness of cell membranes. Calcium exerts a quieting action on nerve cells, thus maintaining normal transmission of nerve impulses. Calcium also activates specific enzymes of the blood-clotting process and those involved in the contraction of the myocardium. Vitamin D must be present in an activated form to promote the absorption of calcium from the small intestine—if not activated, the body will not absorb the calcium.

49. **B** Chapter 44 Rationale: Muscle tremors and cramps are present in mild hypocalcemia. As the calcium level drops, tetany and generalized tonic–clonic seizures occur. The muscles of the heart, lungs, intestines, and skeleton cannot function normally without potassium. However, the calcium value is the most severely outside of its reference range (8.5-10.5mg/dL) and coincides with the symptoms. Choose B.

50. **B** Chapter 44 Rationale: To test for Chvostek's sign, tap your finger over the supramandibular portion of the parotid gland, which is located in the subcutaneous tissue of the cheek. If the upper lip twitches on the side of stimulation, the test is positive.

51. **C** Chapter 44 Rationale: To test for Trousseau's sign, apply a blood pressure cuff to the arm and inflate it until a carpopedal spasm occurs. If no spasm appears in 3 min, the test is negative.

52. **C** Chapter 44 Rationale: Reabsorption of phosphates occurs actively in the proximal convoluted tubule in the presence of sodium. Without sodium, phosphates will not be reabsorbed.

53. **A** Chapter 44 Rationale: Complaints of general malaise, anorexia, and vague muscle weakness may be of chronic or acute onset.

54. **C** Chapter 44 Rationale: The presence of sodium directly affects reabsorption in the proximal tubules. Without sodium, there is no reabsorption of magnesium.

55. **B** Chapter 44 Rationale: Attempts to lower magnesium levels by hemodialysis with a hypomagnesium dialysate have been successful. Loop diuretics may be considered more of a first-line treatment. However, this option is not available. So, choose B.

56. **A** Chapter 44 Rationale: Neuromuscular and central nervous system hyperirritability characterize hypomagnesemia. Muscle tremors, delirium, convulsion, and coma are seen. Positive Chvostek's and Trousseau's signs, tachycardia, increased blood pressure, depressed ST segments, and prolonged QT intervals are also seen.

57. **D** Chapter 43 Rationale: In the fourth mechanism, production and reabsorption of bicarbonate, new bicarbonate ion is manufactured in the distal convoluted tubule as needed. The formula is

		CA		CA		
H_2O	+	CO_2	↔ H_2CO_3 ↔	H^+	+	HCO_3^-
water		carbon dioxide	carbonic acid	hydrogen ion		bicarbonate ion

58. **B** Chapter 44 Rationale: An excessive ingestion of chloride (such as with infusion of large amounts of 0.9% normal saline, or 0.45% saline or lactated ringers) or kidney reabsorption of chloride ions (and excretion of bicarbonate) create hyperchloremic metabolic acidosis.

59. **A** Chapter 45 Rationale: Prerenal AKI is defined as a decreased renal perfusion secondary to renal hypoperfusion, often due to decreased cardiac output.

60. **A** Chapter 45 Rationale: In prerenal failure, urinary sodium (Na^+) is less than 20 mEq/L as the kidneys attempt to conserve sodium and water. Urinary osmolality, which reflects the concentrating ability of the kidney, is elevated. Urinary osmolality is usually greater than 500 mOsm (normal level is 300–900 mOsm). In this patient's case, urinary sodium is 13 and serum osmolality is 1000, which is indicative of prerenal failure.

61. **C** Chapter 44 Rationale: Most cases of hypernatremia are due not to Na^+ disturbances but to fluid disturbances. Hypernatremia may be seen with dehydration. Treatment is centered on giving fluid, not removing sodium.

62. **B** Chapter 44 Rationale: A normal anion gap is less than 15 mEq and is obtained by subtracting bicarbonate and chloride from sodium. Patient 2 has an anion gap of 22, the largest among the 4 patients. Choose B.

63. **B** Chapter 44 Rationale: If an anion gap exceeds 15, a specific type of metabolic acidosis exists. If the anion gap exceeds 15, either a lactic, keto, or chronic renal failure acidosis exists. The anion gap appears to increase because bicarbonate to buffer the acidosis is lost without a simultaneous increase in chloride. In lactic, keto, and chronic renal failure acidosis, anions other than chloride increase to offset the loss of bicarbonate.

64. **A** Chapter 45 Rationale: A serum osmolality more than 500mOsm is consistent with prerenal failure. Normal urinary output is about 0.5 mL/kg/h. In prerenal failure, urine volume is decreased. Decreasing blood pressure and cardiac output are consistent with hypovolemia. Low cardiac filling pressures are also consistent with hypovolemia.

65. **A** Chapter 45 Rationale: Prerenal failure has a number of causes. One major cause is hemorrhage resulting in hypovolemia with fluid and electrolyte imbalance. Correction of the fluid loss is imperative with careful consideration of maintaining appropriate balance of electrolytes.

66. **C** Chapter 45 Rationale: In ATN, when urine output is low, the expected conservation of sodium fails to occur, resulting in a normal urinary sodium level (40–220 mEq/L). Urinary osmolality decreases (<500 mOsm), reflecting the inability of the kidneys to concentrate the urine. Simultaneously, the specific gravity also decreases, usually between 1.008 and 1.012. Minimal to moderate proteinuria is present with an elevated serum BUN and creatinine.

67. **C** Chapter 45 Rationale: Oliguria may or may not be present in AKI. Fifty percent of AKI patients and many ATN patients are anuric. Therefore, urine volume alone is not an adequate guide to renal function. Progressive azotemia (an excess of urea or other nitrogenous bodies in the blood) occurs as a result of decreased GFR in spite of apparently adequate urine output.

68. **C** Chapter 46 Rationale: The most common cause is the lack of or insufficient ADH secretion (eg, diabetes insipidus). The comatose patient is at high risk for hypernatremia, because the thirst mechanism cannot be recognized or expressed. Excessive administration of osmotic diuretics and sodium bicarbonate (in treating lactic acidosis) may also cause an iatrogenic hypernatremia. A serum sodium level above 145 mEq/L is termed hypernatremia.

69. **A** Chapter 45 Rationale: The FeNa is above 1% in ATN. The fractional excretion of sodium (FeNa) is less than 1% in prerenal failure. In prerenal failure, urinary sodium (Na^+) is less than 20 mEq/L as the kidneys attempt to conserve sodium and water.

70. **B** Chapter 45 Rationale: When catheter patency is confirmed, the warmed dialysate is infused, allowed to dwell in the abdomen, usually for 20 to 45 min, and then allowed to drain via gravity as completely as possible. One exchange usually takes about an hour. Turning the patient side to side may enhance the drainage of dialysate.

71. **D** Chapter 45 Rationale: There are a number of instances in which hemodialysis may be used: AKIARF due to trauma or infection, chronic renal failure no longer controlled by medication and diet, when rapid removal of toxins, poisons, and drugs is essential, and when peritoneal dialysis is contraindicated.

72. **B** Chapter 45 Rationale: The purposes of dialysis are to (1) remove the by-products of protein metabolism, including urea, creatinine, and uric acid; (2) remove excess water; (3) maintain or restore the body's buffer system; and (4) maintain or restore the body's concentration of electrolytes.

PART VIII

MULTIORGAN PROBLEMS

Angela Craig

Section Overview

This section will discuss the opportunities to increase survival of the septic patient by

- Encouraging early identification and screening.
- Sharing the evidence from the Surviving Sepsis Campaign.
- Reviewing the latest guidelines for sepsis and septic shock care.

46

Sepsis and Multiorgan Syndrome

CHAPTER OVERVIEW AND OBJECTIVES

Sepsis and multiorgan dysfunction syndrome (MODS) are key parts of the CCRN exam. This chapter, along with toxic ingestions, makes up as much as 14% of the CCRN exam (20 questions) (burns are no longer covered on the exam). This chapter addresses the areas of sepsis and MODS, which may account for anywhere from 5 to 15 questions on the CCRN exam. Because of the relevance of sepsis and MODS to critical care, this is a valuable area to learn about.

Try to understand the major terms and the general sequence of events occurring in sepsis. If you understand the major therapies and symptoms of sepsis, you will probably be adequately prepared for the exam.

After studying this chapter, you should understand the following:

- How to identify and treat sepsis in a timely manner.
- Understand the importance of treating sepsis urgently.
- Understand the pathophysiology of sepsis and septic shock.

"Our arsenals for fighting off bacteria are so powerful, and involve so many different defense mechanisms, that we are more in danger from them than from the invaders. We live in the midst of explosive devices; we are mined!"

This statement from Lewis Thomas is a good introduction to understanding sepsis: how the body responds to an infection and how this response changes help clarify the septic process. Also, a major aid to the understanding, identification, and treatment of sepsis is provided by the Surviving Sepsis Campaign guidelines (www.survivingsepsis.org). This campaign was and is part of an international effort to improve treatment and outcomes in sepsis. This effort was further bolstered with the Centers for Medicare and Medicaid (CMS) adding the first ever sepsis National Core Measure in October of 2015 and continues today.

46.1 SEPSIS

Sepsis is one of the leading causes of increased morbidity and mortality in critical care. It can present in a mild or severe (septic shock) form, with mortalities ranging anywhere from 20% to 80%, depending on the number of organs affected. In this chapter, potential causes of sepsis are presented along with physical symptoms and responses. Current concepts in treating sepsis, as well as controversies over the management of the septic patient, are discussed.

Etiology

Sepsis is defined as a life-threatening organ dysfunction caused by a dysregulated host response to infection. It is not only the direct result of an infection but also reflects an inflammatory response produced by the immune system. Sepsis can originate from any antigen, bacteria, virus, or fungus, although the most common sources are bacterial. The most significant infections are gram-negative bacterial infections (eg, *Pseudomonas aeruginosa*, *Klebsiella*, *Serratia*, and *Escherichia coli*), although gram-positive infections (eg, *Staphylococcus aureus*) are also responsible for sepsis.

The antigen eventually causing sepsis must take hold in tissues and start growing to produce an infectious process. Normally, most infections are controlled by the immune system and further progression does not take place. However, in sepsis, the initial infection progresses to a more advanced state. *The urinary and respiratory systems are the most common sites for initial infections.*

Septic Cascade

From the initial infection, an extension of the infectious response occurs. The extension involves a series of events, primarily an inflammatory response sequence, as well as a direct physiologic response to the infection. Several events occur that characterize the septic process and subsequent inflammatory response.

The exact sequence of events in sepsis is unclear, although one potential scenario is as follows (**Fig. 46-1**). The antigen (eg, bacteria) is recognized by a monocyte, which immediately releases inflammatory mediators. The mediators include factors such as interleukin-1 (IL-1), IL-6, tumor necrosis factor alpha (TNF-α), and tissue factor. These mediators set off a series of responses. The main actions of these responses are to

1. *Initiate the coagulation cascade* to form a clot and seal the antigen in a localized area.
2. Inhibit the body's ability to lyse the clot, at least temporarily until the antigen is destroyed.
3. *Change the endothelial lining to become more permeable*, allowing activated neutrophils to enter the area to destroy the antigen.

For example, the complement system (particularly C3a and C5a) is activated to stimulate neutrophil activity. In addition, platelet activation and aggregation are promoted, perhaps as an attempt to isolate the infection. The neutrophil or other macrophage (eg, monocytes) will initiate a sequence of events also designed to control the antigen. The major immunologic responses are discussed as follows.

Arachidonic Acid Sequence. In response to the infection, macrophage (neutrophil and monocyte) activity (polymorphonuclear

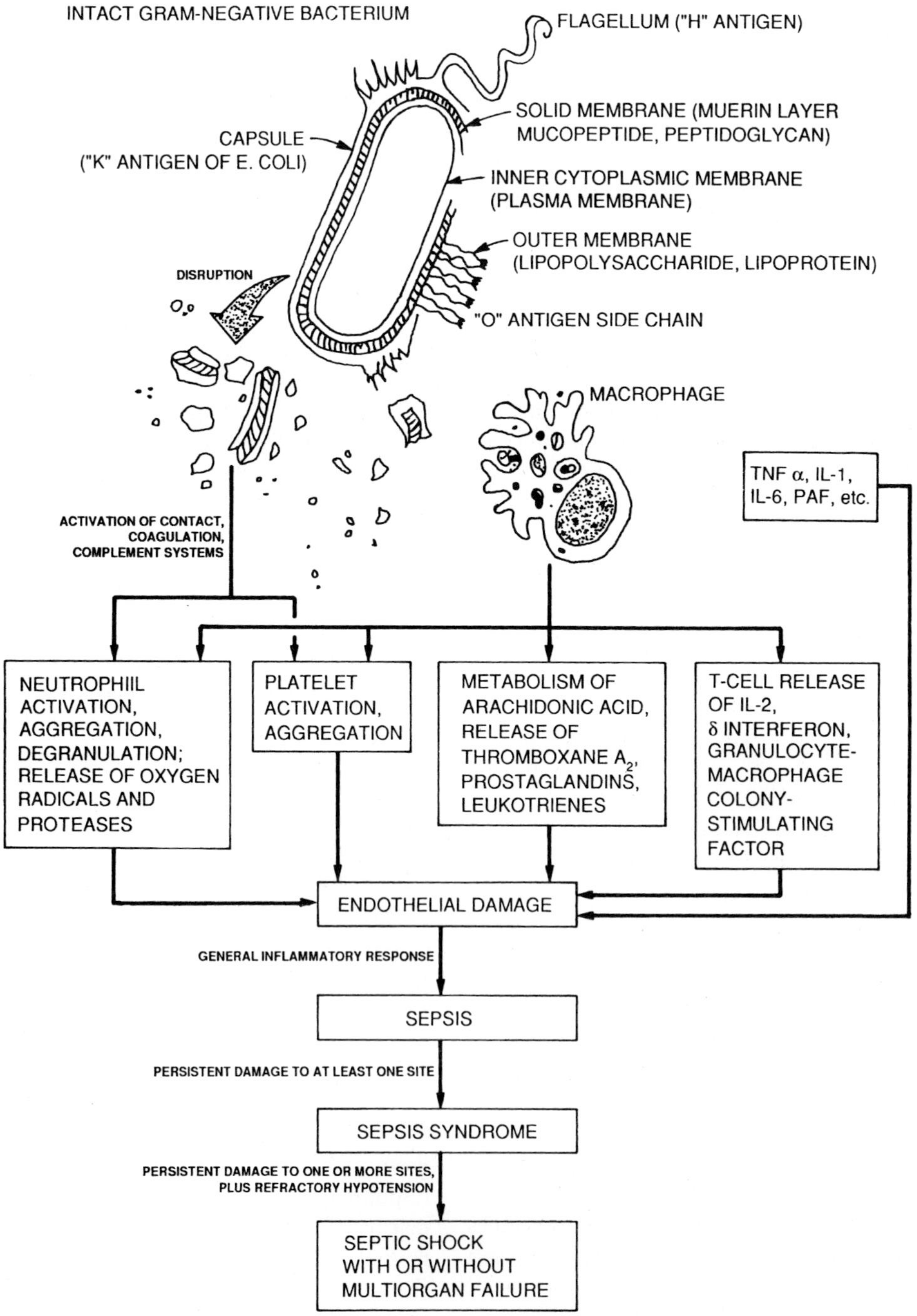

Figure 46-1. The septic response.

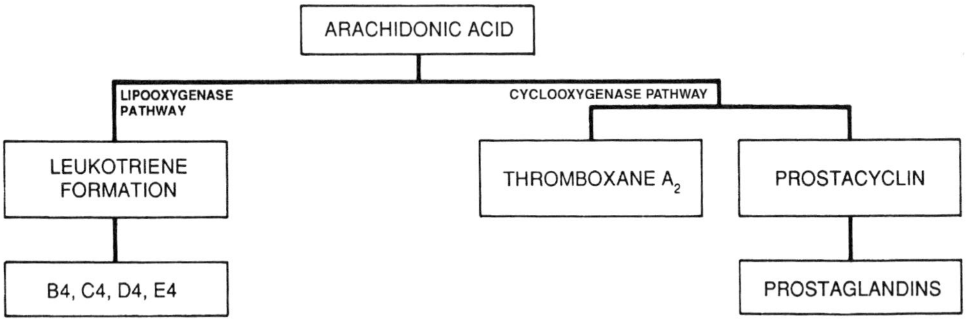

Figure 46-2. Arachidonic acid sequence. Society of Critical Care Medicine. (*Data from Society of Critical Care Medicine. Surviving Sepsis Campaign: International Guidelines for Management of Severe Sepsis and Septic Shock: 2012.* www.survivingsepsis.org.)

leukocytes [PMNs]) in the area increases. PMNs attempt to control the infection through a variety of processes, including the release of highly destructive molecules such as oxygen-free radicals. Another method used by the PMNs involves the breakdown of arachidonic acid. As arachidonic acid is generated, it is further degraded. The degradation of arachidonic acid takes place by either the cyclooxygenase or lipoxygenase pathway (**Fig. 46-2**). From the cyclooxygenase pathway, two important by-products, thromboxane A_2 and prostacyclin (a prostaglandin), are generated. From the lipoxygenase pathway, various leukotrienes (eg, leukotrienes B_4, C_4, D_4, and E_4) are released.

Both leukotrienes and thromboxane A_2 generate a series of reactions, including an increased tendency for platelet aggregation, increased capillary permeability, and vasoconstriction. Prostacyclin (the precursor to specific prostaglandins) produces essentially the opposite responses, that is, a decreased tendency for platelet aggregation, decreased capillary permeability, and vasodilatation.

Downregulation of the Immune/Inflammatory Response. An important aspect of the immune/inflammatory response is the body's ability to neutralize toxic products produced by the immune system. In fact, the immune system is so powerful that in the process of destroying pathogens, it may destroy healthy cells as well. For example, oxygen radicals, once released, will damage or destroy any cell with which they come into contact. The body will attempt to produce neutralizing substances, such as peroxidases for oxygen radicals, to avoid injury to normal tissues. One theory of sepsis holds that the downregulation of the immune system malfunctions and allows normal tissue to be damaged by the immune responses.

T-Cell Response. The macrophage also stimulates T-cell activity by alerting the T cell to the presence of an ingested antigen through markers on its cell surface. The T cell senses these markers and promotes the formation of IL-2. From IL-2, specific interferons as well as granulocyte-macrophage colony-stimulating factor are released. IL-2 is an active cardiovascular modifier. With release of IL-2, the systemic vascular resistance (SVR) decreases and cardiac output increases.

Tumor Necrosis Factor. TNF is thought to be produced in response to a substance such as endotoxin. *TNF stimulates platelet aggregation, increased capillary permeability*, neutrophil activation, and the release of IL-1, IL-6, and IL-8. TNF may have a role in mediating the central response to sepsis, although the exact mechanism for this is unclear. *It is also a pyrogenic, capable of prompting fever, apoptotic cell death, muscle wasting, and inflammation.*

In addition to these responses, the body generates increased quantities of endorphins (releases endogenous opiates). These opiates produce vasodilation (a reduction in SVR) and changes in capillary permeability.

Effect of Immune Response on Endothelial Cells

All the activities described previously are designed to help control the growth of antigens. If properly released, the immune/inflammatory response does not injure normal tissue. However, if the response is not controlled, normal cells can be injured. The most likely cells to be at risk of such injury are the endothelial cells of the blood vessels. *If this endothelial layer is damaged, every organ is threatened* since control of vascular fluid and the supply of oxygen and nutrients may be disrupted.

If the immune response spreads beyond a local level, either because the infection is too great to be controlled or because downregulation fails to occur, the immune response may spread systematically. **It is this systemic spread that may be the first major indicator of a septic process.** This process is called the **systemic inflammatory response syndrome (SIRS)** and is marked by t*achycardia, tachypnea, fever or low temperature, and increased or decreased numbers of white blood cells.*

> QUICK TIP! Even though criteria for sepsis have become more controversial in recent years, it would be helpful to be familiar with SIRS criteria for the exam (See Table 46-1).

Role of Activated Protein C. Protein C is a component of many natural body actions; for example, it is one of the three natural anticoagulant systems in the body. However, it can play a major role in sepsis through other actions. When it is activated, protein C (activated protein C [APC]) inhibits clot formation; allows natural fibrinolysis to occur; and interferes with endothelial cell changes (eg, permeability), neutrophil attraction, and apoptosis (programmed cell death). Protein C levels are deficient in sepsis, likely at a crucial stage.

Extensions of Sepsis. *As the septic process manifests itself, at least one organ will be affected. If the inflammatory response spreads to more than one organ, MODS is likely to occur.* **In addition, if the systemic spread produces hypotension, or elevated**

lactic acid septic shock is likely to occur. Survival from septic shock depends on many factors, a reduced survival being associated with advanced age (>65 years), immunosuppression, or undernourishment.

Clinical Presentations

Sepsis likely occurs in phases, with the **initial phase being marked by signs of systemic inflammatory response system (SIRS) (Table 46-1)**. SIRS criteria are used to trigger the clinician to begin thinking of a potential septic process. Because SIRS is not always related to infectious process, the clinician needs to continue to investigate the case to rule out potential inflammatory, ischemic, or traumatic processes that may be convoluting the patient's condition. **The presence of two SIRS criteria will assist the clinician in this process.**

Additionally, if the patient is septic, from a hemodynamics standpoint, the patient will start to present with *low cardiac output and reduced levels of* $ScvO_2$. As the process continues, *blood lactate will rise as tissue hypoxia develops.* Sepsis is difficult to identify and a biomarker to identify sepsis is desperately needed.

The physical signs of sepsis are generated by several mechanisms. For example, several substances, such as TNF, are directly pyrogenic. Temperature elevation is common in sepsis, although hypothermia can exist. Fever reflects the responses of the immune system to the initial infection and the subsequent inflammatory responses.

The patient generally is tachycardic in response to the systemic hypotension that results from a decrease in SVR secondary to fever and the release of prostaglandins. The activation of the sympathetic nervous system with release of adrenalin in response to the infection is also contributory. Initially this response will increase the cardiac output, but sustained compensatory tachycardia increases the workload of the heart and can lead to myocardial ischemia. This effect is somewhat counter intuitive since sepsis has been demonstrated to produce myocardial depression. The increase in cardiac output is probably a consequence of an increased end-diastolic volume since ejection fraction is usually reduced.

The patient may have pulmonary symptoms reflective of increased extravascular lung fluid secondary to increased capillary permeability (as is seen in acute respiratory distress syndrome). If pulmonary symptoms are present, they may result in refractory hypoxemia (PaO_2 unresponsive to oxygen therapy), generalized crackles heard on auscultation, shortness of breath, and increased production of secretions.

As the septic process continues, any organ system can be affected. For example, a change in level of consciousness may reflect hypoperfusion of the central nervous system or accumulation of toxins in the blood from acute renal or hepatic failure. Physical signs of these organ systems' failures are the same as if the organ had failed for other reasons. Specific signs of individual organ failure can be found in chapters addressing each organ. If the septic process is severe and involves multiple organs, MODS can result.

TABLE 46-1. CRITERIA FOR SEPSIS FOR THE ADULT (Nonpregnant/Laboring)

Infection—Known or Suspected
Inflammatory response to microorganisms
Invasion of normally sterile tissues
PLUS two or more of the following:
Systemic inflammatory response syndrome (SIRS)
Core temperature >38°C or <36°C (>100.4°F or <96.8°F)
Elevated heart rate (>90 bpm)
Respiratory rate >20 breaths/min or $PaCO_2$ <32 mm Hg or mechanical ventilation for acute respiratory process
White blood cell (WBC) count >12,000/mm^3 or <4000/mm^3 or >10% immature neutrophils

Treatment

Treatment of sepsis currently is designed to treat the infectious process, control undesirable immune responses, and provide support to any organ system in failure.

Therapies for Sepsis. The best therapy for sepsis is for clinicians to astutely manage patients to prevent infection from occurring. It is also important to routinely screen for sepsis. However, *if signs and symptoms begin to manifest, the gold standard is to initiate initial resuscitation for sepsis and septic shock within the first hour.* According to the guidelines of the Surviving Sepsis Campaign, the most efficient therapy for sepsis is the implementation of the *hour 1 bundle.* Obtaining a lactic acid level to determine the probability of sepsis and mortality risk is recommended. Blood, urine, and sputum cultures are necessary to identify the infectious agent. If known, the correct antibiotic can be given. If this is unknown, broad antibiotic coverage is given. This treatment frequently employs two or three types of antibiotics—for example, gram-positive coverage, gram-negative coverage, and broad gram-negative and gram-positive coverage. Rapid infusion of intravenous fluids is recommended for patients with sepsis-induced hypotension or hypoperfusion as evidenced by a (serum lactate >2) or poor capillary refill (>3 seconds). Vasopressors should be started when unresponsive to fluid to maintain a mean arterial pressure (MAP) of greater than or equal to 65. Lactate levels should be redrawn, if elevated, at regular intervals until normalized, indicating adequate resuscitation. Fluid should be given only as long as a patient is showing evidence of responsiveness. The sepsis guidelines recommend dynamic measures of fluid responsiveness over static measures such as **central venous pressure (CVP)**. *Dynamic measures of fluid responsiveness are an increase in* ***stroke volume*** *index by 10% after fluid administration or passive leg raise test.*

KEY CLINICAL CONCEPT

The CCRN exam generally does not require that you know the specific type of antibiotic needed. Just knowing "broad spectrum" antibiotic is recommended is sufficient.

Treatments for Sepsis (Table 46-2). The administration of **dobutamine** (or other inotropes) is titrated to achieve an optimal tissue perfusion ($ScvO_2$. If the blood pressure falls and is not maintained by fluids, *vasopressor therapy is used to target an MAP of greater than or equal to 65 mm Hg.* Vasopressor therapy is usually initiated with **norepinephrine (Levophed)**. This is considered the sepsis guideline's first line vasopressor. **Epinephrine** or **dopamine** can be used as an alternative, but it is encouraged to utilize norepinephrine. **For adults with septic**

TABLE 46-2. TREATMENTS FOR SEPSIS

Treatment	Target or Dose	Goals/Comments
Fluid resuscitation	30 mL/kg of balanced crystalloids	Used for sepsis-induced hypoperfusion or septic shock (lactate ≥4 mmoL/L or hypotensive). Goals that are now considered standard of care. Mean arterial pressure (MAP) >65 mm Hg.
Steroids, eg, hydrocortisone	200 mg/day given as 50 mg IV every 6 h or as a continuous infusion	Corticosteroids are not recommended for the treatment of sepsis if adequate fluid resuscitation and vasopressor therapy are able to restore hemodynamic stability. If this is not achievable, guidelines suggest intravenous hydrocortisone.
Glycemic control	Glucose: target range140–180 mg/dL	Guidelines recommend initiating insulin therapy at a glucose level of ≥180 mg/dL Monitoring: Initially, q1–2h After stabilization, q4h
Infusions:		
Norepinephrine Epinephrine		Goal to maintain an MAP ≥ 65 mm Hg.
Vasopressin	0.03 units/min	Goal is to be used as an adjunct to norepinephrine (NE) to maintain MAP ≥ 65 mm Hg or to decrease the dosage of the NE.
Dobutamine		Should be only considered in patients with If cardiac dysfunction with persistent hypoperfusion is present despite adequate volume status and blood pressure.

Evans L, Rhodes A, Alhazzani W, et al. Surviving sepsis campaign: international guidelines for management of sepsis and septic shock 2021. Intensive Care Med. 2021;47(11):181–1247.

KEY CLINICAL CONCEPT

Generally speaking, the goal for glycemic control in medical–surgical critical care patients such as sepsis is to maintain blood glucose <180 mg/dL. This is not to be confused with the "tight glycemic control" goals in cardiac surgery, which are lower.

KEY CLINICAL CONCEPT

The goal for a patient with septic shock is to administer 30 mL/kg of balanced crystalloid fluid, even if the patient initially appears to respond to less fluid.

shock on norepinephrine with inadequate MAP levels guidelines suggest adding vasopressin. Vasopressin has been shown to have a positive effect on blood pressure in septic patients; *however, it is not recommended as a single agent for blood pressure management.* According to the Surviving Sepsis Campaign, if cardiac dysfunction with persistent hypoperfusion is present despite adequate volume status and blood pressure, consider adding **dobutamine** or switching to **epinephrine**.

Corticosteroids. Steroid use in sepsis (such as **hydrocortisone**) is currently restricted to administration only if the patient is hemodynamically unstable after adequate fluid and vasopressor administration. Corticosteroids are contraindicated in the patient that is presenting without shock.

Glycemic Control. Recent research recommends **maintaining a glucose range in the upper limits between 140 and 180 mg/dL to reduce mortality rates in the septic patient.** The patient care team should consider implementing a glycemic control protocol for a patient that has blood sugar more than 180 mg/dL.

Sepsis is a difficult clinical entity to understand and treat. Symptoms are inconsistent and not clear enough to differentiate sepsis from other conditions. Although our understanding of the events that occur in sepsis is improving, treatments are limited in helping improve outcomes. There is great promise for better therapies over the next several years, but the current approach continues to be centered on supportive rather than on curative treatment.

46.2 SEPTIC SHOCK

Septic shock is a continuation of the septic process. In this situation, however, hypotension and or hyperlactatemia develops and is resistant to most therapies. Aggressive fluid resuscitation, vasopressor application and inotropic support may be required to improve perfusion. In septic shock, the likelihood of ameliorating symptoms is limited. Mortality from septic shock is high because of the lack of definitive treatment for the original septic problem.

Septic shock usually presents with *hypotension secondary to a markedly reduced SVR.* The $ScvO_2$ *is elevated because of microcapillary obstruction and poor oxygen utilization at the tissue level.* Cell stunning, specifically mitochondrial dysfunction, is likely one of the many mechanisms for poor utilization of oxygen. Clinically the patient presents with a reduced blood pressure (MAP <65 mm Hg), and or hyperlactatemia, tachycardia, tachypnea, warm skin (due to peripheral vasodilatation), and reduced urine output. It was originally thought that septic shock progressed to a terminal phase in which the cardiac output fell and the SVR increased, although recent evidence suggests that this stage does not necessarily occur prior to death from septic shock.

46.3 MULTIORGAN DYSFUNCTION SYNDROME

As organs fail in sepsis, the term "multiorgan dysfunction" is sometimes used. *There is no real treatment for this condition other than the treatment of each organ.*

Treatment for MODS is supportive of the organs failing, in conjunction with use of any of the therapies described above. It is important to remember that support of an organ is not curative. Consequently, supporting a patient on mechanical ventilation for respiratory failure secondary to sepsis may not improve survival. Perhaps all that is gained is a prolongation of life for several days until the systemic response causes other organs to fail.

KEY CLINICAL CONCEPT

Research suggests that when four or more organ systems are showing sign of failure, risk of mortality can be >80%. This information can be utilized to guide conversations with patients and families regarding end-of-life goals.

Communication with the family is critical. Since survival is poor at this point, it is of paramount importance to understand whether the treatments are aligned with the patient's wishes. Family communication can be led by the nurse and critical care provider and should take place early and throughout this dangerous period.

KEY CONTENT CHECKLIST

- ❒ Always assess/screen for early signs of sepsis.
- ❒ Always ask the question if there is a known/suspected infection, and if so, look to determine if SIRS criteria and organ dysfunction are present, and investigate if criteria met is due to the suspected source.
- ❒ Even though criteria for sepsis have become more controversial in recent years, it would be helpful to be familiar with SIRS criteria for the exam (See Table 46-1).
- ❒ Septic shock usually presents with *hypotension secondary to a markedly reduced SVR.*
- ❒ Gold standard is to initiate initial resuscitation for sepsis and septic shock within the first hour.
- ❒ Antibiotics are the intervention in the sepsis bundle most strongly associated with a mortality benefit.
- ❒ Evidence-based measures of fluid responsiveness are an increase in stroke volume index by 10% after fluid administration or passive leg raise test.
- ❒ Generally speaking, the goal for glycemic control in medical–surgical critical care patients such as sepsis is to maintain blood glucose <180 mg/dL. This is not to be confused with the "tight glycemic control" goals in cardiac surgery, which are lower.
- ❒ The goal for a patient with septic shock is to administer 30 mL/kg of balanced crystalloid fluid, even if the patient initially appears to respond to less fluid.
- ❒ If the blood pressure falls and is not maintained by fluids, vasopressor therapy is used to target a MAP of greater than or equal to 65 mm Hg. Vasopressor therapy is usually initiated with **norepinephrine (Levophed).**
- ❒ Research suggests that when four or more organ systems are showing sign of failure, risk of mortality can be >80%. This information can be utilized to guide conversations with patients and families regarding end-of-life goals.

Review Questions:

Use the following information to answer questions 1 and 2:

A 69-year-old woman is admitted to your unit with probable septic shock after sustaining a ruptured diverticulum in her large intestine. The following information is available:

Blood pressure 80/52 mm Hg
Pulse 121
Respiratory rate 38
Temperature 38°C
Cardiac output 8.9
Cardiac index 5.6
Stroke index 46
PA 24/11
PAOP 8
CVP 2
Pao_2 78
$Paco_2$ 29
pH 7.32
HCO_3^- 16
Lactate 5.1
$ScvO_2$ 81%
Spo_2 95%

1. **Based on this information, which treatment(s) is/are likely to be implemented first?**
   a. Normal saline fluid bolus of 500 mL/30 min and broad-spectrum antibiotics within the first hour of sepsis identification
   b. Dobutamine at 5 μg/kg/min and administration of antipyretics
   c. Normal saline fluid bolus of 300 mL/30 min and administration of antipyretics
   d. All of the above

Answer: A. Rationale: The severe sepsis resuscitation bundle includes serum lactate level, broad-spectrum antibiotics, blood cultures prior to antibiotics, and fluid challenge for hypotension and/or elevated lactate. The only option available that includes only elements of the sepsis bundle is option A. Antipyretics are not associated with improved outcomes in comparison to the bundle, so options B and C can be eliminated. Choose A.

2. **Treatment with which of the following is most likely to reverse the effects of the sepsis?**
   a. Early antibiotic therapy and source control
   b. Ibuprofen
   c. Tight glycemic control
   d. Fluid bolus of either crystalloid or colloidal solutions

Answer: A. Rationale: Antibiotics and source control are interventions most closely associated with mortality benefit in severe sepsis based on the options available. Ibuprofen may be beneficial for symptom management or decreasing metabolic demand; however, nonsteroidal anti-inflammatory drugs (NSAIDs) are not included in the sepsis guidelines and may be harmful to renal function, so eliminate B. Tight glycemic control (serum glucose: 80–110 mg/dL) is not recommended in medical–surgical ICU patients, so eliminate C as well. IV fluids can be helpful in septic shock patients; however, they are not as closely associated with survival as option A. Choose A.

3. **A patient presents to the emergency department and states he has had a cough for a week now and he is short of breath and winded when he walks. Upon assessment, you auscultated crackles in his lower chest area and his oxygen saturation is 90%, RR 32, Temp 102.4. You obtain blood cultures, a lactic acid level, and a complete blood cell (CBC). The white blood cell (WBC) comes back at 13.5. Based on this you know the patient is septic, what should you get started asap?**
   a. Prepare for implementation of the hour 1 bundle Stat.
   b. Give any antibiotic.
   c. Give only 10 mL/kg fluid.
   d. None of these.

Answer: A. Rationale: Administering "any antibiotic" may result in the wrong antibiotic being given, so eliminate B. Since the initial "sepsis dose" fluid challenge is 30 mL/kg, 10 mL/kg of fluid is not correct. We also do not know if the patient is hypotensive, which is criteria for 30 mL/kg, so eliminate C. A is the best, most comprehensive, and evidence-based answer to the scenario (that would also include antibiotics, the intervention most closely associated with mortality benefit in sepsis). Choose A.

REFERENCE

Evans L, Rhodes A, Alhazzani W, et al. Surviving sepsis campaign: International guidelines for management of sepsis and septic shock 2021. *Intensive Care Med.* 2021;47:1181–1247.

47

Toxic Emergencies

CHAPTER OVERVIEW AND OBJECTIVES

The CCRN exam will probably include only one to four questions on toxicology. These are likely to center on the immediate critical care setting, although knowledge of emergency department care may be useful. This section provides a brief but intense review of the area of toxicology. Once again, do not focus on minor details but try to understand the major concepts in assessing and managing the patient with an acute overdose.

After studying this chapter, you should understand the following:

- How and what to assess when you have a suspected toxin ingestion.
- What the antidotes are for multiple toxins.
- The importance of the poison control center and when to notify them.

Toxic emergencies are grouped in four categories: poisonings, overdoses, drug abuse, and alcoholism. It is difficult to know the exact number of toxic ingestions that occur. Reports from poison control centers capture only a portion of toxic ingestions or exposures each year.

47.1 STATISTICS

- According to the Centers for Disease Control and Prevention (CDC), unintentional poisoning is the leading cause of injury death in the United States, comprising nearly 42% of these fatalities in 2020 and surpassing motor vehicle traffic fatalities as the leading cause of injury death in the United States in 2009.
- Provisional data from CDC's National Center for Health Statistics indicate that there were an estimated 100,306 drug overdose deaths in the United States during the 12-month period ending in April 2021, an increase of 28.5% from the 78,056 deaths during the same period the year before. The majority of those cases, approximately 75%, involved an opioid.
- The number of drug overdose deaths has quadrupled since 1999. The continuous rise in prescribing, use, and abuse of opioid drugs and the subsequent increase in opioid-related deaths have come to be known as the opioid epidemic.
- From 1999 to 2016, the drug-poisoning death rates increased for all age groups. In 2016, the drug-poisoning death rates were highest for persons aged 35–44 (35.0 per 100,000), 25–34 (34.6), and 45–54 (34.5).
- In 2016, the age-adjusted death rate was 25.3 for non-Hispanic white persons, 17.1 for non-Hispanic black persons, and 9.5 for Hispanic persons.
- Every year, at least 430 people die in the United States from accidental CO poisoning.
- Approximately 50,000 people in the United States visit the emergency department each year due to accidental CO poisoning.

QUICK TIP! It is not uncommon to see one carbon monoxide case on the exam. The patient often presents with headache, confusion, weakness, nausea, vomiting, and flu-like symptoms. Patients often present in the winter months due to poor indoor ventilation from heating systems. Elevated carboxyhemoglobin (HbCO) levels are identified, and treatment includes 100% O_2 and supportive care.

- Approximately one-half of all poisonings involving teens are classified as suicide attempts.

A *poison* is defined as any substance that, when introduced into an organism, acts chemically on the tissue to produce serious injury or death. There are four routes of entry: ingestion, inhalation, injection, and surface absorption.

Poisonings most commonly involve household products such as petroleum-based agents, cleaning agents, and cosmetics. Medications are the next most frequent and most lethal source, followed by toxic plants and contaminated food. Toxic effects of ingested substances can be delayed or immediate. Delayed effects are dependent on the rate of absorption and metabolism from the gastrointestinal tract. Since most absorption occurs in the small intestine, toxins may remain in the stomach for up to several hours if a large amount of food is present. Medications or other substances that slow gastrointestinal motility may interfere. Some medications or toxins are more rapidly absorbed than others. Immediate effects of a toxin can be seen with the ingestion of corrosive substances such as strong acids or alkalis or with highly toxic and rapidly absorbed toxins such as organophosphates (pesticides) or cyanide.

47.2 ASSESSMENT

Assessment begins with patient history. This should include the five W's:

- Who (patient age and previous medical history, including allergies and current therapies).
- What (inquire about the suspected agent(s) or toxin(s) to which the patient has had access, then obtain management information from local poison control center).
- When (determine the approximate time of ingestion, corroborating with others in contact with the patient).
- Where (it is important to know the surroundings or circumstances to prepare for complications, as in the case of an overdose that takes place in a running car in a garage or in a tub full of water).
- Why (assess the patient's psychiatric stability to account for inaccuracies in the history or the intent of the patient to deliberately mislead). In addition, assess the patient's knowledge about a substance. For example, overconsumption of over-the-counter (OTC) antacids may cause hypercalcemia.

These questions are important tools in assessment because many initial intake histories are incorrect with respect to agent, time, and/or amount.

Patient Assessment/Interventions

In dealing with a suspected toxic ingestion or exposure, it is important to refer to the local poison control center as a guide to identification of the toxin or drug, what associated symptoms to expect, and information on management of toxic exposures. Because many overdose situations involve multiple drugs or substances, it is important to identify those substances that are most likely to produce severe or life-threatening effects. The examination should include vital signs, with a temperature and respiratory rate. Cardiopulmonary stabilization and anticipation of possible deterioration should also occur during initial assessment. Cardiac monitoring, pulse oximetry, and use of a large-bore intravenous line should be initiated.

Respiratory Assessment

Respiratory rate and depth can be affected by a number of agents. *Check for airway patency.* An increased rate and depth can be attributed to *sympathomimetics such as cocaine, amphetamines, or caffeine.* An abnormal rate and pattern may be your first clue to an acid–base disorder. Tachypnea may result in primary alkalosis from *salicylates* or as a compensation for a dangerous metabolic acidosis, which can occur from *ethylene glycol ("anti-freeze"), methanol,* or other agents. Assessment of lung sounds, noting the presence of crackles or wheezes, is an important part of serial assessment in patients who may have aspirated or are experiencing heart failure. Monitor pulse oximetry and blood gas values to ensure appropriate oxygenation. Position the patient with the head of bed more than 30 degrees if tolerated to decrease aspiration risk. Suction as needed to ensure airway clearance.

Cardiovascular Assessment

Evidence of cardiac dysrhythmias, hypotension, or hypertension requires advanced cardiac life support as well as intensive care observation. Continuous cardiac monitoring is required, since life-threatening *dysrhythmias can occur rapidly with such agents as tricyclics, beta-blockers, or cardiac glycosides.* A 12-lead electrocardiogram (ECG), as well as treatment of arrhythmias, may be warranted.

Neurologic Assessment

A depressed level of consciousness is a major complication in the overdose patient. Describe the patient's responses to stimuli; reflexes—presence or absence and type; as well as disturbances in vital signs. Other causes of decreased level of consciousness (trauma, diabetes, hypoglycemia, anoxia, sepsis, etc) should be investigated. The *Glasgow coma scale* is helpful and is commonly used in neurologic assessment.

Seizures are best managed by treating the underlying cause (eg, hypoxia, hypoglycemia, or hyponatremia). **Diazepam, lorazepam, phenytoin**, and **phenobarbital** can be effective in controlling seizures from nonspecific causes or until underlying causes can be determined. *Seizures may be a clue to drug withdrawal*; they may be seen after administration of **naloxone** to a comatose patient who is narcotic-dependent or after the administration of **flumazenil** if the patient is dependent on a benzodiazepine or tricyclic antidepressant.

Gastrointestinal Assessment

Common symptoms associated with gastrointestinal poisoning center around the loss of gastrointestinal fluids and subsequent hypovolemia. Electrolyte imbalances can occur as well. Blood loss can result from irritation of the gastric mucosa or from a Mallory–Weiss tear of the esophagus during protracted vomiting. Gastrointestinal decontamination may be a consideration in the treatment of toxic ingestions. Refer to your hospital policy and procedure manual and poison control center for information in preferred methods of decontamination for the specific toxin involved.

Hepatic and Renal Assessment

Laboratory studies are essential to assess potential damage to hepatic and renal systems. Liver function tests (eg, serum glutamic pyruvic transaminase [SGPT], serum glutamic oxaloacetic transaminase [SGOT], and alkaline phosphatase) are useful in assessing hepatic function.

In assessment of the renal system, urine output, the presence of myoglobinuria or hematuria, as well as laboratory studies (blood urea nitrogen, creatinine, creatine phosphokinase) are significant in determining renal failure that may be due to **rhabdomyolysis**.

Assessment of Skin and Mucous Membranes

Such assessment can provide important clues as to the causative agent. Observe for burns or erosion of oral mucosa as well as cutaneous bullous lesions. Unexplained puncture wounds and/or contusions may be indicative of **snake bites**, **drug abuse**, or trauma.

KEY CLINICAL CONCEPT

- It is not uncommon for a patient with endocarditis and sepsis from IV drug abuse to appear on the exam. Treatment initially consists of supportive care for sepsis. However, if valve vegetation is identified, cardiac surgery if often indicated.
- For snake bite case questions, treatment is usually supportive and administration of the antidote is the priority. This is another example of how they will test to see if you can identify and address underlying causes.

47.3 TREATMENT

The goals in treatment for a known or suspected toxic ingestion are to remove the agent(s), detoxify the patient, and prevent absorption of the suspected agent(s).

Removal of Toxic Agents

Decontamination of Skin and Eyes. For patients with dermal exposures, prompt removal of clothing and thorough washing with mild soap and copious amounts of water are required. Emergency care providers should use protective equipment to prevent contamination by the offending agent. In patients with eye exposures, immediate eye irrigation with normal saline should be done until the ocular pH is 7.0 to 7.3.

Emesis. *Syrup of ipecac is no longer routinely used or recommended to induce vomiting.* Refer to the hospital's policy and procedure and the recommendations from the local poison control center.

Gastric Lavage. Gastric lavage is another method for removal of toxins. It involves the insertion of a large-bore orogastric tube and the instillation and removal of large amounts of water through the tube in order to empty the stomach when a recent ingestion is suspected.

Because gastric lavage is an invasive procedure, it is associated with certain risks and complications. Risks versus benefits should be determined before this procedure is performed. It is important to refer to the Poison Control management and your hospital's policy and procedural manual for contraindications to using gastric lavage. **Airway protection is essential if this procedure is used.**

Cathartics. Cathartics are used to decrease the transit time for any unabsorbed toxin, thereby minimizing absorption in the bowel. Sorbitol is a common cathartic and is an ingredient in most of the activated charcoal preparations used for patients who have ingested toxic substances. Although the use of cathartics is based primarily on empiric and anecdotal evidence, most toxicologists agree with their use as a means of decreasing gastrointestinal transit time for toxins.

Detoxification and Prevention of Absorption

Activated Charcoal. The dry, powder form of activated charcoal is an inert fine black powder. It is tasteless and odorless and has a gritty consistency. Activated charcoal is also available as an aqueous slurry or in a suspension of 20% activated charcoal in 70% sorbitol. It can be given either orally or through a lavage tube. The charcoal slurry tends to be thick and gritty and is not very palatable when administered orally. Whenever lavage is required, it is advantageous to instill the activated charcoal prior to removal of the lavage tube. Activated charcoal is thought to be a safe, inert, nontoxic material. No harmful effects have been shown from exposure of the skin; however, aspiration can be harmful. Although activated charcoal is useful in absorbing many toxins, there are agents that it does not appear to absorb. Refer to the poison control management to determine the recommended use. It is important to remember that activated charcoal absorbs not only toxins but also therapeutic medications. If the toxin requires giving multiple doses of charcoal, activated charcoal *without* a cathartic (sorbitol) should be considered for the additional doses.

Enhanced Elimination

Enhanced elimination of certain drugs may be implemented by making use of certain pharmacokinetic parameters that affect drug excretion. These include forced diuresis (with or without ion trapping), multiple-dose charcoal, dialysis, hemoperfusion, and plasmapheresis.

Forced Diuresis. This method involves enhanced elimination of the agent through urinary excretion. Normally, excretion takes place through glomerular filtration, active tubular secretion, and tubular reabsorption. This method deals with inhibiting tubular reabsorption only by diluting the concentration gradient between the blood and the urine. This will lessen the time during which the agent is exposed to the absorptive sites in the distal tubules.

Ion-Trapping Methods. Ion-trapping methods cause a solution to become more alkaline or acidic, so that the substance is trapped in the kidney and excretion is enhanced. Weak acids are more ionized in an alkaline solution, and weak bases are more ionized in an acidic solution. If a difference in pH occurs across a membrane, ion trapping will occur. **Alkaline diuresis is more commonly used and can be achieved by the administration of sodium bicarbonate in intravenous fluids.** *Usually, sodium bicarbonate (2–3 ampules) is added to each liter of intravenous fluids to achieve a urinary pH of 7.5 or greater.* Refer to your hospital's policy and procedures for specific recommendations. This method is useful for agents that produce metabolic acidosis **(salicylates)**, and careful monitoring of electrolytes is essential in using alkaline diuresis.

Multidose Charcoal. Multiple doses of activated charcoal appear to be effective in enhancing the elimination of drugs that undergo enterohepatic or enterogastric circulation. Activated charcoal without sorbitol should be considered for additional doses. Poison control managements can provide guidance when the use of multiple doses of charcoal is being considered.

Extracorporeal Methods of Elimination Hemodialysis. Hemodialysis can be useful in further clearance of certain substances from the body. It is usually reserved for the patient who has not responded to more conservative and conventional methods.

Antidotes

Certain drugs and toxins have specific antidotes that counteract their harmful effects (**Table 47-1**). *It is best to use an antidote if available, although reversal of certain drugs can precipitate withdrawal symptoms and seizures.* Poison control management can help to identify those toxins that have specific antidotes.

The national number for Poison Control centers is 1-800-222-1222, available 24 hours a day, 7 days a week.

Illegal/Street Drugs

Because of increasing access to and use of illegal drugs, it is important to question the patient and/or family and friends about the patient's recreational use of such substances. A urine drug toxicology screen is necessary to identify patients who have such drugs in their systems (**Table 47-2**).

47.4 AGENTS/TOXINS OF TERRORISM

It is unlikely that many health care facilities will treat patients with exposures to these agents or toxins, due to actual and increasing threats of terrorist events; however, it is important to have a basic awareness of the agents that have either been used in the past or that have the potential for current or future use in terrorist attacks (**Tables 47-3** to **47-6**).

In the event of mass casualty events, whether through acts of individuals or acts of nature, it is important to be able to access your facility's disaster management plan to determine your role in such an event.

TABLE 47-1. COMMON DRUGS AND ANTIDOTES

Drug/Toxin	*Antidote/Dose*	*Comment*
Acetaminophen: also found in combination with other over-the-counter or prescription medications	*N*-acetylcysteine oral or intravenous	Symptoms may not appear until 4–6 h after ingestion
Beta-blockers: eg, atenolol, metoprolol, labetalol	Glucagon: 1–5 mg IV for bradycardia and hypotension	Aggressive cardiac and pulmonary support
Benzodiazepines: eg, diazepam (Valium), clorazepate (Tranxene), alprazolam (Xanax)	Flumazenil: follow pharmacy recommendations	Observe for withdrawal seizures in chronic users
Cardiac glycosides: eg, digoxin	Digibind/DigiFab: follow pharmacy recommendations, based on amount ingested	Used in severe dysrhythmias or with digitoxicity with a K^+ >5–6.0
Carbon monoxide: eg, car fumes, fumes from faulty heating systems	Oxygen: 100% reduces half-life of CO to 1.5 h	Hyperbaric chamber at 3 stm reduces half-life of CO to 23 min
Ethylene glycol, methanol: eg, antifreeze	Ethyl alcohol in conjunction with dialysis Fomepizole (initial dose: 15 mg/kg IVP)	Competes for alcohol dehydrogenase; prevents formation of formic acid and oxalates. Death occurs from severe acidosis
Narcotics/opiates: eg, morphine, codeine, propoxyphene (Darvon), Demerol, heroin	Naloxone 0.01 mg/kg IV Intranasal: 4 or 8 mg ×1 spray IV/IM/SQ: 0.4-2 mg	Frequent repeated doses may be needed, may precipitate acute withdrawal, so should be reserved for severe respiratory depression May repeat doses every 2–3 min then transition to IV drip
Tricyclic antidepressants: eg, amitriptyline (Elavil), protriptyline (Vivactil), doxepin (Sinequan)	Sodium bicarbonate (supportive therapy) Adults: IV: 1–2 mEq/kg; repeat as needed to maintain goal arterial pH; initiation of a-150 mEq/L infusion may be required to maintain alkalosis	Protein binding of tricyclics occurs in an alkalotic pH. Treatment goals include alkalinizing the urine
Warfarin (Coumadin)	Vitamin K; fresh frozen plasma Vitamin K (Phytonadione) PO or IV: follow pharmacy protocol KCentra	Promotes hepatic biosynthesis of prothrombin Dosing based on INR and severity of bleed

TABLE 47-2. COMMON STREET DRUGS

Drug Name(s)	*Drug Class*	*Route of Ingestion*	*Effects*
Heroin (H, horse, monkey, smack)	Opioid/narcotic	Injected, snorted, smoke	CNS depression
Cocaine + heroin (speedball)	Sympathetic stimulant/ opioid	Injected, snorted, smoked	CNS and cardiac stimulation CNS depression
Cocaine (blow, coke, dust, flake girl, snow)	Sympathetic stimulant	Injected, snorted	CNS and cardiac stimulation
Crack: cocaine in rock form (freebase, rock)	Sympathetic stimulant	Smoked	CNS and cardiac stimulation, vasoconstriction (CVA or MI)
Methamphetamine (crank, crystal, ice, meth, speed)	Sympathetic stimulant	Injected, smoked	CNS and cardiac stimulation
MDMA (Adam, ecstasy, X-TC, hug-drug, Molly, love-drug)	Sympathetic stimulant	Ingested, snorted, inserted rectally	CNS and cardiac stimulation
LSD (acid, dragon, red/green dragon, blotters, Zen, microdots, windowpane)	Hallucinogen	Ingested	No specific physical effects; injury or death results from paranoid or violent behavior
PCP (angel dust, crystal, supergrass, ozone, rocket fuel, whack)	Hallucinogen, sedative, paralytic	Ingested, snorted, smoked	CNS and respiratory depression, hypertension, seizures
Rohypnol (roofies; commonly called the date-rape drug)	Sedative/hypnotic	Ingested (often with alcohol)	CNS and cardiac depression, amnesia

TABLE 47-3. BIOLOGIC AGENTS

Agent	*Route of Exposure*	*Symptoms*	*Treatment*
Anthrax (bacteria)	Cutaneous contact, inhalation, ingestion	Blister-like lesions, respiratory distress, severe GI distress	Ciprofloxacin, doxycycline, penicillin, steroids
Brucella (bacteria)	Ingestion, inhalation	Acute febrile illness, respiratory symptoms without obvious signs of pneumonia, GI distress	Doxycycline with streptomycin or rifampin
Pneumonic plague (bacteria)	Inhalation, inoculation (flea bites)	Severe and rapidly progressive respiratory symptoms	Ciprofloxacin, doxycycline, tetracycline
Smallpox (virus)	Inhalation, cutaneous contact	Severe febrile illness, maculopapular rash	Vaccination within 3–4 days of exposure may decrease severity Use of cidofovir is only experimental
Viral encephalitis: various forms	Inhalation	Fever, malaise, seizures	Symptomatic treatment, supportive care

TABLE 47-4. BIOLOGIC TOXINS

Agent	*Route of Exposure*	*Symptoms*	*Treatment*
Botulinum toxin (neurotoxin)	Ingested	Blurred vision, dry mouth, descending flaccid paralysis	Trivalent equine antitoxin from the CDC, symptomatic treatment, supportive care
Ricin (toxin extracted from castor bean)	Ingested, inhaled	Vomiting, diarrhea, rapidly progressive pulmonary edema	Symptomatic treatment, supportive care
Enterotoxin B (*Staphylococcus aureus*)	Ingested, inhaled	Severe GI symptoms, fever, nonproductive cough	Symptomatic treatment, supportive care

TABLE 47-5. CHEMICAL AGENTS

Name	*Route of Exposure*	*Symptoms*	*Treatment*
Sarin, Soman (organophosphates/nerve agents)	Cutaneous contact, inhalation, ingestion	Severe cholinergic effects (lancination, salivation, sweating, pulmonary edema)	Decontamination, anticholinergics (atropine), anticonvulsants
Hydrogen, sulfur mustard (vesicant)	Cutaneous contact, inhalation, ingestion	Intense itching of skin; delayed, painless blister eruption with resulting deep burns; pulmonary edema; severe GI distress	Decontaminate with copious amounts of water, symptomatic treatment
Lewisite (vesicant)	Cutaneous contact, inhaled, ingested	Burns on contact, rapid pulmonary edema, severe GI distress	Initial decontamination with talcum powder or flour to absorb chemical, symptomatic treatment

TABLE 47-6. PULMONARY/ASPHYXIATION AGENTS

Name	*Route of Ingestion*	*Symptoms*	*Treatment*
Ammonia (pulmonary)	Cutaneous contact, inhalation, ingestion	Irritation and burning, respiratory distress, tracheal burns, GI distress	Symptomatic treatment; consider bronchodilators and steroids
Chlorine (pulmonary)	Cutaneous contact, inhalation, ingestion	Corrosive effects, respiratory distress, severe GI distress	Symptomatic treatment
Cyanide (cellular asphyxiation)	Cutaneous contact, inhalation, ingestion	Rapid onset of respiratory distress, nausea/vomiting	Decontamination with copious washing, Cyanokit, containing hydroxocobalamin or Kelocyanor

KEY CONTENT CHECKLIST

- ❒ Working with the Poison Control is essential in making sure the patient is cared for appropriately. Always refer to hospital policy and Poison Control when you are caring for someone with an exposure/poisoning.
- ❒ It is not uncommon to see one carbon monoxide case on the exam. The patient often presents with headache, confusion, weakness, nausea, vomiting, and flu-like symptoms. Patients often present in the winter months due to poor indoor ventilation from heating systems. Elevated HbCO levels are identified, and treatment includes 100% O_2 and supportive care.
- ❒ Cocaine, amphetamines, or caffeine are "sympathomimetics," upregulating the sympathetic nervous system (SNS) ("fight or flight" response).
- ❒ Tachypnea may result in primary alkalosis from salicylates or as a compensation for a dangerous metabolic acidosis.
- ❒ **Ethylene glycol** ("anti-freeze") may cause metabolic acidosis and calcium oxalate crystals to form in the kidneys, inducing renal failure.
- ❒ Dysrhythmias can occur rapidly with such agents as tricyclics, beta-blockers, or cardiac glycosides. A 12-lead ECG may be warranted to monitor for changes.
- ❒ **Alkaline diuresis is more commonly used and can be achieved by the administration of sodium bicarbonate in intravenous fluids.** Usually, sodium bicarbonate (2–3 ampules) is added to each liter of intravenous fluids to achieve a urinary pH of 7.5 or greater to enhance elimination.
- ❒ **Flumazenil** is the reversal agent for benzodiazepines.
- ❒ **Naloxone** is the reversal agent for opioids.
- ❒ Endocarditis and sepsis can result from IV drug abuse. Treatment initially consists of supportive care for sepsis. However, if valve vegetation is identified, cardiac surgery if often indicated.
- ❒ For snake bite case questions, treatment is usually supportive and administration of the antidote is the priority. This is another example of how they will test to see if you can identify and address underlying causes.
- ❒ Syrup of ipecac is no longer routinely used or recommended to induce vomiting.

Review Questions:

1. **A 19-year-old woman is admitted to your unit after an argument with her parents. Her parents state that they found her in her room with an empty bottle of acetaminophen (Tylenol) on her nightstand. Which of the following is the initial treatment for an overdose of acetaminophen?**
   a. Ipecac
   b. Charcoal and intravenous N-acetylcysteine
   c. Dialysis
   d. Lavage and oral N-acetylcysteine

Answer: B. Rationale: The antidote for an acetaminophen overdose is the use of charcoal and intravenous *N*-acetylcysteine. Syrup of ipecac is no longer routinely recommended, eliminating A. Acetaminophen can be dialyzed out of the circulation, however this would require the time and risk associated with central venous access, eliminating C. Lavage may be associated with aspiration, and therefore has a less favorable risk: benefit profile compared to charcoal. Choose B.

2. **A 20-year-old man is admitted to your unit following a suicide attempt after a breakup with his girlfriend. He ingested an unknown drug or drugs and is currently combative but with a reduced level of consciousness. A large-bore nasogastric tube has been inserted in an attempt to lavage his stomach. Which of the following nursing actions should be initiated at this point?**
   a. Protection against aspiration
   b. Intubation and mechanical ventilation
   c. Sedation to reduce the combativeness
   d. All of the above

Answer: A. Rationale: Airway protection is essential in the use of nasogastric lavage as part of prioritization of the "ABCs." There is no other information in the scenarios that suggests respiratory failure requiring intubation, so eliminate B. The patient also has a reduced LOC, so eliminate C. The best answer is A.

REFERENCES

American Family Physician. (September 2015). 76(6), 829–836. www.aafp.org.

Barclay L, Murata P. Acetaminophen may be the leading cause of acute liver failure. *Hepatology*. 2005;42:1252–1254, 1364–1372.

Burns S. *AACN Essentials of Progressive Care Nursing*. 3rd ed. New York, NY: McGraw Hill; 2014.

Burns S. *AACN Essentials of Progressive Care Nursing*. 4th ed. New York, NY: McGraw Hill; 2018.

Centers for Disease Control and Prevention. U.S. Overdose Deaths In 2021 Increased Half as Much as in 2020 - But Are Still Up 15% (cdc.gov).

Centers for Disease Control: National Center for Health Statistics. (March 2016). Poisonings: fact sheet. *http://www.cdc.gov/nchs/data/factsheets/factsheet_drug_poisoning.htm.*

Centers for Disease Control: National Center for Health Statistics. (April 2015). Emergency department visits for drug poisoning: United States, 2008–2011. *http://www.cdc.gov/nchs/products/databriefs/db196.htm.*

Centers for Disease Control: National Center for Injury Prevention and Control (2004). Poisonings: Fact sheet. http://www.cdc.gov/nicpc/factsheets/poisonings.htm. Accessed 12/5/05.

McKinley MG. Alcohol withdrawal syndrome. *Crit Care Nurse*. 2005;25:40–48.

Missouri Department of Health and Senior Services: Center for Emergency Response and Terrorism. *Biological, Chemical and Radiological Terrorism: Basic Information for Medical Professionals*. June 2004 (CD).

Mokhlesi B, Garimella PS, Joffe A, et al. Street drug abuse leading to critical illness. *Intens Care Med*. 2004;30:1526–1536.

Mokhlesi B, Leikin JB, Murray P, et al. Part I: General approach to the intoxicated patient. *Chest*. 2003;123:577–592.

Mokhlesi B, Leikin JB, Murray P, et al. Adult toxicology in critical care: Part II. Specific poisonings. *Chest*. 2003;123:897–922.

National Capital Poison Center. Poison Statistics National Data 2020 | Poison Control.

National Center for Health Statistics Fact Sheet. NCHS Data on Drug-poisoning Deaths (cdc.gov).

Poison Control. Position statistics national data 2014, 2016. http://www.poison.org/poison-statistics-national.

Zimmerman J. Poisonings and overdoses in the intensive care unit: general and specific management issues. *Crit Care Med*. 2003;31:2794–2801.

48

Airway Obstruction

CHAPTER OVERVIEW AND OBJECTIVES

The CCRN exam may include one to four questions on airway obstruction. Airway obstruction might also be addressed in the context of other clinical conditions or situations, such as postextubation. This brief chapter should be adequate to prepare you for the questions on the CCRN exam addressing airway obstruction.

After studying this chapter, you should understand the following:

- The treatment plan for the patient with an upper airway obstruction.
- The strategy for treating a near-drowning patient.
- The importance of airway, breathing, and circulation with any airway compromise.

48.1 UPPER AIRWAY OBSTRUCTION

Upper airway obstruction is *among the highest-priority emergencies* a critical care clinician can encounter. The prompt recognition and treatment of a partially or fully obstructed airway can mean the difference between life and death for the patient. Multiple conditions may be responsible for acute compromise of the upper airway (superior to the primary carina), all of which require prompt diagnosis followed by definitive therapy to reestablish airflow.

QUICK TIP! Be prepared for one to two questions testing whether you are prioritizing the "ABCs," such as prioritizing airway securement first, etc.

Identifying Characteristics

Upper airway obstruction may present either as an obvious life-threatening emergency or in a subtler fashion, depending on the degree of occlusion as well as its cause. *The classic finding in a patient with a partial airway obstruction at or above the larynx is a high-pitched crowing or harsh whistle with inspiration, termed stridor.* In contrast, an intrathoracic obstruction in the trachea is signaled by expiratory stridor due to the natural narrowing of the airway with expiration. Clinically, the obstructed patient may also present with dyspnea, clutching of the throat ("choking sign"), facial swelling, neck vein prominence, pallor or cyanosis, coughing, wheezing, sore throat, altered voice or phonation, dysphagia (difficulty swallowing secretions, which can lead to drooling), or accessory muscle contraction. Foreign-body aspiration is frequently accompanied by paroxysmal coughing. With complete obstruction, the patient is unable to breathe, cough, or speak and rapidly deteriorates to a state of unconsciousness.

Etiology

The underlying causes of upper airway obstruction are varied. As one might expect, foreign-body aspiration is first among these. Infectious processes such as *epiglottitis*, retropharyngeal abscess, laryngeal diphtheria, *Ludwig's angina* (a progressive submaxillary cellulitis that involves the neck and floor of the mouth, frequently following dental disease), tonsillitis, pharyngitis, mononucleosis, fluid secretions, bronchoconstriction, fibrosis, and otitis can all cause asphyxiation by obstruction. More commonly, the infection may erode a blood vessel, causing massive hemorrhage, or a purulent pocket may rupture. Noninfectious laryngeal edema may result from trauma, inhalation of noxious gases, burns, or anaphylactic shock (caused by inhalants, bee stings, drugs, contrast media, blood products), or it **may follow removal of an endotracheal tube**. Neck surgery, trauma, diagnostic procedures (carotid angiography), or erosion of a blood vessel by the invasion of cancerous or infectious cells may result in retropharyngeal hemorrhage.

KEY CLINICAL CONCEPT

The first-line treatment for post-extubation stridor is nebulized epinephrine ("racemic epinephrine")

Clinical Presentation

Patients with airway obstruction may have the following symptoms:

- Hypoxia
- Agitation
- Shortness of breath
- Diaphoresis
- Confusion
- Increase in carbon dioxide levels
- Confusion
- Wheezing

To evaluate the patient labs, such as an arterial blood gas in order to determine oxygenation status to determine what the cause of the obstruction is, assessment of the clinical presentation is warranted.

Treatment

In cases of severe upper airway obstruction, a *mixture of helium and oxygen may be administered* to provide temporary support pending a definitive diagnosis and treatment plan. Severe or complete obstruction requires immediate airway control. Following institution of the *head-tilt and jaw-thrust maneuver to minimize the soft tissue contribution to obstruction*, the larynx and oropharynx must be inspected and any obstructive material (blood, vomitus, foreign matter) removed via suctioning. If adequate ventilation is not then achieved with a bag-valve-mask device driven by 100% oxygen, an airway must be emergently established with the placement of an endotracheal tube or by a tracheostomy or cricothyrotomy.

48.2 NEAR-DROWNING

Near-drowning is defined as a submersion injury after which the patient survives for at least 24 hours. Drowning, on the other hand, is defined as a submersion injury that causes death within 24 hours.

Identifying Characteristics

Although each near-drowning victim presents somewhat differently depending on his or her previous state of health, quantity and type (fresh, salt, chlorinated, polluted) of water aspirated, length of time submerged, and the temperature of the water, there is a predictable sequence of events that occurs during the submersion injury. Initially, the victim begins to cough and gasp as water enters the mouth and nose, which results in a variable amount of water being swallowed. Simultaneously, as water is aspirated into the larynx, laryngospasm develops, which helps to protect the airway from further aspiration of water. Subsequently, the laryngospasm causes asphyxia, which causes the victim to lose consciousness. Hypoxemia then leads to the development of metabolic acidosis. Even though the terminology "wet" and "dry" drowning are no longer accepted terms, it is important to understand what they mean since this description is still used. If the victim dies during the laryngospasm phase, it may be called a "dry" drowning, or suffocation, because a large quantity of water was not aspirated. However, it is estimated that only 10% to 15% of drowning cases are dry drownings. For the other 85% to 90% of victims who aspirate at some point during the submersion injury, the loss of consciousness is thought to cause relaxation of the laryngeal muscles, which allows aspiration of water. However, it is also thought that the hypercarbic or hypoxic drives stimulate inhalation or aspiration of water, thus resulting in a "wet" drowning.

Earlier, it was believed that the inhalation of salt water, with its increased concentration of electrolytes and thus the ability to draw fluid into the lungs, resulted in an electrolyte imbalance and pulmonary edema. Freshwater, on the other hand, was thought to produce hemodilution and hemolysis from the hypotonic fluids. It is now believed that most near-drowning victims do not aspirate sufficient quantities of water to produce these changes. It is thought that it is the amount of aspirated water and not the type of water that results in pulmonary changes during the submersion injury. The aspiration of water decreases pulmonary compliance. Whether surfactant is washed out of the alveoli with freshwater aspiration or is denatured by saltwater entering the alveoli, an intrapulmonary shunt develops and hypoxia occurs. Therefore, the focus of attention with submersion injuries should be the management of hypoxia.

The other inherent problem with submersion injuries is hypothermia. A danger of hypothermia is the development of lethal cardiac dysrhythmias that may result in cardiac arrest. However, hypothermia may be beneficial if it occurs before the development of hypoxia. It is thought to be neuroprotective, as evidenced by those who have survived ice-water submersions for longer than 30 minutes, especially children.

> QUICK TIP! Be familiar with the clinical significance of post-arrest Targeted Temperature Management (TTM) formerly referred to as "hypothermia" and the impact it has on the physiology; however, the exam will not include questions regarding specific post-arrest therapeutic hypothermia protocols.

Treatment

Patient care for the victim of near-drowning includes early endotracheal intubation with the administration of 100% oxygen at 5 to 10 cm positive end-expiratory pressure (PEEP). Early intubation may also protect the airway from the aspiration of gastric contents, which is likely with submersion injuries. In cold-water submersion injuries, cardiac dysrhythmias should be anticipated and aggressively managed. Standard resuscitation protocols should be used in the management of cardiac arrest. Because the metabolic acidosis may be severe, the administration of **sodium bicarbonate** may be warranted. After resuscitation, monitoring for the development of bronchospasm is necessary and the treatment of bronchospasm, if it develops, must be aggressively managed. Hemodynamic monitoring may be necessary in the management of pulmonary edema.

KEY CONTENT CHECKLIST

- ❒ It is important to always remember no matter what the cause of airway pathology, a key objective as the critical care nurse is to prioritize actions associated with airway management. The exam often reinforces the need prioritize the airway in the "ABCs."
- ❒ The classic finding in a patient with a partial airway obstruction at or above the larynx is a high-pitched crowing or harsh whistle with inspiration, termed stridor.
- ❒ The first-line treatment for postextubation stridor is nebulized epinephrine ("racemic epinephrine")
- ❒ Be familiar with the clinical significance of post-arrest targeted temperature management (TTM) formerly referred to as "hypothermia" and the impact it has on the physiology; however, the exam will not include questions regarding specific post-arrest TTM protocols.

Review Questions:

1. **Your patient has just suffered a near-drowning event. After the patient arrives or during transport to the hospital, you can expect which of the following:**
   a. Intubation
   b. Ventilation with 100% FiO_2
   c. PEEP as needed
   d. All of the above

Answer: D. Rationale: The patient will need intubation and then ventilator support with PEEP and high levels of oxygenation. Intubation is likely need for airway protection, and 100% FIO_2 are anticipated due to the pulmonary edema and shunt that are anticipated. Choose D.

2. **Your patient was just extubated you notice he is having difficulty talking and suddenly you hear a sound like stridor coming from him. You should expect what treatment:**
   a. Racemic epinephrine treatment
   b. Stat bronchoscopy
   c. Reintubation Stat
   d. Call the provider

Answer: A. Rationale: Generally speaking, do not select aggressive measures when it is likely that less-invasive measures may be effective. Bronchoscopy and intubation are invasive and above-and-beyond what is required, especially considering the patient had been talking, so eliminate B and C. Calling the provider is only appropriate if no other options are appropriate. Racemic epi addresses the underlying cause, so choose A.

REFERENCES

Burns S. AACN essentials of progressive care nursing. 4th ed. New York, NY: McGraw Hill; 2018.

Chandy D, and Richards D, Drowning (Submersion Injuries) *Up to Date*, September 28, 2022.

Pitt T. *American Association for Respiratory Care.* (12/22/21). Thinking outside intubation, the pros and cons of Heliox Therapy.

PART VIII
Multisystem Organ Dysfunction Practice Exam

Questions 1 and 2 refer to the following scenario:
A 71-year-old man is admitted to the intensive care unit (ICU) with hypotension of unknown origin. His past medical history includes recent surgery for prostate cancer. Because of an initial lack of response to treatment for the hypotension, he has had a fiberoptic pulmonary artery catheter placed. At 0800, he is unresponsive, with a Glasgow Coma Scale score of 4. His skin is warm and dry, and lung sounds reveal generalized crackles. His vital signs and pulmonary artery catheter reveal the information given below for 0800. The physician requests dobutamine to be added to his treatment. One hour after the dobutamine, a repeat set of hemodynamics reveals the information for 0900:

	0800	**0900**
Blood pressure	106/68 mm Hg	114/66 mm Hg
Pulse	101	106
Cardiac output	8.9	9.4
Cardiac index	5.4	5.6
Stroke volume	88	88
PA	42/22	44/23
PAOP	16	16
CVP	12	13
SvO_2	0.86	0.85
PaO_2	67	74
Sao_2	0.92	0.93
$PaCO_2$	36	38
FIO_2	0.70	0.70
PEEP	+10	+10
pH	7.35	7.34
Hb	11	11
Lactate	4.5	4.5

1. **Based on this information, was the addition of dobutamine effective?**
   (A) yes, since an increase in PaO_2 occurred
   (B) yes, since an increased in cardiac output occurred
   (C) no, since the blood pressure did not increase
   (D) no, since the SvO_2 and lactate are unchanged
2. **If tissue oxygenation improved in this patient, which parameters would you most likely see change?**
   (A) decrease in the lactate and SvO_2
   (B) increase in pH
   (C) decrease in PEEP
   (D) increase in SaO_2
3. **A 74-year-old, 66.7-kg woman is in the ICU with the diagnosis of possible sepsis secondary to pneumonia. On admission she was markedly short of breath, with an FIO_2 of 80% and a PaO_2 of 72. She was intubated because of increased work of breathing and placed on assisted mandatory ventilation (AMV), with the following settings:**

FIO_2	80%
PEEP	+8 cm H_2O
Tidal volume (Vt)	400 mL
Ventilator rate	10 breaths per min
Total rate	32 breaths per min
Peak airway pressure	48 cm H_2O

Shortly after admission, she became hypotensive and had a fiberoptic triple-lumen catheter inserted to aid in her management. She is being given lactated Ringer's 30 mL/kg (2 L) over 60 min. Listed below are her first three sets of hemodynamic data and other clinical information:

	0610	**0640**	**0710**
PaO_2	87	78	92
SpO_2	0.98	0.96	0.98
$PaCO_2$	35	32	33
pH	7.33	7.31	7.30
HCO_3^-	21	20	20
Blood pressure	88/52 mm Hg	92/56 mm Hg	90/56 mm Hg
Map	64	68	67
Pulse	114	116	112
Cardiac output	8.6	8.9	9.3
Cardiac index	4.1	4.2	4.7
Stroke volume	75.4	76.7	83
CVP	9	10	10
$ScvO_2$	0.38	0.49	0.71
Lactate	5.6		

Based on the above information, is she improving, deteriorating, or stable?
   (A) improving, based on the stable SpO_2
   (B) stable, based on the blood pressure
   (C) improving, based on the improved $ScvO_2$
   (D) worsening, based on the unchanging CVP
4. **A blood culture report returns for a 73-year-old man who is in the ICU for possible sepsis. The report states that he has *Escherichia coli* (a Gram-negative bacterium) in the blood. He is currently receiving gentamicin, imipenem, and cefoxitin. Based on the report, which drug is likely to have the best effect (most "targeted" effect based on the invading organism)?**
   (A) cefoxitin
   (B) imipenem
   (C) gentamicin
   (D) they all work about the same

Questions 5 and 6 refer to the following scenario:
A 69-year-old woman is admitted to your unit with probable septic shock after sustaining a ruptured diverticulum in her large intestine. The following information is available:

Blood pressure	80/52 mm Hg
MAP	61
Pulse	121
Respiratory rate	38
Temperature	38°C
Cardiac output	8.9
Cardiac index	5.6
Stroke volume	73.6
Stroke index	46
PA	24/11
PAOP	8
CVP	2
PaO_2	78
$PaCO_2$	29
pH	7.32
HCO_3^-	16
Lactate	5.1
$ScvO_2$	81%
SpO_2	95%

5. **Based on this information, which treatment(s) is/are likely to be implemented first?**
   (A) lactated Ringer's fluid bolus of 30 mL/kg min and broad-spectrum antibiotics started within the first hour of sepsis identification
   (B) dobutamine at 5 μg/kg/min and administration of antipyretics
   (C) lactated Ringer's fluid bolus of 300 mL/30 min and administration of antipyretics
   (D) all of the above

6. **Treatment with which of the following is most likely to reverse the effects of the sepsis?**
   (A) Early antibiotic therapy and source control
   (B) ibuprofen
   (C) tight glycemic control
   (D) fluid bolus of either crystalloid or colloidal solutions

7. **A 64-year-old woman is in the ICU with the diagnosis of possible sepsis secondary to a urinary tract infection. Upon admission she was markedly short of breath with a p/f ratio of 96, an FIO_2 of 0.80, and a PaO_2 of 72. She was intubated because of increased work of breathing. Shortly after admission, she became hypotensive and had a triple-lumen oximeter and esophageal Doppler inserted to aid in management. Over the next 2 h, she was aggressively treated with lactated Ringer's fluid bolus (with a subsequent 10-kg weight gain), antibiotics, and dobutamine. Based on the following information, has the therapy been successful to this point?**

	Initial	Hour 1	Hour 2
PaO_2	87	78	92
$PaCO_2$	35	32	37
pH	7.33	7.31	7.33
HCO_3^-	21	20	22
Blood pressure	88/52 mm Hg	92/56 mm Hg	90/56 mm Hg
MAP	64	68	67
Pulse	114	116	112
Cardiac output	8.6	8.9	9.3
Cardiac index	5.1	5.2	5.5
Stroke volume	75.4	76.7	83
CVP	9	10	14
SvO_2	0.55	0.53	0.52
Lactate	4	4.6	4.6

   (A) yes, as illustrated by an increased cardiac index
   (B) yes, as illustrated by an increased PaO_2
   (C) no, as illustrated by an unimproved SvO_2
   (D) no, as illustrated by an increase in CVP

8. **Which group of the following parameters is associated with systemic inflammatory response syndrome (SIRS) criteria that would suggest a positive patient screen for sepsis?**
   (A) Temperature 39.0°C, heart rate 112/min, respiratory rate 18/min, WBC 11,500
   (B) Temperature 39.0°C, heart rate 88/min, respiratory rate 18/min, WBC 11,500
   (C) Temperature 37.8°C, heart rate 88/min, respiratory rate 24/min, WBC 11,500
   (D) Temperature 37.8°C, heart rate 88/min, respiratory rate 18/min, WBC 22,500

9. **A 17-year-old man is admitted to your unit following an electric shock injury. His friends state that he was climbing a sign when a pole he was carrying touched a power line. He fell from the sign and was unresponsive. His friends immediately brought him to the emergency department. Based on the preceding description, which conditions could be anticipated to be present during the first 24 h of ICU admission?**
   (A) cardiac dysrhythmias
   (B) lower fluid requirements since open wounds are small
   (C) little to no pain
   (D) elevated CoHb

10. **Which of the following organs is/are likely to be affected in multisystem organ dysfunction?**
    (A) liver and kidney
    (B) liver and lungs
    (C) kidney and lungs
    (D) all of the above

11. **The effects of tumor necrosis factor, leukotrienes, and thromboxane A_2 are similar in the systemic responses they initiate. Which of the following are consistent with the actions produced by these substances?**
    (A) vasoconstriction and increasing cardiac ejection fraction
    (B) vasoconstriction and promotion of platelet aggregation
    (C) increasing cardiac ejection fraction and promotion of platelet aggregation
    (D) all of the above

12. A 19-year-old woman is admitted to your unit after an argument with her parents. Her parents state that they found her in her room with an empty bottle of acetaminophen (Tylenol) on her nightstand. Which of the following is the initial treatment for an overdose of acetaminophen?

(A) ipecac
(B) charcoal and intravenous *N*-acetylcysteine
(C) dialysis
(D) lavage and oral *N*-acetylcysteine

13. A 20-year-old man is admitted to your unit following a suicide attempt after a breakup with his girlfriend. He ingested an unknown drug or drugs and is currently combative but with a reduced level of consciousness. A large-bore nasogastric tube has been inserted in an attempt to lavage his stomach. Which of the following nursing actions should be initiated at this point?

(A) protection against aspiration
(B) intubation and mechanical ventilation
(C) sedation to reduce the combativeness
(D) all of the above

Questions 14 and 15 refer to the following scenario:

A 47-year-old man is admitted to the hospital following complaint of an infection he developed after stepping on a nail that penetrated his boot. He now has a cellulitis of his right lower leg. During his stay on the medical floor, his level of consciousness has changed and he is now arousable only by deep stimuli. He requires intubation and mechanical ventilation. The following information on laboratory results and vital signs is available:

Blood pressure	88/54 mm Hg
MAP	65
Pulse	126
Respiratory rate	24 (on assisted mandatory ventilation)
Temperature	39°C
PaO_2	78
FIO_2	0.50
HCO_3^-	18
White blood cells	31,000
BUN	38
ALT	433
pH	7.33
$PaCO_2$	32
Hb	13
Creatinine	2.6
AST	512
Alkaline phosphatase	199
Lactic acid	5.4

14. Based on this information, which condition is likely to be developing?

(A) Guillain–Barré syndrome
(B) ARDS
(C) sepsis and multisystem organ dysfunction syndrome (MODS)
(D) amyotrophic lateral sclerosis

15. Treatment for this condition is most likely to include which of the following?

(A) increased intravenous fluids
(B) plasmapheresis
(C) norepinephrine
(D) beta blockers, such as propranolol or esmolol

16. Which of the following are the most characteristic responses of the cardiovascular system initially to sepsis?

(A) increased ejection fraction and increased cardiac output
(B) increased ejection fraction and reduced systemic vascular resistance
(C) increased cardiac output and reduced systemic vascular resistance
(D) all of the above

Question 17 refers to the following scenario:

A 54-year-old woman is in your unit following acute hepatic failure from hepatitis C; she is to be evaluated for a liver transplant and for management of a persistent fever (temperature >39°C). She becomes hypotensive (84/50 mm Hg MAP 61) and tachycardic (130). A fiberoptic pulmonary artery catheter is placed and reveals the following:

Cardiac output	12.9
Cardiac index	7.2
PA	30/12
PAOP	8
CVP	3
SvO_2	0.88

17. Based on the preceding information, which condition would explain her current clinical status?

(A) portal hypertension
(B) left ventricular failure
(C) hypovolemia secondary to loss of plasma proteins
(D) sepsis

PART VIII
Multisystem Organ Dysfunction Practice Exam

Practice Fill-Ins

1. ______________________________
2. ______________________________
3. ______________________________
4. ______________________________
5. ______________________________
6. ______________________________
7. ______________________________
8. ______________________________
9. ______________________________
10. ______________________________
11. ______________________________
12. ______________________________
13. ______________________________
14. ______________________________
15. ______________________________
16. ______________________________
17. ______________________________

PART VIII
Answers

1. **D** Chapter 47 Rationale: The ultimate goal in resuscitating a patient in shock is to optimize delivery and consumption of oxygen and nutrients to the tissues. Based on the data available, this is best measured by the SvO_2 and serum lactate level. From 0800 to 0900, there was essentially no improvement in SvO_2 or lactate was observed, therefore the dobutamine did not contribute to a clinically significant improvement (despite small improvements in BP, PaO_2, and cardiac output). Choose D.
2. **A** Chapter 47 Rationale: The most direct reflection of tissue oxygenation of the options presented is the SvO_2 level, option A. Options B, C, and D would all be positive changes to observe, however the SvO_2 provides the most information regarding oxygen supply and demand balance. Choose A.
3. **C** Chapter 47 Rationale: The parameter that best illustrates the trend in this patient's status is the $ScvO_2$, the parameter summarizing oxygen supply and demand balance. The SpO_2 is more reflective of only oxygen delivery to the tissues, eliminating option A. Like SpO_2, parameters such as blood pressure are late signs of patient changes, eliminating B as well. Central venous pressure (CVP) should never be an overall determining factor in determining patient stability, and is only intended to be a guide for optimizing the stroke volume or cardiac output. Choose C.
4. **C** Chapter 47 Rationale: The cluster technique may be used as an approach to this question. Of the options available, both A and B provide both Gram-positive and Gram-negative antimicrobial coverage, which may help to eliminate them. The only available answer that illustrates focused Gram-negative coverage is gentamicin, option C. Option D is not true. Choose C.
5. **A** Chapter 47 Rationale: The severe sepsis resuscitation bundle includes serum lactate level, broad-spectrum antibiotics, blood cultures prior to antibiotics, and fluid challenge for hypotension and/or elevated lactate. The only option available that includes only elements of the sepsis bundle is option A. Antipyretics are not associated with improved outcomes in comparison to the bundle, so options B and C can be eliminated. Choose A.
6. **A** Chapter 47 Rationale: Antibiotics and source control are interventions most closely associated with mortality benefit in severe sepsis based on the options available. Ibuprofen may be beneficial for symptom management or decreasing metabolic demand, however nonsteroidal anti-inflammatory drugs (NSAIDS) are not included in the sepsis guidelines and may be harmful to renal function, so eliminate B. Tight glycemic control (serum glucose 80–110 mg/dL) is not recommended in medical–surgical ICU patients, so eliminate C as well. IV fluids can be helpful in septic shock patients, however are not as closely associated with survival as option A. Choose A.
7. **C** Chapter 47 Rationale: Of the options available, the SvO_2 is the parameter that best summarizes the patient's supply-and-demand balance for delivering oxygen and nutrients to the tissues. Therefore, in this question it is the best prognostic indicator and reflection of treatment effectiveness. Options A and B focus more on oxygen delivery, which helps eliminate them. The CVP value itself, although used by some during resuscitation, does not correlate with patient outcome. Choose C.
8. **A** Chapter 47 Rationale: Be mindful of questions arranged like this on the exam. Using the vertical technique, line up the parameters for easier visibility and comparison. Remember the SIRS criteria for sepsis include two or more of the following: core temperature more than 38°C or less than 36°C (>100.4°F or <96.8°F); elevated heart rate (>90 bpm or more the two standard deviations above the normal values for age); respiratory rate more than 20 breaths per min or $PaCO_2$ less than 32 mm Hg or mechanical ventilation for acute respiratory process; WBC count more than 12,000/mm^3 or less than 4000/mm^3 or more than 10% immature neutrophils. The only option that fits this criteria is option A.
9. **A** Chapter 50 Rationale: Cardiac dysrhythmias are a major complication occurring after electrical burn injuries, making option A the best answer. Electrical burns carry the potential to be quite extensive despite the possibility of small entry and exit wounds, eliminating option B. Option C may also be eliminated as a possible choice, as the degree of pain largely depends on the depth of the burn. Since no fire or smoke inhalation was observed in this case, option D can be ruled out as well. Choose A.
10. **D** Chapter 47 Rationale: Multisystem organ dysfunction indicates that multiple systems are involved with the patient's pathology. The organ failure will likely be linked to the disease process, the source of infection, or could be secondary to the overall inflammatory cascade affecting organs unrelated to pathology.
11. **B** Chapter 47 Rationale: Both leukotrienes and thromboxane A2 generate a series of reactions, including an increased tendency for platelet aggregation, increased capillary permeability, and vasoconstriction.

12. **B** Chapter 48 Rationale: The antidote for an acetaminophen overdose is the use of charcoal and intravenous *N*-acetylcysteine. Ipeccac is no longer recommended for routine use, and lavage has limited benefit >1 hour after ingestion, eliminating A and D. Acetaminophen is dialyzable, however this is invasive. Choose B.
13. **A** Chapter 48 Rationale: Airway protection is essential in the use of nasogastric lavage. Consulting your organization's policy and procedure is essential when utilizing this intervention. Not enough information is included to be able to confirm if intubation is necessary, and sedation may further his respiratory compromise. A is the answer that best addresses the key priority.
14. **C** Chapter 47 Rationale: The patient is experiencing sepsis and likely MODS. Sepsis is likely due to a suspected source of infection and SIRS criteria being met (HR 126, RR 24, Temp 39°C, and WBC of 31,000). Organ dysfunction is also observed (BP <90, elevated AST/ALT, Creatinine 2.6, and lactate 5.4). Choose C.
15. **A** Chapter 47 Rationale: Treatment of sepsis currently is designed to treat the infectious process, control undesirable immune responses, and provide support to any organ system in failure. Research has shown that fluids, inotropes, and vasopressors have better outcomes if given to improve the tissue perfusion which should normalize $SCVO_2$ levels. Fluids are given, usually at a rate of about 30 mL/kg. Normal $SCVO_2$ is about 70%. Fluids are generally administered before vasopressors, so choose A.
16. **C** Chapter 47 Rationale: The patient generally is tachycardic as a result of an increased cardiac output which is secondary to a decrease in SVR. The increase in cardiac output is probably a consequence of an increased end-diastolic volume, since ejection fraction is usually reduced.
17. **D** Chapter 47 Rationale: The patient is experiencing sepsis. The low CVP of 3 helps eliminate the right-sided congestion of portal hypertension, eliminating A. LV failure would be associated with a low cardiac index, eliminating B. The fever of 39C and infection source of hepatitis C help differentiate plain hypovolemia from sepsis, so choose D.

PART IX

PROFESSIONALISM, ETHICS, AND SYNERGY

Melissa Golombek

49

Professional Caring and Ethical Practice

CHAPTER OVERVIEW AND OBJECTIVES

Professionalism, Ethics, and the Synergy Model make up approximately 20% (up to 30 questions) of the CCRN exam. These questions address the content areas of professional caring, ethical practice, and components of the Synergy Model, which serves as the organizing framework for the CCRN exam. The Synergy Model states that the needs or characteristics of patients and families influence and drive the characteristics or competencies of nurses. Components of the Synergy Model outlined in the blueprint for the CCRN exam relate to the nursing characteristics of the model, which include advocacy/moral agency, caring practices, collaboration, systems thinking, response to diversity, clinical inquiry, and facilitation of learning. **The CCRN exam questions cover *application* of the Synergy Model, not its terminology or model components.**

This chapter contains information related to professionalism, ethical practice, the Synergy Model, and the application of content to clinical care.

After studying this chapter, you should understand the following:

- Describe the elements of professional nursing practice.
- Enhance knowledge related to the ethical principles that guide professional nursing practice.
- Practical application of the Synergy Model into daily practice.

49.1 PROFESSIONALISM IN NURSING

Professional Caring

Professional nursing practice focuses on providing exceptional clinical care, as well as promoting the best outcomes for patients. The goal of professional nursing practice is providing patient- and family-centered care, focused on ensuring the delivery of **individualized care**. *Patient and family needs are prioritized* by the nurse using clinical judgment, reasoning, and critical thinking skills. **This is best characterized when the nurse serves as an advocate**, demonstrates caring practices in support of physical and psychosocial needs, and through the promotion of a healing environment.

To successfully accomplish *patient-centered care*, emphasis on key hallmarks of professional nursing practice is essential. These include quality, safety, multidisciplinary collaboration, and continuity of care coupled with professional accountability, behaviors, and actions. The promotion of these characteristics is achieved through the *incorporation of evidenced-based practices* and instituting interventions to support optimal patient outcomes while providing professional nursing care.

When focusing on providing patient- and family-centered care, it is important to *recognize that each family system is unique* and varies by culture, values, spiritual, health beliefs, communication styles, and previous experience with crisis. Knowledge and *recognition of anxiety and stress*, promoting coping strategies, and meeting the needs of families of critically ill hospitalized patients are essential aspects of patient and family-centered care. The *recognition and acknowledgment of diversity* in patients and families require that the nurse appreciates and incorporates these differences.

In addressing family needs, a focus on the *unique viewpoints* is essential. Research on the needs of families during critical illness has identified that **honesty, reassurance, and hope are essential**. Nursing care during this time should focus on assuring the patient and their family *have their questions answered honestly*, have the most updated knowledge on prognosis and treatment, have a support system established, and are *allowed to be near the patient.*

49.2 ETHICAL PRACTICE

The ethical practice associated with incorporating patient and family-centered care is a critical element to consider. Nurses within critical care play a vital role in upholding their professional values through their clinical practice, education, research, and nursing policy. Several ethical principles guide nursing care, including the principles of respect, autonomy, beneficence, nonmaleficence, and justice.

- Respect for persons focuses on treating patients and families as autonomous agents and remembering that patients with diminished autonomy are entitled to care based upon their stated wishes.
- Autonomy is the duty to maximize the individual's right to make his or her own decisions.
- Beneficence promotes maximizing possible benefits in the provision of patient care. The Hippocratic Oath has long been a fundamental principle of medical ethics and encompasses the philosophy of "do no harm."
- Nonmaleficence identifies the duty to cause no harm.
- Justice is the duty to treat all patients fairly, distributing the risks and benefits of treatment equally.

Professional nursing practice requires that nurses maintain a high awareness around these ethical principles. In daily practice, nurses may encounter situations that require application of these ethical principles. Examples of situations that may arise include

- Code versus no code decision
- Technology versus cost
- Resource allocation and triage decisions
- Informed consent
- Advanced directives and end-of-life care
- Withdrawal of artificial support
- Futility of care
- Quality of life issues

Several strategies for promoting optimal nursing care related to ethics include

- Recognizing that values and beliefs vary not only among different cultures but also within cultures.
- Viewing values and beliefs from different cultures within historical, health care, cultural, and spiritual contexts.
- Awareness of cultural values and biases.
- Cognizance of possible ethical issues in providing care to critically ill patients.
- **Identifying and promoting discussion of ethical issues or dilemmas with members of the healthcare team, the patient, and family.**
- *Promoting appropriate care* for the critically ill including *identification of the need for palliative care.*

Additionally, personal biases, morals, and values must be recognized. It is important that the nurse maintain a high degree of self-awareness around personal beliefs. During these times of crisis, the *nurse should continue to stay focused on providing individualized care* supporting the best possible outcome for the patient and family **with respect to the patient's wishes**.

As ethical challenges are embedded in everyday practices, nurses must continue to define the boundaries of their professional practice with their health care colleagues around ethics. When nurses are unable to have clearly defined boundaries related to ethics, the nurse is likely to experience moral distress. *Moral distress* is the result of nurses being unable to translate their moral choices into action because there are barriers or disagreements related to their own personal values. It is becoming increasingly clear that moral distress is a reality within nursing, and thus the need to strengthen foundational knowledge related to ethics is essential.

49.3 SYNERGY MODEL

The Synergy Model, which was developed in the 1990s, serves as the organizing framework for the CCRN exam and promotes recognition of the value of professional nursing practice, while focusing on the relationship between the nurse, patient, and their family. The result is a model that focuses the dimensions of a nurse's practice on the needs of the patient and their family.

According to the Synergy Model, synergy occurs when the needs and characteristics of a patient, clinical unit, or system drive the nurse's competencies that must be achieved. When there is strong collaboration between the patient and the nurse, the combined effect influences the outcomes, quality of care, and containment of costs. The Synergy Model identifies eight patient needs or characteristics and nursing competencies:

- **Stability:** The ability to maintain a steady state, including physiologic, psychological, emotional, and family or social stability. The stability of a patient is interpreted as minimally, moderately, or highly stable.
- **Complexity:** The intricate interconnectedness of two or more systems (eg, body, family, and social systems). The interpretation of the complexity of the patient should be described by attributing a level 1 as highly complexity (complex patient/family dynamics, atypical presentation), a level 3 as moderately complex (moderately involved patient/family dynamics), or a level 5 as minimally complex (straightforward, typical presentation).
- **Predictability:** The characteristic allowing one to expect a certain trajectory of illness. The predictability of a patient's situation should be described in terms of being not predictable, moderately predictable, or highly predictable.
- **Vulnerability:** A susceptibility to stressors that may affect patient outcomes adversely. A level 1 patient is highly vulnerable and should be considered unprotected and fragile. A patient who is moderately vulnerable and is somewhat protected would be classified as a level 3. Level 5 indicates that the patient is minimally vulnerable and is safe.
- **Resiliency:** The capacity to return to a restorative level of functioning using compensatory and coping mechanisms. The ability to bounce back quickly after an insult. The level of resiliency is described as levels 1 to 5.

  - Level 1 indicates that the patient is minimally resilient and will often be unable to mount a response or has minimal reserves to attempt to mount a response.
  - Level 3 response indicates a moderate level of resilience, and the patient will often be able to initiate some degree of compensation.
  - Level 5 is the highest level of resilience. At this level, the patient is not only able to mount a response but is also able to maintain the response.
- **Participation in decision making:** The extent to which the patient and family engage in decision making is based on a level of 1 to 5. A patient and family have no capacity for decision making, which indicates that they are at a level of 1. The patient and family that have limited decision-making capacity but will seek input or advice from others should be assessed at a level 3. At a level 5, the patient and family have full capacity to make decisions for themselves.
- **Participation in care:** The extent to which the patient or family engages in aspects of care. Participation in care is determined as no participation, moderate level of participation, and fully participative in care.
- **Resource availability:** The resources that the patient/clinical unit/system/community can bring to a situation. These should be assessed along a continuum, recognizing that a level 1 identifies few resources available to the patient and family, and at level 5, there are many resources in place to support the patient and family.

Along with patient characteristics, nursing competencies are a foundational element of the Synergy Model, outlining eight nursing competencies to respond to patient needs to enhance outcomes. According to the American Association of Critical Care Nurses (AACN), these dimensions of nursing practice span the continuum from competent to expert and are defined as follows:

- **Clinical judgment:** "Clinical reasoning, which includes clinical decision-making, critical thinking, and a global grasp of the situation, coupled with nursing skills acquired by integrating formal and experiential knowledge."
- **Clinical inquiry:** "The ongoing process of questioning and evaluating practice and providing informed practice."
- **Caring practices:** "The constellation of nursing activities that create a compassionate, supportive, and therapeutic environment for patients and staff, with the aim of promoting comfort and healing, while preventing unnecessary suffering. Includes, but is not limited to, vigilance, presence, engagement and responsiveness of caregivers, including family and healthcare personnel."
- **Response to diversity:** "The sensitivity to recognize, appreciate, and incorporate differences in the provision of care. Differences may include, but are not limited to, cultural differences, spiritual beliefs, gender, race, ethnicity, lifestyle, socioeconomic status, age, and values."
- **Advocacy and moral agency:** "Working on another's behalf and representing the concerns of the patient/family/colleagues/community and serving as a moral agent in identifying and helping to resolve ethical and clinical concerns within and outside the clinical setting."
- **Facilitation of learning:** "The ability to facilitate, both formally and informally, patient/staff/system/community learning."
- **Collaboration:** "Working with others (patient, family, health-care providers, colleagues, community) in a way that promotes and encourages each person's contributions towards achieving optimal/realistic patient/family goals; involves intra- and interdisciplinary work with colleagues and community."
- **Systems thinking:** "Body of knowledge and tools that allow the nurse to manage whatever environmental and system resources exist for the patient/family and staff, within or across healthcare and non-healthcare systems."

Several assumptions regarding nurses, patients, and families guide the AACN Synergy Model for patient care:

- Patients are biological, psychological, social, and spiritual entities who present at a particular developmental stage. **The whole patient (body, mind, and spirit) must be considered.**
- The patient, family, and community all contribute to providing a context for the nurse–patient relationship.
- Patients can be described by a number of characteristics. *All characteristics are connected and contribute to each other. Characteristics cannot be seen in isolation.*
- Similarly, nurses can be described on several dimensions. The interrelated dimensions paint a profile of the nurse.
- A goal of nursing is to restore a patient to an optimal level of wellness as defined by the patient. *Death can be an acceptable outcome in which the goal of nursing care is to move a patient toward a peaceful death.* Supporting the patient and family should result in the family feeling at ease with the outcome.

The Synergy Model outlines that when patients' characteristics and nurses' competencies synergize, optimal patient outcomes are achieved. Three levels of outcomes are outlined: patient level, unit level, and system level. The Synergy Model helps to promote the measurement of nurse-sensitive outcomes. Based on the model, the outcome of a synergistic relationship is termed "safe passage," which includes helping the patient and family move toward greater self-awareness and self-understanding, competence, and health and/or a peaceful death.

In addition to serving as the organizing framework, the Synergy Model has also been used to describe nursing practice, serve as a framework for nursing interventions and nursing education, and guide advanced practice nursing care.

KEY CONTENT CHECKLIST

The Professional Caring and Ethical Practice questions are often scenario based and often appear as though there is no clear correct answer. However, these key guiding principles will help you achieve success with these questions:

- ❐ Advocate for the patient's wishes/needs whenever possible.
- ❐ Advocate for honesty, transparency, and what is evidence based.
- ❐ When solutions to scenarios are needed, opportunities also include organizing an in-service, performing a literature search (in the absence of evidence), or suggesting a quality improvement project.
- ❐ Honor the patient and family's unique viewpoints, no matter how different (eg, take into consideration the patient's cultural norms or preferences).
- ❐ Bear in mind the age of the patient when identifying solutions. For example, teaching an adolescent about wound care may be challenging due to alterations in body image.
- ❐ Recognize that the patient or family's coping may be limited due to stress.
- ❐ Allow the patient and family to be near the patient whenever possible (as long as it is not disruptive to the patient) (eg, during a cardiac arrest resuscitation).
- ❐ Be mindful in scenarios involving hospital policy; however, be willing to be flexible in an effort to meet the patient's wishes creatively when issues such as hospital policy appear to conflict (eg, visiting hours).
  - However, be mindful of when setting limits with family is in the best interest of the family (eg, visiting hours)
- ❐ Solutions involving a multidisciplinary approach are often strong answers.
- ❐ Refrain from contacting the physician or the unit manager (or chaplain, case manager, etc.) as an answer, unless this option is clearly better than the alternatives (ie, the nurse should be empowered to take an active role to identify solutions).

Review Questions:

1. Which of the following interventions would best help family members to cope with a patient's life-threatening illness?

a. Encouraging the family to participate in patient care
b. Requesting that a chaplain speak with the family
c. Encouraging the family to ask questions
d. Extending visiting hours

Answer: C. Rationale: By encouraging the family to ask questions, the nurse is supporting the family's capacity to cope with the patient's life-threatening illness. The nurse is addressing the families' vulnerability, resiliency, and decision-making ability through this encouragement. A life-threatening illness is not an ideal time to encourage the family to participate in the care, eliminating A. Involving the chaplain may be beneficial. This option in this case takes focus away from the nurses' role, helping to eliminate B as well. Extending visiting hours is more of an indirect, passive intervention than an active one and does not address the underlying issue. Choose C.

2. An older patient with advanced metastatic disease is placed on "do not resuscitate" status but remains in the intensive care unit (ICU) for mechanical ventilatory support because the step-down unit is full. The family asks that an Indian prayer service be held at the patient's bedside. The patient is in a two-bed room with another comatose patient. Which of the following would be the best action for the nurse?

a. Inform the family that the prayer service cannot be conducted.
b. Allow the prayer service to be conducted, as the patient's roommate would not be aware of the event.
c. Arrange to transfer the patient to a single room to facilitate the family's request to hold the service.
d. Since it is near shift change, wait and let the next shift nurse decide.

Answer: C. Rationale: When focusing on providing patient- and family-centered care, it is important to recognize that each family system is unique and varies by culture, values, spiritual beliefs, health beliefs, communication styles, and previous experience with crisis. Knowledge and recognition of anxiety and stress, promoting coping strategies, and meeting the needs of families of critically ill-hospitalized patients are essential aspects of patient-centered care. The recognition and acknowledgment of diversity requires the nurse to appreciate and incorporate these differences while providing care. Additional areas to consider include ethnicity, race, spiritual beliefs, family configuration, socioeconomic status, age, and values.

3. The nurse caring for an older adult that recently sustained a stroke with expressive aphasia could communicate with the patient in writing; this patient expressed his desire to return to his assisted-living facility and receive further treatment there. The nurse contacted the social service department to pursue placement in the facility after discharge.

In doing so, the nurse is exhibiting which of the following competencies?

a. Caring practices
b. Moral agency
c. Advocacy
d. Systems thinking

Answer: C. Rationale: Advocacy: Working on another's behalf and representing the concerns of the patient/family/colleagues/

community, by identifying and helping to resolve ethical and clinical concerns within and outside the clinical setting. While there are elements of caring practices, moral agency, and systems thinking outlined in this example, the primary characteristic is advocacy because the nurse is acting on behalf of the patient.

REFERENCES

Alspach J. *Core Curriculum for Critical Care Nurses.* 6th ed. St. Louis, Missouri; Saunders, 2005.

American Association of Critical-Care Nurses. The AACN Synergy Model of Patient Care. https://www.aacn.org/nursing-excellence/aacn-standards/synergy-model. Accessed January 6, 2024.

American Association of Critical-Care Nurses. AACN standards for establishing and sustaining healthy work environments: a journey to excellence. *Am J Crit Care.* 2005;14(3):187–197.

American Association of Colleges of Nursing. Hallmarks of the Professional Nursing Practice Environment. http://www.aacn.nche.edu/Publications/positions/hallmarks.htm. Accessed August 12, 2009.

Benner P. Relational ethics of comfort, touch, and solace—endangered arts? *Am J Crit Care.* 2004;13(4):346–349.

Benner P. Enhancing patient advocacy and social ethics. *Am J Crit Care.* 2003;12(4):374–375.

Benner P. Creating compassionate institutions that foster agency and respect. *Am J Crit Care.* 2002;11(2):164–166.

Brewer BB, Wojner-Alexandrov AW, Triola N, et al. AACN's synergy model's characteristics of patients: psychometric analysis in a tertiary care health system. *Am J Crit Care.* 2007;16:158–167.

Briggs LA, Kirchhoff KT, Hammes BJ, et al. Patient-centered advance care planning in special patient populations: a pilot study. *J Prof Nurs.* 2004;20(1):47–58.

Cohen SS, Crego N, Cuming RG, et al. The synergy model and the role of clinical nurse specialists in a multihospital system. *Am J Crit Care.* 2002;11:436–446.

Curley MAQ. Patient–nurse synergy: optimizing patients' outcomes. *Am J Crit Care.* 1998;7:64–72.

Curley MAQ. *Synergy: The Unique Relationship Between Nurses and Patients.* Indianapolis, IN: STT; 2007.

Doble RK, Curley MA, Hession-Laband E, et al. Using the Synergy Model to link nursing care to diagnosis-related groups. *Crit Care Nurse.* 2000;20(3):86–92.

Ecklund MM, Stamps DC. The synergy model in clinical practice. *Crit Care Nurse.* 2002;22(4):60–66.

Hardin S, Kaplow R. *Synergy for Clinical Excellence: The AACN Synergy Model for Patient Care.* Boston, MA: Jones and Bartlett; 2005.

Hayes C. The Synergy Model in practice. Strengthening nurses' moral agency. *Crit Care Nurse.* 2000;20(5):90–94.

Jacelon CS, Henneman EA. Profiles in dignity: perspectives on nursing and critically ill older adults. *Crit Care Nurse.* 2004;24(4):30–35.

Jecker NS. Principles and methods of ethical decision making in critical care nursing. *Crit Care Nurs Clin North Am.* 1997;9(1):29–33.

Kirchhoff KT, Beckstrand RL. Critical care nurses' perceptions of obstacles and helpful behaviors in providing end-of-life care to dying patients. *Am J Crit Care.* 2000;9(2):96–105.

Kirchhoff KT, Conradt KL, Anumandla PR. ICU nurses' preparation of families for death of patients following withdrawal of ventilator support. *Appl Nurs Res.* 2003;16(2):85–92.

Kirchhoff KT, Song MK, Kehl K. Caring for the family of the critically ill patient. *Crit Care Clin.* 2004;20(3):453–466.

Lindahl B, Sandman PO. The role of advocacy in critical care nursing: a caring response to another. *Intens Crit Care Nurs.* 1998;14(4):179–186.

Ludwick R, Silva M. Nursing around the world: Cultural values and ethical conflicts. *Online J Issues Nurs.* http://www.nursingworld.org/ojin/ethicol/ethics_4.htm. Accessed July 25, 2009.

Nibert AT. Teaching clinical ethics using a case study family presence during cardiopulmonary resuscitation. *Crit Care Nurse.* 2005;25(1):38–44.

Puntillo KA, Benner P, Drought T, et al. End-of-life issues in intensive care units: a national random survey of nurses' knowledge and beliefs. *Am J Crit Care.* 2001;10(4):216–229.

Reilly T, Humbrecht D. Fostering synergy: a nurse-managed remote telemetry model. *Crit Care Nurse.* 2007;27:22–33.

Rushton, CH. A Blueprint for 21st Century Nursing Ethics: Report of the National Nursing Summary. http://www.bioethicsinstitue.org/nursing-ethics-summit-report.org. Accessed February 28, 2015.

Sigma Theta Tau International. The State of Synergy. Excellence in Nursing Knowledge. http://www.nursingknowledge.org/Portal/main.aspx?pageid =3507&ContentID=55889. Accessed August 10, 2009.

Tracy MF. Assessment of critically ill patients and families. In: Chulay M, Burns S, eds. *AACN Essentials of Critical Care Nursing.* New York, NY: McGraw Hill, 2005:3–15.

Tracy MF. Planning care for critically ill patients and families. In: Chulay M, Burns S, eds. *AACN Essentials of Critical Care Nursing.* New York, NY: McGraw Hill, 2005:17–35.

Truog RD, Cist AF, Brackett SE, et al. Recommendations for end-of-life care in the intensive care unit: The Ethics Committee of the Society of Critical Care Medicine. *Crit Care Med.* 2001;29(12):2332–2348.

PART IX
Synergy Practice Exam

1. **Which of the following is among the most important needs of family members during critical illness?**
   (A) to know the status of transfer plans
   (B) to be near the patient
   (C) to be kept informed
   (D) to participate in treatment decisions
2. **Which ethical principle refers to maximizing possible benefits and minimizing possible harms in providing patient care?**
   (A) respect
   (B) beneficence
   (C) nonmaleficence
   (D) autonomy
3. **Which of the following categories of needs should take priority while caring for the critically ill patient?**
   (A) the needs of the patient
   (B) the needs of the family
   (C) the needs of the nurse
   (D) the needs of the physician
4. **Which of the following interventions would best help family members to cope with a patient's life-threatening illness?**
   (A) encouraging the family to participate in patient care
   (B) requesting that a chaplain speak with the family
   (C) encouraging the family to ask questions
   (D) extending visiting hours
5. **The family of a critically ill patient disagrees with the patient's advance directives and asks the nurse to inform the physician that full aggressive treatment should be given to the patient. Which of the following nursing interventions would be most appropriate?**
   (A) Directly inform the physician of the family's request.
   (B) Inform the family that they will need to discuss this issue with the physician.
   (C) Arrange to have the family meet with the physician to discuss treatment options for the patient.
   (D) Inform the family that the patient's advance directives for comfort care must be honored.
6. **Based on the concepts of the Synergy Model, which of the following is not considered an acceptable outcome of patient care?**
   (A) death
   (B) optimal wellness
   (C) uncertain prognosis
   (D) patient perceptions of a poor outcome
7. **The Hippocratic Oath is a fundamental principle that focuses on what medical ethic?**
   (A) Treat all patients with respect.
   (B) Do no harm.
   (C) Provide care to all patients regardless of their ability to pay.
   (D) Provide the best possible care to patients.
8. **The patient you are caring for has just signed consent for surgery in the morning. Which of the following interventions would ensure that a patient understands and has given informed consent?**
   (A) asking the patient to explain the test/procedure
   (B) giving the patient written instructions for the test/procedure
   (C) verbally informing the patient about the test/procedure
   (D) obtaining the patient's signature on the consent form
9. **An older patient with advanced metastatic disease is placed on "do not resuscitate" status but remains in the intensive care unit (ICU) for mechanical ventilatory support because the step-down unit is full. The family asks that an Indian prayer service be held at the patient's bedside. The patient is in a two-bed room with another comatose patient. Which of the following would be the best action for the nurse?**
   (A) Inform the family that the prayer service cannot be conducted.
   (B) Allow the prayer service to be conducted, as the patient's roommate would not be aware of the event.
   (C) Arrange to transfer the patient to a single room to facilitate the family's request to hold the service.
   (D) Since it is near shift change, wait and let the next shift nurse decide.
10. **Which of the following terms corresponds with serving as a moral agent?**
    (A) collaboration
    (B) systems thinking
    (C) clinical judgment
    (D) advocacy
11. **What ethical principle focuses on the duty to treat all patients fairly, distributing the risks and benefits of treatment equally?**
    (A) nonmaleficence
    (B) autonomy
    (C) respect
    (D) justice

12. A patient who was hospitalized for revision of an arteriovenous fistula for dialysis says that he has been practicing yoga at home daily. He asks the nurse whether there is an area of the hospital where he can go to practice his yoga. Which of the following would be the best nursing action?
(A) Inform the patient he cannot practice yoga while hospitalized.
(B) Tell the patient that the doctor would need to issue an order to allow it.
(C) Consult with the healthcare team to pursue options for the patient to practice yoga.
(D) Help the patient to perform yoga in his room.

13. What is the *least likely* response to a family's initial attempts to manage a critical illness?
(A) denial
(B) stress
(C) acceptance
(D) fear

14. What ethical principle identifies the duty to cause no harm?
(A) nonmaleficence
(B) beneficence
(C) veracity
(D) autonomy

15. The nurse caring for an older adult who recently sustained a stroke with expressive aphasia could communicate with the patient in writing; this patient expressed his desire to return to his assisted-living facility and receive further treatment there. The nurse contacted the social service department to pursue placement in the facility after discharge.

In doing so, the nurse is exhibiting which of the following competencies?
(A) caring practices
(B) moral agency
(C) advocacy
(D) systems thinking

16. A patient has just returned from physical therapy when a family member comes to visit. The patient appears tired. What would be the most appropriate nursing action?
(A) Inform the family member that the patient needs to rest.
(B) Ask the patient whether she wants to have a visitor now.
(C) Make the patient comfortable in bed while they visit with their family member.
(D) Ask the family member if they can come back to visit in an hour.

17. When the night shift nurse questions the routine nursing care of instilling saline during endotracheal suctioning, she is demonstrating which of the following nurse characteristic?
(A) resistance
(B) systems thinking
(C) clinical inquiry
(D) advocacy

18. The modification of visiting hours to accommodate an out-of-town relative is an example of what type of nursing action?
(A) seeking clinical inquiry
(B) meeting family needs
(C) promoting resource availability
(D) reducing patient vulnerability

19. During patient care rounds, the attending physician asks the physical therapist and nurse for input on the best ways to encourage a patient to increase his mobility. The physician is facilitating which clinical competency?
(A) facilitator of learning
(B) clinical inquiry
(C) collaboration
(D) advocacy

20. The Synergy Model holds that caring practices represent the constellation of nursing activities that are responsive to the uniqueness of the patient. Which of the following represents a caring practice?
(A) honesty
(B) presence
(C) truthfulness
(D) veracity

21. A young man involved in a motor vehicle accident was admitted to the ICU several days ago, and has been unresponsive since admission. Testing done today established brain death, and an organ procurement liaison has spoken with the family about organ donation. The family asks that treatment be given for another week until an older sibling can return from the armed forces on extended leave. The nurse can best provide support to the family by which of the following actions?
(A) Inform the family that an extension of care will not be possible.
(B) Call the physician to discuss the requirements for organ donation with the family, including the fact that organ procurement will take place on the next day.
(C) Consult social services to assist with obtaining an emergency medical leave for the sibling.
(D) Notify the family that organ donation will not be possible within their requested time line.

22. A female patient admitted with acute respiratory distress syndrome (ARDS) has become progressively worse despite mechanical ventilation and aggressive medical therapies. Her husband asks that their 9-year-old son be allowed to visit. Which of the following would be the best action by the nurse?
(A) Explain to the husband that visitation in the ICU is limited to adults.
(B) Suggest to the husband that the child might be frightened by the ICU environment and that the husband take a picture of the patient instead.
(C) Allow the son to visit at midnight, when activity on the unit is slow.
(D) Arrange for a patient care conference with the husband and members of the healthcare team to discuss possible options.

23. **A family member visiting a critically ill relative for the first time becomes angry at seeing the patient unable to speak. He shouts at the nurse to come into the room and explain why the patient, who is intubated, cannot speak. Which of the following would be the best action for the nurse?**
    (A) Call security to report the family member.
    (B) Page respiratory therapy to speak to the family member.
    (C) Ask the charge nurse to accompany her into the patient's room to speak with the family member.
    (D) Refuse to speak to the family member until he has calmed down.

24. **A new attending physician is routinely rude to the nursing staff and often refuses to answer their questions. What would be an appropriate nursing action?**
    (A) Inform the physician that his actions are inappropriate.
    (B) Point out the offensive behavior to him the next time it occurs.
    (C) Report the physician to the hospital administrator.
    (D) Ask that the physician attend the next multidisciplinary unit meeting and discuss the unit's philosophy of professional communication.

PART IX
Synergy Practice Exam

Practice Fill-Ins

1. ______________________________
2. ______________________________
3. ______________________________
4. ______________________________
5. ______________________________
6. ______________________________
7. ______________________________
8. ______________________________
9. ______________________________
10. ______________________________
11. ______________________________
12. ______________________________
13. ______________________________
14. ______________________________
15. ______________________________
16. ______________________________
17. ______________________________
18. ______________________________
19. ______________________________
20. ______________________________
21. ______________________________
22. ______________________________
23. ______________________________
24. ______________________________

PART IX
Answers

1. **C** Chapter 49 Rationale: Studies have demonstrated that the needs of families during critical illness include the need for information, honesty, reassurance, and hope are essential. Nursing care during this time should focus on making sure that the patient and their family have their questions answered honestly, have the most updated knowledge on prognosis and treatment, have a support system established, and the family can be near the patient.
2. **B** Chapter 49 Rationale: Beneficence promotes doing no harm by maximizing possible benefits and minimizing possible harms in providing patient care. Respect for persons focuses on treating patients and families as autonomous agents, and remembering that patients with diminished autonomy are entitled to protection. Autonomy is the duty to maximize the individual's right to make their own decisions. Nonmaleficence primarily identifies the duty to cause no harm.
3. **A** Chapter 49 Rationale: The goal of professional nursing practice is to provide the best possible care to the patient. Attention to the needs of the family is also a priority, however the needs of the family do not supersede that of the patient. Choose A.
4. **C** Chapter 49 Rationale: By encouraging the family to ask questions, the nurse is supporting the family's capacity to cope with the patient's life-threatening illness. The nurse is addressing the families' vulnerability, resiliency, and decision-making ability through this encouragement. A life-threatening illness is not an ideal time to encourage the family to participate in the care, eliminating A. Involving the chaplain may be beneficial, this option in this case takes focus away from the nurses' role, helping to eliminate B as well. Extending visiting hours is more of an indirect, passive intervention than an active one and does not address the underlying issue. Choose C.
5. **C** Chapter 49 Rationale: The ethical principle of justice should be applied in this instance. Justice is the duty to treat all patients fairly, distributing the risks and benefits of treatment equally. The physician also has a responsibility to "do no harm" as outlined by the Hippocratic Oath. Option C is the most proactive option for the nurse to take.
6. **D** Chapter 49 Rationale: A goal of nursing is to restore a patient to an optimal level of wellness as defined by the patient. Death can be an acceptable outcome, in which the goal of nursing care is to move a patient toward a peaceful death. Supporting patients and families during the dying process is also a focus of professional nursing practice. The result of practicing in this manner should prevent patient perceptions of a poor outcome.
7. **B** Chapter 49 Rationale: The Hippocratic Oath has long been a fundamental principle of medical ethics and encompasses the philosophy of "do no harm."
8. **A** Chapter 49 Rationale: The nurse must critically assess the patient and family's ability to participate in decision making. A patient that is assessed at a level 1 indicates that the patient and family have no capacity for decision making. Patient and family that have limited decision-making capacity, but will seek input or advice from others should be assessed at a level 3. At a level 5, the patient and family have full capacity and can make decisions for themselves. In this instance, the highest level of decision making would be assessed by "A," having the patient explain the test/procedure back to the nurse.
9. **C** Chapter 49 Rationale: When focusing on providing patient- and family-centered care it is important to recognize that each family system is unique and varies by culture, values, spiritual beliefs, health beliefs, communication styles, and previous experience with crisis. Knowledge and recognition of anxiety and stress, promoting coping strategies, and meeting the needs of families of critically ill hospitalized patients are essential aspects of patient-centered care. The recognition and acknowledgment of diversity requires the nurse to appreciate and incorporate these differences while providing care. Additional areas to consider include ethnicity, race, spiritual beliefs, family configuration, socioeconomic status, age, and values.
10. **D** Chapter 49 Rationale: Advocacy and moral agency: Working on another's behalf and representing the concerns of the patient/family/colleagues/community and serving as a moral agent in identifying and helping to resolve ethical and clinical concerns within and outside the clinical setting.
11. **D** Chapter 49 Rationale: Justice is the duty to treat all patients fairly, distributing the risks and benefits of treatment equally.
12. **C** Chapter 49 Rationale: Knowledge and recognition of anxiety and stress, promotion of coping strategies, and meeting the needs of families of critically ill hospitalized patients are essential aspects of patient and family-centered care. Additionally, promoting the patient's level of resiliency is essential. Resiliency is the capacity to return to a restorative level of functioning using compensatory and coping mechanisms. At the highest level of resiliency, the patient is not only able to mount a response, but is also able to maintain the response. Consider also the action verbs noted—"consult" and "pursue" may be considered

the most proactive and dynamic of the options available, emphasizing the nurses' role in providing the best patient-centered care. Choose C.

13. **C** Chapter 49 Rationale: During this time of crisis, the critical care nurse will be supporting the patient and family to manage their responses to critical illness. These responses may include stress, fear/anxiety, loneliness, powerlessness, anger, depression, and denial. Often "acceptance" is the last phase, and the key word in this question is "initial." Since acceptance is often observed last, it the least likely to manifest initially. Choose C.

14. **A** Chapter 49 Rationale: The principle of nonmaleficence identifies the duty to cause no harm, option A. Beneficence emphasizes maximizing possible benefits for the patient, eliminating B. Veracity emphasizes telling the truth, eliminating C as well. Autonomy is the duty to maximize the individual's right to make his or her own decisions, promoting independence, ruling out D. Choose A.

15. **C** Chapter 49 Rationale: Advocacy: Working on another's behalf and representing the concerns of the patient/family/colleagues/community, by identifying and helping to resolve ethical and clinical concerns within and outside the clinical setting. While there are elements of caring practices, moral agency, and systems thinking outlined in this example, the primary characteristic is advocacy because the nurse is acting on behalf of the patient.

16. **B** Chapter 49 Rationale: The patient and family have full capacity and can make decisions for themselves. In this scenario, the patient is fully capable of making decisions and the nurse is respecting this characteristic related to the patient.

17. **C** Chapter 49 Rationale: Clinical inquiry: The ongoing process of questioning and evaluating practice and providing informed practice. The key word in the scenario provided is that the nurse "questions," hinting that clinical inquiry is the best answer. Choose C.

18. **B** Chapter 49 Rationale: Studies have demonstrated the needs of families during critical illness has identified that the need for information, honesty, reassurance, and hope are essential. Nursing care during this time should focus on assuring that the patient and their family have their questions answered honestly, have the most updated knowledge on prognosis and treatment, have a support system established, and can be near the patient.

19. **C** Chapter 49 Rationale: Collaboration: Working with others (patient, family, healthcare providers, colleagues, community) in a way that promotes and encourages each person's contributions toward achieving optimal/realistic patient/family goals; involves intra- and interdisciplinary work with colleagues and community.

20. **B** Chapter 49 Rationale: The AACN states "Caring practices: The constellation of nursing activities that create a compassionate, supportive, and therapeutic environment for patients and staff, with the aim of promoting comfort and healing, while preventing unnecessary suffering." Includes, but is not limited to, vigilance, presence, engagement and responsiveness of caregivers, including family and healthcare personnel. The "cluster technique" may also be used in this question. Since veracity, truthfulness, and honesty are essentially the same thing, they may be able to be grouped and ruled out as options. Choose B.

21. **C** Chapter 49 Rationale: Systems thinking: Body of knowledge and tools that allow the nurse to manage whatever environmental and system resources exist for the patient/family and staff, within or across healthcare and nonhealthcare systems.

22. **D** Chapter 49 Rationale: Advocacy and moral agency: Working on another's behalf and representing the concerns of the patient/family/colleagues/community and serving as a moral agent in identifying and helping to resolve ethical and clinical concerns within and outside the clinical setting.

23. **C** Chapter 49 Rationale: The nurse must quickly assess the patient and family in this situation. In this scenario, the patient and family member's vulnerability are at risk. Vulnerability: A susceptibility to stressor that may affect patient outcomes adversely. The level of vulnerability should be assessed by the nurse. A level 1 patient is highly vulnerable will be unprotected and fragile. In option C, the nurse is still taking a proactive approach and remains committed to dialoguing with the family member while accompanied by the charge nurse that will likely help deescalate the emotionally charged situation.

24. **D** Chapter 49 Rationale: In this scenario, the nurse must partner systems thinking with respect. Systems thinking: Body of knowledge and tools that allow the nurse to manage whatever environmental and system resources exist for the patient/family and staff, within or across healthcare and nonhealthcare systems. Respect for persons focuses on treating patients and families as autonomous agents, and remembering that patients with diminished autonomy are entitled to protection. A multiprofessional unit meeting is a more interactive approach that may help promote the development of healthcare team relationships and mutual purpose. Choose D.

PART X

BEHAVIOR

Angela Campbell

50

Behavioral and Psychologic Factors in Critical Care

CHAPTER OVERVIEW AND OBJECTIVES

These sections are presented in a brief format, designed to acquaint you with basic fundamentals. The section is not designed to be comprehensive but to help you understand key components that could be addressed on the CCRN exam.

After studying this chapter, you should understand the following:

- Identify the key clinical presentations of depression, substance use and withdrawal, and suicide.
- Identify the key differences between delirium and dementia.
- Describe basic interventions for the behavioral health patient when presenting with a history of abuse, depression, substance use, and suicide/self-harm behaviors.

50.1 ABUSE AND NEGLECT

Although the precise prevalence of abuse is not known because of underreporting, it is estimated that one-half of Americans have experienced violence in their families.. Approximately one in three women and one in four men in the United States will experience some form of physical violence by an intimate partner in their lifetime. Abuse and neglect are found in all religious, cultural, educational, and socioeconomic backgrounds. **Table 50-1** lists categories of abuse and neglect.

Assessment

All aspects of care for the victims of abuse and neglect should be guided by the principles of Trauma-Informed Care, which emphasize safety, trustworthiness, respect for the patient's need for autonomy, inclusion in care, and empowerment. Concerns regarding a patient that may have suffered abuse or neglect must always be discussed in private using empathetic, professional, and nonjudgmental language. Ask *open-ended questions* in an honest and direct manner being mindful of the patient's ability to understand. Be aware of your response to a patient's disclosure, avoiding any display of shock, horror, disapproval, or anger toward the perpetrator or situation. Patients may be less likely to follow treatment recommendations or continue to engage in their care if their experience was distressing.

Intervention

1. It is essential to establish rapport, trust, and confidentiality.
2. If patient is a victim of violence, consider placing patient on a "protective" status in accordance with hospital policy and the patient's wishes.
    a. Ensure *all* staff caring for the patient are aware of and observe protective status.
3. Plan care with consideration to the type of violence your patient has suffered. For example, avoiding the assignment of male care providers may be most appropriate for a rape survivor.
4. Refer the patient to psychiatry for observed symptoms of depression, suicidal ideation, anxiety, and symptoms of acute stress or posttraumatic stress disorder (PTSD).
5. Know your state's reporting requirements and report elder, adolescent, or suspected abuse and neglect to the appropriate protective authority. Reporting abuse or neglect in good faith is immune from prosecution.

TABLE 50-1. CATEGORIES OF ABUSE AND NEGLECT

Types with Examples	*Symptoms/Observations*
Physical: Infliction of physical pain or bodily harm. Biting, burning restraining, slapping, pushing, throwing	1. Injuries inconsistent with stated cause or reason for hospitalization 2. Fractures and bruising at variable stages of healing 3. Explanation of injury is vague, minimized, or avoided. Described as "accident prone" 4. Somatic or stress related conditions, headaches, backaches, and dizziness 5. Changes in behavior, anxiety, withdrawal, overly solicitous, when perpetrator in room 6. Depression 7. Comments on "problems" with spouse/family member
Sexual: Any form of sexual contact or exposure without consent or when victim is unable to consent. It is estimated that 1 in 4 women and 1 in 6 men are sexually abused in childhood. Over one-half of women and almost 1 in 3 men have experienced sexual violence involving physical contact during their lifetimes.	1. Bruising/injury to genitalia 2. Depression, anxiety/panic attacks 3. Symptoms of acute stress or PTSD: Startle, numbing, avoidance, nightmares, insomnia hypervigilance, irritability, anger 4. Fear and anxiety of care procedure 5. Fear of gender of perpetrator
Emotional: Infliction of emotional/mental anguish. Threats, humiliation, intimidation, withholding of affection, controlling, and isolation.	1. Low self-esteem 2. Depression/anxiety 3. Timidity, nervousness around abuser 4. Complacency/helplessness 5. Poor eye contact
Neglect: Failure to provide for physical, developmental, or educational needs.	1. Evidence of starvation or malnutrition 2. Poor hygiene, dirty clothes 3. Lack of medical, dental 4. Ill-fitting clothing/shoes 5. Lacks knowledge of use of routine things, ie, how to use remote control of TV
Economic: Illegal or improper exploitation of money and/or resources of for personal gain or withholding financial support.	1. Evidence of starvation or malnutrition 2. Patient not given needed medications 3. Bills not paid resulting in utilities turned off or foreclosure of home 4. Patient hinting at or complaint that another is controlling their funds/assets

6. Provide the patient with appropriate resources for safety and support on discharge. This may include the patient memorizing resource information to prevent the perpetrator from discovering written materials if they are returning to the same abusive environment.

50.2 DELIRIUM AND DEMENTIA

Definitions

Delirium is a symptom characterized by a sudden disturbance or fluctuation in mental status or level of consciousness with inattention, including changes in behavior and disorganized thinking. Three subtypes of delirium are present: hyperactive, hypoactive, and mixed. *Delirium is differentiated from dementia by observing when an alert patient experiences a gradual, progressive cognitive decline.*

KEY CLINICAL CONCEPT

Be prepared to be able to distinguish the difference delirium and dementia for the exam. Delirium is associated with a rapid onset, fluctuating mental status, inattention, and disorganized thinking (eg, due to drugs, sleep deprivation, etc). In contrast, dementia is slower in onset, chronic, and progressive (eg, due to aging, Parkinson's, etc).

Assessment

One validated test for delirium is the confusion assessment method for the intensive care unit (ICU) (CAM-ICU). Because a primary feature of delirium is inattention in an arousable patient, the CAM-ICU aids clinicians in the assessment of inattention.

Intervention

1. Prevention—identify and eliminate any contributing risk factors.
2. Nonpharmacologic interventions.
3. Pharmacologic interventions.

One of the causes of inability to keep attention is oversedation. The use of sedation scores, such as the Richmond Agitation and Sedation Scale (RASS), can prevent this. For example, in the RASS, a patient should be maintained on sedation at a score of approximately 0 to −2. Subsequently, the evaluation of a patient for an inability to maintain attention should focus on removing any known causes. *Any physiologic causes of inattention should also be addressed.*

Help the patient remain properly oriented through techniques such as providing nonverbal music, assistance with visual and hearing aids, and reorienting the patient as much as possible. As nursing practice allows, maintain consistency in staff and routines. Encourage familiar or personal objects and allow normal television viewing, if possible.

In addition, keep the environment conducive to rest. For example, keep lights dim at night and on during the day and minimize excess staff and other ICU noise. Help the patient to remain active as much as possible during daytime hours.

Of course, any clinical disturbances should be corrected, for example hypotension, hypoperfusion, and hypoxia. *Any correctable clinical problem that could lead to inattentiveness should be addressed as soon as possible.* Pharmacologically, **haloperidol** 2 to 5 mg IVP or IM every 6 hours could be *used to address delirium,* **although addressing the cause is a better solution**. *One side effect of haloperidol is prolongation of the QT with possible development of torsade de pointes (ventricular tachycardia).*

50.3 DEPRESSION

Depression is a mood disorder involving the body, thoughts, and behavior. It affects the way one eats and sleeps, the way one feels about the self, and the way one thinks about once pleasurable activities. At any given time, 10 million Americans suffer from this disabling disorder, which can appear at any age. One in five adults experiences depression at some point in their lives. About 5% of children and adolescents also suffer from this disorder, and it is twice as common in females as in males.

It is estimated that 25% to 33% of medically ill patients have coexisting depression. Unfortunately, depression is often unrecognized and untreated in the medically ill person, in part because the symptoms are attributed to their primary illness. Left untreated, depression complicates care and compounds the pain and suffering of medical illness (**Table 50-2**).

TABLE 50-2. MEDICAL CONDITIONS AND MEDICATIONS THAT MIMIC DEPRESSION

Medical Conditions That Mimic Depression	*Medications That Mimic Depression*
Anemia	CNS depressants
Hepatitis	Benzodiazepines
Mononucleosis	Beta-blockers (such as propranolol)
Hypothyroidism	Calcium channel blockers
Chronic pain/fatigue syndromes	Estrogen
	Fluoroquinolone antibiotics
Hypothyroidism	Statins
Cancer	Accutane
Anemia	Narcotics
Infections	Zovirax
Electrolyte disturbances	CNS depressants (alcohol, benzodiazepines, opioids)
Folate deficiency	Corticosteroids
Neurologic disorders	Contraceptives
Cardiovascular disease	Phenobarbital
Respiratory disease	Brivaracetam
	Levetiracetam
	Perampanel
	Tiagabine
	Topiramate
	Vigabatrin
	Gonadotropin-releasing hormone agonists
	Interferon-α
	Interleukin-2
	Varenicline (Chantix)
	Mefloquine
	Isotretinoin
	Clonidine
	Methyldopa
	Reserpine

Diagnostic Criteria

Diagnostic criteria for depressive disorder would include five or more of the following symptoms nearly every day for most waking hours over the same 2-week period. These symptoms are a change from the person's previous function and are the cause of significant distress or impairment in these areas of function.

1. Depressed, sad mood.
2. Irritability.
3. Anhedonia: decreased interest or pleasure in almost all activities.
4. Significant weight gain or loss (>5% change over 1 month) or change in appetite.
5. Changes in sleep pattern.
6. Increase or decrease in motor activity.
7. Anergia: fatigue, loss of energy, feeling "slowed down."
8. Feelings of worthlessness and (appropriate or inappropriate) guilt. This is especially significant when associated with hyperfocusing or obsessing.
9. Decreased concentration or indecision.
10. Recurrent thoughts of death or suicidal ideation.

Assessment

It is not unusual for a critically ill person to appear depressed during the acute or early recovery stage of an illness. This is described as a "situational depression." As the person recovers and health improves, the depressive symptoms will also improve. If these symptoms persist in spite of improved health, the person may be exhibiting chronic depression and may benefit from treatment.

Intervention

1. If a person has an established history of depression, ensure that the prior medication regime is resumed or appropriately substituted as soon as possible. Some antidepressants may be contraindicated for a new or worsening medical condition and will need to be substituted. For example, the antidepressant bupropion may lower a person's seizure threshold.
2. Request a psychiatric consultation as soon as it is identified that the person is exhibiting symptoms of depression.

3. **Safety of the person is the priority.**
   a. **Ask the patient if he or she is thinking of harming self or ending life.**
   b. *Asking about suicide and self-harm will not increase a person's risk of self-harm and may save their life.*
   c. If the person is expressing suicidal ideation, *continuous observation is indicated* until psychiatric evaluation indicates it is no longer necessary.
4. Other supportive services may help including the person's community support network, hospital chaplain, psychiatric clinical nurse specialist (CNS), and social worker, especially if the person has many social or financial stressors.

50.4 SUBSTANCE USE, DEPENDENCE, AND WITHDRAWAL

Many patients arrive in the ICU with conditions directly or indirectly related to their substance use, dependence, and withdrawal. Prolonged substance use may affect brain functioning and, subsequently, patient behavior. Adequate assessment and intervention can shorten their ICU stay and enhance survival.

Ethyl alcohol (EtOH) is the most commonly abused substance. **Table 50-3** lists commonly abused drugs.

Assessment

All patients should be assessed on admission for current prescription and nonprescription medication use, and history of smoking, substance use, and alcohol use. If the patient discloses use, a more detailed history (substance used, amount, frequency, date last consumed) should be obtained regarding each substance. There are many tools for assessment in the ICU setting.

A few brief questions can reveal problematic alcohol use.

- "Do you sometimes drink beer, wine, or other alcoholic beverages?"
- "On a typical day, how many alcohol drinks do you have?"
- "On average, how many alcohol drinks per week do you have?"
- "When was your last drink?"

Risk factors for withdrawal include—previous history of withdrawal, older age patients, alcohol/substance use history, identified nutritional deficits, comorbid medical conditions, and psychiatric disorders.

In addition to alcohol screening, all patients should be assessed for substance use including urine or serum toxicology screens. In addition to specific substance use, be sure to inquire about duration, frequency, amount, and date of last use.

TABLE 50-3. COMMONLY ABUSED DRUGS OR SUBSTANCES

Category and Name	*Intoxication Effects/Potential Health Consequences*
Depressants	
Barbiturates	
Amytal, Nembutal, Seconal, phenobarbital, Fiorinal	For barbiturates and benzodiazepines taken in greater than prescribed dose, feelings of euphoria and intoxication similar to EtOH/physical dependence and withdrawal syndrome
Benzodiazepines	
Ativan, Librium, Xanax, Valium	Concomitant use with opioids: profound sedation, respiratory depression, coma, and death Abuse, misuse, addictive and withdrawal reactions Amnesia/memory, drowsiness and sedation, paradoxical reaction creating hyperactivity and/or aggressive behavior
Flunitrazepam(Rohypnol) (not FDA approved)	Not approved for medical use in the US, consider "date rape" drug Associated with sexual assaults/amnesia, sedation
Gamma-hydroxybutyric acid (GHB) (Xyrem = Rx)	Considered "date rape" drug/associated with sexual assaults Both sedative and euphoric effects/slowed breathing and heart rate
Dissociative Anesthetics	
Ketamine	Increased heart rate and blood pressure, increase risk cardiac arrhythmia, impaired motor function, memory loss/delirium/hallucinations, respiratory depression/apnea, drug dependence and tolerance, bladder dysfunction (dysuria, frequency, urgency, hematuria, nocturia, hydronephrosis) Laryngospasm (rare)
PCP—phencyclidine	Aggression, panic, hallucinations, violence/mood and cognitive alterations Sedation, immobility, amnesia, analgesia
Hallucinogens	
LSD	Altered states of perception and feeling/flashbacks, hallucinations

(Continued)

TABLE 50-3. COMMONLY ABUSED DRUGS OR SUBSTANCES (*CONTINUED*)

Category and Name	*Intoxication Effects/Potential Health Consequences*
Opioids and Morphine Derivatives	
Codeine, fentanyl, morphine, heroin, oxycodone, hydrocodone	Behavioral: Drowsiness, sedation, slurred speech, impaired memory and attention, psychomotor retardation, confusion Physiologic: pain relief, euphoria constipation, tolerance, physical dependence, withdrawal syndrome, nausea, vomiting, respiratory depression (dose-related), stupor, coma, itching, miosis, hypothermia, bradycardia
Stimulants	
Amphetamines	
Dextroamphetamine, methamphetamine	Increased heart rate, blood pressure, and energy, euphoria/paranoia, weight loss, anxiety, insomnia, irregular heart rate, depression Abuse potential
Cocaine and crack methylenedioxymethamphetamine (MDMA) "ecstasy"	Increased heart rate, blood pressure, euphoria/chest pain, MI, CVA, seizures, paranoia Both hallucinogenic and stimulant effects, increased tactile sensitivity and empathic feelings/ hyperthermia, hypertension, dehydration, renal failure Stimulant and psychedelic, energizing effect
Other	
Inhalants/solvents	Euphoria, stimulation/memory impairment, loss of motor control, muscle weakness, sudden death
Dextromethorphan (in cough and cold medicines)	Distorted visual perceptions, euphoria/impaired motor function and memory
Marijuana/Cannabinoids	Euphoria, relaxation, slowed thinking and reaction time/impaired memory and learning, anxiety, panic attacks, paranoia, withdrawal syndrome Anxiety, euphoria, paranoia, impaired judgment, social withdrawal Impaired motor coordination, tachycardia, xerostomia, conjunctival injection, increased appetite
Alcohol	Disinhibition, euphoria, dysphoria, inappropriate aggressive or sexual behavior, impaired judgment; possibly progressing to somnolence and coma as the blood level increases Blood level concentration dependent: impairment, nausea, vomiting, ataxia, severe dysarthria, amnesia, hypothermia, coma, decreased respiration or respiratory arrest, aspiration, hypotension

- *DEA illicit drug information fact sheets.*
- *Lexicomp (2022).*
- *Paxos C, Teter CJ. Substance-related disorders. In: Chisholm-Burns MA, Schwinghammer TL, Malone PM, Kolesar JM, Bookstaver P, Lee KC. eds.* Pharmacotherapy Principles & Practice. *6th ed. McGraw Hill; 2022. Accessed December 19, 2022. https://ppp-mhmedical-com.cowles-proxy.drake.edu/content.aspx?bookid=3114&sectionid=261474040.*

This information is essential in assessing for intoxication effects and likelihood of withdrawal.

Withdrawal from medications, opioids, and alcohol can result in a variety of physical and psychological signs and symptoms. Monitoring is critical as the impact of withdrawal can be fatal.

Intervention

Alcohol

- Withdrawal is progressive, unless treated.
- Clinical Institute Withdrawal Assessment for Alcohol Scale, Revised (CIWA-Ar) can be utilized for ongoing assessment for those patients who are high risk for alcohol withdrawal.
- Early stages can begin as soon as 3 hours after last drink and can occur up to 7 days after the last drink.
- Onset of withdrawal may be 24 to 72 hours after last drink.
- Early signs and symptoms include anxiety, irritability, problems sleeping, decreased appetite, nausea, elevated heart rate (HR) and blood pressure (BP), hand tremors, sweating.
- Severe withdrawal including delirium tremens (DTs): In addition to previous symptoms, patients experience disorientation to time, place, person, situation, and may experience hypersensitivity to light and noise. Perceptual disturbances can include hallucinations, visual, and/or tactile. The patient's level of consciousness may fluctuate, from lethargy to agitation.
- Withdrawal seizures: Majority occur within first 48 hours, and peak at 24 hours; seizures can occur with or without delirium and are usually generalized tonic–clonic.
- Medications for withdrawal: **Benzodiazepines**, both short or long acting, such as **chlordiazepoxide, diazepam or lorazepam; phenobarbital** and **gabapentin** can also be used.
- **Other treatment interventions:** Adequate hydration (either PO or IV); correction of electrolyte imbalances; multivitamins, thiamine, and folate; monitor vital signs.
- Nursing interventions should focus on patient safety and close monitoring of vital signs, level of consciousness, and mood (see Delirium and Dementia section 50.2).

Pharmacologic Management of Withdrawal

- Signs and symptoms of intoxication and withdrawal are similar to those of alcohol.
- Seizures can occur with or without other signs and symptoms of withdrawal and should always be considered if the person is **benzodiazepine** dependent.
- Patients who take **benzodiazepines** for anxiety, sleep, or panic attacks may have those symptoms emerge during withdrawal.
- Nursing interventions should focus on patient safety and close monitoring of vital signs, level of consciousness, and mood.
- Home medication lists should be rectified and resumed if possible to prevent withdrawal syndromes.
- For known or suspected overdoses, **Romazicon (flumazenil)** will reverse excessive sedation.

Dissociative Anesthetics and Hallucinogens

- Treatment consists of providing a safe environment for patients who may be agitated, violent, or at risk of harming themselves or others.
- Vital signs should be closely monitored for any abnormalities, and treatment should be based on any symptoms.

Opioids and Morphine Derivatives

- For known or suspected overdoses, **naloxone (Narcan)** will reverse excessive sedation and respiratory depression. Use with caution as this medication may have to be repeated, especially if the patient is opioid dependent, has taken an increased dosage of opioids, or if symptoms of withdrawal may be anticipated.
- Unlike alcohol and benzodiazepine/barbiturate withdrawal, opioid withdrawal is seldom life threatening.
- Withdrawal symptoms from heroin and most short-acting opioids begin within 8 to 12 hours after last use and peak at 48 to 72 hours.
- Withdrawal from long-acting opioids such as methadone begins within 24 to 36 hours after last use and peaks at 72 to 96 hours.
- Withdrawal symptoms—autonomic instability including elevated HR and BP, sweating, chills, hot/cold flashes, elevated temperature.
- Other withdrawal symptoms include anxiety, restlessness, irritability, insomnia, muscle aches, bone pain, nausea, vomiting, and diarrhea; intense drug cravings.
- Medications—withdrawal is usually managed in one of three ways—**methadone, clonidine** with or without **benzodiazepines, or buprenorphine**. Opioids given for pain management or other medical reasons will also diminish withdrawal symptoms.
- **Methadone**—prevents withdrawal by binding to mu-opioid receptors displacing shorter acting opioids. Dosage varies depending on amount and duration of use. Withdrawal can usually be completed in 3 to 5 days.
- **Clonidine**—address autonomic instability symptoms. **Benzodiazepines** can be added to address restlessness, irritability, insomnia, and to provide some relief from cravings. **Clonidine** should be held if the patient's BP is less than 90/60.
- **Buprenorphine/naloxone (Suboxone)**—partial mu-opioid agonist. Patients receiving prescribed opioids in ICU setting should not be treated with this medication for withdrawal. The use of benzodiazepines should be used with caution in the patient taking **Suboxone**, as **benzodiazepines** can cause profound respiratory depression in this population.
- Nursing interventions—explain to patients, family members, and/or caregivers that the goal of medications is to diminish withdrawal symptoms, not to remove them completely; help patients differentiate withdrawal symptoms from those of other medical problems; patients' subjective experience of withdrawal may be more intense than objective symptoms.

Stimulants

- Symptomatic treatment of abnormal vital signs, continuous monitoring of patient mood and state of consciousness; close monitoring for seizures and cardiac arrhythmias.
- Providing and maintaining a safe environment as patient behavior indicates.
- Profound dysphoria—often accompanies withdrawal and can lead to suicide attempts or completed suicide. Assess patient for suicidal ideation, **provide for a safe environment**, obtain psychiatric consultation if necessary.

Inhalants/Solvents

- Many different substances can be included in this category; adhesives such as airplane glue; aerosols such as spray paint and computer keyboard cleaner; and cleaning agents such as spot removers.
- It is important to know which substance the patient is using as ingredients may require differing treatments. Treatment may be dependent on what substance is being abused; attempt to obtain as much information as possible about the agent (ie, container to be able to report ingredients to poison control).
- Airway may be compromised by caustic agents. Neurotoxic effects may impair cognition, motor, and sensory involvement.

Dextromethorphan

- See Dissociative Anesthetics and Hallucinogens section.

Marijuana

- Withdrawal syndrome consists of irritability, sleep disturbances, anxiety, restlessness.
- Supportive treatment for symptoms that persist.

Additional Questions or Considerations When Caring for Patients With Opioid Substance Use Disorder

- These patients may be seeking pain relief.
- A complex set of behaviors may be observed; however, take care to avoid labeling the patient. Labeling can lead to judgment and dismissive behaviors in the care team.

- Assessment is very important and should be guided by best practice clinical guidelines, professional ethics, and the patient's presentation.
- Consider what is the current pain management regime for the patient is?
- Are there other ways to explain this behavior?
- What is the patient's level of functioning and quality of life? Adequate pain relief will improve functioning and quality of life for patients.
- *Look for patterns of behavior, not isolated incidences.*

50.5 SUICIDAL IDEATION

Patients may present to the ICU as a result of an attempted suicide or may have suicidal thoughts upon or during their admission. Suicide affects all demographic groups. In 2020, suicide was the 12th leading cause of death overall in the United States, with the loss of over 45,900 individuals. Risk factors include persons 15 to 24 years of age and those older than 65 years. White males and Native Americans have the highest rate of completed suicide. Substance use and psychiatric disorders increase likelihood of suicide. For every 25 persons who attempt, one person completes the suicide attempt.

Assessment

Nurses may be reluctant to address the issue of suicide with patients because they may be concerned it will cause a patient to become suicidal. This is a myth. The topic needs to be openly acknowledged and discussed with patients. *Patients who make direct threats such as "I want to kill myself" or indirect statements such as "I wish I were dead" need to be taken seriously and their thoughts and feelings further explored.* Inquire about previous suicide attempts and what plans the patient has for acting on suicidal thoughts.

If the patient has already acted upon the threat to harm themselves through overdose or poisoning, obtain detailed information as to substances ingested (name, dose, amount, time that has elapsed since the injury). Monitor for signs and symptoms related to the actions taken during the suicide attempt (substance ingestions) and assess any self-inflicted injuries present on admission.

Interventions

1. **Providing for safety is primary concern for patients at high risk for suicide.**
2. An ICU setting provides many means and opportunities for intentional self-harm. Some possible means can be controlled by removing potentially unsafe items, such as not leaving medications accessible to patients. Other means such as IV and oxygen tubing and monitoring wires must be near patients.
3. Close observation and suicide precautions are essential. If a patient is actively trying to harm self, then *one-to-one monitoring/observation is appropriate.*
4. *It is never appropriate to use restraints as a prevention for suicide. Restraints are a last resort for emergent behaviors only.*
5. Psychiatric consultation should be initiated.
6. Various diagnostic testing may be completed based upon the injury (eg, toxicology screen, other laboratory tests, radiographs, computed tomography [CT] scans).
7. Treatments will be employed based upon the mechanism of injury.

KEY CONTENT CHECKLIST

- ❒ Be prepared to be able to distinguish the difference delirium and dementia for the exam. Delirium is associated with a rapid-onset, fluctuating mental status, inattention, and disorganized thinking (eg, due to drugs, sleep deprivation, etc). In contrast, dementia is slower in onset, chronic, and progressive (eg, due to aging, Parkinson's, etc).
- ❒ One side effect of **haloperidol** is prolongation of the QT with possible development of torsade de pointes (ventricular tachycardia).
- ❒ **Benzodiazepines** are not recommended in the treatment for delirium; however, they are first-line treatment for the treatment of alcohol withdrawal.
- ❒ **Romazicon (flumazenil)** is the reversal agent for benzodiazepines.
- ❒ **Naloxone (Narcan)** is the reversal agent for opioids.
- ❒ Nurses may be reluctant to address the issue of suicide with patients because they may be concerned it will cause a patient to become suicidal. This is a myth.
- ❒ Close observation and suicide precautions are essential. If a patient is actively trying to harm self, *one-to-one monitoring/observation is appropriate.*

Review Questions:

1. Which of the following patients with alcohol abuse problems would be most likely to experience withdrawal?

a. A 76-year-old woman with history of depression and liver disease
b. A 30-year-old man who is dependent on heroin
c. A 45-year-old man with gastric ulcers and anxiety disorder
d. A 50-year-old woman with congestive heart failure and diabetes

Answer: A. Rationale: There may be a higher alcohol level in someone with liver disease, and as that level decreases, a patent may experience withdrawal symptoms. Alcohol is more toxic in the aging patient because of changes in metabolism, distribution, and elimination. Aging organs such as the brain and liver are more sensitive to the toxicity of alcohol. Because this patient has depression and liver disease, they may already have a drinking issue and their levels of alcohol may be much higher, making them more susceptible to withdrawal.

2. Which is the key feature of delirium?

a. Fatigue
b. Anxiety
c. Inability to sleep
d. Inattention

Answer: D. Rationale: The hallmark of delirium is an acute fluctuation in consciousness, disorganized thinking, and inattention. The patient may also exhibit confusion and additional cognitive changes.

3. A patient is admitted with diagnosis of alcohol dependence. Which of the following would be most closely associated with the patient is likely experiencing withdrawal?

a. BP 94/66, HR 75, petechiae, piloerection
b. BP 156/94, HR 108 headache, anxiety, tremors, nausea
c. BP 120/74, HR 45, blurred vision, palpitations
d. BP 170/102, HR 57, radiating chest pain, shortness of breath

Answer: B. Rationale: Symptoms in option B are most closely associated with the symptoms on the CIWA scale. Options A and C may be clinically significant, but not associated with the CIWA scale. Option D suggests symptoms that may be more cardiac in origin. Choose B.

REFERENCES

Abuse and Neglect

American Psychiatric Association. *Diagnostic and Statistical Manual of Mental Disorders*. 4th ed. TR. Washington, DC: APA; 2000:467–470.

Responding to Child Sexual Abuse. American Academy of Childhood and Adolescent Psychiatry; July 28, 2004:1–2.

National Center for Trauma Informed Care (NCTIC). Programs &Campaigns, 2015. www.samhsa.gov.

Varcarolis EM. *Foundations of Psychiatric Nursing: A Clinical Approach*. 4th ed. Philadelphia, PA: Saunders; 2002:689–699.

Varcarolis EM. *Psychiatric Nursing Clinical Guide: Assessment Tools and Diagnosis*. Philadelphia, PA: Saunders; 2000:405–420.

Antisocial Personality Disorder

American Psychiatric Association. *Diagnostic and Statistical Manual of Mental Disorders*. 4th ed. TR. Washington, DC: APA; 2000: 701–706.

Chou KR, Lu RB, Chang M. Assaultive behavior by psychiatric in-patients and its related factors. *J Nurs Res*. 2001;9(5):139–151.

Gutmann R. *An Approach to the Aggressive Patient*. Lecture for First Year Psychiatry Residents, July 28, 2009.

Varcarolis EM. *Psychiatric Nursing Clinical Guide: Assessment Tools and Diagnosis*. Philadelphia, PA: Saunders; 2000:100–106.

Delirium and Dementia

Pun BT, Ely EW. The importance of diagnosing and managing ICU delirium. *Chest*. 2007;132(2):124–136. Available at: www.icudelirium.org.

Sona C. Assessing delirium in the ICU. *Crit Care Nurse*. 2009;29:103–105.

Depression

American Psychiatric Association. *Diagnostic and Statistical Manual of Mental Disorders*. 4th ed. TR. Washington, DC: APA; 2000:349.

The Cleveland Clinic, Health Information Center, No. 28, 2004.

Stuart S. *Principles and Practice of Psychiatric Nursing*. St. Louis, MO: Mosby; 1995:414–431.

Varcarolis EM. *Psychiatric Nursing Clinical Guide: Assessment Tools and Diagnosis*. Philadelphia, PA: Saunders; 2000:163.

Substance Abuse/Dependency

American Psychiatric Association DSM-5 Development 2012. http://www.dsm5.org/Pages/Default.aspx.

Martin HA. The possible consequences of combining lorazepam and buprenorphine/naloxone: a case review. *J Emerg Nurs*. 2011 March;37(2):200–202.

McCaffery M, Grimm MA, Pasero C, Ferrell B, Uman GC. On the meaning of "drug seeking." *Pain Manage Nurs*. 2005;6:122–136.

Meier P, Seitz HJ. Age, alcohol metabolism and liver disease. *Curr Opin Clin Nutr Metab Care*. 2008;11(1):21–26.

National Institute on Alcohol Abuse and Alcoholism. *Helping Patients Who Drink Too Much: A Clinician's Guide, Updated 2005 Edition* (NIH Publication No. 07–3769) 2007. http://pubs.niaaa.nih.gov/publications/Practitioner/CliniciansGuide2005/guide.pdf.

National Institute on Alcohol Abuse and Alcoholism. *Rethinking Drinking* (NIH Publication No. 10–3370) 2010. Bethesda, MD. http://pubs.niaaa.nih.gov/publications/RethinkingDrinking/Rethinking_Drinking.pdf.

Developmental Delays

American Psychiatric Association. *Diagnostic and Statistical Manual of Mental Disorders*. 4th ed. TR. Washington, DC: APA; 2000:41–50.

Murphy CC, Boyle C, Schendel D, et al. Epidemiology of mental retardation in children. *Mental Retard Dev Disabl Res Rev*. 1998;4:6–13.

Ricketts RW, et al. Fluoxetine treatment of severe self-injury in young adults with mental retardation. *J Am Acad Childhood Adolescent Psychiatr*. 1993;32(4):865–869.

Tervo R. Identifying patterns of developmental delays can help diagnose neurodevelopment disorders: a pediatric perspective. *Clin Pediatr*. 2003;12(July):1–5.

Failure to Thrive

Blazer DG. Psychiatry and the oldest old. *Am J Psychiatr*. 2000;157:1919.

Golden AG, Daiello LA, Silverman MA, et al. University of Miami division of clinical pharmacology therapeutic rounds: medications used to treat anorexia in the frail elderly. *Am J Ther*. 2003;10:292.

Robertson RG, Montagnini M. Geriatric failure to thrive. *Am Fam Phys*. 2004;70:343.

Rocchiccioli JT, Sanford JT. Revisiting geriatric failure to thrive. *J Gerontol Nurs*. 2009;35(1):18.

Suicidal Behavior

McCaffery M. *Pain: Clinical Manual*. 2nd ed. St. Louis, MO: Mosby; 1999.

McIntosh JL. *USA Suicide: 2006 Final Data*. American Association of Suicidology; 2009. http://www.suicidology.org/c/document_library/get_file?folderId=228&name=DLFE-142.pdf. Accessed 2/7/2010.

U.S. Department of Health and Human Services. *Detoxification and Substance Abuse Treatment: A Treatment Improvement Protocol*. TIP 45. Rockville, MD: U.S. Department of Health and Human Services; 2006.

U.S. Department of Health and Human Services. *Substance Abuse and Suicide Prevention: Evidence and Implications*. Rockville, MD: U.S. Department of Health and Human Services; 2008.

U.S. Department of Health and Human Services, National Institutes of Health, National Institute of Mental Health. (Updated 2021). NIMH Strategic Plan for Research (NIH Publication No. 20-MH-8120). https://www.nimh.nih.gov/health/topics/suicide-prevention.

PART X
Behavior Practice Exam

1. **Which of the following is the most effective safety intervention when caring for suicidal patients?**
   (A) continuous 1:1 observation
   (B) four-point restraints
   (C) removing all potential harmful objects from environment
   (D) asking family to watch the patient
2. **Which of the following patients with alcohol abuse problems would be most likely to experience withdrawal?**
   (A) a 76-year-old woman with history of depression and liver disease
   (B) a 30-year-old man who is dependent on heroin
   (C) a 45-year-old man with gastric ulcers and anxiety disorder
   (D) a 50-year-old woman with congestive heart failure and diabetes
3. **Your patient's last drink was Tuesday at 2200. When would the patient be most likely to experience withdrawal symptoms?**
   (A) Wednesday morning
   (B) Friday morning
   (C) Saturday evening
   (D) Sunday evening
4. **A patient is admitted with diagnosis of alcohol dependence. Which of the following would indicate the patient is likely experiencing withdrawal?**
   (A) B/P 94/66, HR 75, petechiae, piloerection
   (B) B/P 156/94, HR 108 headache, anxiety, tremors, nausea
   (C) B/P 120/74, HR 45, blurred vision, palpitations
   (D) B/P 170/102, HR 57, radiating chest pain, shortness of breath
5. **Which of the following is most important for the nurse to observe for in patients experiencing benzodiazepine withdrawal?**
   (A) paranoia
   (B) hallucinations
   (C) seizures
   (D) irregular heartbeat
6. **In planning care for patients experiencing opioid withdrawal, which of the following is NOT true?**
   (A) Patients are at a high risk for seizures.
   (B) Patients often experience visual and tactile hallucinations.
   (C) Medications are ineffective in treating symptoms.
   (D) Medications are used to diminish, not to alleviate symptoms completely.
7. **Your patient has been requesting increases in dose of opioid pain medications. Staff are concerned that the patient is "drug seeking." Which of the following would be most important in planning care for this patient?**
   (A) Assess for adequacy of pain relief.
   (B) Recommend the doctor change pain medications.
   (C) Request multidisciplinary pain management consultation.
   (D) Recommend the doctor increase opioid dose.
8. **Which is the key feature of delirium?**
   (A) fatigue
   (B) anxiety
   (C) inability to sleep
   (D) inattention
9. **ICU psychosis is which form of delirium?**
   (A) hyperactive
   (B) hypoactive
   (C) mixed
   (D) subclinical
10. **The CAM-ICU is a measure for which condition?**
    (A) dementia
    (B) delirium
    (C) psychosis
    (D) alcohol and barbiturate withdrawal
11. **The RASS (Richmond Agitation and Sedation Score) is a measure for which condition?**
    (A) delirium
    (B) neuromuscular paralysis
    (C) dementia
    (D) adequacy of sedation
12. **Which of the following is a treatment for delirium?**
    (A) haloperidol
    (B) midazolam
    (C) fentanyl
    (D) selenium
13. **Which of the following is a potential side effect of haloperidol?**
    (A) delirium
    (B) prolonged QT
    (C) decreased level of consciousness
    (D) agitation
14. **Which of the following medical conditions can mimic depression?**
    (A) anemia
    (B) asthma
    (C) hyperthyroidism
    (D) steroid abuse

PART X
Behavior Practice Exam

Practice Fill-Ins

1. ______________________________
2. ______________________________
3. ______________________________
4. ______________________________
5. ______________________________
6. ______________________________
7. ______________________________
8. ______________________________
9. ______________________________
10. ______________________________
11. ______________________________
12. ______________________________
13. ______________________________
14. ______________________________

PART X
Answers

1. **A** Chapter 50 Rationale: Continuous 1:1 observation is the most effective way to prevent a patient from suicide since any risk behavior can be prevented or immediately interrupted by the care provider.
2. **A** Chapter 50 Rationale: There may be a higher alcohol level in someone with liver disease, and as that level decreases, a patent may experience withdrawal symptoms. Alcohol is more toxic in the aging patient because of changes in metabolism, distribution, and elimination. Aging organs such as brain and liver are more sensitive to the toxicity of alcohol. Because this patient has depression and liver disease, they may already have a drinking issue and their levels of alcohol may be much higher, making them more susceptible to withdrawal.
3. **A** Chapter 50 Rationale: Alcohol withdrawal symptoms can begin as early as 6 h after the last drink.
4. **B** Chapter 50 Rationale: Symptoms in option B are most closely associated with the symptoms on the CIWA scale. Options A and C may be clinically significant, but not associated with the CIWA scale. Option D suggests symptoms that may be more cardiac in origin. Choose B.
5. **C** Chapter 50 Rationale: Patients withdrawing from benzodiazepines may experience a myriad of symptoms including paranoia, hallucinations, and irregular heartbeat; however, seizures may be life-threatening, and any patient experiencing seizures from withdrawal should be closely monitored for airway protection and safety from bodily harm.
6. **C** Chapter 50 Rationale: A, B, and D are true. Seizures can be life-threatening if a patient is not monitored closely. Padding should be on the bed to protect from bodily injury, and airway supportive equipment should be nearby should a patient need airway support. Medication is supportive and will assist in lessening the severity of the withdrawal symptoms. Option C: this is false.
7. **C** Chapter 50 Rationale: Consulting a pain management team will allow for a (typically multidisciplinary) team of professionals trained in evaluating, diagnosing, and managing pain symptoms. Assessing for adequacy is subjective; recommending a change in medications may lead to the patient asking for an increase in those medications as well, and increasing the opioid dose increases patient's risk for respiratory compromise.
8. **D** Chapter 50 Rationale: The hallmark of delirium is an acute fluctuation in consciousness and inattention. The patient may also exhibit confusion and additional disorganized thinking.
9. **A** Chapter 50 Rationale: ICU psychosis is the perceived most common hyperactive form of delirium. Common behaviors include restlessness, agitation, rapid mood changes. This may be the perceived more common form of delirium because "hypoactive" delirium is often under-recognized or under-appreciated. Bear in mind that the term "ICU psychosis" is becoming more of an outdated term.
10. **B** Chapter 50 Rationale: CAM-ICU is the Confusion Assessment Method developed to assess the presence of delirium.
11. **D** Chapter 50 Rationale: RASS is a tool designed to measure adequacy of the patient's level of sedation in the ICU. Level of sedation is assessed on a scale from combative to unresponsive. It is primarily used on the ventilated patient to avoid over- or undersedation.
12. **A** Chapter 50 Rationale: Haloperidol 2 to 5 mg IVP or IM is frequently used in treating disruptive cognitive symptoms or behaviors during delirium.
13. **B** Chapter 50 Rationale: A serious side effect of haloperidol is prolongation of the QT with possible development of torsade de pointes (ventricular tachycardia).
14. **A** Chapter 50 Rationale: Anemic patients frequently experience fatigue, resulting in a lessening interest in pleasure, poor concentration, insomnia, and irritability, which are all symptoms commonly experienced in depression.

Index

D

E

J

K

L

O

P

Q

T